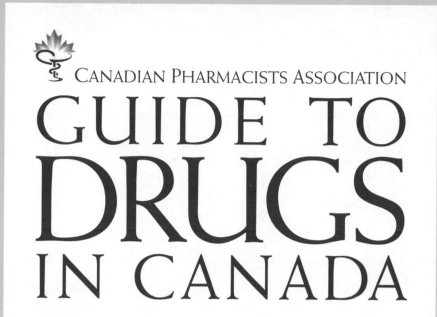

Canadian Pharmacists Association

GUIDE TO DRUGS IN CANADA

CANADIAN PHARMACISTS ASSOCIATION

GUIDE TO DRUGS IN CANADA

EDITOR-IN-CHIEF
Lalitha Raman-Wilms
BSCPHM, PHARMD, FCSHP

THIRD EDITION

CANADIAN PHARMACISTS ASSOCIATION

President Warren Meek, R.Ph, B.Sc.Phm
Executive Director Jeff Poston, PhD, MRPharmS
Senior Director, Digital Publishing Solutions
James de Gaspé Bonar
Editor-in-Chief Carol Repchinsky

Clinical Editors Alka Bhalla, Blair Jarvis,
Barbara Jovaisas, Louise Welbanks,
Sonal Acharya

DORLING KINDERSLEY LIMITED

Editor, Canada Julia Roles
Project Editors, Canada Ian Whitelaw, Julie Whitaker
Production Elizabeth Cherry, Hema Gohil
Photography Gary Ombler
Illustrations Karen Cochrane, Tony Graham,
Mike Johnson, Kevin Marks, Coral Mula,
Lynda Payne, Richard Tibbitts

Editor, India Aakriti Singhal
DTP Coordinator Balwant Singh
DTP Designer Tarun Sharma

Third Canadian edition 2009
Copyright © 1988, 1991, 1994, 1997, 2001, 2004, 2006, 2009 Dorling Kindersley Limited

Dorling Kindersley is represented in Canada by Tourmaline Editions Inc.,
662 King Street West, Suite 304, Toronto, Ontario M5V 1M7

Library and Archives Canada Cataloguing in Publication
Canadian Pharmacists Association guide to drugs in Canada/editor-in-chief,
Lalitha Raman-Wilms. – 3rd ed.
Includes index.

ISBN 978-1-55363-093-7

1. Drugs – Popular works. I. Raman-Wilms, Lalitha
II. Canadian Pharmacists Association   III. Title: Guide to Drugs in Canada.

RM301.15.C35 2008   615'.1   C2008-902480-X

Printed and bound in China by Leo Paper Products Ltd
08 09 10 11 12   8 7 6 5 4 3 2 1

Discover more at
www.dk.com

PREFACE

New developments in drug research move at a tremendous pace, and often generate multiple options for the treatment of various conditions. With more new drugs, and with many patients taking multiple medications, it is important to be vigilant to prevent potential adverse drug events. Increasingly, this vigilance requires that patients and their caregivers be more knowledgeable about the specifics of a particular therapy – which drugs have been prescribed, how they work, what can be expected from the therapy, potential side effects, possible interactions with their other medications, and how to monitor for long-term effectiveness and safety.

The third edition of the Canadian Pharmacists Association *Guide to Drugs in Canada* aims to address these and other questions related to drug therapy by providing factual information in a clear and easy-to-read format. Chapter 1 contains detailed information on what drugs are, how they work in the body, drug use in special risk groups such as children and pregnant women, and information on how best to manage your drug therapy. Chapter 2 is a comprehensive Drug Finder Index that lists generic drug names, as well as brand or product names. The next chapter, on Major Drug Groups, describes how drugs work on the different body systems such as the respiratory system and the heart, and indicates which common drugs are used in conditions affecting these systems. In Chapter 4, detailed profiles of nearly 300 specific drugs are provided. Each drug profile includes information on doses, recommendations on how best to take the medication, available formulations, special precautions, and potential side effects. Information on vitamins, minerals, and supplements, alternative medicines, and the use of drugs in sport and travel are also covered. The glossary and index provide explanations of terminology used in this book, a general index of drugs, as well as useful addresses for health-related organizations and groups.

Our goal is that by providing you with a better understanding of drugs and how they work, and alerting you to early signs of adverse effects, this guide will help you use your medications safely and effectively. This book is not intended to replace advice provided by your physician or pharmacist but, rather, to help you to work in partnership with them. Your healthcare professionals can best explain the reasons why any drug has been prescribed for you and how it may affect you.

We hope that this book will enable you to improve your overall health through informed use of drug therapy.

Lalitha Raman-Wilms, PharmD, FCSHP
Editor-in-Chief

Jeff Poston, PhD, MRPharmS
Executive Director, Canadian Pharmacists Association

CONTENTS

Introduction   8

1 UNDERSTANDING AND USING DRUGS

What are drugs?   12
How drugs are classified   13
How drugs work   14
Methods of administration   17
Drug treatment in special risk groups   20
Drug tolerance and dependence   23
Managing your drug treatment   25

2 DRUG FINDER INDEX

The drug finder   33

3 MAJOR DRUG GROUPS

Brain and nervous system   62
Respiratory system   75
Heart and circulation   81
Gastrointestinal tract   92
Muscles, bones, and joints   101
Allergy   109

Infections and infestations   112
Hormones and endocrine system   126
Nutrition   134
Malignant and immune disease   138
Reproductive and urinary tracts   146
Eyes and ears   155
Skin   160

4   A–Z OF DRUGS

A–Z of medical drugs   172
A–Z of vitamins, minerals,
        and supplements   468
Drugs of abuse   483
Alternative medicine   494
Drugs in sport   496
Medicines and travel   497

5   GLOSSARY AND INDEX

Further information   501
Glossary   503
General index   509

DRUG POISONING EMERGENCY GUIDE 526

INTRODUCTION

The *Guide to Drugs in Canada* has been planned and written to provide clear information and practical advice on drugs and medications in a way that can be readily understood by a non-medical reader. The text reflects current drug usage knowledge and standard medical practice in this country. It is intended to complement and reinforce the advice of your physician and pharmacist.

How the book is structured

The book is divided into five parts. The first part, Understanding and Using Drugs, provides a general introduction to the effects of drugs and gives general advice on practical questions, such as the administration and storage of drugs. The second part, the Drug Finder Index, provides the means of locating information on specific drugs through an index to over 2,000 generic and brand-name drugs. Part 3, Major Drug Groups, will help

you understand the uses and mechanisms of action of the principal classes of drugs. Part 4, the A–Z of Drugs, consists of 292 detailed profiles of commonly prescribed generic drugs, profiles of vitamins, minerals, supplements, drugs of abuse, and information on drugs in sport and travel. Part 5 contains a glossary of drug-related terms (italicized in the text) and a general index.

Finding your way into the book

The information you require, whether on the specific characteristics of an individual drug or on the general effects and uses of a group of drugs, can be easily obtained without prior knowledge of the medical names of drugs or drug classification through one of the two indexes: the Drug Finder or the General Index. The diagram on the facing page shows how you can obtain information throughout the book on the subject concerning you from each of these starting points.

1 UNDERSTANDING AND USING DRUGS

The introductory part of the book, Understanding and Using Drugs, gives a grounding in the fundamental principles underlying the medical use of drugs. Covering such topics as classifications of drugs, mechanisms of action, and the

proper use of medicines, it provides valuable background information that backs up the more detailed descriptions and advice given in Parts 3 and 4. You should read this section before seeking further specific information.

2 DRUG FINDER INDEX

The Drug Finder Index helps you to find information on specific brand-name drugs and generic substances, and lists the drug names alphabetically by both generic and trade names. References are provided to the profiles for individual drugs in Part 4.

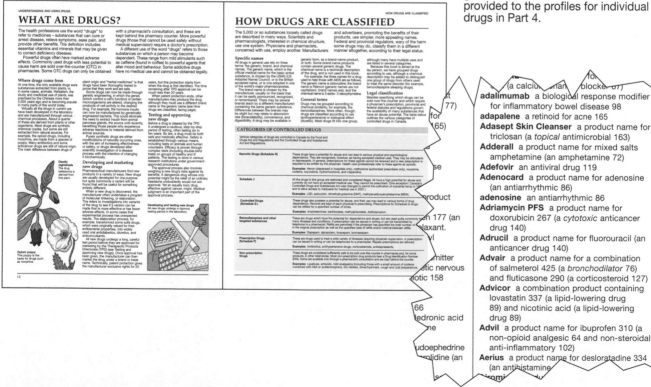

adalimumab a biological response modifier for inflammatory bowel disease 98

adapalene a retinoid for acne 165

Adasept Skin Cleanser a product name for triclosan (a *topical* antimicrobial 163)

Adderall a product name for mixed salts amphetamine (an amphetamine 72)

Adefovir an antiviral drug 119

Adenocard a product name for adenosine (an antiarrhythmic 86)

adenosine an antiarrhythmic 86

Adriamycin PFS a product name for doxorubicin 267 (a *cytotoxic* anticancer drug 140)

Adrucil a product name for fluorouracil (an anticancer drug 140)

Advair a product name for a combination of salmeterol 425 (a *bronchodilator* 76) and fluticasone 290 (a corticosteroid 127)

Advicor a combination product containing lovastatin 337 (a lipid-lowering drug 89) and nicotinic acid (a lipid-lowering drug 89)

Advil a product name for ibuprofen 310 (a non-opioid analgesic 64 and non-steroidal anti-inflammatory 102)

Aerius a product name for desloratadine 334 (an antihistamine

Finding your information

Whether you start by looking up an individual drug or a group of drugs, you will be led by cross-references to relevant information in all parts of the book.

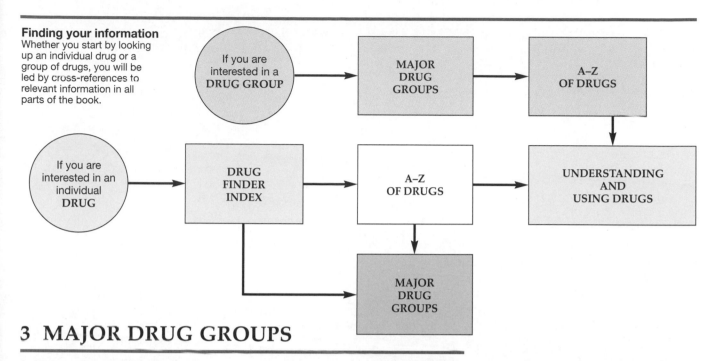

If you are interested in a **DRUG GROUP** → **MAJOR DRUG GROUPS** → **A–Z OF DRUGS**

If you are interested in an individual **DRUG** → **DRUG FINDER INDEX** → **A–Z OF DRUGS** → **UNDERSTANDING AND USING DRUGS**

MAJOR DRUG GROUPS

3 MAJOR DRUG GROUPS

Subdivided into sections dealing with each body system (for example, heart and circulation) or major disease grouping (for example, malignant and immune disease), this part of the book contains descriptions of the principal classes of drugs. Information is given on the uses, actions, effects, and risks associated with each group of drugs and is backed up by helpful illustrations and diagrams. Individual drugs in each group are listed to allow cross-reference to Part 4.

4 A–Z OF DRUGS

This contains profiles of 292 generic drugs, written to a standard format to help you find specific information quickly and easily; cross-references to the relevant major drug groups are provided. Supplementary sections profile vitamins, minerals, supplements, drugs of abuse, alternative medicine, and drugs in sport and travel.

5 GLOSSARY AND INDEX

A glossary of terms explains technical words italicized in the text. The general index enables you to look up references throughout the book.

Adverse reaction
See *Adverse effect*.

Agonist
A term meaning to have a stimulating effect. An agonist drug (often called an activator) is one that binds to a *receptor*, and triggers or increases a particular activity in that cell.

Allergic reaction
An allergic reaction or allergy is one that appears not on first exposure to a drug but on

of the body contain *receptors* like those at which the drug is aimed. The drug molecule may fit other, different receptors well enough to affect them as well. Most of these unwanted effects are dose-related, increasing as the dose is increased, and are commonly referred to as "side effects". Other unwanted adverse effects appear not to be dose-related, such as an *idiosyncrasy* or an *allergic reaction*. See also Adverse effects, p.15.

Analeptic
A drug given in hospital that stimulates breathing. See also Respiratory stimulants (p.72).

Analgesia
Relief of pain, usually by drugs. See also Analgesics (p.64).

Anaphylaxis
A severe reaction to an allergen such as a bee sting or a drug (see Allergy, p.109). Symptoms may include rash, swelling, breathing difficulty, and collapse. See also Anaphylactic shock (p.528).

Antagonist
A term meaning to have an opposing effect. An antagonist drug (often called a blocker) binds to a *receptor* without stimulating cell activity and prevents any other substance from occupying that receptor.

Antioxidant
A substance that delays deterioration due to free radicals (unstable oxygen atoms or radicals are generated by the body's processes and are thought to play a part in aging and disease. Vitamins A, C, and E are antioxidants. See also Vitamins

Antineoplastic
An anticancer drug (p.

Antiperspirant
A substance that is applied to the reduce excess sweating. Antipers

1

UNDERSTANDING AND USING DRUGS

WHAT ARE DRUGS?
HOW DRUGS ARE CLASSIFIED
HOW DRUGS WORK
METHODS OF ADMINISTRATION
DRUG TREATMENT IN SPECIAL RISK GROUPS
DRUG TOLERANCE AND DEPENDENCE
MANAGING YOUR DRUG TREATMENT

WHAT ARE DRUGS?

The health professions use the word "drugs" to refer to medicines – substances that can cure or arrest disease, relieve symptoms, ease pain, and provide other benefits. This definition includes essential vitamins and minerals that may be given to correct deficiency diseases.

Powerful drugs often have marked *adverse effects*. Commonly used drugs with less potential to cause harm are sold over-the-counter (OTC) in pharmacies. Some OTC drugs can only be obtained with a pharmacist's consultation, and these are kept behind the pharmacy counter. More powerful drugs (those that cannot be used safely without medical supervision) require a doctor's prescription.

A different use of the word "drugs" refers to those substances on which a person may become dependent. These range from mild stimulants such as caffeine (found in coffee) to powerful agents that alter mood and behaviour. Some addictive drugs have no medical use and cannot be obtained legally.

Where drugs come from

At one time, the only available drugs were substances extracted from plants, or, in some cases, animals. Herbalism, the study and medicinal use of plants, was practised by the Chinese more than 5,000 years ago and is becoming popular in many parts of the world today.

Virtually all the drugs in current use have been developed in the laboratory and are manufactured through various chemical processes. About a quarter of these are derived from plants or other organisms. Most drugs are synthetic chemical copies, but some are still extracted from natural sources. For example, the opioid drugs, including morphine, are made from a species of poppy. Many antibiotics and some anticancer drugs are still of natural origin. The main difference between drugs of plant origin and "herbal medicines" is that drugs have been thoroughly tested to prove that they work and are safe.

Some drugs can now be made through genetic engineering, in which the genes (which control a cell's function) of certain microorganisms are altered, changing the products of cell activity to the desired drug. For example, the hormone insulin can now be manufactured by genetically engineered bacteria. This could eliminate the need to extract insulin from animal pancreas glands, the source until recently, benefiting those people who experience adverse reactions to material derived from animal sources.

Purely synthetic drugs are either modifications of naturally occurring ones, with the aim of increasing effectiveness or safety, or drugs developed after scientific investigation of a disease process with the intention of changing it biochemically.

Developing and marketing new drugs

Pharmaceutical manufacturers find new products in a variety of ways. New drugs are usually developed for one purpose but quite commonly a variant will be found that will be useful for something entirely different.

When a new drug is discovered, the manufacturer often undertakes a program of molecular tinkering, or elaboration. This refers to investigations into variants of the drug to see if a version can be made that is more effective or has fewer adverse effects. In some cases that experimental process has unexpected results. The elaboration process, for example, transformed some sulfa drugs, which were originally valued for their antibacterial properties, into widely used oral antidiabetics, diuretics, and anticonvulsants.

All new drugs undergo a long, careful test period before they are approved for marketing by the Therapeutic Products Directorate (TPD) (see Testing and approving new drugs). Once approval has been given, the manufacturer can then market the drug under a brand or trade name. Technically, patent protection gives the manufacturer exclusive rights for 20 years, but this protection starts from when the drug is first identified. The time remaining after TPD approval can be much less than 20 years.

When patent protection ends, other manufacturers may produce the drug, although they must use a different brand name or the generic name (see How drugs are classified, facing page).

Testing and approving new drugs

Before a drug is cleared by the TPD it undergoes a cautious, step-by-step period of testing, often lasting six to ten years. By law, a drug must be both safe and medically effective. Safety is established through various means, including tests on animals and human volunteers. Efficacy is proven through complex tests (including *double-blind* trials) on groups of healthy and ill patients. The testing is done in various research institutions under government-approved procedures.

The approval process also involves weighing a new drug's risks against its benefits. A dangerous drug whose only potential might be the relief of an ordinary headache undoubtedly would not win approval. Yet an equally *toxic* drug, effective against cancer, might. Medical judgment is an important part of the approval process.

Deadly nightshade
The drug belladonna is derived from this plant.

Opium poppy
This poppy is the basis for drugs such as morphine.

Developing and testing new drugs
All new drugs undergo a rigorous testing period in the laboratory.

HOW DRUGS ARE CLASSIFIED

The 5,000 or so substances loosely called drugs are described in many ways. Scientists and pharmacologists, interested in chemical structure, use one system. Physicians and pharmacists, concerned with use, employ another. Manufacturers and advertisers, promoting the benefits of their products, use simpler, more appealing names. Federal and provincial regulators, wary of the harm some drugs may do, classify them in a different manner altogether, according to their legal status.

Specific names

All drugs in general use rely on three terms: the generic, brand, and chemical names. The generic name, which is the official medical name for the basic active substance, is chosen by the USAN (US Adopted Name) Council, or is the British accepted name, or is one adopted in one of the world's major pharmacopoeias.

The brand name is chosen by the manufacturer, usually on the basis that it can be easily pronounced, recognized, or remembered. There may be several brands (each by a different manufacturer) containing the same generic substance. Differences between the brands may be slight but may relate to absorption rate (bioavailability), convenience, and digestibility. A drug may be available in generic form, as a brand-name product, or both. Some brand-name products contain several generic drugs. The chemical name is a technical description of the drug, and is not used in this book.

For example, the three names for a drug used to help those with AIDS are as follows. The generic name is zidovudine; the brand name is Retrovir (generic names are not capitalized, brand names are); and the chemical name is 3-azido- 3-deoxythymidine.

General terms

Drugs may be grouped according to chemical similarity, for example, the benzodiazepines. More often, though, drugs are classified according to use (antihypertensive) or biological effect (diuretic). Most drugs fit into one group, although many have multiple uses and are listed in several categories.

Because this book is aimed at the lay person, we have grouped drugs according to use, although a chemical description may be added to distinguish one group of drugs from others used to treat the same disorder (for example, benzodiazepine sleeping drugs).

Legal classification

Besides specifying which drugs can be sold over-the-counter and which require a physician's prescription, provincial and federal statutes and regulations govern the availability of many substances that have an abuse potential. The table below outlines the various categories of controlled drugs in Canada.

CATEGORIES OF CONTROLLED DRUGS

Various categories of drugs are controlled in Canada by the Food and Drugs Act and Regulations and the Controlled Drugs and Substances Act and Regulations.

Narcotic Drugs (Schedule N)	These drugs have a potential for abuse and can lead to serious physical and psychological dependence. They are recognized, however, as having accepted medical uses. They may be stimulants or depressants. In general, prescriptions for these agents cannot be renewed and a new prescription is required to be written by the physician. Health care professionals refer to these agents as opioids. **Examples** Heroin (dispensed in hospitals only), methodone (authorized prescribers only), morphine, codeine, oxycodone, hydromorphone, and meperidine.
Schedule J	All the drugs in this group are restricted and considered illegal. All have a high potential for abuse and currently do not have an accepted medical use. They cannot be prescribed. (One exception: Canada's Controlled Drugs and Substances Act was changed to permit the cultivation of industrial hemp in 1998, and to allow access to marijuana for medical use in 2001.) **Examples** LSD, psilocybin, dimethyltryptamine (DMT), methylenedioxyamphetamine (MDA).
Controlled Drugs (Schedule G)	These drugs also possess a potential for abuse, and their use may lead to various forms of drug dependence. Records are kept of each physician's prescribing. Prescriptions for Schedule G drugs can be refilled for a specified number of times. **Examples** Amphetamines, barbiturates, methylphenidate, diethylpropion.
Benzodiazepines and other targeted substances	These are drugs which have the potential for dependence and abuse, but are used quite commonly for many illnesses and conditions. A prescription can be issued in writing or can be transmitted by telephone to a pharmacist. Refills are permitted if the physician has specified the total number of refills in the original prescription as well as the specified date of refills and/or interval between refills. **Examples** Diazepam, alprazolam, lorazepam, bromazepam.
Prescription Drugs (Schedule F)	These are drugs used to treat a wide variety of illnesses requiring physician supervision. A prescription can be issued in writing or can be telephoned to a pharmacist. Repeat prescriptions are allowed. **Examples** Antibiotics, antihypertensive drugs, corticosteroids, antidepressants.
Non-prescription Drugs	These drugs are considered sufficiently safe to be sold over-the-counter in pharmacies and, for some products, in other retail stores. Most non-prescription drug products bear a Drug Identification Number (DIN). Some are available only through a pharmacist's consultation and are kept behind the counter. **Examples** Laxatives, antacids, mild analgesics (including those with a small amount of codeine combined with ASA or acetaminophen), iron tablets, dimenhydrinate, cough and cold preparations.

HOW DRUGS WORK

Before the discovery of the sulfa drugs in 1935, medical knowledge of drugs was limited to possibly only a dozen or so drugs that had a clear medical value. Most of these were the extracts of plants (such as digitalis, from foxgloves), while others, such as ASA, were chemically closely related to plant extracts (in this case, salicylic acid, from the willow tree). It was soon realized, however, that crude plant extracts had two disadvantages: they were of variable potency, and the same plant could contain a number of different substances with different actions. These might even oppose each other, or cause serious *adverse effects*. Now, thousands of effective drugs are available and scientific knowledge regarding drugs and their actions has virtually exploded.

Today's physician understands the complexity of drug actions in the body, both beneficial and adverse. As a result of extensive research and clinical experience, the doctor and the pharmacist can now also recognize that some drugs interact harmfully with others, or with certain foods and alcohol.

DRUG ACTIONS

While the exact workings of some drugs are not fully understood, medical science provides clear knowledge as to what most of them do once they enter or are applied to the human body. Drugs serve different purposes: sometimes they cure a disease, sometimes they only alleviate symptoms. Their impact occurs in various parts of the anatomy. Although different drugs act in different ways, their actions generally fall into one of three categories.

Replacing chemicals that are deficient

To function normally, the body requires sufficient levels of certain chemical substances. These include vitamins and minerals, which the body obtains from food. A balanced diet usually supplies what is needed. But when deficiencies occur, various deficiency diseases result. Lack of vitamin C causes scurvy, iron deficiency causes anemia, and lack of vitamin D leads to rickets in children and osteomalacia in adults.

Other deficiency diseases arise from a lack of various *hormones* which are the chemical substances produced by glands. Hormones act as internal "messengers". Diabetes mellitus, hypothyroidism, and Addison's disease all result from deficiencies of different hormones.

Deficiency diseases are treated with drugs that replace the substances that are missing or, in the case of some hormone deficiencies, with animal or synthetic replacements.

Interfering with cell function

Many drugs can change the way cells work by increasing or reducing the normal level of activity. Inflammation, for example, is due to the action of certain natural hormones and other chemicals on blood vessels and blood cells . Anti-inflammatory drugs block the action of the inflammatory components or slow their production. Drugs that act in a similar way are used in the treatment of a variety of conditions: hormone disorders, blood clotting problems, and heart and kidney diseases.

Many such drugs do their work by altering the transmission system by which messages are sent from one part of the body to another.

A message – such as to contract a muscle – originates in the brain and enters a nerve cell through its receiving end. The message, in the form of an electrical impulse, travels the nerve cell to the sending end. Here a chemical substance called a *neurotransmitter* is released, conducting the message across the tiny gap (synapse) separating it from an adjacent nerve cell. That process is repeated until the message reaches the appropriate muscle.

Many drugs can alter this process, often by their effect on receptor sites on cells (see left). Some drugs (*agonists*) intensify cell activity, while other drugs (*antagonists*) reduce activity in the cells.

Acting against invading organisms or abnormal cells

Infectious diseases are caused by viruses, bacteria, protozoa, and fungi invading the body. We now have a wide choice of drugs that destroy these microorganisms, either by halting their multiplication or by killing them directly. Other drugs treat disease by killing abnormal cells produced by the human body – cancer cells, for example.

RECEPTOR SITES

Many drugs produce their effects through their action on special sites called *receptors* on the surface of body cells. Natural body chemicals such as *neurotransmitters* bind to these sites, initiating a response in the cell. A cell may have many types of receptors, each of which has an affinity for a different chemical in the body. Drugs may also bind to receptors, either adding to the effect of the body's natural chemicals and enhancing cell response (agonists) or preventing such a chemical from binding to its receptor, and thereby blocking a particular cell response (antagonists).

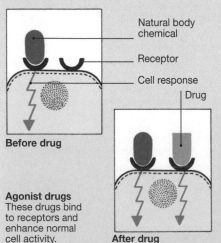

Before drug

Agonist drugs
These drugs bind to receptors and enhance normal cell activity.

After drug

Natural body chemical

Receptor

Cell response

Drug

Before drug

Antagonist drugs
These drugs bind to receptors and block cell activity.

After drug

Natural body chemical

Receptor

Cell response

Drug

THE EFFECTS OF DRUGS

Before a physician selects a drug to be used in the treatment of a sick person, he or she carefully weighs the benefits and the risks. Obviously, the physician expects a positive result from the drug – a cure of the condition or at least the relief of symptoms. At the same time, the physician has to consider the risks, since all drugs are potentially harmful, some of them considerably more so than others.

Reaction time

Some drugs can produce rapid and spectacular relief from the symptoms of disease. Nitroglycerin frequently provides almost immediate relief from the pain of angina; other drugs can quickly alleviate the symptoms of an asthmatic attack. Conversely, some drugs take much longer to produce a response. It may, for example, require several weeks of treatment with an antidepressant drug before a person experiences maximum benefit. This can add to anxiety unless the individual is informed of the possibility of a delay in the onset of beneficial effects.

Adverse effects

The *adverse effects* of a drug (also known as side effects or adverse reactions) are its undesired effects. When drugs are taken, they are distributed throughout the body and their effects are unlikely to be restricted just to the organ or tissue we want them to affect. Other parts of the body contain receptor sites like those the drug is targeting. In addition, the drug molecule may fit other, different receptors well enough to activate or block them too.

For example, *anticholinergic* drugs, given to relieve spasm of the intestinal wall, may also cause blurred vision, dry mouth, and retention of urine. Such effects may gradually disappear as the body becomes used to the drug. If they persist, the dose may have to be reduced, or the time between doses may need to be increased. Reducing the dose will often reduce the severity of the adverse effect for those effects that are called "dose-related".

DOSE AND RESPONSE

People respond in different ways to a drug, and often the dose has to be adjusted to allow for a person's age, weight, or general health. Children and the elderly usually require different doses than adults.

The dose of any drug should be sufficient to produce a beneficial response but not so great that it will cause excessive adverse effects. If the dose is too low, the drug may not have any effect; if it is too high, it will not produce any additional benefits and may produce adverse effects. The aim of drug treatment is to achieve a concentration of drug in the blood or tissue that lies between the lowest effective level and the maximum safe concentration. This is known as the therapeutic range.

For certain drugs the therapeutic range is quite narrow, so the safety/effectiveness margin is small. Other drugs have a much wider therapeutic range.

Wide therapeutic range

Dosage of drugs with a wide therapeutic range can vary considerably without altering the drug's effect. The effect of some drugs can be greater in children and the elderly.

Narrow therapeutic range

Dosage of drugs with a narrow therapeutic range must be carefully calculated to achieve the desired effect without toxicity. Children or the elderly require adjustment in doses.

Adverse effects of some drugs can be quite serious. Such drugs are given because they may be the only treatment for an otherwise fatal disease. But all drugs are chemicals, with a potential for producing serious, *toxic* reactions.

Some adverse effects seem not to be dose-related, and where the effect appears on first use and is unexpected, the phenomenon is called *idiosyncrasy*. People are genetically different and, as a result, their response to drugs differs, perhaps because they lack a particular enzyme or because it is less active than usual. For this reason, not everyone suffers the "common" adverse effects; but, occasionally, a new adverse effect, due to a rare and unsuspected genetic variation, will be discovered only after the drug has been taken by a large number of people.

Other adverse effects that are not dose-related are *allergic reactions*. These reactions do not usually appear on the first exposure to the drug but on a subsequent occasion. The symptoms are similar to those caused by other allergens and, in extreme cases, may cause anaphylactic shock (see p.528).

Beneficial vs. adverse effects

In evaluating the risk/benefit ratio of a prescribed drug, the doctor has to weigh the drug's therapeutic benefit against the possible adverse effects. For example, such side effects as nausea, headache, and diarrhea may result from taking an antibiotic. But the possible risks of these side effects will be considered acceptable if the problem is a life-threatening infection requiring immediate medical treatment. However, such side effects would be considered unacceptable for an over-the-counter drug for the relief of headaches.

Because some people are more at risk from adverse drug reactions than others (particularly those who have a history of drug allergy), the physician normally checks whether there is any reason why a certain drug should not be prescribed (see Drug treatment in special risk groups, p.20). The pharmacist should also verify that the individual has no known contraindications to the drug.

PLACEBO RESPONSE

The word placebo – Latin for "I will please" – is used to describe any chemically inert substance given as a substitute for a drug. Any benefit gained from taking a placebo occurs because the person taking it believes that it will produce good results.

New drugs are almost always tested against a placebo preparation in clinical trials as a way of assessing the efficacy of a drug before it is marketed. The placebo is made to look identical to the active preparation, and the volunteers are not told whether they have been given the active drug or the placebo. Sometimes the physician is also unaware of which preparation an individual has been given. This is known as a *double-blind* trial. In this way, the purely placebo effect can be eliminated and the effectiveness of the drug determined more realistically.

Sometimes the mere taking of a medicine has a psychological effect that produces a beneficial physical response. This type of placebo response can make an important contribution to the overall effectiveness of a chemically active drug. It is most commonly seen with analgesics, antidepressants, and anti-anxiety drugs. Some people, known as placebo responders, are more likely to experience this sort of reaction than the rest of the population.

DRUG INTERACTIONS

When different drugs are taken together, or when a drug is taken in combination with certain foods or with alcohol, effects different from those when the drug is taken alone may be produced. Often, this is beneficial and physicians sometimes make use of interactions to increase the effectiveness of a treatment. Often, more than one drug may be used to treat cancer or high blood pressure.

Other interactions, however, are unwanted and may be harmful. They may occur not only between prescription drugs, but also between prescription and over-the-counter drugs. It is important to read warnings on drug labels and tell your physician and pharmacist if you are taking any preparations – both prescription and over-the-counter, and even herbal or homeopathic remedies.

A drug may interact with another drug or with food or alcohol for a number of reasons (see below).

Altered absorption

Alcohol and some drugs (particularly *opioids* and drugs with an *anticholinergic* effect) slow the digestive process that empties the stomach contents into the intestine. This may delay the absorption, and therefore the effect, of another drug. Other drugs (for example, metoclopramide, an anti-emetic drug) may speed the rate at which the stomach empties and may, therefore, increase the rate at which another drug is absorbed and takes effect. Some drugs also combine with another drug or food in the intestine to form a compound that is not absorbed as readily. This occurs when tetracycline and iron tablets or antacids are taken together. Milk and dairy products also reduce the absorption of tetracycline and some other

Drug absorption in the intestine

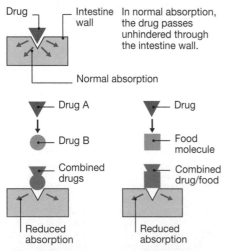

Drug — Intestine wall — In normal absorption, the drug passes unhindered through the intestine wall.

Normal absorption

Drug A → Drug B → Combined drugs — Reduced absorption

Drug → Food molecule → Combined drug/food — Reduced absorption

Absorption of drug (A) may be reduced if it combines with another drug (B).

Absorption of a drug may be reduced if it combines with a food molecule.

EXAMPLES OF IMPORTANT INTERACTIONS

Adverse interactions between drugs may vary from a simple blocking of a drug's beneficial effect to a serious reaction between two drugs that may be life-threatening. Some of the more serious adverse interactions occur between the following:

Drugs that depress the central nervous system (opioids, sedating antihistamines, sleeping drugs, and alcohol). The effects of two or more of these drugs together may be additive, causing dangerous oversedation.

Drugs that lower blood sugar levels and such drugs as sulfonamides and alcohol. The drug interaction increases the effect of blood sugar-lowering drugs, thus further depressing blood sugar levels.

Oral anticoagulants and other drugs, particularly ASA and antibiotics. As these drugs may increase the tendency to bleed, it is essential to check the effects in every case.

Monoamine oxidase inhibitors (MAOIs). Many drugs and foods can produce a severe increase in blood pressure when taken with MAOIs. Such drugs include amphetamines and decongestants; foods include cheese, herring, chocolate, red wine, and beer. Some of the newer MAOIs, however, are much less likely to interact with food and drugs.

---

drugs, such as ciprofloxacin, by combining with the drugs in this manner.

Enzyme effects

Some drugs increase the production of *enzymes* in the liver that break down drugs, while others inhibit or reduce enzyme production. Thus, they affect the rate at which other drugs are activated or inactivated.

Excretion in the urine

A drug may reduce the kidneys' ability to excrete another drug, raising the drug level in the blood and increasing its effect.

Receptor effects

Drugs that act on the same *receptor sites* (p.14) sometimes add to each other's effect on the body, or compete with each other in occupying certain receptor sites. For example, naloxone blocks receptors used by opioid drugs, thereby helping to reverse the effects of opioid poisoning.

Similar or opposite effects

Drugs that produce similar effects (but act on different receptors) add to each others' actions. Often, lower doses are possible as a result, with fewer *adverse effects*. This is common practice in the treatment of high blood pressure and cancer. Antibiotics are given together as the infecting organisms are less likely to develop resistance to the drugs. Drugs with *antagonistic* effects reduce the useful activity of one or both drugs. For example, some antidepressants oppose the effects of anticonvulsants.

Reduced protein binding

Some drugs circulate around the body in the bloodstream with a proportion of the drug attached to the proteins of the blood

---

plasma. The amount of drug attached to the plasma proteins is inactive. If another drug is taken, some of the second drug may also bind to the plasma proteins and displace the first drug; more of the first drug is then active in the body.

Interaction between protein-bound drugs

Blood vessel wall
Free active drug
Protein-bound drug
Protein

Protein-bound drug taken alone
Drug molecules that are bound to proteins in the blood are unable to pass into body tissues. Only free drug molecules are active.

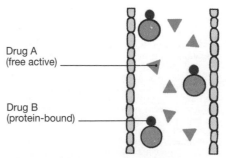

Drug A (free active)

Drug B (protein-bound)

Taken with another protein-bound drug
If a drug (B) with a greater ability to bind with proteins is also taken, drug (A) is displaced, increasing the amount of active drug.

METHODS OF ADMINISTRATION

The majority of drugs must be absorbed into the bloodstream in order for them to reach the site where their effects are needed. The method of administering a drug determines the route it takes to get into the bloodstream and the speed at which it is absorbed into the blood.

When a drug is meant to enter the bloodstream it is usually administered in one of the following ways: through the mouth or rectum, by injection, or by inhalation. Drugs that are implanted under the skin or enclosed in a skin patch also enter the bloodstream. These types are discussed under Slow-release preparations (p.18).

When it is unnecessary or undesirable for a drug to enter the bloodstream in large amounts, it may be applied *topically* so that its effect is limited mainly to the site of the disorder, such as the surface of the skin or mucous membranes (the membranes of the nose, eyes, ears, vagina, or rectum). Drugs are administered topically in a variety of preparations, including creams, sprays, drops, and suppositories. Most inhaled drugs also have a local effect on the respiratory tract.

Very often, a particular drug may be available in different forms. Many drugs are available both as tablets and injectable fluid. The choice between a tablet and an injection depends on a number of factors, including the severity of the illness, the urgency with which the drug effect is needed, the part of the body requiring treatment, and the patient's general state of health, in particular his or her ability to swallow.

The various administration routes are discussed in greater detail below. For a description of the different forms in which drugs are given, see Drug forms (p.19).

ADMINISTRATION BY MOUTH

Giving drugs by mouth is the most common method of administration. Most of the drugs that are given by mouth are absorbed into the bloodstream through the walls of the intestine. The speed at which the drug is absorbed and the amount of active drug that is available for use depend on several factors, including the form in which the drug is given (for example, as a tablet or a liquid) and whether it is taken with food or on an empty stomach. If a drug is taken when the stomach is empty (before meals, for example) it may act more quickly than a drug that is taken after a meal when the stomach is full.

Some drugs (like antacids, which neutralize stomach acidity) are taken by mouth to produce a direct effect on the stomach or digestive tract.

In-mouth administration
Products are available that are placed In the mouth but not swallowed. They are absorbed quickly into the bloodstream through the lining of the mouth, which has a rich supply of blood vessels. Sublingual tablets are placed under the tongue, wafers are placed on the tongue, and buccal tablets are placed in the pouch between the cheek and teeth.

HOW DRUGS PASS THROUGH THE BODY

Most drugs taken by mouth reach the bloodstream by absorption through the wall of the small intestine. Blood vessels supplying the intestine then carry the drug to the liver, where it may be broken down into a form that can be used by the body. The drug (or its breakdown product) then enters the general circulation, which carries it around the body. It may pass back into the intestine before being reabsorbed into the bloodstream. Some drugs are rapidly excreted via the kidneys; others may build up in fatty tissues in the body.

Certain insoluble drugs cannot be absorbed through the intestinal wall and pass through the digestive tract unchanged. These drugs are useful for treating bowel disorders, but if they are intended to have *systemic* effects elsewhere they must be given by intravenous injection.

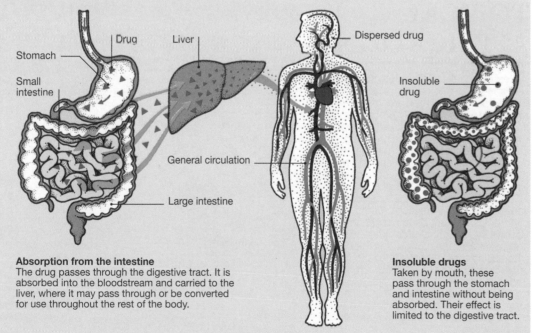

Absorption from the intestine
The drug passes through the digestive tract. It is absorbed into the bloodstream and carried to the liver, where it may pass through or be converted for use throughout the rest of the body.

Insoluble drugs
Taken by mouth, these pass through the stomach and intestine without being absorbed. Their effect is limited to the digestive tract.

RECTAL ADMINISTRATION

INHALATION

Drugs intended to have a *systemic* effect may be given in the form of suppositories inserted into the rectum, from where they are absorbed into the bloodstream. This method may be used to give drugs that might be destroyed by the stomach's digestive juices. It is also sometimes used to administer drugs to people who cannot take medication by mouth, such as those who are suffering from nausea and vomiting.

Drugs may also be given rectally for local effect, either as suppositories (to relieve hemorrhoids) or as enemas (for ulcerative colitis).

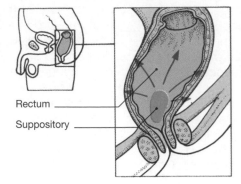

Rectum

Suppository

Drugs may be inhaled to produce a *systemic* effect or a direct local effect on the respiratory tract.

Gases to produce *general anesthesia* are administered by inhalation and are absorbed into the bloodstream through the lungs, producing a general effect on the body, particularly the brain.

Bronchodilators, used to treat certain types of asthma, emphysema, and bronchitis, are a common example of drugs administered by inhalation for their direct effect on the respiratory tract, although some of the active drug also reaches the bloodstream. (See also p.76.)

ADMINISTRATION BY INJECTION

Drugs may be injected into the body to produce a *systemic* effect. One reason for injecting drugs is the rapid response that follows. Other circumstances that call for injection are when: a person is intolerant to the drug when taken by mouth; the drug would be destroyed by the stomach's digestive juices (insulin, for example); or the drug cannot pass through the intestinal walls into the bloodstream. Drug injections may also be given to produce a local effect, as is often done to relieve the pain of arthritis.

The three most common methods of injection – intramuscular, intravenous, and subcutaneous – are described in the illustration (see right). The type of injection depends both on the nature of the drug and the condition being treated.

Muscle | Vein | Skin | Fatty tissue

Intramuscular (IM) injection
The drug is injected into a muscle, usually of the thigh, the upper arm, or the buttock.

Subcutaneous (SC) injection
The drug is injected directly under the surface of the skin.

Intravenous (IV) injection
The drug is injected directly into a vein and therefore directly into the bloodstream. Drugs given by this route act more quickly than drugs given by other types of injection.

TOPICAL APPLICATION

In treating localized disorders such as skin infections and nasal congestion, it is often preferable when a choice is available to prescribe drugs in a form that has a *topical*, or localized, rather than a *systemic* effect. The reason is that it is much easier to control the effects of drugs administered locally and to ensure that they produce the maximum benefit with minimum *adverse effects*.

Topical preparations are available in a variety of forms, from skin creams, ointments, and lotions to nasal sprays, ear and eye drops, bladder irrigations, and vaginal suppositories. It is important when using topical preparations to follow instructions carefully, avoiding a higher dose than recommended or application for longer than necessary. This will help to avoid adverse systemic effects caused by the absorption of larger amounts into the bloodstream.

SLOW-RELEASE AND MODIFIED-RELEASE PREPARATIONS

Some disorders can be treated with specially formulated preparations that can release the active drug slowly. Such preparations may be beneficial when it is inconvenient for a person to visit the physician regularly, or when only small amounts of the drug need to be released into the body. Slow release of drugs can be achieved by *depot injections*, *transdermal patches*, capsules and tablets, and implants. Modified-release tablets and capsules are a more advanced version in which release of the active ingredient is related to time.

Slow-release capsule
Contains pellets of drug in a specially formulated coating.

Outer coating

Drug

Capsule

Transdermal patch
An adhesive, drug-impregnated pad is placed on the skin. The drug passes slowly into the skin.

Transdermal patch

Skin

Drug

Site of incision

Implant

Fatty tissue

Muscle

Implants
A pellet containing the drug is implanted under the skin. By this rarely used method, a drug (usually a hormone) is slowly released into the bloodstream over a period of months.

DRUG FORMS

Most drugs are specially prepared in a form designed for convenience of administration. This helps to ensure that dosages are accurate and that taking the medication is as easy as possible. Inactive ingredients (those with no therapeutic effect) are often added to flavour or colour the medicine, or to improve its chemical stability, extending the period during which it is effective.

The more common drug forms are described in detail below.

Tablets

This contains the drug compressed with other ingredients (see right) into a solid plug. Some are coated with a membrane that allows the drug to be slowly released, to produce a sustained effect; others are composed of granules that are individually layered to give the slow release.

Capsules

The drug is contained in a cylindrically shaped gelatin shell that breaks open after the capsule has been swallowed, releasing the drug. Slow-release capsules contain pellets that dissolve in the gastrointestinal tract, releasing the drug slowly (facing page).

Wafers

The drug is contained in a small wafer, which is placed on the tongue and allowed to dissolve.

Liquids

Some drugs are available in liquid form, the active substance being combined in a solution, suspension, or emulsion with other ingredients – preservatives, solvents, and flavouring or colouring agents. Many liquid preparations should be shaken before use to ensure that the active drug is evenly distributed. If it is not, inaccurate dosages may result.

Mixture

A mixture is one or more drugs, either dissolved to form a solution or suspended in a liquid (often water).

Elixir

An elixir is a solution of a drug in a sweetened mixture of alcohol and water. It is often highly flavoured.

Emulsion

An emulsion is a drug dispersed in oil and water. An emulsifying agent is often included to stabilize the product.

Syrup

A syrup is a concentrated solution of sugar containing the active drug, with flavouring and stabilizing agents added.

Topical skin preparations

These are preparations designed for application to the skin and other surface

WHAT A TABLET CONTAINS

Lubricants (magnesium stearate, purified talc)

Drug

Diluents (sucrose, lactose, sodium chloride)

Disintegrating agents (potato, starch, cocoa butter, tartaric acid, sodium bicarbonate)

Binding agents (acacia, gelatin, glucose, sucrose)

Granulating agents (alcohol, gum, water, starch pastes)

Diluents add bulk. Binders and granulating agents bind the ingredients. Lubricants ensure a smooth surface by allowing the ingredients to flow during the manufacturing process.

Disintegrating agents help the tablet dissolve. A sugar coating or a transparent film protects the surface or modifies the drug's release rate. Dyes and imprints make it recognizable.

tissues of the body. Preservatives are usually included to reduce the growth of bacteria. The most commonly used types of skin preparations are described below. For a more detailed discussion, see Bases for skin preparations, p.160.

Cream

A cream is a non-greasy preparation that is used to apply drugs to an area of the body or to cool or moisten the skin. It is less noticeable than an ointment.

Ointment

An ointment is a greasy preparation used to apply drugs to an area of the body, or as a protective or lubricant layer for the relief of dry skin conditions.

Lotion

A lotion is a solution or suspension applied to unbroken skin to cool and dry the affected area. Some are more suitable for use in hairy areas because they are not as sticky as creams or ointments.

Injection solutions

Solutions used for injections are sterile (germ-free) preparations of a drug that are dissolved or suspended in a liquid. Other chemicals (such as anti-oxidants and buffers) are often added to preserve the stability of the drug or to regulate the acidity or alkalinity of the solution. Most injectable drugs used today are packaged in sterile, disposable syringes. This reduces the chance of contamination. Certain drugs are still available in multiple-dose vials, and a chemical bactericide is added to prevent the growth of bacteria when the needle is reinserted through the rubber

seal. For details on different types, see Administration by injection, facing page.

Suppositories

These are solid, bullet-shaped dosage forms designed for easy insertion into the rectum (rectal suppository) or vagina (vaginal suppository). They contain a drug and an inert (pharmacologically and chemically inactive) substance often derived from cocoa butter or vegetable oil. The drug is gradually released in the rectum or vagina as the suppository dissolves at body temperature.

Eye drops

A sterile drug solution (or suspension) dropped behind the eyelid.

Ear drops

A solution (or suspension) containing a drug introduced into the ear by dropper. Ear drops are usually given to produce an effect on the outer ear canal.

Nasal drops/spray

A solution of a drug for introduction into the nose to produce a local effect.

Inhalers

Aerosol inhalers contain a solution or suspension of a drug under pressure. A valve ensures delivery of a recommended dosage when the inhaler is activated. A mouthpiece facilitates inhalation as the drug is released from the canister. The correct technique is important; the printed instructions should be followed carefully or your physician, pharmacist, or nurse will show you. Aerosol inhalers are used for respiratory conditions such as asthma (see also p.77).

DRUG TREATMENT IN SPECIAL RISK GROUPS

Different people tend to respond in different ways to drug treatment. Taking the same drug, one person may suffer *adverse effects* while another does not. However, physicians know that certain people are always more at risk from adverse effects when they take drugs; the reason is that in those people the body handles drugs differently, or the drug has an atypical effect. Those people at special risk include infants and children, women who are pregnant or breast-feeding, the elderly, and people with long-term medical conditions, especially those who have impaired liver or kidney function.

The reasons that such people may be more likely to suffer adverse effects are discussed in detail on the following pages. Others who may need special attention include those already taking regular medication who may risk complications when they take another drug. Drug interactions are discussed more fully on p.16.

When physicians prescribe drugs for people at special risk, they take extra care to select appropriate medication, adjust dosages, and closely monitor the effects of treatment. If you think you may be at special risk, be sure to tell your physician in case he or she is not fully aware of your particular circumstances. Similarly, if you are buying over-the-counter drugs, you should ask your physician or pharmacist if you think you may be at risk of experiencing any possible adverse effects or hazardous drug interactions.

INFANTS AND CHILDREN

Infants and children need a lower dosage of drugs than adults because children have a relatively low body weight. In addition, because of differences in body composition and the distribution and amount of body fat, as well as differences in the state of development and function of organs such as the liver and kidneys at different ages, children cannot simply be given a proportion of an adult dose as if they were small adults. Dosages need to be calculated in a more complex way, taking into account the child's age and weight. While newborn babies often have to be given very small doses of drugs, older children may need relatively large doses of some drugs compared to the adult dosage.

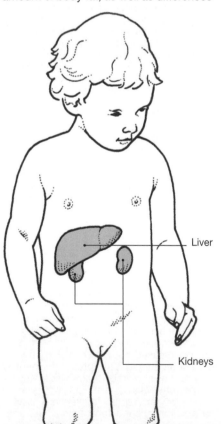

Liver

Kidneys

The liver
The liver's enzyme systems are not fully developed when a baby is born. This means that drugs are not broken down as rapidly as in an adult, and may reach dangerously high concentrations in the baby's body. For this reason, many drugs are not prescribed for babies or are given in very reduced doses. In older children, because the liver is relatively large compared to the rest of the body, some drugs may need to be given in proportionately higher doses.

The kidneys
During the first six months, a baby's kidneys are unable to excrete drugs as efficiently as an adult's kidneys. This may lead to a dangerously high concentration of a drug in the blood. The dose of certain drugs may therefore need to be reduced. Between one and two years of age, kidney function improves, and higher doses of some drugs may then be needed.

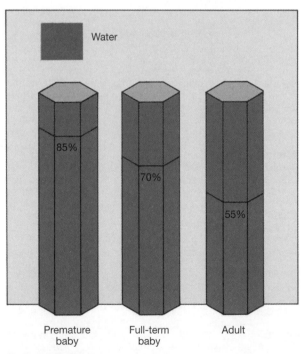

Water

85%

70%

55%

Premature baby

Full-term baby

Adult

Body composition
The proportion of water in the body of a premature baby is about 85 per cent of its body weight, that of a full-term baby is 70 per cent, and that of an adult is only 55 per cent. This means that drugs that stay in the body water will not be as concentrated in an infant's body as in an adult's, unless a higher dose relative to body weight is given.

PREGNANT WOMEN

Great care is needed during pregnancy to protect the fetus so that it develops into a healthy baby. Drugs taken by the mother can cross the placenta and enter the baby's bloodstream. With certain drugs, and at certain stages of pregnancy, there is a risk of developmental abnormalities, retarded growth, or post-delivery problems affecting the newborn baby. In addition, some drugs may affect the health of the mother during pregnancy.

Many drugs are known to have *adverse effects* during pregnancy; others are known to be safe, but in a large number of cases there is no firm evidence to decide on risk or safety. Therefore, the most important rule if you are pregnant or trying to conceive is to consult your physician before taking any prescribed or over-the-counter medication.

Drugs such as marijuana, nicotine, and alcohol should also be avoided during pregnancy. A high daily intake of caffeine should be reduced if possible. Your physician will assess the potential benefits of drug treatment against any possible risks to decide whether or not a drug should be taken. This is particularly important if you need to take medication regularly for a chronic condition such as epilepsy, high blood pressure, or diabetes.

Drugs and the stages of pregnancy

Pregnancy is divided into three three-month stages called trimesters. Depending on the trimester in which they are taken, drugs can have different effects on the mother, the fetus, or both. Some drugs may be considered safe during one trimester, but not during another. Doctors, therefore, often need to substitute one medication for another given during the course of pregnancy and/or labour.

The trimesters of pregnancy

First trimester
During the first three months of pregnancy – the most critical period – drugs may affect the development of fetal organs, leading to congenital malformations. Very severe defects may result in miscarriage.

Second trimester
From the fourth to the sixth month some drugs may retard the growth of the fetus. This may also result in a low birth weight. Other drugs may affect the development of the nervous system.

Third trimester
During the last three months of pregnancy, major risks include breathing difficulties in the newborn baby. Some drugs may also affect labour, causing it to be premature, delayed, or prolonged.

How drugs cross the placenta

The placenta acts as a filter between the mother's bloodstream and that of the baby. It allows small molecules of nutrients to pass into the baby's blood, while preventing larger particles such as blood cells from doing so. Drug molecules are comparatively small and pass easily through the placental barrier.

Wall of uterus · Placenta · Placenta · Umbilical cord

Nutrients · Blood cell · Mother's blood · Drug molecules · Baby's blood · Waste products

BREAST-FEEDING

Milk-producing glands · Nipple · Milk ducts

Blood vessel · Blood · Drug molecule · Milk-producing cells · Breast milk

How drugs pass into breast milk
The milk-producing glands in the breast are surrounded by a network of fine blood vessels. Small molecules of substances such as drugs pass from the blood into the milk. Drugs that dissolve easily in fat may pass across in greater concentrations than other drugs.

Just as drugs may cross from the mother's bloodstream into the baby's through the placenta, they may also pass to the baby from the mother's milk. This means that a breast-fed baby will receive small doses of whatever drugs the mother is taking. In many cases this is not a problem, because the amount of drug that passes into the milk is too small to have any significant effect on the baby. However, some drugs can produce unwanted effects on the baby. Antibiotics may sensitize the infant and consequently prevent their use later in life. Sedative drugs may make the baby drowsy and cause feeding problems. Moreover, some drugs may reduce the amount of milk produced by the mother.

Physicians usually advise breast-feeding women to take only essential drugs. When a mother needs to take regular medication while breast-feeding, her baby may also need to be closely monitored for possible adverse effects.

THE ELDERLY

Older people are particularly at risk when taking drugs. This is partly due to the physical changes associated with aging, and partly because many elderly people need to take several different drugs at the same time. They may also be at risk because they may be unable to manage their treatment properly, or they may lack the information to do so.

Physical changes

Elderly people have a greater risk of accumulating drugs in their body tissues because the liver is less efficient at breaking drugs down and the kidneys are less efficient at excreting them. Because of this, in some cases the normal adult dose will produce side effects, and a smaller dose may be needed to produce a therapeutic effect without the side effects. (See also Liver and kidney disease, below.)

Older people tend to take more drugs than younger people – many take three or more drugs at the same time. Apart from increasing the number of drugs in their systems, adverse drug interactions (see p.16) are more likely.

As people grow older, some parts of the body, such as the brain and nervous system, become more sensitive to drugs, thus increasing the likelihood of adverse reactions from drugs acting on those sites (see right). A similar problem may occur due to changes in the body's ratio of body fat. Although allergic reactions

(see Allergy, p.109) do not become more common due to increasing age, they are more likely because more drugs are prescribed. Accordingly, physicians prescribe more carefully for older people, especially those with disorders that are likely to correct themselves in time.

Incorrect use of drugs

Elderly people often suffer harmful effects from their drug treatment because they may fail to take their medication regularly or correctly. This may happen because they have been misinformed about how to take it or receive vague instructions. Problems arise sometimes because the elderly person cannot remember whether he or she has taken the drug and takes a double dose (see Exceeding the dose, p.30). Problems may also occur because the person is confused; this is not necessarily due to age or illness, but can arise as a result of drug treatment, especially if an elderly person is taking a number of different drugs or a sedative.

Prescriptions for the elderly should be clearly and fully labelled, and/or information about the drug and its use should be provided either for the individual or for the person taking care of him or her. When appropriate, containers with memory aids should be used to dispense the medication in single doses.

Elderly people often find it difficult to swallow medicine in capsule or tablet

Effect of drugs that act on the brain

In young people
There are plenty of receptors to take up the drug as well as natural *neurotransmitters.*

In older people
There are fewer receptors so that even a reduced drug dose may be excessive.

form; they should always take capsules or tablets with a full glass or cup of liquid. A liquid medicine may be prescribed instead.

LIVER AND KIDNEY DISEASE

Long-term illness affects the way in which people respond to drugs. This is especially true of liver and kidney problems. The liver alters the chemical structure of many drugs that enter the body (see How drugs pass through the body, p.17) by breaking them down into simpler substances, while the kidneys excrete drugs in the urine. If the effectiveness of the liver or kidneys is reduced by illness, the action of drugs on the individual can be significantly altered. In most cases, people with liver or kidney disease will be prescribed a smaller number of drugs and lower doses. In addition, certain drugs may, in rare cases, damage the liver or kidneys. For

example, tetracycline can cause kidney failure in those with poor kidney function. A physician may be reluctant to prescribe such a drug to someone with already reduced liver or kidney function in order to avoid the risk of further damage.

Drugs and liver disease

Severe liver diseases, such as cirrhosis and hepatitis, affect the way the body breaks down drugs. This can lead to a dangerous accumulation of certain drugs in the body. People suffering from these diseases should consult their physician before taking any medication (including over-the-counter drugs) or alcohol. Many

drugs must be avoided completely, since they could cause coma in someone with liver damage.

Drugs and kidney disease

People with poor kidney function are at risk from drug side effects. There are two reasons for this. First, drugs build up in the system because smaller amounts are excreted in urine. Second, kidney disease can cause protein loss through the urine, which lowers the level of protein in the blood. Some drugs bind to blood proteins, and if there are fewer protein molecules, a greater proportion of drug becomes free and active in the body.

Drug passing through body

Normal liver and kidneys
Drugs are processed in the liver before being excreted by the kidneys.

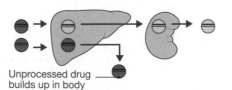

In liver damage
The liver cannot process sufficient drug and this builds up in the body tissues.

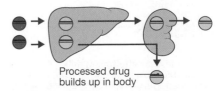

In kidney damage
The kidneys cannot excrete the processed drug in the urine and drug levels in the body rise.

DRUG TOLERANCE AND DEPENDENCE

In the course of treatment with many common drugs, the body acquires the ability to adapt to the drug's effect. This response is known as tolerance. As a result, the drug dose has to be increased to achieve the same effect as before. Tolerance is not always associated with dependence (often called addiction), which is the compulsion to continue taking a drug in order to experience a desired effect, or in order to avoid the unpleasant effects that occur when it is not taken. Dependence is almost always confined to drugs which act on the brain and nervous system, such as opiates, tobacco, and alcohol.

TOLERANCE

Drug tolerance occurs as the body adapts to a drug's actions. A person taking the drug needs larger and larger doses to achieve the original effect and as the dose increases, so too do the risks of toxic effects and dependence. Although people can develop a tolerance to many drugs, it is a dangerous characteristic of virtually all the drugs of dependence.

How tolerance develops

Drug tolerance can develop through a variety of different mechanisms, many of which are not fully understood. In some cases, the liver becomes more efficient at breaking the drug down to an inactive form. In other cases, the drug receptors adapt to the presence of the drug, In yet other cases, the drug exhausts the body's supply of chemicals necessary to produce a response.

Tolerance to one particular drug may result in the reduced effect of a drug that has similar properties or is processed in the body in the same way. This is known as cross tolerance. For example, a regular drinker, who can tolerate high levels of alcohol (a depressant), can have a dangerous tolerance to other depressants such as sleeping drugs and anti-anxiety drugs. While cross-tolerance can often cause problems, it sometimes has a beneficial effect in allowing a substance with a less addictive potential to replace the original drug. For example, the symptoms of alcohol withdrawal can be controlled by the anti-anxiety drug diazepam, which is also a depressant.

Tolerance to some drugs has its benefits. A person can develop tolerance to the side effects of a drug while still benefiting from its useful effects. For example, many people taking antidepressants find that side effects such as dry mouth slowly disappear, with the primary action of the drug continuing (see below).

Increasing drug tolerance has dangers. A person who has developed tolerance to a drug may keep raising the dose to sometimes toxic levels in order to achieve the desired effect.

Effects of tolerance

Development of tolerance
A gradually increasing dose of the drug is needed to produce the desired effect as tolerance develops over time.

Beneficial effect of tolerance
During treatment with many drugs, the unwanted side effects decrease with time, while the desired effect of the drug is maintained.

DEPENDENCE

Drug dependence is defined as the compulsive use of a substance resulting in physical, psychological, or social harm to the user, with continued use despite the harm.

Drug dependence (now widely preferred as a term to the word addiction) applies far more widely than most people realize. It is usually thought of in association with the use of illegal drugs, such as heroin, or with excessive intake of alcohol. But millions of people are dependent on other drugs, including stimulants – such as caffeine found in coffee and tea, and nicotine in tobacco – and certain prescription medicines, such as analgesics, sleeping drugs, amphetamines, and tranquillizers.

Psychological and physical dependence

Drug dependence, implying that a person is reliant on the continued use of a substance with potential for abuse, is of two types. Psychological dependence is an emotional state of craving for a drug whose presence has a desired effect on the mind, or whose absence has an undesired effect. Physical dependence, which often accompanies psychological dependence, involves physiological adaptation to a medicine or alcohol that is characterized by severe physical disturbances – withdrawal symptoms – during a period of abstinence. Some drugs, such as laxatives, can produce physical dependence.

Drugs that cause dependence

Many people who need to take regular medication worry that they may become dependent on their drugs. In fact, only a few groups of drugs produce physical or psychological dependence, and most of them are substances that alter mood or behaviour. Such drugs include heroin and the *opioid* analgesics such as morphine and meperidine, sleeping and anti-anxiety drugs (benzodiazepines and barbiturates), depressants (alcohol), and nervous system stimulants (cocaine, caffeine, amphetamines, and nicotine).

Antidepressant drugs do not cause psychological dependence. When a depressive illness has been treated effectively, drugs can usually be stopped

DEPENDENCE continued

without any problems, although some people may experience physical withdrawal symptoms if drugs are stopped suddenly. Consult the drug profile in Part 4 of this book to discover the dependence rating of any drug you are taking.

The use of nicotine, in the form of tobacco, and of opioid analgesics, whether controlled or uncontrolled, invariably produces physical dependence if taken regularly over a period of time. However, it is also true that not all regular users of alcohol become alcoholics. There is much argument over the definition of an alcoholic. A widely used definition is: a person who has experienced physical, psychological, social, or occupational impairment as a consequence of habitual, excessive consumption of alcohol.

Recognizing the dangers of drug dependence

Factors that determine a person's risk of developing physical dependence include the characteristics of the drug itself, the strength and frequency of doses, and the duration of use. However, the presence of these factors does not always result in dependence. Psychological and physiological factors that are unique to each individual also enter into the equation, and there may be other, as yet unknown, factors involved. For example, when the use of opioid analgesics is

DRUG MISUSE

The term is defined as any use of drugs that causes physical, psychological, economic, legal, or social harm to the user, or to persons who may be affected by the user's behaviour. Drug abuse commonly refers to taking drugs obtained illegally (such as heroin), but may also be used to describe the misuse of drugs generally obtainable legally (nicotine, alcohol), and to drugs obtainable through a physician's prescription only (everything from sleeping drugs and tranquillizers to analgesics and stimulants).

The misuse of prescription drugs deserves more attention than it usually receives. The practice can include the personal use of drugs left over from a previous course of treatment, the sharing with others of drugs that have been prescribed for yourself, the deliberate deception of physicians, the forgery of prescriptions, and the theft of drugs from pharmacies. All of these practices can have dangerous consequences. Careful

attention to the advice in the section on Managing your drug treatment (p.25) will help to avoid inadvertent misuse of drugs. The dangers associated with abuse of individual drugs are discussed under Drugs of abuse (pp.483–493).

Commonly misused drugs

Alcohol	Mescaline
Amphetamines	Nicotine
Barbiturates	Nitrates
Benzodiazepines	Opioids (including
Cocaine (including	heroin and
crack)	methadone
Ecstasy	Phencyclidine
GHB	Solvents
Ketamine	
Khat	
Lysergide (LSD)	
Cannabis	

restricted to the short-term relief of pain in a medical setting or long-term use in patients with cancer, dependence is rare. Yet there is a high risk of physical dependence when these drugs, or other drugs of abuse, are taken for non-medical reasons. There is also a risk in some cases of low-dose use when the drug is continued over a long period (e.g. with

benzodiazepines, p.67). No one can say for sure exactly what leads a person to drug-dependent behaviour. A person's psychological and physical make-up are thought to be factors, as well as his or her social environment, occupational pressures, and outlook on life.

The indiscriminate use of certain prescription drugs can also cause drug dependence. Benzodiazepine drugs can produce dependence, and this is one reason why physicians today discourage the use of any drug to induce sleep or calm anxiety for more than a few weeks. Appetite suppressants (see p.72) require close medical supervision. Amphetamines are no longer prescribed as appetite suppressants because of the frequency with which they are abused.

Treating drug dependence

Treatment for drug dependence can only be effective if the person is sufficiently motivated. There are two parts to treatment. The first part, detoxification, can take different forms. In some cases, if it is possible to do so, abstinence may be abruptly imposed. Sometimes, the drug may be gradually withdrawn or other safer substances substituted. For example, methadone (p.346) is substituted for heroin. Physical or mental withdrawal symptoms may need close monitoring, for instance, withdrawal from depressants such as barbiturates or alcohol may result in convulsions. Once the drug has been cleared from the body, the second part of treatment is directed at preventing a recurrence. This can involve psychological therapies to tackle the initial cause of the dependence, such as social problems. Psychotherapy, counselling, and support organizations, such as Alcoholics Anonymous, may all play a role in the rehabilitation of the alcoholic or addict.

SYMPTOMS OF WITHDRAWAL

These can range from the mild (sneezing, sweating) to the serious (vomiting, confusion) to the extremely serious (fits, coma). Alcohol withdrawal may be associated with delirium tremens, very occasionally fatal. Withdrawal from benzodiazepines can sometimes involve hallucinations and fits. But under medical guidance, withdrawal symptoms can be

relieved with doses of the original drug, or with less addictive substitutes.

Withdrawal symptoms occur because the body has adapted to the action of the drug (see Drug tolerance, p.23). When a drug is continuously present, the body may stop the release of a natural chemical necessary to normal function, like endorphins (below).

Pain and heroin withdrawal

Normal brain
When no drug is present, natural substances called endorphins inhibit the transmission of pain signals.

Effect of heroin
Heroin occupies the same receptors in the brain as endorphins, suppressing production of endorphins.

Heroin withdrawal
Abrupt withdrawal of heroin leaves the brain without a buffer to pain signals, even from minor stimuli.

MANAGING YOUR DRUG TREATMENT

A prescribed drug does not automatically produce a beneficial response. For a drug to have maximum benefit, it must be taken as directed by your physician, pharmacist, or manufacturer. It is estimated that two out of every five people for whom a drug is prescribed do not take it properly, if at all. The reasons include failure to understand or remember instructions, fear of adverse reactions, and lack of motivation, often arising from the disappearance of symptoms.

It is your responsibility to take a prescribed drug at the correct time, and in the manner stipulated. To do this, you need to know where to obtain

information about the drug (see Questioning your physician, p.26) and to make certain that you fully understand the instructions.

The following pages describe the practical aspects of drug treatment, from obtaining a prescription and buying over-the-counter drugs to storing drugs and disposing of old medications safely. Problems caused by mismanaging drug treatment – overdosing, underdosing, or stopping the drug altogether – and long-term drug treatment are dealt with on pp.28–31. Information regarding specific drugs is given in Part 4.

OVER-THE-COUNTER DRUGS

Over-the-counter drugs are those for which a prescription is not required. All are available from pharmacies (many only from pharmacies).

It is generally accepted that over-the-counter drugs are suitable for self-treatment and are unlikely to produce serious adverse reactions if taken as directed. But, as with all medicines, they can be harmful if they are misused. The ease with which they can be purchased is no guarantee of their absolute safety. For this reason, the same precautions should be taken when using any over-the-counter medicine as when using a drug prescribed by your physician.

Using over-the-counter drugs

A number of minor ailments and problems, ranging from coughs and colds to minor cuts and bruises, can be adequately dealt with by taking or using over-the-counter medicines. However, when using these treatments, you must be sure to read the directions on the label and follow them carefully, particularly those advising on dosage and under what circumstances a physician should be consulted. Most over-the-counter drugs are clearly labelled. They may warn of conditions under which the drug should not be taken, or advise you to consult a doctor if symptoms persist.

The pharmacist is a good source of information about over-the-counter drugs and can usually tell you what is suitable for your complaint. He or she can also determine when an over-the-counter drug may not be effective and can warn you if self-treatment or prolonged treatment is not advisable. When consulting the pharmacist regarding over-the-counter drugs, you should inform him or her if you are taking prescription drugs for any other illnesses.

It is important to speak to your physician before buying over-the-counter drugs for children. Some symptoms, such as

diarrhea in young children, should be treated only by a physician since they may be caused by a serious condition.

Buying over-the-counter medications
Various drugs are available over-the-counter, ranging from cough medicines to eye drops. Your pharmacist can help you to select the appropriate medication.

Eye preparations

Medicated creams, lotions, and powders

Cough and cold treatments

Laxatives

Analgesics

Antacids

PRESCRIPTION DRUGS

Drugs prescribed by a physician are not necessarily "stronger" or more likely to have side effects than those you can buy without prescription. Indeed, physicians often prescribe drugs that are also available over-the-counter (OTC). Drugs that are available only on prescription are drugs whose safe use is difficult to ensure without medical supervision.

When a physician prescribes a drug, he or she usually starts treatment at the normal dosage for the disorder being treated. The dosage may later be adjusted (lowered or increased) if the drug is not producing the desired effect or if you experience adverse side effects. The physician may also decide to switch to an alternative drug that may be more effective at treating the disorder.

Prescribing generic and brand-name drugs

When writing a prescription for a drug, the physician often has a choice between a generic and a brand-name product. Although the active ingredient is the same, two versions of the same drug may act in slightly different ways, as each manufacturer may formulate their product differently. They may also look different. Generic drugs are often cheaper than brand-name products. For this reason, certain brand-name products are not available on certain drug plans. These are factors that a physician must consider when writing a prescription.

Community pharmacists usually need to consider which drug is covered on your plan and may consult with you in substituting a generic name drug. Physicians may indicate "no substitution" on the prescription if they feel that the brand name product would be most suitable for treatment.

If you are prescribed a generic drug, the pharmacist is free to dispense whatever version of this drug is available. This means that your regular medication may vary in appearance each time you renew your prescription. If your medication does look different, always check with your pharmacist to reassure yourself that it is the correct drug.

Hospital pharmacies often dispense only generic versions of certain drugs. Therefore, if you are in hospital, the regular medication you receive may look different from that which you are used to at home.

Your prescription

Prescriptions usually have the same information. Your name and address will be listed, and the name of the medication you are being prescribed. The prescription will also state the dose or strength of the medication to be prescribed, how much to take (the number of tablets or amount of liquid), and how frequently it should be taken.

The prescription informs the pharmacist of the amount of the drug to be dispensed, and the information that should be put on the label.

In some cases, your physician will indicate that the prescription can be refilled a certain number of times without having to obtain a repeat prescription. The pharmacist will record this information. When your supply of the drug is exhausted, you can return to the pharmacist to obtain a refill without having to get a new prescription. If treatment needs to be continued after the set number of refills have been prescribed, you will have to see your physician again. He or she will decide if a repeat prescription is necessary, or if the treatment should be altered.

Your physician's signature, phone number, and address are included on the prescription, so that the pharmacist can contact him or her if there is a query about the drug to be prescribed.

Usually, you will receive a Patient Information Leaflet, which gives details about the drug, its adverse effects, whether it is safe for you, when not to use it, and so on. Compare this with your physician's instructions, and ask the pharmacist about any differences. You should also consult with the pharmacist if the label on your medication differs from the information on the prescription.

It is advisable for you to obtain all of your prescription drugs from the same pharmacist or at least from the same pharmacy, so that your pharmacist can advise you about any particular problems you may have, and keep supplies of any unusual drugs you may be taking.

If you need to take drugs that are prescribed by more than one physician, or by your dentist in addition to your physician, the pharmacist is able to call attention to possible harmful interactions. Physicians do ask if you are taking other medicines before prescribing, but your regular pharmacist provides valuable additional advice.

Questioning your physician

Countless surveys unmistakably point to lack of information as the most common reason for failure of drug treatment. Responses such as "The doctor is too busy to be bothered with a lot of questions" or "The doctor will think I'm stupid if I ask that" recur over and over. Be certain you understand the instructions for a drug before leaving your physician's office, and don't leave with any questions unanswered.

It is a good idea to make a list of the questions you may want to ask before your visit, and to make notes while you are there about what you are told (see page 31). It is not uncommon to forget some of the instructions your physician gives you during a consultation. You can check your instructions from the physician with the pharmacist.

Know what you are taking

Your physician should tell you the generic or brand name of the drug he or she is prescribing, and exactly what condition or symptom it has been prescribed to treat.

As well as telling you the name of the drug prescribed, your physician should explain what dose you should take, how often to take it, and whether the prescription should be repeated. Be certain you understand the instructions about how and when to take the drug (see also Taking your medication, facing page). For example, does four times a day mean four times during the time you are awake, or four times in 24 hours? Ask your physician how long the treatment should last; some medications cause harmful effects if you stop taking them abruptly, or do not have beneficial effects unless the full course of drug treatment is completed.

To help you remember, the label on your dispensed medicine may repeat the instructions, and the pharmacist may give you a patient information leaflet that will give you detailed information about the drug. The pharmacist can also help by answering your questions, if you have forgotten to ask the physician.

Risks and special precautions

All drugs have *adverse effects* (see The effects of drugs, p.15), and you should know what these are. Ask your physician what the possible adverse effects of the drug are and what you should do if they occur. Also ask if there are any foods or other drugs you should avoid during treatment, whether the drug can cause drowsiness, and if you can drink alcohol while taking the drug.

PRESCRIPTION TERMS

ac before meals	**pc** after meals
ad lib freely	**PM** evening
AM morning	**po** by mouth
bid twice a day	**prn** as needed
c with	**qid** four times
cap capsule	a day
cc cubic centimetre	**s** without
ext for external use	**sr** slow release
gtt drops	**stat** at once
mg milligrams	**tab** tablet
ml millilitres	**tid** three times
nocte at night	a day
top apply topically	**ud** use as directed
x times	

TAKING YOUR MEDICATION

Among the most important aspects of managing your drug treatment is knowing how often the drug is to be taken. Should it be taken on an empty stomach? With food? Mixed with something? Specific instructions on such points are given in the individual drug profiles in Part 4.

When to take your drugs

Certain drugs, such as analgesics and drugs for migraine, are taken only as necessary, when warning symptoms occur. Others are meant to be taken regularly at specified intervals. The prescription or label instructions can be confusing, however. For instance, does four times a day mean once every six hours out of 24 – at 8 am, 2 pm, 8 pm, and 2 am? Or does it mean take at four equal intervals during waking hours – morning, lunchtime, late afternoon, and bedtime? The latter is usually the case, but you need to ask your physician or pharmacist for precise directions.

The actual time of day that you take a drug is generally flexible, so you can normally schedule your doses to fit your daily routine. This has the additional advantage of making it easier for you to remember to take your drugs. For example, if you are to take the drug three times during the day, it may be most convenient to take the first dose at 7 am, the second at 3 pm, and the third at 11 pm, while it may be more suitable for another person on the same regimen to take the first dose at 8 am, and so on. You must, however, establish with your pharmacist or your physician whether the drug should be taken with food, in which case you would probably need to take it with your breakfast, lunch, and dinner. Try to take your dose at the recommended intervals; if you take them too close

Four times a day?

Midnight

A

Sleeping hours

6pm — 6am

Scheduled dose

Noon

Midnight

B

6pm — 6am

Noon

Waking hours

Check with your physician whether your prescription means (A) take your drug 4 times a day during waking hours, or (B) take 4 times over a 24-hour period.

TIPS ON TAKING MEDICINES

● Whenever possible, take capsules and tablets while standing up or in an upright sitting position, and take them with water. If you take them when you are lying down, or without enough water, it is possible for the capsules or tablets to become stuck in the esophagus. This can delay the action of the drug and may damage the esophagus.

● Always measure your dose carefully, using a 5ml spoon or an accurate measure such as a dropper, children's medicine spoon, or oral syringe.

● When taking liquid medicines, shake the bottle before measuring each dose, or you may take improper dosages if the active substance has risen to the top or settled at the bottom of the bottle.

● A drink of cold water taken immediately before and after an unpleasantly flavoured medicine will often hide the taste.

together, the risk of side effects occurring is increased.

If you are taking several different drugs, ask your doctor or pharmacist if they can be taken together, or if they must be taken at different times in order to avoid any adverse effects or reduced effectiveness caused by an interaction between them.

How to take your drugs

If your prescription specifies taking your drug with food – or without food – it is very important to follow this instruction if you are to get the maximum benefit from your treatment.

Certain drugs, such as ampicillin and captopril, should be taken on an empty stomach (usually one to two hours before eating) so they will be absorbed more quickly into the bloodstream; others, such as ibuprofen, metronidazole, and allopurinol, should be taken with food to avoid stomach irritation. Similarly, you should comply with any instructions to avoid particular foods. Milk and dairy products may inhibit the absorption of some drugs, such as tetracycline; fruit juices can break down certain antibacterial drugs in the stomach and thereby decrease their effectiveness; alcohol is best avoided with many drugs. (See also Drug interactions, p.16.)

In some cases, when taking diuretics, for example, you may be advised to eat foods rich in potassium. But do not take potassium supplements unless you are advised to do so by your physician (see Potassium, p.460). If you use any of the salt substitutes (all of which contain potassium), remember to tell your doctor.

GIVING MEDICINES TO CHILDREN

A number of over-the-counter medicines are specifically prepared for children. Many other medicines have labels that give both adult's and children's dosages. For the purposes of drug labelling, anyone 12 years of age or under is considered a child.

When giving over-the-counter medicines to children, you should always follow the instructions on the label exactly and under no circumstances exceed the dosage recommended for a child. Never give a child even a small amount of a medicine intended for adult use without the advice of your physician.

Do not deceive your child about the medicine, such as pretending that tablets are sweets or that liquid medicines are soft drinks. Never leave a child's medicine within reach; he or she may be tempted to take an extra dose in order to hasten recovery.

27

MISSED DOSES

Missing a dose of your medication can be a problem only if you are taking the drug as part of a regular course of treatment. Missing a drug dose is not uncommon and it is not a cause for concern in most cases. The missed dose may sometimes produce a recurrence of symptoms or a change in the action of the drug, so you should know what to do when you have forgotten to take your medication. Ask your pharmacist how to deal with missed doses. For advice on individual drugs, consult the drug profile in Part 4.

Additional measures

With some drugs, the timing of doses depends on how long the actions of the drugs last. When you miss a dose, the amount of drug in your body is lowered, and the effect of the drug may be diminished. You may therefore have to take other steps to avoid unwanted consequences. For example, if you are taking an oral contraceptive and you forget to take one pill at your usual time, you should take the pill as soon as you remember, and for the next week use another form of contraception.

If you miss more than one dose of any drug you are taking regularly, you should tell your physician. Missed doses are especially important with insulin and drugs for epilepsy.

If you frequently forget to take your medication, you should tell your physician. He or she may be able to simplify your treatment schedule by prescribing a preparation that contains several drugs, or a preparation that releases the drug slowly into the body over time, and only needs to be taken once or twice daily.

REMEMBERING YOUR MEDICATION

If you take several different drugs, it is useful to draw up a chart to remind yourself of when each drug should be taken. This will also help anyone who looks after you, or a physician who is unfamiliar with your treatment.

The example given here is of a dosage chart for an elderly woman suffering from arthritis and a heart condition who has trouble sleeping. Her physician has prescribed the following treatment:

Hydrochlorothiazide (a diuretic to counter fluid retention), one 25mg tablet in the morning.

Amiloride (another diuretic to counter the potassium loss caused by hydrochlorothiazide), two 5mg tablets in the morning.

Ibuprofen (for arthritis), three 400mg tablets daily with meals.

Verapamil (to treat heart condition), three 80mg tablets a day.

Zopiclone (a sleeping drug), one 5mg tablet at bedtime.

Dosage Chart

8am	1pm
2 x Amiloride	1 x Ibuprofen
1 x Ibuprofen	1 x Verapamil
1 x Verapamil	
1 x Hydrochlorothiazide	

7pm	11pm
1 x Ibuprofen	1 x Verapamil
	1 x Zopiclone

Pill box
Using a pill box is a handy way of making sure you take your tablets in the right order. There is a strip for each day of the week, and compartments for morning, afternoon, evening, and bedtime. Ask your pharmacist about strategies to help you remember to take your medicines.

ENDING DRUG TREATMENT

As with missed doses, ending drug treatment too soon can be a problem when you are taking a regular course of drugs. With medication that you take as required, you can stop treatment as soon as you feel better.

Advice on stopping individual drugs is given in the drug profiles in Part 4. Some general guidelines for ending drug treatment are given below.

Risks of stopping too soon

Suddenly stopping drug treatment before completing your course of medication may cause the original condition to recur or lead to other complications, including withdrawal symptoms. The disappearance of the symptoms does not necessarily mean that a disorder is cured. Even if you feel better, do not stop taking the drug unless your physician advises you to do so. People taking antibiotics often stop too soon, but the full course of treatment prescribed should always be followed.

Adverse effects

Do not stop taking a medication simply because it produces unpleasant side effects. Many adverse effects disappear or become bearable after a while. But if they do not, check with your physician, who may want to reduce the dosage of the drug gradually or, alternatively, substitute another drug that does not produce the same side effects.

Gradual reduction

While many medications can be stopped abruptly, others need to be reduced gradually to prevent a reaction when treatment ends. This is the case with long-term corticosteroid therapy (see right) as well as with *dependence*-inducing drugs.

Phased reduction of corticosteroids

■ Corticosteroid drug

■ Natural adrenal hormone

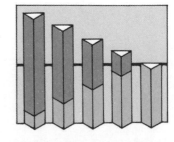

Normal hormone level

Corticosteroid drugs suppress production in the body of natural adrenal hormones. A phased reduction of the dosage allows levels of the natural hormones to revert to normal. The last stages of withdrawal are made very slowly.

STORING DRUGS

Once you have completed a medically directed course of treatment, you should not keep any unused drugs. But most families will want to keep a supply of remedies for indigestion, headaches, colds, and so forth. Such medicines should not be used if they show any signs of deterioration, or if their period of effectiveness has expired (see When to dispose of drugs, right).

How to store drugs

All drugs, including cough medicines, iron tablets, and oral contraceptives, should be kept out of the reach of children. If you are in the habit of keeping your medicines where you will see them as a reminder to take them, leave an empty medicine container out instead, and put the drug itself safely out of reach.

Over-the-counter and prescription drugs should normally be stored in the container in which you purchased them. If it is necessary to put them into other containers, such as special containers designed for the elderly, make sure you keep the original container with the label, as well as any separate instructions, for future reference.

Make certain that caps and lids are replaced and tightly closed after use; loose caps may leak and spill, or hasten deterioration of the drug.

Where to store drugs

The majority of drugs should be stored in a cool, dry place out of direct sunlight, even those in plastic containers or tinted glass. Room temperature, away from sources of direct heat, is suitable for most medicines. A few drugs should be stored in the refrigerator. Storage information for individual drugs is given in the drug profiles in Part 4.

Wall cabinets that can be locked are ideal for storing drugs, as long as the cabinet itself is located in a cool, dry place and not, as often happens, in the bathroom, which is frequently warm and humid.

WHEN TO DISPOSE OF DRUGS

Old drugs should be returned to the pharmacist for proper disposal. Always dispose of:

● Any drug that is past its expiry date.

● ASA and acetaminophen tablets that smell of vinegar.

● Tablets that are chipped, cracked, or discoloured, and capsules that have softened, cracked, or stuck together.

● Liquids that have thickened or discoloured, or that taste or smell different in any way from the original product.

● Tubes that are cracked, leaky, or hard.

● Ointments and creams that have changed odour, or changed appearance by discolouring, hardening, or separating.

● Any liquid needing refrigeration that has been kept for over two weeks.

LONG-TERM DRUG TREATMENT

Many people require regular, prolonged treatment with one or more drugs. People who suffer from chronic or recurrent disorders often need lifelong treatment with drugs to control symptoms or prevent complications. Antihypertensive drugs for high blood pressure and insulin or oral antidiabetic drugs for diabetes mellitus are familiar examples. Many other disorders take a long time to cure; for example, people with tuberculosis usually need at least six months' treatment with antituberculous drugs. Long-term drug treatment may also be necessary to prevent a condition from occurring, and will have to be taken for as long as the individual is at risk. Antimalarial drugs are a good example.

Possible adverse effects

You may worry that taking a drug for a long period will reduce its effectiveness or that you will become dependent on it. However, *tolerance* develops only with a few drugs; most medicines continue to have the same effect indefinitely without necessitating an increase in dosage or change in drug. Similarly, taking a drug for more than a few weeks does not normally create dependence.

Changing drug treatment

If you are taking a drug regularly, you will need to know what to do if something else occurs to affect your health. If you wish to become pregnant, for example, you should ask your physician right away if it is preferable to continue on your regular medicine or switch to another less likely to affect your pregnancy. If you contract a new illness, for which an additional drug is prescribed, your regular treatment may be altered.

There are a number of other reasons for changing a drug. You may have had an adverse reaction, or an improved preparation may have become available.

Adjusting to long-term treatment

You should establish a daily routine for taking your medication in order to reduce the risk of a missed dose. Usually you should not stop taking your medication, even if there are side effects, without consulting your physician (see Ending drug treatment, facing page). If you fear possible side effects from the drug, discuss this with your physician.

Many people deliberately stop their drugs because they feel well or their symptoms disappear. This can be dangerous, especially with a disease like high blood pressure, which has no noticeable symptoms. Stopping treatment may lead to a recurrence or worsening of a disease. If you are uncertain about why you have to keep taking a drug, ask your physician.

Only a few drugs require an alteration in habits. Some drugs should not be taken with alcohol; with a few drugs you should avoid certain foods. If you require a drug that makes you drowsy, you should not drive a car or operate dangerous equipment.

If you are taking a drug that should not be stopped suddenly or that may interact with other drugs, it is a good idea to carry a warning card or bracelet, a MedicAlert for example. Such information might be essential for emergency medical treatment in an accident.

Monitoring treatment

If you are on long-term treatment, you need to visit your physician for periodic check-ups. He or she will check your underlying condition and monitor any adverse effects of treatment. Levels of the drug in the blood may be measured. With insulin, in addition to checks with the physician, you need to monitor blood and/or urine levels each day.

If a drug is known to cause damage to an organ, tests may be done to check the function of the organ. For example, blood and urine tests to check kidney function, or a blood count to check the bone marrow, may be indicated.

Medical check-ups
Blood pressure is commonly checked in people on long-term drug treatment.

EXCEEDING THE DOSE

Most people associate drug overdoses with attempts at suicide or the fatalities and near fatalities brought on by abuse of street drugs. However, drug overdoses can also occur among people who deliberately or inadvertently exceed the stated dose of a drug that has been prescribed for them by their physician.

A single extra dose of most drugs is unlikely to be a cause for concern, although accidental overdoses can create anxiety in the individual and his or her family, and may cause overdose symptoms, which can appear in a variety of different forms.

Overdose of some drugs, however, is potentially dangerous even when the dose has been exceeded by only a small amount. Each of the drug profiles in Part 4 gives detailed information on the consequences of exceeding the dose, symptoms to look out for, and what to do. Each drug has an overdose danger rating of low, medium, or high, which are described fully on p.174.

Taking an extra dose
People sometimes exceed the stated dose in the mistaken belief that by increasing dosage they will obtain more

Effects of repeated overdose
Repeated overdose of a drug over an extended period may lead to a build-up of high levels of the drug in the body, especially if liver or kidney function is reduced.

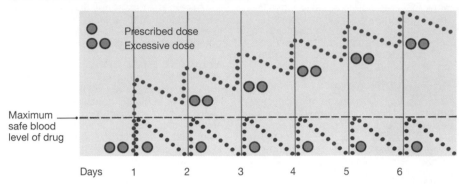

immediate action or a more effective cure. This action is a particular risk with *tolerance*-inducing drugs (see Drug tolerance and dependence, p.23). Others exceed their dose accidentally, by miscalculating the amount or forgetting that the dose has already been taken.

Taking extra doses is often a problem in the elderly, who may repeat their dose through forgetfulness or confusion. This is

a special risk with medicines that cause drowsiness (see also p.22).

In some cases, especially when liver or kidney function is impaired, the drug builds up in the blood because the body cannot break down and excrete the extra dose quickly enough, so that symptoms of poisoning may result. Symptoms of excessive intake may not be apparent for many days.

When and how to get help
If you are not sure whether or not you have taken your medicine, think back and check again. If you honestly cannot remember, assume that you have missed the dose and follow the advice given in the individual drug profiles in Part 4 of this book. If you cannot find your drug, consult your physician. Make a note to use some system in the future which will help you remember to take your medicine.

If you are looking after an elderly person on regular drug treatment who suddenly develops unusual symptoms such as confusion, drowsiness, or unsteadiness, consider the possibility of an inadvertent drug overdose and consult the physician as soon as possible.

Deliberate overdose
While many cases of drug overdose are accidental or the result of a mistaken belief that increasing the dose will enhance the benefits of drug treatment, sometimes an excessive amount of a drug is taken with the intention of causing harm or even as a suicide attempt. Whether or not you think a dangerous amount of a drug has been taken, deliberate overdoses of this kind should always be brought to the attention of your doctor. Not only is it necessary to ensure that no physical harm has occurred as a result of the overdose, but the psychological condition of a person who takes such action may indicate the need for additional medical help, especially when the person is elderly, has a physical illness, or is known to suffer from depression.

THE EFFECT OF DRUG OVERDOSE ON THE BODY

The effect of drug overdose on the body depends on the type of drug involved. Some drugs produce an exaggeration of the desired effect, for instance overdose of tranquillizers leads to unconsciousness. With many drugs, the toxic overdose effects are unrelated to the action or side effects of the drug when it is taken in normal doses.

Heart and circulation
Some antidepressants, cause severe, and possibly fatal, arrhythmias in overdose.

Heart muscle

Liver
Fatal liver damage can occur with as few as 20 tablets of acetaminophen. Treatment can prevent damage but must be given within 12 hours of taking the drug.

Liver

Gallbladder

Stomach

Small intestine

Stomach and intestines
Iron overdose causes bleeding in the digestive tract. An overdose of NSAIDs causes ulceration of the stomach and intestines.

Respiratory centre

Brain
Depression of the respiratory centre in the brain is common with overdose of barbiturates and tranquillizers. ASA in overdose can result in convulsions.

Kidney

Ureter

Bladder

Kidney
An overdose of NSAIDs, particularly in people who have impaired kidney function, can result in kidney failure.

Prescribed dose
Excessive dose

Maximum safe blood level of drug

Days 1 2 3 4 5 6

DOs AND DON'Ts

On this page you will find a summary of the most important practical points concerning the management of your drug treatment. The advice is arranged under general headings, explaining the safest methods of storing drugs and following treatment, whether it is a prescribed medicine or an over-the-counter drug. This information is equally applicable whether you are taking medicine yourself or supervising the drug treatment of someone in your care.

At the physician's office

DO
● Tell your physician about drugs you are already taking: prescription, over the counter, street drugs, and herbal or natural products.
● Tell your physician if you are pregnant, intending to become pregnant, or breast-feeding.
● Tell your physician about any allergic reactions you have experienced to past drug treatments.
● Tell your physician if you have a current health problem or if you think you might be at risk from drug treatment.

● Ask your physician how your prescribed medication will help you and when you will know it is working.
● Make sure you understand the reasons why you have been prescribed a particular drug and how long you will need to take it. People who do not understand the reasons for their treatment often fail to take their prescribed drug correctly.

DON'T
▼ Leave your physician's office before you have a clear understanding of how and when to take your drug.

At the pharmacy

DO
● Ask your pharmacist's advice about over-the-counter drugs if you are not sure what you should buy, or if you think you may react adversely to a drug.
● Try to see the same pharmacist or use the same pharmacy to obtain your regular prescriptions.
● Be sure you know the name of the drug you have been prescribed. If you are getting a repeat prescription and your physician has specified that you should always use the same brand, make sure the brand is correct.

● Make sure you understand what is on the drug label.
● Ask the pharmacist to put your drug in a container with an easy-to-remove cap if you have difficulty using child-resistant containers.
● Ask the pharmacist if the medication will interact with any other drugs you are taking, foods, or vitamins.

DON'T
▼ Send children to the pharmacy to get your medicine for you.

Giving medicines to children

DO
● Check the dose on the label carefully before giving medicines to children.
● Make sure over-the-counter preparations you give to children under 16 years old do not contain ASA.

DON'T
▼ Pretend to children that medicines are sweets or soft drinks.
▼ Give any medicines to children under the age of five, except on the advice of your physician.

Taking your drug

DO
● Make sure that your drug will not make you drowsy or otherwise affect your ability before you drive or perform difficult or dangerous tasks.
● Read the label carefully and do what it says. This is equally important with all types of drugs, creams, and lotions as well as drugs taken by mouth.
● Finish the drug treatment your physician prescribes for you.
● Consult your physician for advice if you experience side effects.

DON'T
▼ Take any prescribed or over-the-counter drugs without first consulting your physician if you are pregnant or trying to conceive.
▼ Offer your medicine to other people or take medicine that has been prescribed for someone else (even if the symptoms are the same).

Food, drink, and drugs of abuse

DO
● Check with your physician and phamacist whether it is safe to take alcohol with the drugs you are prescribed.
● Check that there are no foods you should avoid.
● Follow the timing of your drugs with respect to meals, when instructed to do so by your physician or pharmacist.

DON'T
▼ Take drugs (except those prescribed by your physician) or alcohol if you are pregnant or trying to conceive. They may adversely affect the unborn baby.
▼ Take drugs of abuse under any circumstances.

Storing drugs

DO
● Take care to store drugs in a cool, dry place and protect them from light or refrigerate them, if advised to do so.
● Keep all drugs, including seemingly harmless ones such as cough preparations, locked away out of the reach of children.
● Check your medicine chest regularly in case other members of the family have left their unwanted drugs in it, and to make sure that none of the normal supplies are out of date.

● Keep drugs in their original containers with the original instructions to avoid confusion.

DON'T
▼ Keep drugs you no longer need at home. When you have stopped taking a prescribed drug, take it to your pharmacist to dispose of it unless it is part of your family's first aid kit.

2

DRUG FINDER INDEX

THE DRUG FINDER

THE DRUG FINDER

This section contains the names of approximately 2,000 individual drug products and substances. It provides a quick and easy reference for readers interested in learning about a specific drug or medication. There is no need for you to know whether the item is a brand name or a generic name, or whether it is a prescription or an over-the-counter drug; all types of drug are listed.

What it contains

The drugs are listed alphabetically and include all major generic drugs and many less widely used substances. A broad range of brand names, as well as many vitamins and minerals, are also included. This comprehensive selection reflects the wide diversity of products available in Canada for the treatment and prevention of disease. Inclusion of a drug or product does not imply endorsement by the publishers or the CPhA, nor does the exclusion of any particular drug or product indicate their disapproval.

How the references work

Entries with an upper case letter are the product names of drugs. References are to the pages in Part 4, containing the drug profiles of each principal generic drug, and to the section in Part 3 that describes the relevant drug group, as appropriate. For products that contain a combination of drugs or substances, page references are given for each drug. Some entries for generic drugs that do not have a full profile in Part 4 have a brief description here. Certain technical terms within the entries are printed in italics to indicate that they are defined in the Glossary (pp.503–508).

A

abacavir an antiretroviral drug for HIV/AIDS 144

abatacept a biological response modifier for rheumatoid arthritis 103

abciximab an antiplatelet drug 90

Abelcet a product name for amphotericin B 191 (an antifungal 124)

Abenol a product name for acetaminophen 177 (an non-opioid analgesic 64)

acarbose 176 (an oral antidiabetic 128)

Accolate a product name for zafirlukast (a leukotriene antagonist for asthma 77)

Accutane Roche a product name for isotretinoin 319 (a drug for acne 165)

acebutolol a beta blocker 83

acetaminophen 177 (a non-opioid analgesic 64)

acetazolamide a carbonic anhydrase inhibitor diuretic 85 and drug for glaucoma 156

Acetazone Forte a combination product containing codeine 242 (an opioid analgesic 64) with acetaminophen 177 (an analgesic p.64) and a muscle relaxant.

Acetoxyl a product name for benzoyl peroxide 204 (a drug for acne 167)

acetylcholine a chemical neurotransmitter that stimulates the parasympathetic nervous system 62 and is used as a miotic 158

acetylcysteine a mucolytic 80

acetylsalicylic acid *see* ASA

acitretin a drug for psoriasis 166

Aclasta a product name for zoledronic acid (a drug used for treatment of bone disorders 108)

Actifed a product name for pseudoephedrine 404 (a decongestant 79) and triprolidine (an antihistamine 111)

Activase a product name for alteplase (a thrombolytic drug 91)

Actonel a product name for risedronate 417 (a drug for bone disorders 108)

Actonel Plus a combination product with risedronate 417 (a drug for bone disorders 108) and calcium 469 (a mineral 152)

Actos a product name for pioglitazone 390 (a drug for diabetes 128)

Acular a product name for ketorolac (a non-steroidal anti-inflammatory 102)

acyclovir 178 (an antiviral 119)

Adalat XL a product name for nifedipine 368 (a calcium channel blocker 87)

adalimumab a biological response modifier for inflammatory bowel disease 98

adapalene a retinoid for acne 165

Adasept Skin Cleanser a product name for triclosan (a *topical* antimicrobial 163)

Adderall a product name for mixed salts amphetamine (an amphetamine 72)

Adefovir an antiviral drug 119

Adenocard a product name for adenosine (an antiarrhythmic 86)

adenosine an antiarrhythmic 86

Adriamycin PFS a product name for doxorubicin 267 (a *cytotoxic* anticancer drug 140)

Adrucil a product name for fluorouracil (an anticancer drug 140)

Advair a product name for a combination of salmeterol 425 (a *bronchodilator* 76) and fluticasone 290 (a corticosteroid 127)

Advicor a combination product containing lovastatin 337 (a lipid-lowering drug 89) and nicotinic acid (a lipid-lowering drug 89)

Advil a product name for ibuprofen 310 (a non-opioid analgesic 64 and non-steroidal anti-inflammatory 102)

Aerius a product name for desloratadine 334 (an antihistamine 110)

Airomir a product name for salbutamol 424 (a *bronchodilator* 76)

Akineton a product name for biperiden (an *anticholinergic* for *parkinsonism* 71)

Alcomicin a product name for gentamicin 298 (an *antibiotic* 110)

Aldactazide a product name for a combination of spironolactone 433 (a potassium-sparing diuretic 85) and hydrochlorothiazide 306 (a thiazide diuretic 85)

Aldactone a product name for spironolactone 433 (a potassium-sparing diuretic 85)

alendronate 179 (a drug for treatment of bone disorders 108)

Alertec a product name for modafinil (a drug used in narcolepsy 72)

Alesse a product name for levonorgestrel 328 (a female sex hormone 133 and oral contraceptive 149) and ethinyl estradiol 278 (an estrogen 133)

alfacalcidol vitamin D 481 (a vitamin 135)

alfuzosin a drug used in urinary disorders 154

alginates/alginic acid 180 (substances extracted from brown seaweed used to protect stomach and esophagus from acid reflux (antacids 94)

Alka-Seltzer Morning Relief a combination product with ASA 194 (a non-opioid analgesic 64) and caffeine

Alkeran a product name for melphalan (an anticancer drug 140)

allantoin a uric acid derivative. Applied *topically*, is said to encourage healing of minor wounds

Allegra a product name for fexofenadine (an antihistamine 110)

Allerdryl a product name for diphenhydramine 259 (an antihistamine 110, anti-emetic 74, and antipruritic 161)

Alloprin a generic company version of allopurinol 181 (a drug for gout 105)

allopurinol 181 (a drug for gout 105)

almotriptan a drug for migraine 73

Alomide a product name for lodoxamide (a drug for allergy 109)

ALPHAGAN–APO-SOTALOL

Alphagan a product name for brimonidine (a drug for glaucoma 156)

alpha tocopheryl vitamin E 481 (a vitamin 135)

alprazolam 182 (a benzodiazepine anti-anxiety drug 67)

alprostadil 183 a prostaglandin used for male impotence 152

Altace a product name for ramipril 412 (an ACE inhibitor 100)

Altace HCT a product name for combination of hydrochlorothiazide 306 (a thiazide diuretic 85) and ramipril 412 (an ACE inhibitor 84)

alteplase a thrombolytic 91

Alti-Beclomethasone a product name for beclomethasone 203 (a corticosteroid 127)

aluminum acetate an *astringent* used for inflammation of the skin or outer ear canal 159

aluminum hydroxide 184 (an antacid 94)

Alvesco a product name for ciclesonide (an inhaled corticosteroid 127 used in asthma 78)

amantadine 185 (an antiviral 119 and drug used for *parkinsonism* 71)

Amaryl a product name for glimepiride 300 (an oral antidiabetic 128)

AmBisome a product name for amphotericin B 191 (an antifungal124)

Amcinonide a *topical* corticosteroid 162

Amerge a product name for naratriptan (a drug for migraine 73)

amethocain a local *anesthetic* 64

Ametop a product name for tetracaine (also known as amethocain, a local *anesthetic* 64)

amikacin an *antibiotic* 114

Amikin a product name for amikacin (an aminoglycoside *antibiotic* 114)

amiloride 186 (a potassium-sparing diuretic 85)

aminobenzoic acid an ingredient of sunscreens 169

aminophylline 448 (a *bronchodilator* 76)

amiodarone 187 (an anti-arrhythmic 86)

amitriptyline 188 (a tricyclic antidepressant 68)

amlodipine 189 (a calcium channel blocker 87)

ammonium chloride a drug that increases urine acidity 154

amoxicillin 190 (a penicillin *antibiotic* 114)

amoxicillin/clavulinic acid a combination of amoxicillin 190 (a penicillin *antibiotic* 114) and clavulinic acid (a substance given with it to make amoxicillin more effective)

Amphojel a product name for aluminum hydroxide 184 (an antacid 94)

amphotericin B 191 (an antifungal 124)

ampicillin a penicillin *antibiotic* 116

amprenavir a drug for HIV/AIDS 144

Anafranil a product name for clomipramine 236 (a tricyclic antidepressant 68)

Anakinra 192 an immunomodulatory drug for rheumatoid arthritis 103

Anaprox a product name for naproxen 366 (a non-steroidal anti-inflammatory 102)

anastrozole 193 (an anticancer drug 140)

Andriol a product name for testosterone 446 (a male sex hormone 132)

Androcur a product name for cyproterone (a synthetic sex hormone used for acne 165, cancer of the prostate 140, and male sexual disorders 132)

Androderm a product name for testosterone 446 (a male sex hormone 132)

AndroGel a product name for testosterone 446 (a male sex hormone 132)

Ansaid a product name for flurbiprofen (a non-steroidal anti-inflammatory 102)

Anthraforte a product name for anthralin (a drug used in psoriasis 166)

anthralin a drug used in psoriasis 166

Anthranol a product name for anthralin (a drug used in psoriasis 166)

Anthrascalp a product name for anthralin (a drug used in psoriasis 166)

antihemophilic factor a blood protein used to promote blood clotting in hemophilia 90

Anugesic-HC a combination drug with hydrocortisone 308 (a corticosteroid 127 and antipruritic 161) and other drugs

Anusol a product-name preparation for hemorrhoids 101 containing zinc sulfate

Anuzinc HC Plus a combination drug with hydrocortisone 308 (a corticosteroid 127 and antipruritic 161) and other drugs

Anzemet a product name for dolasetron (an antiemetic 74)

Apo-Acetaminophen a generic company version of acetaminophen 177 (an non-opioid analgesic 64)

Apo-Acyclovir a generic company version of acyclovir 178 (an antiviral 119)

Apo-Allopurinol a generic company version of allopurinol 181 (a drug for gout 105)

Apo-Alpraz a generic company version of alprazolam 182 (a benzodiazepine anti-anxiety drug 67)

Apo-Alpraz TS a generic company version of alprazolam 182 (a benzodiazepine anti-anxiety drug 67)

Apo-Amitriptyline a generic company version of amitriptyline 188 (a tricyclic antidepressant 68)

Apo-Amoxi a generic company version of amoxicillin 190 (a penicillin *antibiotic* 114)

Apo-Amoxi-Clav a generic company version of amoxicillin/clavulinic acid (a combination of amoxicillin 190 (a penicillin *antibiotic* 114) and clavulinic acid (a substance given with it to make amoxicillin more effective)

Apo-Atenolol a generic company version of atenolol 195 (a beta blocker 83)

Apo-Azathioprine a generic company version of azathioprine 200

Apo-Baclofen a generic company version of baclofen 202 (a muscle relaxant 106)

Apo-Benztropine a generic company version of benztropine (an *anticholinergic* for *parkinsonism* 71)

Apo-Bromocriptine a generic company version of bromocriptine 210 (a pituitary agent 131 and drug for *parkinsonism* 71)

Apo-Buspirone a generic company version of buspirone 214 (anti-anxiety drug 67)

Apo-Capto a generic company version of captopril 216 (an ACE inhibitor 84)

Apo-Carbamazepine a generic company version of carbamazepine 217 (an anticonvulsant 70)

Apo-Cefaclor a generic company version of cefaclor (a cephalosporin *antibiotic* 114)

Apo-Cefuroxime a generic company version of cefuroxime 218 (a cephalosporin antibiotic 114)

Apo-Cephalex a generic company version of cephalexin 220 (a cephalosporin *antibiotic* 114)

Apo-Cetirizine a generic company version of cetirizine 221 (an antihistamine 110)

Apo-Chlorax a generic company version of a combination product of chloriazepoxide (a benzodiazepine anti-anxiety drug 67) with an *anticholinergic*

Apo-Chlordiazepoxide a generic company version of chlordiazepoxide 223 (a benzodiazepine anti-anxiety drug 67)

Apo-Chlorpromazine a generic company version of chlorpromazine 226 (a phenothiazine antipsychotic 69 and anti-emetic 74)

Apo-Chlorpropamide a generic company version of chlorpropamide (a drug for diabetes 128)

Apo-Chlorthalidone a generic company version of chlorthalidone (a thiazide diuretic 85)

Apo-Cimetidine a generic company version of cimetidine 228 (an antiulcer drug 95)

Apo-Citalopram a generic version of citalopram 231 (an antidepressant 68)

Apo-Clindamycin a generic company version of clindamycin 233 (an antibiotic 114)

Apo-Clomipramine a generic company version of clomipramine 236 (a tricyclic antidepressant 68)

Apo-Clonazepam a generic company version of clonazepam 237 (a benzo-diazepine anti-anxiety drug 67 and anticonvulsant 70)

Apo-Clonidine a generic company version of clonidine (an antihypertensive 88)

Apo-Clorazepate a generic company version of clorazepate (a benzodiazepine anti-anxiety drug 67)

Apo-Cloxi a generic company version of cloxacillin 240 (a penicillin *antibiotic* 114)

Apo-Clozapine a generic company version of clozapine 241 (an antipsychotic 69)

Apo-Cyclobenzaprine a generic company version of cyclobenzaprine (a muscle relaxant 106)

Apo-Desipramine a generic company version of desipramine (a tricyclic antidepressant 68)

Apo-Diazepam a generic company version of diazepam 253 (a benzodiazepine anti-anxiety drug 67, sedative 67, muscle relaxant 106, and anticonvulsant 70)

Apo-Diclo a generic company version of diclonefac 254 (a non-steroidal anti-inflammatory 102)

Apo-Diflunisal a generic company version of diflunisal (a non-steroidal anti-inflammatory 102)

Apo-Diltiaz a generic company version of diltiazem 257 (an antihypertensive 88 and calcium channel blocker 87)

Apo-Dipivefrin a generic company version of dipivefrin (a *sympathomimetic* for glaucoma 156)

Apo-Divalproex a generic company version of divalproex (an anticonvulsant 70)

Apo-Domperidone a generic company version of domperidone 263 (an anti-emetic 74)

Apo-Doxazosin a generic company version of doxazosin 266 (a sympatholytic antihypertensive 88)

Apo-Doxepin a generic company version of doxepin (a tricyclic antidepressant 68)

Apo-Doxy a generic company version of doxycycline 268 (a tetracycline *antibiotic* 114)

Apo-Erythro-ES a generic company version of erythromycin 274 (an *antibiotic* 114)

Apo-Erythromycin a generic company version of erythromycin 274 (an *antibiotic* 114)

Apo-Fenofibrate a generic company version of fenofibrate (a lipid-lowering drug 89)

Apo-Feno-Micro a generic company version of fenofibrate (a lipid-lowering drug 89)

Apo-Fluconazole a generic company version of fluconazole 286 (an antifungal drug 124)

Apo-Flunisolide a generic company version of flunisolide (a corticosteroid 127)

Apo-Fluoxetine a generic company version of fluoxetine 287 (an antidepressant 68)

Apo-Fluphenazine a generic company version of fluphenazine (an phenothiazine antipsychotic 69)

Apo-Flurazepam a generic company version of flurazepam (a benzodiazepine sleeping drug 66)

Apo-Flurbiprofen a generic company version of flurbiprofen (a non-steroidal anti-inflammatory 102)

Apo-Flutamide a generic company version of flutamide 289 (an anticancer drug 140)

Apo-Fluvoxamine a generic name for fluvoxamine 291 (an antidepressant 68)

Apo-Gabapentin a generic company version of gabapentin 294 (an anticonvulsant 70)

Apo-Gain a generic company version of minoxidil 358 (an antihypertensive 88)

Apo-Gemfibrozil a generic product name for gemfibrozil 297 (a lipid-lowering drug 89)

Apo-Glimepiride a generic company version of glimepiride 300 (a drug used in diabetes 128)

Apo-Haloperidol a generic company version of haloperidol 304 (an antipsychotic 69)

Apo-Hydroxyzine a generic company version of hydroxyzine (an antihistamine used as an anti-anxiety drug 67)

Apo-Ibuprofen a generic company version of ibuprofen 310 (a non-opioid analgesic 64 and non-steroidal anti-inflammatory 102)

Apo-Imipramine a generic company version of imipramine 311 (a tricyclic antidepressant 68)

Apo-Indapamide a generic company version of indapamide 312 (a thiazide-like diuretic 85)

Apo-Ipravent a generic company version of ipratropium bromide 315 (a *bronchodilator* 76)

Apo-ISDN a generic company version of isosorbide dinitrate 318 (a nitrate *vasodilator* 84 and anti-angina drug 87)

Apo-Keto a generic company version of ketoprofen 321 (a non-steroidal anti-inflammatory 102)

Apo-Ketoconazole a generic company version of ketoconazole 320 (an antifungal 124)

Apo-Ketotifen a generic company version of ketotifen (a drug used in asthma 77)

Apo-lactulose a generic company version of lactulose 322 (an osmotic laxative 97)

Apo-levobunolol a generic company version of levobunolol (a beta blocker 83 and drug for glaucoma 156)

Apo-Levocarb a generic company version of levodopa/carbidopa 326 (a combination of levodopa 326 and carbidopa for *parkinsonism* 71)

Apo-Loperamide a generic company version of loperamide 332 (an antidiarrheal 96)

Apo-Loratadine a generic company version of loratadine 334 (an antihistamine 110)

Apo-Lorazepam a generic company version of lorazepam 335 (a benzodiazepine anti-anxiety drug 67 and sleeping drug 66)

Apo-Lovastatin a generic company version of lovastatin 337 (a lipid-lowering drug 89)

Apo-Loxapine a generic company version of loxapine (an antipsychotic 69)

Apo-Metformin a generic company version of metformin 346 (a drug for diabetes 128)

Apo-Methyldopa a generic company version of methyldopa 350 (an antihypertensive 88)

Apo-Metoclop a generic company version of metoclopramide 353 (a gastrointestinal motility regulator and anti-emetic 74)

Apo-Metoprolol a generic company version of metoprolol 354 (a beta blocker 83)

Apo-Methotrimeprazine a generic company version of methotrimeprazine (a phenothiazine antipsychotic 69)

Apo-Minocycline a generic company version of minocycline 357 (a tetracycline *antibiotic* 114)

Apo-Misoprostol a generic company version of misoprostol 360 (an antiulcer drug 95)

Apo-Moclobemide a generic company version of moclobemide 361 (an antidepressant 68)

Apo-Nabumetone a generic company version of nabumetone (a non-steroidal anti-inflammatory 102)

Apo-Naproxen SR a generic company version of naproxen 366 (a non-steroidal anti-inflammatory 102)

Apo-Nifed a product name for nifedipine 368 (a calcium channel blocker 87)

Apo-Nifed PA a generic company version of nifedipine 368 (a calcium channel blocker 87)

Apo-Nortriptyline a generic company version of nortriptyline (a tricyclic antidepressant 68)

Apo-Orciprenaline a generic company version of orciprenaline (a *bronchodilator* 76)

Apo-Oxazepam a generic company version of oxazepam 380 (a benzodiazepine anti-anxiety drug 67)

Apo-Oxtriphylline a generic company version of oxtriphylline (a *bronchodilator* 76)

Apo-Pen VK a generic company version of penicillin V 384 (a penicillin *antibiotic* 114)

Apo-Perphenazine a generic company version of perphenazine (a phenothiazine antipsychotic 69)

Apo-Pioglitazone a generic company version of pioglitazone 390 (a drug for diabetes 128)

Apo-Piroxicam a generic company version of piroxicam 391 (a non-steroidal anti-inflammatory 102)

Apo-Pravastatin a generic company version of Pravastatin 394 (a lipid-lowering drug 89)

Apo-Prazo a generic company version of prazosin (a sympatholytic antihypertensive 88)

Apo-Prednisone a generic company version of prednisone 395 (a corticosteroid 127)

Apo-Primidone a generic company version of primidone (an anticonvulsant 70)

Apo-Procainamide a generic company version of procainamide (an anti-arrhythmic 86)

Apo-Prochlorperazine a generic company version of prochlorperazine 397 (a phenothiazine anti-emetic 74 and antipsychotic 69)

Apo-Propafenone a generic company version of propafenone (an anti-arrhythmic 86)

Apo-Propranolol a generic company version of propranolol 402 (a beta blocker 83)

Apo-Quinidine a generic company version of quinidine 409 (an anti-arrhythmic drug 86)

Apo-Salvent a generic company version of salbutamol 424 (a *bronchodilator* 76)

Apo-Salvent-HFA a generic company version of salbutamol 424 (a *bronchodilator* 76)

Apo-Selegiline a generic company version of selegiline 426 (a drug for *parkinsonism* 71)

Apo-Sertraline a generic company version of sertraline 427 (an antidepressant 68)

Apo-Sotalol a generic company version of sotalol 432 a beta blocker 83

APO-SULFATRIM–CALCIUM D 500

Apo-Sulfatrim a generic company version of sulfamethoxazole/trimethoprim – a sulfonamide antibacterial 117 combined with trimethoprim 457

Apo-Sulfinpyrazone a generic company version of sulfinpyrazone (a drug for gout 105)

Apo-Sulin a generic company version of sulindac (a non-steroidal anti-inflammatory 102)

Apo-Temazepam a generic company version of temazepam 440 (a benzodiazepine sleeping drug 66)

Apo-Tenoxicam a generic company version of tenoxicam (a non-steroidal anti-inflammatory 102)

Apo-Terazosin a generic company version of terazosin 442 (a sympatholytic antihypertensive 88)

Apo-Terbinafine a generic company version of terbinafine 443 (an antifungal 124)

Apo-Tetra a generic company version of tetracycline 447 (an *antibiotic* 114 and antimalarial 123)

Apo-Theo LA a generic company version of theophylline 448 (a *bronchodilator* 76)

Apo-Thioridazine a generic company version of thioridazine (an antipsychotic 69)

Apo-Tiaprofenic a generic company version of tiaprofenic acid (a non-steroidal anti-inflammatory 102)

Apo-Trazodone a generic company version of trazodone (an antidepressant 68)

Apo-Trazodone D a generic company version of trazodone (an antidepressant 68)

Apo-Triazo a generic company version of temazepam 440 (a benzodiazepine sleeping drug 66)

Apo-Trifluoperazine a generic company version of trifluoperazine 456 (a phenothiazine antipsychotic 69)

Apo-Trihex a generic company version of trihexyphenidyl (a drug for *parkinsonism* 71)

Apo-Trimethroprim a generic company version of trimethroprim 457 (an antibacterial 117)

Apo-Trimip a generic company version of trimipramine (a tricyclic antidepressant 68)

Apo-Zopiclone a generic company version of zopiclone 467 (a sleeping drug 66)

apraclonidine a drug for glaucoma 156

Aprepitant an anti-emetic 74

Apresoline a product name for hydralazine (an antihypertensive 102)

aprotinin an antifibrinolytic 90 used to promote blood clotting

Aptivus a product name for tipranavir (an antiretroviral drug used in the treatment of HIV and AIDS 144)

Aranesp a product name for darbepoetin 275 (a kidney hormone 126 used for anemia due to kidney failure).

Arava a product name for leflunomide (an antirheumatic drug 103)

Aricept a product name for donepezil 264 (a drug for Alzheimer's disease 71)

Arimidex a product name for anastrozole 193 (an anticancer drug 140)

Aristocort a product name for triamcinolone (a corticosteroid 127)

Aristospan a product name for triamcinolone (a corticosteroid 127)

Arixtra a product name for fondaparinux (an anticoagulant 91)

Arthrotec a product-name combination drug containing diclofenac 254 (a non-steroidal anti-inflammatory drug 102) and misoprostol 360 (an antiulcer drug 95)

ASA 194 (a non-opioid analgesic 64 and antiplatelet drug 90)

Asacol a product name for mesalamine/5-ASA 345 (a drug for inflammatory bowel disease 98)

Asaphen a product name for ASA 194 (a non-opioid analgesic 64 and antiplatelet drug 90)

Asaphen EC a product name for ASA 194 (a non-opioid analgesic 64 and antiplatelet drug 90)

ascorbic acid vitamin C 480 (a vitamin 135)

Aspirin a product name for ASA 193 (a non-opioid analgesic 64 and antiplatelet drug 90)

Aspirin Backache a combination product with ASA 194 (a non-opioid analgesic 64) and methocarbamol (a muscle relaxant 106)

Atacand a product name for candesartan (a vasodilator 84 and an antihypertensive drug 88)

Atarax a product name for hydroxyzine (an antihistamine used as an anti-anxiety drug 67)

Atasol a product name for acetaminophen 177 (an non-opioid analgesic 64)

Atazanavir an antiretroviral drug for HIV infection and AIDS 144

atenolol 195 a beta blocker 83

Ativan a product name for lorazepam 335 (a benzodiazepine anti-anxiety drug 67 and sleeping drug 66)

atomoxatine 196 (a drug used to treat hyperactivity 72)

atorvastatin 197 a lipid-lowering drug 89

atovaquone an antiprotozoal 122 and antimalarial 123

Atripla a product combination product containing emtricitabine, tenofovir disoproxil, and efavirenz 269 (drugs used in HIV and immune deficiency 144)

atropine 198 (an *anticholinergic* for irritable bowel syndrome 98 and a mydriatic 158)

Atrovent a product name for ipratropium bromide 315 (a *bronchodilator* 76)

attapulgite 199 (an adsorbent used as an antidiarrheal 96)

auranofin an antirheumatic 103

Avalide a combination drug containing irbesartan 316 (a vasodilator 84 and antihypertensive drug 88) and hydrochlorothiazide 306 (a diuretic 85)

Avamys a product name for fluticasone 290 (a corticosteroid 127)

Avandamet a combination drug with rosiglitazone 422 (a drug for diabetes 128) and metformin 346 (a drug for diabetes 128)

Avandia a product name for rosiglitazone 422 (a drug for diabetes 128)

Avandryl a combination drug with rosiglitazone 422 (a drug for diabetes 128) and glimepiride 300 (a drug for diabetes 128)

Avapro a product name for irbesartan 316 (a *vasodilator* 84 and antihypertensive drug 88)

Avastin a product name for bevacizumab (a monoclonal antibody 140)

Avelox a product name for moxifloxacin 365 (an antibacterial 117)

avobenzone an ingredient of sunscreens 169

Avodart a product name for dutasteride (a drug used in urinary disorders 154)

Avonex a product name for interferon beta-1a 314 (a drug used in multiple sclerosis)

Axert a product name for almotripton (a drug for migraine 73)

azatadine an antihistamine 110

azathioprine 200 (an antirheumatic 103 and immunosuppressant 143)

Azilect a product name for rasagiline 414 (a drug used for parkinsonism 71)

azithromycin 201 (an *antibiotic* 114)

Azopt a product name for brinzolamide (a drug for glaucoma 156)

B

Baciguent a product name for bacitracin (an *antibiotic* 114)

bacitracin an *antibiotic* 114

baclofen 202 (a muscle relaxant 106)

Bactigras a product name for chlorhexidine (a skin antiseptic 163)

Bactroban a product name for mupirocin (an antibacterial for skin infections 163)

Balminil Codeine Night-Time and Expectorant a combination drug with ammonium chloride (an expectorant 80), codeine 242 (an opioid analgesic 64), and diphenhydramine 259 (an antihistamine 110)

Balminil DM a product name for dextromorphan 252 (a cough suppressant 80)

Balminil DM-D-E a combination product containing guafenesin (an expectorant 80) and dextromorphan 252 (a cough suppressant)

Baraclude a product name for entecavir (an antiviral 119)

Basalgel a product name for aluminum hydroxide 184 (an antacid 94)

basiliximab an immunosuppressant 143

beclomethasone 203 (a corticosteroid 127)

Beech Nut Cough Drops Honey-Lemon a lozenge with eucalyptus and menthol

Beech Nut Cough Drops Menthol a lozenge with eucalyptus and menthol

Beech Nut Cough Drops Wild Cherry a lozenge with eucalyptus and menthol

belladonna an *antispasmodic anticholinergic* for irritable bowel syndrome 98

Bellergal Spacetabs a product name for ergotamine 273 (a drug for migraine 73) with belladonna (an *antispasmodic*), and pentobarbital (a barbiturate sedative 66)

Benadryl a product name for diphenhydramine 259 (an antihistamine 110, anti-emetic 74, and antipruritic 161)

Benoxyl a product name for benzoyl peroxide 204 (a drug for acne 165)

benserazide a drug used to enhance the effect of levodopa 326 (a drug for *parkinsonism* 71)

Bentylol a product name for dicyclomine 255 (a drug for irritable bowel syndrome 98)

Benuryl a product name for probenecid 397 (a drug for gout 105)

Benylin DM a product name for dextromorphan 252 (a cough suppressant 80)

Benylin DM-E Extra Strength a combination product containing guafenesin (an expectorant 80) and dextromorphan 252 (a cough suppressant)

Benylin First Defence Syrup a syrup with menthol and echinacea

Benzac AC a product name for benzoyl peroxide 204 (a drug for acne 165)

Benzac W Wash a product name for benzoyl peroxide 204 (a drug for acne 165)

Benzaclin a product name for a combination product of clindamycin 233 (an antibiotic 114) and benzoyl peroxide 204 (a drug for acne 165)

Benzalip-SR a product name for bezafibrate 207 (a lipid-lowering drug 89)

Benzamycin a combination of benzoyl peroxide 204 (a drug for acne 165) and erythromycin 274 (an *antibiotic* 114)

benzocaine a local *anesthetic* 64

benzophones an ingredient of sunscreens 169

benzoyl peroxide 204 (a drug for acne 165)

benztropine an *anticholinergic* for *parkinsonism* 71

Benztropine Mesylate a product name for benztropine (an *anticholinergic* for *parkinsonism* 71)

Benztropine Omega a product name for benztropine (an *anticholinergic* for *parkinsonism* 71)

benzylpenicillin see penicillin G (a penicillin *antibiotic* 114)

Berotec a product name for fenoterol (a *sympathomimetic bronchodilator* 76)

beta-carotene vitamin A 479 (a vitamin 135 and food additive)

Betadine Topical a product name for povidone-iodine (a skin antiseptic 163)

Betagan a product name for levobunolol (a beta blocker 83 and drug for glaucoma 56)

betahistine 205 (an antivertigo 74)

Betaject a product name for betamethasone 206 (a corticosteroid 127)

Betaloc a product name for metoprolol 354 (a beta blocker 83)

Betaloc Durules a product name for metoprolol 354 (a beta blocker 83)

betamethasone 206 (a corticosteroid 127)

Betaseron a product name for interferon beta-1b 314. (a drug used in multiple sclerosis)

betaxolol a beta blocker 83 also used in glaucoma 156

bethanechol a para*sympathomimetic* for urinary retention 154

Betnesol a product name for beta-methasone 206 (a corticosteroid 127)

Betoptic S a product-name drug for glaucoma 156 containing betaxolol

Bevacizumab a monoclonal antibody 140

bezafibrate 207 (a lipid-lowering drug 89)

Biaxin a product name for clarithromycin 232 (a macrolide *antibiotic* 114)

Biaxin BID a product name for clarithromycin 232 (a macrolide *antibiotic* 114)

Biaxin XL a product name for clarithromycin 232 (a macrolide *antibiotic* 114)

bimatoprost a drug for glaucoma 156

biotin 469 (a vitamin 135)

Biquin Durules a product name for quinidine 409 (an anti-arrhythmic drug 86)

bisacodyl 208 (a laxative 97)

Bismutal a product name combination of bismuth (a metal given in compound form for gastric and duodenal ulcers 95 that is also used for sore throats) and guaifenesin (an expectorant 80)

bismuth a metal given in compound form for gastric and duodenal ulcers 95 and is also used for sore throats

Blephamide a product name for a combination of prednisolone 395 (a corticosteroid 127) and sulfacetamide (a sulfonamide antibacterial 117) for use in the eye

Bonamine a product name for meclizine (an antihistamine used as an anti-emetic drug 74)

Botox a product name for botulinum toxin type A 209 (a muscle relaxant 106)

Botox Cosmetic a product name for botulinum toxin type A 209 (a muscle relaxant 106)

botulinum toxin 209 (a muscle relaxant 106)

bretylium an anti-arrhythmic 86

Bretylium Tosylate a product name for bretylium (an anti-arrhythmic 86)

Brevibloc a product name for esmolol (a beta blocker 83)

Brevicon 0.5/35 a product-name oral contraceptive 149 containing ethinyl estradiol 278 and norethindrone 371

Bricanyl Turbuhaler a product name for terbutaline 444 (a *bronchodilator* 76 and drug used in labour 153)

brimonidine a drug for glaucoma 156

brinzolamide a drug for glaucoma 156

bromocriptine 210 (a pituitary agent 131 and drug for *parkinsonism* 71)

brompheniramine an antihistamine 110

buclizine an antihistamine 110 used for motion sickness

budesonide 211 a corticosteroid 127

bumetanide 212 (a loop diuretic 85)

bupivacaine a long-lasting local *anesthetic* 64 used in labour 153

bupropion 213 (an antidepressant 68 used as an aid when stopping smoking in addition to counselling)

Burinex a product name for bumetanide 212 (a loop diuretic 85)

Buro-Sol a combination of aluminum (an *astringent* used for inflammation of the skin or outer ear canal 163) and benzethonium chloride

buserelin a drug for menstrual disorders 148

BuSpar a product name for buspirone 214 (an anti-anxiety drug 67)

buspirone 214 (a non-benzodiazepine anti-anxiety drug 67)

butaconazole an antifungal 124

C

cabergoline a drug to treat infertility 152 or to stop milk production in women who do not want to breast-feed, also used for Parkinson's disease 71

Caduet a product name for combination product containing amlodipine 189 (a calcium channel blocker 87) and atorvastatin 197 (a lipid-lowering drug 89)

Caelyx a product name for doxorubicin 267 (a *cytotoxic* anticancer drug 140)

Cafergot a product name for ergotamine 273 (a drug for migraine 73) with caffeine (a stimulant 72)

Cafergot-PB a product name for ergotamine 273 (a drug for migraine 73) with belladonna (an *antispasmodic* drug), caffeine (a stimulant 72), and pentobarbital (a barbiturate sedative 66)

caffeine a stimulant 72 in coffee, tea, and cola, added to some analgesics 64

calamine a substance containing zinc carbonate (an antipruritic 161) used to soothe irritated skin

calcifediol vitamin D 481 (a vitamin 135)

Calcimar a product name for calcitonin (a drug for bone disorders 108)

calcipotriol 215 (a drug for psoriasis 166)

Calcite 500 a product name for calcium carbonate (a calcium salt (a mineral 137) used as an antacid 94)

Calcite D-500 a combination product with calcium carbonate (a calcium salt (a mineral 137) used as an antacid 94) and vitamin D 481

calcitonin a drug for bone disorders 108

calcitriol vitamin D 481 (a vitamin 135)

calcium 469 (a mineral 152)

Calcium 500 a product name for calcium carbonate (a calcium salt (a mineral 137) used as an antacid 94)

calcium acetate calcium 469 (a mineral 152)

calcium carbonate a calcium salt (a mineral 137) used as an antacid 94

calcium chloride calcium 469 (a mineral 152)

Calcium D 500 a combination product with calcium carbonate (a calcium salt (a mineral 137) used as an antacid 94) and vitamin D 481 (a vitamin 135)

CALCIUM GLUCONATE–CYPROTERONE

calcium gluconate calcium 469 (a mineral 152)

Calcium Oyster Shell a product name for calcium carbonate (a calcium salt (a mineral 137) used as an antacid 94)

Caltine a product name for calcitonin (a drug for bone disorders 108)

camphor a *topical* antipruritic 161

Camptosar a product name for irinotecan (an anticancer drug 140)

Cancidas a product name for caspofungin (an antifungal drug 124)

Candesartan a vasodilator 84 and an antihypertensive drug 88

Candistatin a product name for nystatin 373 (an antifungal 124)

Canesten a product name for clotrimazole 239 (an antifungal 124)

cannabidiol an analgesic (64) used in multiple sclerosis

Capex shampoo a product name for fluocinolone (a *topical* corticosteroid 162)

Capoten a product name for captopril 216 (an ACE inhibitor 84)

capreomycin an antituberculous drug 118

captopril 216 (an ACE inhibitor 84)

carbachol a drug used for its miotic effect in glaucoma 156 and as a para*sympathomimetic*

Carbachol a product name for carbachol (a drug used for its miotic effect in glaucoma 156 and as a para*sympathomimetic*)

carbamazepine 217 (an anticonvulsant 70)

carbidopa a substance that enhances the therapeutic effect of levodopa 326 (a drug for *parkinsonism* 71)

carbocysteine a mucolytic 95

Carbolith a product name for lithium 331 (a drug for mania 69)

carboplatin an anticancer drug 140

Cardizem a product name for diltiazem 257 (an antihypertensive 88 and calcium channel blocker 87)

Cardizem CD a product name for diltiazem 257 (an antihypertensive 88 and calcium channel blocker 87)

Cardura a product name for doxazosin 266 (a sympatholytic antihypertensive 88)

carnitine an amino acid used as a nutritional supplement 134

cascara a laxative 97

caspofungin an antifungal drug 124

castor oil a stimulant laxative 97

Catapres a product name for clonidine (an antihypertensive 88)

Caverject a product name for alprostadil 183 (a prostaglandin used for male impotence 134, 152)

Cedocard SR a product name for isosorbide dinitrate 318 (a nitrate *vasodilator* 84 and anti-angina drug 87)

cefaclor a cephalosporin *antibiotic* 114

cefadroxil a cephalosporin *antibiotic* 114

cefamandole a cephalosporin *antibiotic* 114

cefazolin an *antibiotic* 114

cefepime an *antibiotic* 114

cefixime a cephalosporin *antibiotic* 114

Cefizox a product name for ceftizoxime (a cephalosporin *antibiotic* 114)

Cefotan a product name for cefotetan (a cephalosporin *antibiotic* 114)

cefotaxime a cephalosporin *antibiotic* 114

cefoxitin a cephalosporin *antibiotic* 114

cefprozil an *antibiotic* 114

ceftazidime a cephalosporin *antibiotic* 114

Ceftin a product name for Cefuroxime axetil 218 (a cephalosporin *antibiotic* 115)

ceftriaxone an *antibiotic* 114

Cefuroxime 218 (a cephalosporin *antibiotic* 114)

Cefzil a product name for cefprozil (an antibiotic 114)

Celebrex a product name for celecoxib 219 (a non-steroidal anti-inflammatory 102)

celecoxib 219 a non-steroidal anti-inflammatory 102

Celestone a product name for betamethasone 206 (a corticosteroid 127)

Celexa a product name for citalopram 231 (a tricyclic antidepressant 68)

CellCept a product name for mycophenolate mofetil (an immunosuppressant 143)

Celontin a product name for methsuximide (an anticonvulsant 70)

Celsentri a product name for Maraviroc (an antiretroviral drug used in the treatment of HIV and AIDS 144)

cephalexin 220 (a cephalosporin *antibiotic* 114)

Cerebyx a product name for fosphenytoin 388 (an anticonvulsant 70)

C.E.S. a product name for conjugated estrogens 244 (a female sex hormone 133)

Cesamet a product name for nabilone (an anti-emetic 74)

cetirizine 221 (an antihistamine 110)

cetrimide a skin antiseptic 163

Champix a product name for varenicline 460 (a drug used in smoking cessation)

Cheracol a product name for a combination product containing codeine 242 (an opioid analgesic 64) and cough/cold medications

chloral hydrate a sleeping drug 66

chlorambucil an anticancer drug 140 used for chronic lymphocytic leukemia and lymphatic and ovarian cancers, and as an immunosuppressant 143 for rheumatoid arthritis 103

chloramphenicol 222 (an *antibiotic* 114)

chlordiazepoxide 223 (a benzodiazepine anti-anxiety drug 67)

chlorhexidine a skin antiseptic 179

Chloromycetin a product name for chloramphenicol 222 (an *antibiotic* 114)

chloroquine 224 (an antimalarial 123 and antirheumatic 103)

chlorpheniramine 225 (an antihistamine 110)

chlorpromazine 226 (a phenothiazine antipsychotic 69 and anti-emetic 74)

chlorpropamide a drug for diabetes 128

chlorthalidone a thiazide diuretic 85

Chlor-Tripolon a product name for chlorpheniramine 225 (an antihistamine 110)

Chlor-Tripolon N.D. a combination of loratadine 334 (an antihistamine 110) and pseudoephedrine 404 (a decongestant 79)

Choledyl a product name for oxtriphylline (a *bronchodilator* 76)

cholestyramine 227 (a lipid-lowering drug 89)

chromium 470 (a mineral 137)

Cialis a product name for tadalafil (a drug used for the treatment of sexual impotence 152)

Cicatrin a combination of bacitracin (an *antibiotic* 114), amino acids, and neomycin

ciclesonide an inhaled corticosteroid 127 used in asthma 78

Ciclopirox an antifungal drug 124

Ciloxan a product name for ciprofloxacin 229 (a quinolone antibacterial 117)

cimetidine 228 (an anti-ulcer drug 95)

Cipralex a product name for escitalopram (an antidepressant 68)

Cipro a product name for ciprofloxacin 229 (an antibacterial 117)

Ciprodex a combination product containing ciprofloxacin 229 (an antibacterial 117) and dexamethasone 251 (a corticosteroid 127) used in ear infections

ciprofloxacin 229 (an antibacterial 117)

Cipro HC a combination of ciprofloxacin 229 (an antibacterial 117) and hydrocortisone 308 (a corticosteroid 127) used in ear infections

cisplatin 230 (an anticancer drug 140)

citalopram 231 (a tricyclic antidepressant 68)

Citrate 600 a product name for calcium carbonate used as an antacid 94

Citro-Mag a product name for magnesium citrate (an osmotic laxative 97)

Claforan a product name for cefotaxime (a cephalosporin *antibiotic* 114)

clarithromycin 232 (a macrolide *antibiotic* 114)

Claritin a product name for loratadine 334 an antihistamine 110

Claritin Allergic Congestion Relief a product name product containing oxymetazoline (a *topical* decongestant 79)

Claritin Extra a combination of loratadine 334 (an antihistamine 110) and pseudoephedrine 404 (a decongestant 79)

Claritin Eye Allergy Relief a product name product containing oxymetazoline (a *topical* decongestant 79)

Claritin Liberator a combination of loratadine 334 (an antihistamine 110) and pseudoephedrine 404 (a decongestant 79)

Claritin Skin Itch Relief a product name for hydrocortisone 308 (a corticosteroid 127 and antipruritic 161)

Clarus a generic version of isotretinoin 319 (a drug for acne 165)

clavulinic acid a substance given with amoxicillin 190 (a penicillin *antibiotic* 114) to make it more effective

Clavulin a product name for amoxicillin/ clavulinic acid (a combination of amoxicillin 190 (a penicillin *antibiotic* 114) and clavulinic acid (a substance given with it to make amoxicillin more effective))

clemastine an antihistamine 110

clindamycin 233 a lincosamide *antibiotic* 114

Clindets a product name for topical clindamycin 233 (a lincosamide antibiotic 114)

Clindoxyl a product name for a combination product of clindamycin 233 (an antibiotic 114) and benzoyl peroxide 204 (a drug for acne 165)

clioquinol an antibacterial 117 and antifungal 124

Clioquinol a product name for clioquinol (an antibacterial 117 and antifungal drug 124)

clobazam a benzodiazepine drug used as an anticonvulsant 70

clobetasol 234 (a *topical* corticosteroid drug 162)

clobetasone a *topical* corticosteroid 162

Clomid a product name for clomiphene 235 (a drug for infertility 152)

clomiphene 235 (a drug for infertility 152)

clomipramine 236 (a tricyclic antidepressant 68)

clonazepam 237 (a benzodiazepine anti- anxiety drug 67 and anticonvulsant 70)

Clopixol a product name for zuclopenthixol (an antipsychotic drug 69)

Clopixol-Acuphase a product name for zuclopenthixol (an antipsychotic 69)

Clopixol-Depot a product name for zuclopenthixol (an antipsychotic 69)

clonidine an antihypertensive drug 88

clopidogrel 238 (an antiplatelet drug 90)

Clotrimaderm a product name for clotrimazole 239 (an antifungal 124

clotrimazole 239 (an antifungal 124)

cloxacillin 240 (a penicillin *antibiotic* 114)

clozapine 241 (an antipsychotic 69)

Clozaril a product name for clozapine 241 (an antipsychotic 69)

CoActifed Tablets a combination product containing codeine 242 (an opioid analgesic 64) and cough/cold medications.

coal tar a substance for psoriasis 166 and eczema 167

Coated Aspirin a product name for ASA 194 (a non-opioid analgesic 64 and antiplatelet drug 90)

cocaine a local *anesthetic* 64 and drug of abuse 488

codeine 242 (an opioid analgesic 64, cough suppressant 80, and antidiarrheal 96)

Codeine Contin a product name for codeine 242 (an opioid analgesic 64)

Codeine Phosphate a product name for codeine 242 (an opioid analgesic 64)

co-enzyme Q$_{10}$ a supplement 470

CO Fluoxetine a product name for fluoxetine 287 (a tricyclic antidepressant 68)

Cogentin a product name for benztropine (an *anticholinergic* for *parkinsonism* 71)

Co-Glimepiride a generic company version of glimepiride 300 (a drug used in diabetes 128)

Colace a product name for docusate sodium 262 (a stool softener, laxatives 97)

colchicine 243 (a drug for gout 105)

colecalciferol vitamin D 481 (a vitamin 135)

colestipol a lipid-lowering drug 89

colistin an *antibiotic* 114

collodion a substance that dries to form a sticky film, protecting broken skin

Combigan a product name for a combination of brimonidine (an alpha adrenergic receptor agonist used in glaucoma 156) and timolol 449 (a beta blocker 83 and drug for glaucoma 156)

Combivent a product name for a combination of salbutamol 424 and ipratropium bromide 315 (both *bronchodilator*s 90)

Comtan a product name for entacapone (a drug for *parkinsonism* 71)

Concerta a product name for methylphenidate 351 (a drug used to treat hyperactivity in children 72)

Condyline a product name for podophyllotoxin (a drug for genital warts 135)

Congest a product name for conjugated estrogens 244 (a female sex hormone 133)

conjugated estrogens 244 (a female sex hormone 133 and drug for bone disorders 108)

Contac Cold 12 Hour Relief Non Drowsy a product name for pseudoephedrine 404 (a decongestant 79)

Contact Head and Chest Congestion a combination product containing guafenesin (an expectorant 80) and pseudoephedrine 404 (a decongestant)

Co-Pioglitazone a generic company version of pioglitazone 390 (a drug for diabetes 128)

copper 471 (a mineral 137)

Cordarone a product name for amiodarone 187 (an anti-arrhythmic 86)

Cortate a product name for hydrocortisone 308 (a corticosteroid 127 and antipruritic 161)

Cortef a product name for hydrocortisone 308 (a corticosteroid 127)

Cortenema a product name for hydrocortisone 308 (a corticosteroid 127)

corticotropin a pituitary hormone 131

Cortifoam a product name for hydro- cortisone 308 (a corticosteroid 127)

Cortimyxin ointment a combination of polymyxin B (a skin antiseptic 163) and bacitracin zinc (an *antibiotic* 114), hydrocortisone 308 (a corticosteroid 127 and antipruritic 161) and neomycin (an *antibiotic* 114)

cortisol an old name for hydrocortisone 308

cortisone a corticosteroid 127

Cortisone acetate a product name for cortisone (a corticosteroid 127)

Cortisporin ointment a combination of polymyxin B (a skin antiseptic 163), bacitracin zinc (an *antibiotic* 114), hydrocortisone 308 (a corticosteroid 127 and antipruritic 161), and neomycin (an *antibiotic* 114)

Cortoderm a product name for hydrocortisone 308 (a corticosteroid 127 and antipruritic 161)

Cosopt a combination of dorzolamide 265 (a carbonic anhydrase inhibitor for glaucoma 156) and timolol 449 (a beta blocker 83)

co-trimoxazole 245 a combination of sulfamethoxazole/trimethoprim (a sulfonamide antibacterial 117 combined with trimethoprim 457)

Coumadin a product name for warfarin 463 (an anticoagulant 90)

Coversyl a product name for perindopril 385 (an ACE inhibitor 84)

Coversyl Plus a combination of perindopril 385 (an ACE inhibitor 84) and indapamide 312 (a thiazide-like diuretic 85)

Coversyl Plus LD a product name for a combination of indapamide 312 (a thiazide- like diuretic 85) and perindopril 385 (an ACE inhibitor 84)

Cozaar a product name for losartan 336 (an antihypertensive 88)

Creon a product name for pancreatin (a preparation of pancreatic enzymes 114)

Crestor a product name for rosuvastatin 423 (a lipid-lowering drug 89)

Crinone a product name for progesterone (a female sex hormone 133)

Crixivan a product name for indinavir (a drug for HIV/AIDS 144)

Cromolyn a product name for sodium cromoglycate 431 (an anti-allergy drug 109 used to prevent asthma attacks 77)

crotamiton an antipruritic 161 and antiparasitic 164 for scabies

Crystapen a product name for benzylpenicillin (a penicillin *antibiotic* 114)

Cubicin a product name for daptomycin (an antibacterial 117)

Cuprimine a product name for penicillamine (an antirheumatic 103)

cyanocobalamin vitamin B12 480 (a vitamin 135)

cyclizine an antihistamine 110 used as an anti-emetic 74

Cyclogyl a product name for cyclopentolate (an *anticholinergic* mydriatic 158)

Cyclomen a product name for danazol 248 (a drug for menstrual disorders 148)

cyclopentolate an *anticholinergic* mydriatic 158

cyclophosphamide 246 (an anticancer drug 140)

cyclosporine 247 (an immunosuppressant 143)

Cyklokapron a product name for tranexamic acid (an antifibrinolytic used to promote blood clotting 90)

cyproheptadine an antihistamine 111

cyproterone a synthetic sex hormone used for acne 165, cancer of the prostate 140, and male sexual disorders 134

CYTARABINE–ERGOCALCIFEROL

cytarabine a drug for leukemia 140

Cytomel a product name for liothyronine (a thyroid hormone 130)

Cytovene a product name for ganciclovir (an antiviral 119)

Cytoxan a product name for cyclophosphamide 246 (an anticancer drug 140)

D

daclizumab an immunosuppressant 143

Dalacin C a product name for clindamycin 233 (a lincosamide *antibiotic* 114)

dalfopristin an *antibiotic* 114

Dalmacol a product name combination product with doxylamine (a sleeping drug 66) and a cough suppressant 80

dalteparin 305 (an anticoagulant 91)

danazol 248 (a drug for menstrual disorders 148)

Dantrium a product name for dantrolene (a muscle relaxant 106)

dantrolene tizanidine a muscle relaxant 106

dapsone an antibacterial 117

Daptomycin an antibiotic drug 114

Daraprim a product name for pyrimethamine 407 (an antimalarial 123)

darbepoetin 275 (a kidney hormone 126 used for anemia due to kidney failure)

darifenacin 249 (a drug for urinary disorders 154)

darunavir an antiretroviral drug used in the treatment of HIV and AIDS 144

Darvon-N a product name for propoxyhene (an opioid analgesic 64)

Daypro a product name for oxaprozin (a non-steroidal anti-inflammatory 102)

Deca-Durabolin a product name for nandrolone (an anabolic steroid 134)

Delatestryl a product name for testosterone 446 (a male sex hormone 132)

Delavirdine an antiretroviral drug used in the treatment of HIV and AIDS 144

Delestrogen a product name for estradiol 276 (an estrogen 133)

Demerol a product name for meperidine (an opioid analgesic 64 and drug used in labour 153)

Denavir a product name for penciclovir (an antiviral 119)

Denorex a product name for coal tar (a substance for psoriasis 166 and eczema 167)

Depakene a product name for valproic acid 458 (an anticonvulsant 70)

DepoCyt a product name for cytarabine (a drug for leukemia 140)

Depo-Medrol a product name for methyl-prednisolone 352 (a corticosteroid 127)

Depo-Provera a product name for medroxyprogesterone 339 (a female sex hormone 133)

Depo-Testosterone a product name for testosterone 446 (a male sex hormone 132)

Derma-Smooth/FS a product name for fluocinolone (a *topical* corticosteroid 162)

Dermovate a product name for clobetasol 234 (a *topical* corticosteroid 162)

desipramine a tricyclic antidepressant 68

desloratadine 334 (an antihistamine 110)

desmopressin 250 (a pituitary hormone 131 used for diabetes insipidus 128)

desogestrel a progestin 133

desonide a *topical* corticosteroid 127

Desoxi a product name for desoximetasone (a *topical* corticosteroid 162)

desoximetasone a *topical* corticosteroid 162

Desquam-X a product name for benzoyl peroxide 204 (a drug for acne 165)

Desyrel a product name for trazodone (an antidepressant 68)

Desyrel Dividose a product name for trazodone (an antidepressant 68)

Detrol a product name for tolterodine 452 (an *anticholinergic* and *antispasmodic* for urinary disorders 154)

dexamethasone 251 (a corticosteroid 127 used as anti-emetic 74)

dextroamphetamine an amphetamine 72

dexedrine a product name for dextroamphetamine (an amphetamine 72)

dextromethorphan 252 (a cough suppressant 80)

Diabeta a product name for glyburide 301 (an oral antidiabetic drug 128)

Diamicron a product name for gliclazide 299 (an oral antidiabetic 128)

Diamicron MR a product name for gliclazide 299 (an oral antidiabetic 128)

diamorphine see heroin

Diamox a product name for acetazolamide (a carbonic anhydrase inhibitor diuretic 85)

Diane-35 a combination of cyproterone (a synthetic sex hormone used to treat acne 165, cancer of the prostate 140, and male sexual disorders 134) and ethinyl estradiol 278 (an estrogen 133)

Diastat a product name for diazepam 253 (a benzodiazepine anti-anxiety drug 67, sedative 64, muscle relaxant 106, and anticonvulsant 70)

Diazemuls a product name for diazepam 253 (a benzodiazepine anti-anxiety drug 67, sedative 64, muscle relaxant 106, and anticonvulsant 70)

diazepam 253 (a benzodiazepine anti-anxiety drug 67, sedative 64, muscle relaxant 106, and anticonvulsant 70)

Diclectin a product name combination product with doxylamine (a sleeping drug 66) and pyroxidine 477 (vitamin B6)

diclofenac 254 (a non-steroidal anti-inflammatory 102)

dicyclomine 255 (a drug for irritable bowel syndrome 98)

didanosine an antiretroviral drug for HIV infection and aids 144

Didrocal a product containing tablets of etidronate 279 (a drug for bone disorders 108) and calcium 469 (a mineral 137)

Didronel a product name for etidronate 279 (a drug for bone disorders 108)

diethylcarbamazine an anthelmintic 125

diethylstilbestrol previously known as stilboestrol (a female sex hormone 133)

Differin a product name for adapalene (a retinoid for acne 165)

Diflucan a product name for fluconazole 286 (an antifungal 124)

diflucortolone a *topical* corticosteroid 162

diflunisal a non-steroidal anti-inflammatory 102

digoxin 256 (a digitalis drug 82)

Digoxin Injection C.S.D. a product name for digoxin 256 (a digitalis drug 82)

dihydroergotamine a drug for migraine 73

Dihydroergotamine Mesylate Injection a product name for dihydroergotamine (a drug for migraine 73)

dihydrotachysterol vitamin D 481 (a vitamin 135)

Dilantin a product name for phenytoin 388 (an anticonvulsant 70)

Dilaudid a product name for hydromorphone 309 (an opioid analgesic 64 used in the management of pain)

diloxanide an antiprotozoal 122 for amoebic dysentery

diltiazem 257 (an antihypertensive 88 and calcium channel blocker 87)

dimenhydrinate 258 (an antiemetic 74 and an anti-vertigo drug 74)

dimercaprol an antidote for heavy metal poisoning

Dimetapp Cold Liquid a product name combination product with phenylephrine (a decongestant 79) and brompheniramine (an antihistamine 110)

Dimetapp-C Syrup a product name combination product with phenylephrine (a decongestant 79) and codeine 242 (a cough suppressant 80)

Dimetapp Daytime Cold a combination product with pseudoephedrine 404 (a decongestant 79) and acetaminophen 177 (an analgesic 64)

Dimetapp Oral Infant Cold Drops a product name combination product with phenylephrine (a decongestant 79) and brompheniramine (an antihistamine 110)

Dimetane Expectorant -DC a product name for hydrocodone 307 (an opioid used in cough preparations 94)

dimethyl sulfoxide a drug to treat bladder inflammation

dinoprost a prostaglandin used to terminate pregnancy 167

dinoprostone a prostaglandin used to terminate pregnancy 167

Diophenyl-T a combination of tropicamide (an *anticholinergic* mydriatic 158) and phenylephrine

Diovan a product name for valsartan 459 (a vasodilator 84 and antihypertensive 88)

Diovan-HCT a product name for a combination of valsartan 459 (a vasodilator 84 and antihypertensive 88) with hydrochlorothiazide 306 (a diuretic 85)

Diovol a combination product with aluminum hydroxide 184 and magnesium hydroxide 338 (both antacids 94)

Diovol Plus a combination product with aluminum hydroxide 184 (an antacid 94), magnesium hydroxide 338 (an antacid 94), and simethicone (an antiflatulent 98)

Dipentum a product name for olsalazine (a drug for ulcerative colitis 98)

diphenhydramine 259 (an antihistamine 110, anti-emetic 74, and antipruritic 161)

diphenoxylate 260 an opioid antidiarrheal 96

diphenylpyraline an antihistamine 110

Diprolene Glycol a product name for betamethasone 206 (a corticosteroid 127)

Diprosalic a product-name skin preparation containing betamethasone 206 (a corticosteroid 127) and salicylic acid (a keratolytic 165)

Diprosone a product name for betamethasone 206 (a corticosteroid 127)

dipyridamole 261 (an antiplatelet drug 89)

disopyramide an anti-arrhythmic 86

dithranol a drug for psoriasis 166

Ditropan a product name for oxybutynin 381 (an *anticholinergic* and *anti-spasmodic* for urinary disorders 154)

Ditropan XL a product name for oxybutynin 381 (an *anticholinergic* and *antispasmodic* for urinary disorders 154)

divalproex an anticonvulsant 70

Dixarit a product name for clonidine (an antihypertensive 88)

Doak Oil a product name for coal tar (a substance for psoriasis 166 and eczema 167)

docetaxel an anticancer drug 140)

docusate sodium 262 (a stool softener, laxatives 97)

dolasetron an antiemetic 74

Dom-Indapamide a generic company version of indapamide 312 (a thiazide-like diuretic 85)

Dom Lindane a product name for lindane (also called gamma benzene hexachloride), a drug used for pediculosis and scabies 164

domperidone 263 (an anti-emetic 74)

donepezil 264 (a drug for Alzheimer's disease 71)

dopamine a drug for heart failure, kidney failure, and shock

dornase alfa a drug for cystic fibrosis 80

dorzolamide 265 (a carbonic anhydrase inhibitor for glaucoma 156)

Dostinex a product name for cabergoline (a drug to treat infertility 152 or to stop milk production in women who do not want to breast-feed, also used for Parkinson's disease 71)

Dovobet a product name for a combination of calcipotriol 215 (a drug for psoriasis 166) and betamethasone 206 (a corticosteroid 127)

Dovonex a product name for calcipotriol 215 (a drug for psoriasis 166)

doxazosin 266 (a sympatholytic antihypertensive 88)

doxepin a tricyclic antidepressant 68

doxorubicin 267 (a *cytotoxic* anticancer drug 140)

doxycycline 268 (a tetracycline *antibiotic* 114)

doxylamine succinate an antihistamine 110

Doxylar a product name for doxycycline 268 (a tetracycline *antibiotic* 114)

Drisdol a product name for ergocalciferol (a vitamin 135)

Dristan Long Lasting Nasal Mist/Spray a product name for oxy-metazoline (a *topical* decongestant 79)

Dristan N.D. a combination product containing pseudoephedrine 404 (a decongestant 79) and acetaminophen 177 (an analgesic 64)

Dristan Decongestant a product name combination product containing ibuprofen 310 (a non-steroidal anti-inflammatory 102), acetaminophen 177 (an analgesic 64) and pseudoephedrine 404 (a decongestant 79)

dronabinol an anti-emetic 74

drospirenone a synthetic progestin 133

Dulcolax a product name for bisacodyl 208 laxative 97)

Duofilm a product name for salicylic acid (a keratolytic for treating acne 165, dandruff 168, psoriasis 166, and warts)

Duovent a product name for fenoterol with ipratropium bromide 315 (both *bronchodilators* 76)

Duragesic a product name for fentanyl 283 (an opioid analgesic 64 used in the management of pain)

Duralith a product name for lithium 331 (a drug for mania 69)

Duricef a product name for cefadroxil (a cephalosporin *antibiotic* 114)

dutasteride a drug used in urinary disorders 154

E

Ebixa a product name for memantine 343 (a drug for dementia 71)

econazole an antifungal 124

Ecostatin a product name for econazole (an antifungal 124)

edrophonium a drug for diagnosis of myasthenia gravis 107

EES a product name for erythromycin 274 (an *antibiotic* 114)

efavirenz 269 (a drug for HIV and immune deficiency 144)

Effexor a product name for venlafaxine 461 (an antidepressant 68)

Effexor XR a product name for venlafaxine 461 (an antidepressant 68)

Efudex a product name for fluorouracil (an anticancer drug 140)

eletriptan a drug for migraine 73

Elocom a product name for mometasone 362 (a *topical* corticosteroid 162)

Eltor 120 a product name for pseudoephedrine 404 (a decongestant 79)

Eltroxin a product name for levothyroxine 329 (a thyroid hormone 130)

Emend a product name for aprepitant (an anti-emetic 74)

EMLA Cream a combination product with lidocaine and prilocaine (both local *anesthetics* 64)

EMLA Patch a combination product with lidocaine and prilocaine (both local *anesthetics* 64)

Emocort a product name for hydrocortisone 308 (a corticosteroid 127 and antipruritic 161)

emtricitabine an antiretroviral drug used in the treatment of HIV and AIDS 144

Emtriva a product name for emtricitabine (an antiretroviral drug used in the treatment of HIV and AIDS 144)

Enablex a product name for darifenacin 249 (a drug for urinary disorders 154)

enalapril 270 (a *vasodilator* 84 and antihypertensive 88)

Enbrel a product name for etanercept (a biological response modifier for rheumatoid arthritis 103)

Endantadine a product name for amantadine 185 (an antiviral 119 and drug used for *parkinsonism* 71)

Endocet a product name for oxycodone (an opioid analgesic 64)

enfuvirtide a drug for HIV/AIDS 144

Enlon a product name for edrophonium (a drug for diagnosis of myasthenia gravis 107)

enoxaparin 300 (an anticoagulant 91)

Entacapone a drug for *parkinsonism* 71

entecavir an antiviral drug 119

Entocort a product name for budesonide 211 (a corticosteroid 143)

Entrophen a product name for ASA 193 (a non-opioid analgesic 64 and antiplatelet drug 90)

ephedrine 271 (a *bronchodilator* 76 and decongestant 79)

Ephedrine Sulfate a product name for ephedrine 271 (a *bronchodilator* 76 and decongestant 79)

epinephrine 272 (a *bronchodilator* 76 and drug for glaucoma 156)

EpiPen a product name for epinephrine 272 (an anti-allergy drug 109)

epirubicin a *cytotoxic* anticancer drug 140

Epival a product name for valproic acid 458 (an anticonvulsant 70)

Epival ER a product name for divalproex (an anticonvulsant 70)

epoprostenol a prostaglandin used for its vasodilator effects 84

Eprex a product name for erythropoietin 275 (a kidney hormone 126 used for anemia due to kidney failure)

Ergamisol a product name for levamisole (an anthelmintic 125)

ergocalciferol vitamin D 481 (a vitamin 135)

ERGODRYL–GEN-TERBINAFINE

Ergodryl a product name for ergotamine 273 (a drug for migraine 73) with caffeine (a stimulant 72), and diphenhydramine 259 (an antihistamine 110 and antiemetic 74)

ergometrine another name for ergonovine (a uterine stimulant 153)

ergonovine a uterine stimulant 153

Ergonovine maleate a product name for ergonovine (a uterine stimulant 153)

ergotamine 273 (a drug for migraine 73)

ertapenem an *antibiotic* 114

Erybid a product name for erythromycin 274 (an *antibiotic* 114)

Eryc a product name for erythromycin 274 (an *antibiotic* 114)

Erythro Base a product name for erythromycin 274 (an *antibiotic* 114)

erythromycin 274 (an *antibiotic* 114)

erythropoietin 275 (a kidney hormone 126 used for anemia due to kidney failure). Also known as epoetin

escitalopram an antidepressant 68

esmolol a beta blocker 83

Estalis a product name for a combination product containing estradiol 276 (an estrogen 135)

Estalis-Sequi a product-name combination oral contraceptive 149 containing estradiol 276 and norethindrone 371

Estar a product name for coal tar (a substance for psoriasis 166 and eczema 167)

Estrace a product name for estradiol 276 (an estrogen 135)

Estracomb a product-name oral contraceptive 149 containing estradiol 276 and norethindrone 371

Estraderm a product name for estradiol 276 (an estrogen 133)

estradiol 276 (an estrogen 133)

Estring a product name for estradiol 276 (an estrogen 133)

Estrogel a product name for estradiol 276 (an estrogen 133)

estrone estropipate an estrogen 133

etanercept a biological response modifier for rheumatoid arthritis 103

ethambutol 277 (an antituberculous drug 118)

ethinyl estradiol 278 (a female sex hormone 133 and oral contraceptive 149**)**

ethopropazine a drug used for parkinsonism 71

ethosuximide an anticonvulsant 70

Ethynodiol diacetate an estrogen 151

Etibi a product name for ethambutol 277 (an antituberculous drug 118)

etidronate 279 (a drug for bone disorders 108)

etodolac a non-steroidal anti-inflammatory 102

etomidate a drug for induction of general anesthesia

Etonogestrel a progestin 151

etoposide a drug for cancers of the lung, lymphatic system, and testes 140

eucalyptus a cough medication 80

Euflex a product name for flutamide 289 (an anticancer drug 140)

Euglucon a product name for glyburide 301 (an oral antidiabetic drug 128)

Eumovate a product name for clobetasone (a *topical* corticosteroid 162)

Eurax a product name for crotamiton (an antipruritic 162)

Evista a product name for raloxifene 411 (a selective estrogen receptor modulator 133 for osteoporosis 108)

Evra a product name for a transdermal contraception containing norelgestromin and ethinyl estradiol 278 (female sex hormones 133)

Exdol-8 a combination product containing codeine 242 (an opioid analgesic 64) with acetaminophen 177 (an analgesic 64) and caffeine

Exdol-15 a combination product containing codeine 242 (an opioid analgesic 64) with acetaminophen 177 (an analgesic 64), and caffeine

Exdol-30 a combination product containing codeine 242 (an opioid analgesic 64) with acetaminophen 177 (an analgesic 64), and caffeine

Exelon a product name for rivastigmine 420 (a drug for Alzheimer's disease 71)

ezetimibe 280 (a cholesterol-lowering drug 89)

Ezetrol a product name for ezetimibe 280 (a cholesterol lowering drug 89)

F

5-ASA also called mesalamine 345 (a drug for inflammatory bowel disease 98)

famciclovir 281 (an antiviral 119)

famotidine 282 (an anti-ulcer drug 95)

Famvir a product name for famciclovir 281 (an antiviral 119)

felodipine a calcium channel blocker 87 and an antihypertensive 88

Femara a product name for letrozole (an anticancer drug 140)

FemHRT a product-name oral contraceptive 149 containing ethinyl estradiol 278 and norethindrone 371

fenofibrate a lipid-lowering drug 89

fenoprofen a non-steroidal anti-inflammatory 102

fenoterol a *sympathomimetic bronchodilator* 76

fentanyl 283 (an opioid analgesic 64 used in the management of pain)

Ferrlecit a product name for sodium ferric gluconate complex, an intravenous iron preparation 473 (a mineral 137)

ferrous fumarate iron 473 (a mineral 137)

ferrous gluconate iron 473 (a mineral 137)

ferrous sulfate iron 473 (a mineral 137)

fexofenadine an antihistamine 110

filgrastim 284 (a blood growth stimulant)

finasteride 285 (a drug for benign prostatic hypertrophy)

Fiorinal-C a combination product containing codeine 242 (an opioid analgesic 64) with ASA 193, bultalbital (a barbiturate sleeping drug p.66), and caffeine.

Flagyl a product name for metronidazole 355 (an antibacterial 117 and antiprotozoal 122)

Flagystatin a combination of metronidazole 355 (an antibacterial 117 and antiprotozoal 122) and nystatin 373 (an antifungal 124)

flavoxate a urinary *antispasmodic* 154

flecainide an anti-arrhythmic 86

Flexeril a product name for cyclobenzapine (a muscle relaxant 106)

Flolan a product name for epoprostenol (a prostaglandin used for its vasodilator effects 84)

Flomax a product name for tamsulosin 439 (an alpha-blocking drug for prostate disorders 134)

Flonase a product name for fluticasone 290 (a corticosteroid 127)

Florazole ER a product name for metronidazole 355 (an antibacterial 117 and antiprotozoal 122)

Florinef a product name for fludrocortisone (a corticosteroid 127)

Flovent Diskus a product name for fluticasone 290 (a corticosteroid 127)

Flovent HFA a product name for fluticasone 290 (a corticosteroid 127)

Fluanxol a product name for flupentixol 288 (an antipsychotic 69)

Fluanxol Depot a product name for flupentixol 288 (an antipsychotic 69)

fluconazole 286 (an antifungal 124)

flucytosine an antifungal 124

fludrocortisone a corticosteroid 127

flumazenil an antidote for benzodiazepine overdose

flumethasone a corticosteroid 127

flunarizine a calcium channel blocker used in the prevention of migraine 73

flunisolide a corticosteroid 127

fluocinolone a *topical* corticosteroid 162

fluocinonide a *topical* corticosteroid 162

Fluoderm a product name for fluocinolone (a *topical* corticosteroid 162)

fluoride 471 (a mineral 137)

fluorometholone a corticosteroid 127 for eye disorders

fluorouracil an anticancer drug 140

Fluotic a product name for fluoride 457 (a mineral 137)

fluoxetine 287 (an antidepressant 68)

flupentixol 288 (an antipsychotic 69 used in depression 68)

fluphenazine an phenothiazine antipsychotic 69

Fluphenazine Omega a product name for fluphenazine (an phenothiazine antipsychotic 69)

flurazepam a benzodiazepine sleeping drug 66

flurbiprofen a non-steroidal anti-inflammatory 102

flutamide 289 (an anticancer drug 140)

fluticasone 290 (a corticosteroid 127)
fluvastatin a lipid-lowering drug 89
fluvoxamine 291 (an antidepressant 68)
folic acid 472 (a vitamin 135)
folinic acid a vitamin 135
follitropin alpha a drug for infertility 152
follitropin beta a drug for treatment of infertility 152
fondaparinux an anticoagulant 91
Foradil a product name for formoterol 292 (a *bronchodilator* 76)
formoterol 292 (a *bronchodilator* 76)
Fortaz a product name for ceftazidime (a cephalosporin *antibiotic* 114)
Forteo a product name for teriparatide 445 (a drug for osteoporosis 108)
Fortovase a product name for saquinivir (a drug for HIV/AIDS 144)
Fosamax a product name for alendronate 179 (a drug for bone disorders 108)
Fosamprenavir a drug for HIV/AIDS 144
Fosavance a combination product with alendronate 179 (a drug for treatment of bone disorders 108) and vitamin D 481 (a vitamin 135)
fosfomycin tromethamine an *antibiotic* 114
fosinopril an ACE inhibitor 98
fosphenytoin 388 (an anticonvulsant 70)
Fragmin a product name for LMWH (low molecular weight heparin) 305 (an anticoagulant 91)
framycetin a *topical* aminoglycoside *antibiotic* 114 used for the treatment of ear, eye, and skin infections
Fraxiparine a product name for LMWH (low molecular weight heparin) 305 (an anticoagulant 91)
Frisium a product name for clobazam (a benzodiazepine drug used as a anticonvulsant 70)
Froben SR a product name for flurbiprofen (a non-steroidal anti-inflammatory drug 102)
FSH follicle-stimulating hormone (a natural hormone for infertility 166)
Fucidin a product name for fusidic acid (an *antibiotic* 114)
Fucidin H a product name for a combination drug with hydrocortisone 308 (a corticosteroid 127 and antipruritic 161) and other drugs
Fucithalmic a product name for fusidic acid (an *antibiotic* 114)
Fulvicin U/F a product name for griseofulvin (an antifungal 124)
Fungizone Intravenous a product name for amphotericin B 191 (an antifungal 126)
furosemide 293 (a loop diuretic 85)
fusidic acid an *antibiotic* 114
Fuzeon a product name for enfuvirtide (a drug for HIV/AIDS 144)

G

gabapentin 294 (an anticonvulsant 70)
galantamine 295 (a drug for Alzheimer's disease 71)

gamma benzene hexachloride also called lindane; used in the treatment of pediculosis and scabies 164
ganciclovir an antiviral 119
ganirelix a drug for treatment of infertility 152
Garamycin a product name for gentamicin 298 (an aminoglycoside *antibiotic* 114)
Gardasil a product name for human papilloma virus (HPV), used in prevention of cervical cancer 139
Gasulsol a product name combination product containing aluminum hydroxide 184 (an antacid 94) and magnesium trisilicate (an antacid 94)
gatifloxacin 296 (an antibacterial drug 117)
Gaviscon Heartburn Relief Formula a combination product with alginic acid 180 (used to protect stomach and esophagus from acid reflux) and magnesium carbonate (an antacid 94)
Gelusil a combination product with aluminum hydroxide 184 and magnesium hydroxide 338 (both antacids 94)
gemfibrozil 297 (a lipid-lowering drug 89)
G**Gen-Acyclovir** a generic company version of acyclovir 178 (an antiviral 119)
Gen-Alprazolam a generic company version of alprazolam 182 (a benzodiazepine anti-anxiety drug 67)
Gen-Amantadine a generic company version of amantadine 185 (an antiviral 119 and drug used for *parkinsonism* 71)
Gen-Amoxicillin a generic company version of amoxicillin 190 (a penicillin *antibiotic* 114)
Gen-Atenolol a generic company version of atenolol 195 (a beta blocker 83)
Gen-Azathioprine a generic company version of azathioprine 200 (an antirheumatic 103 and immunosuppressant 143)
Gen-Baclofen a generic company version of baclofen 202 (a muscle relaxant 106)
Gen-Buspirone a generic company version of buspirone 214 (an anti-anxiety drug 67)
Gen-Carbamazepine a generic company version of carbamazepine 217 (an anticonvulsant 70)
Gen-Cimetidine a generic company version of cimetidine 228 (an antiulcer drug 95)
Gen-Clindamycin a generic company version of clindamycin 233 (an antibiotic 114)
Gen-Clobetasol a generic company version of clobetasol 234 (a *topical* corticosteroid 162)
Gen-Clomipramine a generic company version of clomipramine 236 (a tricyclic antidepressant 68)
Gen-Clonazepam a generic company version of clonazepam 237 (a benzodiazepine anti-anxiety drug 67 and anticonvulsant 70)
Gen-Cyclobenzaprine a generic company version of cyclobenzaprine (a muscle relaxant 106)
Gen-Cyproterone a generic company version of cyproterone (a synthetic sex hormone used for acne 165, cancer of the prostate 140, and male sexual disorders 134)

Gen-Diltiazem a generic company version of diltiazem 257 (an antihypertensive 88 and calcium channel blocker 87)
Gen-Doxazosin a generic company version of doxazosin 266 (a sympatholytic antihypertensive 88)
Gen-Fenofibrate Micro a generic company version of fenofibrate (a lipid-lowering drug 89)
Gen-Fluoxetine a generic company version of fluoxetine 287 a tricyclic antidepressant 68)
Gen-Gemfibrozil a generic company version of gemfibrozil 297 (a lipid-lowering drug 89)
Gen-Gliclazide a generic company version of gliclazide 299 (an oral antidiabetic 128)
Gen-Indapamide a generic company version of indapamide 312 (a thiazide-like diuretic 85)
Gen-Ipratropium a product name for ipratropium bromide 315 (a *bronchodilator* 76)
Gen-Lovastatin a generic company version of lovastatin 337 (a lipid-lowering drug 89)
Gen-Medroxy a generic company version of medroxyprogesterone 339 (a female sex hormone 133)
Gen-metformin a generic company version of metformin 346 (a drug for diabetes 128)
Gen-Metoprolol a product name for metoprolol 354 (a beta blocker 83)
Gen-Minocycline a generic company version of minocycline 357 (a tetracycline *antibiotic* 114)
Gen-Mirtazapine a generic product name for mirtazapine 359 (an antidepressant 68)
Gen-Nabumetone a generic company version of nabumetone (a non-steroidal anti-inflammatory 102)
Gen-Nortriptyline a generic company version of ortriptyline (a tricyclic antidepressant 68)
Gen-Oxybutynin a generic company version of oxybutynin 381 (an *anticholinergic* and *antispasmodic* for urinary disorders 154)
Gen-Pioglitazone a generic company version of pioglitazone 390 (a drug for diabetes 128)
Gen-Piroxicam a product name for piroxicam 391 (a non-steroidal anti-inflammatory 102)
Gen-Salbutamol a generic company version of salbutamol 424 (a *bronchodilator* 76)
Gen-Selegiline a generic company version of selegiline 426 (a drug for *parkinsonism* 71)
Gen-Sertraline a generic company version of sertraline 427 (an antidepressant 68)
Gen-Sotalol a generic company version of sotalol 432 a beta blocker 83
gentamicin 298 (an aminoglycoside *antibiotic* 114)
Gen-Temazepam a product name for temazepam 440 (a benzodiazepine sleeping drug 66)
Gen-Terbinafine a generic company version of terbinafine 443 (an antifungal 124)

GENTLAX–LITHANE

Gentlax a product name for bisacodyl 208 (a laxative 97)

Gentlax.S a combination product name for bisacodyl 208 and docusate 262 (a laxative 97)

Gen-Trazodone a generic company version of trazodone (an antidepressant 68)

Gen-Triazolam a generic company version of temazepam 440 (a benzodiazepine sleeping drug 66)

Gen-Valproic a generic company version of valproic acid 458 (an anticonvulsant 70)

Gen-Verapamil a generic company version of verapimil 462 (an antihypertensive 88 and calcium channel blocker 87)

Gen-Zopiclone a product name for zopiclone 467 (a sleeping drug 66)

Gleevec a product name for imatinib (an anticancer drug 140)

gliclazide 299 (an oral antidiabetic 128)

glimepiride 300 (an oral antidiabetic 128)

glucagon a pancreatic hormone for hypoglycemia 126

Glucobay a product name for acarbose 176 (an oral antidiabetic 128)

GlucoNorm a product name for repaglinide 415 (a drug for diabetes 128)

Glucophage a product name for metformin 346 (a drug for diabetes 128)

glucosamine 472 a supplement

glyburide 301 (an oral antidiabetic drug 128)

gold sodium thiomalate a drug for rheumatoid arthritis 103

gonadorelin a drug for infertility 152

gonadotropin, human chorionic 302 (a drug for infertility 152)

Gonal-F a product name for follitropin alpha (a drug for infertility 152)

goserelin 303 (a female sex hormone 133 and anticancer drug 140, also used for menstrual disorders 148 and infertility 152)

gramicidin an aminoglycoside *antibiotic* 114 for eye, ear, and skin infections

granisetron an antiemetic 74

Gravol Preparations a product name for dimenhydrinate 258 (an antiemetic 74 and an anti-vertigo drug 74)

griseofulvin an antifungal 124

growth hormone somatropin (pituitary hormones 131)

guaifenesin an expectorant 80

Gynazole-I a product name for butaconzole (an antifungal 124)

H

halcinonide a *topical* corticosteroid 162

Halcion a product name for triazolam (a benzodiazepine sleeping drug 66)

halobetasol a *topical* corticosteroid 162

Halog a product name for halcinonide (a *topical* corticosteroid 162)

haloperidol 304 (an antipsychotic 69)

Haloperidol LA a product name for haloperidol 304 (an antipsychotic 69)

Haloperidol-LA Omega a product name for haloperidol 304 (an antipsychotic 69)

halothane a gas used to induce general anesthesia

Hepalean a product name for heparin 305 (an anticoagulant 91)

Hepalean-Lok a product name for heparin 305 (an anticoagulant 91)

heparin 305 (an anticoagulant 91)

Heparin Leo a product name for heparin 305 (an anticoagulant 91)

Hepsera a product name for adefovir (an antiviral 119)

Heptovir a product name for lamivudine 466 (an antiretroviral used for HIV/AIDS 144)

herceptin a product name for trastuzumab (an anticancer drug 140)

heroin diamorphine (an opioid 492)

Herplex-D a product name for idoxuridine (an antiviral 119)

hexachlorophene a skin antiseptic 163

Histanil a product name for promethazine 401 (an antihistamine 110 and anti-emetic 74)

homatropine a mydriatic 158

Hp-PAC a combination of clarithromycin 232 (a macrolide *antibiotic* 114), amoxicillin 190 (an *antibiotic* 114) and lansoprazole 324 (an antiulcer drug 95)

Humalog a product name for insulin lispro (a drug for diabetes 128)

Humatrope a product name for somatropin, a pituitary hormone 131 (a synthetic pituitary hormone 131)

Humira a product name for adalimumab (a biological response modifier for inflammatory bowel disease 98)

Humulin a product name for insulin lente (a drug for diabetes 128)

Humulin N a product name for insulin NPH (a drug for diabetes 128)

hyaluronidase helps injections penetrate tissues

Hycodan a product name for hydrocodone 307 (an opioid used in cough preparations 80)

Hycomine a product name combination product with phenylephrine (a decongestant 79), ammonium chloride (an expectorant 80), hydrocodone 307 (a cough suppressant 80), and pyrilamine maleate (an antihistamine 110)

Hycomine-S a product name combination product with phenylephrine (a decongestant 79), ammonium chloride (an expectorant 80), hydrocodone 307 (a cough suppressant 80), and pyrilamine maleate (an antihistamine 110)

Hycort a product name for hydrocortisone 308 (a corticosteroid 127 and anti-pruritic 161)

Hyderm a product name for hydrocortisone 308 (a corticosteroid 127 and antipruritic 161)

hydralazine an antihypertensive 88

hydrochlorothiazide 306 (a thiazide diuretic 85)

hydrocodone 307 (a cough suppressant 80)

hydrocortisone 308 (a corticosteroid 127 and antipruritic 161)

Hydromorph Contin a product name for hydromorphone 309 (an opioid analgesic 64 used in the management of pain)

hydromorphone 309 (an opioid analgesic 64 used in the management of pain)

Hydromorphone HP a product name for hydromorphone 309 (an opioid analgesic 64 used in the management of pain)

Hydromorphone HP Forte a product name for hydromorphone 309 (an opioid analgesic 64 used in the management of pain)

hydroxocobalamin vitamin B12 480 (a vitamin 135)

hydroxychloroquine an antimalarial 123 and antirheumatic drug 103

hydroxyzine an antihistamine used as an anti-anxiety drug 67

Hygroton a product name for chlortalidone (a thiazide diuretic 101)

Hypurin insulin a product name for insulin derived from pork 129

Hytrin a product name for terazosin 442 (a sympatholytic antihypertensive 88)

I

ibuprofen 310 (a non-opioid analgesic 64 and non-steroidal anti-inflammatory 102)

ibutulide an anti-arrhythmic 86

ichthammol a substance in skin preparations for eczema 167

idoxuridine an antiviral 119

imatinib an anticancer drug 140

Imdur a product name for isosorbide mononitrate 318 (a nitrate *vasodilator* 84 and anti-angina drug 87)

imipenem-cilastin an *antibiotic* 114

imipramine 311 (a tricyclic antidepressant 68)

Imitrex a product name for sumatriptan 437 (a drug for migraine 73)

Imodium a product name for loperamide 332 (an antidiarrheal 96)

Imovane a product name for zopiclone 467 (a sleeping drug 66)

Imuran a product name for azathioprine 200 (an antirheumatic 103 and immunosuppressant 143)

indapamide 312 (a thiazide-like diuretic 85)

Inderal-LA a product name for propranolol 402 (a beta blocker 83)

indinavir a drug for HIV/AIDS 144

Indocid P.D.A. a product name for indomethacin (a non-steroidal anti-inflammatory 102)

indomethacin a non-steroidal anti-inflammatory 102

infliximab a biological response modifier for rheumatoid arthritis 103 and Crohn's disease 98

Innohep a product name for LMWH 305 (an anticoagulant 91)

inosiplex an antiviral 119

insulin 313 (a drug for diabetes 128)

insulin aspart a drug for diabetes 128

insulin detemir a drug for diabetes 128

insulin glargine a drug for diabetes 128

insulin NPH a drug for diabetes 128

insulin ultralente a drug for diabetes 128

Intal a product name for sodium cromoglycate 431 (an anti-allergy drug 109 used to prevent asthma attacks 77)

interferon 314 (an antiviral 119 and anticancer drug 140)

Interferon alfa-2b an antiviral 119 and anticancer drug 140

Interferon beta-1a a drug used in multiple sclerosis

Interferon beta-1b a drug used in multiple sclerosis

Intron-A a product name for interferon alfa-2b (an antiviral 119 and anticancer drug 140)

Invirase a product name for saquinavir (a drug for HIV/AIDS 144)

iodine 473 (a mineral 137)

iopidine a product name for apraclonidine (a drug for glaucoma 156)

ipecac a drug used to induce vomiting in drug overdose and poisoning, also used as an expectorant 80

ipratropium bromide 315 (a *bronchodilator* 76)

irbesartan 316 (a *vasodilator* 84 and antihypertensive drug 88)

irinotecan an anticancer drug 140

iron 473 (a mineral 137)

Isentress a product name for raltegravir (an antiretroviral drug used in the treatment of HIV and AIDS 144)

isoflurane a volatile liquid inhaled as a general *anesthetic*

isoniazid 317 (an antituberculous drug 134)

isoproterenol a *sympathomimetic*

Isoproterenol Hydrochloride a product name for isoproterenol (a *sympathomimetic*)

Isoptin a product name for verapimil 462 (an antihypertensive 88 and calcium channel blocker 87)

Isopto Atropine a product name for atropine 198 (an *anticholinergic* mydriatic 158)

Isopto Carbachol a product name for carbachol eye drops (a miotic for glaucoma 156)

Isopto Carpine a product name for pilocarpine 389 (a miotic for glaucoma 156)

Isopto Homatropine a product name for homatropine (a mydriatic 158)

isosorbide dinitrate 318 (a nitrate *vasodilator* 84 and anti-angina drug 87)

isosorbide mononitrate 318 (a nitrate *vasodilator* 84 and anti-angina drug 87)

Isotamine a product name for isoniazid 317 (an antituberculous drug 134)

isotretinoin 319 (a drug for acne 165)

itraconazole an antifungal 124

JK

Januvia a product name for sitagliptin (a drug for diabetes 128)

Kadian a product name for morphine 364 (an opioid analgesic 64)

Kaletra a product name for lopinavir/ritonavir 333 (a drug for HIV and immune deficiency 144)

Kaolin see attapulgite

Kaopectate a product name for attapulgite 199 (an adsorbent used as an anti-diarrheal 96)

Kefzol a product name for cefazolin (a cephalosporin *antibiotic* 114)

Kenalog a product name for triamcinolone (a corticosteroid 127)

Keppra a product name for levetiracetam (an anticonvulsant 70)

ketamine a drug used to induce general anesthesia, also a drug of abuse 489

Ketek a product name for telithromycin (an antibiotic 114)

ketoconazole 320 (an antifungal 124)

Ketoderm a product name for ketoconazole 320 (an antifungal 124)

ketoprofen 321 (a non-steroidal anti-inflammatory 102)

ketorolac a non-steroidal anti-inflammatory 102

ketotifen a drug used in asthma 77

Kineret a product name for anakinra 192 (an immunomodulatory drug for rheumatoid arthritis 103)

K-Lyte a product name for potassium citrate (a drug used in the treatment of low potassium)

Koffex DM a product name for dextromorphan 252 (a cough suppressant 80)

Kwellada-P a product name for permethrin 386 (a *topical* antiparasitic 164)

Kytril a product name for granisetron (an antiemetic 74)

L

lactic acid an ingredient in preparations for warts, emollients, and vaginal suppositories

lactulose 322 (an osmotic laxative 113)

Lamictal a product name for lamotrigine 323 (an anticonvulsant 70)

Lamisil a product name for terbinafine 443 (an antifungal 124)

lamivudine 466 (an antiretroviral drug used for HIV/AIDS 144)

lamotrigine 323 (an anticonvulsant 70)

Lanoxin a product name for digoxin 256 (a digitalis drug 82)

lansoprazole 324 (an anti-ulcer drug 95)

Lariam a product name for mefloquine 340 (an antimalarial 123)

Lasix a product name for furosemide 293 (a loop diuretic 85)

latanoprost 325 (a drug for glaucoma 156)

Leflunomide an antirheumatic drug 103

Lescol a product name for fluvastatin (a lipid-lowering drug 89)

letrozole an anticancer drug 140

Leukeran a product name for chlorambucil (an anticancer drug 140 used for chronic lymphocytic leukemia and lymphomas)

Levaquin a product name for levofloxacin 327 (an antibacterial 117)

Levetiracetam an anticonvulsant 70

Levitra a product name for vardenafil (a drug used for the treatment of sexual impotence 152)

levobunolol a beta blocker 83 and drug for glaucoma 156

levocabastine a *topical* antihistamine 110

levodopa 326 (a drug for *parkinsonism* 71)

levodopa/benserazide a combination of levodopa 326 and benserazide for *parkinsonism* 71

levodopa/carbidopa 326 (a combination of levodopa 326 and carbidopa for *parkinsonism* 71)

levofloxacin 327 (an antibacterial 117)

levonorgestrel 328 (a female sex hormone 133 and oral contraceptive 149)

levothyroxine previously known as thyroxine 329 (a thyroid hormone 130)

Levsin a product name for hyoscine (an *antispasmodic* drug 96)

Librax a product name for a combination product of chlordiazepoxide 223 (a benzodiazepine anti-anxiety drug 67) with an *anticholinergic*

Lidemol a product name for fluocinonide (a *topical* corticosteroid 162)

Lidex a product name for fluocinonide (a *topical* corticosteroid 162)

lldocalne a local *anesthetic* 64 and anti-arrhythmic 86

Lidocaine Parenteral a product name for lidocaine (a local *anesthetic* 64 and anti-arrhythmic 86)

Lidodan Endotracheal a product name for lidocaine (a local *anesthetic* 64 and anti-arrhythmic 86)

Lin-Buspirone a generic company version of buspirone 214 (an anti-anxiety drug 67)

lindane also called gamma benzene hexachloride; used in the treatment of pediculosis and scabies 164

linezolid an *antibiotic* 114

Lipidil EZ a product name for fenofibrate (a lipid-lowering drug 89)

Lipidil-Micro a product name for fenofibrate (a lipid-lowering drug 89)

Lipidil Supra a product name for fenofibrate (a lipid-lowering drug 89)

Lipitor a product name for atorvastatin 197 (a lipid-lowering drug 89)

Lioresal a product name for baclofen 202 (a muscle relaxant 106)

liothyronine a thyroid hormone 130

liquid paraffin a lubricating agent used as a laxative and in artificial tear preparations

lisinopril 330 (an ACE inhibitor 84)

Lithane a product name for lithium 331 (a drug for mania 69)

LITHIUM–NARCAN

lithium 331 (a drug for mania 69)

Livostin a product name for levocabastine (an antihistamine 110)

LMWH 305 (an anticoagulant 91)

Locacorten Vioform a combination of clioquinol (an antibacterial 117 and antifungal 124) and flumethasone (a corticosteroid 127)

Iodoxamide an anti-allergy drug 109

Loestrin a product-name oral contraceptive 149 containing ethinyl estradiol 278 and norethindrone 371

Lomine a product name for dicyclomine 255 (a drug for irritable bowel syndrome 98)

Lomotil a product name for diphenoxylate 260 (an opioid antidiarrheal 96) and atropine 198

Loniten a product name for minoxidil 358 (an antihypertensive 88)

loperamide 332 (an antidiarrheal 96)

Lopid a product name for gemfibrozil 297 (a lipid-lowering drug 89)

lopinavir/ritonavir 333 (a drug for HIV/AIDS 144)

Lopresor a product name for metoprolol 354 (a cardioselective beta blocker 83)

loratadine 334 (an antihistamine 110)

lorazepam 335 (a benzodiazepine anti-anxiety drug 67 and sleeping drug 66)

losartan 336 (an antihypertensive 88)

Losec a product name for omeprazole 375 (an antiulcer drug 95)

Lotriderm a product-name product containing betamethasone 206 (a corticosteroid 127) and clotrimazole 239 (an antifungal 124)

lovastatin 337 (a lipid-lowering drug 89)

Lovenox a product name for LMWH 305 (an anticoagulant 91)

Lovenox HP a product name for LMWH 305 (an anticoagulant 91)

Low molecular weight heparin see LMWH

Loxapac a product name for loxapine (an antipsychotic 69)

loxapine an antipsychotic 69

Lozide a product name for indapamide 312 a thiazide-like diuretic 85

Lugol's solution an iodine 473 solution for overactive thyroid gland

Lumigan a product name for bimatoprost (a drug for glaucoma 156)

lutein 474 a natural supplement

Lutrepulse a product name for gonadorelin (a drug for infertility 152)

Luvox a product name for fluvoxamine 291 (an antidepressant 68)

Lyderm a product name for fluocinonide (a *topical* corticosteroid 162)

Lyrica a product name for pregabalin 396 (an anticonvulsant 70)

M

Maalox a combination product with aluminum hydroxide 184 and magnesium hydroxide 338 (both antacids 94)

Maalox Antacid with Anti-Gas a combination product with aluminum hydroxide 184 (an antacid 94), magnesium hydroxide 338 (an antacid 94), and simethicone (an antiflatulent 98)

Maalox Antacid with Anti-Gas Extra Strength a combination product with aluminum hydroxide 184 (an antacid 94), magnesium hydroxide 338 (an antacid 94), and simethicone (an antiflatulent 98)

Maalox Quick Dissolve a product name for calcium carbonate (a calcium salt and a mineral 137 used as an antacid 94)

Maalox TC a combination product with aluminum hydroxide 184 and magnesium hydroxide 338 (both antacids 94)

magnesium 474 (a mineral 137)

magnesium carbonate an antacid 94

magnesium citrate an osmotic laxative 97

magnesium hydroxide 338 (an antacid 94 and laxative 97)

magnesium oxide an antacid 94

magnesium sulfate an osmotic laxative 97

magnesium trisilicate an antacid 94

Malarone a combination of proguanil and atovaquone 400 (both antimalarials 123)

Manerix a product name for moclobemide 361 (a reversible MAOI antidepressant 68)

mannitol an osmotic diuretic 85

maprotiline an antidepressant 68

Maraviroc an antiretroviral drug used in the treatment of HIV and AIDS 144

Marcaine a product name for bupivacaine local *anesthetic* 64 used in labour 153)

Marinol a product name for dronabinol (an anti-emetic 74)

Marvelon a product-name oral contraceptive 149 containing ethinyl estradiol 278 and desogestrel (a progestin 135)

Maxidex a product name for dexamethasone 251 (a corticosteroid 127)

Maxitrol a product name for dexamethasone 251 (a corticosteroid 127) with neomycin and polymyxin B (both *antibiotics* 114)

Maxalt a product name for rizatriptan 421 (a drug for migraine 73)

Maxalt RPD a product name for rizatriptan 421 (a drug for migraine 73)

mebendazole an anthelmintic 125

meclizine an antihistamine used as an anti-emetic drug 74

Medrol a product name for methylprednisolone 352 (a corticosteroid 127)

medroxyprogesterone 339 (a female sex hormone 133 and anticancer drug 140)

mefloquine 340 (an antimalarial 123)

Mefoxin a product name for cefoxitin (a cephalosporin *antibiotic* 114)

Megace a product name for megestrol 341 (a female sex hormone 133 and anticancer drug 140)

Megace OS a product name for megestrol 341 (a female sex hor-mone 135 and anticancer drug 140)

megestrol 341 (a female sex hormone 133 and anticancer drug 140)

meloxicam 342 (a non-steroidal anti-inflammatory 102)

melphalan an alkylating agent for multiple myeloma 140

memantine 343 a drug for dementia 71

menadiol vitamin K 482 (a vitamin 135)

menotropins a drug for infertility 152

menthol an alcohol from mint oils used as an inhalation and *topical* anti-pruritic 161

menthyl anthranilate an ingredient of sunscreens 169

mepacrine an antiprotozoal 122 for giardiasis

meperidine an opioid analgesic 64 and drug used in labour 153

mepivacaine a local anesthetic 64

Mepron a product name for atovaquone (an antimalarial 123)

mercaptopurine 344 (an anticancer drug 140)

Meridia a product name for sibutramine 428 (an appetite suppressant and nervous system stimulant 72)

meropenem an *antibiotic* 114

Mersyndol with Codeine a combination product with doxylamine (a drug used to aid sleep 66), acetaminophen 177 (an analgesic 64), and codeine 242 (an opioid analgesic 64)

mesalamine/5-ASA 345 see 5-ASA

Mesasal a product name for 5-ASA 345 (a drug for inflammatory bowel disease 98)

M-Eslon a product name for morphine 364 (an opioid analgesic 64)

Mestinon a product name for pyridostigmine 406 (a drug for myasthenia gravis 107)

Mestinon-SR a product name for pyridostigmine 406 (a drug for myasthenia gravis 107)

Metadol a product name for methadone 347 (an opioid used in the maintenance treatment of opioid-dependent individuals and as an analgesic 64 in acute and chronic pain)

Metamucil a fiber laxative containing psyllium 405 (laxative 97)

metformin 346 (a drug for diabetes 128)

methadone 347 (an opioid used in the maintenance treatment of opioid-dependent individuals and as an analgesic 64 in acute and chronic pain)

methazolamide a drug used in glaucoma 156

methenamine a drug for urinary tract infections 154

methimazole an antithyroid drug 130

methocarbamol a muscle relaxant 106

methotrexate 348 (an antimetabolite anticancer drug 140)

methotrimeprazine a phenothiazine antipsychotic 69

Methoxacet-C a combination product containing codeine 242 (an opioid analgesic 64) with acetaminophen 177 (an analgesic p.64) and a muscle relaxant 106

Methoxisal a combination product with ASA 194 (a non-opioid analgesic 64) and methocarbamol (a muscle relaxant 106)

methoxsalen a drug used in the treatment of psoriasis (166) and atopic dermatitis

Methsuximide an anticonvulsant 70

methylcellulose 349 (a laxative 97, and artificial tear preparation 158)

methyldopa 350 (an antihypertensive 88)

methylphenidate 351 (a drug used to treat hyperactivity in children 72)

methylprednisolone 352 (a corticosteroid 127)

methyl salicylate a topical analgesic 64 for muscle and joint pain

methysergide a drug to prevent migraine 73

metoclopramide 353 (a gastrointestinal motility regulator and anti-emetic 74)

Metoclopramide Omega a product name for metoclopramide 353 (a gastrointestinal motility regulator and anti-emetic 74)

metolazone a thiazide-like diuretic 85

metoprolol 354 (a beta blocker 83)

Metreton a combination of prednisone 395 (a corticosteroid 127), chlorpheniramine 225 (an antihistamine 110), and vitamin C 480 (a vitamin 135)

MetroCream a product name for metronidazole 355 (an antibacterial 117 and antiprotozoal 122)

MetroGel a product name for *topical* metronidazole 355 (an antibacterial 117)

metronidazole 355 (an antibacterial 117 and antiprotozoal 122)

Mevacor a product name for lovastatin 337 (a lipid-lowering drug 89)

mexiletine an anti-arrhythmic 86

mexoryl SX an ingredient of sunscreens 169

Miacalcin NS a product name for calcitonin (a drug for bone disorders 108)

micafungin an antifungal 124

Micardis a product name for telmisartan (a vasodilator 84 and antihypertensive 88)

Micatin a product name for miconazole 356 (an antifungal 124)

miconazole 356 (an antifungal 124)

Micozole a product name for miconazole 356 (an antifungal 124)

Micronor a product-name oral contraceptive 149 containing norethindrone 371

Midamor a product name for amiloride 186 (a potassium sparing diuretic 85)

Midol Regular a combination product with ASA 194 (a non-opioid analgesic 64) and caffeine

Migranal a product name for dihydroergotamine (a drug for migraine 73)

mineral oil a lubricant laxative 97

Minestrin a product-name oral contraceptive 149 containing ethinyl estradiol 278 and norethindrone 371

Minims Atropine a product name for atropine 198 (an *anticholinergic* mydriatic 158)

Minims Cyclopentolate a product name for cyclopentolate (an *anticholinergic* mydriatic 158)

Minims Phenylephrine a product name for phenylephrine (a decongestant eye drop 79)

Minims Tetracaine a product name for tetracaine (also known as amethocain, a local anesthetic 64)

Minims Tropicamide a product name for tropicamide (a mydriatic 158)

Minipress a product name for prazosin (a sympatholytic antihypertensive 88)

Minitram a product name for nitroglycerin 370 (an anti-angina drug 87)

Minocin a product name for minocycline 357 (a tetracycline *antibiotic* 114)

minocycline 357 (a tetracycline *antibiotic* 114)

Min-Ovral a product name for levonorgestrel 328 (a female sex hormone 133 and oral contraceptive 149) and ethinyl estradiol 278 (an estrogen 135)

minoxidil 358 (an antihypertensive drug 88 and treatment for hair loss 168)

Mintezol a product name for tiabendazole (an anthelmintic 125)

Miostat a product name for carbachol (a miotic drug used in glaucoma 156 and a para*sympathomimetic*)

Mirapex a product name for pramipexole 393 (a drug for *parkinsonism* 71)

Mirena a product name for levonorgestrel 328 (a female sex hormone 133 and oral contraceptive 149)

mirtazapine 359 (an antidepressant 68)

misoprostol 360 (an antiulcer drug 95)

Mobicox a product name for meloxicam 342 (a non-steroidal anti-inflammatory 102)

moclobemide 361 a reversible MAOI antidepressant 68

modafinil a drug used in treatment of narcolepsy

Modecate a product name for fluphenazine (a phenothiazine antipsychotic 69)

Mogadon a product name for nitrazepam 369 (a benzodiazepine sleeping drug 80)

molybdenum a mineral 137 required in minute amounts in the diet, poisonous if ingested in large quantities

mometasone 362 (a *topical* corticosteroid 162)

Monistat a product name for miconazole 356 (an antifungal 124)

montelukast 363 (a leukotriene antagonist for asthma 77)

Monurol a product name for fosfomycin tromethamine (an *antibiotic* 114)

morphine 364 (an opioid analgesic 64)

Morphine Sulfate a product name for morphine 364 (an opioid analgesic 64)

M.O.S. a product name for morphine 364 (an opioid analgesic 64)

Motrin a product name for ibuprofen 310 (a non-steroidal anti-inflammatory 102)

moxifloxacin 365 (an antibacterial 117)

MS Contin a product name for morphine 364 (an opioid analgesic 64)

MSD Enteric Coated ASA a product name for ASA 194 (a non-opioid analgesic 64 and antiplatelet drug 90)

MS-IR a product name for morphine 364 (an opioid analgesic 64)

Mucaine a product name for aluminum hydroxide 184 (an antacid 94)

mupirocin an antibacterial for skin infections 163

MUSE a product name for alprostadil 183 (a prostaglandin used for male impotence 134, 152)

Mycamine a product name for micafungin (an antifungal 124)

Mycobutin a product name for rifabutin (an antituberculosis drug 118)

mycophenolate mofetil an immunosuppressant 143

Mycostatin a product name for nystatin 373 (an antifungal 124)

Mydfrin a product name for phenylephrine (used as a mydriatic 158)

Mydriacil a product name for tropicamide (a mydriatic 158)

Mylanta Double Strength Plain a combination product with aluminum hydroxide 184 (an antacid 94) and magnesium hydroxide 338 (an antacid 94)

Mylanta Extra Strength a combination product with aluminum hydroxide 184 (an antacid 94), magnesium hydroxide 338 (an antacid 94), and simethicone (an antiflatulent 98)

Myocet a product name for doxorubicin 267 (a *cytotoxic* anticancer drug 140)

Myochrysine a product name for gold sodium thiomalate (an antirheumatic 117)

Myotonachol a product name for bethanechol (a parasympathomimetic for urinary retention 154)

Mysoline a product name for primidone (an anticonvulsant 70)

N

nabilone an anti-emetic 74

nabumetone a non-steroidal anti-inflammatory 102

nadolol a beta blocker 97

nadroparin 305 (an anticoagulant 91)

nafarelin a drug for menstrual disorders 148

nalbuphine an opioid analgesic 64

Nalcrom a product name for sodium cromoglycate 431 (an anti-allergy drug 109)

Nalfon a product name for fenoprofen (a non-steroidal anti-inflammatory 102)

naloxone an antidote for opioid 507 poisoning

naltrexone a drug used in formally opioid dependent individuals; also used in alcohol dependence

nandrolone an anabolic steroid 134

Naprosyn a product name for naproxen 366 (a non-steroidal anti-inflammatory 102)

naproxen 366 (a non-steroidal anti-inflammatory 102)

naratriptan a drug for migraine 73

Narcan a product name for naloxone (an antidote for opioid 490 poisoning)

NARDIL–NU-CLONAZEPAM

Nardil a product name for phenelzine (an MAOI antidepressant 68)

Nasacort AQ a product name for triamcinolone (a corticosteroid 127)

Nasonex a product name for mometasone 362 (a *topical* corticosteroid 162)

nateglinide a drug for diabetes 128

Navane a product name for thiothixene (an antipsychotic 69)

Nebcin a product name for tobramycin (an aminoglycoside *antibiotic* 114)

nedocromil a drug used to prevent asthma attacks 77

nelfinavir an antiretroviral drug for HIV/AIDS 144

Neo-Laryngobis a product name for bismuth (a metal given in compound form to treat gastric and duodenal ulcers 95 that is also used for sore throats)

Neo-Medrol Acne Lotion a combination product with methylprednisolone 352 (a corticosteroid 127), neomycin (an *antibiotic* 114), aluminum chlorhydroxide, and sulfur

neomycin an aminoglycoside *antibiotic* 114 used in ear drops 175

Neoral a product name for cyclosporine 247 (an immunosuppressant 143)

neostigmine a drug for myasthenia gravis 107

NeoStrata Canada Blemish Spot Gel a product name for salicylic acid (a keratolytic for acne 165, dandruff 168, psoriasis 166, and warts)

Neo-Synephrine Parenteral a product name for phenylephrine (used as a vasoconstrictor)

Nerisalik a combination of diflucortolone (a *topical* corticosteroid 162) with alicyclic acid

Nerisone a product name for diflucortolone (a *topical* corticosteroid 162)

Neulasta a product name for pegfilgrastim (a blood stimulant)

Neuleptil a product name for pericyazine (an antipsychotic 69)

Neupogen a product name for filgrastim 284 (a blood growth stimulant)

Neurontin a product name for gabapentin 294 (an anticonvulsant 70)

nevirapine an antiretroviral drug for HIV/AIDS 144

niacin 475 (a vitamin 135)

niacinamide another name for niacin 475 (a vitamin 135)

Nicoderm a product name for nicotine 367 (used in smoking cessation)

Nicorette a product name for nicotine 367 (used in smoking cessation)

nicotinamide a B vitamin 475 (a vitamin 135)

nicotine 367

nicotinic acid see niacin; *a* lipid-lowering drug 103 and vitamin 135

nicotinyl alcohol tartrate niacin 475 (a vitamin 135)

NidaGel a product name for metronidazole 355 (an antibacterial 117 and antiprotozoal 122)

Nidazol a product name for metronidazole 355 (an antibacterial 117 and antiprotozoal 122)

nifedipine 368 (a calcium channel blocker 87)

nitrazepam 369 (a benzodiazepine sleeping drug 66 and anticonvulsant 70)

Nitrazodon a product name for nitrazepam 369 (a benzodiazepine sleeping drug 66)

Nitro-Dur a product name for nitroglycerin 370 (an anti-angina drug 87)

nitrofurantoin an antibacterial 117

nitroglycerin 370 (an anti-angina drug 87)

Nitrol a product name for nitroglycerin 370 (an anti-angina drug 87)

Nitrolingual Pumpspray a product name for nitroglycerin 370 (an anti-angina drug 87)

Nitrostat a product name for nitroglycerin 370 (an anti-angina drug 87)

nitrous oxide *anesthetic* gas

Nix a product name for permethrin 386 (a *topical* antiparasitic 164)

nizatidine an antiulcer drug 95

Nizoral a product name for ketoconazole 320 (an antifungal 124)

nonacog alfa a synthetic form of factor IX to promote blood clotting

nonoxynol '9' a spermicidal agent

noradrenaline see norepinephrine

Norelgestromin a progestin 151

norepinephrine a drug similar to epinephrine 272 used to raise the blood pressure during shock

norethindrone 371 (a female sex hormone 133 and oral contraceptive 149)

Norflex a product name for orphenadrine 378 (an *anticholinergic* muscle relaxant 106)

norfloxacin 372 (an antibacterial 117)

Norgesic Forte a product name for a combination product containing orphenadrine 378 (a muscle relaxant 106), ASA 194 (a non-opioid analgesic 64) and caffeine

norgestimate a progestin (133) used as an oral contraceptive 149

norgestrel a progestin 135

Noritate a product name for metronidazole 355 (an antibacterial 117 and antiprotozoal 122

Norpramin a product name for desipramine (a tricyclic antidepressant 68)

nortriptyline a tricyclic antidepressant 68

Norvasc a product name for amlodipine 189 (an anti-hypertensive 88 and calcium channel blocker 87)

Novahistex DH a combination product with phenylephrine (a decongestant 79) and hydrocodone 307 (a cough suppressant 80)

Novahistine DH a combination product with phenylephrine (a decongestant 79) and hydrocodone 307 (a cough suppressant 80)

Novamoxin a product name for amoxicillin 190 (an *antibiotic* 114)

Novasen a product name for ASA 194 (a non-opioid analgesic 64 and antiplatelet drug 90)

Novo-Alprazol a generic company version of alprazolam 182 (a benzodiazepine anti-anxiety drug 67)

Novo-Amiodarone a generic company version of amiodarone 187 (an antiarrhythmic 88)

Novo-Atenol a generic company version of atenolol 195 (a beta blocker 83)

Novo-Azathioprine a generic company version of azathioprine 200

Novo-Buspirone a generic company version of buspirone 214 (an anti-anxiety drug 67)

Novo-Carbamaz a generic company version of carbamazepine 217 (an anticonvulsant 70)

Novo-Cefaclor a generic company version of cefaclor (a cephalosporin *antibiotic* 114)

Novo-Chloroquine a generic company version of chloroquine 224 (an antimalarial 123 and antirheumatic 103)

Novo-Chlorpromazine a generic company version of chlorpromazine 226 (a phenothiazine antipsychotic 69 and anti-emetic 74)

Novo-Cholamine a generic company version of cholestyramine 227 (a lipid-lowering drug 89)

Novo-Clindamycin a generic company version of clindamycin 233 (an antibiotic 114)

Novo-Clobetasol a generic company version of clobetasol 234 (a *topical* corticosteroid 162)

Novo-Clobazam a product name for clobazam (a benzodiazepine drug used as a anticonvulsant 70)

Novo-Clonazepam a generic company version of clonazepam 237 (a benzodiazepine anticonvulsant 70)

Novo-Clonidine a generic company version of clonidine (an antihypertensive 88)

Novo-Clopamine a generic company version of clomipramine 236 (a tricyclic antidepressant 68)

Novo-Clopate a generic company version of clorazepate (a benzodiazepine anti-anxiety drug 67)

Novo-Cloxin a generic company version of cloxacillin 240 (a penicillin *antibiotic* 114)

Novo-Cycloprine a generic company version of cyclobenzaprine (a muscle relaxant 106)

Novo-Cyproterine a product name for cyproterone (a synthetic sex hormone used for acne 165, cancer of the prostate 140, and male sexual disorders 132)

Novo-Desipramine a generic company version of desipramine (a tricyclic antidepressant 68)

Novo-Difenac a generic company version of diclonefac 250 (a non-steroidal anti-inflammatory 102)

Novo-Diflunisal a generic company version of diflunisal (a non-steroidal anti-inflammatory 102)

Novo-Diltiazem a generic company version of diltiazem 257 (an antihypertensive 88 and calcium channel blocker 87)

Novo-Divalproex a generic company version of divalproex (an anticonvulsant 70)

Novo-Domperidone a generic company version of domperidone 263 (an anti-emetic 74)

Novo-Doxazosin a generic company version of doxazosin 266 (a sympatholytic antihypertensive 88)

Novo-Doxepin a generic company version of doxepin (a tricyclic antidepressant 68)

Novo-Doxylin a generic company version of doxycycline 268 (a tetracycline *antibiotic* 114)

Novo-Fluoxetine a generic company version of fluoxetine 287 (a tricyclic antidepressant 68)

Novo-Flutamide a generic company version of flutamide 289 (an anticancer drug 140)

Novo-Fluprofen a generic company version of flurbiprofen (a non-steroidal anti-inflammatory 102)

Novo-Fluvoxamine a generic company version of fluvoxamine 291 (an antidepressant 68)

Novo-Gabapentin a generic company version of gabapentin 294 (an anticonvulsant 70)

Novo-Gemfibrozil a generic company version of gemfibrozil 297 (a lipid-lowering drug 89)

Novo-Gesic C8 a combination product containing codeine 242 (an opioid analgesic 64) with acetaminophen 177 (an analgesic 64), and caffeine.

Novo-Gesic C-15 a combination product containing codeine 242 (an opioid analgesic 64) with acetaminophen 177 (an analgesic 64), and caffeine.

Novo-Gliclazide a product name for gliclazide 299 (an oral antidiabetic 128)

Novo-Hydroxyzin a generic company version of hydroxyzine (an antihistamine used as an anti-anxiety drug 67)

Novo-Ipramide a generic company version of ipratropium bromide 315 (a *bronchodilator* 76)

Novo-Ketoconazole a generic company version of ketoconazole 320 (an antifungal 124)

Novo-Ketotifen a generic company version of ketotifen (a drug used in asthma 77)

Novo-Levodicarbidopa a generic company version of levodopa/carbidopa 326 (a combination of levodopa 326 and carbidopa for *parkinsonism* 71)

Novo-Levobunolol a generic company version of levobunolol (a beta blocker 83 and drug for glaucoma 156)

Novo-Lexin a generic company version of cephalexin 220 (a cephalosporin *antibiotic* 114)

Novolin ge NPH a product name for insulin NPH (a drug for diabetes 128)

Novo-Loperamide a generic company version of loperamide 332 (an antidiarrheal 96)

Novo-Lorazem a generic company version of lorazepam 335 (a benzodiazepine anti-anxiety drug 67 and sleeping drug 66)

Novo-Maprotiline a generic company version of maprotiline (an antidepressant 68)

Novo-Medrone a generic company version of medroxyprogesterone 339 (a female sex hormone 133)

Novo-Metformin a product name or metformin 346 (drug for diabetes 128)

Novo-Methacin a generic company version of indomethacin (a non-steroidal anti-inflammatory 102)

Novo-Metoprol a generic company version of metoprolol 354 (a beta blocker 83)

Novo-Mexiletine a generic company version of mexiletine (an anti-arrhythmic 86)

Novo-Minocycline a generic company version of minocycline 357 (an *antibiotic* 114)

Novo-Misoprostol a generic company version of misoprostol 360 (an anti-ulcer drug 95)

Novo-Moclobemide a generic company version of moclobemide 361 (an antidepressant 68)

Novo-Naprox a generic company version of naproxen 366 (a non-steroidal anti-inflammatory 102)

Novo-Nifedin a product name for nifedipine 368 (a calcium channel blocker 87)

Novo-Nortriptyline a generic company version of nortriptyline (a tricyclic antidepressant 68)

Novo-Oxybutynin a generic company version of oxybutynin 381 (an *anticholinergic* and *antispasmodic* for urinary disorders 154)

Novo-Pen-VK a generic company version of penicillin V 384 (a penicillin *antibiotic* 114)

Novo-Peridol LA a generic company version of haloperidol 304 (an antipsychotic 69)

Novo-Pirocam a generic company version of piroxicam 391 (a non-steroidal anti-inflammatory 102)

Novo-Prazin a generic company version of prazosin (a sympatholytic antihypertensive 88)

Novo-Profen a generic company version of ibuprofen 310 (a non-opioid analgesic 64 and non-steroidal anti-inflammatory 102)

Novo-Purol a generic company version of allopurinol 181 (a drug for gout 105)

Novo Rapid a product name for insulin aspart (a drug for diabetes 128)

Novo-Salmol a generic company version of salbutamol 424 (a *bronchodilator* 76)

Novo-Selegiline a generic company version of selegiline 426 (a drug for *parkinsonism* 71)

Novo-Sertraline a generic company version of sertraline 427 (an antidepressant 68)

Novo-Sotalol a generic company version of sotalol 432 (a beta blocker 83)

Novo-Spiroton a generic company version of spironolactone 433 (a potassium-sparing diuretic 85)

Novo-Spirozine a generic product name for combination of spironolactone 433 (a potassium-sparing diuretic 85) and hydrochlorothiazide 306 (a thiazide diuretic 85)

Novo-Sundac a generic company version of sulindac (a non-steroidal anti-inflammatory 102)

Novo-Temazepam a generic company version of temazepam 440 (a benzodiazepine sleeping drug 66)

Novo-Terazosin a generic company version of terazosin 442 (a sympatholytic antihypertensive 88)

Novo-Terbinafine a generic company version of terbinafine 443 (an antifungal 124)

Novo-Tetra a generic company version of tetracycline 447 (an *antibiotic* 114)

Novo-Theophyl SR a generic company version of theophylline 448 (a *bronchodilator* 76)

Novo-Tiaprofenic a generic company version of tiaprofenic acid (a non-steroidal anti-inflammatory 102)

Novo-Trazodone a generic company version of trazodone (an antidepressant 68)

Novo-Trimel a generic company version of co-trimoxazole 245 (a combination of (sulfamethoxazole (a sulfonamide antibacterial 117) and trimethoprim 457

Novo-Tripramine a generic company version of trimipramine (a tricyclic antidepressant 68)

Novo-Valproic a generic company version of valproic acid 458 (an anticonvulsant 70)

Novo-Veramil a generic company version of verapimil 462 (an antihypertensive 88 and calcium channel blocker 87)

Novo-Zopiclone a generic company version of zopiclone 467 (a sleeping drug 66)

Nozinan a product name for methotrimeprazine (an antipsychotic 69)

Nu-Acyclovir a generic company version of acyclovir 178 (an antiviral 119)

Nu-Alpraz a generic company version of alprazolam 182 (a benzodiazepine anti-anxiety drug 67)

Nu-Amoxi a generic company version of amoxicillin 190 (a penicillin *antibiotic* 114)

Nu-Ampi a generic company version of ampicillin (a penicillin *antibiotic* 114)

Nu-Atenol a generic company version of atenolol 195 (a beta blocker 83)

Nu-Baclo a generic company version of baclofen 202 (a muscle relaxant 106)

Nubain a product name for nalbuphine (an opioid analgesic 64)

Nu-Buspirone a generic company version of buspirone 214 (an anti-anxiety drug 67)

Nu-Cefaclor a generic company version of cefaclor (a cephalosporin *antibiotic* 114)

Nu-Cephalex a generic company version of cephalexin 220 (a cephalosporin *antibiotic* 114)

Nu-Clonazepam a generic company version of clonazepam 237 (a benzodiazepine anti-anxiety drug 67 and anticonvulsant 70)

NU-CLONIDINE–PIROXICAM

Nu-Clonidine a product name for clonidine (an antihypertensive 88)

Nu-Cloxi a generic company version of cloxacillin 240 (a penicillin *antibiotic* 114)

Nu-Cotrimox a product name for co-trimoxazole 245

Nu-Cyclobenzaprine a generic company version of cyclobenzaprine (a muscle relaxant 106)

Nu-Desipramine a generic company version of desipramine (a tricyclic antidepressant 68)

Nu-Diclo a generic company version of diclonefac 250 (a non-steroidal anti-inflammatory 102)

Nu-Diflunisal a generic company version of diflunisal (a non-steroidal ßßßßanti-inflammatory 102)

Nu-Diltiaz a generic company version of diltiazem 257 (an antihypertensive 88 and calcium channel blocker 87)

Nu-Divalproex a product name for divalproex (an anticonvulsant 70)

Nu-Doxycycline a product name for doxycycline 268 (a tetracycline *antibiotic* 114)

Nu-Fenofibrate a generic company version of fenofibrate (a lipid-lowering drug 89)

Nu-Fluoxetine a generic company version of fluoxetine 287 (a tricyclic antidepressant 68)

Nu-Flurbiprofen a generic company version of flurbiprofen (a non-steroidal anti-inflammatory 102)

Nu-Fluvoxamine a generic company version of fluvoxamine 291 (an antidepressant 68)

Nu-Gemfibrozil a generic company version of gemfibrozil 297 (a lipid-lowering drug 89)

Nu-Ibuprofen a generic company version of ibuprofen 310 (a non-opioid analgesic 64 and non-steroidal anti-inflammatory 102)

Nu-Indo a generic company version of indomethacin (a non-steroidal anti-inflammatory 102)

Nu-Ipratropium a generic company version of ipratropium bromide 315 (a *bronchodilator* 76)

Nu-Ketoprofen a generic company version of ketoprofen 321 (a non-steroidal anti-inflammatory 102)

Nu-Levocarb a generic company version of levodopa/carbidopa 326 (a combination of levodopa 326 and carbidopa used in the treatment of *parkinsonism* 71)

Nu-Loraz a generic company version of lorazepam 335 (a benzodiazepine anti-anxiety drug 67 and sleeping drug 66)

Nu-Loxapine a generic company version of loxapine (an antipsychotic 69)

Nu-Megestrol a generic company version of megestrol 341 (a female sex hormone 133 and anticancer drug 140)

Nu-Metoclopramide a product name for metoclopramide 353 (a gastrointestinal motility regulator and anti-emetic 74)

Nu-Metop a generic company version of metoprolol 354 (a beta blocker 83)

Nu-Moclobemide a generic company version of moclobemide 361 (an antidepressant 68)

Nu-Naprox a generic company version of naproxen 366 (a non-steroidal anti-inflammatory 102)

Nu-Nifed a generic company version of nifedipine 368 (a calcium channel blocker 87)

Nu-Nifedipine-PA a product name for nifedipine 368 (a calcium channel blocker 87)

Nu-Nortriptyline a generic company version of nortriptyline (a tricyclic antidepressant 68)

Nu-Oxybutyn a product name for oxybutynin 381 (an *anticholinergic* and *antispasmodic* for urinary disorders 154

Nu-Pen-VK a generic company version of penicilin V 377 (a penicillin *antibiotic* 114)

Nu-Pirox a generic company version of piroxicam 391 (a non-steroidal anti-inflammatory 102)

Nu-Pravastatin a generic company version of pravastatin 394 (a lipid-lowering drug 89)

Nu-Prazo a generic company version of prazosin (a sympatholytic antihypertensive 88)

Nu-Prochlor a generic company version of prochlorperazine 397 (a phenothiazine anti-emetic 74 and antipsychotic 69)

Nu-Propranolol a generic company version of propranolol 402 (a beta blocker 83)

Nu-Salbutamol a generic company version of salbutamol 424 (a *bronchodilator* 76)

Nu-Selegiline a generic company version of selegiline 426 (a drug for *parkinsonism* 71)

Nu-Sotalol a generic company version of sotalol 432 (a beta blocker 83)

Nu-Sulfinpyrazone a generic company version of sulfinpyrazone (a drug for gout 105)

Nu-Sulindac a generic company version of sulindac (a non-steroidal anti-inflammatory 102)

Nu-Temazepam a product name for temazepam 440 (a benzodiazepine anti-anxiety drug 67 and sleeping drug 66)

Nu-Terazosin a generic company version of terazosin 442 (a sympatholytic antihypertensive 88)

Nu-Tetra a generic company version of tetracycline 447 (an *antibiotic* 114 and antimalarial 123)

Nu-Tiaprofenic a generic company version of tiaprofenic acid (a non-steroidal anti-inflammatory 102)

Nu-Trazodone a generic company version of trazodone (an antidepressant 68)

Nu-Trazodone-D a generic company version of trazodone (an antidepressant 68)

Nu-Trimipramine a generic company version of trimipramine (a tricyclic antidepressant 68)

Nutropin a product name for somatropin, a pituitary hormone 131 (a synthetic pituitary hormone 131)

Nu-Valproic a product name for valproic acid 458 (an anticonvulsant 70)

Nu-Verap a generic company version of verapimil 462 (an antihypertensive 88 and calcium channel blocker 87)

Nu-Zopiclone a product name for zopiclone 467 (a sleeping drug 66)

Nyaderm a product name for nystatin 373 (an antifungal 124)

nystatin 373 (an antifungal 124**)**

Nytol a product name for diphenhydramine 259 used as a sleep aid (an antihistamine 110, anti-emetic 74, and antipruritic 161)

O

octocrylene an ingredient of sunscreens 169

octoxynol a spermicidal agent

octreotide a synthetic pituitary hormone 131 used to relieve symptoms of cancer of the pancreas

Ocufen a product name for flurbiprofen (a non-steroidal anti-inflammatory 102)

Oesclim a product name for estradiol 276 (an estrogen 135)

ofloxacin an antibacterial 117

Ogen a product name for estropipate (an estrogen 135)

olanzapine 374 (an antipsychotic 69)

olopatadine an antihistamine 111

olsalazine a drug for ulcerative colitis 98

omalizumab a monoclonal antibody 140

omega-3 fatty acids 475 a supplement

omeprazole 375 (an anti-ulcer drug 95)

ondansetron 376 (an anti-emetic 74)

opium an extract of poppy seeds; basis for opioid analgesics 64

Opticrom a product name for sodium cromoglycate 431 (an anti-allergy drug 109)

Optimine a product name for azatadine (an antihistamine 110)

Optimyxin ointment a combination of polymyxin B and bacitracin zinc (both *antibiotics* 114)

Oracort a product name for triamcinolone (a corticosteroid 127)

Orap a product name for pimozide (an antipsychotic 69)

orciprenaline a *bronchodilator* 76

Orencia a product name for abatacept (a biological response modifier 103)

Orgalutran a product name for ganirelix (a drug for infertility 152)

orlistat 377 (a drug that blocks the action of enzymes that digest fats)

orphenadrine 378 (an *anticholinergic* muscle relaxant 106)

Ortho 0.5/35 a product-name oral contraceptive 149 containing ethinyl estradiol 278 (an estrogen 133 and oral contraceptive 149) and norethindrone 371 (a progestin 133)

Ortho 7/7/7 a product-name oral contraceptive 149 containing ethinyl estradiol 278 (an estrogen 133 and norethindrone 371 (a progestin 133)

Ortho-Cept a product-name oral contraceptive 149 containing ethinyl estradiol 278 (an estrogen 133) and desogestrel (a progestin 133)

Ortho-Novum a product-name oral contraceptive 149 containing mestranol (an estrogen 133 and oral contraceptive 149) and norethindrone 371 (a progestin 133)

Os-Cal a product name for calcium carbonate (a calcium salt (a mineral 137) used as an antacid 94)

oseltamavir 379 (an anitiviral drug 119)

Ostoforte a product name for ergocalciferol (a vitamin 135)

Otrivin a product name for xylometazoline 464 (a decongestant 79)

Ovol a product name for simethicone (an antiflatulent 98)

oxaprozin a non-steroidal anti-inflammatory 102

oxazepam 380 (a benzodiazepine anti-anxiety drug 67)

oxcarbazepine an anticonvulsant 70

Oxeze Turbuhaler a product name for formoterol 292 (a *bronchodilator* 76)

Oxipar Lotion a product name for coal tar (a substance for psoriasis 166 and eczema 167)

oxprenolol a beta blocker 97

Oxsoralen a product name for methoxsalen a drug used in the treatment of psoriasis (166) and atopic dermatitis

Oxsoralen-Ultra a product name for methoxsalen a drug used in the treatment of psoriasis (166) and atopic dermatitis

oxtriphylline a *bronchodilator* 76

oxybenzone a sunscreen 169

oxybuprocaine a local anesthetic 64

oxybutynin 381 (an *anticholinergic* and *antispasmodic* for urinary disorders 154)

oxycodone an opioid analgesic 64

OxyContin a product name for oxycodone (an opioid analgesic 64)

Oxyderm a product name for benzoyl peroxide 204 (a drug for acne 165)

Oxy.IR a product name for oxycodone (an opioid analgesic 64)

oxymetazoline a *topical* decongestant 79

oxymorphone an opioid analgesic 64

oxytocin an uterine stimulant 153

Oxytrol a product name for oxybutynin 381 (an anticholinergic and antispasmodic for urinary disorders 154)

Ozonol a combination of zinc and phenol used topically for minor burns and skin irritation

P

paclitaxel an anticancer drug 140

padimate-O an ingredient of sunscreens 169

palivizumab an antiviral drug 119

pamidronate a drug for bone disorders 108

pancrealipase a preparation of pancreatic enzymes 100

Pancrease a product name for pancrelipase (a preparation of pancreatic enzymes 100)

pancreatin a preparation of pancreatic enzymes 100

panthenol pantothenic acid 476 (a vitamin 135)

PANTO IV a product name for pantoprazole 382 (an anti-ulcer drug 95)

Pantoloc a product name for pantoprazole 382 (an anti-ulcer drug 95)

pantoprazole 382 (an anti-ulcer drug 95)

pantothenic acid 476 (a vitamin 135)

papaverine a muscle relaxant 106

paraldehyde an anticonvulsant 84 used for status epilepticus

Paraplatin-AQ a product name for carboplatin (an anticancer drug 140)

Parlodel a product name for bromocriptine 210 (a pituitary agent 131 and drug for *parkinsonism* 71)

Parnate a product name for tranylcypromine (an MAOI antidepressant 68)

paroxetine 383 (an antidepressant 68)

Parsitan a product name for ethopropazine (drug for parkinsonism 71)

Parvolex a product name for acetylcysteine (a mucolytic 94)

Patanol a product name for olopatadine (an antihistamine 111)

Paxil a product name for paroxetine 383 (an antidepressant 68)

Pediapred a product name for prednisolone 395 (a corticosteroid 127)

Pediatrix a product containing acetaminophen 177 (an analgesic 64)

Pediazole a combination of erythromycin 274 (an *antibiotic* 114) and sulfisoxazole (an *antibiotic* 114)

Pegetron a combination of ribavirin (an antiviral 119) and peginterferon alfa-2b (an antiviral 119)

peginterferon alfa-2a a biological response modifier used in hepatitis B and C 119

peginterferon alfa-2b a biological response modifier used in hepatitis C 119

Peg-Intron a product name for peginterferon alfa-2b (an antiviral 119)

Penbritin a product name for ampicillin (a penicillin *antibiotic* 114)

penciclovir an antiviral 119

penicillamine an antirheumatic 103

penicillin *antibiotic*s 114

penicillin G a penicillin *antibiotic* 114

penicillin V 384 (a penicillin *antibiotic* 114)

Penlac a product name for ciclopirox (an antifungal 124)

Pentacarinat a product name for pentamidine (an antiprotozoal 122)

pentamidine an antiprotozoal 122

Pentamycetin a product name for chloramphenicol 222 (an *antibiotic* 114)

Pentasa a product name for 5-ASA 345 (a drug for inflammatory bowel disease 98)

pentazocine an opioid analgesic 64

pentoxifylline a *vasodilator* 98 used to improve blood flow to the limbs in peripheral vascular disease

Pepcid a product name for famotidine 282 (an anti-ulcer drug 95)

Pepcid Complete a combination product name containing famotidine 282 (an anti-ulcer drug 95), calcium carbonate 137, and magnesium hydroxide 338 (an antacid 94)

Pepto-Bismol product-name preparation for diarrhea 96 and upset stomach 94

Percocet a product name for oxycodone (an opioid analgesic 64) and acetaminophen 177 (a non-opioid analgesic 64)

Percodan a product name for oxycodone (an opioid analgesic 64) and ASA (a non-opioid analgesic 64)

Pergonal a product name for menotropins (a drug for infertility 152)

pericyazine an antipsychotic 69

Peridex a product name for chlorhexidine (a skin antiseptic 163)

perindopril 385 (an ACE inhibitor 84)

permethrin 386 (a *topical* antiparasitic 164)

perphenazine a phenothiazine antipsychotic 69

Persantine a product name for dipyridamole 261 (an antiplatelet drug 89)

Peru balsam an antiseptic 163 for hemorrhoids

Pharmorubicin PFS a product name for epirubicin (a *cytotoxic* anticancer drug 140)

Phazyme a product name for simethicone (an antiflatulent 98)

phenelzine an MAOI antidepressant 68

phenobarbital 387 (a barbiturate anticonvulsant 70)

phenol an antiseptic used in throat lozenges and sprays 163

phentolamine an antihypertensive 102

phenylephrine a decongestant 79

phenytoin 388 (an anticonvulsant 70)

Phillips Preparations a product name for magnesium hydroxide 338 (an antacid 94)

pHisoHex a product name for hexachlorophene (a skin antiseptic 163)

PHL-Cholestyramine Light a generic version of cholestyramine 227 (a lipid-lowering drug 89)

PHL-Procyclidine a generic company version of procyclidine 399 (an anticholinergic for *parkinsonism* 71)

phosphorus a mineral 137

Phyllocontin a product name for aminophylline 448 (a *bronchodilator* 76)

phytomenadione vitamin K 482 (a vitamin 135)

pilocarpine 389 (a miotic for glaucoma 156)

Pilopine HS a product name for pilocarpine 389 (a miotic for glaucoma 156)

pimozide an antipsychotic 69

pioglitazone 390 (a drug for diabetes 128)

piperacillin a penicillin *antibiotic* 114

piperazine an anthelmintic 125

piperonyl butoxide used to treat pediculosis and scabies 164

Piportil L4 a product name for pipotiazine (an antipsychotic 69)

pipotiazine an antipsychotic 69

Pipracil a product name for piperacillin (a penicillin *antibiotic* 114)

piroxicam 391 (a non-steroidal anti-inflammatory 102)

PIZOTIFEN–RATIO-IPRATROPIUM UDV

pizotifen 392 (a drug for migraine 73)

Plan B a product name for levonorgestrel 328 (a female sex hormone 133) used as emergency contraception

Plaquenil a product name for hydroxychloroquine (an antimalarial 123 and antirheumatic 103)

Plavix a product name for clopidogrel 238 (an antiplatelet drug 90)

Plendil a product name for felodipine (an antihypertensive 88 and calcium channel blocker 87)

PMS-Atenolol a generic company version of atenolol 195 (a beta blocker 83)

PMS-Baclofen a generic company version of baclofen 202 (a muscle relaxant 106)

PMS-Bezafibrate a generic company version of bezafibrate 207 (a lipid-lowering drug 89)

PMS-Bromocriptine a generic company version of bromocriptine 210 (a pituitary agent 131 and drug for *parkinsonism* 71)

PMS-Buspirone a generic company version of buspirone 214 (an anti-anxiety drug 67)

PMS-Cefaclor a generic company version of cefaclor (a cephalosporin *antibiotic* 114)

PMS-Chloral Hydrate a generic company version of chloral hydrate (a sleeping drug 66)

PMS-Clonazepam a generic company version of clonazepam 237 (a benzodiazepine anticonvulsant 70)

PMS-Desipramine a generic company version of desipramine (a tricyclic antidepressant 68)

PMS-Dexamethasone a generic company version of dexamethasone 251 (a corticosteroid 127)

PMS-Diclofenac a generic company version of diclonfenac 254 (a non-steroidal anti-inflammatory 102)

PMS-Dipivefrin a generic company version of dipivefrin (a *sympathomimetic* for glaucoma 156)

PMS-Dopazide a generic company version of methyldopa 350 (an antihypertensive 889) and hydrochlorothiazide 306 (a thiazide diuretic 85)

PMS-Fluoxetine a generic company version of fluoxetine 287 (a tricyclic anti-depressant 68)

PMS-Fluphenazine a generic company version of fluphenazine (an phenothiazine antipsychotic 69)

PMS-Flutamide a product name for flutamide 289 (an anticancer drug 140)

PMS-Fluvoxamine a generic company version of fluvoxamine 291 (an antidepressant 68)

PMS-Gabapentin a generic company version of gabapentin 294 (an anticonvulsant 70)

PMS-Gemfibrozil a generic company version of gemfibrozil 297 (a lipid-lowering drug 89)

PMS Hydroxyzine a generic company version of hydroxyzine (an antihistamine used as an anti-anxiety drug 67)

PMS-Indapamide a generic company version of indapamide 312 (a thiazide-like diuretic 85)

PMS-Isoniazid a generic company version of isoniazid 317 (an antituberculous drug 134)

PMS-lactulose a generic company version of lactulose 322 (an osmotic laxative 113)

PMS Lindane Lotion a generic company version of Lindane (also called gamma benzene hexachloride) used to treat pediculosis and scabies 164

PMS-Levobunolol a generic company version of levobunolol (a beta blocker 83 and drug for glaucoma 156)

PMS-Loperamide a generic company version of loperamide 332 (an antidiarrheal 96)

PMS-Loxapine a generic company version of loxapine (an antipsychotic 69)

PMS-Mefenamic Acid a generic company version of mefenamic acid (a non-steroidal anti-inflammatory 102)

PMS-Methylphenidate a generic company version of methylphenidate 351 (a drug for hyperactivity in children 72)

PMS-Metoprolol-B a generic company version of metoprolol 354 (a beta blocker 83)

PMS-Moclobemide a generic company version of moclobemide 361 (an antidepressant 68)

PMS-Nortriptyline a generic company version of nortriptyline (a tricyclic antidepressant 68)

PMS-Nystatin a generic company version of nystatin 373 (an antifungal 124)

PMS-Oxybutynin a generic company version of oxybutynin 381 (an *anticholinergic* and *antispasmodic* for urinary disorders 154)

PMS-Sodium Cromoglycate a generic company version of sodium cromoglycate 431 (an anti-allergy drug 109 used to prevent asthma attacks 77)

PMS-Sotalol a generic company version of sotalol 432 a beta blocker 83

PMS-Temazepam a generic company version of temazepam 440 (a benzodiazepine anti-anxiety drug 67 and sleeping drug 66)

PMS-Terazosin a generic company version of terazosin 442 (a sympatholytic antihypertensive 88)

PMS-Terbinafine a generic company version of terbinafine 443 (an antifungal 124)

PMS-Tiaprofenic a generic company version of tiaprofenic acid (a non-steroidal anti-inflammatory 102)

PMS-Trazodone a generic company version of trazodone (an antidepressant 68)

PMS-Valproic Acid a product name for valproic acid 458 (an anticonvulsant 70)

podophyllin a *topical* treatment for genital warts

Polycitra-K a product name for potassium citrate (a drug used in the treatment of low potassium)

polymyxin B an *antibiotic* 114, 159

Polysporin ear drops a product name combination of polymyxin B and gramiacidin (both *antibiotics* 114, 159)

Polysporin ointment a product name combination of polymyxin B and bacitracin zinc (both *antibiotics* 114)

polyvinyl alcohol an ingredient of artificial tear preparations 160

Pontocaine a product name for tetracaine (also known as amethocain, a local anesthetic 64)

posaconazole an antifungal drug 124

potassium 476 (a mineral 137)

potassium bicarbonate an antacid 94

potassium citrate a drug used in the treatment of low potassium

potassium iodide a drug used for overactive thyroid before surgery

potassium permanganate a skin antiseptic 163

povidone-iodine a skin antiseptic 163

pralidoxime mesylate antidote for organophosphorus poisoning

pramipexole 393 (a drug for *parkinsonism* 71)

Pramox HC a combination drug with hydrocortisone 308 (a corticosteroid 127 and antipruritic 161) and pramoxine (a local anesthetic 64)

Pramoxine a local anesthetic 161

Pravachol a product name for pravastatin 394 (a lipid-lowering drug 89)

Pravasa a product name for a combination of pravastatin 394 (a lipid-lowering drug 89) and acetylsalicylic acid (ASA) 194 (an analgesic 64 and an antiplatelet drug 90)

pravastatin 394 (a lipid-lowering drug 89)

praziquantel an anthelmintic 125 for tapeworms

prazosin a sympatholytic antihypertensive 88 also used to relieve urinary obstruction 154

Pred Forte a product name for prednisolone 395 (a corticosteroid 127)

Pred Mild a product name for prednisolone 395 (a corticosteroid 127)

Prednicarbate a *topical* corticosteroid 162

prednisone 395 (a corticosteroid 127)

prednisolone the active form of prednisone 395 (a corticosteroid 127)

pregabalin 396 (an anticonvulsant 70)

Pregnyl a product name for gonadotrophin, human chorionic 302 (a drug for infertility 152)

Premarin a product name for conjugated estrogens 244 (a female sex hormone 133)

Premplus a product name for a combination of conjugated estrogens 244 and medroxyprogesterone 339 (female sex hormones 133)

Prevacid a product name for lansoprazole 324 (an anti-ulcer drug 95)

Prevex HC a product name for hydrocortisone 308 (a corticosteroid 127 and antipruritic 161)

Prezista a product name for darunavir (an antiretroviral drug used in the treatment of HIV and AIDS 144)

prilocaine a local *anesthetic* 64

primaquine an antimalarial 123 and antiprotozoal 122

Primaquine sulfate a product name for primaquine (an antimalarial 123 and antiprotozoal 122

Primaxim a product name for imipenem (an *antibiotic* 114) with cilastatin (used to make imipenem more effective)

primidone an anticonvulsant 70

Prinivil a product name for lisinopril 330 (an ACE inhibitor 98)

probenecid 397 (a uricosuric for gout 105)

Probeta a combination of levobunolol (a beta blocker 83 and drug for glaucoma 156) and dipivefrin (a *sympathomimetic* for glaucoma 156)

procainamide an anti-arrhythmic 86

Procan-SR a product name for procainamide (an anti-arrhythmic 86)

prochlorperazine 398 (a phenothiazine anti-emetic 74 and antipsychotic 69)

Proctodan HC a combination drug with hydrocortisone 308 (a corticosteroid 127 and antipruritic 161) and pramoxine (a local anesthetic 64)

Proctofoam HC a combination drug with hydrocortisone 308 (a corticosteroid 127 and antipruritic 161) and other drugs

procyclidine 399 (an *anticholinergic* for *parkinsonism* 71)

Procytox a product name for cyclophos-phamide 246 (an anticancer drug 140)

Prodium Plain a fiber laxative containing psyllium 405 (laxative 97)

Prodium Plus a fiber laxative containing psyllium 405 (laxative 97) and senna (a stimulant laxative 97)

Profasi HP a product name for gonadotrophin, human chorionic 302 (a drug for infertility 152)

progesterone a female sex hormone 133

progestin a female sex hormone 133

Prograf a product name for tacrolimus (an immunosuppressant 143)

proguanil 400 (an antimalarial 123)

Prolopa a product name for levodopa/ benserazide (a combination of levodopa 326 and benserazide for *parkinsonism* 71)

Proloprim a product name for tri-methroprim 444 (an antibacterial 117)

promethazine 401 (an antihistamine 110 and anti-emetic 74)

Prometrium a product name for progesterone (a female sex hormone 133)

Pronestyl-SR a product name for procainamide (an anti-arrhythmic 86)

propafenone an anti-arrhythmic 86

Propecia a product name for finasteride 285 (a drug for benign prostatic hypertrophy)

Propine a product name for dipivefrin (a *sympathomimetic* for glaucoma 156)

propoxyphene an opioid analgesic 64

propranolol 402 (a beta blocker 83)

propylthiouracil 403 (an antithyroid drug 130)

Propyl-Thyracil a product name for propylthiouracil 403 (an antithyroid drug 130)

Proscar a product name for finasteride 285 (a drug for benign prostatic hypertrophy)

Prostin VR a product name for alprostadil 183 (a prostaglandin used for male impotence 134, 152)

protirelin test of thyroid function

Protopic a product name for tacrolimus (an immunosuppressant 143)

Provera a product name for medroxyprogesterone 339 (a female sex hormone 133)

Proviodine a product name for povidone-iodine (a skin antiseptic 163)

Prozac a product name for fluoxetine 287 (an antidepressant 68)

pseudoephedrine 404 (a decongestant 79)

Pseudofrin a product name for pseudoephedrine 404 (a decongestant 79)

Psyllium 405 (a laxative 97)

Pulmicort a product name for budesonide 211 (a corticosteroid 127)

Pulmozyme a product name for dornase alfa (a drug for cystic fibrosis 80)

Puregon a product name for follitropin beta (a drug for infertility 152)

Purinethol a product name for mercaptopurine 344 (an anticancer drug 140)

pyrantel a drug used in the treatment of intestinal worms, such as pinworms (125)

pyrazinamide an antituberculous drug 118

pyridostigmine 406 (a drug for myasthenia gravis 107)

pyridoxine another name for vitamin B6 477 (a vitamin 135)

pyrimethamine 407 (an antimalarial 123)

pyrvinium pamoate a drug used in the treatment of pinworms (125)

Q

quetiapine 408 (an antipsychotic 69)

quinapril an ACE inhibitor 98

quinidine 409 (an anti-arrhythmic drug 86)

quinidine sulfate quinidine 409 (an anti-arrhythmic drug 86)

quinine 410 (an antimalarial 123 and muscle relaxant 106)

Quinine-Odan a product name for quinine 410 (an antimalarial 123 and muscle relaxant 106)

Qvar a product name for beclomethasone 203 (a corticosteroid 127)

R

radioactive iodine see iodine

Ralivia a product name for tramadol 454 (an opioid analgesic 64)

raloxifene 411 (a selective estrogen receptor modulator 133 for osteoporosis 108)

raltegravir an antiretroviral drug used in the treatment of HIV and AIDS 144

ramipril 412 (an ACE inhibitor 98)

R and C II Shampoo/Conditioner a product name for piperonyl butoxide (used in the treatment of pediculosis and scabies 164)

R and C II Spray a product name for piperonyl butoxide (used in the treatment of pediculosis and scabies 164)

ranitidine 413 (an anti-ulcer drug 95)

rasagiline 414 (used for parkinsonism 71)

ratio-Aclavulanate a product name for amoxicillin/clavulinic acid (a combination of amoxicillin 190 (a penicillin *antibiotic* 114) and clavulinic acid (a substance given with it to make amoxicillin more effective)

ratio-Amiodarone a generic company version of amiodarone 187 (an antiarrhythmic 86)

ratio-Atenolol a generic company version of atenolol 195 (a beta blocker 83)

ratio-Baclofen a generic company version of baclofen 202 (a muscle relaxant 106)

ratio-Brimonidine a product name for brimonidine (a drug for glaucoma 156)

ratio-Buspirone a generic company version of buspirone 214 (an anti-anxiety drug 67)

ratio-Calmydone a combination of doxylamine (an antihistamine 110), hydrocodone 307 (a cough suppressant 80), and etafedrine (a decongestant 79)

ratio-Clindamycin a generic company version of clindamycin 233 (an *antibiotic* 114)

ratio-Clobazam a generic company version of clobazam (a benzodiazepine drug used as a anticonvulsant 70)

ratio-Clobetasol a generic company version of clobetasol 234 (a *topical* corticosteroid 162)

ratio-Clonazepam a generic company version of clonazepam 237 (a benzodiazepine anticonvulsant 70)

ratio-Codeine a generic company version of codeine 242 (an opioid analgesic 64)

ratio-Colchicine a generic company version of colchicine 243 (a drug for gout 105)

ratio-Coristex-DH a combination product with phenylephrine (a decongestant 79) and hydrocodone 307 (a cough suppressant 80)

ratio-Cyclobenzapine a generic company version of cyclobenzapine (a muscle relaxant 106)

ratio-Desipramine a generic company version of desipramine (a tricyclic antidepressant 68)

ratio-Dexamethasone a generic company version of dexamethasone 251 (a corticosteroid 127)

ratio-Doxazosin a generic company version of doxazosin 266 (a sympatholytic antihypertensive 88)

ratio-Flunisolide a generic company version of flunisolide (a corticosteroid 127)

ratio-Fluoxetine a generic company version of fluoxetine 287 (an antidepressant 68)

ratio-Fluvoxamine a generic company version of fluvoxamine 291 (an antidepressant 68)

ratio-Gentamicin a generic company version of gentamicin 298 (an *antibiotic* 114)

ratio-Indomethacin a generic company version of indomethacin (a non-steroidal anti-inflammatory 102)

ratio-Ipratropium UDV a generic company version of ipratropium bromide 315 (a *bronchodilator* 76)

RATIO-LOVASTATIN–SULCRATE

ratio-Lovastatin a generic company version of lovastatin 337 (a lipid-lowering drug 89)

ratio-Methotrexate a generic company version of methotrexate 348 (an antimetabolite anticancer drug 140)

ratio-methylphenidate a generic company version of methylphenidate 351 (a drug for hyperactivity in children 72)

ratio-Morphine a generic company version of morphine 364 (an opioid analgesic 64)

ratio-MPA a generic company version of medroxyprogesterone 339 (a female sex hormone 133)

ratio-Nortriptyline a generic company version of nortriptyline (a tricyclic antidepressant 68)

ratio-Nystatin a generic company version of nystatin 373 (an antifungal 124)

ratio-Oxycodone a generic company version of oxycodone (an opioid analgesic 64)

ratio-Prednisolone a generic company version of prednisolone 395 (a corticosteroid 127)

ratio-Salbutamol HFA a generic company version of salbutamol 424 (a *bronchodilator* 76)

ratio-Sertraline a generic company version of sertraline 427 (an antidepressant 68)

ratio-Terazosin a generic company version of terazosin 442 (a sympatholytic antihypertensive 88)

ratio-Theo-Brone a combination of theophylline 448 (a *bronchodilator* 76), potassium iodide, guaifenesin (an expectorant 80), and mepyramine maleate

ratio-Topilene a generic company version of betamethasone 206 (a corticosteroid 127)

ratio-Trazodone a generic company version of trazodone (an antidepressant 68)

ratio-Triacomb a combination of nystatin 373 (a drug for fungal infections 124), gramicidin and neomycin sulfate (both *antibiotic*s 114), and triamcinolone acetonide (a corticosteroid 127)

ratio-Valproic a generic company version of valproic acid 458 (an anticonvulsant 70)

ratio-Zopiclone a generic company version of zopiclone 467 (a sleeping drug 66)

Reactine a product name for cetirizine 221 (an antihistamine 110)

Rebif a product name for interferon beta-1a (a drug used for the treatment of multiple sclerosis)

Rectogel HC a product name combination product with hydrocortisone 308 (a corticosteroid 127), benzocaine (an *anesthetic* 64), and zinc sulfate monohydrate

Rejuva-A a product name for tretinoin (a drug for acne 165)

Relenza a product name for zanamivir 465 (an antiviral drug 119)

Relpax a product name for eletriptan (a drug for migraine 73)

Remeron a product name for mirtazapine 359 (an antidepressant 68)

Remicade a product name for infliximab (a biological response modifier for rheumatoid arthritis 103 and Crohn's disease 98)

Reminyl a product name for galantamine 295 (a drug used for the treatment of Alzheimer's disease 71)

Renedil a product name for felodipine (an antihypertensive 88 and calcium channel blocker 87)

Renova a product name for tretinoin (a drug for acne 165)

repaglinide 415 (a drug for diabetes 128)

ReQuip a product name for ropinirole (a drug for *parkinsonism* 71)

Rescriptor a product name for delavirdine (an antiretroviral drug used in the treatment of HIV and AIDS 144)

resorcinol a keratolytic mainly for acne 165

Restoril a product name for temazepam 440 (a benzodiazepine sleeping drug 66)

Retin-A a product name for tretinoin (a drug for acne 165)

Retin-A Micro a product name for tretinoin (a drug for acne 165)

retinoic acid vitamin A 479 (a vitamin 135)

retinol vitamin A 479 (a vitamin 135)

Retrovir a product name for zidovudine 466 (an antiretroviral drug used for the treatment of HIV infection and AIDS 144)

Revatio a product name for sildenafil 429 (drug for impotence 152)

Reyataz a product name for atazanavir (an antiretroviral drug for HIV infection and AIDS 144)

Rhinocort Aqua a product name for budesonide 211 (a corticosteroid 143)

Rhodacine a product name for indomethacin (a non-steroidal anti-inflammatory 102)

Rho-Nitro Pumpspray a product name for nitroglycerin 370 (an anti-angina drug 87)

Rhovane a product name for zopiclone 467 (a sleeping drug 66)

Rhoxal-loperamide a generic company version of loperamide 332 (an antidiarrheal drug 96)

Rhoxal-Sotalol a generic company version of sotalol 432 (a beta blocker 83)

Rhythmol a product name for propafenone (an anti-arrhythmic 86)

ribavirin an antiviral 119

riboflavin 477 (a vitamin 135)

Ridaura a product name for auranofin (a drug used for the treatment of rheumatoid arthritis 117)

rifabutin an antituberculous drug 118

rifampin 416 (an antituberculous drug 118)

Rifater a combination of isoniazid 317 (an antituberculous drug 118) and rifampin 416 (an antituberculous drug 118)

Rimso-50 a product name for dimethyl sulfoxide (a drug for urinary infection 154)

risedronate 417 (a drug for bone disorders 108)

Risperdal a product name for risperidone 418 (an antipsychotic 69)

risperidone 418 (an antipsychotic 69)

Ritalin a product name for methylphenidate 351 (a drug for hyperactivity in children 72)

Ritalin SR a product name for methylphenidate 351 (a drug for hyperactivity in children 72)

ritodrine a uterine muscle relaxant 167

Rituxan a product name for rituximab 419 (an anticancer drug 140)

rituximab 419 (an anticancer drug 140)

Riva-Loperamide a generic company version of loperamide 332 (an antidiarrheal 96)

Rivanase AQ a product name for beclomethasone 203 (a corticosteroid 143)

rivastigmine 420 (a drug for Alzheimer's disease 71)

Rivotril a product name for clonazepam 237 (a benzodiazepine anticonvulsant 84)

rizatriptan 421 (drug for migraine 73)

Robaxacet-8 a combination product containing codeine 242 (an opioid analgesic 64) with acetaminophen 177 (an analgesic 64) and methocarbomal (a muscle relaxant 106)

Robaxin a product name for methocarbamol (a muscle relaxant 106)

Robaxisal a combination of ASA 194 (a non-opioid analgesic 64) and methocarbamol (a muscle relaxant 106)

Robaxisal Extra Strength a combination product with ASA 194 (a non-opioid analgesic 64) and methocarbamol (a muscle relaxant 106)

Robitussin DM a product name combination product containing guafenesin (an expectorant 80) and dextromorphan 252 (a cough suppressant)

Robitussin Honey Cough DM a product name for dextromorphan 252 (a cough suppressant 80)

Rocaltrol a product name for calcitriol 481 (a vitamin 135)

Rofact a product name for rifampin 416 (an antituberculous drug 118)

Rogaine a product name for minoxidil 358 (an antihypertensive 88) used for hair regrowth

Ropinirole a drug for *parkinsonism* 71

rosiglitazone 422 (a drug for diabetes 128)

rosuvastatin 423 (a lipid-lowering drug 89)

Royvac a product name combination product with bisacodyl 208 and magnesium citrate (laxatives 97)

Rythmodan a product name for disopyramide (an anti-arrhythmic 86)

Rythmodan-LA a product name for disopyramide (an anti-arrhythmic 86)

S

642 Tablets a product name for propoxyphene (an opioid analgesic 64)

Sabril a product name for vigabatrin (an anticonvulsant 70)

Saizen a product name for somatropin, a pituitary hormone 131 (a synthetic pituitary hormone 131)

Salagen a product name for pilocarpine 389 (used in the treatment of dry mouth and dry eyes)

Salazopyrin a product name for sulfasalazine 436 (a drug for inflammatory bowel disease 98 and an antirheumatic 103)

Salazopyrin En-Tabs a product name for sulfasalazine 436 (a drug for inflammatory bowel disease 98 and an antirheumatic 103)

salbutamol 424 (a *bronchodilator* 76)

salicylic acid a keratolytic for acne 165, dandruff 168, psoriasis 166, and warts.

salmeterol 425 (a *bronchodilator* 76)

Salofalk a product name for 5-ASA 345 (a drug for inflammatory bowel disease 98)

Sandimmune IV a product name for cyclosporine 247 (an immunosuppressant 143)

Sandomigran a product name for pizotifen 392 (a drug for migraine 73)

Sandomigran DS a product name for pizotifen 392 (a drug for migraine 73)

Sandostatin a product name for octrotide (a synthetic pituitary hormone 131 used to relieve symptoms of cancer of the pancreas)

Sandostatin LAR a product name for octrotide (a synthetic pituitary hormone 131 used to relieve symptoms of cancer of the pancreas)

Sandoz Glimepiride a generic company version of glimepiride 300 (a drug used in diabetes 128)

Sandoz Pioglitazone a generic company version of pioglitazone 390 (a drug for diabetes 128)

Sansert a product name for methysergide (a drug for migraine 73)

Saquinavir a drug for HIV/AIDS 144

Sarna HC a product name for hydrocortisone 308 (a corticosteroid 127 and antipruritic 161)

Sativex a product name combination product with cannabidiol and delta-9-tetrahydrocannabinol (cannabis sativa extract) (an analgesic used in multiple sclerosis 64)

Scabene Aerosol a product name for piperonyl butoxide (used in the treatment of pediculosis and scabies 164)

scopolamine a drug for prevention of nausea and vomiting 74

Sebcur a product name for salicylic acid (a keratolytic for acne 165, dandruff 168, psoriasis 166, and warts)

Sebivo a product name for telbivudine (an antiviral 119)

Select 1/35 a product-name oral contraceptive 149 containing ethinyl estradiol 278 and norethindrone 371

selegiline 426 (a drug for severe *parkinsonism* 71)

selenium 478 (a mineral 137)

selenium sulfide a substance for skin inflammation 163 and dandruff 168

Selsun a product-name dandruff shampoo 168 containing selenium sulfide

senna a stimulant laxative 97

Sensorcaine a product name for bupivacaine (a local *anesthetic* 64 used in labour 153)

Sensorcaine with Epinephrine a product name for a combination of epinephrine 272 and bupivacaine (a local *anesthetic* 64)

Septra a product name for cotrimoxazole 242 (sulfamethoxazole/trimethoprim – a sulfonamide antibacterial 117 combined with trimethoprim 457)

Serc a product name for betahistine 205 (a drug for Ménière's disease 74)

Serevent a product name for salmeterol 425 (a *bronchodilator* 76)

Serophene a product name for clomiphene 235 (a drug for infertility 152)

Seroquel a product name for quetiapine 408 (an antipsychotic 69)

Serostim a product name for somatropin, a pituitary hormone 131 (a synthetic pituitary hormone 131)

sertraline 427 (an antidepressant 68)

Sibelium a product name for flunarizine (a calcium channel blocker used in the prevention of migraine 73)

sibutramine 428 (an appetite suppressant and nervous system stimulant 72)

Sildenafil 429 (a drug used for the treatment of sexual impotence 152)

silver sulfiadiazine a *topical* antibacterial 117 used to prevent infection in burns

simethicone an antiflatulent 98

Simply Sleep a product name for diphenhydramine 259 (an antihistamine 110, anti-emetic 74, and antipruritic 161)

simvastatin 430 (a lipid-lowering drug 89)

Simulect a product name for basiliximab (an immunosuppressant 143)

Sinemet a product name for levodopa/carbidopa 326 (a combination of levodopa 326 and carbidopa for *parkinsonism* 71)

Singulair a product name for montelukast 363 (a leukotriene antagonist for asthma 77)

Sinomet CR a product name for levodopa/carbidopa 326 (a combination of levodopa 326 and carbidopa for *parkinsonism* 71)

Sinutab with Codeine a combination product containing codeine 242 (an opioid analgesic 64) pseudoephedrine 404 (a decongestant 79), acetaminophen 177 (an analgesic 64), and chlorpheniramine 225 (an antihistamine 110)

Sinutab Sinus and Allergy a combination product with pseudoephedrine 404 (a decongestant 79), acetaminophen 177 (an analgesic 64), and chlorpheniramine 225 (an antihistamine 110)

sitagliptin a drug for diabetes 128

Slow-Fe a product name for iron 473 (a mineral 137)

Slow-Fe Folic a product name for folic acid 472 (a vitamin 135) with iron 473 (a mineral 137)

Slow-K a product name for potassium 476 (a mineral 137)

sodium 478 (a mineral 137)

sodium cellulose phosphate an agent used to reduce levels of calcium 462 in the blood

sodium chloride common salt, a source of sodium 478 (a mineral 137)

sodium cromoglycate 431 (an anti-allergy drug 109 used to prevent asthma attacks 77)

sodium ferric gluconate an intravenous iron preparation 473 (a mineral 137)

sodium fluoride 471 (a mineral 137)

Sofracort a combination of dexamethasone 251 (a corticosteroid 127), framycetin (an *antibiotic* 114) and gramicidin (an *antibiotic* 114)

Soframycin a product name for framycetin (an *antibiotic* 114)

sofra-Tulle a product name for framycetin (an *antibiotic* 114)

solifenacin a drug used in urinary disorders 154

Solugel a product name for benzoyl peroxide 204 (a drug for acne 165)

Solu-Medrol a product name for methyl-prednisolone 352 (a corticosteroid 127)

Soluver a product name for salicylic acid (a keratolytic for acne 165, dandruff 168, psoriasis 166, and warts)

Somatostatin a drug used in the management of esophageal variceal bleeding

somatropin a synthetic pituitary hormone 131

Soriatane a product name for acitretin (a drug for psoriasis 166)

sotalol 432 (a beta blocker 83)

Spiriva a product name for tiotropium 450 (a *bronchodilator* 76)

spironolactone 433 (a potassium-sparing diuretic 85)

Sporanox a product name for itraconazole (an antifungal 124)

Spriafil a product name for posaconazole (an antifungal 124)

Starlix a product name for nateglinide (a drug for diabetes 128)

stavudine an antiretroviral drug for HIV/AIDS 144

Stieva-A a product name for tretinoin (a drug for acne 165)

Stilamine a product name for somatostatin (a drug used in the management of esophageal variceal bleeding)

stilboestrol see diethylstilbestrol (a female sex hormone 133)

Strattera a product name for atomoxatine 196 (a drug for hyperactivity 72)

Streptase a product name for streptokinase 434 (a thrombolytic 91)

streptokinase 434 (a thrombolytic 91)

streptomycin an antituberculous drug 118 and aminoglycoside *antibiotic* 114

sucralfate 435 (an ulcer-healing drug 95)

Sudafed Decongestant 12 Hour a product name for pseudoephedrine 404 (a decongestant 79)

Sulcrate a product name for sucralfate 435 (an ulcer-healing drug 95)

SULFACETAMIDE–VERMOX

sulfacetamide a sulfonamide antibacterial 117
sulfadiazine a sulfonamide antibacterial 117
sulfamethoxazole a sulfonamide antibacterial 117 combined with trimethoprim 457 in co-trimoxazole 245
sulfasalazine 436 (a drug for inflammatory bowel disease 98 and an antirheumatic 103)
sulfinpyrazone a drug for gout 105
sulindac a non-steroidal anti-inflammatory 102
sumatriptan 437 (a drug for migraine 73)
Supeudol a product name for oxycodone (an opioid analgesic 64)
Suprax a product name for cefixime (a cephalosporin antibiotic 114)
Suprefact a product name for buserelin (a drug for menstrual disorders 148)
Suprefact Depo a product name for buserelin (a drug used in the treatment of menstrual disorders 148)
Surgam a product name for tiaprofenic acid (a non-steroidal anti-inflammatory 102)
Surgam SR a product name for tiaprofenic acid (a non-steroidal anti-inflammatory 102)
Surmontil a product name for trimipramine (a tricyclic antidepressant 68)
Sustiva a product name for efavirenz 269 (a drug for HIV and immune deficiency 144)
Symbicort Turbuhaler a product name for a combination of formoterol 292 (a bronchodilator 76) and budesonide 211 (a corticosteroid 127)
Symmetrel a product name for amantadine 185 (an antiviral 119 and drug for parkinsonism 71)
Synagis a product name for palivizumab (an antiviral drug 119)
Synalar a product name for fluocinolon (a topical corticosteroid 162)
Synarel a product name for nafarelin (a drug for menstrual disorders 148)
Synphasic a product-name oral contraceptive 149 containing ethinyl estradiol 278 (an estrogen 133) and norethindrone 371 (a progestin 133)
Synthroid a product name for levothyroxine 329 (a thyroid hormone 130)

T

222 Tablets a combination product containing codeine 242 (an opioid analgesic 64) and caffeine.
282/292 Tablets a combination product containing codeine 242 (an opioid analgesic 64) and caffeine.
282 MEP C8 a combination product containing codeine 242 (an opioid analgesic 64) and caffeine.
tacrolimus an immunosuppressant 143
tadalafil a drug used for the treatment of sexual impotence 152
Talwin a product name for pentazocine (an opioid analgesic 64)
Tambocor a product name for flecainide (an anti-arrhythmic 86)

Tamiflu a product name for oseltamavir 379 (an antiviral drug 119)
Tamofen a product name for tamoxifen 438 (an anticancer drug 140)
tamoxifen 438 (an anticancer drug 140)
tamsulosin 439 (an alpha-blocking drug for prostate disorders 134)
Tapazole a product name for methimazole (an antithyroid drug 130)
Tardan a combination of triclosan (a topical antimicrobial 161), coal tar, and salicyclic acid
Tarka a product name for verapamil 462 (an antihypertensive 88 and calcium channel blocker 87) and trandolapril (an antihypertensive and an ACE inhibitor 88)
Taro-Sone a product name for betamethasone 206 (a corticosteroid 127)
Taxol a product name for paclitaxel (an anticancer drug 140)
Taxotere a product name for docetaxel (an anticancer drug 140)
Tazidime a product name for ceftazidime (a cephalosporin antibiotic 114)
tazarotene a retinoid (see vitamin A 479) for psoriasis 166
tazobactam an antibiotic 114
Tazocin a product name for piperacillin (an antibiotic 114) with tazobactam (a substance that increases the effectiveness of piperacillin)
Tazorac a product name for tazarotene (a retinoid (see vitamin A 479) for psoriasis 166)
Tears Naturale a product-name artificial tear preparation containing hydroxypropylmethylcellulose
Tebrazid a product name for pyrazinamide (an antituberculous drug 118)
Tegretol a product name for carbamazepine 217 (an anticonvulsant 70)
telbivudine an antiviral drug 119
telithromycin an antibiotic 114
telmisartan a vasodilator 84 and an antihypertensive drug 88
Telzir a product name for fosamprenavir (a drug for HIV/AIDS 144)
temazepam 440 (a benzodiazepine sleeping drug 66)
Tempra a product name for acetaminophen 177 (an analgesic 64)
tenecteplase 441 (a thrombolytic drug 91)
tenofovir a drug for HIV/AIDS 144
Tenoretic a product name product with a combination of chlorthalidone (a thiazide diuretic 85) and atenolol 195 (a beta blocker 83)
Tenormin a product name for atenolol 195 (a beta blocker 83)
tenoxicam a non-steroidal anti-inflammatory 102
Tequin a product name for gatifloxacin 296 (an antibacterial drug 117)
Terazol a product name for terconazole (an antifungal 124)
terazosin 442 (a sympatholytic antihypertensive 88)
terbinafine 443 (an antifungal 124)

terbutaline 444 (a sympathomimetic bronchodilator 76 and uterine muscle relaxant 153)
terconazole an antifungal drug 124
teriparatide 445 (a drug used in osteoporosis 108)
Tersaseptic a product name for triclosan (a topical antimicrobial 161)
testosterone 446 (a male sex hormone 132)
tetracaine also known as amethocain, a local anesthetic 64
tetracycline 447 (an antibiotic 114 and antimalarial 123)
Theolair a product name for theophylline 448 (a bronchodilator 76)
theophylline 448 (a bronchodilator 76)
thiamine 479 (a vitamin 135)
thiopental a fast-acting barbiturate used to induce general anesthesia
thiothixene an antipsychotic 69
Tiamol a product name for fluocinonide (a topical corticosteroid 162)
tiaprofenic acid a non-steroidal anti-inflammatory 102
Tiazac a product name for diltiazem 257 (an antihypertensive 88 and calcium channel blocker 87)
ticarcillin an antibiotic 114
tigecycline an antibiotic 114
Tilade a product name for nedocromil (a drug for asthma 77)
timolol 449 (a beta blocker 83 and drug for glaucoma 156)
Timoptic a product name for timolol 449 (a beta blocker 83 and drug for glaucoma 156)
Timoptic-XE a product name for timolol 449 (a beta blocker 83 and drug for glaucoma 156)
tinidazole an antibacterial 117 and antiprotozoal 122
tinzaparin 305 (an anticoagulant 91)
tiotropium 450 (a bronchodilator 76)
tipranavir an antiretroviral drug used in the treatment of HIV and AIDS 144
titanium dioxide an ingredient of sunscreens 169
tizanidine 451 (an antispastic agent 106)
TNKase a product name for tenecteplase 441 (a thrombolytic drug 91)
TOBI a product name for tobramycin (an antibiotic 114)
Tobradex a combination of dexamethasone 251 (a corticosteroid 127) and tobramycin (an antibiotic 114)
tobramycin an aminoglycoside antibiotic 114
tocopherol vitamin E 481 (a vitamin 135)
tocopheryl acetate vitamin E 481 (a vitamin 135)
Tofranil a product name for imipramine 311 (a tricyclic antidepressant 68)
tolnaftate an antifungal 124
tolterodine 452 (an anticholinergic and antispasmodic for urinary disorders 154)
Topamax a product name for topiramate 453 (an anticonvulsant 70, a drug for migraine 73)

Topicort a product name for desoximetasone (a *topical* corticosteroid 162)

topiramate 453 (an anticonvulsant 70, a drug for migraine 73)

Topsyn a product name for fluocinonide (a *topical* corticosteroid 162)

Tramacet a combination product containing tramadol 454 (an opioid analgesic 64) with acetaminophen 177 (an analgesic 64)

tramadol 454 (an opioid analgesic 64)

tranexamic acid an antifibrinolytic used to promote blood clotting 90

Transderm-Nitro a product name for nitroglycerin 370 (an anti-angina drug 87)

Trans-Plantar a product name for salicylic acid (a keratolytic for acne 165, dandruff 168, psoriasis 166, and warts)

Trans Ver Sal a product name for salicylic acid (a keratolytic for acne 165, dandruff 168, psoriasis 166, and warts)

tranylcypromine an MAOI antidepressant 68

trastuzumab an anticancer drug 140

Travatan a product name for travoprost (a drug for glaucoma 156)

travoprost a drug for glaucoma 156

trazodone an antidepressant 68

Trelstar a product name for triptorelin (a drug for menstrual disorders 148)

Trental a product name for pentoxifylline (a *vasodilator* 98)

tretinoin a drug for acne 165

triamcinolone a corticosteroid 127

Triaderm a product name for triamcinolone (a corticosteroid 127)

Triaminic Pediatric Oral Cold Drops a product name for pseudoephedrine 404 (a decongestant 79)

triamterene 455 (a potassium-sparing diuretic 85)

Triatec-8 a combination product containing codeine 242 (an opioid analgesic 64) with acetaminophen 177 (an analgesic 64), and caffeine.

Triatec-30 a combination product containing codeine 242 (an opioid analgesic 64) with acetaminophen 177 (an analgesic 64).

Triavil a product name for a combination drug containing amitriptyline 188 (a tricyclic antidepressant 68) and perphenazine (a phenothiazine antipsychotic)

triclosan a *topical* antimicrobial 161

Tridural a product name for tramadol 454 (an opioid analgesic 64)

trifluoperazine 456 (a phenothiazine antipsychotic 69)

trifluridine an antiviral drug 119

Trilafon a product name for perphenazine (a phenothiazine antipsychotic 69)

Trileptal a product name for oxcarbazepine (an anticonvulsant 70)

trimeprazine an antihistamine 124

trimethoprim 457 (an antibacterial 117)

trimipramine a tricyclic antidepressant 68

Trinalin a combination of azatadine (an antihistamine 110) and pseudoephedrine 404 (a decongestant 79)

Triphasil a product name for an oral contraceptive containing levonorgestrel 328 (a progestin 133 and oral contraceptive 149) and ethinyl estradiol 278 (an estrogen 133)

triptorelin a drug for menstrual disorders 148

tropicamide a mydriatic 158

Trosec a product name for trospium (a drug used in urinary disorders 154)

trospium a drug used in urinary disorders 154

Trusopt a product name for dorzolamide 265 (a carbonic anhydrase inhibitor for glaucoma 156)

Truvada a product name combination of emtricitabine and tenofovir (drugs used for HIV and AIDS 144)

tryptophan an antidepressant 68

T-Stat a combination of erythromycin 274 (an *antibiotic* 114) and ethyl alcohol

Tussionex a combination product with hydrocodone 307 (an opioid cough supressant 80) and phenyltoloxamine (an antihistamine 110)

Tygacil a product name for tigecycline (an antibiotic 114)

Tylenol a product name for acetaminophen 177 (an analgesic 64)

Tylenol Allergy Sinus a combination product with pseudoephedrine 404 (a decongestant 79), acetaminophen 177 (an analgesic 64), and chlorpheniramine 225 (an antihistamine 110)

Tylenol Cold Suspension Children's a combination product containing pseudoephedrine 404 (a decongestant 79), acetaminophen 177 (an analgesic 64), and chlorpheniramine 225 (an antihistamine 110)

Tylenol Elixir with Codeine a combination product containing codeine 242 (an opioid analgesic 64) with acetaminophen 177 (an analgesic 64)

Tylenol No. 1 a combination product containing codeine 242 (an opioid analgesic 64) with acetaminophen 177 (an analgesic 64), and caffeine

Tylenol No.1 Forte a combination product containing codeine 242 (an opioid analgesic 64) with acetaminophen 177 (an analgesic 64), and caffeine

Tylenol No. 2 with Codeine a combination product containing codeine 242 (an opioid analgesic 64) with acetaminophen 177 (an analgesic 64), and caffeine

Tylenol No. 4 with Codeine a combination product containing codeine 242 (an opioid analgesic 64) with acetaminophen 177 (an analgesic 64)

U

Ultradol a product name for etodolac (a non-steroidal anti-inflammatory drug 102)

Ultramop capsules a product name for methoxsalen (a drug used in the treatment of psoriasis (166) and atopic dermatitis)

Ultramop lotion a product name for methoxsalen (a drug used in the treatment of psoriasis (166) and atopic dermatitis)

Uniphyl a product name for theophylline 448 (a *bronchodilator* 76)

Unisom a product name for diphenhydramine 259 (an antihistamine 110, anti-emetic 74, and antipruritic 161)

Unisom-2 a product name for doxylamine succinate (a drug used to aid sleep 66, and an antihistamine 110)

Urispas a product name for flavoxate (a urinary *antispasmodic* 154)

urofollitropin a drug for pituitary disorders 147

Uromax a product name for oxybutynin 381 (a drug used in urinary disorders 154)

Urso a product name for ursodiol (a drug for cholestatic liver disease 100)

ursodeoxycholic acid a substance present in bile used to treat gallstones 100

Ursodiol a drug for cholestatic liver disease 100

V

Vagifem a product name for estradiol 276 (an estrogen 135)

valacyclovir an antiviral 119

Valcyte a product name for valganciclovir (an antiviral 144 used for cytomegalovirus)

valganciclovir an antiviral 144 used for cytomegalovirus

Valisone a product name for betamethasone 206 (a corticosteroid 127)

Valium Roche Oral a product name for diazepam 253 (a benzodiazepine anti-anxiety drug 67, sedative 64, muscle relaxant 106, and anticonvulsant 70)

valproic acid 458 (an anticonvulsant 70)

valsartan 459 (a vasodilator 84 and antihypertensive drug 88)

Valtrex a product name for valacyclovir (an antiviral 119)

Vancocin a product name for vancomycin (an *antibiotic* 114)

vancomycin an *antibiotic* 114

vardenafil a drug used for the treatment of sexual impotence 152

varenicline 460 (a drug used in smoking cessation)

Vasotec a product name for enalapril 270 (a *vasodilator* 84 and anti-hypertensive 88)

venlafaxine 461 (an antidepressant 68)

Ventodisks a product name for salbutamol 424 (a *bronchodilator* 76)

Ventolin a product name for salbutamol 424 (a *bronchodilator* 76)

Vepesid a product name for etoposide (an anticancer drug 140)

Veramil a product name for verapamil 462 (an antihypertensive 88 and calcium channel blocker 87)

verapamil 462 (an antihypertensive 88 and calcium channel blocker 87)

Vermox a product name for mebendazole (an anthelmintic 125)

VESANOID–ZYVOXAM

Vesanoid a product name for tretinoin (a drug for acne 165)

Vesicare a product name for solifenacin (a drug used for urinary disorders 154)

Vfend a product name for variconazole (an antifungal drug 124)

Viaderm-K.C. a product name combination of nystatin 373 (an antifungal 124), gramicidin and neomycin sulfate (both *antibiotic*s 114), and triamcinolone acetonide (a corticosteroid 127)

Viagra a product name for sildenafil 429 (a drug for impotence 134, 152)

Vibramycin a product name for doxycycline 268 (a tetracycline *antibiotic* 114)

Vibramycin-D a product name for doxycycline 268 (a tetracycline *antibiotic* 114)

Vibra-Tabs a product name for doxycycline 268 (a tetracycline *antibiotic* 114)

Videx a product name for didanosine (an antiretroviral drug used in the treatment of HIV infection and AIDS 144)

vigabatrin an anticonvulsant 70

Vigamox a product name for moxifloxacin 365 (an antibacterial 117)

vinblastine a drug used in cancer treatment 140

vincristine a drug used in cancer treatment 140

Vioform Hydrocortisone a product name combination of clioquinol (an antibacterial 117 and antifungal 124) and hydrocortisone 308 (a corticosteroid 127)

Virazole a product name for ribivirin (an antiviral 119)

Viread a product name for tenofovir (a drug for HIV/AIDS 144)

Viroptic a product name for trifluridine (an antiviral 119)

Visine Workplace Eye Drops a product name product containing oxymetazoline (a *topical* decongestant 79)

vitamin A 479 (a vitamin 135)

Vitamin A Acid a product name for tretinoin (a drug for acne 165)

vitamin B complex (see vitamins 135)

vitamin B1 another name for thiamine 479 (a vitamin 135)

vitamin B2 another name for riboflavin 477 (a vitamin 135)

vitamin B6 another name for pyridoxine 477 (a vitamin 135)

vitamin B12 480 (a vitamin 135)

vitamin C another name for ascorbic acid 480 (a vitamin 135)

vitamin D 481 (a vitamin 135)

vitamin E 481 (a vitamin 135)

vitamin K 482 (a vitamin 135)

Voltaren a product name for diclonefac 254 (a non-steroidal anti-inflammatory 102)

Voltaren Ophtha a product name for diclonefac 254 (a non-steroidal anti-inflammatory 102 used as eye drops)

voriconazole an antifungal drug 124

W

warfarin 463 (an anticoagulant 90)

Wellbutrin SR a product name for bupropion 213 (an antidepressant 68 used as an aid when stopping smoking in addition to counselling)

Westcort a product name for hydrocortisone 308 (a corticosteroid 127 and antipruritic 161)

X

Xalatan a product name for latanoprost 325 (a drug for glaucoma 156)

Xanax a product name for alprazolam 182 (a benzodiazepine anti-anxiety drug 67)

Xanax TS a product name for alprazolam 182 (a benzodiazepine anti-anxiety drug 67)

Xatral a product name for alfuzosin (an alpha-adrenergic blocker for prostate disorders 148)

Xenical a product name for orlistat 377 (a drug that blocks the action of enzymes that digest fats)

Xolair a product name for omalizumab (a monoclonal antibody 140)

Xylocaine a product name for lidocaine (a local *anesthetic* 64)

Xylocaine Jelly 2% a product name for lidocaine (a local *anesthetic* 64 and anti-arrhythmic 86)

Xylocaine Parenteral with Epinephrine a product name for a combination of epinephrine 272 and lidocaine (a local *anesthetic*)

Xylocard a product name for lidocaine (a local *anesthetic* 64 and anti-arrhythmic 86)

xylometazoline 464 (a *topical* decongestant 79)

Y

Yasmin a product name for oral contraceptive 149 containing drospirenone (a progestin 151) and ethinyl estradiol 278 (an estrogen 133)

Z

Zaditen a product name for ketotifen (a drug used to prevent asthma 77)

zafirlukast a leukotriene antagonist for asthma 77

Zanaflex a product name for tizanidine 451 (a muscle relaxant 106)

zanamivir 465 (an antiviral drug 119)

Zantac a product name for ranitidine 413 (an anti-ulcer drug 95)

Zarontin a product name for ethosuximide (an anticonvulsant 70)

ZeaSorb AF a product name for tolnaftate (an antifungal 124)

Zenapax a product name for daclizumab (an immunosuppressant 142)

Zestoretic a product name for lisinopril 330 (an ACE inhibitor 98) and hydrochlorothiazide 306 (a diuretic 101)

Zestril a product name for lisinopril 330 (an ACE inhibitor 98)

zidovudine (AZT) 466 (an antiretroviral for HIV infection and AIDS 144)

zinc 482 (a mineral 137)

Zincofax a product name for zinc oxide (a soothing agent 163)

zinc oxide a soothing agent 163

zinc pyrithione an antimicrobial with antibacterial 117 and antifungal properties used for dandruff

zinc sulfate zinc 482 (a mineral 137)

Zithromax a product name for azithromycin 201 (an *antibiotic* 114)

Zocor a product name for simvastatin 430 (a lipid-lowering drug 89))

Zofran a product name for ondansetron 376 (an anti-emetic 74)

Zofran ODT a product name for ondansetron 376 (an anti-emetic 74)

Zoladex a product name for goserelin 303 (a female sex hormone 133 and anticancer drug 140)

Zoladex LA a product name for goserelin 303 (a female sex hormone 133 and anticancer drug 140)

zoledronic acid a drug for treatment of bone disorders 108

zolmitriptan a drug for migraine 73

Zoloft a product name for sertraline 427 (an antidepressant 68)

Zomig a product name for zolmiptran (a drug for migraine 73)

Zomig Rapimelt a product name for zolmiptran (a drug for migraine 73)

Zopiclone 467 (a sleeping drug 66)

Zovirax a product name for acyclovir 178 (an antiviral 119)

Z-PAK a product name for azithromycin 201 (an *antibiotic* 114)

Zuclopenthixol an antipsychotic 69

Zyban a product name for bupropion 213 (an antidepressant 68 used as an aid when stopping smoking in addition to counselling)

Zyloprim a product name for allopurinol 181 (a drug for gout 105)

Zyprexa a product name for olanzapine 374 (an antipsychotic 69)

Zyprexa Zydis a product name for olanzapine 374 (an antipsychotic 69)

Zytram a product name for tramadol 454 (an opioid analgesic 64)

Zyvoxam a product name for linezolid (an *antibiotic* 114)

PART

3

MAJOR DRUG GROUPS

BRAIN AND NERVOUS SYSTEM
RESPIRATORY SYSTEM
HEART AND CIRCULATION
GASTROINTESTINAL TRACT
MUSCLES, BONES, AND JOINTS
ALLERGY
INFECTIONS AND INFESTATIONS
HORMONES AND ENDOCRINE SYSTEM
NUTRITION
MALIGNANT AND IMMUNE DISEASE
REPRODUCTIVE AND URINARY TRACTS
EYES AND EARS
SKIN

BRAIN AND NERVOUS SYSTEM

The human brain contains over 100 billion nerve cells (neurons). These nerve cells receive electrochemical impulses from everywhere in the body. They interpret these impulses and send responsive signals back to various glands and muscles. The brain functions continuously as a switchboard for the human communications system. At the same time, it serves as the seat of emotions and mood, of memory, personality, and thought. Extending from the brain is an additional cluster of nerve cells that forms the spinal cord. Together, these two elements comprise the central nervous system.

Radiating from the central nervous system is the peripheral nervous system, which has three parts. One branches off the spinal cord and extends to skin and muscles throughout the body. Another, in the head, links the brain to the eyes, ears, nose, and taste buds. The third is a semi-independent network called the autonomic, or involuntary, nervous system. This is the part of the nervous system that controls unconscious body functions such as breathing, digestion, and glandular activity (see facing page).

Signals traverse the nervous system by electrical and chemical means. Electrical impulses carry signals from one end of a neuron to the other. To cross the gap between neurons, chemical *neurotransmitters* are released from one cell to bind on to the *receptor* sites of nearby cells. *Excitatory* transmitters stimulate action; *inhibitory* transmitters reduce it.

What can go wrong

Disorders of the brain and nervous system may manifest as illnesses that show themselves as physical impairments, such as epilepsy or strokes, or as mental and emotional impairments (for example, schizophrenia or depression).

Illnesses causing physical impairments can result from different types of disorder of the brain and nervous system. Death of nerve cells resulting from poor circulation can result in paralysis, while electrical disturbances of certain nerve cells cause the fits of epilepsy. Temporary changes in blood circulation within and around the brain are thought to cause migraine. Parkinson's disease is caused by a lack of dopamine, a neurotransmitter that is produced by specialized brain cells.

The causes of disorders that trigger mental and emotional impairment are not known, but these illnesses are thought to result from the defective functioning of nerve cells and neurotransmitters. The nerve cells may be underactive, overactive, or poorly coordinated. Alternatively, mental and

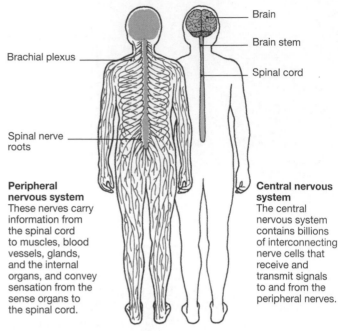

Peripheral nervous system
These nerves carry information from the spinal cord to muscles, blood vessels, glands, and the internal organs, and convey sensation from the sense organs to the spinal cord.

Central nervous system
The central nervous system contains billions of interconnecting nerve cells that receive and transmit signals to and from the peripheral nerves.

How nerve signals are transmitted
A nerve signal is an electrical impulse produced by chemical reactions on the surface of the cell body of a neuron (nerve cell). The signal is transmitted by a neurotransmitter, released from the ends of a nerve fibre, that binds to a receptor on the neighbouring cell body. This, in turn, transmits the signal to another neuron or triggers a response in a muscle or organ.

emotional impairment may be due to too much or too little neurotransmitter in one area of the brain.

Why drugs are used

By and large, the drugs described in this section do not eliminate nervous system disorders. Their function is to correct or modify the communication of the signals that traverse the nervous system. By doing so they can relieve symptoms or restore normal functioning and behaviour. In some cases, such as anxiety and insomnia, drugs are used to

AUTONOMIC NERVOUS SYSTEM

The autonomic, or involuntary, nervous system governs the actions of the muscles of the organs and glands. Such vital functions as heart beat, salivation, and digestion continue without conscious direction, whether we are awake or asleep.

The autonomic system is divided into two parts, the effects of one generally balancing those of the other. The *sympathetic* nervous system has an *excitatory* effect. It widens the airways to the lungs, for example, and increases the flow of blood to the arms and legs. The *parasympathetic* system, by contrast, has an opposing effect. It slows the heart rate and redirects blood from the limbs to the gut.

Although the functional pace of most organs results from the interplay between the two systems, the muscles surrounding the blood vessels respond only to the signals of the sympathetic system. Whether a vessel is dilated or constricted is determined by the relative stimulation of two sets of receptor sites: alpha sites and beta sites.

Neurotransmitters

The parasympathetic nervous system depends on the neurotransmitter acetylcholine to transmit signals from one cell to another. The sympathetic nervous system relies on adrenaline and noradrenaline, products of the adrenal glands and neurons that act as both hormones and neurotransmitters.

Drugs that act on the sympathetic nervous system

The drugs that stimulate the sympathetic nervous system are called adrenergics (or sympathomimetics, see chart). They either promote the release of adrenaline and noradrenaline or mimic their effects. Drugs that interfere with the action of the sympathetic nervous system are called sympatholytics. Alpha blockers act on alpha receptors; beta blockers act on beta receptors (see also Beta blockers, p.83).

Drugs that act on the parasympathetic nervous system

Drugs that stimulate the parasympathetic nervous system are called cholinergics (or parasympathomimetics), and drugs that oppose its action are called anticholinergics. Many prescribed drugs have anticholinergic properties (see chart, right).

Effects of stimulation of the autonomic nervous system

	Sympathetic	Parasympathetic
Heart	The rate and strength of the heart beat are increased.	The rate and strength of the heart beat are reduced.
Blood vessels in skin	These are constricted by stimulation of alpha receptors.	No effect.
Pupils	The pupils are dilated.	The pupils are constricted.
Airways	The bronchial muscles relax and widen the airways.	The bronchial muscles contract and narrow the airways.
Intestines	Activity of the muscles of the intestinal wall is reduced.	Activity of the muscles of the intestinal wall is increased.
Bladder	The bladder wall relaxes and the sphincter muscle contracts.	The bladder wall contracts and the sphincter muscle relaxes.
Salivary glands	Secretion of thick saliva increases.	Secretion of watery saliva increases.
Pancreas	Insulin secretion is increased (beta receptors) or reduced (alpha receptors).	Insulin secretion is increased.

Drugs that act on the autonomic nervous system

	Sympathetic	Parasympathetic
Stimulated by		
Natural neurotransmitters	Epinephrine (adrenaline) Norepinephrine (noradrenaline)	Acetylcholine
Drugs	Adrenergic drugs (including alpha agonists, beta agonists) Sympathomimetics	Cholinergic drugs Parasympathomimetics
Blocked by		
Drugs	Alpha blockers (antagonists) Beta blockers (antagonists)	Anticholinergic drugs

lower the level of activity in the brain. In other disorders – depression, for example – drugs are given to encourage the opposite effect, increasing the level of activity.

Drugs that act on the nervous system are also used for conditions that outwardly have nothing to do with nervous system disorders. Migraine headaches, for example, are often treated with drugs that cause the autonomic nervous system to send out signals constricting the dilated blood vessels that cause the migraine.

MAJOR DRUG GROUPS

Analgesics
Sleeping drugs
Anti-anxiety drugs
Antidepressant drugs
Antipsychotic drugs
Anticonvulsant drugs

Drugs for parkinsonism
Drugs for dementia
Nervous system stimulants
Drugs for migraine
Anti-emetics
Anti-vertigo

ANALGESICS

Analgesics are drugs that relieve pain. Pain is not a disease but a symptom, long-term relief depends on treatment of the underlying cause. For example, toothache can be relieved by drugs but can be cured only by appropriate dental treatment. If the underlying disorder is irreversible, such as some rheumatic conditions, long-term analgesic treatment may be necessary.

Damage to body tissues as a result of disease or injury is detected by nerve endings that transmit signals to the brain. The interpretation of these sensations can be affected by the psychological state of the individual, so that pain is worsened by anxiety and fear, for example. Often a reassuring explanation of the cause of discomfort makes pain easier to bear and may even relieve it altogether. Anti-anxiety drugs (see p.67) are helpful when pain is accompanied by anxiety, and some of these drugs are also used to reduce painful muscle spasms. Antidepressant drugs (see p.68) act to block the transmission of impulses signalling pain and are particularly useful for nerve pains (neuralgia), which do not always respond to analgesics. Other medications used to treat nerve pains include anticonvulsant drugs (see p.70) like valproic acid, gabapentin, or pregabalin.

Types of analgesics

Analgesics are divided into the opioids (with similar properties to drugs derived from opium, such as morphine) and non-opioids. Non-opioids include all the other analgesics, including acetaminophen and non-steroidal anti-inflammatory drugs (NSAIDs), the most well known of which is ASA. Non-opioids are less powerful painkillers than opioids. Local anesthetics are also used to relieve pain (see below).

Opioid drugs and acetaminophen act directly on the brain and spinal cord to alter the perception of pain. Opioids act like the endorphins, hormones naturally produced in the brain that stop the cell-to-cell transmission of pain sensation. NSAIDs prevent stimulation of the nerve endings at the site of the pain and also act centrally.

When pain is treated under medical supervision, it is common to start with acetaminophen or an NSAID; if neither provides adequate pain relief, they may be combined. A mild opioid (for example, codeine) may also be used. If the less powerful drugs are ineffective, a strong opioid such as morphine may be given. As there is now a wide variety of oral analgesic formulations, injections are seldom necessary to control even the most severe pain.

When treating pain with an over-the-counter preparation, for example, taking ASA for a headache, you should seek medical advice if pain persists for longer than 48 hours, recurs, or is worse or different from previous pain.

Non-opioid analgesics

Acetaminophen

This analgesic is believed to act by reducing the production of chemicals called prostaglandins in the brain. It does not affect prostaglandin production in the rest of the body, so it does not reduce inflammation, although it can reduce fever. Acetaminophen can be used for everyday aches and pains, such as headaches and joint pains. It is given as a liquid to treat pain and reduce fever in children.

As well as being the most widely used analgesic, it is one of the safest when taken correctly. It does not usually irritate the stomach and allergic reactions are rare. However, an overdose can cause severe and possibly fatal liver or kidney damage.

SITES OF ACTION

Acetaminophen and the opioid drugs act on the brain and spinal cord to reduce pain perception. Non-steroidal anti-inflammatory drugs (NSAIDs) act at the site of pain to prevent the stimulation of nerve endings and on the spinal cord to decrease pain perception.

Acetaminophen and the opioid drugs act on the brain and spinal cord

NSAIDs act at the site of pain

NSAIDs AND DIGESTIVE TRACT IRRITATION

NSAIDs can cause irritation, even ulceration and bleeding, of the stomach and duodenum, so they are best taken after a meal. NSAIDs are not usually given to people with stomach ulcers. An NSAID may be combined with an anti-ulcer drug (see p.111). Alternatively, a COX-2 selective inhibitor may be used.

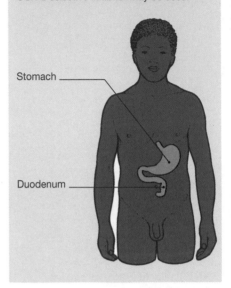

Stomach

Duodenum

Its toxic potential may be increased in heavy drinkers or those who are malnourished.

Non-steroidal anti-inflammatory drugs (NSAIDs): ASA (acetylsalicylic acid)
Used for many years to relieve pain and reduce fever, ASA also acts to reduce inflammation by blocking the production of prostaglandins, which contribute to the swelling and pain in inflamed tissue (see Action of analgesics, facing page). ASA is useful for headaches, toothaches, mild rheumatic pain, sore throat, and discomfort caused by feverish illnesses. Given regularly, it can also relieve the pain and inflammation of chronic rheumatoid arthritis (see Antirheumatic drugs, p.103).

LOCAL ANESTHETICS

These drugs are used to prevent pain, usually in minor surgical procedures, for example, dental treatment and stitching cuts. They can also be injected into the space around the spinal cord to numb the lower half of the body. This is called spinal or epidural anesthesia and can be used for some major operations in people who are not fit for a general anesthetic. Epidural anesthesia is also used during childbirth.

Local anesthetics block the passage of nerve impulses at the site of administration, deadening all feeling conveyed by the nerves they come into contact with. They do not, however, interfere with consciousness. Local anesthetics are usually given by injection, but they can also be applied to the skin, the mouth and other areas lined with mucous membrane (such as the vagina), or the eye to relieve pain. Some local anesthetics are formulated for injection together with epinephrine (adrenaline). Epinephrine constricts the blood vessels and prevents the local anesthetic from being removed. This action prolongs the anesthetic's effect.

Local anesthetic creams are often used to numb the skin before injections in children and people with a fear of needles.

ASA is found in combination with other substances in a variety of medicines (see Cold cures, p.80). It is also used in some individuals to prevent heart attacks and stroke since ASA helps to prevent abnormal clotting of blood (see Drugs that affect blood clotting, p.90). For this reason, it is not suitable for people whose blood does not clot normally.

ASA in the form of soluble tablets, dissolved in water before being taken, is absorbed into the bloodstream more quickly, thereby relieving pain faster than tablets. Soluble ASA is not, however, less irritating to the stomach lining.

ASA is available in many forms, all of which have a similar effect, but because the amount of ASA in a tablet of each type varies, it is important to read the package for the correct dosage. It is not recommended for children aged under 16 years with flu-like symptoms because its use has been linked to Reye's syndrome, which is a very rare but potentially fatal liver and brain disorder.

Other non-steroidal anti-inflammatory drugs (NSAIDs)

These drugs can relieve both pain and inflammation. NSAIDs are related to ASA and also work by blocking the production of *prostaglandins* in the brain. They are most commonly used to treat muscle and joint pain and may also be prescribed for other types of pain including menstrual pain. For further information on these drugs, see p.102.

Combined analgesics

Mild opioids, such as codeine, are often found in combination preparations with non-opioids, such as acetaminophen or NSAIDs. These mixtures may add the advantages of analgesics that act on the brain to the benefits of those acting at the site of pain. Another advantage of combining analgesics is that the reductions in dose of the components may reduce the side effects of the preparation. Combinations can be helpful in reducing the number of tablets taken during long-term treatment.

Opioid analgesics

These drugs are related to opium, an extract of poppy seeds. They act directly on several sites in the central nervous system to block the transmission of pain signals (see Action of analgesics, above). Because they act directly on the parts of the brain where pain is perceived, opioids are the strongest analgesics and are therefore used to treat the pain arising from surgery, serious injury, and cancer. These drugs are particularly valuable for relieving severe pain during terminal illnesses. In addition, their ability to produce a state of relaxation and euphoria is often of help in relieving the stress that accompanies severe pain.

ACTION OF ANALGESICS

Cause of pain
Damage to tissue (due to injury or infection, for example) leads to the production of chemicals, called prostaglandins, which act on nerve endings so that a signal is passed along a series of nerve cells to the brain, where the signal is interpreted as pain by brain cells.

Brain

Pain signal

Nerve ending

Brain cells

Prostaglandins

Damaged cell

Pain signal received by brain cell and interpreted

Action of non-opioids
These drugs block production of prostaglandins. As a result, the nerve endings cannot be stimulated, so no pain signal passes to the brain.

Opioid

Opioid receptor

Pain signal blocked

Action of opioids
Normally the pain signal is transmitted between brain cells. Opioids combine with receptors on brain cells (opioid receptors), blocking transmission of pain signals within the brain and also in the spinal cord.

Brain cell

Morphine is the best known of the opioid analgesics. Others include oxycodone and meperidine. The use of these powerful opioids is strictly controlled because they produce feelings of euphoria, which can lead to abuse and addiction. However, when these powerful opioids are given under medical supervision to treat severe pain, the risk of addiction is negligible.

Opioid analgesics may prevent clear thought and cloud consciousness. Other possible adverse effects include nausea, vomiting, constipation, drowsiness, and depressed breathing. When they are taken in overdose, these drugs may induce a deep coma and lead to fatal breathing difficulties.

In addition to the powerful opioids, there are some less powerful analgesics in this group that are used to relieve mild to moderate pain. They include hydrocodone, codeine, and diphenoxylate. Their normally unwanted side effects of depressing respiration and causing constipation make them useful as cough suppressants (p.80) and as anti-diarrheal drugs (p.96).

COMMON DRUGS

Opioids	NSAIDs (see p.102)
Cannabis Sativa	ASA ✳
Extract	Diclofenac ✳
(Cannabidiol,	Etodolac
Delta-9-tetrahydro-	Flurbiprofen
cannabinol)	Ibuprofen ✳
Codeine ✳	Indomethacin
Fentanyl ✳	Ketoprofen ✳
Hydromorphone ✳	Ketorolac
Methadone ✳	Mefenamic acid ✳
Meperidine	Meloxicam ✳
Morphine ✳	Naproxen ✳
Oxycodone	Oxaprozin
Pentazocine	Piroxicam ✳
Tramadol ✳	
	Other non-opioids
Cox-2 Selective	Acetaminophen ✳
Inhibitor	
Celecoxib ✳	✳ See Part 4

SLEEPING DRUGS

Difficulty in getting to sleep or staying asleep (insomnia) has many causes. Most people suffer from sleepless nights from time to time, usually as a result of a temporary worry or discomfort from a minor illness. Persistent sleeplessness can be caused by psychological problems including anxiety or depression, or by pain arising from a physical disorder.

Why they are used

For occasional bouts of sleeplessness, simple, common remedies to promote relaxation – for example, taking a warm bath or a hot milk drink before bedtime – are usually the best form of treatment. Sleeping drugs (also known as hypnotics) are normally prescribed only when these self-help remedies have failed, and when lack of sleep is beginning to affect your general health. These drugs are used to re-establish the habit of sleeping. They should be used in the smallest dose and for the shortest possible time (not more than three weeks). It is best not to use sleeping tablets every night (see Risks and precautions). Do not use alcohol to get to sleep as it can cause disturbed sleep and insomnia. Long-term treatment of sleeplessness depends on resolving the underlying cause of the problem.

How they work

Most sleeping drugs promote sleep by depressing brain function. The drugs interfere with chemical activity in the brain and nervous system by reducing communication between nerve cells. This leads to reduced brain activity,

TYPES OF SLEEPING DRUGS

Benzodiazepines These are the most commonly used class of sleeping drugs as they have comparatively few *adverse effects* and are relatively safe in overdose. They are also used to treat anxiety (see facing page).

Chloral derivatives These drugs effectively promote sleep but are used little now.

Other non-benzodiazepine sleeping drugs Zopiclone works in a similar way to benzodiazepines. It is not intended for long-term use and withdrawal symptoms have been reported.

Antihistamines Widely used to treat allergic symptoms (see p.109), antihistamines such as diphenhydramine also cause drowsiness. They are sometimes used to promote sleep but can cause adverse effects and are not recommended in some individuals, including older people.

Antidepressant drugs Some of these drugs may be used to promote sleep in depressed people (see p.68), as well as being effective in treating underlying depressive illness.

allowing you to fall asleep more easily, but the nature of the sleep is affected by the drug. The main class of sleeping drugs, the benzodiazepines, is described on the facing page.

How they affect you

A sleeping drug rapidly produces drowsiness and slowed reactions. Some people find that the drug makes them appear to be drunk, their speech slurred, especially if they delay going to bed after taking their dose. Most people find they usually fall asleep within one hour of taking the drug.

Because the sleep induced by drugs is not the same as normal sleep, many people find they do not feel as well rested by it as by a night of natural sleep. This is the result of suppressed brain activity. Sleeping drugs also suppress the sleep

during which dreams occur; both dream sleep and non-dream sleep are essential for a good night's sleep (see The effects of drugs on sleep patterns, below).

Some people experience a variety of "hangover" effects the following day. Some benzodiazepines may produce minor side effects, such as daytime drowsiness, dizziness, and unsteadiness, that can impair the ability to drive or operate machinery. Elderly people are likely to become confused, and selection of an appropriate drug is important.

Risks and special precautions

Sleeping drugs become less effective after the first few nights and there may be a temptation to increase the dose. Apart from the antihistamines, most sleeping drugs can produce psychological and physical dependence (see p.23) when taken regularly for more than a few weeks, especially if they are taken in larger-than-normal doses.

When sleeping drugs are suddenly withdrawn, anxiety, convulsions, and hallucinations sometimes occur. Vivid dreams and nightmares may be a problem because the time spent in dream sleep increases. Sleeplessness will recur and may lead to a temptation to use the drugs again. Gradual withdrawal of these drugs is important. Anyone who wishes to stop taking sleeping drugs, particularly after prolonged use, should seek his or her physician's advice to prevent these withdrawal symptoms from occurring.

THE EFFECTS OF DRUGS ON SLEEP PATTERNS

Normal sleep can be divided into three types: light sleep, deep sleep, and dream sleep. The proportion of time spent in each type of sleep changes with age and is altered by sleeping drugs. Dramatic changes in sleep patterns also occur in the first few days following abrupt withdrawal of sleeping drugs after regular, prolonged use.

Normal sleep Young adults spend most sleep time in light sleep with roughly equal proportions of dream and deep sleep.

Drug-induced sleep has less dream sleep and less deep sleep with relatively more light sleep.

Sleep following drug withdrawal There is a marked increase in dream sleep following withdrawal of drugs used regularly for a long time.

- Dream sleep
- Deep sleep
- Light sleep

COMMON DRUGS

Benzodiazepines
Flurazepam
Lorazepam ✳
Nitrazepam ✳
Oxazepam ✳
Temazepam ✳
Triazolam

Chloral derivatives
Chloral hydrate

Other non-benzodiazepine sleeping drugs
Zopiclone ✳

✳ See Part 4

ANTI-ANXIETY DRUGS

A certain amount of stress can be beneficial, providing a stimulus to action. But too much will often result in anxiety, which might be described as fear or apprehension not caused by real danger.

Clinically, anxiety arises when the balance of certain chemicals in the brain is disturbed. The fearful feelings increase brain activity, stimulating the sympathetic nervous system (see p.63), and often triggering physical symptoms such as shaking, palpitations, and headaches.

Why they are used

Anti-anxiety drugs (also called anxiolytics) are prescribed for short-term relief of severe anxiety and nervousness caused by psychological problems. But these drugs cannot resolve the causes. Tackling the underlying problem through counselling and perhaps psychotherapy offers the best hope of a long-term solution. The drugs are also used to relax people before uncomfortable medical procedures.

There are several types of drugs for relieving anxiety: benzodiazepines, beta blockers, antidepressants and buspirone. Antidepressants, such as SSRIs (see p.68), are most widely used for generalized anxiety disorder, as are others such as venlafaxine and clomipramine. These are also helpful in other types of anxiety-related conditions such as obsessive-compulsive and panic disorders. Benzodiazepines are also effective, although these are more commonly used early on for a short period to promote relaxation. Their sedative effects also help relieve insomnia, which often accompanies anxiety (see also Sleeping drugs, opposite). Buspirone, a non-benzodiazepine drug, is also an option in generalized anxiety disorders. These drugs are commonly prescribed for people who feel excessively anxious in certain situations, such as interviews or public appearances.

How they work

Benzodiazepines and related drugs

These drugs depress activity in the part of the brain that controls emotion by promoting the action of the *neurotransmitter* gamma-aminobutyric acid (GABA) which binds to neurons, blocking transmission of electrical impulses and thus reducing communication between brain cells. Benzodiazepines increase the inhibitory effect of GABA on brain cells (see Action of benzodiazepines and related drugs, above), preventing the excessive brain activity that causes anxiety. Buspirone is different from other anti-anxiety drugs; it binds mainly to serotonin (another neurotransmitter) receptors and does not cause drowsiness. Its effect is not felt for at least two weeks after starting treatment.

Beta blockers

The physical symptoms of anxiety are produced by an increase in the activity

ACTION OF BENZODIAZEPINES AND RELATED DRUGS

Action on the brain
The reticular activating system (RAS) in the brain stem controls the level of mental activity by stimulating higher centres of the brain controlling consciousness. Benzodiazepines and related drugs depress the RAS, relieving anxiety. In larger doses they depress the RAS sufficiently to cause drowsiness and sleep.

Higher centres of brain

Stimulation of brain | RAS | Brain stem

GABA
GABA receptor
Brain cell
Benzo-diazepine
Benzo-diazepine receptor
Cell activity inhibited

Action on brain cells in the RAS
Brain cell activity is normally inhibited by GABA, a chemical that binds to specialized cell *receptors*. Brain cells also have receptors for benzodiazepines. The drug binds to its receptor and promotes the inhibitory effect of GABA, thereby depressing brain cell activity in the RAS.

of the sympathetic nervous system. Sympathetic nerve endings release a chemical transmitter called norepinephrine (noradrenaline) that stimulates the heart, digestive system, and other organs. Beta blockers block the action of noradrenaline in the body, reducing the physical symptoms of anxiety. For more information on beta blockers, see p.83.

How they affect you

Benzodiazepines and related drugs reduce feelings of restlessness and agitation, slow mental activity, and often produce drowsiness. They are said to reduce motivation and, if they are taken in large doses, may lead to apathy. They also have a relaxing effect on the muscles, and some benzodiazepines are used specifically for that purpose (see Muscle relaxants, p.106).

Minor *adverse effects* of these drugs include dizziness and forgetfulness. People who need to drive or operate potentially dangerous machinery should be aware that their reactions may be slowed. Because the brain soon becomes tolerant to, and dependent on, their effects, benzo-diazepines are usually effective for only a few weeks at a time.

Beta blockers reduce the physical symptoms associated with anxiety, which may promote greater mental calmness. As they do not cause drowsiness they are safer for people who need to drive.

Risks and special precautions

The benzodiazepines are safe for most people and are not likely to be fatal in overdose unless combined with alcohol and other substances. The main risk is psychological and physical dependence, especially for regular users or when larger-than-average doses have been used. For this reason, they are usually given for courses of two weeks or less. If used for a longer period, they should be withdrawn gradually under medical supervision. If they are stopped suddenly, withdrawal symptoms, such as excessive anxiety, nightmares, and restlessness, may occur.

Benzodiazepines have been abused for their sedative effect, and are therefore prescribed with caution for people with a history of drug or alcohol abuse.

COMMON DRUGS

Benzodiazepines
Alprazolam *
Chlordiazepoxide *
Clonazepam *
Diazepam *
Lorazepam *
Oxazepam *

Other
Buspirone *

Beta blockers
Atenolol *
Metoprolol *
Propranolol *

Antidepressants
Citalopram
Clomipramine *
Desipramine
Paroxetine *
Sertraline *
Venlafaxine *

* See Part 4

ANTIDEPRESSANT DRUGS

Occasional moods of discouragement or sadness are normal and usually pass quickly. But more severe depression, accompanied by despair, lethargy, loss of sex drive, and often poor appetite, may call for medical attention. Such depression can arise from life stresses such as the death of someone close, an illness, or sometimes from no apparent cause.

Three main types of drugs are used to treat depression: tricyclic antidepressants (TCAs), selective serotonin re-uptake inhibitors (SSRIs), and monoamine oxidase inhibitors (MAOIs) (see Types of antidepressant, below). Lithium, a metallic element, is used to treat bipolar disorder (see Antimanic drugs, facing page). It is sometimes used with an antidepressant drug for treating resistant depression. Several other antidepressants may be prescribed, including venlafaxine, maprotiline, mirtazapine, or trazodone.

Why they are used
Minor depression does not usually require drug treatment. Cognitive behavioural therapy, support and help in coming to terms with the cause of the depression is often all that is needed. Moderate or severe depression usually requires drug treatment, which is effective in most cases. Antidepressant drugs may have to be taken for many months. Treatment should not be stopped too soon because symptoms are likely to reappear if it is. When treatment is stopped, the dose should be gradually reduced over several weeks because withdrawal symptoms may occur if they are stopped suddenly.

How they work
Depression is thought to be caused by a reduction in the level of certain chemicals in the brain called *neurotransmitters*, which affect mood by stimulating brain cells. Antidepressants increase the level of these *excitatory* neurotransmitters. See Action of antidepressants (right).

Tricyclics (TCAs)
TCAs and venlafaxine block the re-uptake of the neurotransmitters serotonin and norepinephrine (noradrenaline), increasing neurotransmitter levels at receptors.

Selective serotonin re-uptake inhibitors (SSRIs)
SSRIs act by blocking the re-uptake of only one neurotransmitter, serotonin.

Monoamine oxidase inhibitors (MAOIs)
MAOIs act by blocking the breakdown of neurotransmitters, mainly serotonin and norepinephrine (noradrenaline).

How they affect you
The antidepressant effect of these drugs starts after 10 to 14 days treatment and it may be six to eight weeks before the full effect is seen. However, side effects may happen at once. *Tolerance* to these usually occurs and treatment should be continued.

Risks and special precautions
Ongoing monitoring of individuals with depression, by their physician and other care providers, with regards to feelings of self-harm is important. Overdose can be dangerous: tricyclics can produce coma, fits, and disturbed heart rhythm, which may be fatal; MAOIs can also cause muscle spasms and even death. Both are prescribed with caution for people with heart problems or epilepsy.

Monoamine oxidase inhibitors taken with certain drugs or foods rich in tyramine (for example, cheese, meat, yeast extracts, and red wine) can produce a dramatic rise in blood pressure, with headache or vomiting. People taking MAOIs are given a list of prohibited drugs and foods. However, moclobemide is a reversible inhibitor of MAOI-A and strict dietary precautions are not required at standard doses. Because of this adverse interaction, MAOIs are used much less frequently today. SSRIs or tricyclics are prescribed in preference.

TYPES OF ANTIDEPRESSANT

Treatment usually begins with either a TCA or an SSRI.

Tricyclic antidepressants (TCAs)
Some TCAs, such as amitriptyline, cause drowsiness, which is useful for sleep problems in depression. TCAs also cause *anticholinergic* effects, including blurred vision, a dry mouth, and difficulty urinating.

Selective serotonin re-uptake inhibitors (SSRIs)
The SSRIs generally have fewer *side effects* than TCAs. The main unwanted effects of the SSRIs are nausea and vomiting. Anxiety, headache, and restlessness may also occur at the beginning of treatment.

Monoamine oxidase inhibitors (MAOIs)
These are especially effective in people who are anxious as well as depressed, or who suffer from phobias.

COMMON DRUGS

Tricyclics
Amitriptyline *
Clomipramine *
Desipramine
Doxepin
Imipramine *
Nortriptyline
Trimipramine

SSRIs
Citalopram *
Escitalopram
Fluoxetine *
Fluvoxamine *
Paroxetine *
Sertraline *

MAOIs
Moclobemide *
Phenelzine
Tranylcypromine

Other drugs
Bupropion *
Maprotiline
Mirtazapine *
Trazodone
Venlafaxine *

* See Part 4

ACTION OF ANTIDEPRESSANTS

Normally, the brain cells release sufficient quantities of excitatory chemicals (known as neurotransmitters) to stimulate neighbouring cells. The neurotransmitters are constantly reabsorbed into the brain cells where they are broken down by an enzyme called monoamine oxidase. In depression, fewer neurotransmitters are released. The levels of neurotransmitters in the brain are raised by antidepressant drugs.

- Monoamine oxidase
- Nerve ending
- Neurotransmitters reabsorbed
- Receptor
- Brain cell stimulated

Normal brain activity
In a normal brain neurotransmitters are constantly being released, reabsorbed, and broken down.

Brain activity in depression
The brain cells release fewer neurotransmitters than normal, leading to reduced stimulation.

- Brain cell poorly stimulated

- Drug blocks reabsorption of neurotransmitter

Action of TCAs and SSRIs
TCA and SSRI drugs increase the levels of neurotransmitters by blocking their reabsorption.

- Drug blocks enzyme

Action of MAOIs
MAOIs increase the neurotransmitter levels by blocking the action of the enzyme (monoamine oxidase) that breaks them down.

ANTIPSYCHOTIC DRUGS

Psychosis is a term used to describe mental disorders that prevent the sufferer from thinking clearly, recognizing reality, and acting rationally. These disorders include schizophrenia and manic depression. The precise causes of these disorders are unknown, although a number of factors, including stress, heredity, and brain injury, may be involved. Temporary psychosis can also arise as a result of alcohol withdrawal or the abuse of mind-altering drugs (see Drugs of abuse, p.483). A variety of drugs is used to treat psychotic disorders (see Common drugs, below), most of which have similar actions and effects. One exception is lithium, which is particularly useful for bipolar disorder (see Antimanic drugs, right).

Why they are used

A person with a psychotic illness may recover spontaneously, and so a drug will not always be prescribed. Long-term treatment is started only when normal life is seriously disrupted. Antipsychotic drugs (sometimes called neuroleptics) do not cure the disorder, but they do help to control symptoms.

By controlling the symptoms of psychosis, antipsychotic drugs make it possible for most sufferers to live in the community and be admitted to hospital only for acute episodes.

The drug given to a particular individual depends on the nature of his or her illness and the expected *adverse effects* of that drug. Drugs differ in the amount of sedation produced; the need for sedation also influences the choice of drug.

Antipsychotics may also be given to calm or sedate a highly agitated or aggressive person, whatever the cause. Some antipsychotic drugs also have a powerful action against nausea and vomiting (see p.71), and are therefore sometimes used as premedication before a person has surgery.

How they work

It is thought that some forms of mental illness are caused by an increase in communication between brain cells due to overactivity of an *excitatory* chemical called dopamine. This may disturb normal thought processes and produce abnormal behaviour. Dopamine combines with *receptors* on the brain cells. Antipsychotic drugs reduce the transmission of nerve signals by binding to these receptors, thereby making the brain cells less sensitive to dopamine (see Action of antipsychotics, below). Some new antipsychotic drugs, such as clozapine and risperidone, also bind to receptors for the chemical serotonin.

How they affect you

Because antipsychotics depress the action of dopamine, they can disturb its balance with another chemical in the brain, acetylcholine. If an imbalance occurs, extrapyramidal side effects (EPSE) may appear. These include restlessness, disorders of movement, and parkinsonism (see Drugs for parkinsonism, p.71).

In these circumstances, a change in medication to a different type of antipsychotic may be necessary. If this is not possible, an anticholinergic drug (see p.71) may be prescribed.

Antipsychotics may block the action of noradrenaline, another neurotransmitter in the brain. This lowers the blood pressure, especially when you stand up, causing dizziness. This effect on noradrenaline may also prevent ejaculation.

Risks and special precautions

It is important to continue taking these drugs even if all symptoms have gone, because the symptoms are controlled only by taking the prescribed dose.

Because antipsychotic drugs can have permanent as well as temporary side effects, the minimum necessary dosage is used. This minimum dose is found by

starting with a low dose and increasing it until the symptoms are controlled. Sudden withdrawal after more than a few weeks can cause nausea, sweating, headache, and restlessness. Therefore, the dose is reduced gradually when treatment needs to be stopped.

The most serious long-term risk of antipsychotic treatment is a disorder known as *tardive dyskinesia*, which may develop after one to five years. This consists of repeated jerking movements of the mouth, tongue, and face, and sometimes of the hands and feet.

The condition is less common with the newer antipsychotics (atypical antipsychotics) than the older drugs (typical antipsychotics).

How they are administered

Antipsychotics may be given by mouth as tablets, capsules, or syrup, or by injection. They can also be given in the form of a *depot injection* which releases the drug slowly over several weeks. This is helpful for people who might forget to take their drugs or who might take an overdose.

ANTIMANIC DRUGS

Changes in mood are normal, but when a person's mood swings become grossly exaggerated, with peaks of elation or mania alternating with troughs of depression, it becomes an illness known as manic depression. It is usually treated with lithium, a drug that reduces the intensity of the mania, lifts the depression, and lessens the frequency of mood swings. Because it may take three weeks before the lithium starts to work, an antipsychotic may be prescribed with lithium at first to give immediate relief of symptoms.

Lithium can be toxic if levels of the drug in the blood rise too high. Regular checks on the blood concentration of lithium should therefore be carried out during treatment. Symptoms of lithium poisoning include blurred vision, twitching, vomiting, and diarrhea (see p.331).

ACTION OF ANTIPSYCHOTICS

Brain activity is partly governed by the action of a chemical called dopamine, which transmits signals between brain cells. In psychotic illness the brain cells release too much dopamine, resulting in excessive stimulation. The antipsychotic drugs help to reduce the adverse effects of excess dopamine.

Dopamine activity in psychosis
Dopamine activity is excessive, causing overstimulation.

- Dopamine
- Dopamine receptor
- Stimulation

Dopamine activity blocked by drugs
Antipsychotic drugs occupy dopamine receptors and prevent the effects of excess dopamine being felt.

- Drugs

COMMON DRUGS

First generation antipsychotics	Second generation (atypical) antipsychotics
Chlorpromazine ✳	Clozapine ✳
Flupenthixol ✳	Olanzapine ✳
Fluphenazine	Quetiapine ✳
Haloperidol ✳	Risperidone ✳
Loxapine	Ziprasidone
Methotrimeprazine	
Perphenazine	**Antimanic drugs**
Pimozide	Carbamazepine ✳
Pipotiazine	Divalproex
Thiothixene	Lithium ✳
Trifluoperazine ✳	
Zuclopenthixol	

✳ See Part 4

ANTICONVULSANT DRUGS

Electrical signals from nerve cells in the brain are normally finely coordinated to produce smooth movements of arms and legs, but these signals can become irregular and chaotic, and trigger the disorderly muscular activity and mental changes that are characteristic of a seizure (also called a fit or convulsion). The most common cause of seizures is the disorder known as epilepsy, which is caused by brain disease or injury. In patients with epilepsy, a fit may be triggered by an outside stimulus such as a flashing light. Seizures can also result from the *toxic* effects of certain drugs and, in young children, by a high temperature.

Anticonvulsant drugs are used both to reduce the risk of an epileptic seizure and to stop one that is in progress.

Why they are used

Isolated convulsions seldom require drug treatment, but anticonvulsant drugs are the usual treatment for controlling seizures that are caused by epilepsy. These drugs permit most people with epilepsy to lead a normal life.

ACTION OF ANTICONVULSANTS

Normally, the electrical activity of the brain is under good control. If an area of the brain is electrically unstable and there is an uncontrolled discharge of electrical impulses, epilepsy may occur (see Types of epilepsy, right). Anticonvulsants stabilize the electrical activity of brain cells, thus reducing the liklihood of a seizure.

Normal brain activity

- Brain
- Normal electrical activity
- Spinal cord

Brain activity in a fit

- Uncontrolled electrical activity
- Electrical signals to body cause fit

Drug action on brain activity

- Anticonvulsant stabilizes excess electrical activity

Most people with epilepsy need to take anticonvulsants on a regular basis to prevent seizures. Usually a single drug is used, and treatment continues until there have been no attacks for at least two years. The particular drug prescribed depends on the type of epilepsy (see Types of epilepsy, right). If one drug is not effective, a different anticonvulsant will be tried. Occasionally, it is necessary to take a combination of drugs. A person can suffer seizures even when on treatment. A prolonged seizure can be halted by injection of diazepam or a similar drug.

How they work

Brain cells bring about body movement by electrical activity that passes through the nerves to the muscles. In an epileptic seizure, uncontrolled electrical activity starts in one part of the brain and spreads to other parts, causing uncontrolled stimulation of brain cells. Most anticonvulsants have an *inhibitory* effect on brain cells and damp down electrical activity, preventing the excessive build-up that causes epileptic seizures (see Action of anticonvulsants, left).

How they affect you

Ideally, the only effect an anticonvulsant should have is to reduce or prevent epileptic seizures. Unfortunately, no drug prevents seizures without potentially affecting normal brain function, leading to poor memory, inability to concentrate, lack of coordination, and lethargy. It is important, therefore, to find a dosage sufficient to prevent seizures without causing unacceptable side effects. The dose has to be carefully tailored to the individual. It is usual to start with a low dose of a selected drug and to increase it gradually until a balance is achieved between the control of seizures and the occurrence of side effects, many of which wear off after the first weeks of treatment.

Blood tests are used to monitor levels of some anticonvulsants in the body as an aid to dose adjustment. Finding the correct dose may take several months.

Risks and special precautions

Each anticonvulsant drug has its own specific *adverse effects* and risks. In addition, some affect the liver's ability to break down other drugs (see Drug interactions, p.16) and so may influence the action of other drugs you are taking. Physicians try to prescribe the minimum number of anticonvulsants needed to control the person's seizures in order to reduce the risk of such interactions.

Some anticonvulsants have risks for a foetus – if you wish to become pregnant, discuss the risks and whether to change your medication, with your physician. People taking anticonvulsants need to take their medicine regularly as prescribed. If the anticonvulsant levels in the body are allowed to fall suddenly,

TYPES OF EPILEPSY

The selection of anticonvulsant (antieileptic) drug depends on the type of epilepsy, the age of the patient, and his or her particular response to individual drug treatment.

Generalized epilepsy In this form of epilepsy, there is a widespread disturbance of the electrical activity in the brain and loss of consciousness occurs at the outset. In its simplest form, a momentary loss of consciousness occurs during which the sufferer may stare into space. This is called an absence seizure, and mainly affects children. Convulsions do not occur.

Another form of generalized epilepsy causes a brief jerk of a limb (myoclonus).

The most severe type is a tonic-clonic (grand mal) seizure, which is characterized by loss of consciousness, and convulsions that may last for a few minutes. Sufferers may have one or more of these types of generalized epilepsy.

Valproic acid, lamotrigine, carbamazepine, topiramate, phenytoin, or the benzodiazepines are normally used for these types of epilepsy.

Partial (focal) epilepsy This type of epilepsy is caused by an electrical disturbance in only one part of the brain. The result is a disturbance of function, such as an abnormal sensation or movement of a limb, without loss of consciousness. Known as a simple partial seizure, this may precede a more serious attack associated with loss of consciouness (complex partial seizure), which may in turn progress to a generalized convulsive seizure.

Carbamazepine, lamotrigine, or phenytoin may be prescribed for this type of epilepsy.

Status epilepticus Repeated epileptic attacks without full recovery between them, or a single attack lasting more than 10 minutes, is called status epilepticus and it requires emergency treatment.

seizures are very likely to occur. The dose should not be reduced or the treatment stopped, except on the advice of a doctor.

If, for any reason, anticonvulsant drug treatment needs to be stopped, the dose should be reduced gradually. People on anticonvulsant therapy are advised to carry an identification tag giving full details of their condition and treatment (see p.29).

COMMON DRUGS

Carbamazepine *
Clobazam
Clonazepam *
Diazepam *
Divalproex
Ethosuximide
Fosphenytoin
Gabapentin *
Lamotrigine *
Levetiracetam
Lorazepam *
Methsuximide

Nitrazepam *
Oxcarbazepine
Phenobarbital *
Phenytoin *
Primidone
Topiramate *
Valproic acid *
Vigabatrin

| * See Part 4 |

DRUGS FOR PARKINSONISM

Parkinsonism is a general term used to describe shaking of the head and limbs, muscular stiffness, an expressionless face, and inability to control or initiate movement. It is caused by an imbalance of chemicals in the brain; the effect of acetylcholine is increased by a reduction in the action of dopamine.

Parkinsonism has a variety of causes, but the most common is Parkinson's disease, degeneration of the dopamine-producing cells in the brain. Other causes include the *side effects* of certain drugs, notably antipsychotics (see p.69), and narrowing of the blood vessels in the brain.

Why they are used

Drugs can relieve the symptoms of parkinsonism but, unfortunately, the degeneration of brain cells in Parkinson's disease cannot be halted, although drugs can minimize symptoms for many years.

How they work

Drugs to treat parkinsonism restore the balance between the chemicals dopamine and acetylcholine. They fall into two main groups: those that reduce the effect of acetylcholine *(anticholinergic* drugs) and those that boost the effect of dopamine.

Anticholinergics combine with *receptors* on brain cells, preventing acetylcholine from binding to them. This action reduces acetylcholine's relative overactivity and restores the balance with dopamine.

Dopamine cannot pass from the blood to the brain, and therefore cannot be given to boost its levels in the brain. Levodopa (L-dopa), the chemical from which it is naturally produced in the brain, is combined with carbidopa or benserazide to prevent it from being converted to dopamine before it reaches the brain. Amantadine (also used as an antiviral, see p.119) boosts levels of dopamine in the brain by stimulating its release. The action

of dopamine can also be boosted by other drugs, including bromocriptine, pergolide, pramipexole, or ropinirole, which mimic the action of dopamine.

Choice of drug

Anticholinergics are often effective in the early stages of Parkinson's disease and are used to treat parkinsonism due to anti-psychotic drugs, which have dopamine-blocking properties. L-dopa is usually given when the disease impairs walking. Its effectiveness usually wanes after two to five years, in which case other dopamine-boosting drugs may also be prescribed.

ACTION OF DRUGS FOR PARKINSONISM

Normal movement depends on a balance in the brain between dopamine and acetylcholine, which combine with receptors on brain cells. In parkinsonism, there is less dopamine present, with the result that acetylcholine is relatively overactive. The balance between acetylcholine and dopamine may be restored by anticholinergic drugs, which combine with the receptor for acetylcholine to block the action of acetylcholine on the brain cell, or by dopamine-boosting drugs, which increase the level of dopamine activity in the brain.

Normal chemical balance
Normally dopamine and acetylcholine are balanced.

Chemical imbalance in parkinsonism
If dopamine activity is low, acetylcholine is overactive.

Action of anticholinergic drugs
Anticholinergic drugs displace acetylcholine and restore balance.

Action of dopamine-boosting drugs
These drugs increase dopamine activity and restore balance.

COMMON DRUGS

Dopamine-boosting drugs
Amantadine *
Bromocriptine *
Entacapone
Ethopropazine
Levodopa/
 benserazide *
Levodopa/
 carbidopa *
Pramipexole *
Rasagiline *

Ropinirole
Selegiline *

Anticholinergic drugs
Benztropine
Procyclidine *
Trihexyphenidyl

* See Part 4

DRUGS FOR DEMENTIA

Dementia is a decline in mental function that is severe enough to affect normal social or occupational activities. It can be sudden and irreversible, for example due to a stroke or a head injury. It can also develop gradually and may be a feature of a number of disorders, including poor circulation in the brain, multiple sclerosis, and Alzheimer's disease. Much research on Alzheimer's disease, which is the most common cause of dementia, is ongoing.

Why they are used

Drugs called acetylcholinesterase inhibitors (AchIs) have been found to improve the symptoms of dementia in Alzheimer's disease, although they do not prevent its long-term progression. Memantine, a new drug which is a N-methyl-D-aspartate

(NMDA) receptor antagonist, may be used in conjunction with an AchI.

How they work

In healthy people, acetylcholinesterase (an enzyme in the brain) breaks down the *neurotransmitter* acetylcholine, balancing its levels and limiting its effects. In Alzheimer's disease, there is a deficiency of acetylcholine. AchIs block the action of the enzyme acetylcholinesterase, raising brain levels of acetylcholine, thus increasing the patient's alertness and slowing the rate of deterioration.

How they affect you

Drug treatment is started at a low dose following an assessment by a specialist of mental function. The dosage is increased

gradually to minimize *side effects*. Any improvements should begin to appear in about 3 weeks. Assessment is repeated after 3 months to see if the treatment has been beneficial. About half of those people treated show some improvement.

Risks and special precautions

It is important to continue taking these drugs because there is a gradual loss of improvement after they are stopped.

COMMON DRUGS

Acetylcholinesterase inhibitors
Donepezil *
Galantamine *
Rivastigmine *

Other
Memantine *

* See Part 4

NERVOUS SYSTEM STIMULANTS

A person's state of mental alertness varies throughout the day and is under the control of chemicals in the brain, some of which are depressant, causing drowsiness, and others that are stimulant, heightening awareness.

It is thought that an increase in the activity of the depressant chemicals may be responsible for a condition called narcolepsy, which is a tendency to fall asleep during the day for no obvious reason. In this case, the nervous system stimulants are administered to increase wakefulness. These drugs include the amphetamines (usually dextroamphetamine), the related drug methylphenidate, and modafinil. Amphetamines are used less often these days because of the risk of dependence. A common home remedy for increasing alertness is caffeine, a mild stimulant that is present in coffee, tea, and cola. Respiratory stimulants related to caffeine are used to improve breathing (see right).

Why they are used

In adults who suffer from narcolepsy, some of these drugs prevent excessive drowsiness during the day. Stimulants do not cure narcolepsy and, since the disorder usually lasts throughout the sufferer's lifetime, may have to be taken indefinitely. Methylphenidate, mixed salts amphetamine, or dextroamphetamine are sometimes given to children suffering from attention deficit hyperactivity disorder (ADHD). Stimulants were once used as part of the treatment for obesity because reduced appetite is a *side effect* of amphetamines but they are no longer thought appropriate for weight reduction. Diet is now the main treatment, together with orlistat or sibutramine if necessary.

Caffeine is added to some analgesics to counteract the effects of caffeine withdrawal which can cause headaches, but no clear medical justification exists for this.

Apart from their use in narcolepsy, nervous system stimulants are not useful in the long term because the brain soon develops *tolerance* to them.

How they work

The level of wakefulness is controlled by a part of the brain stem called the reticular activating system (RAS). Activity in this area depends on the balance between chemicals, some of which are *excitatory* (including norepinephrine (noradrenaline)) and some *inhibitory*, such as gamma aminobutyric acid (GABA). Stimulants promote release of noradrenaline, increasing activity in the RAS and other parts of the brain, so raising alertness.

How they affect you

In adults, the central nervous system stimulants taken in the prescribed dose for narcolepsy increase wakefulness, thereby allowing normal concentration and

RESPIRATORY STIMULANTS

Some stimulants (for example, aminophylline and theophylline) act on the part of the brain – the respiratory centre – that controls respiration. They are sometimes used in hospitals to help people who have difficulty breathing, mainly very young babies and adults with severe chest infections.

thought processes to occur. They may also reduce appetite and cause tremors. In hyperactive children, they reduce the general level of activity to a more normal level and increase the attention span.

Risks and special precautions

Some people, especially the elderly or those with previous psychiatric problems, are particularly sensitive to stimulants and may experience adverse effects, even when the drugs are given in comparatively low doses. They need to be used with caution in children because they can retard growth if taken for prolonged periods. An excess of these drugs given to a child may depress the nervous system, producing drowsiness or even loss of consciousness. Palpitations may also occur. These medications are generally not recommended in those with an overactive thyroid, high blood pressure, or abnormalities of the heart or heart disease. Modafinil is generally not recommended for use in children.

These drugs reduce the level of natural stimulants in the brain, so after regular use for a few weeks a person may become physically dependent on them for normal function. If they are abruptly withdrawn, the excess of natural inhibitory chemicals in the brain depresses central nervous system activity, producing withdrawal symptoms. These may include lethargy, depression, increased appetite, and difficulty staying awake.

Stimulants can produce overactivity in the brain if used inappropriately or in excess, resulting in extreme restlessness, sleeplessness, nervousness, or anxiety. They also stimulate the sympathetic branch of the autonomic nervous system (see p.63), causing shaking, sweating, and palpitations. More serious risks of exceeding the prescribed dose are fits and a major disturbance in mental functioning that may result in delusions and hallucinations. Because these drugs have been abused, amphetamines and methylphenidate are classified as controlled drugs (see pp.13 and 483).

ACTION OF NERVOUS SYSTEM STIMULANTS

Wakefulness is controlled by a part of the brain stem called the reticular activating system (RAS).

Normal brain activity
When the brain is functioning normally, signals from the RAS stimulate the upper parts of the brain, which control thought processes and alertness.

Brain activity in narcolepsy
In narcolepsy, the level of signals from the RAS is greatly reduced.

Normal brain activity restored
Central nervous system stimulants act on the RAS to increase the level of stimulatory signals to the brain.

COMMON DRUGS

Nervous system stimulants	Mixed salts amphetamine
Dextroamphetamine	Modafinil
Methylphenidate *	
	* See Part 4

DRUGS USED FOR MIGRAINE

Migraine is a term applied to recurrent severe headaches affecting only one side of the head and caused by changes in the blood vessels around the brain and scalp. They may be accompanied by nausea and vomiting and sometimes preceded by warning signs, usually an impression of flashing lights or numbness and tingling in the arms. Occasionally, speech may be impaired, or the attack may be disabling. The cause of migraine is unknown, but an attack may be triggered by a blow to the head, physical exertion, certain foods and drugs, or emotional factors such as excitement, tension, or shock. A family history of migraine also increases the chance of an individual suffering from it.

Why they are used

Drugs are used either to relieve symptoms or to prevent attacks. Different drugs are used in each approach, but none cures the underlying disorder. However, a susceptibility to migraine headaches can clear up spontaneously, and if you are taking drugs regularly, your physician may recommend that you stop them after a few months to see if this has happened.

In most people, migraine headaches can be relieved by a mild analgesic (painkiller), for example, acetaminophen, ibuprofen, or ASA, or a stronger one like naproxen, ergotamine, or a triptan (see Analgesics, p.64). If nausea and vomiting accompany the migraine, tablets may not be absorbed sufficiently from the gut. Absorption can be increased if drugs are taken as soluble tablets in water or with an anti-emetic.

Some drugs used to relieve attacks can be given by injection, inhaler, nasal spray, or suppository. Preparations that contain caffeine should be avoided since headaches may be caused by excessive use or on stopping treatment. 5HT$_1$ *agonist* drugs (triptans, such as sumatriptan) are used if analgesics are not effective. Ergotamine is used less often now.

The factors that trigger an individual's attacks should be identified and avoided. Anti-anxiety drugs are not usually prescribed if stress is a precipitating factor because of the potential for dependence. If the attacks occur more often than once a month, drugs to prevent migraine may be taken every day. Drugs used to prevent migraine are betablockers (such as propranolol, see p.83), calcium channel blockers (such as flunarizine and verapamil), antidepressants (such as amitriptyline, see p. 68) and pizotifen (an antihistamine and serotinin blocker). Methysergide is not commonly used because of its serious side effects.

How they work

A migraine attack begins when blood vessels surrounding the brain constrict (become narrower), producing the typical migraine warning signs. The constriction

ACTION OF DRUGS USED FOR MIGRAINE

Migraine is caused by the action of chemicals in the bloodstream on blood vessels surrounding the brain and in the scalp. In the first stage of a migraine attack, the blood vessels surrounding the brain constrict, causing warning signs (below left). In the second stage, the blood vessels in the scalp dilate, causing a severe headache (below right).

Skin
Bone
Blood vessel in scalp
Blood vessels surrounding brain
Brain

Constricted blood vessel

Preventing migraine
Migraine-preventing drugs block the action of chemicals that cause constriction of the blood vessels surrounding the brain.

Dilated blood vessel

Stopping an attack
Ergotamine and 5HT$_1$ agonists taken during a migraine attack return the dilated blood vessels in the scalp to their normal size.

is thought to be caused by certain chemicals found in food or produced by the body. The neurotransmitter serotonin causes large blood vessels in the brain to constrict. Pizotifen and propranolol block the effect of chemicals on blood vessels and thereby prevent attacks (see Action of drugs used for migraine, above).

The next stage of a migraine attack occurs when blood vessels in the scalp and around the eyes dilate (widen). As a result, chemicals called prostaglandins are released, producing pain. ASA and acetaminophen relieve this pain by blocking prostaglandins. Ergotamine and 5HT$_1$ agonists relieve pain by narrowing dilated blood vessels in the scalp.

How they affect you

Each drug has its own *adverse effects*. 5HT$_1$ agonists may cause chest tightness and drowsiness. Ergotamine may cause drowsiness, tingling sensations in the skin, cramps, and weakness in the legs, and vomiting may be made worse. Pizotifen may cause drowsiness and weight gain. For effects of beta blockers such as propranolol, see p.402, and for analgesics, see p.64.

Risks and special precautions

5HT$_1$ agonists should not usually be used by those with high blood pressure, angina, or coronary heart disease. Ergotamine

can damage blood vessels by prolonged overconstriction so it should be used with caution by those with poor circulation. Excessive use can lead to dependence and many adverse effects, including headache. You should not take more than your physician advises in any one week.

How they are administered

These drugs are usually taken by mouth as tablets or capsules. Sumatriptan can also be taken as an injection and zolmitriptan and sumatriptan are available as a nasal spray. Ergotamine can be taken orally or as an injection.

COMMON DRUGS

Drugs to prevent migraine
Amitriptyline ✴
Atenolol ✴
Flunarizine
Methysergide
Metoprolol ✴
Nadolol
Pizotifen ✴
Propranolol ✴
Topiramate ✴
Valproic acid ✴
Verapamil ✴

5HT$_1$ agonists
Almotriptan
Eletriptan
Frovatriptan
Naratriptan
Rizatriptan ✴
Sumatriptan ✴
Zolmitriptan

Other drugs to relieve migraine
Acetaminophen ✴
ASA ✴
Dihydroergotamine
Ergotamine ✴
Ibuprofen ✴

✴ See Part 4

ANTI-EMETICS

Drugs used to treat or prevent vomiting or nausea are known as anti-emetics. Vomiting is a reflex action for getting rid of harmful substances, but it may also be a symptom of disease. Vomiting and nausea are often caused by a digestive tract infection, travel sickness, pregnancy, or vertigo (a balance disorder involving the inner ear). They can also occur as a *side effect* of some drugs, especially those used for cancer, radiation therapy, or general anesthesia.

Commonly used anti-emetics include metoclopramide, domperidone, cyclizine, haloperidol, ondansetron, granisetron, prochlorperazine, and promethazine. The phenothiazine and butyrophenone drug groups are also used as antihistamines (see p.110) and prescribed to treat some types of mental illness (see Antipsychotic drugs, p.69). Corticosteroids like dexamethasone may also be used in the prevention of chemotherapy related nausea and vomiting.

Why they are used

Physicians usually diagnose the cause of vomiting before prescribing an anti-emetic because vomiting may be due to a digestive tract infection or some other condition of the abdomen that might require treatment such as surgery. Treating only the vomiting and nausea might delay diagnosis, correct treatment, and recovery. Anti-emetics may be taken to prevent travel sickness (using one of the antihistamines), vomiting resulting from anticancer (see p.140) and other drug treatments (metoclopramide, haloperidol, domperidone, ondansetron, and prochlorperazine), to help the nausea in vertigo (see right), and occasionally to relieve cases of severe vomiting during pregnancy. You should not take an anti-emetic during pregnancy except on medical advice. No anti-emetic drug should be taken for longer than a couple of days without consulting your physician.

How they work

Nausea and vomiting occur when the vomiting centre in the brain is stimulated by signals from three places in the body: the digestive tract, the part of the inner ear controlling balance, and the brain itself via thoughts and emotions and via its chemoreceptor trigger zone, which responds to harmful substances in the blood. Anti-emetic drugs may act at one or more of these places (see Action of anti-emetics, left). Some help the stomach to empty its contents into the intestine. A combination may be used that works at different sites and has an additive effect.

How they affect you

As well as treating vomiting and nausea, many anti-emetic drugs may make you feel drowsy. However, for preventing travel sickness on long journeys, a sedating antihistamine may be an advantage.

Some anti-emetics (in particular, the phenothiazines and antihistamines) can block the parasympathetic nervous system (see p.63), causing dry mouth, blurred vision, or difficulty in passing urine. The phenothiazines may also lower blood pressure, leading to dizziness or fainting.

Risks and special precautions

As some antihistamines can make you drowsy, it may be advisable not to drive while taking them. Phenothiazines, butyrophenones, and metoclopramide can produce uncontrolled movements of the face and tongue, so they are used with caution in people with *parkinsonism*.

VERTIGO AND MÉNIÈRE'S DISEASE

Vertigo is a spinning sensation in the head, which is often accompanied by nausea and vomiting. It is usually caused by a disease affecting the organ of balance in the inner ear. Anti-emetic drugs are prescribed to relieve the symptoms.

Ménière's disease is a disorder in which excess fluid builds up in the inner ear, causing vertigo, noises in the ear, and gradual deafness. It is usually treated with betahistine, prochlorperazine, or an anti-anxiety drug (see p.67). A diuretic (see p.85) may also be given in order to reduce the excess fluid in the ear.

ACTION OF ANTI-EMETICS

The vomiting reflex, in which the muscles of the stomach contract to expel the stomach contents, is triggered when the vomiting centre in the brain is stimulated by signals arising in the stomach, the inner ear, or in parts of the brain.

Brain

Inner ear

Signal to vomiting centre

Stomach

Signal to stomach

5HT₃ antagonists block signals from the stomach to vomiting centre

Vomiting centre

Signal from blood

Chemoreceptor trigger

Signal to stomach

Drug acts on chemoreceptor trigger

Drug acts on vomiting centre

Phenothiazines, butyrophenones and 5HT₃ antagonists prevent the chemoreceptor trigger from stimulating vomiting.

Antihistamines reduce the sensitivity of the vomiting centre.

COMMON DRUGS

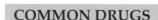

Antihistamines
Dimenhydrinate ✳
Hydroxyzine
Meclizine
Promethazine ✳

Phenothiazines
Chlorpromazine ✳
Perphenazine
Prochlorperazine ✳
Trifluoperazine ✳

Anti-vertigo
Betahistine ✳

5HT₃ antagonists
Dolasetron
Granisetron
Ondansetron ✳

Butyrophenones
Haloperidol ✳

Other drugs
Aprepitant
Dexamethasone ✳
Dronabinol
Metoclopramide ✳
Nabilone
Scopolamine

✳ See Part 4

RESPIRATORY SYSTEM

The respiratory system consists of the lungs and the passageways, such as the trachea and bronchi, by which air reaches them. Through the process of inhaling and exhaling air – breathing – the body is able to obtain the oxygen necessary for survival, and to expel carbon dioxide, which is the waste product of the basic human biological processes.

What can go wrong

Difficulty in breathing may be due to narrowing of the air passages, from spasm, as in asthma and bronchitis, or from swelling of the linings of the air passages, as in bronchiolitis and bronchitis. Breathing difficulties may also be due to an infection of the lung tissue, as in pneumonia and bronchitis, or to damage to the small air sacs (alveoli) from emphysema or from inhaled dusts or moulds, which cause pneumoconiosis and farmer's lung. Smoking and air pollution can affect the respiratory system in many ways, leading to diseases such as lung cancer and bronchitis.

Sometimes difficulty in breathing may be due to congestion of the lungs from heart disease, to an inhaled object such as a peanut, or to infection or inflammation of the throat. Symptoms of breathing difficulties often include a cough and a tight feeling in the chest.

Why drugs are used

Drugs with a variety of actions are used to clear the air passages, soothe inflammation, and reduce the production of mucus. Some can be bought without a prescription as single-ingredient or combined-ingredient preparations, often with an analgesic.

Decongestants (p.79) reduce the swelling inside the nose, thereby making it possible to breathe more freely. If the cause of the congestion is an allergic response, an antihistamine (p.110) is often recommended to relieve symptoms or to prevent attacks. Infections of the respiratory tract are usually treated with antibiotics (p.114).

Bronchodilators are drugs that widen the bronchi (p.76). They are used to prevent and relieve asthma attacks. Corticosteroids (p.127) reduce inflammation in the swollen inner layers of the airways. They are used to prevent asthma attacks. Other drugs, such as sodium cromoglycate, may be used for treating allergies and preventing asthma attacks but they are not effective once an asthma attack has begun.

A variety of drugs are used to relieve a cough, depending on the type of cough involved. Some drugs make it easier to eliminate phlegm; others suppress the cough by inhibiting the cough reflex.

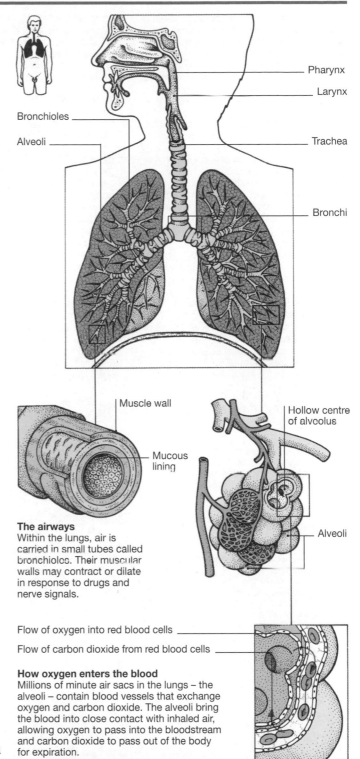

Pharynx

Larynx

Bronchioles

Alveoli

Trachea

Bronchi

Muscle wall

Mucous lining

Hollow centre of alveolus

Alveoli

The airways
Within the lungs, air is carried in small tubes called bronchioles. Their muscular walls may contract or dilate in response to drugs and nerve signals.

Flow of oxygen into red blood cells

Flow of carbon dioxide from red blood cells

How oxygen enters the blood
Millions of minute air sacs in the lungs – the alveoli – contain blood vessels that exchange oxygen and carbon dioxide. The alveoli bring the blood into close contact with inhaled air, allowing oxygen to pass into the bloodstream and carbon dioxide to pass out of the body for expiration.

MAJOR DRUG GROUPS

Bronchodilators
Drugs for asthma
Decongestants
Drugs to treat coughs

See also sections on Allergy (p.109) and Infections (p.112)

BRONCHODILATORS

Chronic Obstructive Pulmonary Disease (COPD) affects airways (both large and small) and the lung tissue. Air entering the lungs passes through narrow tubes called bronchioles. In asthma and COPD the bronchioles become narrower, either as a result of contraction of the muscles in their walls, or as a result of mucus congestion. This narrowing of the bronchioles obstructs the flow of air into and out of the lungs and causes breathlessness.

Bronchodilators are prescribed to widen the bronchioles and improve breathing. There are three main groups of bronchodilators: *sympathomimetics*, *anticholinergics*, and xanthine drugs, which are related to caffeine. They are all used for relief of symptoms, and do not affect the underlying disease process. Anticholinergics are thought to be more effective in, and are used particularly for, COPD. In asthma, they are less effective, and are usually prescribed as additional therapy when control with other drugs is inadequate. Sympathomimetics or Beta$_2$-agonists are the mainstay of asthma treatment, and are also frequently used in COPD. Xanthines have been used for many years, both for asthma and bronchitis.

They usually need precise adjustment of dosage to be effective while avoiding side effects. This makes them more difficult to use, and they are reserved for people whose condition cannot be controlled by other bronchodilators alone.

Why they are used

Bronchodilators help to dilate the bronchioles of people suffering from asthma and COPD. However, they are of little benefit to those suffering from severe COPD.

Bronchodilators can either be taken when they are needed in order to relieve an attack of breathlessness that is in progress, or on a regular basis to prevent such attacks from occurring. Some people find it helpful to take an extra dose of their bronchodilator immediately before undertaking any activity likely to provoke an attack of breathlessness.

A patient who requires treatment with a Beta$_2$-agonist inhaler more than once daily should see his or her physician about preventative treatment with an inhaled corticosteroid.

Beta$_2$-agonist drugs are mainly used for the rapid relief of breathlessness; anticholinergic and xanthine drugs are used long term.

How they work

Bronchodilator drugs act by relaxing the muscles surrounding the bronchioles. Beta$_2$-agonist and anticholinergic drugs achieve this by interfering with nerve signals passed to the muscles through the autonomic nervous system (see p.63). Xanthine drugs are thought to relax the muscle in the bronchioles by a direct effect on the muscle fibres, but their precise action is not known.

Bronchodilator drugs usually improve breathing within a few minutes of administration. Corticosteroids usually start to increase the sufferer's capacity for exercise within a few days, and most people find that the frequency of their attacks of breathlessness is reduced.

Because Beta$_2$-agonist drugs stimulate a branch of the autonomic nervous system that controls heart rate, they may sometimes cause palpitations and trembling. Typical side effects of anticholinergic drugs include dry mouth, blurred vision, and difficulty in passing urine. However, when used in an inhaler, these effects are rarely reported. Xanthine drugs may cause headaches and nausea.

Risks and special precautions

Since most bronchodilators are not taken by mouth, but inhaled, they do not usually cause serious side effects. However, because of their possible effect on heart rate, xanthine and Beta$_2$-agonist drugs need to be prescribed with caution to people with heart problems, high blood pressure, or an overactive thyroid gland. Smoking tobacco and drinking alcohol increase excretion of xanthines from the body, reducing their effects. Stopping smoking after being stabilized on xanthine may result in a rise in blood concentration, and an increased risk of side effects. It is advisable to stop smoking before starting treatment. The anticholinergic drugs may not be suitable for people with urinary retention or those who have a tendency to glaucoma.

ACTION OF BRONCHODILATORS

When the bronchioles are narrowed following contraction of the muscle layer and swelling of the mucous lining, the passage of air is impeded. Bronchodilators act on the nerve signals that govern muscle activity. Sympatho-mimetics or Beta$_2$-agonists enhance the action of neurotransmitters that encourage muscle relaxation. Anticholinergics block the neurotransmitters that trigger muscle contraction and reduce production of mucus. Xanthines promote muscle relaxation by a direct effect on the muscles.

- Trachea
- Lung
- Bronchi
- Bronchioles
- Diaphragm

Normal bronchioles
The muscle surrounding the bronchioles is relaxed, thus leaving the airway open.

Asthma attack
The bronchiole muscle contracts and the lining swells, narrowing the airway.

After drug treatment
The muscles relax, thereby opening the airway, but the lining remains swollen.

COMMON DRUGS

Sympathomimetics
Fenoterol
Formoterol *
Salbutamol *
Salmeterol *
Terbutaline *

Xanthines
Aminophylline *
Oxtriphylline
Theophylline *

Anticholinergics
Ipratropium *
Tiotropium *

| * See Part 4 |

DRUGS FOR ASTHMA

Asthma is a chronic lung disease characterized by episodes in which the bronchioles constrict due to over-sensitivity. The attacks are usually, but not always, reversible; asthma is also known as reversible airways obstruction. About 5 per cent of adults and 10 per cent of children have the disease. Sometimes the inflammation causing the constriction is due to an identifiable allergen in the atmosphere, such as house dust mites, but often there is no obvious trigger. Breathlessness is the main symptom. Wheezing, coughing, and chest tightness are common. Asthma sufferers often have attacks during the night and wake up with breathing difficulty. The illness varies in severity, and it can be life threatening.

There are a number of drugs that are used in the control of asthma. Where drugs are needed only to control an occasional attack (relievers), a sympathomimetic bronchodilator will probably be used in inhaler form. When the patient needs continuous preventative treatment (preventers/controllers) there are a number of choices: often an inhaled corticosteroid or sodium cromoglycate may be used (with a sympathomimetic inhaler if attacks persist). More severe cases may require higher dose cortico-steroids or the addition of a long-acting sympathomimetic bronchodilator. If this is not adequate, a high dose corticosteroid will be used with an anticholinergic drug, or theophylline, or these in combination with others already tried. There are also leukotriene antagonists, which may be used when corticosteroids cannot be used in an individual; they are less effective in severe cases when patients are taking high doses of other drugs. Some people who suffer from very severe asthma may need such large doses of corticosteroids that tablets have to be taken. In those who still have asthma symptoms while on inhaled corticosteroids, omalizumab can help reduce the number of asthma attacks. Omalizumab blocks IgE, which is a naturally occurring substance in the body that plays a role in asthma. Antihistamines were prescribed for asthma in the past but this has not proved to be a successful treatment.

Why they are used

In asthma, the airways (bronchioles) constrict making it difficult to get air in or out of the lungs. Bronchodilators (sympathomimetics, anticholinergics, and theophylline) relax the constricted muscles around the bronchioles (p.76). Short-acting sympathomimetics act almost immediately when inhaled and are used to provide relief of symptoms during an attack, and in more severe cases the long-acting sympathomimetics may be used to help with continuous protective cover. Anticholinergic drugs do not act as rapidly as the sympathomimetics. They are used for continuous prevention. Theophylline/aminophylline must be given by mouth or injection; the tablets are used for regular continuous dosing, and the injection is used in hospital to gain control of severe asthma. Drugs that are not bronchodilators, such as corticosteroids and leukotriene receptor antagonists (see p.78), are not useful for dealing with an acute attack of asthma, but they are effective for long-term protection.

Antihistamines have been tried in the treatment of asthma, but although they are useful for other allergic conditions, they are not very effective in asthma. One antihistamine-like drug, ketotifen, is sometimes given but is not widely used.

How they work

Inhaling a drug directly into the lungs is the best way of getting benefit without excessive side effects. A selection of devices for delivering the drug into the airways is illustrated below.

Inhalers or puffers release a small dose when they are pressed, but require some skill to use effectively. A large hollow plastic "spacer" can help you to inhale your drug more easily. Insufflation cartridges deliver larger amounts of drug than inhalers and are easier to use because the drug is taken in as you breathe normally.

Nebulizers pump compressed air through a solution of drug to produce a fine mist that is inhaled through a face mask. They deliver large doses of the drug to the lungs, rapidly relieving breathing difficulty.

Bronchodilators act by relaxing the muscles surrounding the bronchioles (see p.76). Corticosteroids are used for their anti-inflammatory properties. By suppressing airway inflammation they reduce the swelling inside the bronchioles, complementing the relaxation of the walls by the bronchodilators in opening up the tubes. Reducing the inflammation also reduces the amount of mucus produced, and this again helps to clear the airways.

DIFFERENT TYPES OF INHALER

Inhalers are used to deliver drugs to relieve or prevent the symptoms of asthma. A wide range of different types of inhaler is available and the most commonly prescribed ones are shown here. Many people are prescribed a reliever and a preventer drug and these may come in different types of inhaler, depending on the drugs that are given. Although every inhaler works on the same broad principle to deliver the drug directly to the bronchioles through a mouthpiece, there are individual differences in the actions required.

Therefore, it is important to read the instructions carefully and practise using the inhaler before you need it in an emergency. Some inhalers are activated by taking in a breath, and these may be easier for some people to use. If you have trouble operating an inhaler, you can ask your physician for a spacer device (see p.78); this requires less coordination between releasing the drug and breathing in, and is particularly suitable for children and the elderly. Always check how to use your particular device with the pharmacist.

Mouthpiece

Accuhaler

Mouthpiece

Turbuhaler

Mouthpiece

Metered-dose

DRUGS FOR ASTHMA continued

HOW TO USE A SPACER

A spacer is a large, hollow plastic device that has a mouthpiece at one end and a slot for an inhaler at the other; it can be split in two for easy cleaning and transporting. A spacer is ideal for groups such as children and the elderly as it avoids special breathing techniques and allows the patient to breathe in the drug at a normal rate. For small children and the very sick, the mouthpiece can be fitted with a mask that covers the mouth and nose. It is important to clean the spacer once a week to rid it of static electricity because this can reduce the amount of drug that reaches the airways.

1 Click the two halves of the spacer together securely. Remove the cap from the inhaler's mouthpiece and shake the inhaler.

2 Push the mouthpiece of the inhaler into the slot at the blunt end of the spacer. Breathe out as deeply as possible; prepare to place the spacer in your mouth.

3 Press the canister to release a dose of the drug. Breathe in, hold breath for 10 seconds, breathe out into the spacer, and repeat. Another dose can be taken.

HOW TO USE A METERED-DOSE INHALER

The metered-dose inhaler is one of the most commonly prescribed devices for treating asthma, and is used to deliver a range of drugs. It is easy to use, and it takes only a matter of seconds for the drug to reach the airways and relieve breathing. Practise the technique before you need to use the inhaler in an emergency.

1 Remove the cap from the mouthpiece and shake the inhaler. Breathe out gently. Get ready to place the mouthpiece in the mouth.

2 Tilt back the head, breathe in slowly and deeply, and at the same time press the canister. Hold breath for 10 seconds.

Corticosteroids usually start to increase the sufferer's capacity for exercise within a few days, and most people find that the frequency of their attacks is reduced.

Leukotrienes occur naturally in the body; they used to be called "slow-reacting substances". They are chemically related to the prostaglandins, but much more potent in producing an inflammatory reaction; they are also much more potent than histamine at causing broncho-constriction. Leukotrienes seem to play an important part in asthma. Drugs have been developed that block their receptors (leukotriene receptor antagonists) and therefore reduce the inflammation and bronchoconstriction of asthma. Cromoglycate acts by stabilizing mast cells in the lungs, preventing them from releasing histamine, leukotrienes, and other inflammation-causing chemicals.

Risks and special precautions

The drugs taken by inhalation act locally and are used in much lower doses than would be needed as tablets. They do not commonly cause serious side effects, although the dry powder inhalations can cause a reflex bronchospasm as the powder hits the lining of the airways; this can be avoided by using a short-acting sympathomimetic first. Inhaled cortico-steroids may encourage fungal growth in the mouth and throat (thrush). This can be minimized by using a spacer and/or by rinsing the mouth with water after each use. High doses of inhaled steroids may suppress adrenal gland function, reduce bone density, and increase the risk of glaucoma. Sympathomimetics and

theophylline taken by mouth may affect heart rate, and should be prescribed with caution to people with heart problems, high blood pressure, or an overactive thyroid gland. The effects of theophylline may last longer if you have a viral infection, heart failure, or liver cirrhosis. The drugs also interact with many other drugs. The anticholinergic drugs must be used with caution in patients who have prostate problems or urinary retention. Leukotriene receptor antagonists may produce a syndrome with several potentially serious effects including worsening lung function and heart complications.

COMMON DRUGS

Sympathomimetics
Fenoterol
Formoterol *
Salbutamol *
Salmeterol *
Terbutaline *

Anticholinergics
Ipratropium *
Tiotropium *

Leukotriene antagonists
Montelukast *
Zafirlukast

Xanthines
Aminophylline *
Oxtriphylline
Theophylline *

Corticosteroids
Beclomethasone *
Budesonide *
Ciclesonide
Fluticasone *
Prednisolone/
   prednisone *

IgE blocker
Omalizumab

Other drugs
Sodium
   cromoglycate *
Krtotifen

* See Part 4

DECONGESTANTS

The usual cause of a blocked nose is swelling of the delicate mucous membrane that lines the nasal passages and excessive production of mucus as a result of inflammation. This may be caused by an infection (for example, a common cold) or it may be caused by an allergy (for example, to pollen), a condition known as allergic rhinitis or hay fever. Congestion can also occur in the sinuses (the air spaces in the skull), resulting in sinusitis. Decongestants are drugs that reduce swelling of the mucous membrane and suppress the production of mucus, helping to clear blocked nasal passages and sinuses. Antihistamines counter the allergic response in allergy-related conditions (see p.110). If the symptoms are persistent, either topical corticosteroids (see p.127) or sodium cromoglycate (p.431) may be preferred. For children under 2 years of age, consult a physician or pharmacist before using a cough or cold product.

Why they are used

Decongestants aren't necessary for most common colds and blocked noses. Simple home remedies, for example, steam inhalation, possibly with the addition of an aromatic oil – such as menthol or eucalyptus – are often effective. Decongestants are used when such measures are ineffective or when there is a particular risk from untreated congestion – for example, in people who suffer from recurrent middle-ear or sinus infections.

Decongestants are available in the form of drops or sprays applied directly into the nose or they can be taken by mouth. Small quantities of decongestant drugs are added to many over-the-counter cold remedies (see p.80).

How they work

When the mucous membrane lining the nose is irritated by infection or allergy, the blood vessels supplying the membrane become enlarged. This leads to fluid accumulation in the surrounding tissue and encourages the production of larger-than-normal amounts of mucus.

Most decongestants belong to the *sympathomimetic* group of drugs that stimulate the sympathetic branch of the

ACTION OF DECONGESTANTS

Normal nasal passages
The lining of the nasal passages consists of a layer of mucus-producing cells (the mucous membrane) supplied by blood vessels. The walls of the blood vessels contain nerve endings that, when stimulated, cause the vessels to constrict.

Sinus

Lining

Nasal passage

Mucus

Nasal passage

Blood vessels

Mucous membrane

Congested nasal lining
When the blood vessels enlarge in response to infection or irritation, increased amounts of fluid pass into the mucous membrane, which swells and produces more mucus.

Effect of decongestants
Decongestants enhance the action of chemicals that stimulate constriction of the blood vessels. Narrowing of the blood vessels reduces swelling and mucus production.

autonomic nervous system (see p.63). One effect of this action is to constrict the blood vessels, reducing swelling of the lining of the nose and sinuses.

How they affect you

When applied topically in the form of drops or sprays, these drugs start to relieve congestion within a few minutes. Decongestants by mouth take a little longer to act, but their effect may also last

longer. Used in moderation, topical decongestants have few *adverse effects*, because they are not absorbed by the body in large amounts. Used for too long or in excess, topical decongestants can, after giving initial relief, do more harm than good, causing a "rebound congestion" (see left). This effect can be prevented by taking the minimum effective dose and by using decongestant preparations only when absolutely necessary. Decongestants taken by mouth do not cause rebound congestion but are more likely to cause other side effects.

REBOUND CONGESTION

This can happen when decongestant nose drops and sprays are withdrawn or overused. The result is a sudden increase in congestion due to widening of the blood vessels in the nasal lining because blood vessels are no longer constricted by the decongestant.

Congestion before drug treatment

Congestion after stopping drug treatment

COMMON DRUGS

Used topically	Taken by mouth
Ephedrine ✳	Ephedrine ✳
Oxymetazoline	Phenylephrine
Phenylephrine ✳	Pseudoephedrine ✳
Xylometazoline ✳	

✳ See Part 4

DRUGS TO TREAT COUGHS

Coughing is a natural response to irritation of the lungs and air passages, designed to expel harmful substances from the respiratory tract. Common causes of coughing include infection of the respiratory tract (for example, bronchitis or pneumonia), inflammation of the airways caused by asthma, or exposure to certain irritant substances such as smoke or chemical fumes. Depending on their cause, coughs may be productive – that is, phlegm-producing – or they may be dry.

In most cases, coughing is a helpful reaction that assists the body in ridding itself of excess phlegm and substances that irritate the respiratory system; suppressing the cough may actually delay recovery. However, repeated bouts of coughing can be distressing, and may increase irritation of the air passages. In such cases, medication to ease the cough may be recommended.

There are two main groups of cough remedies, according to whether the cough is productive or dry.

Productive coughs

Mucolytics and expectorants are sometimes recommended for productive coughs when simple home remedies such as steam inhalation have failed to "loosen" the cough and make it easier to cough up phlegm. Mucolytics alter the consistency of the phlegm, making it less sticky and easier to cough up. These are often given by inhalation. However, there

is little evidence that they are effective. Dornase alfa may be given to people who suffer from cystic fibrosis; the drug, given by inhalation via a nebulizer, is an enzyme that improves lung function by thinning the mucus. Expectorant drugs are taken by mouth to loosen a cough. There is some evidence that guaifenesin is effective. Expectorants are included in many over-the-counter cough remedies.

Dry coughs

In dry coughs there is no advantage to be gained from promoting the expulsion of phlegm. Drugs used for dry coughs are given to suppress the coughing mechanism by calming the part of the brain that governs the coughing reflex. Antihistamines are often given for mild coughs, particularly in children. Dextromethorphan (DM) is used in many over-the-counter cough products. For persistent coughs, mild opioid drugs such as codeine may be prescribed (see also Analgesics, p.64). All cough suppressants have a generally sedating effect on the brain and nervous system and commonly cause drowsiness and other *side effects*.

Selecting a cough medication

There is a bewildering variety of over-the-counter medications available for the treatment of coughs. Most consist of a syrupy base to which active ingredients and flavourings are added. Many contain a number of different active ingredients,

COLD CURES

Many preparations are available over-the-counter to treat different symptoms of the common cold. The main ingredient in most preparations is a mild analgesic, such as ASA or acetaminophen, accompanied by a decongestant (p.79), an antihistamine (p.110), and sometimes caffeine. Often the dose of each added ingredient is too low to provide any benefit. There is no evidence that vitamin C (see p.480) speeds recovery, but zinc supplements (see p.482) may be effective in shortening the cold's duration.

While some people find these drugs help to relieve symptoms, over-the-counter "cold cures" do not alter the course of the illness. Most doctors recommend using a product with a single analgesic, as the best way of alleviating symptoms. Other decongestants or antihistamines may be taken if needed. These medicines are not harmless: take care to avoid overdose if using different brands.

sometimes with contradictory effects: it is not uncommon to find an expectorant (for a productive cough) and a decongestant included in the same preparation.

It is important to select the correct type of medication for your cough to avoid the risk that you may make your condition worse. For example, using a cough suppressant for a productive cough may prevent you getting rid of excess infected phlegm and may delay your recovery. It is best to choose a preparation with a single active ingredient that is appropriate for your type of cough. Diabetics may need to select a sugar-free product. If you are in any doubt about which product to choose, ask your physician or pharmacist for advice. Since there is a danger that use of over-the-counter cough remedies to alleviate symptoms may delay the diagnosis of a more serious underlying disorder, it is important to seek medical advice for any cough that persists for longer than a few days or if a cough is accompanied by additional symptoms such as fever or blood in the phlegm. For children under 2 years of age, a physician or pharmacist should be consulted before using a cough or cold product.

ACTION OF COUGH REMEDIES

Cough remedies are divided into two main groups: those that alter the consistency or production of phlegm (mucolytics and expectorants); and those that suppress the coughing reflex (opioid and non-opioid cough suppressants). Mucolytics are usually given by inhalation and act directly on the lungs and airways. Expectorants are taken by mouth, and are supposed to help bring up phlegm. Cough suppressants are taken by mouth and they act on the coughing centre in the brain.

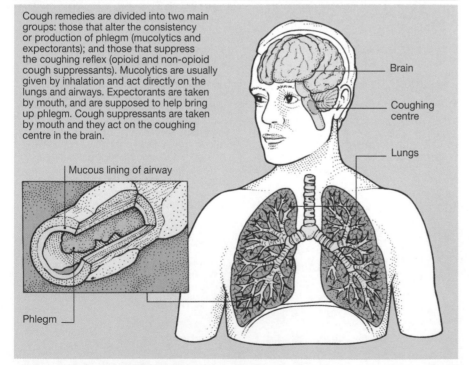

Mucous lining of airway

Phlegm

Brain

Coughing centre

Lungs

COMMON DRUGS

Expectorants
Guaifenesin

Mucolytics
Dornase alfa

Steam inhalation
Eucalyptus
Menthol

Opioid cough suppressants
Codeine ✳
Hydrocodone ✳

Non-opioid cough suppressants
Antihistamines (see p.110)
Dextromethorphan ✳

✳ See Part 4

HEART AND CIRCULATION

The blood transports oxygen, nutrients, and heat, contains chemical messages in the form of drugs and hormones, and carries away waste products for excretion by the kidneys. It is pumped by the heart to and from the lungs, and then in a separate circuit to the rest of the body, including the brain, digestive organs, muscles, kidneys, and skin.

What can go wrong
The efficiency of the circulation may be impaired by weakening of the heart's pumping action (heart failure) or irregularity of heart rate (arrhythmia). In addition, the blood vessels may be narrowed and clogged by fatty deposits (atherosclerosis). This may reduce blood supply to the brain, the extremities (peripheral vascular disease), or the heart muscle (coronary heart disease), causing angina. These last disorders can be complicated by the formation of clots that may block a blood vessel. A clot in the arteries supplying the heart muscle is known as coronary thrombosis; a clot in an artery inside the brain is the most frequent cause of stroke.

One common circulatory disorder is abnormally high blood pressure (hypertension), in which the pressure of circulating blood on the vessel walls is increased for reasons not yet fully understood. One factor may be loss of elasticity of the vessel walls (arteriosclerosis). Several other conditions, such as migraine and Raynaud's disease, are caused by temporary alterations to blood vessel size.

Why drugs are used
Because those suffering from heart disease often have more than one problem, several drugs may be prescribed at once. Many act directly on the heart to alter the rate and rhythm of the heart beat. These are known as anti-arrhythmics and include beta blockers and digoxin.

Other drugs affect the diameter of the blood vessels, either dilating them (vasodilators) to improve blood flow and reduce blood pressure, or constricting them (vasoconstrictors).

Drugs may also reduce blood volume and fat levels, and alter clotting ability. Diuretics (used in the treatment of hypertension and heart failure) increase the body's excretion of water. Lipid-lowering drugs reduce blood cholesterol levels, thereby minimizing the risk of atherosclerosis. Drugs to reduce blood clotting are administered if there is a risk of abnormal blood clots forming in the heart, veins, or arteries. Drugs that increase clotting are given when the body's natural clotting mechanism is defective.

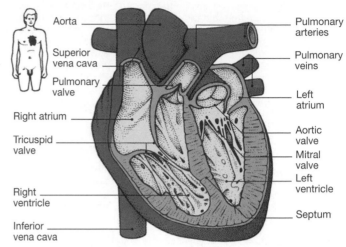

The heart
The heart is a pump with four chambers. The atrium and ventricle on the left side pump oxygenated blood to the body, while the chambers on the right pump deoxygenated blood to the lungs. Backflow of blood is stopped by valves at the chamber exits.

How blood circulates
Deoxygenated blood is carried to the heart from all parts of the body. It is then pumped to the lungs, where it becomes oxygenated. The oxygenated blood returns to the heart and from there is pumped throughout the body.

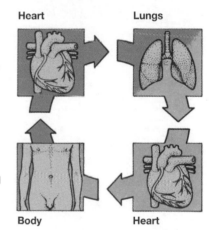

- Deoxygenated blood
- Oxygenated blood

Arteries
Arteries carry blood away from the heart. Muscle walls contract and dilate in response to nerve signals.

Veins
Veins carry blood back to the heart. The walls are less elastic than artery walls.

MAJOR DRUG GROUPS

Digitalis	Anti-angina drugs
Beta blockers	Antihypertensive drugs
Vasodilators	Lipid-lowering drugs
Diuretics	Drugs that affect blood
Anti-arrhythmics	clotting

DIGITALIS

Digitalis is the collective term for the naturally occurring substances (also called cardiac glycosides) that are found in the leaves of plants of the foxglove family and used to treat certain heart disorders.

The principal drug in this group is digoxin. Digoxin dosage is usually adjusted to a therapeutic drug level in the blood (see also Risks and special precautions, below).

Why it is used

Digoxin does not cure heart disease but improves the heart's pumping action and so relieves many of the symptoms that result from poor heart function. It is useful for treating conditions in which the heart beats irregularly or too rapidly (notably in atrial fibrillation, see Anti-arrhythmic drugs, p.86), when it pumps too weakly (in congestive heart failure), or when the heart muscle is damaged and weakened following a heart attack.

Digoxin can be used for a short period when the heart is working poorly, but in many cases it has to be taken indefinitely. Its effect does not diminish with time. In cases of heart failure, this digitalis drug is often given together with a diuretic drug (see p.85).

How it works

The normal heart beat results from electrical impulses generated in nerve tissue within the heart. These impulses cause the heart muscle to contract and pump blood to the body. Digoxin reduces the flow of electrical impulses in the heart, therefore making the heart contract more slowly.

The force with which the heart muscle contracts depends on chemical changes in the heart muscle. By promoting these chemical changes, digoxin increases the force of muscle contraction each time the heart is stimulated. This compensates for the loss of power that occurs when some of the muscle is damaged following a heart attack. The stronger heart beat increases blood flow to the kidneys. This leads to increased urine production and therefore helps to remove the excess fluid that often accumulates as a result of heart failure.

How it affects you

Digoxin relieves the symptoms of heart failure – fatigue, breathlessness, and swelling of the legs – and increases your capacity for exercise. The frequency with which you need to pass urine is also increased initially.

Risks and special precautions

Digoxin can be *toxic* and, if blood levels of digoxin rise too high, the symptoms of digitalis poisoning may be produced. These symptoms include excessive tiredness, confusion, loss of appetite, nausea, vomiting, visual disturbances, and diarrhea. If such symptoms occur during treatment with digoxin, it is important to report them to your physician promptly.

Digoxin is normally removed from the body by the kidneys; if kidney function is impaired, the drug is more likely to accumulate in the body and cause toxic side effects.

Digoxin is more toxic when blood potassium levels are low. Potassium deficiency is commonly caused by diuretic drugs, therefore people taking these drugs as well as digoxin need to have the effects of both the drugs and their blood potassium levels carefully monitored. Potassium supplements may be required.

ACTION OF DIGITALIS

The heart beat is triggered by electrical impulses that are generated by the pacemaker, a small mass of nerve tissue in the right atrium. Electrical signals are passed from the pacemaker to the atrio-ventricular node. From here a wave of impulses spreads throughout the heart muscle, causing it to contract and pump blood to the body. The pumping action of the heart can become weak if the heart muscle is damaged or if the heart beat is too fast, as in atrial fibrillation. In this condition (shown right), rapid signals from the pacemaker trigger fast and inefficient contractions of both the atria and the ventricles.

Pacemaker

Atrio-ventricular node

Heart muscle

Right ventricle

Left ventricle

Abnormally rapid heart beat (rate: 120/minute)

The effect of digitalis
The digitalis drug digoxin reduces the flow of electrical impulses through the atrioventricular node so that the ventricles contract less often. In addition, by promoting the chemical changes in muscle cells necessary for muscular contraction, this drug increases the force with which the heart muscle contracts and thereby improves the efficiency of each heart beat.

Drug

Slowed heart beat (rate: 80/minute)

COMMON DRUGS

Digoxin *

* See Part 4

BETA BLOCKERS

Beta blockers are drugs that interrupt the transmission of stimuli through the beta *receptors* of the body. Since the actions they block originate in the adrenal glands (and elsewhere) they are also sometimes called beta adrenergic blocking agents. Used mainly in heart disorders, these drugs are occasionally prescribed for other conditions.

Why they are used

Beta blockers are used for treating angina (see p.87), hypertension (see p.88), and irregular heart rhythms (see p.86). They are also given after a heart attack to reduce the likelihood of abnormal heart rhythms or further damage to the heart muscle. These drugs are also prescribed to improve heart function in heart muscle disorders, known as cardiomyopathies.

Beta blockers may also be given to prevent migraine headaches (see p.73), or to reduce the physical symptoms of anxiety (see p.67). The drugs may also be given to control symptoms of an overactive thyroid gland. A beta blocker is sometimes given in the form of eye drops in glaucoma to lower the fluid pressure inside the eye (see p.156).

How they work

By occupying the beta receptors, beta blockers nullify the stimulating action of norepinephrine (noradrenaline), the main "fight or flight" hormone. As a result, they reduce the force and speed of the heart

THE USES AND EFFECTS OF BETA BLOCKERS

Blocking the transmission of signals through beta receptors in different parts of the body produces a wide variety of benefits and side effects depending on the disease being treated. The illustration (right) shows the main areas and body systems affected by the action of beta blockers.

Brain
Dilation of the blood vessels surrounding the brain is inhibited, so preventing migraine.

Eye
Beta blocker eye drops reduce fluid production and so lower pressure inside the eye.

Lungs
Constriction of the airways may provoke breathlessness in asthmatics or those with chronic bronchitis.

Heart
Slowing of the heart rate and reduction of the force of the heart beat reduces the workload of the heart, helping to prevent angina and abnormal heart rhythms. But this action may worsen heart failure.

Blood vessels
Constriction of the blood vessels may cause coldness of the hands and feet.

Muscles
Muscle tremor due to anxiety or to over activity of the thyroid gland is reduced.

Blood pressure
This is lowered because the rate and force at which the heart pumps blood into the circulatory system is reduced.

beat and prevent the dilation of the blood vessels surrounding the brain and leading to the extremities. The effect of this "beta blockade" in a variety of disorders is shown in the box above.

How they affect you

Beta blockers are taken to treat angina. They reduce the frequency and severity of attacks. As part of the treatment for hypertension, beta blockers help to lower blood pressure and thus reduce the risks that are associated with this condition. Beta blockers help to prevent severe attacks of arrhythmia, in which the heart beat is wild and uncontrolled.

Because beta blockers affect many parts of the body, they often produce minor *side effects*. By reducing heart rate and air flow to the lungs, they may reduce capacity for strenuous exercise, although this is unlikely to be noticed by somebody whose physical activity was previously limited by heart problems. Many people experience cold hands and feet while taking these drugs as a result of the reduction in the blood supply to the limbs. Reduced circulation can also lead to temporary impotence during treatment.

Risks and special precautions

The main risk of beta blockers is that of provoking breathing difficulties as a result of their blocking effect on beta receptors in the lungs. Cardioselective beta blockers, which act principally on the heart, are thought to be less likely than non-cardioselective ones to cause such problems. But all beta blockers are prescribed with caution for people who

have asthma, bronchitis, or other forms of respiratory disease.

Beta blockers are not commonly prescribed for people who have poor circulation in the limbs because they reduce the flow of blood and may aggravate such conditions. They may be given, very cautiously, to people who are subject to heart failure because they may further reduce the force of the heart beat. Diabetics who need to take beta blockers should be aware that they may notice a change in the warning signs of low blood sugar; in particular, they may find that symptoms such as palpitations and tremor are suppressed.

Beta blockers should not be stopped suddenly after prolonged use; this may provoke a sudden and severe recurrence of symptoms of the original disorder, even a heart attack. The blood pressure may also rise markedly. When treatment with beta blockers needs to be stopped, it should be withdrawn gradually under medical supervision.

BETA RECEPTORS

Signals from the sympathetic nervous system are carried by noradrenaline, a *neurotransmitter* produced in the adrenal glands and at the ends of the sympathetic nerve fibres. Beta blockers stop the signals from the neurotransmitter.

Neurotransmitter

Beta blocker

Types of beta receptor
There are two types of beta receptor: beta 1 and beta 2. Beta 1 receptors are located mainly in the heart muscle; beta 2 receptors are found both in the airways and blood vessels. Cardioselective drugs act mainly on beta 1 receptors; non-cardioselective drugs act on both types of receptor.

▲ Beta 1 receptors
▼ Beta 2 receptors

COMMON DRUGS

Cardioselective	Non-cardioselective
Acebutolol	Carvedilol
Atenolol *	Labetalol
Betaxolol	Nadolol
Bisoprolol	Oxprenolol
Esmolol	Pindolol
Metoprolol *	Propranolol *
	Sotalol *
	Timolol *

* See Part 4

VASODILATORS

Vasodilators are drugs that widen blood vessels. Their most obvious use is to reverse narrowing of the blood vessels when this leads to reduced blood flow and, consequently, a lower oxygen supply to parts of the body. This problem occurs in angina, when narrowing of the coronary arteries reduces blood supply to the heart muscle. Vasodilators are also often used to treat high blood pressure (hypertension).

Why they are used

Vasodilators improve the blood flow and thus the oxygen supply to areas of the body where they are most needed. In angina, dilation of the blood vessels throughout the body reduces the force with which the heart needs to pump and thereby eases its workload (see also Anti-angina drugs, p.87). Specifically, ACE Inhibitors are helpful in treating congestive heart failure.

Because blood pressure is dependent partly on the diameter of blood vessels, vasodilators are often helpful in treating hypertension (see p.88).

In peripheral vascular disease, narrowed blood vessels in the legs cannot supply sufficient blood to the extremities, often leading to pain in the legs during exercise. Unfortunately, because the vessels are narrowed by atherosclerosis, vasodilators have little effect.

Vasodilator drugs have also been used to treat senile dementia, in the hope of increasing the supply of oxygen to the brain. The benefits of this treatment have not yet been proved.

How they work

Vasodilators widen the blood vessels by relaxing the muscles surrounding them. They achieve this either by affecting the action of the muscles directly (nitrates, hydralazine, and calcium channel blockers) or by interfering with the nerve signals that govern contraction of the

blood vessels (alpha blockers). ACE inhibitors act by blocking the activity of an enzyme in the blood. The enzyme is responsible for producing angiotensin II, a powerful vasoconstrictor (see box below).

How they affect you

As well as relieving the symptoms of the disorders for which they are taken, vasodilators can have many minor *side effects* related to their action on the circulation. Flushing and headaches are common at the start of treatment. Dizziness and fainting may also occur as a result of lowered blood pressure. Dilation of the blood vessels can also

cause fluid build-up, leading to swelling, particularly of the ankles.

Risks and special precautions

The major risk is that blood pressure may fall too low. Therefore vasodilator drugs are prescribed with caution for people with unstable blood pressure. It is also advisable to sit or lie down after taking the first dose of a vasodilator drug.

ACTION OF VASODILATORS

The diameter of blood vessels is governed by the contraction of the surrounding muscle. The muscle contracts in response to signals from the sympathetic nervous system (p.63). Vasodilators encourage the muscles to relax, thus increasing the size of blood vessels.

Constricted blood vessel **Dilated blood vessel**

Muscle band

Where they act
Each type of vasodilator acts on a different part of the mechanism controlling blood vessel size in order to prevent contraction of the surrounding layer of muscles.

Nerves – Alpha blockers interfere with nerve signals to the muscles.

Muscle layer – Nitrates and calcium channel blockers act directly on the muscle to inhibit contraction.

Blood – ACE inhibitors block enzyme activity in the blood (see box below).

ACE INHIBITORS

The ACE (angiotensin-converting enzyme) inhibitors are powerful vasodilators. They act by blocking the action of an enzyme in the bloodstream that is responsible for converting a chemical called angiotensin I into angiotensin II. Angiotensin II encourages constriction of the blood vessels, and its absence permits them to dilate (see right).

Angiotensin II

Angiotensin I | ACE

Before drug
Angiotensin I is converted by the enzyme into angiotensin II. The blood vessel constricts.

Drug

Drug action
ACE inhibitors block enzyme activity, thereby preventing the formation of angiotensin II. The blood vessel dilates.

COMMON DRUGS

ACE inhibitors
Benazepril
Captopril ✳
Cilazapril
Enalapril ✳
Fosinopril
Lisinopril ✳
Perindopril ✳
Quinapril
Ramipril ✳
Trandolapril

Alpha blockers
Doxazosin ✳
Prazosin
Terazosin ✳

Nitrates
Nitroglycerin ✳
Isosorbide dinitrate/
  mononitrate ✳

Calcium channel blockers
Amlodipine ✳
Diltiazem ✳
Felodipine
Nifedipine ✳
Verapamil ✳

Angiotensin II blockers
Candesartan
Eprosartan
Irbesartan ✳
Losartan ✳
Telmisartan
Valsartan ✳

Other drugs
Hydralazine
Minoxidil ✳

✳ See Part 4

DIURETICS

Diuretic drugs help to turn excess body water into urine. As the urine is expelled, two disorders are relieved: the tissues become less water-swollen (edema) and the heart action improves because it has to pump a smaller volume of blood. There are several classes of diuretics, each of which has different uses, modes of action, and effects (see Types of diuretic, below). But all diuretics act on the kidneys, the organs that govern the water content of the body.

Why they are used

Diuretics are most commonly used in the treatment of high blood pressure (hypertension). By removing a larger amount of water than usual from the bloodstream, the kidneys reduce the total volume of blood circulating. This drop in volume causes a reduction of the pressure within the blood vessels (see Antihypertensive drugs, p.88).

Diuretics are also widely used to treat heart failure in which the heart's pumping mechanism has become weak. In the treatment of this disorder, they remove fluid that has accumulated in the tissues and lungs. The resulting drop in blood volume reduces the work of the heart.

Other conditions for which diuretics are often prescribed include nephrotic syndrome (a kidney disorder that causes edema), cirrhosis of the liver (in which fluid may accumulate in the abdominal cavity), and premenstrual syndrome (when hormonal activity can lead to fluid retention and bloating).

Less commonly, diuretics are used to treat glaucoma (see p.156) and Ménière's disease (see p.74).

How they work

The kidneys' normal filtration process takes water, salts (mainly potassium and sodium), and waste products out of the bloodstream. Most of the salts and water are returned to the bloodstream, but some are expelled from the body together with the waste products in the urine. Diuretics interfere with this filtration process by reducing the amounts of sodium and water taken back into the

ACTION OF DIURETICS

As blood passes through the kidney, water, sodium and potassium salts, and waste products are filtered out of the bloodstream. Most of the water and filtered salts are then reabsorbed by the bloodstream from the tubule; the remainder is excreted as urine.

By blocking the movement of sodium back into the bloodstream, diuretics prevent the reabsorption of water, so that more is expelled from the body as urine. Different diuretic drugs act on different parts of the tubule (see right).

Artery   Kidney tubule

Vein

Kidney

Diuretic action in the kidney tubule

Water, salts, and waste removed from blood in the glomerulus.

Sodium and water reabsorbed. Blocked by **osmotics.**

Sodium and water reabsorbed. Potassium lost. Blocked by **potassium-sparing diuretics.**

Water, sodium, and potassium reabsorbed. Blocked by **thiazides.**

Water, sodium, and potassium reabsorbed. Blocked by **loop diuretics.**

Urine to the bladder

bloodstream, thus increasing the volume of urine produced. Modifying the filtration process in this way means that the water content of the blood is reduced; less water in the blood causes excess water present in the tissues to be drawn out and eliminated in urine.

How they affect you

All diuretics increase the frequency with which you need to pass urine. This is most noticeable at the start of treatment. People who have suffered from edema may notice that swelling – particularly of the ankles – is reduced, and those with heart failure may find that breathlessness is relieved.

Risks and special precautions

Diuretics can cause blood chemical imbalances, of which a fall in potassium levels (hypokalemia) is the most common. Hypokalemia can cause confusion, weakness, and trigger abnormal heart rhythms (especially in people taking digitalis drugs). Potassium supplements or a potassium-sparing diuretic usually corrects the imbalance. A diet that is rich in potassium (containing plenty of fresh fruits and vegetables) may be helpful.

Some diuretics may raise blood levels of uric acid, increasing the risk of gout. They may also raise blood sugar levels, causing problems for diabetics.

TYPES OF DIURETIC

Thiazides The diuretics most commonly prescribed, thiazides may lead to potassium deficiency and they are, therefore, often given together with a potassium supplement or in conjunction with a potassium-sparing diuretic (see right).

Loop diuretics These fast-acting, powerful drugs increase the output of urine for a few hours, and are therefore sometimes used in emergencies. They may cause excessive loss of potassium, which may need to be countered as for thiazides. Large doses may disturb hearing.

Potassium-sparing diuretics These mild diuretics are usually used in conjunction with a thiazide or a loop diuretic to prevent excessive potassium loss.

Osmotic diuretics Prescribed only rarely, these drugs are used to maintain the flow of urine through the kidneys after surgery or injury, and to reduce pressure rapidly within fluid-filled cavities.

Acetazolamide This mild diuretic drug is used principally in the treatment of glaucoma (see p.156).

COMMON DRUGS

Loop diuretics
Bumetanide *
Furosemide *

Potassium-sparing diuretics
Amiloride *
Spironolactone *
Triamterene *

Thiazides
Chlorthalidone
Hydrochlorothiazide *
Indapamide *
Metolazone

Others
Ethacrynic acid

* See Part 4

ANTI-ARRHYTHMICS

The heart contains two upper and two lower chambers, which are known as the atria and ventricles (see p.81). The pumping actions of these two sets of chambers are normally coordinated by electrical impulses that originate in the pacemaker and then travel along conducting pathways so that the heart beats with a regular rhythm. If this coordination breaks down, the heart will beat abnormally, either irregularly, or faster or slower than usual. The general term for abnormal heart rhythm is arrhythmia.

Arrhythmias may occur as a result of a birth defect, coronary heart disease, or other less common heart disorders. A variety of more general conditions, including overactivity of the thyroid gland, and certain drugs – such as caffeine and *anticholinergic* drugs – can also disturb heart rhythm.

SITES OF DRUG ACTION

Anti-arrhythmic drugs either slow the flow of electrical impulses to the heart muscle, or inhibit the muscle's ability to contract. Beta blockers reduce the ability of the pacemaker to pass electrical signals to the atria. Digoxin reduces the passage of signals from the atrioventricular node. Calcium channel blockers interfere with the ability of the heart muscle to contract by impeding the flow of calcium into muscle cells. Other drugs, such as quinidine and disopyramide, reduce the sensitivity of muscle cells to electrical impulses.

Aorta

Pacemaker

Pulmonary arteries

Atria

Heart muscle

Ventricles

Atrioventricular node

A broad selection of drugs is used to regulate heart rhythm, including beta blockers, the digitalis drug digoxin, and calcium channel blockers. Other drugs used are disopyramide, procainamide, and quinidine.

Why they are used

Minor disturbances of heart rhythm are common and do not usually require drug treatment. However, if the pumping action of the heart is seriously affected, the circulation of blood throughout the body may become inefficient, and drug treatment may be necessary.

Drugs may be taken to treat individual attacks of arrhythmia, or they may be taken on a regular basis to prevent or control abnormal heart rhythms. The particular drug prescribed depends on the type of arrhythmia to be treated, but because people differ in their response, it may be necessary to try several in order to find the most effective one. When the arrhythmia is sudden and severe, it may be necessary to inject a drug immediately to restore normal heart function.

How they work

The heart's pumping action is governed by electrical impulses under the control of the sympathetic nervous system (see Autonomic nervous system, p.63). These signals pass through the heart muscle, causing the two pairs of chambers – the atria and ventricles – to contract in turn (see Sites of drug action, left).

All anti-arrhythmic drugs alter the conduction of electrical signals in the heart. However, each drug or drug group has a different effect on the sequence of events controlling the pumping action. Some block the transmission of signals to the heart (beta blockers); some affect the way in which signals are conducted within the heart (digoxin); others affect the response of the heart muscle to the signals received (calcium channel blockers, disopyramide, procainamide, and quinidine).

How they affect you

These drugs usually prevent symptoms of arrhythmia and may restore a regular heart rhythm. Although they do not prevent all arrhythmias, they usually reduce the frequency and severity of any symptoms.

Unfortunately, as well as suppressing arrhythmias, many of these drugs tend to depress normal heart function, and may produce dizziness on standing up, or increased breathlessness on exertion. Mild nausea and visual disturbances are also fairly frequent. Verapamil can cause constipation, especially when it is prescribed in high doses. Disopyramide may interfere with the parasympathetic nervous system (see p.63), resulting in a number of *anticholinergic* effects.

TYPES OF ARRHYTHMIA

Atrial fibrillation In this common type of arrhythmia, the atria contract irregularly at such a high rate that the ventricles cannot keep pace. It is treated with digoxin, calcium channel blockers such as verapamil, or a beta blocker.

Ventricular tachycardia In this condition, abnormal electrical activity in the ventricles causes them to contract rapidly. Regular treatment with quinidine, disopyramide, or procainamide is usually given. Amiodarone may be used if these are not effective.

Supraventricular tachycardia This condition occurs when extra electrical impulses arise in the pacemaker or atria. These extra impulses stimulate the ventricles to contract rapidly. Attacks may disappear on their own without treatment, but drugs such as adenosine, digoxin, verapamil, or propranolol may be given.

Heart block When impulses are not conducted from the atria to the ventricles, the ventricles start to beat at a slower rate. Some cases of heart block do not require treatment. For more severe heart block accompanied by dizziness and fainting, it is usually necessary to fit the patient with an artificial pacemaker.

Risks and special precautions

These drugs may further disrupt heart rhythm under certain circumstances and therefore they are used only when the likely benefit outweighs the risks.

Quinidine can be *toxic* if an overdose is taken, resulting in a syndrome called cinchonism, which includes disturbed hearing, giddiness, and impaired vision (even blindness). Because some people are particularly sensitive to this drug, a test dose is usually given before regular treatment is started.

Amiodarone may accumulate in the tissues over time, and may lead to light-sensitive rashes, changes in thyroid function, and lung problems.

COMMON DRUGS

Beta blockers
Propranolol *
Sotalol *
(see also p.83)

Calcium channel blockers
Diltiazem *
Verapamil *

Digitalis
(see also p.82)
Digoxin *

Other drugs
Amiodarone *
Bretylium
Disopyramide
Flecainide
Ibutilide
Lidocaine
Mexiletine
Procainamide
Propafenone
Quinidine *

* See Part 4

ANTI-ANGINA DRUGS

Angina is chest pain, or chest discomfort, produced when the heart muscle receives insufficient oxygen. Women may not always feel pain, just chest tightness with some shortness of breath. Angina is usually caused by narrowing of the blood vessels (coronary arteries) that transport blood and oxygen to the heart muscle.

In the most common type of angina (classic angina), narrowing of the coronary arteries results from deposits of fat – called atheroma – on the walls of the arteries. Symptoms usually occur during emotional stress or physical exertion. In variant angina, the arteries are narrowed by contraction (spasm) of the muscle fibres in the artery walls, and pain may also occur at rest.

Atheroma deposits build up more rapidly in the arteries of smokers and people who eat a high-fat diet. This is why, as a basic component of angina treatment, doctors recommend giving up smoking and changing the diet. Overweight people are also advised to lose weight to reduce the demands placed on the heart. While such changes in lifestyle often produce an improvement in symptoms, drug treatment to relieve angina is also often necessary.

The drugs used to treat angina include beta blockers, nitrates, and calcium channel blockers.

Why they are used

Frequent episodes of angina can be disabling and, if left untreated, can lead to an increased risk of a heart attack. Drugs can be used both to relieve angina attacks and to reduce their frequency. People who suffer from only occasional episodes are usually prescribed a rapid-acting drug to take at the first signs of an attack, or before an activity that is known to bring on an attack. A rapid-acting nitrate – nitroglycerin – is usually prescribed for this purpose.

If attacks become more frequent or more severe, regular preventative treatment may be advised. Beta blockers, long-acting nitrates, and calcium channel blockers are used as regular medication to prevent attacks. The introduction of adhesive patches to administer nitrates through the patient's skin has extended the duration of action of nitroglycerin, making treatment easier.

Drugs can often control angina for many years, but they cannot cure the disorder. When severe angina cannot be controlled by drugs, surgery to increase the blood flow to the heart may be recommended.

How they work

Nitrates and calcium channel blockers dilate blood vessels by relaxing the muscle layer in the blood vessel walls (see also Vasodilators, p.84). Blood is more easily pumped through the dilated vessels, reducing the strain on the heart.

Beta blockers reduce heart muscle stimulation during exercise or stress by interrupting signal transmission in the heart. Decreased heart muscle stimulation means less oxygen is required, reducing the risk of angina attacks. For further information on beta blockers, see p.83.

How they affect you

Treatment with one or more of these medicines usually effectively controls angina. Drugs to prevent attacks allow sufferers to undertake more strenuous activities without provoking pain, and if an attack does occur, nitrates usually provide effective relief.

ACTION OF ANTI-ANGINA DRUGS

Anginal pain occurs when the heart muscle runs short of oxygen as it pumps blood round the circulatory system. Nitrates, calcium channel blockers, and potassium channel openers reduce the heart's work by dilating blood vessels. Beta blockers impede the stimulation of heart muscle, reducing its oxygen requirement, thus relieving angina.

Before drug
Body tissues
Blood vessels of body
Lungs
Reduced blood flow
Heart

After drug
Improved blood flow
Drug

These drugs do not usually cause serious *adverse effects*, but they can produce a variety of minor symptoms. By dilating blood vessels throughout the body, the nitrates and calcium channel blockers can cause dizziness (especially when standing) and may cause fainting. Other possible side effects are headaches at the start of treatment, flushing of the skin (especially of the face), and ankle swelling. Beta blockers often cause cold hands and feet, and sometimes they may produce tiredness and a feeling of heaviness in the legs.

CALCIUM CHANNEL BLOCKERS

The passage of calcium through special channels into muscle cells is an essential part of the mechanism of muscle contraction (see right). These drugs prevent movement of calcium in the muscles of the blood vessels and so encourage them to dilate (see far right). The action helps to reduce blood pressure and relieves the strain on the heart muscle in angina by making it easier for the heart to pump blood throughout the body (see Action of anti-angina drugs, above right). Verapamil also slows the passage of nerve signals through the heart muscle. This can be helpful for correcting certain arrhythmias.

Before drug
Muscle
Constricted blood vessel
Muscle cell
Calcium
Calcium channel

After drug
Dilated blood vessel
Blocked calcium
Drug blocks calcium channel

COMMON DRUGS

Beta blockers
(see p.83)

Calcium channel blockers
Amlodipine
Diltiazem *
Felodipine
Nifedipine *
Verapamil *

Nitrates
Isosorbide dinitrate/
    mononitrate *
Nitroglycerin *

Other drugs
ASA *
Simvastatin *
Heparin/LMWH *

* See Part 4

ANTIHYPERTENSIVE DRUGS

Blood pressure is the force exerted by the blood against the walls of the arteries. Two measurements are taken: one indicates force while the heart's ventricles are contracting (systolic pressure). This reading is a higher figure than the other one, which measures the blood pressure during ventricle relaxation (diastolic pressure). Blood pressure varies among individuals and normally increases with age. If a person's blood pressure is higher than normal on at least three separate occasions, a physician may diagnose the condition as hypertension.

Blood pressure may be elevated as a result of an underlying disorder, which the physician will try to identify. Usually, however, it is not possible to determine a cause. This condition is referred to as essential hypertension.

Although hypertension does not usually cause any symptoms, severely raised blood pressure may produce headaches, palpitations, and general feelings of ill-health. It is important to reduce high blood pressure because it can have serious consequences, including stroke, heart attack, heart failure, and kidney damage. Certain groups are particularly at risk from high blood pressure. These risk groups include diabetics, smokers, people with pre-existing heart damage, and those whose blood contains a high level of fat. High blood pressure is more common among black people than among whites, and in countries, such as Japan, where the diet is high in salt.

A small reduction in blood pressure may be brought about by reducing weight, exercising regularly, and avoiding an excessive amount of salt in the diet. But for more severely raised blood pressure, one or more antihypertensive drugs may be prescribed. Several classes of drugs have antihypertensive properties, including the centrally acting antihypertensives, diuretics (p.85), beta blockers (p.83), calcium channel blockers (p.87), ACE (angiotensin-converting enzyme) inhibitors (p.84), and alpha blockers. See also Vasodilators, p.84.

Why they are used

Antihypertensive drugs are prescribed when diet, exercise, and other simple remedies have not brought about an adequate reduction in blood pressure, and your physician sees a risk of serious consequences if the condition is not treated. These drugs do not cure hypertension and may have to be taken indefinitely. However, it is sometimes possible to taper off drug treatment when blood pressure has been reduced to a normal level for a year or more.

How they work

Blood pressure depends not only on the force with which the heart pumps blood, but also on the diameter of blood vessels and the volume of blood in circulation: blood pressure is increased either if the vessels are narrow or if the volume of blood is high. Antihypertensive drugs lower blood pressure either by dilating the blood vessels or by reducing blood volume. Antihypertensive drugs work in different ways and some have more than one action (see Action of antihypertensive drugs, left).

Choice of drug

Drug treatment depends on the severity of hypertension. At the beginning of treatment for mild or moderately high blood pressure, a single drug is used. A thiazide diuretic is often chosen for initial treatment, but it is also increasingly common to use a beta blocker, a calcium channel blocker, or an ACE inhibitor. If a single drug does not reduce the blood pressure sufficiently, a diuretic in combination with one of the other drugs may be used. Some people who have moderate hypertension require a third drug, in which case a vasodilator, centrally acting antihypertensive, or alpha blocker, may also be prescribed.

Severe hypertension is usually controlled with a combination of several drugs, which may need to be given in high doses. Your physician may need to try a number of drugs before finding a combination that controls blood pressure without unacceptable *side effects*.

How they affect you

Treatment with antihypertensive drugs relieves symptoms such as headache and palpitations. However, since most people with hypertension have few, if any, symptoms, side effects may be more noticeable than any immediate beneficial effect. Some antihypertensive drugs may cause dizziness and fainting at the start of treatment because they can sometimes cause an excessive fall in blood pressure. It may take a while for your physician to determine a dosage that avoids such effects. For detailed information on the adverse effects of drugs used to treat hypertension, consult the individual drug profiles in Part 4.

Risks and special precautions

Since your physician needs to know exactly how treatment with a particular drug affects your hypertension – the benefits as well as the side effects – it is important for you to keep using the antihypertensive medication as prescribed, even though you may feel the problem is under control. Sudden withdrawal of some of these drugs may cause a potentially dangerous rebound increase in blood pressure. To stop treatment, the dose needs to be reduced gradually under medical supervision.

ACTION OF ANTI-HYPERTENSIVE DRUGS

Each type of antihypertensive drug acts on a different part of the body to lower blood pressure.

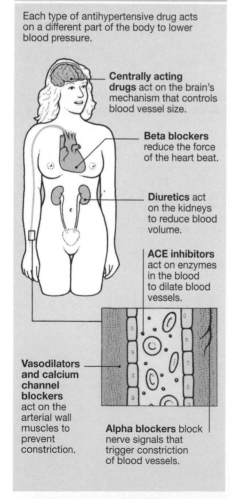

Centrally acting drugs act on the brain's mechanism that controls blood vessel size.

Beta blockers reduce the force of the heart beat.

Diuretics act on the kidneys to reduce blood volume.

ACE inhibitors act on enzymes in the blood to dilate blood vessels.

Vasodilators and calcium channel blockers act on the arterial wall muscles to prevent constriction.

Alpha blockers block nerve signals that trigger constriction of blood vessels.

COMMON DRUGS

ACE inhibitors (see p.84)

Beta blockers (see p.83)

Calcium channel blockers (see p.87)
Amlodipine *
Diltiazem *
Felodipine
Nifedipine *
Verapamil *

Centrally acting antihypertensives
Clonidine
Methyldopa *

Diuretics (see p.85)

Alpha blockers
Doxazosin *
Prazosin
Terazosin *

Vasodilators (see p.84)

* See Part 4

LIPID-LOWERING DRUGS

The blood contains several types of fats, or lipids. They are necessary for normal body function but can be damaging if present in excess, particularly saturated fats such as cholesterol. The main risk is atherosclerosis, in which fatty deposits called atheroma build up in the arteries, restricting and disrupting the flow of blood. This can increase the likelihood of the formation of abnormal blood clots, leading to potentially fatal disorders such as stroke and heart attack.

For most people, cutting down the amount of fat in the diet is sufficient to reduce the risk of atherosclerosis. For others, and for those with an inherited tendency to high levels of fat in the blood (hyperlipidemia or dyslipidemia), lipid-lowering drugs may also be prescribed.

Why they are used

Lipid-lowering drugs are generally given only when dietary measures have failed. The drugs may be given at an earlier stage to individuals at increased risk of atherosclerosis – such as diabetics and people already suffering from circulatory disorders. The drugs may remove existing atheroma in the blood vessels and prevent accumulation of new deposits.

For maximum benefit, these drugs are used in conjunction with a low-fat diet and a reduction in other risk factors such as obesity and smoking. The choice of drug depends on the type of lipid causing problems, so a full medical history, examination, and laboratory analysis of blood samples are needed before drug treatment is given.

How they work

Cholesterol and triglycerides are two of the major fats in the blood. One or both may be raised, influencing the choice of lipid-lowering drug. Ezetimibe prevents the absorption of cholesterol from the bowel. Drugs like cholestyramine act on bile salts, which contain a large amount of cholesterol and are normally released into the bowel to aid digestion before being reabsorbed into the blood. Drugs that bind to bile salts reduce cholesterol levels by blocking their reabsorption, allowing them to be lost from the body.

Other drugs act on the liver. Fibrates and niacin can reduce the level of cholesterol and triglycerides. Statins lower blood cholesterol. Fish oil preparations reduce blood triglycerides, but they may raise cholesterol levels.

Lipid-lowering drugs do not correct the underlying cause of raised levels of fat in the blood, so it is usually necessary to continue with diet and drug treatment indefinitely. Stopping treatment usually leads to a return of high blood lipid levels.

How they affect you

Because dyslipidemia and atherosclerosis are usually without symptoms, you are unlikely to notice any short-term benefits from these drugs. Rather, the aim of treatment is to reduce long-term complications. There may be minor *side effects* from some of these drugs.

By increasing the amount of bile in the digestive tract, several drugs can cause gastrointestinal disturbances such as nausea and constipation or diarrhea, especially at the start of treatment. Statins appear to be well tolerated and are widely used to lower cholesterol levels when diet alone does not work.

Risks and special precautions

Drugs that bind to bile salts can limit absorption of some fat-soluble vitamins, so vitamin supplements may be needed. Fibrates can increase susceptibility to gallstones and occasionally upset the balance of fats in the blood. Statins are used with caution in people with reduced kidney or liver function, and monitoring of blood samples is often advised.

ACTION OF LIPID-LOWERING DRUGS

Lipid-lowering drugs reduce the levels of fats in the blood by interfering with the absorption of bile salts in the bowel, or by altering the way in which the liver converts fatty acids in the blood into different types of lipids.

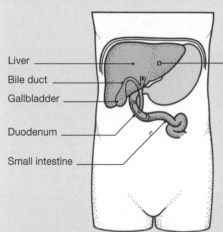

Liver
Bile duct
Gallbladder
Duodenum
Small intestine

Blood
Fatty acid
Liver cell
Enzyme
Lipid

Drugs that act on the liver
Fatty acids in the blood are normally converted into lipids by enzyme activity in the liver (above). Several drugs alter the way fatty acids are taken into the liver cells and others alter the enzyme activity in the liver to prevent the manufacture of lipids.

Drugs that bind to bile salts
Bile is produced by the liver and released into the small intestine via the bile duct to aid digestion. Salts in the bile carry large amounts of cholesterol and are normally reabsorbed from the intestine into the bloodstream during digestion (right). Some drugs bind to bile salts in the intestine and prevent their reabsorption (far right). This action reduces the levels of bile salts in the blood, and triggers the liver to convert more cholesterol into bile salts, thus reducing blood cholesterol levels.

Before drug

After drug

Bile salts
Small intestine
Blood vessel
Bile salt bound to drug

COMMON DRUGS

Fibrates Bezafibrate ✳ Fenofibrate Gemfibrozil ✳	**Nicotinic acid** Niacin ✳
Statins Atorvastatin ✳ Fluvastatin Lovastatin ✳ Pravastatin ✳ Rosuvastatin ✳ Simvastatin ✳	**Drugs that bind to bile salts** Cholestyramine ✳ Colestipol **Other drugs acting on the liver** Omega-3 acid ethyl esters ✳ Omega-3 marine triglycerides
Cholesterol absorption inhibitor Ezetimibe ✳	✳ See Part 4

DRUGS THAT AFFECT BLOOD CLOTTING

When bleeding occurs from injury or surgery, the body normally acts swiftly to stem the flow by sealing the breaks in the blood vessels. This occurs in two stages – first, when cells called platelets accumulate as a plug at the opening in the blood vessel wall, and then when these platelets produce chemicals that activate clotting factors in the blood to form a protein called fibrin. Vitamin K plays an important role in this process (see The clotting mechanism, below). An *enzyme* in the blood called plasmin ensures that clots are broken down when the injury has been repaired.

Some disorders interfere with this process, either preventing clot formation or creating clots uncontrollably. If the blood does not clot, there is a danger of excessive blood loss. Inappropriate development of clots may block the supply of blood to a vital organ.

Drugs used to promote blood clotting

Fibrin formation depends on the presence in the blood of several clotting-factor proteins. When Factor VIII is absent or at low levels, an inherited disease called hemophilia exists; the symptoms almost always appear only in males. Factor IX deficiency causes another bleeding condition called Christmas disease, named after the person in whom it was first identified. Lack of these clotting factors can lead to uncontrolled bleeding or excessive bruising following even minor injuries.

Regular drug treatment for hemophilia is not normally required. However, if severe bleeding or bruising occurs, a concentrated form of the missing factor, extracted from normal blood, may be injected in order to promote clotting and thereby halt bleeding. Injections may need to be repeated for several days after injury.

It is sometimes useful to promote blood clotting in non-hemophiliacs when bleeding is difficult to stop (for example, after surgery). In such cases, blood clots are sometimes stabilized by reducing the action of plasmin with an antifibrinolytic (or hemostatic) drug like tranexamic acid; this is also occasionally given to hemophiliacs before minor surgery such as tooth extraction.

A tendency to bleed may also occur as a consequence of vitamin K deficiency (see the box below).

Drugs used to prevent abnormal blood clotting

Blood clots normally form only as a response to injury. In some people, however, there is a tendency for clots to form in the blood vessels without apparent cause. Disturbed blood flow occurring as a result of the presence of fatty deposits – atheroma – inside the blood vessels increases the risk of the formation of this type of abnormal clot (or thrombus). In addition, a portion of a blood clot (known as an embolus) formed in response to injury or surgery may sometimes break off and be removed in the bloodstream. The likelihood of this happening is increased by long periods of little or no activity. When an abnormal clot forms, there is a risk that it may become lodged in a blood vessel, thereby blocking the blood supply to a vital organ such as the brain or heart.

THE CLOTTING MECHANISM

When a blood vessel wall is damaged, platelets accumulate at the site of damage and form a plug (1). Platelets clumped together release chemicals that activate blood clotting factors (2). These factors together with vitamin K act on a substance called fibrinogen and convert it to fibrin (3). Strands of fibrin become enmeshed in the platelet plug to form a blood clot (4).

1

Vessel wall — — Platelet plug

2 — — Blood clotting factor

3

Fibrinogen — — Fibrin

4

Blood clot

VITAMIN K

Vitamin K is required for the production of several blood clotting factors. It is absorbed from the intestine in fats, but some diseases of the small intestine or pancreas cause fat to be poorly absorbed. As a result, the level of vitamin K in the circulation is low, causing impaired blood clotting. A similar problem sometimes occurs in newborn babies due to an absence of the vitamin. Injections of phytomenadione, a vitamin K preparation, are used to restore normal levels.

ACTION OF ANTIPLATELET DRUGS

Blood vessel

Atheroma

Platelet clump

Platelet

Before drug
Where the blood flow is disrupted by an atheroma in the blood vessels, platelets tend to clump together.

Antiplatelet drug

After drug
Antiplatelet drugs reduce the ability of platelets to stick together and so prevent clot formation.

Three main types of drugs are used to prevent and disperse clots: antiplatelet drugs, anticoagulants, and thrombolytics.

Antiplatelet drugs

Taken regularly by people with a tendency to form clots in the fast-flowing blood of the heart and arteries, these drugs are also given to prevent clots from forming after heart surgery. They reduce the tendency of platelets to stick together when blood flow is disrupted (see Action of antiplatelet drugs, above).

The most widely used antiplatelet drug is ASA (see also Analgesics, p.64). This drug has an antiplatelet action even when given in much lower doses than would be necessary to reduce pain. In these low doses *adverse effects* that may occur when ASA is given in pain-relieving doses are unlikely. Other antiplatelet drugs are clopidogrel and dipyridamole.

Anticoagulants

Anticoagulant drugs help to maintain normal blood flow in people who are at risk from clot formation. They can either prevent the formation of blood clots in the veins or stabilize an existing clot so that it does not break away and become a circulation-stopping embolism. All of the anticoagulant drugs reduce the activity of certain blood clotting factors, although the mode of action of each drug differs (see Action of anticoagulant drugs, right). However, these medicines do not dissolve the clots that have already formed: these clots are treated with thrombolytic drugs (below).

Anticoagulants fall into two groups: those that are given by intravenous injection and act immediately, and those that are given by mouth and take effect after a few days.

Injected anticoagulants
Heparin is the most widely used drug of this type and it is used mainly in hospital during or after surgery. In addition, it is also given during kidney dialysis to prevent clots from forming in the dialysis equipment. Because heparin cannot be taken by mouth, it is less suitable for long-term treatment in the home.

A number of synthetic injected anticoagulants called low molecular weight heparins (LMWH) have recently been developed. Some act for a longer time than heparin. Others are alternatives for people who react adversely to heparin.

Oral anticoagulants
Warfarin is the most widely used of the oral anticoagulants. These drugs are mainly prescribed to prevent the formation of clots in veins and in the chambers of the heart – they are less likely to prevent the formation of blood clots in arteries. Oral anticoagulants may be given after injury or surgery (in particular, heart valve replacement) when there is a high risk of embolism. They are also given long term as a preventative treatment to people at risk from strokes. A common problem experienced with these drugs is that

ACTION OF ANTICOAGULANT DRUGS

Anticoagulant drugs block the action of certain blood clotting factors that convert fibrinogen into fibrin, the protein that binds platelets into blood clots.

Before drug   **After drug**

overdosage may lead to bleeding from the nose or gums, or in the urinary tract. For this reason, the dosage needs to be carefully calculated; regular blood tests are performed to ensure that the clotting mechanism is correctly adjusted.

The action of oral anticoagulant drugs may be affected by many other drugs It may therefore be necessary to alter the dosage of anticoagulant when other drugs also need to be given. People who have been prescribed oral anticoagulants should carry a warning list of drugs that they should not be given. In particular, none of the anticoagulants should be taken with ASA except on the direction of a physician.

Thrombolytics
Also known as fibrinolytics, these drugs are used to dissolve clots that have already formed. They are usually given in hospital intravenously to clear a blocked blood vessel – for example, in coronary thrombosis. The sooner they are given after the start of symptoms, the more

likely they are to reduce the size and severity of a heart attack. Thrombolytic drugs may be given either intravenously or directly into the blocked blood vessel. The main thrombolytics are streptokinase and alteplase, which act by increasing the blood level of plasmin, the enzyme that breaks down fibrin (see Action of thrombolytic drugs, below). When given promptly, alteplase appears to be tolerated better than streptokinase.

The most common problems with use of these drugs are increased susceptibility to bleeding and bruising, and allergic reactions to streptokinase, such as rashes, breathing difficulty, or general discomfort. Once streptokinase has been given, patients are given a card indicating this, because further treatment with the same drug may be less effective.

COMMON DRUGS

Blood clotting factors	**Injected anticoagulants**
Factor VIIa	Antithrombin III
Factor VIII	Dalteparin ✳ (see
Factor IX	Heparin)
	Danaparoid
Antifibrinolytic or haemostatic drugs	Enoxaparin ✳
Aprotinin	Epoprostenol
Tranexamic acid	Fondaparinux
	Heparin ✳
Vitamin K	Lepirudin
Phytonadione	Nadroparin
	Tinzaparin
Antiplatelet drugs	
Abciximab	**Thrombolytic drugs**
ASA ✳	Alteplase
Clopidogrel ✳	Reteplase
Dipyridamole ✳	Streptokinase ✳
Eptifibatide	Tenecteplase ✳
Ticlopidine	
Tirofiban	**Oral anticoagulant**
	Warfarin ✳

✳ See Part 4

ACTION OF THROMBOLYTIC DRUGS

Before drug
When platelets accumulate in a blood vessel and are reinforced by strands of fibrin, the resultant blood clot, which is known as a thrombus, cannot be dissolved either by antiplatelet drugs or anticoagulant drugs.

After drug
Thrombolytic drugs boost the action of plasmin, an enzyme in the blood that breaks up the strands of fibrin that bind the clot together. This allows the accumulated platelets to disperse and restores normal blood flow.

GASTROINTESTINAL TRACT

The gastrointestinal tract, also known as the digestive or alimentary tract, is the pathway through which food passes as it is processed to enable the nutrients it contains to be absorbed for use by the body. It consists of the mouth, esophagus, stomach, duodenum, small intestine, large intestine (including the colon and rectum), and anus. In addition, a number of other organs are involved in the digestion of food: the salivary glands in the mouth, the liver, pancreas, and gallbladder. These organs, together with the gastrointestinal tract, form the digestive system.

The digestive system breaks down the large, complex chemicals – proteins, carbohydrates, and fats – present in the food we eat into simpler molecules that can be used by the body (see also Nutrition, p.134). Undigested or indigestible material, together with some of the body's waste products, pass to the large intestine, and, when a sufficient mass of such matter has accumulated, it is expelled from the body as faeces.

What can go wrong

Inflammation of the lining of the stomach or intestine (gastroenteritis) is usually the result of an infection or parasitic infestation. Damage may also be done by the inappropriate production of digestive juices, leading to minor complaints like acidity and major disorders like peptic ulcers. The lining of the intestine can be damaged by abnormal functioning of the immune system (inflammatory bowel disease). The rectum and anus can become painful and irritated by damage to the lining, tears in the skin at the opening of the anus (anal fissure), or enlarged veins (hemorrhoids).

The most frequently experienced gastrointestinal complaints – constipation, diarrhea, and irritable bowel syndrome – usually occur when something disrupts the normal muscle contractions that propel food residue through the bowel.

Why drugs are used

Many drugs for gastrointestinal disorders are taken by mouth and act directly on the digestive tract without first entering the bloodstream. Such drugs include certain antibiotics and other drugs used to treat infestations. Some antacids for peptic ulcers and excess stomach acidity, and the bulk-forming agents for constipation and diarrhea, also pass through the system unabsorbed.

However, for many disorders, drugs with a *systemic* effect are required, including anti-ulcer drugs, *opioid* antidiarrheal drugs, and some of the drugs for inflammatory bowel disease.

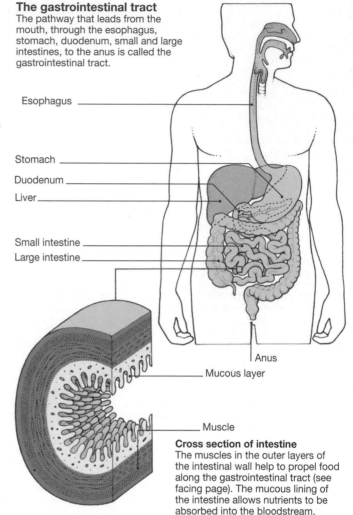

The gastrointestinal tract
The pathway that leads from the mouth, through the esophagus, stomach, duodenum, small and large intestines, to the anus is called the gastrointestinal tract.

Esophagus

Stomach

Duodenum

Liver

Small intestine

Large intestine

Anus

Mucous layer

Muscle

Cross section of intestine
The muscles in the outer layers of the intestinal wall help to propel food along the gastrointestinal tract (see facing page). The mucous lining of the intestine allows nutrients to be absorbed into the bloodstream.

Pancreas
The pancreas produces *enzymes* that digest fats, carbohydrates, and proteins into simpler substances. Pancreatic juices neutralize acidity of the stomach contents.

Gallbladder
Bile produced by the liver is stored in the gallbladder and released into the small intestine. Bile assists the digestion of fats by reducing them to smaller units that are more easily acted upon by digestive enzymes.

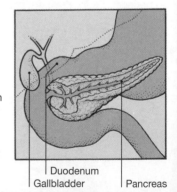

Duodenum

Gallbladder

Pancreas

MAJOR DRUG GROUPS

Antacids
Anti-ulcer drugs
Antidiarrheal drugs
Laxatives
Drugs for inflammatory bowel disease

Drugs for rectal and anal disorders
Drug treatment for gallstones

The lining of the gastrointestinal tract

The lining of the different sections of the gastrointestinal tract varies according to the function of that part, depending, for example, on whether its principal role is to secrete digestive juices or to absorb nutrients.

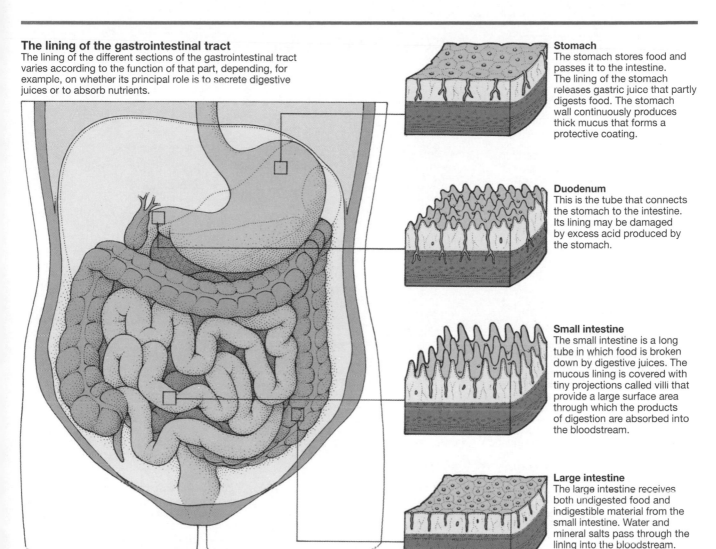

Stomach
The stomach stores food and passes it to the intestine. The lining of the stomach releases gastric juice that partly digests food. The stomach wall continuously produces thick mucus that forms a protective coating.

Duodenum
This is the tube that connects the stomach to the intestine. Its lining may be damaged by excess acid produced by the stomach.

Small intestine
The small intestine is a long tube in which food is broken down by digestive juices. The mucous lining is covered with tiny projections called villi that provide a large surface area through which the products of digestion are absorbed into the bloodstream.

Large intestine
The large intestine receives both undigested food and indigestible material from the small intestine. Water and mineral salts pass through the lining into the bloodstream.

MOVEMENT OF FOOD THROUGH THE GASTROINTESTINAL TRACT

Food is propelled through the gastrointestinal tract by rhythmic waves of muscular contraction called peristalsis. The illustration shows how peristaltic contractions of the bowel wall push food through the intestine.

Muscle contraction in the tract is controlled by the autonomic nervous system (p.63) and is therefore easily disrupted by drugs that either stimulate or inhibit the activity of the autonomic nervous system. Excessive peristaltic action may cause diarrhea; slowed peristalsis may cause constipation.

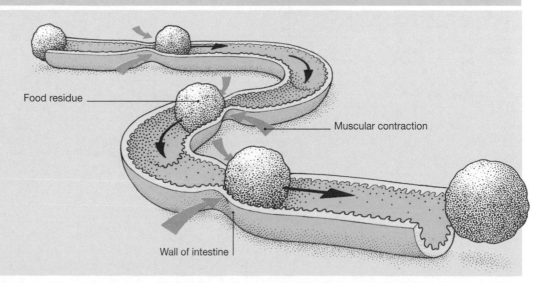

Food residue

Muscular contraction

Wall of intestine

ANTACIDS

Digestive juices in the stomach contain acid and *enzymes* that break down food before it passes into the intestine. The wall of the stomach is normally protected from the action of digestive acid by a layer of mucus that is constantly secreted by the stomach lining. Problems arise when the stomach lining is damaged or too much acid is produced and eats away at the mucous layer.

Excess acid that leads to discomfort, commonly referred to as indigestion, may result from anxiety, overeating or eating certain foods, coffee, alcohol, or smoking. Some drugs, notably ASA and non-steroidal anti-inflammatory drugs, can irritate the stomach lining and even cause ulcers to develop.

Antacids are used to neutralize acid and thus relieve pain. They are simple chemical compounds that are mildly alkaline, and some also act as chemical buffers. Their chalky taste is often disguised with flavourings.

Why they are used

Antacids may be needed when simple remedies (a change in diet or a glass of milk) fail to relieve indigestion. They are especially useful one to three hours after meals to neutralize after-meal acid surge.

Doctors prescribe these drugs in order to relieve dyspepsia (pain in the chest or upper abdomen caused by or aggravated by acid) in disorders such as inflammation or ulceration of the esophagus, stomach lining, and duodenum. Antacids usually relieve pain resulting from ulcers in the esophagus, stomach, or duodenum within a few minutes. Regular treatment with antacids reduces the acidity of the stomach, thereby encouraging the healing of any ulcers that may have formed.

How they work

By neutralizing stomach acid, antacids prevent inflammation, relieve pain, and

ACTION OF ANTACIDS

Excess acid in the stomach may eat away at the layer of mucus that protects the stomach. When this occurs, or when the mucous lining is damaged, for example, by an ulcer, stomach acid comes into contact with the underlying tissues, causing pain and inflammation (right). Antacids combine with stomach acid to reduce the acidity of the digestive juices. This helps to prevent pain and inflammation, and allows the mucous lining to repair itself (far right).

Acid   Drug

Mucus

Mucous lining

Stomach wall

Before drug
Acid damages mucous layer of stomach lining.

After drug
Acid is neutralized by antacid action.

allow the mucous layer and lining to mend. When used in the treatment of ulcers, they prevent acid from attacking damaged stomach lining and so allow the ulcer to heal.

How they affect you

If antacids are taken according to the instructions, they are usually effective in relieving abdominal discomfort caused by acid. The speed of action, dependent on the ability to neutralize acid, varies. Their duration of action also varies; the short-acting drugs may have to be taken quite frequently.

Although most antacids have few serious *side effects* when used only occasionally, some may cause diarrhea, and others may cause constipation (see Types of antacids, below).

Risks and special precautions

Antacids should not be taken to prevent abdominal pain on a regular basis except under medical supervision, as they may suppress the symptoms of stomach cancer. Your physician is likely to want to arrange tests such as endoscopy or barium X-rays before prescribing long-term treatment.

Antacids can interfere with the absorption of other drugs. If you are taking a prescription medicine, you should check with your physician or pharmacist before taking an antacid.

TYPES OF ANTACIDS

Aluminum compounds These drugs have a prolonged action and are widely used, especially for the treatment of indigestion and dyspepsia. They may cause constipation, but this is often countered by combining this type of antacid with one that contains magnesium. Aluminum compounds can interfere with the absorption of phosphate from the diet, causing weakness and bone damage if taken in high doses over a long period.

Magnesium compounds Like the aluminum compounds, these have a prolonged action. In large doses they can cause diarrhea, and in people who have impaired kidney function, a high blood magnesium level may build up, causing weakness, lethargy, and drowsiness.

Sodium bicarbonate This antacid, the only sodium compound used as an antacid, acts quickly, but its effect soon passes. It reacts

with stomach acids to produce gas, which may cause bloating and belching. Sodium bicarbonate is not advised for people with heart or kidney disease, as it can lead to the accumulation of water (edema) in the legs and lungs, or serious changes in the acid-base balance of the blood.

Combined preparations Antacids may be combined with other substances called alginates and antifoaming agents. Alginates are intended to float on the contents of the stomach and produce a neutralizing layer to subdue acid that can otherwise rise into the esophagus, causing heartburn.

Antifoaming agents (usually simethicone) are intended to relieve flatulence. In some preparations a local anesthetic is combined with the antacid to relieve discomfort in esophagitis. The value of these additives is dubious.

COMMON DRUGS

Antacids
Aluminum
  hydroxide *
Calcium carbonate
Magnesium
  hydroxide *
Magnesium
  trisilicate
Sodium
  bicarbonate

Antifoaming agent
Simethicone

Other drugs
Alginates/alginic
  acid *

* See Part 4

ANTI-ULCER DRUGS

Normally, the linings of the esophagus, stomach, and duodenum are protected from the irritant action of stomach acids or bile by a thin covering layer of mucus. If this is damaged, or if large amounts of stomach acid are formed, the underlying tissue may become eroded, causing a peptic ulcer. An ulcer often leads to abdominal pain, vomiting, and changes in appetite. The most common type of ulcer occurs just beyond the stomach, in the duodenum. The exact cause of peptic ulcers is not understood, but a number

of risk factors have been identified, including heavy smoking, the regular use of ASA or similar drugs, and family history. An organism found in almost all patients who have peptic ulcers, *Helicobacter pylori*, is now believed to be the main causative agent.

The symptoms caused by ulcers may be relieved by an antacid (see facing page), but healing is slow. The usual treatment is with an anti-ulcer drug, such as an H$_2$ blocker, a proton pump inhibitor, bismuth, or sucralfate, combined

with antibiotics to eradicate the *Helicobacter pylori* infection which seems to cause many ulcers.

Why they are used
Anti-ulcer drugs are used to relieve symptoms and heal the ulcer. Untreated ulcers may erode blood vessel walls or perforate the stomach or duodenum.

Until recently, drugs could heal ulcers but not cure them. However, eradication of *Helicobacter pylori* by a proton pump inhibitor, or rantidine bismuth citrate combined with two antibiotics (triple therapy), may provide a cure in one to two weeks. Surgery is reserved for complications such as obstruction, perforation, hemorrhage, and when there is a possibility of cancer.

How they work
Drugs protect ulcers from the action of stomach acid, allowing the tissue to heal. H$_2$ blockers, misoprostol, and proton pump inhibitors reduce the amount of acid released; bismuth and sucralfate form a protective coating over the ulcer. Bismuth also has an antibacterial effect. It is combined with an H$_2$ blocker in ranitidine bismuth citrate.

How they affect you
These drugs begin to reduce pain in a few hours and usually allow the ulcer to heal in four to eight weeks. They produce few side effects, although H$_2$ blockers can cause confusion in the elderly. Bismuth and sucralfate may cause constipation; misoprostol, diarrhea; and proton pump inhibitors, either constipation or diarrhea. Triple therapy is given for one or two weeks. If *Helicobacter pylori* is eradicated, maintenance therapy should not be necessary. Sucralfate is usually prescribed for up to 12 weeks, and bismuth and misoprostol for four to six weeks. As they may mask symptoms of stomach cancer, H$_2$ blockers and proton pump inhibitors are normally prescribed only when tests have ruled out this disorder.

ACTION OF ANTI-ULCER DRUGS

Proton pump inhibitors
Acid secretion by the cells lining the stomach depends on an *enzyme* system (also known as the proton pump) that transports hydrogen ions across the cell walls. Omeprazole, lansoprazole, and

similar drugs work by blocking the proton pump. They can stop stomach acid production until a new supply of the enzyme can be made by the body and, therefore, have a long duration of action.

The proton pump
This enzyme system transports hydrogen ions across the cell wall into the stomach, thereby stimulating acid secretion.

The action of proton pump inhibitors
Proton pump inhibitors block the enzyme system, stopping the transport of hydrogen ions and, thus, the secretion of acid.

H$_2$ blockers
Histamine is a chemical released by mast cells (see Allergies, p.109) that can produce a number of effects in different parts of the body. In the stomach, histamine stimulates H$_2$ receptors, causing acid production. To control stomach acid production, a class of

antihistamine drugs was developed that acts by blocking the H$_2$ receptors. These drugs are known as H$_2$ blockers to distinguish them from antihistamines used for allergic disorders (see p.110), which are sometimes called H$_1$ blockers because they block H$_1$ receptors.

The action of histamine on the stomach
Histamine binds to specialized H$_2$ receptors and stimulates acid-producing cells in the stomach wall to release acid.

The action of H$_2$ blockers
H$_2$ blockers occupy H$_2$ receptors, preventing histamine from triggering the production of acid. This allows the mucous lining to heal.

Sucralfate and bismuth
Sucralfate forms a coating over the ulcer, protecting it from the action of stomach acid and allowing it to heal. Bismuth may stimulate production of *prostaglandins* or bicarbonate, and also kills the bacteria that are thought to cause most peptic ulcers. Bismuth is used in triple therapy with antibiotics to cure ulcers.

COMMON DRUGS

Proton pump inhibitors	Other drugs
Esomeprazole	Antacids (see p.94)
Lansoprazole ✻	Antibiotics (see p.114)
Omeprazole ✻	Bismuth subsalicylate
Pantoprazole ✻	Misoprostol ✻
Rabeprazole	Sucralfate ✻

H$_2$ blockers
Cimetidine ✻
Famotidine ✻
Nizatidine
Ranitidine ✻

✻ See Part 4

ANTIDIARRHEAL DRUGS

Diarrhea is an increase in the fluidity and frequency of bowel movements. In some cases diarrhea protects the body from harmful substances in the intestine by hastening their removal. The most common causes are viral infection, food poisoning, and parasites. But it also occurs as a symptom of other illnesses. It can be a *side effect* of some drugs and may follow radiation therapy for cancer. Diarrhea may also be caused by anxiety.

An attack of diarrhea usually clears up quickly without medical attention. The best treatment is to abstain from food and to drink plenty of clear fluids. Rehydration solutions containing sugar as well as potassium and sodium salts are widely recommended for preventing dehydration and chemical imbalances, particularly in children. You should consult your physician if: the condition does not improve within 48 hours; the diarrhea contains blood; severe abdominal pain and vomiting are present; you have just returned from a foreign country; or if the diarrhea occurs in a small child or an elderly person.

Severe diarrhea can impair absorption of drugs, and anyone taking a prescribed drug should seek advice from a physician or pharmacist. A woman taking oral contraceptives may need additional contraceptive measures (see p.149).

The main types of drugs used to relieve non-specific diarrhea are *opioids*, and bulk-forming and *adsorbent* agents. Antispasmodic drugs may also be used to relieve accompanying pain (see Drugs for irritable bowel syndrome, below).

Why they are used

An antidiarrheal drug may be prescribed to provide relief when simple remedies are not effective, and once it is certain the diarrhea is neither infectious nor *toxic*.

Opioid drugs are the most effective antidiarrheals. They are used when the diarrhea is severe and debilitating. The bulking and adsorbent agents have a

ACTION OF ANTIDIARRHEAL DRUGS

Opioid antidiarrheals
These drugs reduce the transmission of nerve signals to the intestinal muscles, thus reducing muscle contraction. This allows more time for water to be absorbed from the food residue and therefore reduces the fluidity as well as the frequency of bowel movements.

Bowel contents
Bowel wall

Before drug
Rapid bowel contraction prevents water from being absorbed.

After drug
Slowed bowel action allows more water to be absorbed.

Bulk-forming agents
These preparations contain particles that swell up as they absorb water from the large intestine. This makes the feces firmer and less fluid. It is thought that bulk-forming agents may absorb irritants and harmful chemicals along with excess water.

Bulk-forming agent

Water

Water is attracted by bulk-forming agent.

Bulk-forming agent swells as water is absorbed.

milder effect and are often used when it is necessary to regulate bowel action over a prolonged period – for example, in people with colostomies or ileostomies.

How they work

Opioids decrease the muscles' propulsive activity so that fecal matter passes more slowly through the bowel.

Bulk-forming agents and adsorbents absorb water and irritants present in the bowel, thereby producing larger and firmer stools at less frequent intervals.

How they affect you

Drugs that are used to treat diarrhea reduce the urge to move the bowels.

Opioids and antispasmodics may relieve abdominal pain. All antidiarrheals may cause constipation if used in excess.

Risks and special precautions

Used in relatively low doses for a limited period of time, the opioid drugs are unlikely to produce adverse effects. However, these drugs should be used under medical supervision when diarrhea is caused by an infection, since they may slow the elimination of microorganisms from the intestine. All antidiarrheals should be taken with plenty of water. It is important not to take a bulk-forming agent together with an opioid or antispasmodic drug, because a bulky mass could form and obstruct the bowel.

DRUGS FOR IRRITABLE BOWEL SYNDROME

Irritable bowel syndrome (IBS) is a common stress-related condition in which the normal coordinated waves of muscular contraction responsible for moving the bowel contents smoothly through the intestines become strong and irregular, often causing pain, and associated with diarrhea or constipation.

Symptoms are often relieved by adjusting the amount of fibre in the diet, although medication may also be required. Bulk-forming agents may be given to regulate the consistency of the bowel contents. Tegaserod may be used for symptomatic treatment of constipation associated with IBS. If pain is severe, an antispasmodic drug may be prescribed. These *anticholinergic* drugs reduce the transmission of nerve signals to the bowel wall, thus preventing spasm.

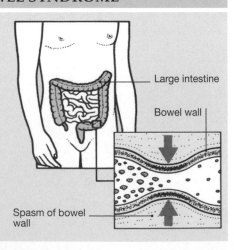

Large intestine

Bowel wall

Spasm of bowel wall

COMMON DRUGS

Antispasmodics
Atropine ✳
Dicyclomine ✳
Scopolamine

Opioids
Codeine ✳
Diphenoxylate ✳
Loperamide ✳

Bulk-forming agents and adsorbents
Attapulgite ✳
Bismuth subsalicylate
Ispaghula
Psyllium ✳

Antibacterials
Ciprofloxacin ✳
Co-trimoxazole ✳

✳ See Part 4

LAXATIVES

When your bowels do not move as frequently as usual and the feces are hard and difficult to pass, you are suffering from constipation. The most common cause is lack of sufficient fibre in your diet; fibre supplies the bulk that makes the feces soft and easy to pass. The simplest remedy is more fluid and a diet that contains plenty of foods that are high in fibre, but laxative drugs may also be used.

Ignoring the urge to defecate can also cause constipation, because the feces become dry, hard to pass, and too small to stimulate the muscles that propel them through the intestine.

Certain drugs may be constipating: for example, *opioid* analgesics, tricyclic antidepressants, and antacids containing aluminium. Some diseases, such as hypothyroidism (underactive thyroid gland) and scleroderma (a rare disorder of connective tissue characterized by the hardening of the skin), can also lead to constipation.

The onset of constipation in a middle-aged or elderly person may be an early symptom of bowel cancer. Consult your physician about any persistent change in bowel habit.

Why they are used

Since prolonged use is harmful, laxatives should be used for very short periods only. They may prevent pain and straining in people suffering from either hernias or hemorrhoids (p. 99). Physicians may prescribe laxatives for the same reason after childbirth or abdominal surgery. Laxatives are also used to clear the bowel before investigative procedures such as colonoscopy. They may be prescribed for patients who are elderly or bedridden because lack of exercise can often lead to constipation.

How they work

Laxatives act on the large intestine – by increasing the speed with which fecal matter passes through the bowel, or increasing its bulk and/or water content.

ACTION OF LAXATIVES

Bulk-forming agents
Taken after a meal, these agents are not absorbed as they pass through the digestive tract. They contain particles that absorb many times their own volume of water. By doing so, they increase the bulk of the bowel movements and thus encourage bowel action.

Bowel wall

Bulk-forming agent swollen with water

Fecal matter

Stimulant laxatives
These laxatives are thought to encourage bowel movements by acting on nerve endings in the wall of the intestines that trigger contraction of the intestinal muscles. This speeds the passage of fecal matter through the large intestine, allowing less time for water to be absorbed. Thus feces become more liquid and are passed more frequently.

Increased contractions speed passage of fecal matter

Before drug

After drug

Stimulants cause the bowel muscles to contract, increasing the speed at which fecal matter goes through the intestine. Bulk-forming laxatives absorb water in the bowel, thereby increasing the volume of feces, making them softer and easier to pass. Lactulose also causes fluid to accumulate in the intestine. Osmotic laxatives act by keeping water in the bowel, and thereby make the bowel movements softer. This also increases the bulk of the feces and enables them to be passed more easily. Lubricant liquid paraffin preparations make bowel movements softer and easier to pass

without increasing their bulk. Prolonged use can interfere with absorption of some essential vitamins.

Risks and special precautions

Laxatives can cause diarrhea if taken in overdose, and can make constipation worse if overused. The most serious risk of prolonged use of most laxatives is developing dependence on the laxative for normal bowel action. Use of a laxative should therefore be discontinued as soon as normal bowel movements have been re-established. Children should not be given laxatives except in special circumstances on the advice of a doctor.

TYPES OF LAXATIVES

Bulk-forming agents These are relatively slow acting but are less likely than other laxatives to interfere with normal bowel action. Only after consultation with your physician should they be taken for constipation accompanied by abdominal pain because of the risk of intestinal obstruction.

Stimulant (contact) laxatives These are for occasional use when other treatments have failed or when rapid onset of action is needed. Stimulant laxatives should not normally be used for longer than a week as they can cause abdominal cramps and diarrhea.

Softening agents These are often used when hard bowel movements cause pain on defecation – for example, when hemorrhoids

are present, or after surgery when straining must be avoided. Liquid paraffin was once popular but can cause *side effects* and has generally been replaced by sodium docusate. and for the relief of fecal impaction (blockage of the bowel by fecal material).

Osmotic laxatives Salts such as Epsom salts (magnesium sulfate) may be used to evacuate the bowel before surgery or investigative procedures. They are not normally used for the long-term relief of constipation because they can cause chemical imbalances in the blood.

Lactulose is an alternative to bulk-forming laxatives for the long-term treatment of chronic constipation. It may cause stomach cramps and flatulence but is usually well tolerated.

COMMON DRUGS

Stimulant laxatives
Bisacodyl ✳
Cascara
Castor oil
Sennosides

Bulk-forming agents
Bran
Psyllium ✳

Softening agents
Docusate sodium ✳
Glycerin
Liquid paraffin

Osmotic laxatives
Lactulose ✳
Magnesium citrate
Magnesium hydroxide ✳
Magnesium sulfate
Sodium acid phosphate

Lubricant laxative
Mineral oil

✳ See Part 4

DRUGS FOR INFLAMMATORY BOWEL DISEASE

Inflammatory bowel disease is the term used for disorders in which inflammation of the intestinal wall causes recurrent attacks of abdominal pain, general feelings of ill-health, and frequently diarrhea, with blood and mucus present in the feces. Loss of appetite and poor absorption of food may often result in weight loss.

There are two main types of inflammatory bowel disease (IBD): Crohn's disease (CD) and ulcerative colitis (UC). In Crohn's Disease (also called regional enteritis), any part of the digestive tract may become inflamed, although the small intestine is the most commonly affected site. In ulcerative colitis, it is the large intestine (colon) that becomes inflamed and ulcerated, often producing bloodstained diarrhea (see right).

The exact cause of these disorders is unknown, although stress-related, dietary, infectious, and genetic factors may all be important.

Establishing a proper diet and a less stressful lifestyle may help to alleviate these conditions. Bed rest during attacks is also advisable. However, these simple measures alone do not usually relieve or prevent attacks, and drug treatment is often necessary.

Three types of drug are used to treat inflammatory bowel disease: corticosteroids (p.127), immunosuppressants (p.143), and aminosalicylate anti-inflammatory drugs such as sulfasalazine. Nutritional supplements (used especially for Crohn's disease) and antidiarrheal drugs (p.96) may also be used. Surgery to remove damaged areas of the intestine may be needed in severe cases.

SITES OF BOWEL INFLAMMATION

The two main types of bowel inflammation are ulcerative colitis and Crohn's disease. The former occurs in the large intestine. Crohn's disease can occur anywhere along the gastrointestinal tract, but it most often affects the small intestine.

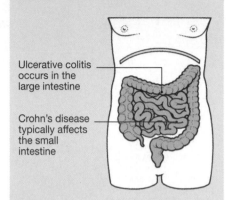

Ulcerative colitis occurs in the large intestine

Crohn's disease typically affects the small intestine

Why they are used

Drugs help control symptoms and prevent complications of IBD, especially perforation of the intestinal wall. Aminosalicylates are used to treat acute attacks of UC and CD, and they may be continued as maintenance therapy. With severe bowel inflammation, a course of corticosteroids may be presecribed, particularly during a sudden flare-up. Once symptoms are controlled, an immunosuppressant drug may be prescribed to prevent a relapse.

How they work

Corticosteroids and sulfasalazine damp down the inflammatory process, allowing the damaged tissue to recover. They act in different ways to prevent migration of white blood cells into the bowel wall, which may be responsible in part for the inflammation of the bowel. New drugs such as infliximab and adalimumab act by blocking the actions of a substance called tumor necrosis factor-alpha or TNF-alpha, which causes inflammation in the body.

How they affect you

Taken to treat attacks, these drugs relieve symptoms within a few days, and general health improves gradually over a period of a few weeks. Aminosalicylates usually provide long-term relief from the symptoms of inflammatory bowel disease.

Treatment with an immunosuppressant drug may take several months before the condition improves; and regular blood tests to monitor possible drug *side effects* are often required.

Risks and special precautions

Immunosuppressant and corticosteroid drugs can cause serious adverse effects and are only prescribed when potential benefits outweigh the risks involved.

The side effects of corticosteroids can be reduced by the use of budesonide in a topical preparation that releases the drug at the site of inflammation.

It is important to continue taking these drugs as instructed because stopping them abruptly may cause a sudden flare-up of the disorder. Physicians usually supervise a gradual reduction in dosage when such drugs are stopped, even when they are given as a short course for an attack. Antidiarrheal drugs should not be taken on a routine basis because they may mask signs of deterioration or cause sudden bowel dilation or rupture.

How they are administered

Antidiarrheal drugs are usually taken in the form of tablets, although mild ulcerative colitis in the last part of the large intestine may be treated with suppositories or an enema containing a corticosteroid or aminosalicylate.

ACTION OF DRUGS IN ULCERATIVE COLITIS

The most common form of inflammatory bowel disease is ulcerative colitis. It affects the large intestine, causing ulceration of the lining and producing pain and violent blood-stained diarrhea. It is often treated with cortico-steroids and aminosalicylates.

Large intestine

Bowel wall
Ulcerated area
Prostaglandins

White blood cell | Corticosteroid drug
Blood vessel | Aminosalicylate drug

Before drug
Damage to the intestinal lining provokes the formation of chemicals known as prostaglandins, which trigger the migration of white blood cells into the ulcerated area. The accumulation of white blood cells in the bowel wall causes inflammation.

Drug action
Aminosalicylate drugs pass into the ulcerated area from inside the bowel. They prevent prostaglandins from forming in the damaged tissue. Corticosteroids in the bloodstream reduce the ability of white blood cells to pass into the bowel wall.

COMMON DRUGS

Corticosteroids
Betamethasone *
Budesonide *
Hydrocortisone *
Methylprednisolone *
Prednisolone/
  prednisone *

Immunosuppressants
Azathioprine *
Cyclosporine *
Mercaptopurine *
Methotrexate *

Aminosalicylates
5-Aminosalicylic
  Acid (5-ASA)
Olsalazine
Sulfasalazine *

Other drugs
Adalimumab
Infliximab
Metronidazole *

$\boxed{* \text{ See Part 4}}$

DRUGS FOR RECTAL AND ANAL DISORDERS

The most common disorder affecting the rectum (the last part of the large intestine) and anus (the opening from the rectum) is hemorrhoids, commonly known as piles. They occur when hemorrhoidal veins become swollen or irritated, often as a result of prolonged local pressure such as that caused by a pregnancy or a job requiring long hours of sitting. Hemorrhoids may cause irritation and pain, especially on defecation. The condition is aggravated by constipation and straining during defecation. In some cases hemorrhoids may bleed and occasionally clots form in the swollen veins, leading to severe pain, a condition called thrombosed hemorrhoids.

Other common disorders affecting the anus include anal fissure (painful cracks in the anus) and pruritus ani (itching around the anus). Anal disorders of all kinds occur less frequently in people who have soft, bulky stools.

A number of both over-the-counter and prescription-only preparations are available for the relief of such disorders.

Why they are used

Preparations for relief of hemorrhoids and anal discomfort fall into two main groups: creams or suppositories that act locally to relieve inflammation and irritation, and measures that relieve constipation, which contributes to the formation of, and the discomfort from, hemorrhoids and anal fissure.

Preparations from the first group often contain a soothing agent with *antiseptic*, *astringent*, or *vasoconstrictor* properties. Ingredients of this type include zinc oxide or sulfate, bismuth, hamamelis (witch hazel), and phenylephrine or naphazoline. Some of these products include a mild local anesthetic (see p.64)

DISORDERS OF THE RECTUM AND ANUS

The rectum and anus form the last part of the digestive tract. Common conditions affecting the area include swelling of the veins around the anus (hemorrhoids), cracks in the anus (anal fissure), and inflammation or irritation of the anus and surrounding area (pruritus ani).

Anal fissure

Hemorrhoid

Pruritus ani

such as benzocaine, dibucaine, or pramoxine. A physician may also prescribe an ointment containing a corticosteroid to relieve inflammation around the anus (see Topical corticosteroids, p.162).

People who suffer from hemorrhoids or anal fissure are generally advised to include in their diets plenty of fluids and fibre-rich foods, such as fruits, vegetables, and whole grain products, both to prevent constipation and to ease defecation. A mild bulk-forming or softening laxative may also be prescribed (see p.97).

Neither of these treatments can shrink large hemorrhoids, although they may provide relief while anal fissures heal naturally. Severe, persistently painful hemorrhoids that continue to be troublesome in spite of these measures

may need to be removed surgically or, more commonly, by banding with specially applied small rubber bands (see below left).

How they affect you

The treatments described above usually relieve discomfort, especially during defecation. Most people experience no adverse effects, although preparations containing local anesthetics may cause irritation or even a rash in the anal area. It is rare for ingredients in locally acting preparations to be absorbed into the body in sufficient quantities to cause generalized *side effects*.

The main risk is that self-treatment of hemorrhoids may delay diagnosis of bowel cancer. It is therefore always wise to consult your physician if symptoms of hemorrhoids are present, especially if you have noticed bleeding from the rectum or a change in bowel habits.

SITES OF DRUG ACTION

The illustration below shows how and where drugs for the treatment of rectal disorders act to relieve symptoms.

Fecal matter

Laxatives
These act in the large intestine to soften and ease the passage of feces.

Creams and suppositories
Vasoconstrictors and astringents reduce the swelling and restrict blood supply, helping to relieve hemorrhoids. Local anesthetics numb pain signals from the anus. Topical corticosteroids relieve inflammation.

Banding treatment
A small rubber band is applied tightly to a hemorrhoid, thereby blocking off its blood supply. The hemorrhoid will eventually wither away.

Rubber band

Hemorrhoid

COMMON DRUGS

Soothing and astringent agents
Aluminium acetate
Bismuth
Zinc oxide

Vasoconstrictors
Ephedrine *

Topical corticosteroids
Hydrocortisone *

Local anesthetics
(see p.64)

Laxatives
(see p.97)

* See Part 4

DRUG TREATMENT FOR GALLSTONES

The formation of gallstones is the most common disorder of the gallbladder, which is the storage and concentrating unit for bile, a digestive juice produced by the liver. During digestion, bile passes from the gallbladder via the bile duct into the small intestine, where it assists in the digestion of fats. Bile is composed of several ingredients, including bile acids, bile salts, and bile pigments. It also has a significant amount of cholesterol, which is dissolved in bile acid. If the amount of cholesterol in the bile increases, or if the amount of bile acid is reduced, a proportion of the cholesterol cannot remain dissolved, and under certain circumstances this excess accumulates in the gallbladder as gallstones.

Gallstones may be present in the gallbladder for years without causing symptoms. However, if they become lodged in the bile duct they cause pain and block the flow of bile. If the bile accumulates in the blood, it may cause an attack of jaundice, or the gallbladder may become infected and inflamed.

Drug treatment with ursodeoxycholic acid, also known as ursodiol, is only effective against stones made principally of cholesterol (some contain other substances), and even these take many months to dissolve. Therefore, surgery and ultrasound have become widely used, as techniques have improved. Surgery and ultrasound treatments are always used to remove stones blocking the bile duct.

Why they are used
Even if you have not experienced any symptoms, once gallstones have been diagnosed your physician may advise treatment because of the risk of blockage of the bile duct. Drug treatment is usually preferred to surgery for small cholesterol stones or when there is a possibility that surgery may be risky.

How they work
Ursodeoxycholic acid is a substance that is naturally present in bile. It acts on chemical processes in the liver to regulate the amount of cholesterol in the blood by controlling the amount that passes into the bile. Once the cholesterol level in the bile is reduced, the bile acids are able to start dissolving the stones in the gallbladder. To achieve maximum effect,

DIGESTION OF FATS

The digestion of fats (or lipids) in the small intestine is assisted by the action of bile, a digestive juice produced by the liver and stored in the gallbladder. A complex sequence of chemical processes enables fats to be absorbed through the intestinal wall, broken down in the liver, and converted for use in the body. Cholesterol, a lipid present in bile, plays an important part in this chain.

2 Bile salts act on fats to enable them to pass from the small intestine into the bloodstream, either directly or via the lymphatic system.

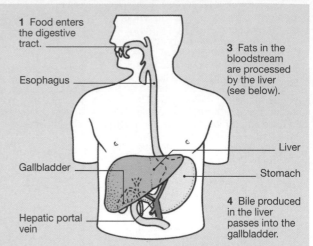

1 Food enters the digestive tract.

Esophagus

3 Fats in the bloodstream are processed by the liver (see below).

Liver

Gallbladder

Stomach

Hepatic portal vein

4 Bile produced in the liver passes into the gallbladder.

How fats are processed in the liver

Fat molecules are broken down in the liver into fatty acids and glycerol. Glycerol, as well as some of the fatty acids, pass back into the bloodstream. Other fatty acids are used to form cholesterol, some of which in turn is used to make bile salts. Unchanged cholesterol is dissolved in the bile, which then passes into the gallbladder.

Fat molecule   Glycerol   Cholesterol   Bile salts

Fatty acids   To gallbladder

To bloodstream

ursodeoxycholic acid treatment usually needs to be accompanied by adherence to a low-cholesterol, high-fibre diet.

How they affect you
Drug treatment may often take years to dissolve gallstones completely. You will not, therefore, feel any immediate benefit from the drug, but you may have some minor *side effects*, the most usual of which is diarrhea. If this occurs, your physician may adjust the dosage. The effect of drug treatment on the gallstones is usually monitored at regular intervals by means of ultrasound or X-ray examinations.

Even after successful treatment with drugs, gallstones often recur when the

drug is stopped. In some cases drug treatment and dietary restrictions may be continued even after the gallstones have dissolved, to prevent a recurrence.

Although the drug reduces cholesterol in the gallbladder, it increases the level of cholesterol in the blood because it reduces its excretion in the bile. Physicians therefore prescribe it with caution to people who have atherosclerosis (fatty deposits in the blood vessels). The drug is not usually given to people who have liver disorders because it can interfere with normal liver function. Surgical or ultrasound treatment is used for those with liver problems.

AGENTS USED IN DISORDERS OF THE PANCREAS

The pancreas releases certain *enzymes* into the small intestine that are necessary for digestion of a range of foods. If the release of pancreatic enzymes is impaired (caused by, for example, chronic pancreatitis or cystic fibrosis), enzyme replacement therapy may be necessary. Replacement of enzymes does not cure the underlying disorder, but it restores normal digestion. Pancreatic enzymes should

be taken just before or with meals, and usually take effect immediately. Your physician will probably advise you to eat a diet that is high in protein and carbohydrates and low in fat.

Pancreatin, the generic name for those preparations containing pancreatic enzymes, is extracted from pig pancreas. Treatment must be continued indefinitely as long as the pancreatic disorder persists.

COMMON DRUGS

Drug for gallstones
Ursodeoxycholic acid (Ursodiol)

Drug for cholestatic liver disease
Ursodeoxycholic acid (Ursodiol)

Pancreatic enzymes
Pancreatin

MUSCLES, BONES, AND JOINTS

The basic architecture of the human body relies on 206 bones, over 600 muscles, and a complex assortment of ligaments, tendons, and cartilage that enable the body to move with remarkable efficiency.

What can go wrong

Although tough, these structures often suffer damage. Muscles, tendons, and ligaments can be strained or torn by violent movement, causing inflammation, making the affected tissue swollen and painful. Joints, especially those that bear the body's weight – hips, knees, ankles, and vertebrae – are prone to wear and tear. The cartilage covering the bone ends may tear, causing inflammation and pain. Some may develop osteoarthritis as a result of cartilage damage. Joint damage also occurs in rheumatoid arthritis, which is an autoimmune disorder. Gout, in which uric acid crystals form in some joints may cause inflammation, a condition known as gouty arthritis.

The muscles and joints can also suffer nerve injury or degeneration, altering nerve control over muscle contraction. Myasthenia gravis, in which transmission of signals between nerves and muscles is reduced, affects muscle control. Bones may also be weakened by vitamin, mineral, or hormone deficiencies.

Why drugs are used

An analgesic or an anti-inflammatory drug provides pain relief in most of these conditions. For severe inflammation, a doctor may inject a drug with a more powerful anti-inflammatory effect, such as a corticosteroid, into the affected site. In progressive rheumatoid arthritis, antirheumatic drugs may halt the disease's progression and relieve symptoms. Glucosamine (p.472), a natural health product, has been tried in osteoarthritis.

Drugs that help to eliminate excess uric acid from the body are often prescribed to treat gout. Muscle relaxants that inhibit transmission of nerve signals to the muscles are used to treat muscle spasm. Drugs that increase nervous stimulation of the muscle are prescribed for myasthenia gravis. Bone disorders in which the mineral content of the bone is reduced are treated with supplements of minerals, vitamins, hormones, and other drugs.

MAJOR DRUG GROUPS

- Non-steroidal anti-inflammatory drugs
- Antirheumatic drugs
- Locally acting corticosteroids
- Drugs for gout
- Muscle-relaxant drugs
- Drugs used for myasthenia gravis
- Drugs for bone disorders

Muscles that control body movement are attached to the bones by tendons.

Tendon

Bones act as levers, which are worked by muscles: when the muscle contracts, movement occurs at the joint.

Friction between the ends of two bones is reduced by the cartilage that covers each bone end.

Cartilage

Joints are held together by bands of tough fibrous tissue known as ligaments.

Ligament

Muscle fibre bundle

Muscle fibril

Longitudinal canal

Transverse canal

Muscle
Each muscle is made of thick bundles of fibres: each bundle in turn is made of fibrils. Tiny nerves and blood vessels enable the muscle to function.

Bone
Long bones, such as the femur, contain a network of longitudinal and transverse canals to carry blood, nerves, and lymph vessels through the bone.

NON-STEROIDAL ANTI-INFLAMMATORY DRUGS

These drugs are used to relieve the pain, stiffness, and inflammation of painful conditions affecting the muscles, bones, and joints. NSAIDs are called "non-steroidal" to distinguish them from corticosteroid drugs (see p.127), which also decrease inflammation.

Why they are used

NSAIDs are widely prescribed for the treatment of osteoarthritis, rheumatoid arthritis, and other rheumatic conditions. They do not alter the progress of these diseases, but reduce inflammation and thus relieve pain and swelling of joints.

The response to the various drugs in this group varies between individuals. It is sometimes necessary to try several different NSAIDs before finding the one that best suits a particular individual.

NSAIDs do not change the progress of a disease. Medications called DMARDS are used in rheumatoid arthritis to decrease disease progression (see facing page).

NSAIDs are also commonly prescribed to relieve back pain, headaches, gout (p.105), menstrual pain (p.148), mild pain following surgery, and pain from soft tissue injuries, such as sprains and strains (see also Analgesics, p.64).

How they work

Prostaglandins are chemicals released by the body at the site of injury. They are responsible for producing inflammation and pain following tissue damage. NSAIDs block an enzyme, cyclo-oxygenase (COX) which is involved in the production of prostaglandins, and thus reduce pain and inflammation (see p.65).

How they affect you

NSAIDs are rapidly absorbed from the digestive system and most start to relieve pain within an hour. When used regularly they reduce pain, inflammation, and stiffness and may restore or improve the function of a damaged or painful joint.

Most NSAIDs are short acting and need to be taken a few times a day in order to provide optimal relief from pain. Some need to be taken only twice daily. Others, such as piroxicam, are very slowly eliminated from the body and are effective when taken once a day.

Risks and special precautions

Most NSAIDs carry a low risk of serious adverse effects although nausea, indigestion, and altered bowel action are common. However, the main risk from NSAIDs is that, occasionally, they can cause ulcers and bleeding in the stomach or duodenum. They should therefore be avoided by people who have suffered from peptic ulcers.

Most NSAIDs are not recommended during pregnancy or for breast-feeding mothers. Caution is also advised for those with kidney or liver abnormalities or with a

ACTION OF NSAIDs IN OSTEOARTHRITIS

Non-steroidal anti-inflammatory drugs (NSAIDs) are often prescribed to diminish the pain and stiffness associated with osteoarthritis, a disorder in which, typically, a weight-bearing joint such as the hip is damaged by wear and tear or other factors.

Pelvis

Cartilage

Fluid

Head of femur

Damaged cartilage

Inflamed joint tissues

Before treatment
The protective layers of cartilage surrounding the joint are worn away and the joint becomes inflamed and painful.

Drug

Reduced inflammation

Effect of NSAIDs
NSAIDs reduce inflammation and may thus relieve pain, but damage to the joint remains and symptoms are likely to worsen or recur if the drug is stopped.

history of hypersensitivity to other drugs.

NSAIDs may impair blood clotting and are, therefore, prescribed with caution for people with bleeding disorders or who are taking drugs that reduce blood clotting.

Anti-ulcer drugs

An NSAID may cause bleeding when its antiprostaglandin action occurs in the digestive tract. To protect against this side effect, proton-pump inhibitors (PPIs) and misoprostol are used. Misoprostol is sometimes combined with the NSAID.

COX-2 selective inhibitors

NSAIDs block two types of COX enzymes, COX-1 and COX-2, at different sites in the body. Blocking COX-1 leads to the stomach irritation of NSAIDs, while blocking COX-2 leads to the anti-inflammatory effect. As a result, one class of NSAIDs, COX-2 selective inhibitors, was developed to block COX-2 only. Thus, the benefits of NSAIDs can be obtained with less risk of stomach pain,

peptic ulcers, or intestinal bleeding. Celecoxib is a COX-2 selective inhibitor, and is useful in people at risk of stomach problems, but should be used cautiously in those with kidney or heart disease.

COMMON DRUGS

ASA *	Mefenamic acid *
Diclofenac *	Meloxicam *
Diflunisal	Nabumetone
Etodolac	Naproxen *
Flurbiprofen	Oxaprozin
Ibuprofen *	Piroxicam *
Indomethacin	Sulindac
Ketoprofen *	Tenoxicam
Ketorolac	Tiaprofenic acid

COX-2 selective inhibitor
Celecoxib *

* See Part 4

ANTIRHEUMATIC DRUGS

These drugs are used in the treatment of various rheumatic disorders, the most crippling and deforming of which is rheumatoid arthritis (RA), an autoimmune disease in which the body's immune system causes damage of its own joint tissue. The disease causes pain, stiffness, and swelling of the joints that, over many months, can lead to deformity. Flare-ups of RA also cause a general feeling of being unwell, fatigue, and loss of appetite.

Treatments for RA include drugs, rest, changes in diet, physiotherapy, and immobilization of joints. RA cannot yet be cured, although with treatment, disability can be prevented. It sometimes subsides spontaneously for prolonged periods.

Why they are used

The aim of drug treatment is to relieve the symptoms of pain and stiffness, maintain mobility, and prevent deformity. There are two main forms of drug treatment for RA: one to alleviate symptoms, and the second to modify, halt, or slow the underlying disease process. Drugs in the first category include ASA (p.194) and the other non-steroidal anti-inflammatory drugs (NSAIDs, facing page). These drugs are usually prescribed for early relief of pain and inflammation.

The second category of drugs, called disease-modifying antirheumatic drugs (DMARDs) are also started early in the disease, as these drugs may prevent any further joint damage and disability. They are usually prescribed in moderate to severe disease and can have potentially severe adverse effects. For individuals with aggressive, debilitating arthritis, biologic agents called Biological Response Modifiers (BRM) may be considered. These target specific components of the body's immune system and can reduce inflammation. BRMs are administered by injection and may need to be given daily, weekly, or every 2 weeks, depending on the agent. There are important health cautions in using these, which needs to be discussed with your physician. BRMs are generally expensive. Corticosteroids (p.127) are sometimes used in the

THE EFFECTS OF ANTIRHEUMATIC DRUGS

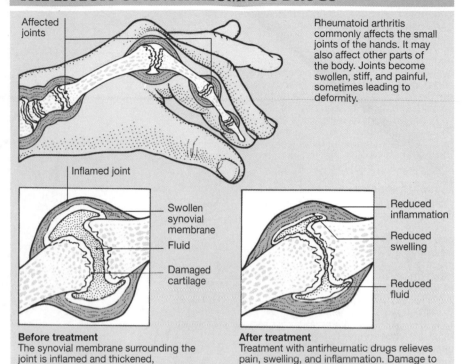

Rheumatoid arthritis commonly affects the small joints of the hands. It may also affect other parts of the body. Joints become swollen, stiff, and painful, sometimes leading to deformity.

Affected joints

Inflamed joint

Swollen synovial membrane
Fluid
Damaged cartilage

Reduced inflammation
Reduced swelling
Reduced fluid

Before treatment
The synovial membrane surrounding the joint is inflamed and thickened, producing increased fluid within the joint. The surrounding tissue is inflamed and joint cartilage is damaged.

After treatment
Treatment with antirheumatic drugs relieves pain, swelling, and inflammation. Damage to cartilage and bone may be halted so that further deformity is minimized.

treatment of RA, but only for limited periods because these drugs depress the immune system, thereby increasing susceptibility to infection.

How they work

It is not known precisely how most antirheumatic drugs slow the disease process. Some may reduce the body's immune response (see Immunosuppressant drugs, p.143). Antirheumatic drugs prevent damage to the cartilage and bone, reducing progressive deformity and disability. The effectiveness of each drug varies with the individual response.

How they affect you

These drugs are generally slow acting; it may be weeks or even months before benefit is noticed. NSAID treatment is usually continued until remission occurs. Prolonged treatment with antirheumatic drugs can cause a marked improvement in symptoms. Arthritic pain is relieved, joint mobility increased, and general symptoms of ill health fade.

Some side effects may be noticed before any beneficial effect is evident, so patience is required. Severe adverse effects may necessitate abandoning the treatment.

TYPES OF ANTIRHEUMATIC DRUGS (DMARDs)

Hydroxychloroquine Originally developed to treat malaria (see p.123), this drug is less effective than penicillamine or gold. Since prolonged use may cause eye damage, regular eye checks are needed.

Immunosuppressants These are prescribed if other drugs do not provide relief and if RA is severe and disabling. Regular observation and blood tests must be carried out because immunosuppressants can cause severe complications.

Sulfasalazine Used mainly for ulcerative colitis (p.98), sulfasalazine was first introduced to treat RA and is effective in some cases.

Gold-based drugs These are believed to be the most effective and may be given orally or by injection for many years. Side effects can include a rash and digestive disturbances. Gold may sometimes damage the kidneys, which recover on stopping treatment; regular urine tests are usually carried out. It can suppress blood cell production in bone marrow, so periodic blood tests are also carried out.

Penicillamine This drug may be used when RA is worsening, or when gold cannot be given. Improvement in symptoms may take 3 to 6 months. It has similar side effects to gold, and periodic blood and urine tests are usually performed.

COMMON DRUGS

Immunosuppressants
Azathioprine ✳
Cyclosporine ✳
Cyclophosphamide ✳
Leflunomide
Methotrexate ✳

NSAIDs
(see facing page)

Gold-based drugs
Auranofin
Sodium aurothiomalate (Myochrysine)

Biological Response Modifiers
Abatacept
Adalimumab
Anakinra ✳
Ketorolac
Etanercept
Infliximab
Rituximab ✳

Other drugs
Hydroxychloroquine
Minocyline
Penicillamine
Prednisone ✳
Sulfasalazine ✳

✳ See Part 4

LOCALLY ACTING CORTICOSTEROIDS

The adrenal glands, which lie on the top of the kidneys, produce a number of important hormones. Among these are the corticosteroids, so named because they are made in the outer part (cortex) of the glands. The corticosteroids play an important role, influencing the immune system and regulating the carbohydrate and mineral *metabolism* of the body. A number of drugs that mimic the natural corticosteroids have been developed.

These drugs have many uses and are discussed in detail under Corticosteroids (p.127). This section concentrates on those corticosteroids injected into an affected site to treat joint disorders.

Why they are used

Corticosteroids given by injection are particularly useful for treating joint disorders – notably rheumatoid arthritis and osteoarthritis – when one or only a few joints are involved, and when pain and inflammation have not been relieved by other drugs. In such cases, it is possible to relieve symptoms by injecting each of the affected joints individually. Corticosteroids may also be injected to relieve pain and inflammation caused by strained or contracted muscles, ligaments, and/or tendons – for example, in frozen shoulder or tennis elbow. They may also be given for bursitis, tendinitis, or swelling that is compressing a nerve. Corticosteroid injections are sometimes used in order to relieve pain and stiffness sufficiently to permit physiotherapy.

How they work

Corticosteroid drugs have two important actions that are believed to account for their effectiveness. They block the production of prostaglandins – chemicals responsible for triggering inflammation and pain – and depress the accumulation and activity of the white blood cells that cause the inflammation (below). Injection concentrates the corticosteroids, and their effects, at the site of the problem, thus giving the maximum benefit where it is most needed.

How they affect you

Corticosteroids usually produce dramatic relief from symptoms when the drug is injected into a joint. Often a single injection is sufficient to relieve pain and swelling, and to improve mobility. When used to treat muscle or tendon pain, they may not always be effective because it is difficult to position the needle so that the drug reaches the right spot. In some cases, repeated injections are necessary.

Because these drugs are concentrated in the affected area, rather than being dispersed in significant amounts in the body, the generalized *adverse effects* that sometimes occur when corticosteroids are taken by mouth are unlikely. Minor side effects, such as loss of skin pigment at the injection site, are uncommon. Occasionally, a temporary increase in pain (steroid flare) may occur. In such cases, rest, local application of ice, and analgesic medication may relieve the condition. Sterile injection technique is critically important.

COMMON INJECTION SITES

Corticosteroids are often injected into joints affected by osteo- and rheumatoid arthritis. Joints commonly treated in this way are knee, shoulder, and finger joints.

Shoulder joint

Finger joints

Knee joint

ACTION OF CORTICOSTEROIDS ON INFLAMED JOINTS

Inflamed joint tissue

White blood cell

Blood vessel

Inflamed tissue
Inflammation occurs when disease or injury causes large numbers of white blood cells to accumulate in the affected area. In joints this leads to swelling and stiffness.

Reduced inflammation

Drug

Action of corticosteroids
Corticosteroids, when injected into the area, permeate the joint lining (synovial membrane), blocking prostaglandin production and preventing white blood cells accumulating.

COMMON DRUGS

Dexamethasone ✷   Prednisolone/
Hydrocortisone ✷   prednisone ✷
Methylprednisolone ✷   Triamcinolone

✷ See Part 4

DRUGS FOR GOUT

Gout is a disorder that arises when the blood contains increased levels of uric acid, which is a by-product of normal body *metabolism*. When its concentration in the blood is excessive, uric acid crystals may form in various parts of the body, especially in the joints of the foot (most often the big toe), the knee, and the hand, causing intense pain and inflammation known as gouty arthritis. Crystals may form as white masses, known as tophi, in soft tissue, and in the kidneys as stones. Attacks of gouty arthritis can recur, and may lead to damaged joints and deformity. Kidney stones can cause kidney damage.

An excess of uric acid can be caused either by increased production or by decreased elimination by the kidneys, which remove it from the body. The disorder tends to run in families and is far more common in men than women. The risk of attack is increased by high alcohol intake, the consumption of certain foods (red meat, sardines, anchovies, and offal

such as liver, brains, and sweetbreads), and obesity. In susceptible individuals, an attack may be triggered by drugs such as thiazide diuretics (see p.85) or anticancer drugs (see p.140), or excessive drinking. Changes in diet and a reduction in the consumption of alcohol may be an important part of treatment.

Drugs used to treat acute attacks of gouty arthritis include non-steroidal anti-inflammatory drugs (NSAIDs, see p.102), and colchicine. Sometimes, corticosteroids may be injected into a joint to decrease inflammation. Other drugs, which lower the blood level of uric acid, are used for the long-term prevention of gout. These include the uricosuric drugs (probenecid and sulfinpyrazone), as well as allopurinol. ASA is not prescribed for pain relief because it slows the excretion of uric acid.

Why they are used

Drugs may be prescribed either to treat an attack of gout or to prevent recurrent

attacks that could lead to deformity of affected joints and kidney damage. The NSAIDs and colchicine are both used to treat an attack of gout and should be taken as soon as an attack begins. Because colchicine is relatively specific in relieving the pain and inflammation arising from gout, doctors sometimes administer it in order to confirm their diagnosis of the condition before prescribing an NSAID.

If symptoms recur, your physician may advise long-term treatment with either allopurinol or a uricosuric drug. One of these drugs must usually be taken indefinitely. Since they can trigger attacks of gout at the beginning of treatment, colchicine is sometimes given with these drugs for a few months.

How they work

Allopurinol reduces the level of uric acid in the blood by interfering with the activity of xanthine oxidase, an *enzyme* involved in the production of uric acid in the body. Both sulfinpyrazone and probenecid increase the rate at which uric acid is excreted by the kidneys. The process by which colchicine reduces inflammation and relieves pain is not understood. The actions of NSAIDs are described on p.102.

How they affect you

Drugs used in the long-term treatment of gout are usually successful in preventing attacks and joint deformity. However, response may be slow.

Colchicine can disturb the digestive system, causing abdominal pain and diarrhea, which your physician can control by prescribing other drugs.

Risks and special precautions

Since they increase the output of uric acid through the kidneys, uricosuric drugs can cause uric acid crystals to form in the kidneys. They are not, therefore, usually prescribed for those people who already have kidney problems. In such cases, allopurinol may be preferred. It is always important to drink plenty of fluids while taking drugs for gout in order to prevent kidney crystals from forming. Regular blood tests to monitor levels of uric acid in the blood may be required.

ACTION OF URICOSURIC DRUGS

Uric acid is removed from the blood by the kidneys and excreted in the urine. Excess uric acid, caused by increased production or impaired kidney function, requires treatment with uricosuric drugs, which increase the rate at which uric acid is expelled.

Kidney tubule (enlarged)

Kidney

Blood vessels

Blood flow

Ureter (to bladder)

Uric acid and gouty arthritis

Gouty arthritis occurs when uric acid crystals form in a joint, often a toe, knee, or hand, causing inflammation and pain. This is the result of excessively high levels of uric acid in the blood. In some cases this is caused by overproduction of uric acid, while in others it is the result of reduced excretion of uric acid by the kidneys.

Uric acid

Blood vessels

Drug

Before drug treatment
Excess uric acid from the kidney tubule is reabsorbed into the surrounding blood vessels. This leads to the formation of uric acid crystals, which can cause gouty arthritis.

After drug treatment
By blocking the reabsorption of uric acid into the blood vessels, the amount of uric acid excreted in the urine is increased.

COMMON DRUGS

Drugs to treat attacks	Drugs to prevent attacks
Colchicine *	Allopurinol *
Methylprednisolone *	Probenecid*
NSAIDs (see p.102)	Sulfinpyrazone

Drugs to treat high uric acid caused by cytotoxic drugs
Allopurinol *

* See Part 4

MUSCLE RELAXANTS

Several drugs are available to treat muscle spasm – the involuntary, painful contraction of a muscle or a group of muscles that can stiffen an arm or leg, or make it nearly impossible to straighten your back. There are various causes. It can follow an injury, or come on without warning. It may also be brought on by a disorder such as osteoarthritis, the pain in the affected joint triggering abnormal tension in a nearby muscle.

Spasticity is another form of muscle tightness seen in some neurological disorders, such as multiple sclerosis, stroke, or cerebral palsy. Spasticity can sometimes be helped by physiotherapy but in severe cases drugs may be used to relieve symptoms.

Why they are used

Muscle spasm resulting from direct injury is usually treated with a non-steroidal anti-inflammatory drug (see p.102) or an analgesic. However, if the spasm is severe, a muscle relaxant may also be tried for a short period.

In spasticity, the sufferer's legs may become so stiff and uncontrollable that walking unaided is impossible. In such cases, a drug may be used to relax the muscles. Relaxation of the muscles often permits physiotherapy to be given for longer-term relief from spasms.

The muscle relaxant botulinum toxin may be injected locally to relieve muscle spasm in small groups of accessible muscles, such as those around the eye or in the neck.

How they work

Muscle-relaxant drugs work in one of several ways. The centrally acting drugs damp down the passage of the nerve signals from the brain and spinal cord that cause muscles to contract, thus reducing excessive stimulation of muscles as well as unwanted muscular contraction. Tizanidine stimulates the alpha receptors in the blood vessels. Dantrolene reduces

SITES OF ACTION OF MUSCLE RELAXANTS

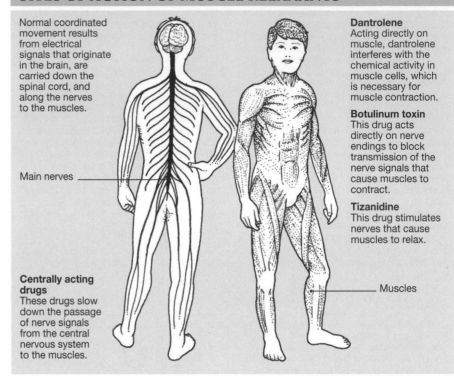

Normal coordinated movement results from electrical signals that originate in the brain, are carried down the spinal cord, and along the nerves to the muscles.

Main nerves

Centrally acting drugs
These drugs slow down the passage of nerve signals from the central nervous system to the muscles.

Dantrolene
Acting directly on muscle, dantrolene interferes with the chemical activity in muscle cells, which is necessary for muscle contraction.

Botulinum toxin
This drug acts directly on nerve endings to block transmission of the nerve signals that cause muscles to contract.

Tizanidine
This drug stimulates nerves that cause muscles to relax.

Muscles

the sensitivity of the muscles to nerve signals. When injected locally, botulinum toxin prevents transmission of impulses between nerves and muscles.

How they affect you

Drugs taken regularly for a spastic disorder of the central nervous system usually reduce stiffness and improve mobility. They may restore the use of the arms and legs when this has been impaired by muscle spasm.

Unfortunately, most centrally acting drugs can have a generally depressant effect on nervous activity and produce

drowsiness, particularly at the beginning of treatment. Too high a dosage can excessively reduce the muscles' ability to contract and can therefore cause weakness. For this reason, the dosage needs to be carefully adjusted to find a level that controls symptoms but which, at the same time, maintains sufficient muscle strength.

Risks and special precautions

The main long-term risk associated with centrally acting muscle relaxants is that the body becomes dependent. If the drugs are withdrawn suddenly, the stiffness may become worse than before drug treatment.

Rarely, dantrolene can cause serious liver damage. Anyone who is taking this drug should have his or her blood tested regularly to assess liver function.

Unless used very cautiously, botulinum toxin can paralyse unaffected muscles, and might interfere with functions such as speech and swallowing.

ACTION OF CENTRALLY ACTING DRUGS

Centrally acting muscle relaxants restrict passage of nerve signals to the muscles by occupying a proportion of the *receptors* in the central nervous system that are normally used by *neurotransmitters* to transmit such impulses. Reduced nervous stimulation allows the muscles to relax; however, if the dose of the drug is too high, this action may give rise to excessive muscle weakness.

Before drug

Contracted muscle fibre

Nerve signal

Neurotransmitter

After drug

Relaxed muscle fibre

Drug occupies receptor

COMMON DRUGS

Centrally acting drugs
Baclofen *
Cyclobenzaprine
Diazepam *

Methocarbamol
Orphenadrine *

Other drugs
Botulinum toxin type A *
Dantrolene
Tizanidine *

| * See Part 4 |

DRUGS USED FOR MYASTHENIA GRAVIS

Myasthenia gravis is a disorder that occurs when the immune system (see p.138) becomes defective and produces antibodies that disrupt the signals being transmitted between the nervous system and muscles that are under voluntary control. As a result, the body's muscular response is progressively weakened. The first muscles to be affected are those controlling the eyes, eyelids, face, pharynx, and larynx, with muscles in the arms and legs becoming involved as the disease progresses. The disease is often linked to a disorder of the thymus gland, which is the source of the destructive antibodies concerned.

Various methods can be used in the treatment of myasthenia gravis, including the removal of the thymus gland (called a thymectomy) or temporarily clearing the blood of antibodies using a procedure known as plasmapheresis. Drugs that improve muscle function, principally neostigmine and pyridostigmine, may be prescribed. They may be used alone or together with other drugs that depress the immune system – usually azathioprine (see Immunosuppressant drugs, p.143) or corticosteroids (see p.127).

THE EFFECTS OF MYASTHENIA GRAVIS

Myasthenia gravis initially causes weakness of the muscles in the face and throat, affecting the muscles around the eyes and the mouth. In the later stages, arms and legs may be affected.

Early stages

Late stages

The thymus gland Located in the upper part of the chest, this gland is thought to be partly responsible for the abnormal antibody activity in this disease.

Principal muscles affected

Why they are used

Drugs that improve the muscle response to nerve impulses have several uses. One such drug, edrophonium, acts very quickly and, once administered, it brings about a dramatic improvement in the symptoms. This effect is used to confirm the diagnosis of myasthenia gravis. However, because of its short duration of action, edrophonium is not used for long-term treatment. Pyridostigmine and neostigmine are preferred for long-term treatment, especially when surgery to remove the thymus gland is not feasible or does not provide adequate relief.

These drugs may be given following surgery to counteract the effects of a muscle-relaxant drug given prior to certain surgical procedures.

How they work

Normal muscle action occurs when a nerve impulse triggers a nerve ending to release a *neurotransmitter*, which combines with a specialized *receptor* on the muscle cells and causes the muscles to contract. In myasthenia gravis, the body's immune system destroys many of these receptors, so that the muscle is less responsive to nervous stimulation. Drugs used to treat the disorder increase the amount of neurotransmitter at the nerve ending by blocking the action of an *enzyme* that normally breaks it down. Increased levels of the neurotransmitter permit the remaining receptors to function more efficiently (see Action of drugs used for myasthenia gravis, below).

How they affect you

These drugs usually restore the muscle function to a normal or near-normal level, particularly when the disease takes a mild form. Unfortunately, the drugs can produce unwanted muscular activity by enhancing the transmission of nerve impulses elsewhere in the body.

Common side effects include vomiting, nausea, diarrhea, and muscle cramps in the arms, legs, and abdomen.

Risks and special precautions

Muscle weakness can suddenly worsen even when it is being treated with drugs. Should this occur, it is important not to take larger doses of the drug in an attempt to relieve the symptoms, since excessive levels can interfere with the transmission of nerve impulses to muscles, causing further weakness. The administration of other drugs, including some antibiotics, can also markedly increase the symptoms of myasthenia gravis. If your symptoms suddenly become worse, consult your physician.

ACTION OF DRUGS USED FOR MYASTHENIA GRAVIS

Normal nerve transmission Muscles contract when a neurotransmitter (acetylcholine) binds to receptors on muscle cells. An enzyme breaks down acetylcholine.

Enzyme / Acetylcholine (neurotransmitter) / Receptor / Nerve signals transmitted / Muscle cell

In myasthenia gravis Abnormal antibody activity destroys many receptors, reducing stimulation of the muscle cells and weakening the muscle action.

Antibody

Drug action Anticholinesterase drugs block enzyme action, increasing acetylcholine and prolonging the muscle cell response to nervous stimulation.

Drug acts on enzyme / Nerve signals transmitted

COMMON DRUGS

Azathioprine *
Corticosteroids (see p.127)
Edrophonium

Neostigmine
Pyridostigmine *

* See Part 4

DRUGS FOR BONE DISORDERS

Bone is a living structure. Its hard, mineral quality is created by the action of the bone cells. These cells continuously deposit and remove phosphorus and calcium, stored in a honeycombed protein framework called the matrix. Because the rates of deposit and removal (the bone metabolism) are about equal in adults, the bone mass remains fairly constant.

Removal and renewal is regulated by hormones and influenced by a number of factors, notably the level of calcium in the blood, which depends on the intake of calcium and vitamin D from the diet, the actions of various hormones, plus everyday movement and weight-bearing stress. When normal bone metabolism is altered, various bone disorders result.

Osteoporosis

In osteoporosis, the strength and density of bone are reduced. Such wasting occurs when the rate of removal of mineralized bone exceeds the rate of deposit. In most people, bone density decreases very gradually from the age of 30. But bone

loss can dramatically increase when a person is immobilized for a period, an important cause of osteoporosis in elderly people. Hormone deficiency is another important cause, commonly occurring in women with lowered estrogen levels after the menopause or removal of the ovaries. It also occurs in disorders in which there is excess production of adrenal or thyroid hormones and can result from long-term treatment with corticosteroid drugs.

People with osteoporosis often have no symptoms, but, if the vertebrae become so weakened that they are unable to bear the body's weight, they may collapse spontaneously or after a minor accident. Subsequently, the individual suffers from back pain, reduced height, and a round-shouldered appearance. Osteoporosis also leads to fracture of the arm, leg, or hip.

Most doctors emphasize the need to prevent the disorder by an adequate intake of protein and calcium and by regular exercise throughout adult life. Estrogen supplements during and after the menopause may be used to prevent

osteoporosis in older women. (See Hormone replacement therapy, p.133.)

Drug treatment can help prevent further deterioration and help fractures to heal. For people whose diet is deficient in calcium or vitamin D, supplements may be prescribed. However, these are of limited value on their own. Drugs that inhibit removal of calcium from the bones are usually prescribed for osteoporosis, along with adequate calcium and vitamin D intake. In the past, the hormone calcitonin was used, but it has now been largely superseded by drugs such as etidronate and alendronate. These drugs, known as bisphosphonates, bind very tightly to bone matrix, preventing its removal by bone cells. Bisphosphonates may be administered daily or as a weekly dose. A newer bisphosphonate, zoledronic acid, is administered once yearly.

Osteomalacia and rickets

In osteomalacia – called rickets when it affects children – lack of vitamin D leads to loss of calcium, resulting in softening of the bones. It causes pain and tenderness and there is a risk of fracture and bone deformity. In children, growth is retarded.

Osteomalacia is most commonly caused by a lack of vitamin D. This can result from an inadequate diet, inability to absorb the vitamin, or insufficient exposure of the skin to sunlight (the action of the sun on the skin produces vitamin D inside the body). People who are at special risk include those whose absorption of vitamin D is impaired by an intestinal disorder, such as Crohn's disease or celiac disease. People with dark skins living in Northern Europe are also susceptible. Chronic kidney disease is an important cause of rickets in children and of osteomalacia in adults, since healthy kidneys play an essential role in the body's metabolism of vitamin D.

Long-term relief depends on treating the underlying disorder where possible. In rare cases, treatment may be lifelong.

Vitamin D

A number of substances that are related to vitamin D may be used in the treatment of bone disorders. These drugs include alfacalcidol, calcitriol, and ergocalciferol. The one prescribed depends on the underlying problem (see also page 481).

BONE WASTING

Normal bone
Regulated by hormones, bone cells constantly renew the hard mineralized tissue in the bone matrix with minerals from the blood.

Active bone cells

Matrix

Hormone

Healthy bone cell | Mineral

Bone cell wasted by lack of hormones

Damage to bone cell halted by drug

Drug

In osteoporosis
Hormonal disturbance leads to wasting of active bone cells. The bones become less dense and more fragile. Drug treatment with hormone and mineral supplements usually only prevents further bone loss.

Bone cell softened by lack of mineral

Bone cell restored by drug

Drug

In osteomalacia
Deficiency of calcium or vitamin D causes softening of the bone tissue. The bones become weaker and sometimes deformed. Drug treatment with vitamin D and minerals usually restores bone strength.

COMMON DRUGS

Bisphosphonates	Other drugs
Alendronate *	Calcitonin
Etidronate *	Calcitriol
Risedronate *	Conjugated
Zoledronic acid	estrogens *
	Ergocalciferol
Supplements	Raloxifene *
Calcium carbonate *	Teriparatide *
Calcium citrate	
Vitamin D *	* See Part 4

ALLERGY

Allergy, which is a hypersensitivity to certain substances, is a extreme reaction of the body's immune system. Through a variety of mechanisms (see Malignant and immune disease, p.138), the immune system protects the body by eliminating foreign substances that it does not recognize, such as microorganisms (bacteria or viruses).

One way in which the immune system acts is through the production of *antibodies*. When the body encounters a particular foreign substance (or allergen) for the first time, one type of white blood cell, the lymphocyte, produces antibodies that attach themselves to another type of white blood cell, the mast cell. If the same substance is encountered again, the allergen binds to the antibodies on the mast cells, causing the release of chemicals known as mediators.

The most important mediator is histamine. This can produce a rash, swelling, narrowing of the airways, and a drop in blood pressure. Although these effects are important in protecting the body against infection, they may also be triggered inappropriately in an allergic reaction.

What can go wrong
One of the most common allergic disorders, hay fever, is caused by an allergic reaction to inhaled grass pollen leading to allergic rhinitis – swelling and irritation of the nasal passages and watering of the nose and eyes. Other substances, such as house-dust mites, animal fur, and feathers, may cause a similar reaction in susceptible people.

Asthma, another allergic disorder, may result from the action of leukotrienes rather than histamine. Other allergic conditions include urticaria (hives) or other rashes (sometimes in response to a drug), some forms of eczema and dermatitis, and allergic alveolitis (farmer's lung). Anaphylaxis is a serious systemic allergic reaction (p.512) that occurs when an allergen reaches the bloodstream.

Why drugs are used
Antihistamines and drugs that inhibit mast cell activity are used to prevent and treat allergic reactions. Other drugs minimize allergic symptoms, such as decongestants (p.79) to clear the nose in allergic rhinitis, bronchodilators (p.76) to widen the airways of those with asthma, and corticosteroids applied to skin affected by eczema (p.167).

MAJOR DRUG GROUPS

Antihistamines	Corticosteroids (see p.127)
Leukotriene antagonists	

Allergic response
Lymphocytes produce antibodies to allergens and these attach to mast cells. If the allergen enters the body again, it binds to the antibodies, and the mast cells release histamine.

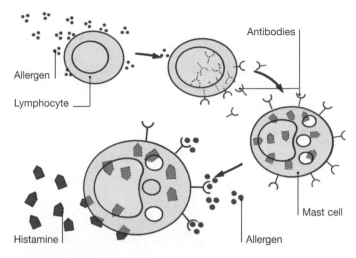

Histamine and histamine receptors
Histamine, released in response to injury or the presence of allergens, acts on H_1 *receptors* in the skin, blood vessels, nasal passages, and airways, and on H_2 receptors in the stomach lining, salivary glands, and lacrimal (tear) glands. It provokes dilation of blood vessels, inflammation and swelling of tissues, and narrowing of the airways. In some cases a reaction called anaphylactic shock may occur, caused by a dramatic fall in blood pressure, which may lead to collapse. Antihistamine drugs block the H_1 receptors, and H_2 blockers block the H_2 receptors (see also Antihistamines, p.110, and Anti-ulcer drugs, p.95).

Histamine acts on two types of receptor: H_1 and H_2. Each type is found in different body tissues.

Histamine can cause the airways to constrict.

Production of stomach acid is increased.

Blood vessels dilate.

The skin may itch and become inflamed.

H_1 receptor

H_2 receptor

ANTIHISTAMINES

Antihistamines are the most widely used drugs in the treatment of allergic reactions of all kinds. They can be subdivided according to their chemical structure, each subgroup having slightly different actions and characteristics (see table on facing page). Their main action is to counter the effects of histamine, one of the chemicals released in the body when there is an allergic reaction. (For a full explanation of the allergy mechanism, see p.109.)

Histamine is also involved in other body functions, including blood vessel dilation and constriction, contraction of muscles in the respiratory and gastrointestinal tracts, and the release of digestive juices in the stomach. The antihistamine drugs described here are also known as H_1 blockers because they only block the action of histamine on certain *receptors*, known as H_1 receptors. Another group of antihistamines, known as H_2 blockers, is used in the treatment of peptic ulcers (see Anti-ulcer drugs, p.97).

Some antihistamines have a significant *anticholinergic* action. This has benefits in a variety of conditions, but it also accounts for certain undesired side effects.

Why they are used

Antihistamines relieve allergy-related symptoms when it is not possible or practical to prevent exposure to the substance that has provoked the reaction. They are most commonly used in the prevention of allergic rhinitis (hay fever), the inflammation of the nose and upper airways that results from an allergic reaction to a substance such as pollen, house dust, or animal fur. Antihistamines are more effective when taken before the start of an attack. If they are taken only after an attack has begun, beneficial effects may be delayed.

Antihistamines are not usually effective in asthma caused by similar allergens because the symptoms of this allergic disorder are not solely caused by the action of histamine, but are likely to be the result of more complex mechanisms. Antihistamines are usually the first drugs to be tried in the treatment of allergic disorders but there are alternatives that can be prescribed (see below).

Antihistamines are also prescribed to relieve the itching, swelling, and redness that are characteristic of allergic reactions involving the skin – for example, urticaria (hives), eczema, and other forms of dermatitis. Irritation from chickenpox may be reduced by these drugs. Allergic reactions to insect stings may also be reduced by antihistamines. Applied as drops, antihistamines can reduce inflammation and irritation of the eyes and eyelids in allergic conjunctivitis.

An antihistamine is often included as an ingredient in cough and cold preparations (see p.80), when the anticholinergic effect of drying mucus secretions and their sedative effect on the coughing mechanism may be helpful.

Because most antihistamines have a depressant effect on the brain, they are sometimes used to promote sleep, especially when discomfort from itching is disturbing sleep (see also Sleeping drugs, p.66). The depressant effect of antihistamines on the brain also extends to the centres that control nausea and vomiting. Antihistamines are therefore often effective for preventing and controlling these symptoms (see Anti-emetics, p.74).

Occasionally, antihistamines are used to treat fever, rash, and breathing difficulties that may occur in adverse reactions to blood transfusions and allergic reactions to drugs. Promethazine may also be used as *premedication* to provide sedation and to dry secretions during surgery, particularly in children.

How they work

Antihistamines block the action of histamine on H_1 receptors. These are found in various body tissues, particularly the small blood vessels in the skin, nose, and eyes. This helps prevent the dilation of the vessels, thus reducing the redness, watering, and swelling. The anticholinergic action of these drugs also contributes to this effect by reducing the secretions from tear glands and nasal passages.

SITES OF ACTION

Antihistamines act on a variety of sites and systems throughout the body. Their main action is on the muscles surrounding the small blood vessels that supply the skin and mucous membranes. They also act on the airways in the lungs and on the brain.

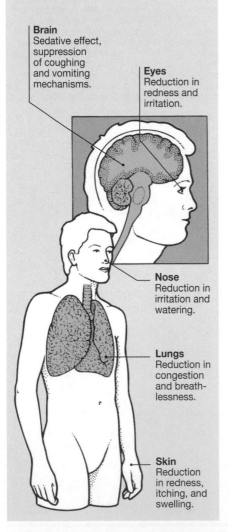

Brain
Sedative effect, suppression of coughing and vomiting mechanisms.

Eyes
Reduction in redness and irritation.

Nose
Reduction in irritation and watering.

Lungs
Reduction in congestion and breathlessness.

Skin
Reduction in redness, itching, and swelling.

OTHER ALLERGY TREATMENTS

Sodium cromoglycate
This drug (p.431) prevents the release of histamine from mast cells (see p.109) in response to exposure to an allergen, thus preventing the physical symptoms of allergies. It is given as eye drops for the prevention of allergic conjunctivitis or hay fever conjunctivitis.

Leukotriene antagonists
Like histamines, leukotrienes are substances that occur naturally in the body and seem to play an important part in asthma. Montelukast (p.363), known as a leukotriene antagonist, has been developed to prevent asthma attacks. It is not a bronchodilator and will not relieve an existing attack (see Drugs for asthma, p.78).

Corticosteroids
These are used to treat allergic rhinitis and asthma. They are given by inhaler, which use much lower doses than tablets.

Desensitization
This may be tried in conditions such as allergic rhinitis due to pollen sensitivity and insect venom hypersensitivity, when avoidance, antihistamines, and other treatments have not been effective and tests have shown one or two specific allergens to be responsible. Desensitization often provides incomplete relief and can be time consuming.

Treatment involves giving a series of injections containing gradually increasing doses of an extract of the allergen. The way in which this prevents allergic reactions is not understood. Perhaps controlled exposure triggers the immune system into producing increasing levels of antibodies so that the body no longer responds dramatically when the allergen is encountered naturally.

Desensitization must be carried out under medical supervision because it can provoke a severe allergic response. It is important to remain near emergency medical facilities for at least one hour after each injection.

COMPARISON OF ANTIHISTAMINES

Although antihistamines have broadly similar effects and uses, differences in their strength of anticholinergic action and the amount of drowsiness they produce, as well as in their duration of action, affect the uses for which each drug is commonly selected. The table indicates the main uses of some of the common antihistamines and gives an indication of the relative strengths of their anticholinergic and sedative effects and of their duration of action.

- ● Drug used
- ■ Strong
- ◰ Medium
- □ Minimal
- ▲ Long (over 12 hours)
- ◮ Medium (6–12 hours)
- △ Short (4–6 hours)

Drugs	Common uses						Actions and effects		
	Allergic rhinitis	Skin allergy	Sedation	Premedication	Nausea/vomiting	Cough/cold remedies	Drowsiness	Anticholinergic action	Duration of action
Azatadine	●	●					■	◰	▲
Brompheniramine	●	●				●	◰	◰	△
Cetirizine	●	●					□	□	▲
Chlorpheniramine	●	●	●			●	◰	■	△
Cyproheptadine	●	●					◰	◰	△
Desloratadine	●	●					□	□	▲
Diphenhydramine			●		●	●	■	■	△
Fexofenadine	●	●					□	□	▲
Hydroxyzine		●	●				■	◰	△
Loratadine	●	●					□	□	▲
Promethazine	●	●	●	●		●	■	■	◮

Some antihistamine drugs pass from the blood into the brain. In the brain, the blocking action of the antihistamines on histamine activity may produce general sedation and depression of various brain functions, including the vomiting and coughing mechanisms.

How they affect you

Antihistamines frequently cause a degree of drowsiness and may adversely affect coordination, leading to clumsiness.

Some of the newer drugs have little or no sedative effect (see table above).

Anticholinergic side effects, including dry mouth, blurred vision, and difficulty passing urine, are common. Most side effects diminish with continued use and can often be helped by an adjustment in dosage or a change to a different drug.

Risks and special precautions

It may be advisable to avoid driving or operating machinery while taking antihistamines, particularly those that are more likely to cause drowsiness (see table above). The sedative effects of alcohol, sleeping drugs, opioid analgesics, and anti-anxiety drugs can also be increased by antihistamines.

In high doses, or in children, some antihistamines can cause excitement, agitation, and even, in extreme cases, hallucinations and convulsions. Abnormal heart rhythms have occurred after high doses with some antihistamines or when drugs that interact with them, such as antifungals and antibiotics, have been taken at the same time. Heart rhythm problems may also affect people with liver disease, electrolyte disturbances, or abnormal heart activity. A person who has these conditions, or who has glaucoma or prostate trouble, should seek medical advice before taking antihistamines because their various drug actions may make such conditions worse.

ANTIHISTAMINES AND ALLERGIC RHINITIS

Before drug treatment
In allergic rhinitis, histamine released in response to an allergen acts on histamine receptors and produces dilation of the blood vessels supplying the lining of the nose, leading to swelling and increased mucus production. There is also irritation that causes sneezing, and often redness and watering of the eyes.

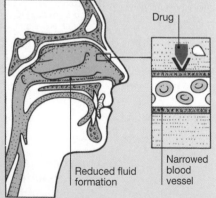

After drug treatment
Antihistamine drugs prevent histamine from attaching to histamine receptors, thereby preventing the body from responding to allergens. Over a period of time, the swelling, irritation, sneezing, and watery discharge are reduced, and further contact with the allergen responsible usually produces only minor allergic symptoms.

COMMON DRUGS

Generally non-sedating
Cetirizine *
Desloratadine *
Fexofenadine
Loratadine *

Sedating
Azatadine
Brompheniramine
Chlorpheniramine *
Clemastine
Cyproheptadine
Diphenhydramine *
Hydroxyzine *
Promethazine *

Anti-allergic eye preparations
Emedastine
Ketotifen
Levocabastine
Lodoxamide
Nedocromil
Olopatadine
Sodium cromoglycate *

✳ See Part 4

INFECTIONS AND INFESTATIONS

The human body provides a suitable environment for the growth of many types of microorganisms, including bacteria, viruses, fungi, yeasts, and protozoa. It may also become the host for animal parasites such as insects, worms, and flukes.

Microorganisms (microbes) exist all around us and can be transmitted from person to person in many ways: direct contact, inhalation of infected air, and consumption of contaminated food or water (see Transmission of infection, facing page). Not all microorganisms cause disease; many types of bacteria exist on the skin surface or in the bowel without causing ill effects, while others cannot live either in or on the body.

Normally the immune system protects the body from infection. Invading microbes are killed before they can multiply in sufficient numbers to cause serious disease. (See also Malignant and immune disease, p.138.)

What can go wrong

Infectious diseases occur when the body is invaded by microbes. This may be caused by the body having little or no natural immunity to the invading organism, or the number of invading microbes being too great for the body's immune system to overcome. Serious infections can occur when the immune system does not function properly or when a disease weakens or destroys the immune system, as occurs in AIDS (acquired immune deficiency syndrome).

Infections (such as childhood infectious diseases or those with flu-like symptoms) can cause generalized illness or they may affect a specific part of the body (as in wound infections). Some parts are more susceptible to infection than others – respiratory tract infections are relatively common, whereas bone and muscle infections are rare.

Some symptoms are the result of damage to body tissues by the infection, or by *toxins* released by the microbes. In other cases, the symptoms result from the body's defence mechanisms.

Most bacterial and viral infections cause fever. Bacterial infections may also cause inflammation and pus formation in the affected area.

Why drugs are used

Treatment of an infection is necessary only when the type or severity of symptoms shows that the immune system has not overcome the infection.

Bacterial infection can be treated with antibiotic or antibacterial drugs. Some of these drugs actually kill the infecting bacteria, whereas others merely prevent them from multiplying.

Types of infecting organisms
Bacteria
A typical bacterium (right) consists of a single cell that has a protective wall. Some bacteria are aerobic – that is, they require oxygen – and therefore are more likely to infect surface areas such as the skin or respiratory tract. Others are anaerobic and multiply in oxygen-free surroundings such as the bowel or deep puncture wounds.

Nucleus

Cell wall

Cocci (spherical) *Streptococcus* (above) can cause sore throats and pneumonia.

Bacilli (rod-shaped) *Mycobacterium tuberculosis* (above) causes tuberculosis.

Spirochaete (spiral-shaped) This group includes bacteria that cause syphilis and gum infections.

Viruses
These infectious agents are smaller than bacteria and consist simply of a core of genetic material surrounded by a protein coat. A virus can multiply only in a living cell by using the host tissue's replicating material.

Protein coat

Viral genetic material

Protozoa
These single-celled parasites are slightly bigger than bacteria. Many protozoa live in the human intestine and are harmless. However, some types cause malaria, sleeping sickness, and dysentery.

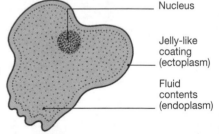

Nucleus

Jelly-like coating (ectoplasm)

Fluid contents (endoplasm)

Unnecessary use of antibiotics may result in the development of resistant bacteria.

Some antibiotics can be used to treat a broad range of infections, while others are effective against a particular type of bacterium or in a certain part of the body. Antibiotics are most commonly given by mouth, or by injection in severe infections, but they may be applied topically for a local action.

Antiviral drugs are used for severe viral infections that threaten body organs or survival. Antivirals may

How bacteria affect the body

Bacteria can cause symptoms of disease in two principal ways: first, by releasing toxins that harm body cells; second, by provoking an inflammatory response in the infected tissues.

Effects of toxins

The invading bacterium gives off poisons (toxins) that attack the body cell.

The toxins emanating from the bacterium break through the cell structure and destroy the cell.

Inflammatory response

White blood cells of the immune system attack the bacterium directly by releasing inflammatory substances and, later, antibodies.

A side effect of this attack of the immune system on the bacterium is damage to, and inflammation of, the body's own cells.

Transmission of infection

Infecting organisms can enter the human body through a variety of routes, including direct contact between an infected person and someone else, and eating or inhaling infected material.

Droplet infection
Coughing and sneezing spread infected secretions.

Insects
Insect bites may transmit infection.

Physical contact
Everyday contact may spread infection.

Sexual contact
Certain infections and infestations may be spread by genital contact.

Food
Many infecting organisms can be ingested in food.

Water
Infections can be spread in polluted water.

be used in topical preparations, given by mouth, or administered in hospital by injection.

Other drugs used in the fight against infection include antiprotozoal drugs for protozoal infections such as malaria; antifungal drugs for infection by fungi and yeasts, including *Candida* (thrush); and anthelmintics to eradicate worm and fluke infestations. Cases of infestation by skin parasites are usually treated with the topical application of insecticides (see p.164).

INFESTATIONS

Invasion by parasites that live on the body (such as lice) or in the body (such as tapeworms) is known as infestation. Since the body lacks strong natural defences against infestation, antiparasitic treatment is necessary. Infestations are often associated with tropical climates and poor standards of hygiene.

Tapeworms and roundworms live in the intestines and may cause diarrhea and anemia. Roundworm eggs may be passed in feces. Hookworm larvae in infected soil usually enter the body through the skin. Tapeworms may grow to 9m (30 feet) and infection occurs through undercooked meat containing larvae.

Flukes are of various types. The liver fluke (acquired from infected vegetation) lives near the bile duct in the liver and can cause jaundice. A more serious type (which lives in small blood vessels supplying the bladder or intestines) causes schistosomiasis and is acquired from contact with infected water.

Lice and scabies spread by direct contact. Head, clothing, and pubic lice need human blood to survive and die away from the body. Dried feces of lice on clothing spread typhus by infecting wounds or being inhaled. Scabies (caused by a tiny mite that does not carry disease) makes small, itchy tunnels in the skin.

Life cycle of a worm

Many worms have a complex life cycle. The life cycle of the worm that causes the group of diseases known as filariasis is illustrated below.

A mosquito ingests the filarial larvae and bites a human, thereby transmitting the larvae.

The mature larvae enter the lymph glands and vessels and reproduce there, often causing no ill effects.

Infected mosquitoes

Mature larvae

Adult worms

The infestation is spread by mosquitoes biting infected people and restarting the cycle.

The larvae grow into adult worms, which release larvae into the bloodstream.

MAJOR DRUG GROUPS

Antibiotics and antibacterial drugs (including antituberculosis drugs)
Antiviral drugs
Vaccines and immunizations

Antiprotozoal drugs (including antimalarial drugs)
Antifungal drugs
Anthelmintic drugs

ANTIBIOTICS

Antibiotics are one of the most commonly prescribed drugs. These drugs are usually safe and effective in the treatment of bacterial disorders ranging from minor infections, like conjunctivitis, to life-threatening diseases like pneumonia, meningitis, and septicemia. They are similar in function to the antibacterial drugs (see p.117), but the early antibiotics all had a natural origin in moulds and fungi, although most antibiotics are now synthesized.

Since 1941, when the first antibiotic, penicillin, was introduced, many different classes have been developed. Each one has a different chemical composition and is effective against a particular range of bacteria. None is effective against viral infections (see Antiviral drugs, p.119).

Some of the antibiotics have a broad spectrum of activity against a wide variety of bacteria. Others are used in the treatment of infection by only a few specific organisms. For a description of each common class of antibiotic, see Classes of antibiotics p.116.

Why they are used

We are surrounded by bacteria – in the air we breathe, on the mucous membranes of our mouth and nose, on our skin, and in our intestines – but we are protected, most of the time, by our immunological defences. When these break down, or when bacteria already present migrate to a vulnerable new site, or when harmful

ANTIBIOTIC RESISTANCE

The increasing use of antibiotics in the treatment of infection has led to resistance in certain types of bacteria to the effects of particular antibiotics. This resistance to the drug usually occurs when bacteria develop mechanisms of growth and reproduction that are not disrupted by the effects of the antibiotics. In other cases, bacteria produce *enzymes* that neutralize the antibiotics.

Antibiotic resistance may develop in a person during prolonged treatment when a drug has failed to eliminate the infection quickly. The resistant strain of bacteria is able to multiply, thereby prolonging the illness.

It may also infect other people, and result in the spread of resistant infection. One particularly important example is methicillin-resistant staphylococcus aureus, which resists most antibiotics but can be treated with other drugs such as vancomycin.

Doctors try to prevent the development of antibiotic resistance by selecting the drug most likely to eliminate the bacteria present in each individual case as quickly and as thoroughly as possible. Failure to complete a course of antibiotics that has been prescribed by your physician increases the likelihood that the infection will recur in a resistant form.

bacteria not usually present invade the body, infectious disease sets in.

The bacteria multiply uncontrollably, destroying tissue, releasing toxins, and, in some cases, threatening to spread via the bloodstream to such vital organs as the heart, brain, lungs, and kidneys. The symptoms of infectious disease vary widely, depending on the site of the infection and the type of bacteria.

Confronted with a sick person and suspecting a bacterial infection, the physician should identify the organism causing the disease before prescribing any drug. However, tests to analyse blood, sputum, urine, stool, or pus usually take 24 hours or more. In the meantime, especially if the person is in discomfort

or pain, the physician usually makes a preliminary drug choice, something of an educated guess as to the causative organism. In determining this "empirical treatment", as it is called, the physician is guided by the site of the infection, the nature and severity of the symptoms, the likely source of infection, and the prevalence of any similar illnesses in the community at that time.

In such circumstances, pending laboratory identification of the trouble-making bacteria, the physician may initially prescribe a broad-spectrum antibiotic, which is effective against a wide variety of bacteria. As soon as tests provide more exact information, he or she may switch the person to the recommended antibiotic treatment for the identified bacteria. In some cases, more than one antibiotic is prescribed, to be sure of eliminating all strains of bacteria.

In most cases, antibiotics can be given by mouth. However, in serious infections when high blood levels of the drug are needed rapidly, or when a type of antibiotic is needed that cannot be given by mouth, the drug may be given by injection. Antibiotics are also included in *topical* preparations for localized skin, eye, and ear infections (see also Anti-infective skin preparations, p.163, and Drugs for ear disorders, p.159).

How they work

Depending on the type of drug and the dosage, antibiotics are either bactericidal, killing organisms directly, or bacteriostatic, halting the multiplication of bacteria and enabling the body's natural defences to overcome the remaining infection.

Penicillins and cephalosporins are bactericidal, destroying bacteria by preventing them from making normal cell walls; most other antibiotics act inside the bacteria by interfering with the chemical activities essential to their life cycle.

How they affect you

Antibiotics stop most common types of infection within days. Because they do not relieve symptoms directly, you may be

ACTION OF ANTIBIOTICS

Penicillins and cephalosporins
Drugs from these groups are bactericidal – that is, they kill bacteria. They interfere with the chemicals needed by bacteria to form normal cell walls (right). The cell's outer lining disintegrates and the bacterium dies (far right).

Bacterium

Drug

Cell wall

Disintegrating cell wall

Other antibiotics
These drugs alter chemical activity inside the bacteria, thereby preventing the production of proteins that the bacteria need to multiply and survive (right). This may have a bactericidal effect in itself, or it may prevent reproduction (bacteriostatic action) (far right).

Drug

Protein

Unformed protein

USES OF ANTIBIOTICS

The table below shows which common drugs in each class of antibiotic are used for the treatment of infections in different parts of the body. For the purposes of comparison, this table also includes (in the Other drugs category) some antibacterial drugs that are discussed on page 117. This table is not intended to be used as a guide to prescribing but indicates the possible applications of each drug. Some drugs have a wide range of possible uses; this table concentrates on the most common ones.

Antibiotic / Site of infection	Ear, nose, throat, and mouth	Respiratory tract	Skin and soft tissue	Gastrointestinal tract	Eye	Kidney and urinary tract	Brain and nervous system	Heart and blood	Bones and joints	Genital tract
Penicillins										
Amoxicillin	●	●	●			●		●	●	
Amoxicillin/clavulinic acid	●	●	●			●			●	
Ampicillin	●	●	●			●	●		●	
Cloxacillin	●		●					●	●	
Penicillin G	●	●	●				●	●	●	
Penicillin V	●	●	●							
Cephalosporins										
Cefaclor	●	●				●				
Cefazolin		●	●			●			●	
Cefotaxime		●		●			●	●		
Cefoxitin		●	●			●				
Cefprozil	●	●	●							
Cefuroxime	●	●	●							●
Cephalexin		●	●			●				
Macrolides										
Azithromycin	●	●	●							
Clarithromycin	●	●	●	●						
Erythromycin	●	●	●	●	●				●	●
Tetracyclines										
Doxycycline	●	●				●				
Tetracycline	●	●			●	●				●
Aminoglycosides										
Amikacin		●	●			●	●		●	
Gentamicin		●	●	●	●	●		●	●	
Tobramycin		●	●	●		●			●	
Sulfonamide combination										
Co-trimoxazole		●				●				
Other drugs										
Clindamycin		●	●	●					●	
Fusidic acid		●						●	●	
Metronidazole	●	●	●				●	●	●	
Nitrofurantoin						●				
Trimethoprim		●	●			●				
Vancomycin				●				●		
Quinolones										
Ciprofloxacin		●	●			●				●
Levofloxacin		●								
Moxifloxacin		●								
Norfloxacin						●				

ANTIBIOTICS continued

advised to take other medication, such as analgesics (see p.64), to relieve pain and fever until the antibiotics take effect.

It is important to complete the course of medication as it has been prescribed by your physician, even if all your symptoms have disappeared. Failure to do this can lead to a resurgence of the infection in an antibiotic-resistant form (see Antibiotic resistance, p.114).

Most antibiotics used in the home do not cause any adverse effects if taken in the recommended dosage. In people who do experience adverse effects, nausea and diarrhea are among the more common ones (see also individual drug profiles in Part 4). Some people may be sensitive to certain types of

antibiotics, which can result in a variety of serious adverse effects.

Risks and special precautions

Most antibiotics used for short periods outside a hospital setting are safe for most people. The most common risk, especially with cephalosporins and penicillins, is a severe allergic reaction that can cause rashes and sometimes swelling of the face and throat. If this occurs, the drug should be stopped and medical advice sought immediately. If you have had a previous allergic reaction to an antibiotic, all other drugs in that class and related classes should be avoided. It is important to inform your physician and your pharmacist if you have suffered an adverse reaction to treatment with an antibiotic (with the exception of minor bowel disturbances).

Another risk of antibiotic treatment, especially if it is prolonged, is that the balance among microorganisms normally inhabiting the body may be disturbed. Antibiotics may destroy the bacteria that normally limit the growth of Candida, a yeast that is often present in the body in small amounts. This can lead to overgrowth of Candida (thrush) in the mouth, vagina, or bowel, and an antifungal drug (p.124) may be needed. A rarer, but more serious, result of disruption of normal bacterial activity in the body is a disorder known as pseudomembranous colitis, in which bacteria that are resistant to the antibiotic multiply in the bowel, causing violent,

bloody diarrhea. This potentially fatal disorder can occur with any antibiotic, but is more commonly reported with the lincosamides.

COMMON DRUGS

Aminoglycosides
Amikacin
Gentamicin *
Neomycin
Streptomycin
Tobramycin

Cephalosporins
Cefaclor
Cefadroxil
Cefazolin
Cefotaxime
Cefoxitin
Cefprozil
Ceftriaxone
Cefuroxime *
Ceftazidime
Cephalexin *

Lincosamides
Clindamycin *

Macrolides
Azithromycin *
Clarithromycin *
Erythromycin *

Penicillins
Amoxicillin *
Ampicillin
Cloxacillin *
Penicillin G
Penicillin V *
Piperacillin
Ticarcillin/
  clavulinic acid

Tetracyclines
Doxycycline *
Tetracycline *
Tigecycline

Other drugs
Chloramphenicol *
Daptomycin
Fosfomycin
  Tromethamine
Fusidic acid
Imipenem-cilastin
Linezolid
Meropenem
Metronidazole *
Rifampin *
Sulfamethoxazole/
  trimethoprim *
Telithromycin
Trimethoprim *
Vancomycin *

* See Part 4

DRUG TREATMENT FOR MENINGITIS

Meningitis is inflammation of the meninges (the membranes surrounding the brain and spinal cord) and is caused by both bacteria and viruses. Bacterial meningitis can kill previously well individuals within hours.

If bacterial meningitis is suspected, intra-venous antibiotics are needed immediately and admission to hospital is arranged.

In cases of bacterial meningitis caused by Haemophilus influenzae or Neisseria meningitidis, close contacts of these patients are advised to have a preventative course of antibiotics, usually rifampin.

CLASSES OF ANTIBIOTICS

Penicillins
The first antibiotic drugs to be developed, penicillins are still widely used to treat many common infections. Some penicillins are not effective when they are taken by mouth and therefore have to be given by injection in hospital. Unfortunately, certain strains of bacteria are resistant to penicillin treatment, and other drugs may have to be substituted. Penicillins often cause allergic reactions.

Cephalosporins
These are broad-spectrum antibiotics similar to the penicillins. They are often used when penicillin treatment has proved ineffective. Some cephalosporins can be given by mouth, but others are only given by injection. About 10 per cent of people who are allergic to penicillins may be allergic to cephalosporins. Some cephalosporins can occasionally damage the kidneys, particularly if used with aminoglycosides. Another serious, although rare, adverse effect of a few cephalosporins is that they occasionally interfere with normal blood clotting, leading to abnormally heavy bleeding, especially in the elderly.

Macrolides
Erythromycin is the most common drug in this group. It is a broad-spectrum antibiotic that is often prescribed as an alternative to penicillins or cephalosporins. Erythromycin is also effective against certain diseases, such as Legionnaires' disease (a rare type of

pneumonia), that cannot be treated with other antibiotics. The main risk with erythromycin is that it can occasionally impair liver function.

Tetracyclines
These have a broader spectrum of activity than other classes of antibiotic. However, increasing bacterial resistance (see Antibiotic resistance, p.114) has limited their use, although they are still widely prescribed. As well as being used for the treatment of infections, tetracyclines are also used in the long-term treatment of acne, although this application is probably not related to their antibacterial action. A major drawback to the use of tetracycline antibiotics in young children and in pregnant women is that they are deposited in developing bones and teeth.

With the exception of doxycycline, drugs from this group are poorly absorbed through the intestines, and when given by mouth they have to be administered in high doses in order to reach effective levels in the blood. Such high doses increase the likelihood of diarrhea as a side effect. The absorption of tetracyclines can be further reduced by interaction with calcium and other minerals. Drugs from this group should not therefore be taken with iron tablets or milk products. Tetracyclines deteriorate and may become poisonous with time, so leftover tablets or capsules should always be discarded.

Aminoglycosides
These potent drugs are effective against a broad range of bacteria. However, they are not

as widely used as some other antibiotics since they have to be given by injection and they have potentially serious side effects. Their use is therefore limited to hospital treatment of serious infections. They are often given with other antibiotics. Possible adverse effects include damage to the kidneys and the nerves in the ear and severe skin rashes.

Lincosamides
The lincosamide clindamycin is not commonly used as it is more likely to cause serious disruption of bacterial activity in the bowel than other antibiotics. It is mainly reserved for the treatment of bone, joint, abdominal, and pelvic infections that do not respond well to other antibiotics. Clindamycin is also used topically for acne and vaginal infections.

Quinolones (see p.117)
These drugs are often called antibacterials because they are derived from chemicals rather than living organisms. Quinolones have a broad spectrum of activity. They are used in the treatment of urinary and respiratory infections, and are widely effective in acute diarrheal diseases, including that caused by salmonella, as well as in the treatment of enteric fever.

The absorption of quinolones is reduced by antacids containing magnesium and aluminium. They are well tolerated but should be avoided by epileptics, as they may rarely cause convulsions, and by children, as studies have shown that they may damage joints.

ANTIBACTERIAL DRUGS

This broad classification of drugs comprises agents that are similar to the antibiotics (p.114) in function but dissimilar in origin. The original antibiotics were derived from living organisms, for example, moulds and fungi. Antibacterials were developed from chemicals. The sulfonamides were the first drugs to be given for the treatment of bacterial infections and provided the mainstay of the treatment of infection before penicillin (the first antibiotic) became generally available. Increasing bacterial resistance and the development of antibiotics that are more effective and less *toxic* have reduced the use of sulfonamides.

Why they are used

Sulfonamides are especially useful for treating urinary tract infections because high concentrations of the drug reach the urine. They are also used for middle ear infections, although their use is limited due to resistance.

Trimethoprim is used for chest and urinary tract infections. The drug is also combined with sulfamethoxazole as co-trimoxazole.

Antibacterials used for tuberculosis are discussed on p.118. Others, sometimes classified as antimicrobials, include metronidazole, prescribed for a variety of genital infections and for some serious infections of the abdomen, pelvic region, heart, and central nervous system. Other antibacterials are used to treat urinary infections. These include nitrofurantoin and drugs in the quinolone group (see facing page) used to cure or prevent recurrent urinary tract infections. The quinolones are effective against a broad spectrum of bacteria. More potent relatives of nalidixic acid include norfloxacin, used to treat urinary tract infections, and ciprofloxacin,

ACTION OF SULFONAMIDES

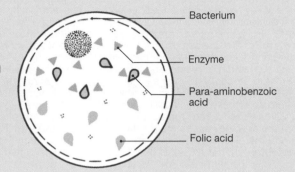

Before drug treatment
Folic acid, a chemical that is necessary for the growth of bacteria, is produced within bacterial cells by an *enzyme* that acts on a chemical called para-aminobenzoic acid.

- Bacterium
- Enzyme
- Para-aminobenzoic acid
- Folic acid

After drug treatment
Sulfonamides interfere with the release of the enzyme. This prevents folic acid from being formed. The bacterium is therefore unable to function properly and dies.

- Drug
- Dying bacterium

levofloxacin, and ofloxacin. These drugs are all used to treat many serious bacterial infections.

How they work

Most antibacterials function by preventing growth and multiplication of bacteria (see also Action of antibiotics, p.114, and Action of sulfonamides, above).

How they affect you

Antibacterials usually take several days to eliminate bacteria. During this time your physician may recommend additional medication to alleviate pain and fever. Possible side effects of sulfonamides include loss of appetite, nausea, a rash, and drowsiness.

Risks and special precautions

Like antibiotics, most antibacterials can cause allergic reactions in susceptible people. Possible symptoms that should always be brought to your physician's attention include rashes and fever. If such symptoms occur, a change to another drug is likely to be necessary.

Treatment with sulfonamides carries a number of serious, but uncommon risks. Some drugs in this group can cause crystals to form in the kidneys, a risk that can be reduced by drinking adequate amounts of fluid during prolonged treatment. Because sulfonamides may also occasionally

damage the liver, they are not usually prescribed for people with impaired liver function. There is also a slight risk of damage to bone marrow, lowering the production of white blood cells and thereby increasing the chances of a serious infection. Sulfonamides are therefore not prescribed for prolonged periods. Liver function and blood composition are often monitored during unavoidable long-term treatment.

DRUG TREATMENT FOR HANSEN'S DISEASE

Hansen's disease, better known as leprosy, is a bacterial infection caused by *Mycobacterium leprae*. It is rare in Canada, but relatively common in parts of Africa, Asia, and Latin America.

The disease progresses slowly, first affecting the peripheral nerves and causing loss of sensation in the hands and feet. This leads to frequent unnoticed injuries or burns and consequent scarring. Later, the nerves of the face may also be affected.

Treatment uses three drugs together to prevent the development of resistance. Usually, dapsone, rifampin, and clofazimine will be given for at least 2 years. If one of these cannot be used, then a second line drug (ofloxacin, minocycline, or clarithromycin) might be substituted. Complications during treatment sometimes require the use of prednisone, ASA, chloroquine, or even thalidomide.

COMMON DRUGS

Quinolones
Ciprofloxacin *
Gemifloxacin
Levofloxacin *
Moxifloxacin *
Norfloxacin *
Ofloxacin

Sulfonamides
Co-trimoxazole
(Sulfamethoxazole/
trimethoprim) *

Urinary antiseptic
Nitrofurantoin *

Other drugs
Clindamycin *
Metronidazole *
Trimethoprim *

---

* See Part 4

ANTITUBERCULOUS DRUGS

Tuberculosis is an infectious bacterial disease acquired, often in childhood, by inhaling the tuberculosis bacilli present in the spray caused by a sneeze or cough from someone who is actively infected. It may also be acquired from infected cow's milk. The disease usually starts in a lung and takes one of two forms: either primary infection or reactivated infection.

In 90 to 95 per cent of those with a primary infection, the body's immune system suppresses the infection but does not kill the bacilli. They remain alive but dormant and may cause the reactivated form of the disease. After they are reactivated, the tuberculosis bacilli may spread via the lymphatic system and bloodstream throughout the body (see Sites of infection, below).

The first symptoms of the primary infection may include a cough, fever, tiredness, night sweats, and weight loss. Tuberculosis is confirmed through clinical investigations, which may include a chest X-ray, isolation of the bacilli from the person's sputum, and a positive reaction – localized inflammation – to the Mantoux test, an injection of tuberculin (a protein extracted from tuberculosis bacilli) into the skin.

The gradual emergence in adults of the destructive and progressive form of tuberculosis is caused by the reactivated infection. It occurs in 5 to 10 per cent of those who have had a previous primary infection. Another form, reinfection tuberculosis, occurs when someone with

the dormant, primary form is reinfected. This type of tuberculosis is clinically identical to the reactivated form. Reactivation is more likely in those people whose immune system is suppressed, such as the elderly, those on corticosteroids or other immunosuppressant drugs, and those who have HIV/AIDS. Reactivation tuberculosis may be difficult to identify because the symptoms may start in any part of the body seeded with the bacilli. It is most often first seen in the upper lobes of the lung, and is frequently diagnosed after a chest X-ray. The early symptoms may be identical to those of primary infection: a cough, night sweats, tiredness, fever, and weight loss.

If left untreated, tuberculosis continues to destroy tissue, spreading throughout the body and eventually causing death. It was one of the most common causes of death in developed countries until the 1940s but the disease is now on the increase again worldwide. Vulnerable groups are people with suppressed immune systems and the homeless.

Why they are used
A person who has been diagnosed as having tuberculosis is likely to be treated with three or four antituberculous drugs. This helps to overcome the risk of drug-resistant strains of the bacilli emerging (see Antibiotic resistance, p.114).

The standard drug combination for the treatment of tuberculosis consists of rifampin, isoniazid, and pyrazinamide. In areas where there is a high prevalence of drug-resistant tuberculosis ethambutol may be added. However, other drugs may be substituted if the initial treatment fails or if drug sensitivity tests indicate that the bacilli are resistant to these drugs.

The standard duration of treatment for a newly diagnosed tuberculosis infection is a six-month regimen as follows: isoniazid, rifampin, pyrazinamide with or without ethambutol depending on susceptibility of bacteria, daily for two months, followed by isoniazid and rifampin for four months. The duration of treatment can be extended from nine months to up to two years in people at particular risk, such as those with a suppressed immune system.

Corticosteroids may be added to the treatment in specific situations, if the patient does not have a suppressed immune system, to reduce the amount of tissue damage.

Both the number of drugs required and the long duration of treatment may make treatment difficult, particularly for those who are homeless. To help with this problem, supervised administration of treatment is available when required, both in the community and in hospital.

Tuberculosis infection in patients with HIV infection or AIDS is treated with the standard antituberculous drug regimen.

SITES OF INFECTION

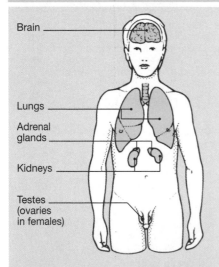

Brain

Lungs

Adrenal glands

Kidneys

Testes (ovaries in females)

Tuberculosis usually affects only part of one lung at first. However, later outbreaks usually spread to both lungs and may also affect the kidneys, leading to pyelonephritis; the adrenal glands, causing Addison's disease; and the membranes surrounding the brain, which may lead to meningitis. The testes (in men) and the ovaries (in women) may also be affected.

TUBERCULOSIS PREVENTION

A vaccine prepared from an artificially weakened strain of cattle tuberculosis bacteria can provide immunity from tuberculosis by provoking the development of natural resistance to the disease (see Vaccines and immunization, p.120). The BCG (Bacille Calmette-Guérin) vaccine is a form of tuberculosis bacillus that provokes the body's immune response but does not cause the illness because it is not infectious. The vaccine is given to some children between the ages of 10 and 14 years who are shown to have no natural immunity when given a skin test. BCG vaccination may be given to newborn babies if, for example, someone in the family has tuberculosis.

How it is done
The vaccine is usually injected into the upper arm. A small pustule usually appears 6–12 weeks later, by which time the person can be considered immune.

How they work
Antituberculous drugs act in the same way as antibiotics, either by killing bacilli or preventing them from multiplying (see Action of antibiotics, p.114).

How they affect you
Although the drugs start to combat the disease within days, benefits of drug treatment are not usually noticeable for a few weeks. As the infection is eradicated, the body repairs the damage caused by the disease. Symptoms such as fever and coughing gradually subside, and appetite and general health improve.

Risks and special precautions
Antituberculous drugs may cause adverse effects (nausea, vomiting, and abdominal pain), and they occasionally lead to serious allergic reactions. When this happens, another drug is substituted.

Rifampin and isoniazid may affect liver enzymes; isoniazid may adversely affect the nerves as well. Ethambutol can cause changes in colour vision. Dosage is carefully monitored, especially in children, the elderly, and those with reduced kidney function.

COMMON DRUGS

Ethambutol *	Rifabutin
Isoniazid *	Rifampin *
Pyrazinamide	Streptomycin

* See Part 4

ANTIVIRAL DRUGS

Viruses are simpler and smaller organisms than bacteria and are less able to sustain themselves. These organisms can survive and multiply only by penetrating body cells (see Action of antiviral drugs, right). Because viruses perform few functions independently, medicines that disrupt or halt their life cycle without harming human cells have been difficult to develop.

There are many different types of virus, and viral infections cause illnesses with various symptoms and degrees of severity. Common viral illnesses include the cold, influenza and flu-like illnesses, cold sores, and the usual childhood diseases such as chickenpox and mumps. Throat infections, pneumonia, acute bronchitis, gastroenteritis, and meningitis are often, but not always, caused by a virus.

Fortunately, the natural defences of the body are usually strong enough to overcome infections such as these, with drugs given to ease pain and lower fever. However, the more serious viral diseases, such as pneumonia and meningitis, need close medical supervision.

Another difficulty with viral infections is the speed with which the virus multiplies. By the time symptoms appear, the viruses are so numerous that antiviral drugs have little effect. Antiviral agents must be given early in the course of a viral infection or they may be used prophylactically (as a preventative). Some viral infections can be prevented by vaccination (see p.120).

Why they are used

Antiviral drugs are helpful in the treatment of various conditions caused by the herpes virus: cold sores, encephalitis, genital herpes, chickenpox, and shingles.

Acyclovir is applied *topically* to treat outbreaks of cold sores, herpes eye infections, and genital herpes. They can reduce the severity and duration of an outbreak, but they do not eliminate the infection permanently. The drugs acyclovir, famciclovir, and valacyclovir are given by mouth or, under exceptional circumstances by injection, to prevent chickenpox or severe, recurrent attacks of the herpes virus infections in those people who are already weakened by other conditions.

Influenza may sometimes be prevented by amantadine, oseltamivir, or zanamivir. These antivirals are also used in treating it.

The interferons are proteins produced by the body and involved in the immune response and cell function. Interferon alpha and beta are effective in reducing the activity of hepatitis B and hepatitis C. Peginterferon alfa-2a, telbivudine, laminidine, entacavir, and adefovir are also used to treat hepatitis B, and peginterferon alfa and ribavirin for hepatitis C.

Ganciclovir is sometimes used for cytomegalovirus (CMV). Respiratory syncytial virus (RSV) has been treated with ribavirin, and prevented by palivizumab. Drug treatment for AIDS is discussed on p.144.

ACTION OF ANTIVIRAL DRUGS

In order to reproduce, a virus requires a living cell. The invaded cell eventually dies and the new viruses are released, spreading and infecting other cells. Most antiviral drugs act to prevent the virus from using the host cell's genetic material, DNA, to multiply. Unable to divide, the virus dies and the spread of infection is halted.

Before drug

Host cell DNA

Virus

Host cell

Virus enters body cell.

Virus uses host cell's DNA to reproduce.

Host cell dies and new viruses are released.

After drug

Drug

Virus enters cell that has absorbed an antiviral drug.

Cell DNA is altered by drug action and virus cannot use it.

Virus dies and spread of infection is thereby halted.

How they work

Some antiviral drugs, such as idoxuridine, act by altering the cell's genetic material (DNA) so that the virus cannot use it to multiply. Other drugs stop multiplication of viruses by blocking enzyme activity within the host cell. Halting multiplication prevents the virus from spreading to uninfected cells and improves symptoms rapidly. However, in herpes infections, it does not eradicate the virus from the body. Infection may therefore flare up on another occasion.

Amantadine has a different action: it prevents the virus from entering the cells. It is therefore most effective when it is given as a *prophylactic*, before the infection has spread widely.

How they affect you

Topical antiviral drugs usually start to act immediately. Providing that the treatment is applied early enough, an outbreak of herpes can be cut short. Symptoms usually clear up within two to four days.

Antiviral ointments may cause irritation and redness. Antiviral drugs given by mouth or injection can occasionally cause nausea and dizziness.

Risks and special precautions

Because some of these drugs may affect the kidneys adversely, they are prescribed with caution for people with reduced kidney function. Some antiviral drugs can adversely affect the activity of normal body cells, particularly those in the bone marrow. Idoxuridine is, for this reason, available only for topical application.

COMMON DRUGS

Acyclovir *	Peginterferon alfa-2a
Adefovir	
Amantadine *	Peginterferon alfa-2b
Entecavir	
Famciclovir *	Penciclovir
Ganciclovir	Ribavirin
Idoxuridine	Telbivudine
Interferon alfa-2b *	Trifluridine
Lamivudine *	Valacyclovir
Oseltamivir *	Valganciclovir
Palivizumab	Zanamivir *

* See Part 4	See also Drugs for HIV, p.144

VACCINES AND IMMUNIZATION

Many infectious diseases, including most of the common viral infections, occur only once during a person's lifetime. The reason is that the antibodies produced in response to the disease remain afterwards, prepared to repel any future invasion as soon as the first infectious germs appear. The duration of such immunity varies, but it can last a lifetime.

Protection against many infections can now be provided artificially by the use of vaccines derived from altered forms of the infecting organism. These vaccines stimulate the immune system in the same way as a genuine infection, and provide lasting, active immunity. Because each type of microbe stimulates the production of a specific antibody, a different vaccine must be given for each disease.

Another type of immunization, called passive immunization, relies on giving antibodies (see Immune globulins, below).

Why they are used

Some infectious diseases cannot be treated effectively or are so serious that prevention is the best course. Routine immunization not only protects the individual but may gradually eradicate the disease completely, as with smallpox.

Newborn babies receive antibodies for many diseases from their mothers, but this protection lasts only for about three months. Most children from 2 months to 15 years are vaccinated against common childhood infectious diseases. In addition, travellers to many countries, especially in the tropics, are advised to be vaccinated against the diseases common in those regions. Rabies, yellow fever, and hepatitis B vaccines may be required for remote areas.

Effective lifelong immunization can sometimes be achieved by a single dose of the vaccine. However, in many cases reinforcing doses, commonly called booster shots, are needed later in order to maintain reliable immunity.

Vaccines do not provide immediate protection against infection and it may be

ACTIVE AND PASSIVE IMMUNIZATION

Active immunization

Injected vaccine
Blood

Before infection
A vaccine containing altered forms of the infection is injected.

Antibody formation
The vaccine causes antibodies to form against the infection.

Antibodies

Infecting organism attacked by antibodies

Immunity
Invasion of the body by a similar organism causes antibodies to form as a result of the vaccine and eliminate the infection.

Passive immunization

Injected antibodies

Infecting organisms

After infection
Passive immunization is needed when the infection has entered the blood.

Infecting organism attacked by antibodies

Immune globulin injection
A serum containing antibodies (immune globulin) extracted from donated blood is injected. This helps the body to fight the infection.

up to four weeks before full immunity is able to develop. When immediate protection from infectious disease is needed – for example, following exposure to infection – it may be necessary to establish passive immunity with immune globulins (see below).

How they work

Vaccines provoke the immune system into creating antibodies that help the body to resist specific infectious diseases. Many vaccines (known as live vaccines) are made from artificially weakened forms of the disease-causing germ. But even these weakened germs are effective in stimulating sufficient growth of antibodies. Other vaccines rely either on inactive (or killed) disease-causing germs, or inactive derivatives of these germs, but their effect on the immune system remains the same. Effective antibodies are created, thereby establishing active immunity.

How they affect you

The degree of protection varies among different vaccines. Some provide reliable lifelong immunity; others may not give full protection against a disease, or the effects may last for as little as six months. Influenza vaccines usually protect only against the variety of virus causing the latest outbreak of flu. New varieties appear during most years.

Any vaccine may cause side effects but they are usually mild and soon disappear. The most common reactions are a red, slightly raised, tender area at the site of injection, and a slight fever or a flu-like illness lasting for one or two days.

Risks and special precautions

Serious reactions are rare and, for most children, the risk is far outweighed by the protection given. Children who have had fits (seizures) may be advised against

IMMUNE GLOBULINS

Antibodies, which can result from exposure to snake and insect venom as well as infectious disease, permeate the serum of the blood (the part remaining after the red cells and clotting agents are removed). The concentrated serum of people who have survived diseases or poisonous bites is called immune globulin, and, given by injection, it creates passive immunity. Immune globulin from blood donated by a wide cross-section of donors is likely to contain antibodies to most common diseases. Specific immune globulins against rare diseases or toxins are derived from the blood of selected donors likely to have high levels of antibodies to that disease. These are called hyperimmune globulins. Some

immune globulins are extracted from horse blood following repeated doses of the toxin.

Because immune globulins do not stimulate the body to produce its own antibodies, their effect is not long-lasting and diminishes progressively over three or four weeks. Continued protection requires repeated injections of immune globulins.

Adverse effects from immune globulins are uncommon. Some people are sensitive to horse globulins, and about a week after the injection they may experience a reaction known as serum sickness, with fever, a rash, joint swelling, and pain. This usually ends in a few days but should be reported to your physician before any further immunization.

vaccinations for pertussis (whooping cough) or measles. Children who have any infection more severe than a common cold will not be given any routine vaccination until they have recovered.

Live vaccines should not be given during pregnancy because they can affect the developing baby, nor should they be given to people whose immune systems are weakened by disease or drug treatment. It is also advisable for those taking high doses of corticosteroids (p.127) to delay their vaccinations until the end of drug treatment.

The risk of high fever following the DPT (combined diphtheria, pertussis, and tetanus) vaccine can be reduced by giving acetaminophen at the time of vaccination. The pertussis vaccine may rarely cause a mild seizure (fit), which is brief, usually associated with fever, and stops without treatment. Children who have experienced such fits recover completely without neurological or developmental problems.

COMMON VACCINATIONS

Disease	Age at which vaccination is given	How given	General information
Diphtheria	2 months, 4 months, 6 months, 18 months, 4–6 years.	Injection	Infants: given with tetanus and pertussis vaccines. In later life immunity may diminish. Adults: booster every 10 years.
Tetanus	2 months, 4 months, 6 months, 18 months, 4–6 years.	Injection	Infants: given with diphtheria and pertussis. Protection lasts 5–10 years. Booster shots given for injuries likely to result in tetanus infection. Adults: booster every 10 years.
Acellular pertussis	2 months, 4 months, 6 months, 18 months, 4–6 years.	Injection	Preferable to use products in which diptheria toxin is combined with acellular pertussis. Preschool booster. Adults: give one dose as Tdap if not previously received.
Polio	2 months, 4 months, 6 months, 18 months, 4–6 years.	By mouth	Many physicians may recommend a booster every 10 years, especially if primary series during childhood is not complete, and especially for people who are travelling to countries where polio is still prevalent. Single booster dose recommended for those at high risk of exposure.
Haemophilus influenzae type b (Hib)	2 months, 4 months, 6 months, 18 months.	Injection	Routinely given in infancy to prevent serious disease up to the age of 4 years.
Rubella (German measles)	12 months and at 18 months or 4–6 years.	Injection	Given in infancy with measles and mumps vaccines (MMR). Rubella is important because it can damage the fetus if it affects a woman in early pregnancy.
Measles	12 months and at 18 months or 4–6 years.	Injection	Given with mumps and rubella vaccines (MMR) in infancy.
Mumps	12 months and at 18 months or 4–6 years.	Injection	Given with measles and rubella vaccines (MMR) in infancy.
Influenza	Recommended for all children 6–23 months. Also children and adults of any age who are at risk of serious illness or death if they develop influenza and their household carers, health care workers, as well as those wishing to be protected against influenza, and all adults 65 years of age and over.	Injection	Long-term immunity against all forms of influenza is impossible. Annual vaccinations are needed to protect against the latest strains. Also given to individuals capable of transmitting influenza to those at high risk (e.g. health care workers). Safe in pregnant and breast-feeding women.
Hepatitis A	Single dose for people any age who are at risk. Booster 6–12 months after initial shot.	Injection	Given to people travelling to areas of poor hygiene or where hepatitis infection is likely and to those exposed at school or work.
Hepatitis B	3 inoculations any age, with the second and third shots 1 and 6 months after the first.	Injection	Efficacy is checked by a blood test. Recommended for "at risk" groups, such as health-care providers, intravenous drug users, and long-stay travellers. Adolescents (11–15 years) may be given a 2-dose regimen of adult formulation.
Pneumococcal pneumonia	2 months, 4 months, 6 months, and at 12–15 months of age (pneumococcal conjugate vaccine). Single dose for people any age who are at risk and adults 65 years of age and over (pneumococcal polysaccharide).	Injection	Given to persons at risk of contracting pneumococcal pneumonia. This includes people who have had their spleen removed, immunodeficient persons, or those with chronic liver or lung disease or diabetes mellitus.
Meningococcal meningitis A + C	Single dose for people any age who are at risk. Schedule depends on age of individual.	Injection	Given to persons at risk of contracting meningitis; for example to travellers to the "Meningitis belt" of tropical and subtropical countries where there is a high risk of meningitis infection, also contacts of cases in Canada.
Meningococcal meningitis C	2 months, 4 months, 6 months (less than 2 years old).	Injection	Given in infancy to protect against one of the most common types of childhood meningitis.
Typhoid	Single dose for people any age who are at risk.	Injection	Travellers to areas with poor sanitation.

ANTIPROTOZOAL DRUGS

Protozoa are single-celled organisms that are present in soil and water. They may be transmitted to or between humans through contaminated food or water, sexual contact, or insect bites. There are many types of protozoal infection, each of which causes a different disease depending on the organism involved. Trichomoniasis, toxoplasmosis, cryptosporidium, giardiasis, and pneumocystis pneumonia are probably the most common protozoal infections. The rarer infections are usually contracted as a result of exposure to infection in another part of the world.

Many types of protozoa infect the bowel, causing diarrhea and generalized symptoms of ill-health. Others may infect the genital tract or skin. Some protozoa may penetrate vital organs such as the lungs, brain, and liver. Prompt diagnosis and treatment are important in order to limit the spread of the infection within the body and, in some cases, prevent it from spreading to other people. Increased attention to hygiene is an important factor in controlling the spread of the disease.

A variety of medicines is used in the treatment of these diseases. Some, such as metronidazole and tetracycline, are also commonly used for their antibacterial action. Others, such as pentamidine, are rarely used except in treating specific protozoal infections.

How they affect you

Protozoa are often difficult to eradicate from the body. Drug treatment may therefore need to be continued for several months in order to eliminate the infecting organisms completely and thus prevent recurrence of the disease. In addition, unpleasant side effects such as nausea, diarrhea, and abdominal cramps are often unavoidable because of the limited choice of drugs and the need to maintain dosage levels that will effectively cure the disease. For detailed information on the risks and adverse effects of individual antiprotozoal drugs, consult the appropriate drug profile in Part 4.

The table below describes the principal protozoal diseases, the organisms that cause them, and some of the drugs used in their treatment. Malaria, which is probably the most common protozoal disease in the world today, is discussed on the facing page.

SUMMARY OF PROTOZOAL DISEASES

Disease	Protozoan	Description	Drugs
Amoebiasis (amoebic dysentery)	*Entamoeba histolytica*	Infection of the bowel and sometimes of the liver and other organs. Usually transmitted in contaminated food or water. Major symptom is violent, sometimes bloody, diarrhea.	Metronidazole
Balantidiasis	*Balantidium coli*	Infection of the bowel, specifically the colon. Usually transmitted through contact with infected pigs. Possible symptoms include diarrhea and abdominal pain.	Tetracycline Metronidazole Iodoquinol
Cryptosporidiosis	*Cryptosporidium*	Infection of the bowel, also occasionally of the respiratory tract and bile ducts. Symptoms include diarrhea and abdominal pain.	No specific drugs but paromomycin and azithromycin may be effective.
Giardiasis (lambliasis)	*Giardia lamblia*	Infection of the bowel. Usually transmitted in contaminated food or water but may also be spread by some types of sexual contact. Major symptoms are general ill health, diarrhea, flatulence, and abdominal pain.	Metronidazole
Leishmaniasis	*Leishmania*	A mainly tropical and subtropical disease caused by organisms spread through sandfly bites. It affects the mucous membranes of the mouth, nose, and throat, and may in its severe form invade organs such as the liver.	Paromomycin Pentamidine Amphotericin
Pneumocystis pneumonia	*Pneumocystis carinii*	Potentially fatal lung infection that usually affects only those with reduced resistance to infection, such as AIDS sufferers. The symptoms include cough, breathlessness, fever, and chest pain.	Atovaquone Co-trimoxazole Pentamidine
Toxoplasmosis	*Toxoplasma gondii*	Infection is usually spread via cat feces or by eating undercooked meat. Although usually symptomless, infection may cause generalized ill-health, mild fever, and eye inflammation. Treatment is necessary only if the eyes are involved or if the patient is immunosuppressed (such as in AIDS). It may also pass from mother to baby during pregnancy, leading to severe disease in the fetus.	Pyrimethamine with sulfadiazine or with azithromycin, clarithromycin, or clindamycin Spiramycin (during pregnancy)
Trichomoniasis	*Trichomonas vaginalis*	Infection most often affects the vagina, causing irritation and an offensive discharge. In men, infection may occur in the urethra. The disease is usually sexually transmitted.	Metronidazole
Trypanosomiasis	*Trypanosoma*	African trypanosomiasis (sleeping sickness) is spread by the tsetse fly and causes fever, swollen glands, and drowsiness. South American trypanosomiasis (Chagas' disease) is spread by assassin bugs and causes inflammation, enlargement of internal organs, and infection of the brain.	Pentamidine (sleeping sickness) Primaquine (Chagas' disease)

ANTIMALARIAL DRUGS

Malaria is one of the main killing diseases in the tropics (see map below). It is most likely to affect people who live in or travel to such places.

The disease is caused by protozoa (see also facing page) whose life cycle is far from simple. The malaria parasite, which is called *Plasmodium*, lives in and depends on the female *Anopheles* mosquito during one part of its life cycle. It lives in and depends on human beings during other parts of its life cycle.

Transferred to humans in the saliva of the female mosquito as she penetrates ("bites") the skin, the malaria parasite enters the bloodstream and settles in the liver, where it multiplies asexually.

Following its stay in the liver, the parasite (or plasmodium) enters another phase of its life cycle, circulating in the bloodstream, penetrating and destroying red blood cells, and reproducing again. If the plasmodia then transfer back to a female *Anopheles* mosquito via another "bite", they breed sexually, and are again ready to start a human infection.

Following the emergence of plasmodia from the liver, the symptoms of malaria occur: episodes of high fever and profuse sweating alternate with equally agonizing episodes of shivering and chills. One of the four strains of malaria, *Plasmodium falciparum*, can produce a single severe attack that can be fatal unless treated.

The others cause recurrent attacks, sometimes extending over many years.

A number of drugs are available for preventing malaria, the choice depending on the region in which the disease can be contracted and the resistance to the commonly used drugs. In most areas, *Plasmodium falciparum* is resistant to chloroquine (see Choice of drugs, below). In all regions, three drugs are commonly used for treating malaria: quinine, mefloquine, and Malarone.

Why they are used

The medical response to malaria takes three forms: prevention, treatment of attacks, and the complete eradication of the plasmodia (radical cure).

For someone planning a trip to an area where malaria is prevalent, drugs are given that destroy the parasites in the liver. Dosing begins one week (2–3 weeks for mefloquine) before the traveller arrives in the malarial area and should continue for four to six weeks after return from the area.

Drugs such as mefloquine can produce a radical cure but chloroquine does not. After chloroquine treatment of non-falciparum malaria, a 14- to 21-day course of primaquine is administered. Although highly effective in destroying plasmodia in the liver, the drug is weak against the plasmodia in the blood. Primaquine is recommended only after a

person leaves the malarial area because of the high risk of reinfection.

How they work

Taken to prevent the disease, the drugs kill the plasmodia in the liver, preventing them from multiplying. Once plasmodia have multiplied, the same drugs may be used in higher doses to kill plasmodia that re-enter the bloodstream. If these drugs are not effective, primaquine may be used to destroy any plasmodia that are still present in the liver.

How they affect you

The low doses of antimalarial drugs taken for prevention rarely produce noticeable effects. Drugs taken for an attack usually begin to relieve symptoms within a few hours. Most of them can cause nausea, vomiting, and diarrhea. Quinine can cause disturbances in vision and hearing. Mefloquine can cause sleep disturbance, dizziness, and difficulties in coordination.

Risks and special precautions

When drugs are given to prevent or cure malaria, the full course of treatment must be taken. No drugs give long-term protection; a new course of treatment is needed for each journey.

Most of these drugs do not produce severe adverse effects, but primaquine can cause the blood disorder hemolytic anemia, particularly in people with glucose-6-phosphate dehydrogenase (G6PD) deficiency. Blood tests are taken before treatment to identify susceptible individuals. Mefloquine is not prescribed for those who have had psychological disorders or convulsions.

Other protective measures

Because *Plasmodium* strains continually develop resistance to the available drugs, prevention using drugs is not absolutely reliable. Protection from mosquito bites is of the highest priority. Such protection includes the use of insect repellents and mosquito nets impregnated with permethrin insecticide, as well as covering any exposed skin after dark.

CHOICE OF DRUGS

The parts of the world in which malaria is prevalent (illustrated on the map, right), and travel to which may make antimalarial drug treatment advisable, can be divided into six zones. The table below indicates the drug(s) currently used for the prevention of malaria in each zone. As prevalent strains of malaria change very rapidly, you must always seek specific medical advice before travelling to these areas.

Zone	Countries	Recommended antimalarial drugs for prevention
1	North Africa and the Middle East	Chloroquine, plus proguanil in areas of chloroquine resistance
2	Sub-Saharan Africa	Mefloquine, or chloroquine with proguanil, or doxycycline, or Malarone
3	South Asia	Mefloquine, or chloroquine with proguanil, or doxycycline, or Malarone
4	Southeast Asia	Mefloquine in high-risk areas, or chloroquine with proguanil; doxycycline or Malarone in mefloquine-resistant areas
5	Oceania	Mefloquine, or doxycycline, or Malarone
6	Latin America	Central America except Panama: chloroquine or proguanil. Panama and South America: mefloquine, or doxycycline, or Malarone in high-risk areas, or chloroquine with proguanil

COMMON DRUGS

Drugs for prevention	Drugs for treatment
Chloroquine ✳	Chloroquine ✳
Doxycycline ✳	Mefloquine ✳
Hydroxychloroquine	Primaquine
Mefloquine ✳	Proguanil with
Primaquine	atovaquone ✳
Proguanil ✳	Pyrimethamine✳
Proguanil with	Quinine ✳
atovaquone ✳	

✳ See Part 4

ANTIFUNGAL DRUGS

We are continually exposed to fungi – in the air we breathe, the food we eat, and the water we drink. Fortunately, most of them cannot live in the body, and few are harmful. But some can grow in the mouth, skin, hair, or nails, causing irritating or unsightly changes, and a few can cause serious and possibly fatal disease. The most common fungal infections are caused by the tinea group. These include tinea pedis (athlete's foot), tinea cruris (jock itch), tinea corporis (ringworm), and tinea capitis (scalp ringworm). Caused by a variety of organisms, they are spread by direct or indirect contact with infected humans or animals. Infection is encouraged by warm, moist conditions.

Problems may also result from the proliferation of a fungus normally present in the body; the most common example is excessive growth of *Candida*, a yeast that causes thrush infection of the mouth, vagina, and bowel. It can also infect other organs if it spreads through the body via the bloodstream. Overgrowth of *Candida* may occur in people taking antibiotics (p.114) or oral contraceptives (p.149), in pregnant women, or in those with diabetes or immune system disorders such as AIDS.

Superficial fungal infections – those that attack only the outer layer of the skin and mucous membranes – are relatively common and, although irritating, do not usually present a threat to general health. Internal fungal infections – for example, of the lungs, heart, or other organs – are rare, but may be serious and prolonged.

As antibiotics and other antibacterial drugs have no effect on fungi and yeasts, a different type of drug is needed. Drugs for fungal infections are either applied *topically* to treat minor infections of the skin, nails, and mucous membranes, or they are given by mouth or injection to eliminate serious fungal infections of the internal organs and nails.

Why they are used

Drug treatment is necessary for most fungal infections since they rarely improve alone. Measures such as careful washing and drying of affected areas may help but are not a substitute for antifungal drugs. The use of over-the-counter preparations to increase the acidity of the vagina is not usually effective.

Fungal infections of the skin and scalp are usually treated with a cream or shampoo. Drugs for vaginal thrush are most commonly applied in the form of vaginal suppositories or cream applied with a special applicator. For very severe or persistent vaginal infections, fluconazole or itraconazole may be given as a short course by mouth. Mouth infections are usually eliminated by lozenges dissolved in the mouth or an antifungal solution or gel applied to the affected areas. When *Candida* infects the bowel, an antifungal drug that is not absorbed into the bloodstream, such as nystatin, is given in tablet form. For severe or persistent infections of the nails, either griseofulvin or terbinafine are given by mouth until the infected nails have grown out.

In the rare cases of fungal infections affecting internal organs, such as the blood, the heart, or the brain, potent drugs such as fluconazole and itraconazole are given by mouth, or amphotericin and flucytosine are given by injection. These drugs pass into the bloodstream to fight the fungi.

ACTIONS OF ANTIFUNGAL DRUGS

Stage one
The drug acts on the wall of the fungal cell.

Stage two
The drug damages the cell wall and the cell contents leak out. The cell dies.

How they work

Most antifungals alter the permeability of the fungal cell's walls. Chemicals needed for cell life leak out and the fungal cell dies.

How they affect you

The speed with which antifungal drugs provide benefit varies with the type of infection. Most fungal or yeast infections of the skin, mouth, and vagina improve within a week. The condition of nails affected by fungal infections improves only when new nail growth occurs, which takes months. *Systemic* infections of the internal organs can take weeks to cure.

Antifungal drugs applied topically rarely cause side effects, although they may irritate the skin. However, treatment by mouth or injection for systemic and nail infections may produce more serious side effects. Amphotericin, injected in cases of life-threatening, systemic infections, can cause potentially dangerous effects, including kidney damage.

CHOICE OF ANTIFUNGAL DRUG

The table below shows the range of uses for some antifungal drugs. The particular drug chosen in each case depends on the precise nature and site of the infection. The usual route of administration for each drug is also indicated.

Drug	Infection									Administration		
---	Esophageal thrush	Cryptococcal meningitis	Skin ringworm	Scalp ringworm	Nail infection	Mouth thrush	Vaginal thrush	Candida of the skin	Systemic candida	Topical	Injection	Oral
Amphotericin B	●	●			●	●	●		●	●	●	●
Ciclopirox				●						●		
Clotrimazole			●	●		●	●	●		●		
Fluconazole	●	●					●	●			●	●
Flucytosine	●	●						●			●	●
Griseofulvin			●	●	●							●
Ketoconazole	●		●	●			●	●	●	●		●
Miconazole							●	●		●		●
Nystatin						●	●			●		●
Terbinafine			●	●	●							●

COMMON DRUGS

Amphotericin B ✳ Miconazole ✳
Caspofungin Nystatin ✳
Ciclopirox Posaconazole
Clotrimazole ✳ Terbinafine ✳
Econazole Terconazole
Fluconazole ✳ Tolnaftate
Flucytosine Voriconazole
Griseofulvin
Itraconazole
Ketoconazole ✳
Micafungin

| ✳ See Part 4 |

ANTHELMINTIC DRUGS

Anthelmintics are drugs that are used to eliminate the many types of worm (helminths) that can enter the body and live there as parasites, producing a general weakness in some cases and serious harm in others. The body may be host to many different worms (see Choice of drug, below). Most species spend part of their life cycle in another animal, and the infestation is often passed on to humans in food contaminated with the eggs or larvae. In some cases, such as hookworm, larvae enter the body through the skin. Larvae or adults may attach themselves to the intestinal wall and feed on the bowel contents; others feed off the intestinal blood supply, causing *anemia*. Worms can also infest the bloodstream or lodge in the muscles or internal organs.

Many people have worms at some time during their life, especially during childhood; most can be effectively eliminated with anthelmintic drugs.

Why they are used

Most common worms cause only mild symptoms and usually do not pose a serious threat to general health. Anthelmintic drugs are usually necessary, however, because the body's natural defences against infection are not effective against most worm infestations. Certain types of infestation must always be treated since they can cause serious complications. In some cases, such as threadworm infestation, physicians may recommend anthelmintic treatment for the whole family to prevent reinfection. If worms have invaded tissues and formed cysts, they may have to be removed surgically. Laxatives are given with some anthelmintics to hasten expulsion of worms from the bowel. Other drugs may be prescribed to ease symptoms or to compensate for any blood loss or nutritional deficiency.

How they work

The anthelmintic drugs act in several ways. Many of them kill or paralyse the worms, which pass out of the body in the faeces. Others, which act *systemically*, are used to treat infection in the tissues.

Many anthelmintics are specific for particular worms, and the physician must identify the nature of the infection before selecting the most appropriate treatment (see Choice of drug, below). Most of the common intestinal infestations are easily treated, often with only one or two doses of the drug. However, tissue infections may require more prolonged treatment.

How they affect you

Once the drug has eliminated the worms, symptoms caused by infestation rapidly disappear. Taken as a single dose or a short course, anthelmintics do not usually produce side effects. However, treatment can disturb the digestive system, causing abdominal pain, nausea, and vomiting.

COMMON DRUGS

Mebendazole
Piperazine
Praziquantel

CHOICE OF DRUG

Threadworm (*enterobiasis*)
A common worm infection, particularly among young children. The worm lives in the intestine, but it travels to the anus at night to lay eggs. This causes itching; scratching leaves eggs on the fingers, usually under the fingernails. These eggs are transferred to the mouth, often by sucking the fingers or eating food with unwashed hands. Keeping nails short and good hygiene, including washing the hands after using the toilet and before each meal, and an early morning bath to remove the eggs, are all important elements in the eradication of infection.
Drugs Mebendazole, piperazine. All members of the family should be treated simultaneously.

Common roundworm (*ascariasis*)
The most common worm infection worldwide. Transmitted to humans in contaminated raw food or in soil. Infects the intestine. The worms are large and dense clusters of them can block the intestine.
Drugs Levamisole, mebendazole, piperazine

Tropical threadworm (*strongyloidiasis*)
Occurs in the tropics and southern Europe. Larvae from contaminated soil penetrate skin, pass into the lungs, and are swallowed into the gut.
Drugs Albendazole, ivermectin

Whipworm (*trichuriasis*)
Mainly occurs in tropical areas as a result of eating contaminated raw vegetables. Worms infest the intestines.
Drug Mebendazole

Hookworm (*uncinariasis*)
Mainly found in tropical areas. Worm larvae penetrate skin and pass via the lymphatic system and bloodstream to the lungs. They then travel up the airways, are swallowed, and attach themselves to the intestinal wall, where they feed off the intestinal blood supply.
Drug Mebendazole

Pork roundworm (*trichinosis*)
Transmitted in infected undercooked pork. Initially worms lodge in the intestines, but larvae may invade muscle to form cysts that are often resistant to drug treatment and may require surgery.
Drug Mebendazole

Toxocariasis (*visceral larva migrans*)
Usually occurs as a result of eating soil or eating with fingers contaminated with dog or cat feces. Eggs hatch in the intestine and may travel to the lungs, liver, kidney, brain, and eyes. Treatment is not always effective.
Drug Mebendazole

Creeping eruption (*cutaneous larva migrans*)
Mainly occurs in tropical areas and coastal areas of southeastern United States as a result of skin contact with larvae from cat and dog feces. Infestation is usually confined to the skin.
Drug Ivermectin

Filariasis (including onchocerciasis and loiasis)
Tropical areas only. Infection by this group of worms is spread by bites of insects that are carriers of worm larvae or eggs. May affect the lymphatic system, blood, eyes, and skin.
Drug Ivermectin

Flukes
Sheep liver fluke (*fascioliasis*) is indigenous to the United Kingdom. Infestation usually results from eating watercress grown in contaminated water. Mainly affects the liver and biliary tract. Flukes found in other countries may infect the lungs, intestines, or blood.
Drug Praziquantel

Tapeworms (including beef, pork, fish, and dwarf tapeworms)
Depending on the type may be carried by cattle, pigs, or fish and transmitted to humans in undercooked meat. Most types affect the intestines. Larvae of the pork tapeworm may form cysts in muscle and other tissues.
Drug Praziquantel

Hydatid disease (*echinococciasis*)
Eggs are transmitted in dog faeces. Larvae may form cysts over many years, commonly in the liver. Surgery is the usual treatment for cysts.
Drug Albendazole

Bilharzia (*schistosomiasis*)
Occurs in polluted water in tropical areas. Larvae may be swallowed or penetrate the skin; they migrate to the liver: adult worms live in the bladder.
Drug Praziquantel

Some drugs may not be readily available; check with your physician.

HORMONES AND ENDOCRINE SYSTEM

The endocrine system is a collection of glands located throughout the body that produce *hormones* and release them into the bloodstream. Each endocrine gland produces one or more hormones, each of which governs a particular body function, including growth and repair of tissues, sexual development and reproductive function, and the body's response to stress.

Most hormones are released continuously from birth, but the amount produced fluctuates with the body's needs. Others are produced mainly at certain times – for example, growth hormone is released mainly during childhood and adolescence. Sex hormones are produced by the testes and ovaries from puberty onwards (see p.146).

Many endocrine glands release their hormones in response to triggering hormones produced by the pituitary gland. The pituitary releases a variety of pituitary hormones, each of which, in turn, stimulates the appropriate endocrine gland to produce its hormone.

A "feedback" system usually regulates blood hormone levels: if the blood level rises too high, the pituitary responds by reducing the amount of stimulating hormone produced, thereby allowing the blood hormone level to return to normal.

What can go wrong

Endocrine disorders, usually resulting in too much or too little of a particular hormone, have a variety of causes. Some are congenital in origin; others may be caused by autoimmune disease (including some forms of diabetes mellitus), malignant or benign tumours, injury, or certain drugs.

Why drugs are used

Natural hormone preparations or their synthetic versions are often prescribed to treat deficiency. Sometimes drugs are given to stimulate increased hormone production in the endocrine gland, such as oral antidiabetic drugs, which act on the insulin-producing cells of the pancreas. When too much hormone is produced, drug treatment may reduce the activity of the gland.

Hormones or related drugs are also used to treat certain other conditions. Corticosteroids related to adrenal hormones are prescribed to relieve inflammation and to suppress immune system activity (see p.143). Several types of cancer are treated with sex hormones (see p.140). Female sex hormones are used as contraceptives (see p.149) and to treat menstrual disorders (see p.148).

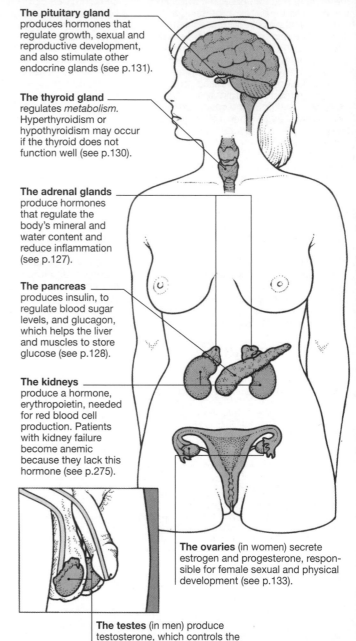

The pituitary gland produces hormones that regulate growth, sexual and reproductive development, and also stimulate other endocrine glands (see p.131).

The thyroid gland regulates *metabolism*. Hyperthyroidism or hypothyroidism may occur if the thyroid does not function well (see p.130).

The adrenal glands produce hormones that regulate the body's mineral and water content and reduce inflammation (see p.127).

The pancreas produces insulin, to regulate blood sugar levels, and glucagon, which helps the liver and muscles to store glucose (see p.128).

The kidneys produce a hormone, erythropoietin, needed for red blood cell production. Patients with kidney failure become anemic because they lack this hormone (see p.275).

The ovaries (in women) secrete estrogen and progesterone, responsible for female sexual and physical development (see p.133).

The testes (in men) produce testosterone, which controls the development of male sexual and physical characteristics (see p.132).

MAJOR DRUG GROUPS

Corticosteroids
Drugs used in diabetes
Drugs for thyroid disorders
Drugs for pituitary disorders
Male sex hormones
Female sex hormones

CORTICOSTEROIDS

Corticosteroid drugs – often referred to simply as steroids – are derived from, or are synthetic variants of, the natural corticosteroid *hormones* formed in the outer part (cortex) of the adrenal glands, situated on top of each kidney. Release of these hormones is governed by the pituitary gland (see p.131).

Corticosteroids may have either mainly glucocorticoid or mainly mineralocorticoid effects. Glucocorticoid effects include the maintenance of normal levels of sugar in the blood and the promotion of recovery from injury and stress. Main mineralocorticoid effects are the regulation of the balance of mineral salts and the water content of the body. When present in large amounts, they reduce inflammation and suppress allergic reactions and immune activity. They are distinct from another group of steroid hormones, the anabolic steroids (see p.132). Although corticosteroids have broadly similar actions to each other, they vary in their relative strength and duration of action. The mineralocorticoid effects of these drugs also vary in strength.

ADVERSE EFFECTS OF CORTICOSTEROIDS

Corticosteroids are effective and useful drugs that often provide benefit in cases where other drugs are ineffective. However, long-term use of high doses can lead to a variety of unwanted effects on the body, as shown below.

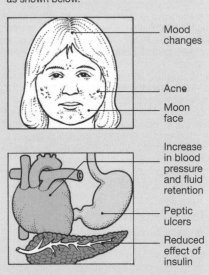

Mood changes

Acne

Moon face

Increase in blood pressure and fluid retention

Peptic ulcers

Reduced effect of insulin

Fat pad on back

Muscle wasting

Osteo-porosis

Easy bruising

Why they are used

Corticosteroid drugs are used primarily for their effect in controlling inflammation, whatever its cause. Topical preparations containing corticosteroids are often used for the treatment of many inflammatory skin disorders (see p.162). These drugs may also be injected directly into a joint or around a tendon to relieve inflammation caused by injury or disease (see p.104). However, when local administration of the drug is either not possible or not effective, corticosteroids may be given systemically, either by mouth or by intravenous injection.

Corticosteroids are commonly part of the treatment of many disorders in which inflammation is thought to be caused by excessive or inappropriate activity of the immune system. These disorders include inflammatory bowel disease (p.98), rheumatoid arthritis (p.103), glomerulonephritis (a kidney disease), and some rare connective tissue disorders, such as systemic lupus erythematosus. In these conditions corticosteroids relieve symptoms and may also temporarily halt the disease.

Corticosteroids may be given regularly by mouth or inhaler to treat asthma, although they are not effective for the relief of asthma attacks in progress (see Bronchodilators, p.76 and Drugs for asthma, p.78).

An important use of oral corticosteroids is to replace the natural hormones that are deficient when adrenal gland function is reduced, as in Addison's disease. In these cases, the drugs most closely resembling the actions of the natural hormones are selected and a combination of these may be used.

Some cancers of the lymphatic system (lymphomas) and the blood (leukemias) may also respond to corticosteroid treatment. These drugs are also widely used to prevent or treat rejection of organ transplants, usually in conjunction with other drugs, such azathioprine (see Immunosuppressants, p.143).

How they work

Given in high doses, corticosteroid drugs reduce inflammation by blocking the action of chemicals called prostaglandins that are responsible for triggering the inflammatory response. These drugs also temporarily suppress the immune system by reducing the activity of certain types of white blood cells.

How they affect you

Corticosteroid drugs often produce a dramatic improvement in symptoms. Given systemically, corticosteroids may also act on the brain to produce a heightened sense of well-being and, in some people, a sense of euphoria. Troublesome day-to-day side effects are rare. Long-term corticosteroid treatment, however, carries a number of serious risks for the patient.

Risks and special precautions

In the treatment of Addison's disease, corticosteroids can be considered as "hormone replacement therapy", with drugs replacing the natural hormone hydrocortisone. Because replacement doses are given, the adverse effects of high-dose corticosteroids do not occur.

Drugs with strong mineralocorticoid effects, such as fludrocortisone, may cause water retention, swelling (especially of the ankles), and an increase in blood pressure. Because corticosteroids reduce the effect of insulin, they may create problems in diabetics, and may even give rise to diabetes in susceptible individuals. They also increase the risk of peptic ulcers, especially when given concurrently with non-steroidal anti-inflammatory drugs (NSAIDs).

Because corticosteroids suppress the immune system, they increase susceptibility to infection. They also suppress symptoms of infectious disease. People who are taking corticosteroids should avoid exposure to chickenpox or shingles, but if they catch either disease, acyclovir tablets may be prescribed. With long-term use, corticosteroids may cause a variety of adverse effects (see left). Physicians try to avoid long-term use of corticosteroids drugs to children because prolonged use may retard growth.

Long-term use of corticosteroids suppresses the production of the body's own corticosteroid hormones. For this reason, treatment that lasts for more than a few weeks should be withdrawn gradually to give the body time to adjust. If the drug is stopped abruptly, the lack of corticosteroid hormones may lead to sudden collapse.

People taking corticosteroids by mouth for longer than one month are advised to carry a warning card. If someone who is taking steroids long-term has an accident or serious illness, his or her defences against shock may need to be quickly strengthened with extra hydrocortisone, administered intravenously.

COMMON DRUGS

Beclomethasone *	Flunisolide
Betamethasone *	Fluocinolone
Budesonide *	Fluocinonide
Clobetasol *	Fluticasone *
Clobetasone	Halcinonide
Cortisone	Halobetasol
Desonide	Hydrocortisone *
Desoximetasone	Methyl-
Dexamethasone *	prednisolone *
Diflucortolone	Mometasone *
Fludrocortisone	Prednisolone/
Flumethasone	prednisone *
	Triamcinolone

* See Part 4

DRUGS USED IN DIABETES

The body obtains most of its energy from glucose, a simple form of sugar made in the intestine from the breakdown of starch and other sugars. Insulin, one of the hormones produced in the pancreas, enables body tissues to take up glucose from the blood, either to use it for energy or to store it. In diabetes mellitus, insulin production is defective. This results in reduced uptake of glucose by the tissues and thus the glucose level in the blood rises abnormally. A high blood glucose level is medically known as hyperglycemia.

There are two main types of diabetes mellitus. Type 1 diabetes usually appears in young people, 50 per cent of cases occurring around the time of puberty. The insulin-secreting cells in the pancreas are gradually destroyed. An autoimmune condition (where the body recognizes its pancreas as "foreign" and tries to eliminate it) or a childhood viral infection is the most likely cause. Although the decline in insulin production is slow, the condition often appears suddenly, brought on by periods of stress (for example, infection or puberty) when the body's insulin requirements are high. Symptoms of Type 1 diabetes include extreme thirst, increased urination, lethargy, and weight loss. This type of diabetes is fatal if it is left untreated.

In Type 1 diabetes, insulin treatment is the only treatment option. It has to be continued for life. Several types of insulin are available, which are broadly classified by their duration of action (short-, medium-, and long-acting).

Type 2 or maturity-onset diabetes, appears at an older age (usually over 40) and tends to come on much more gradually – there may be a delay in its diagnosis for several years because of the gradual onset of symptoms. In this type of diabetes, the levels of insulin in the blood are usually high initially. However, the cells of the body are resistant to the effects of insulin and have a reduced glucose uptake despite the high insulin levels. This results in hyperglycemia. Obesity is the most common cause of Type 2 diabetes.

ADMINISTRATION OF INSULIN

The non-diabetic body produces a background level of insulin, with additional insulin being produced as required during meals. The insulin delivery systems that are currently available cannot mimic this precisely. In people with Type 1 diabetes, short-acting insulin is usually given before meals, and a medium-acting insulin is given either before the evening meal or at bedtime. Insulin pen injectors are particularly useful for administration during the day because they are discreet and easy to carry and use. In patients with Type 2 diabetes who require insulin, a mixture of short- and medium-acting insulin may be given twice a day. Special pumps that deliver continuous subcutaneous insulin appear to have no advantage over multiple subcutaneous injections. Some new types of insulins called "insulin analogues" (e.g. Insulin lispro) may be better at mimicking the insulin-producing behaviour of the normal pancreas.

Duration of action of types of insulin

— Short-acting insulin   — Medium-acting insulin   — Long-acting insulin

Effective range

Hours   5   10   15   20   25   30   35   40

In both types of diabetes, an alteration in diet is vital. A healthy diet consisting of a low-fat, high-fibre, low simple sugar (cakes, sweets) and high complex sugar (pasta, rice, potatoes) intake is advised. In Type 2 diabetes, a reduction in weight alone may be sufficient to lower the body's energy requirements and restore blood glucose to normal levels. If an alteration in diet fails, oral antidiabetic drugs, such as metformin, acarbose, or sulfonylureas, are prescribed. Insulin may need to be given to people with Type 2 diabetes if the above treatments fail, or in pregnancy, during severe illness, and before the patient undergoes any surgery requiring a general anesthetic.

Importance of treating diabetes

If diabetes is left untreated, the continuous high blood glucose levels damage various parts of the body. The major problems are caused by the build-up of atherosclerosis in arteries, which narrows the vessels, reducing the flow of blood. This can result in heart attacks, blindness, kidney failure, reduced circulation in the legs, and even gangrene. The risk of these conditions is greatly reduced with treatment. Careful control of diabetes in young people, during puberty and afterwards, is of great importance in reducing possible long-term complications. Good diabetic control before conception reduces the chance of miscarriage or abnormalities in the baby.

How antidiabetic drugs work

Insulin treatment directly replaces the natural hormone that is deficient in diabetes mellitus. Animal-sourced (commonly pork) and biosynthetic human insulins are available, with more patients using the human insulins. Human and porkinsulins are the most widely available. When transferring between animal and human insulin, alteration of the dose may be required.

Insulin cannot be given by mouth because it is broken down in the digestive tract before it reaches the bloodstream. Regular injections are therefore necessary (see Administration of insulin, above).

ACTION OF SULFONYLUREA DRUGS

Insulin

Islet cell

Before drug treatment
In Type 2 diabetes, the islet cells of the pancreas secrete insufficient insulin to meet the body's needs.

Drug

After drug treatment
The drug stimulates the islet cells to release increased amounts of insulin.

Sulfonylurea oral antidiabetic drugs encourage the pancreas to produce insulin. They are therefore effective only when some insulin-secreting cells remain active, and this is why they are ineffective in the treatment of Type 1 diabetes. Metformin alters the way in which the body *metabolizes* sugar. Acarbose slows digestion of starch and sugar. Both slow the increase in blood sugar that occurs after a meal. Nateglinide and repaglinide stimulate insulin release. Pioglitazone and rosiglitazone reduce the body's resistance to insulin.

Insulin treatment and you

The insulin requirements in diabetes vary greatly between individuals and also depend on physical activity and calorie intake. Hence, insulin regimens are tailored to each person's particular needs, and the diabetic is encouraged to take an active role in his or her own management.

A regular record of home blood glucose monitoring should be kept. This is the basis on which insulin doses are adjusted, preferably by diabetics themselves.

A person with diabetes should learn to recognize the warning signs of hypoglycemia or low blood sugar. A hypoglycemic event may be induced by giving insulin under medical supervision. The symptoms of sweating, faintness, or palpitations are produced but disappear with the administration of glucose, so a diabetic should always carry glucose tablets or sweets. Recurrent "hypos" at specific times of the day or night may

require a reduction of insulin dose. Rarely, undetected low glucose levels may lead to coma. The injection of glucagon (a substance that raises blood glucose) rapidly reverses this. A relative may be instructed how to perform this procedure.

Repeated injection at the same site may disturb the fat layer beneath the skin, producing either swelling or dimpling. This alters the rate of insulin absorption and can be avoided by regularly rotating injection sites.

Insulin requirements are increased during illness and pregnancy. During an illness, the urine should be checked for ketones, which are produced when there is insufficient insulin to permit the normal uptake of glucose by the tissues. If high ketone levels occur in a diabetic's urine during an illness, urgent medical advice should be sought. The combination of high blood sugars, high urinary ketones, and vomiting is a diabetic emergency and the person should be taken to an Emergency department without delay.

Exercise increases the body's need for glucose, and therefore extra calories should be taken prior to exertion. The effects of vigorous exercise on blood sugar levels may last up to 18 hours, and the subsequent (post-exercise) doses of insulin may need to be reduced by 10–25 per cent to avoid hypoglycemia.

It is advisable for diabetics to carry a card or bracelet detailing their condition and treatment. This may be useful in a medical emergency.

SITES OF INJECTION

The shaded areas indicate suitable sites for the injection of insulin.

Antidiabetic drugs and you

The sulfonylureas may lower the blood glucose too much, causing a condition called hypoglycemia. This condition can be avoided by starting treatment with low doses of these drugs and ensuring that food intake is regular. Rarely, these drugs cause a decrease in the blood cell count, a rash, or intestinal or liver disturbances. Interactions may occur with other drugs, so your physician should be informed of your treatment before prescribing any medicines for you.

Unlike the sulfonylureas, metformin does not cause hypoglycemia. Its most common side effects are nausea, weight loss, abdominal distension, and diarrhea. Metformin should not be used in people with liver, kidney, or heart problems. Acarbose does not cause hypoglycemia if used on its own. However, the tablets must be taken with the first mouthful of food at mealtimes.

COMMON DRUGS

Sulfonylurea drugs	Insulins cont.
Chlorpropamide	Lente (pork)
Gliclazide ✳	Lispro
Glimepiride ✳	NPH
Glyburide ✳	bio
Tolbutamide	
Antiobesity agent	
Orlistat ✳	
Other drugs	
Acarbose ✳	
Glucagon	
Insulins	
As	

MONITORING BLOOD GLUCOSE

Diabetics need to check either their blood or urine glucose level at home. Blood tests give the most accurate results and are usually recommended.

There are a variety of devices that can measure blood glucose to help monitor diabetes. These meters, called glucometers, measure the blood sugar level in a drop of blood obtained from a finger prick.

Glucometers can be purchased at most pharmacies. If you have diabetes, ask your diabetes educator, physician, or pharmacist which meter would be best for you. You should also ask for training on how to use the chosen meter properly. Your physician may be able to recommend a Diabetes Education Centre, which can provide support and training.

1 Prick your finger to give a large drop of blood.

2 Touch the blood on to the test pads of the testing strip.

3 Within 120 seconds insert the strip into the meter. Your reading (e.g. 6.8) will appear after 120 seconds.

DRUGS FOR THYROID DISORDERS

The thyroid gland produces the *hormone* thyroxine, which regulates the body's *metabolism*. During childhood, thyroxine is essential for normal physical and mental development. Calcitonin, also produced by the thyroid, regulates calcium metabolism and is used as a drug for certain bone disorders (p.108).

Hyperthyroidism

In this condition (often called thyrotoxicosis), the thyroid is overactive and produces too much thyroxine. Women are more commonly affected than men.

ACTION OF DRUGS FOR THYROID DISORDERS

Thyroid hormone production
Iodine combines with other chemicals (precursors) in the thyroid gland to make thyroid hormones.

Iodine

Thyroid precursor

Thyroid hormone

Thyroid hormone

Normal output of thyroid hormones
Thyroid output is normally regulated according to the body's needs.

After drug

Drug

Before drug

Action of antithyroid drugs
In hyperthyroidism, antithyroid drugs partly reduce the production of thyroid hormones by preventing iodine from combining with thyroid precursors in the thyroid gland.

Before drug **After drug**

Synthetic thyroid hormone

Action of thyroid hormones
In hypothyroidism, when the thyroid gland is underactive, supplements of synthetic thyroid hormones restore normal.

Symptoms include anxiety, palpitations, weight loss, increased appetite, heat intolerance, diarrhea, and menstrual disturbances. Graves' disease is the most common form of hyperthyroidism. It is an autoimmune disease in which the body produces antibodies that stimulate the thyroid to produce excess thyroxine. Patients with Graves' disease may develop abnormally protuberant eyes (exophthalmos) or a swelling involving the skin over the shins (pretibial myxedema). Hyperthyroidism can be caused by a benign single tumour of the thyroid or a pre-existing multinodular goitre. Rarely, an overactive thyroid may follow a viral infection, a condition called thyroiditis. Inflammation of the gland leads to the release of stored thyroxine.

Management of hyperthyroidism

There are three possible treatments for hyperthyroidism: antithyroid drugs, radioactive iodine, and surgery. The most commonly used antithyroid drug is methimazole. This drug inhibits the formation of thyroid hormones and reduces their levels to normal over a period of about 4–8 weeks. In the early stage of treatment a beta blocker (p.83) may be prescribed to control symptoms. This should be stopped once thyroid function returns to normal. Long-term methimazole is usually given for 18 months to prevent relapse. A "block and replace" regimen may also be used. In this treatment, the thyroid gland is blocked by high doses of methimazole and thyroxine is added when the level of thyroid hormone in the blood falls below normal.

Methimazole may produce minor side effects such as nausea, vomiting, skin rashes, or headaches. Rarely, the drug may reduce the white blood cell count. Propylthiouracil may be used as an alternative antithyroid drug.

Radioactive iodine is frequently chosen as a first-line therapy, especially in the elderly, and is the second choice if hyperthyroidism recurs following use of methimazole. It acts by destroying thyroid tissue. Hypothyroidism occurs in up to 80 per cent of people within 20 years after treatment. Long-term studies show radioactive iodine to be safe, but its use should be avoided during pregnancy.

Surgery is a third-line therapy. Its use may be favoured for patients with a large goitre, particularly if it causes difficulty in swallowing or breathing. Exophthalmos may require corticosteroids (p.127) as it does not respond to other treatments.

Hypothyroidism

This is a condition resulting from too little thyroxine. Sometimes it may be caused by an autoimmune disorder, in which the body's immune system attacks the

---

TREATMENT FOR GOITRE

A goitre is a swelling of the thyroid gland. It may occur only temporarily, during puberty or pregnancy, or it may be due to an abnormal growth of thyroid tissue that requires surgical removal. It may rarely be brought about by iodine deficiency. This last cause is treated with iodine supplements (see also p.473).

Goitre

Normal size of thyroid gland

thyroid gland. Other cases may follow treatment for hyperthyroidism. In newborn babies, hypothyroidism may be the result of an inborn *enzyme* disorder. In the past, it also arose from a deficiency of iodine in the diet.

The symptoms of adult hypothyroidism develop slowly and include weight gain, mental slowness, dry skin, hair loss, increased sensitivity to cold, and heavy menstrual periods. In babies, low levels of thyroxine cause permanent mental and physical retardation and, for this reason, babies are tested for hypothyroidism within a week of birth.

Management of hypothyroidism

Lifelong oral treatment with synthetic thyroid hormones (thyroxine (levothyroxine), or liothyronine) is the only option. Blood tests are performed regularly to monitor the treatment and permit dosage adjustments. In the elderly, as well as people with heart disease, gradual introduction of thyroxine is used to prevent heart strain.

In severely ill patients, thyroid hormone may be given by injection. This method of administration may also be used to treat newborn infants with low levels of thyroxine.

Symptoms of thyrotoxicosis may appear if excess thyroxine replacement is given. Otherwise, no adverse events occur since treatment is adjusted to replace the natural hormone that the body should produce itself.

COMMON DRUGS

Drugs for hypothyroidism	Drugs for hyperthyroidism
Liothyronine	Iodine ✱
Levothyroxine (thyroxine) ✱	Methimazole ✱
	Metopolol ✱
	Propranolol ✱
	Propylthiouracil ✱
	Radioactive iodine

✱ See Part 4

DRUGS FOR PITUITARY DISORDERS

The pituitary gland, which lies at the base of the brain, produces a number of *hormones* that regulate physical growth, *metabolism*, sexual development, and reproductive function. Many of these hormones act indirectly by stimulating other glands, such as the thyroid, adrenal glands, ovaries, and testes, to release their own hormones. A summary of the actions and effects of each pituitary hormone is given below.

An excess or a lack of one of the pituitary hormones may produce serious effects, the nature of which depends on the hormone involved. Abnormal levels of a particular hormone may be caused by a pituitary tumour, which may be treated surgically, with radiotherapy, or with drugs. In other cases, drugs may be used to correct the hormonal imbalance.

The more common pituitary disorders that can be treated with drugs are those involving growth hormone, antidiuretic hormone, prolactin, adrenal hormones, and the gonadotrophins. The first three are discussed below. For information on the use of drugs to treat infertility arising from inadequate levels of gonadotrophins, see p.152. Lack of corticotrophin, leading to inadequate production of adrenal hormones, is usually treated with corticosteroids (see p.127).

Drugs for growth hormone disorders

Growth hormone (somatotropin) is the principal hormone required for normal growth in childhood and adolescence.

Lack of growth hormone impairs normal physical growth. Physicians administer hormone treatment only after tests have proven that a lack of this hormone is the cause of the disorder. If treatment is started at an early age, regular injections of somatropin, a synthetic form of natural growth hormone, administered until the end of adolescence usually allow normal growth and development to take place.

Less often, the pituitary produces an excess of growth hormone. In children this can result in pituitary gigantism; in adults, it can produce a disorder known as acromegaly. This disorder, which is usually the result of a pituitary tumour, is characterized by thickening of the skull, face, hands, and feet, and enlargement of some internal organs.

The pituitary tumour may either be surgically removed or destroyed by radiotherapy. In the frail or elderly, drugs such as bromocriptine and octreotide are used to reduce growth hormone levels. Octreotide is also used as an adjunctive treatment before surgery and in those with increased growth hormone levels occurring after surgery. People who have undergone surgery and/or radiotherapy may require long-term replacement with other hormones (such as sex hormones, thyroid hormone, or corticosteroids).

Drugs for diabetes insipidus

Antidiuretic hormone (also known as ADH or vasopressin) acts on the kidneys, controlling the amount of water retained in the body and returned to the blood.

A lack of ADH is usually caused by damage to the pituitary, and this in turn causes diabetes insipidus. In this rare condition, the kidneys cannot retain water and large quantities pass into the urine. The chief symptoms of diabetes insipidus are constant thirst and the production of large volumes of urine.

Diabetes insipidus is treated with ADH or a related synthetic drug, desmopressin. These replace naturally produced ADH and may be given by injection or in the form of a nasal spray. Chlorpropamide may be used to treat mild cases; it works by increasing ADH release from the pituitary and by sensitizing the kidneys to the effect of ADH.

Alternatively, a thiazide diuretic (such as chlorthalidone) may be prescribed for mild cases (see Diuretics, p.85). The usual effect of such drugs is to increase urine production, but in diabetes insipidus they have the opposite effect, reducing water loss from the body.

Drugs used to reduce prolactin levels

Prolactin, also called lactogenic hormone, is produced in both men and women. In women, prolactin controls the secretion of breast milk following childbirth. The function of this hormone in men is not understood, although it appears to be necessary for normal sperm production.

The disorders associated with prolactin are all concerned with overproduction. High levels of prolactin in women can cause lactation that is unassociated with pregnancy and birth (galactorrhea), lack of menstruation (amenorrhea), and infertility. If excessive amounts are produced in men, the result may be galactorrhea, impotence, or infertility.

Some drugs, notably methyldopa, estrogen, and the phenothiazine antipsychotics, can raise the prolactin level in the blood. More often, however, the increased prolactin results from a pituitary tumour and is usually treated with bromocriptine or cabergoline. These drugs inhibit prolactin production.

THE EFFECTS OF PITUITARY HORMONES

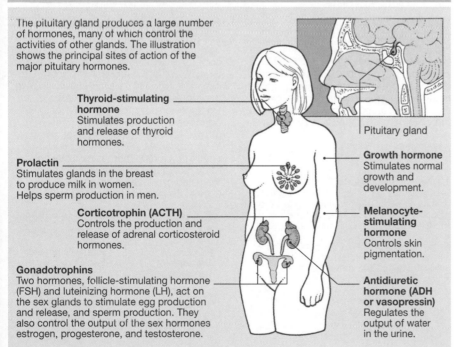

The pituitary gland produces a large number of hormones, many of which control the activities of other glands. The illustration shows the principal sites of action of the major pituitary hormones.

Thyroid-stimulating hormone
Stimulates production and release of thyroid hormones.

Prolactin
Stimulates glands in the breast to produce milk in women. Helps sperm production in men.

Corticotrophin (ACTH)
Controls the production and release of adrenal corticosteroid hormones.

Gonadotrophins
Two hormones, follicle-stimulating hormone (FSH) and luteinizing hormone (LH), act on the sex glands to stimulate egg production and release, and sperm production. They also control the output of the sex hormones estrogen, progesterone, and testosterone.

Pituitary gland

Growth hormone
Stimulates normal growth and development.

Melanocyte-stimulating hormone
Controls skin pigmentation.

Antidiuretic hormone (ADH or vasopressin)
Regulates the output of water in the urine.

COMMON DRUGS

Drugs for growth hormone disorders
Bromocriptine ✳
Octreotide
Somatostatin
Somatropin

Drugs for diabetes insipidus
Carbamazepine ✳
Chlorpropamide
Chlorthalidone
Desmopressin ✳
Vasopressin (ADH)

Drugs to reduce prolactin levels
Bromocriptine ✳
Cabergoline

✳ See Part 4

MALE SEX HORMONES

Male sex hormones – androgens – are responsible for the development of male sexual characteristics. The principal androgen is testosterone, which in men is produced by the testes from puberty onwards. Women produce testosterone in small amounts in the adrenal glands, but its exact function in the female body is not known.

Testosterone has two major effects: an androgenic effect and an anabolic effect. Its androgenic effect is to stimulate the appearance of the secondary sexual characteristics at puberty, such as the growth of body hair, deepening of the voice, and an increase in genital size. Its anabolic effects are to increase muscle bulk and accelerate growth rate.

There are a number of synthetically produced derivatives of testosterone that produce varying degrees of the androgenic and anabolic effects mentioned above. Derivatives that have a mainly anabolic effect are known as anabolic steroids (see box below).

Testosterone and its derivatives have been used under medical supervision in both men and women to treat a number of conditions.

Why they are used

Male sex hormones are mainly given to men to promote the development of male sexual characteristics when hormone production is deficient. This may be the result of an abnormality of the testes or of inadequate production of the pituitary hormones that stimulate the testes to release testosterone.

A course of treatment with male sex hormones is sometimes prescribed for adolescent boys in whom the onset of puberty is delayed by pituitary problems. The treatment may also help to stimulate development of secondary male sexual characteristics and to increase sex drive (libido) in adult men who are producing inadequate testosterone levels. However, this type of hormone treatment has been found to reduce the production of sperm. (For information on the drug treatment of male infertility, see p.152.)

EFFECTS OF MALE SEX HORMONES

Anabolic effects
These are the tissue-building effects of male sex hormones.

Increase in muscle size

Increased muscle bulk
Anabolic hormones promote development of muscles, especially of the upper body.

Pelvis

Growing end of femur

Bone growth
Anabolic hormones increase bone density. They also halt growth of the bone ends.

Androgenic effects
These are the effects of male sex hormones on the development of secondary male sexual characteristics.

Voice changes
Androgenic hormones cause enlargement of the larynx and, thus, deepen the voice.

Facial hair

Larynx

Facial and body hair
Androgenic hormones stimulate hair growth on face and body areas.

Penis

Testis

Genital development
Androgenic hormones stimulate enlargement of the testes and penis.

Androgens may also be prescribed for women to treat certain types of cancer of the breast and uterus (see Anticancer drugs, p.140). Testosterone can be given by injection, capsules, patches, or pellets that are surgically inserted.

How they work

Taken in low doses as part of replacement therapy when natural production is low, male sex hormones act in the same way as the natural hormones. In adolescents suffering from delayed puberty, hormone treatment produces both androgenic and anabolic effects (above), initiating the development of secondary sexual

characteristics over a few months; full sexual development usually takes place over three to four years. When sex hormones are given to adult men, the effects on physical appearance and libido may begin to be felt within a few weeks.

Risks and special precautions

The main risks with these drugs occur when they are given to boys with delayed puberty and to women with breast cancer. Given to initiate the onset of puberty, they may stunt growth by prematurely sealing the growing ends of the long bones. Doctors normally try to avoid prescribing hormones in these circumstances until growth is complete. High doses given to women have various masculinizing effects, including increased facial and body hair, and a deeper voice. The drugs may also produce enlargement of the clitoris, changes in libido, and acne.

ANABOLIC STEROIDS

Anabolic steroids are synthetically produced variants that mimic the anabolic effects of the natural hormones. They increase muscle bulk and body growth.

Doctors occasionally prescribe anabolic steroids and a high-protein diet to promote recovery after serious illness or major surgery. The steroids may also help to increase the production of blood cells in some forms of anemia and to reduce itching in chronic obstructive jaundice.

Anabolic steroids have been widely abused by athletes because these drugs speed up

the recovery of muscles after a session of intense exercise. This enables the athlete to go through a more demanding daily exercise programme, which results in a significant improvement in muscle power. The use of anabolic steroids by athletes to improve their performance is condemned by doctors and athletic organizations because of the risks to health, particularly for women. The side effects range from acne and baldness to fluid retention, reduced fertility in men and women, hardening of the arteries, a long-term risk of liver disease, and certain forms of cancer.

COMMON DRUGS

Primarily androgenic
Testosterone ✳

Primarily anabolic
Nandrolone

Anti-androgens
Cyproterone
Finasteride ✳

✳ See Part 4

FEMALE SEX HORMONES

There are two types of female sex hormones: estrogen and progesterone. In women, these hormones are secreted by the ovaries from puberty until the menopause. Each month, the levels of estrogen and progesterone fluctuate, producing the menstrual cycle (see p.148). During pregnancy, estrogen and progesterone are produced by the placenta. The adrenal gland also makes small amounts of estrogen. Production of estrogen and progesterone is regulated by the two gonadotrophin hormones (FSH and LH) produced by the pituitary gland (see p.131).

Estrogen is responsible for the development of female sexual characteristics, including breast development, growth of pubic hair, and widening of the pelvis. Progesterone prepares the lining of the uterus for implantation of a fertilized egg. This hormone is also important for the maintenance of pregnancy.

Synthetic forms of these hormones are used medically to treat a number of conditions and are known as estrogens and progestins.

Why they are used

The best-known use of estrogens and progestins is in oral contraceptives. These drugs are discussed on p.149. Other uses include the treatment of menstrual disorders (p.148) and certain hormone-sensitive cancers (p.140). This page discusses the drug treatments that are used for natural hormone deficiency.

Hormone deficiency

Deficiency of female sex hormones may occur as a result of deficiency of gonadotrophins caused by a pituitary disorder or by abnormal development of the ovaries (ovarian failure). This may lead to the absence of menstruation and lack of sexual development. If tests show a deficiency of gonadotrophins, preparations of these hormones may be prescribed (see p.152). These trigger the release of estrogen and progesterone from the ovaries. If pituitary function is normal and ovarian failure is diagnosed as the cause of hormone deficiency, estrogens and progestins may be given as supplements. In this situation, these supplements ensure development of normal female sexual characteristics but cannot stimulate ovulation.

Menopause

A decline in levels of estrogen and progesterone occurs naturally after the menopause, when the menstrual cycle ceases. The sudden reduction in levels of estrogen often causes distressing symptoms. Various options are available for the management of these, including hormone replacement therapy (HRT). HRT can also delay some of the long-term consequences of reduced estrogen levels, such as osteoporosis (p.108). A balance between the benefits and risk for individual women must be considered, however, because there can be a slight increase in risk of breast

cancer and thrombosis. It should be used with caution, especially in women with heart disease. When dryness of the vagina is a particular problem, a cream containing an estrogen drug may be prescribed. It is used together with a progestin unless the woman has had a hysterectomy, in which case the estrogen alone is used. Some women with very severe symptoms respond poorly to oral drugs and may be helped by estrogen implants. Hormone replacement therapy may also be prescribed for women who have undergone a premature menopause as a result of surgical removal of the ovaries or radiotherapy for ovarian cancer.

How they affect you

Hormones given to treat ovarian failure or delayed puberty take three to six months to produce a noticeable effect on sexual development. Taken for menopausal symptoms, they can dramatically reduce the number of hot flushes within a week.

Both estrogens and progestins can cause fluid retention, and estrogens may also cause nausea, vomiting, breast tenderness, headache, dizziness, and depression. Progestins may cause "breakthrough" bleeding between menstrual periods. In the comparatively low doses used to treat these disorders, side effects are unlikely.

Risks and special precautions

The use of estrogens and progestins as replacement in ovarian failure carries few risks for otherwise healthy young women. Because estrogens increase the risk of hypertension (raised blood pressure), thrombosis (abnormal blood clotting), and breast cancer, there are risks associated with long-term HRT in older women. Treatment is prescribed with caution for women who have heart or circulatory disorders, and in those who are overweight or smoke. Your physician may order regular breast cancer checks. Estrogens may also trigger the onset of diabetes mellitus or aggravate blood sugar control in diabetic women.

EFFECTS OF HORMONE REPLACEMENT THERAPY (HRT)

Besides alleviating the symptoms of the menopause, such as hot flashes and vaginal dryness, HRT has a beneficial effect in preventing osteoporosis (p.108). Benefits must, however, be weighed against a slightly increased risk of breast cancer.

Bones
HRT reduces the thinning of bone that occurs in osteoporosis and thus protects against fractures.

Breasts
There is a slightly increased risk of breast cancer with long-term use of HRT, especially in older women.

Reproductive organs
Thinning of the vaginal tissues leading to painful intercourse can be prevented by HRT.

COMMON DRUGS

Estrogens
Conjugated
  estrogens *
Ethinyl estradiol *
Estrone
Estropipate

Progestins
Desogestrel
Drospirenone
Levonorgestrel *
Medroxyprogesterone
  acetate *
Norethindrone *
Norgestimate
Norgestrel
Progesterone

* See Part 4

NUTRITION

Food provides energy (as calories) and materials called nutrients needed for growth and renewal of tissues. Protein, carbohydrate, and fat are the three major nutrient components of food. Vitamins and minerals are found only in small amounts in food, but are just as important for normal function of the body. Fibre, found only in foods from plants, is needed for a healthy digestive system.

During digestion, large molecules of food are broken down into smaller molecules, releasing nutrients that are absorbed into the bloodstream. Carbohydrate and fat are then *metabolized* by body cells to produce energy. They may also be incorporated with protein into the cell structure. Each metabolic process is promoted by a specific *enzyme* and often requires the presence of a particular vitamin or mineral.

Why drugs are used

Dietary deficiency of essential nutrients can lead to illness. In poorer countries where there is a shortage of food, marasmus (resulting from lack of food energy) and kwashiorkor (from lack of protein) are common. In the developed world, however, excessive food intake leading to obesity is more common. Nutritional deficiencies in developed countries result from poor food choices and usually stem from a lack of a specific vitamin or mineral, such as in iron-deficiency anemia.

Some nutritional deficiencies may be caused by an inability of the body to absorb nutrients from food (malabsorption) or to utilize them once they have been absorbed. Malabsorption may be caused by lack of an enzyme or an abnormality of the digestive tract. Errors of metabolism are often inborn and are not yet fully understood. They may be caused by failure of the body to produce the chemicals required to process nutrients for use.

Why supplements are used

Deficiencies such as kwashiorkor or marasmus are usually treated by dietary improvement and, in some cases, food supplements, rather than drugs. Vitamin and mineral deficiencies are usually treated with appropriate supplements. Malabsorption disorders may require changes in diet or long-term use of supplements. Metabolic errors are not easily treated with supplements or drugs, and a special diet may be the main treatment.

The preferred treatment of obesity is reduction of food intake, altered eating patterns, and inceased exercise. When these methods are not effective, and the *body mass index (BMI)* is 30 or more, an anti-obesity drug may be used.

Major food components

Proteins
Vital for tissue growth and repair. In meat and dairy products, cereals, and pulses. Moderate amounts required.

Carbohydrates
A major energy source, stored as fat when taken in excess. In cereals, sugar, and vegetables. Starchy foods preferable to sugar.

Fats
A concentrated energy form that is needed only in small quantities. In animal products such as butter and in plant oils.

Fibre (non-starch polysaccharides)
The indigestible part of any plant product that, although it contains no nutrients, adds bulk to feces.

Absorption of nutrients
Food passes through the mouth, esophagus, and stomach to the small intestine. The lining of the small intestine secretes many enzymes and is covered by tiny projections (villi) that enable nutrients to pass into the blood.

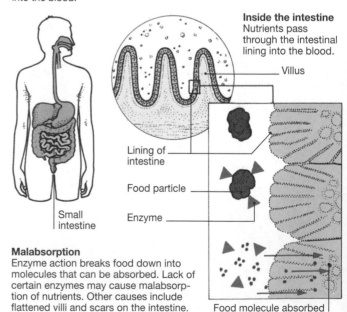

Inside the intestine
Nutrients pass through the intestinal lining into the blood.

Villus

Lining of intestine

Food particle

Enzyme

Small intestine

Food molecule absorbed

Malabsorption
Enzyme action breaks food down into molecules that can be absorbed. Lack of certain enzymes may cause malabsorption of nutrients. Other causes include flattened villi and scars on the intestine.

MAJOR DRUG GROUPS

Vitamins

VITAMINS

Vitamins are complex chemicals that are essential for a variety of body functions. With the exception of vitamin D, the body cannot manufacture these substances itself and therefore we need to include them in our diet. There are 13 major vitamins: A, C, D, E, K, and the B complex vitamins – thiamine (B_1), riboflavin (B_2), niacin (B_3), pantothenic acid (B_5), pyridoxine (B_6), and cobalamin (B_{12}), folic acid, and biotin. Most vitamins are required in very small amounts and each vitamin is present in one or more foods (see Main food sources of vitamins, p.136). Vitamin D is also produced in the body when the skin is exposed to sunlight. Vitamins fall into two groups, depending on whether they dissolve in fat or water (see Fat-soluble and water-soluble vitamins, p.137).

A number of vitamins (such as vitamins A, C, and E) have now been recognized as having strong antioxidant properties. Antioxidants neutralize the effect of free radicals, substances produced during the body's normal processes that may be potentially harmful if they are not neutralized. Free radicals are believed to play a role in cardiovascular disease, aging, and cancer.

A balanced diet that includes a variety of different types of food is likely to contain adequate amounts of all the vitamins. Inadequate intake of any vitamin over an extended period can lead to symptoms of deficiency. The nature of these symptoms depends on the vitamin concerned.

A doctor may recommend taking supplements of one or more vitamins in a variety of circumstances: to prevent vitamin deficiency occurring in people who are considered at special risk, to treat symptoms of deficiency, and in the treatment of certain medical conditions.

Why they are used
Preventing deficiency
Most people in Canada obtain sufficient quantities of vitamins in their diet, and it is therefore not usually necessary to take additional vitamins in the form of supplements. People who are unsure if their present diet is adequate are advised to look at the table on p.136 to check that foods that are rich in vitamins are eaten regularly. Vitamin intake can often be boosted simply by increasing the quantities of fresh foods and raw fruit and vegetables in the diet. Certain groups in the population are, however, at increased

risk of vitamin deficiency. These include people who have an increased need for certain vitamins that may not be met from dietary sources – in particular, women who are pregnant or breast-feeding, and infants and young children. The elderly, who may not be eating a varied diet, may also be at risk. Strict vegetarians, vegans, and others on restricted diets may not receive adequate amounts of all vitamins.

In addition, people who suffer from disorders in which absorption of nutrients from the bowel is impaired, or who need to take drugs that reduce the absorption of vitamins (for example, some types of lipid-lowering drugs), are usually given additional vitamins.

In these cases, the physician is likely to advise supplements of one or more vitamins. Although most preparations are available without a prescription, it is important to seek specialist advice before starting a course of vitamin supplements, so that a proper assessment is made of your individual requirements.

Vitamin supplements should not be used as a general tonic to improve well-being – they are not effective for this purpose – nor should they ever be used as a substitute for a balanced diet.

PRIMARY FUNCTIONS OF VITAMINS

The role of vitamins in the body is not yet fully understood; much of our knowledge is based on the evidence that is provided by symptoms occurring as a result of deficiency of a particular vitamin. Most vitamins have been found to have a number of important actions on one or more body systems or functions. Many are involved in the activity of *enzymes* (substances that promote or enable biochemical reactions in the body). The illustration below indicates the organs and body systems on which each vitamin has its principal effect.

Brain and nervous system
Folic acid, pyridoxine, pantothenic acid, thiamine, vitamin B_{12}, vitamin C

Eyes
Riboflavin, vitamin A

Blood vessels
Vitamin E

Lungs
Vitamin A, vitamin E

Heart
Thiamine, vitamin E

Adrenal hormones
Pantothenic acid, riboflavin, vitamin C

Fertility
Folic acid, vitamin A

Skin
Niacin, pyridoxine, riboflavin, vitamin A, vitamin E

Muscles
Pyridoxine, thiamine, vitamin E

Connective tissue
Vitamin C

Teeth and gums
Vitamin A, vitamin C, vitamin D

Digestion
Pantothenic acid, pyridoxine

Bones
Vitamin A, vitamin C, vitamin D

Metabolism
Biotin, folic acid, niacin, pantothenic acid, pyridoxine, riboflavin, thiamine, vitamin B_{12}, vitamin E

Growth
Folic acid, vitamin A, vitamin B_{12}

Immune system
Vitamin C

Blood
Folic acid, pantothenic acid, pyridoxine, vitamin B_{12}, vitamin E, vitamin K

VITAMINS continued

MAIN FOOD SOURCES OF VITAMINS AND MINERALS

The table below indicates which foods are especially good sources of particular vitamins and minerals. Ensuring that you regularly select foods from a variety of categories helps to maintain adequate intake for most people, without a need for supplements. It is important to remember that processed and overcooked foods are likely to contain fewer vitamins than fresh, raw, or lightly cooked foods.

Vitamins

	Red meat	Poultry	Liver	Milk	Cheese	Butter/margarine	Eggs	Fish	Cereals and bread	Green vegetables	Root vegetables	Pulses/legumes	Nuts	Fruit	Other	Notes
Biotin			●				●					●	●			Especially peanuts. Cauliflower and mushrooms are good sources.
Folic acid			●				●			●					●	Wheat germ and mushrooms are rich sources.
Niacin as nicotinic acid	●	●	●				●	●				●	●			Protein-rich foods such as milk and eggs contain tryptophan, which can be converted to niacin in the body.
Pantothenic acid			●				●	●								Each food group contributes some pantothenic acid.
Pyridoxine	●	●	●				●	●	●							Especially white meat (poultry), fish, and wholemeal cereals.
Riboflavin			●	●	●		●	●		●	●				●	Found in most foods.
Thiamine	●		●					●		●	●					Brewer's yeast, wheat germ, and bran are also good sources.
Vitamin A		●	●	●	●	●	●			●	●				●	Fish liver oil, dark green leafy vegetables such as spinach, and orange or yellow-orange vegetables and fruits such as carrots, apricots, and peaches, are especially good sources of vitamin A.
Vitamin B$_{12}$	●		●	●	●		●	●								Obtained only from animal products, especially liver and red meat.
Vitamin C										●	●				●	Especially citrus fruits, tomatoes, potatoes, broccoli, strawberries, and melon.
Vitamin D				●		●	●	●								Fish liver oils, margarine, and milk are the best sources, but the vitamin is also produced when the skin is exposed to sunlight.
Vitamin E						●	●		●	●		●	●			Vegetable oils, wholemeal cereals, and wheat germ are the best sources.
Vitamin K									●	●						Found In small amounts in fruits, seeds, root vegetables, dairy and meat products.

Minerals

	Red meat	Poultry	Liver	Milk	Cheese	Butter/margarine	Eggs	Fish	Cereals and bread	Green vegetables	Root vegetables	Pulses/legumes	Nuts	Fruit	Other	Notes
Calcium				●	●				●			●	●			Dark green leafy vegetables, soya bean products, and nuts are good non-dairy alternatives. Also present in hard, or alkaline, water supplies.
Chromium	●			●					●	●						Especially unrefined wholemeal cereals.
Copper	●	●	●				●	●	●			●	●			Especially shellfish, wholemeal cereals, and mushrooms.
Fluoride								●								Primarily obtained from fluoridated water supplies. Also in seafood and tea.
Iodine				●	●		●	●								Provided by "iodized" table salt, but adequate amounts can be obtained without using table salt from dairy products, saltwater fish, and bread.
Iron	●	●	●				●	●	●							Especially liver, red meat, and enriched or whole grains.
Magnesium				●			●	●	●			●	●			Dark green leafy vegetables such as spinach are rich sources. Also present in alkaline water supplies.
Phosphorus	●	●	●	●	●		●	●	●	●	●	●	●		●	Common food additive. Large amounts found in some carbonated beverages.
Potassium									●	●		●			●	Best sources are fruits and vegetables, especially oranges, bananas, and potatoes.
Selenium	●		●	●			●	●								Seafood is the richest source. Amounts in most foods are variable, depending on soil where plants were grown and animals grazed.
Sodium	●	●	●	●	●	●	●	●	●	●	●	●	●	●	●	Sodium is present in all foods, especially table salt, processed foods, potato crisps, crackers, and pickled, cured, or smoked meats, seafood, and vegetables. Also present in "softened" water.
Zinc	●				●		●	●				●				Highest amounts in wholemeal breads and cereals.

Vitamin deficiency

It is rare for a diet to be completely lacking in a particular vitamin. But if intake of a particular vitamin is regularly lower than the body's requirements, over a period of time the body's stores of vitamins may become depleted and symptoms of deficiency may begin to appear. In Canada, vitamin deficiency disorders are most common among malnourished individuals and alcoholics. Deficiencies of water-soluble vitamins are more likely since most of these are not stored in large quantities in the body. For descriptions of individual deficiency disorders, see the appropriate vitamin profile in Part 4.

Dosages of vitamins prescribed to treat vitamin deficiency are likely to be larger than those used to prevent deficiency. Medical supervision is required when correcting vitamin deficiency.

Other medical uses of vitamins

Various claims have been made for the value of vitamins in the treatment of medical disorders other than vitamin deficiency. High doses of vitamin C have been said to be effective in the prevention and treatment of the common cold, but such claims are not yet proved; zinc, however, may be helpful for this purpose. Vitamin and mineral supplements do not improve IQ in well-nourished children, but quite small dietary deficiencies can cause poor academic performance.

Certain vitamins have recognized medical uses apart from their nutritional role. Vitamin D has long been used to treat bone-wasting disorders (p.108). Niacin is sometimes used as a lipid-lowering drug (p.89). Derivatives of vitamin A (retinoids) are an established part of the treatment for severe acne (p.165).

MINERALS

Minerals are elements – the simplest form of substances – many of which are essential in trace amounts for normal metabolic processes. A balanced diet usually contains all of the minerals that the body requires; mineral deficiency diseases, except iron-deficiency anemia, are uncommon.

Dietary supplements are necessary only when a physician has diagnosed a specific deficiency or as part of the prevention or treatment of a medical disorder. Physicians often prescribe minerals for people with intestinal diseases that reduce the absorption of minerals from the diet. Iron supplements are often advised for pregnant or breast-feeding women, and iron-rich foods are recommended for infants over six months.

Much of the general advice given for vitamins also applies to minerals: taking supplements unless under medical direction is not advisable, exceeding the body's daily requirements is not beneficial, and large doses may be harmful.

CALCULATING DAILY VITAMIN REQUIREMENTS

Everyone needs a minimum amount of each vitamin for maintenance of health. The amount may vary with age, sex, and whether a woman is pregnant or breast-feeding. Guidelines for assessing the nutritional value of diets are called Recommended Daily Allowances (RDA), and are based on the amount of a nutrient that is enough, or more than enough, for 97 per cent of people. Those consuming much less than the RDA on a daily basis may not be consuming less than their needs but the risk of doing so is increased.

The current RDA (see table below) were set by Health Canada.

Daily reference nutrient intakes of vitamins for adults (aged 19–50)

| Vitamin (unit) | Recommended Daily Allowance | | |
	Men	Women	Pregnancy and breast-feeding
Biotin (mcg)	30	30	30–35
Folic acid as folate (mcg)	400	400	500–600
Niacin (mg)	16	14	17–18
Pantothenic acid (mg)	5	5	6–7
Pyridoxine (mg)	1.3	1.3	1.9–2.0
Riboflavin (mg)	1.3	1.1	1.4–1.6
Thiamine (mg)	1.2	1.1	1.4
Vitamin A (mcg)	900	700	770–1300
Vitamin B_{12} (mcg)	2.4	2.4	2.6–2.8
Vitamin C (mg)	90	75	85–120
Vitamin D (mcg) [1]	5	5	5
Vitamin E (mg)	15*	15*	15–19*

*as alpha-tocophenol [1] adequate intake

Many women who suffer from pre-menstrual syndrome take pyridoxine (vitamin B_6) supplements to relieve their symptoms. See also Drugs for menstrual disorders, p.148.

Risks and special precautions

Vitamins are essential for health, and supplements can be taken without risk by most people. It is important, however, not to exceed the recommended dosage, particularly in the case of fat-soluble vitamins, which may accumulate in the body. Dosage needs to be carefully calculated, taking into account the degree of deficiency, the dietary intake, and the duration of treatment. Overdosage has at best no therapeutic value and at worst it may incur the risk of serious harmful effects. Multivitamin preparations containing a large number of different vitamins are widely available. Fortunately, the amounts of each vitamin contained in each tablet are not usually large and are not likely to be harmful unless the dose is greatly exceeded. Single vitamin supplements can be harmful because an excess of one vitamin may increase requirements for others; hence, they should be used only on medical advice. For specific information on each vitamin, see Part 4, pp.468–482.

FAT-SOLUBLE AND WATER-SOLUBLE VITAMINS

Fat-soluble vitamins
Vitamins A, D, E, and K are absorbed from the intestine into the bloodstream together with fat (see also How drugs pass through the body, p.17). Deficiency of these vitamins may occur as a result of any disorder that affects the absorption of fat (for example, celiac disease). These vitamins are stored in the liver and reserves of some of them may last for several years. Taking an excess of a fat-soluble vitamin for a long period may cause it to build up to a harmful level in the body. Ensuring that foods rich in these vitamins are regularly included in the diet usually provides a sufficient supply without the risk of overdosage.

Water-soluble vitamins
Vitamin C and the B vitamins dissolve in water. Most are stored in the body for only a short period and are rapidly excreted by the kidneys if taken in higher amounts than the body requires. Vitamin B_{12} is the exception; it is stored in the liver, which may hold up to six years' supply. For these reasons, foods containing water-soluble vitamins need to be eaten daily. They are easily lost in cooking, so uncooked foods containing these vitamins should be eaten regularly. An overdose of water-soluble vitamins does not usually cause toxic effects, but adverse reactions to large dosages of vitamin C and pyridoxine (vitamin B_6) have been reported.

MALIGNANT AND IMMUNE DISEASE

New cells are continuously needed by the body to replace those that wear out and die naturally and to repair injured tissue. Usually the rate at which cells are created is carefully regulated. However, abnormal cells that multiply uncontrollably are sometimes formed. They may form lumps of abnormal tissue. These tumours are usually confined to one place and cause few problems; these are benign growths, such as warts. In other types of tumour the cells may invade or destroy the structures around it, and abnormal cells may spread to the rest of the body, forming metastatic tumours. These are malignant growths, also called cancers.

Opposing tumour growth is the body's immune system. This recognizes invading bacteria and viruses, and also transplanted tissue and cells that have become cancerous as foreign. The immune system relies on different types of white blood cells produced in the lymph glands and the bone marrow. They respond to foreign cells in a variety of ways, which are described on the facing page.

What can go wrong

A single cause for cancer has not been identified, and an individual's risk of developing cancer may depend upon both genetic predisposition and exposure to external risk factors, known as carcinogens. These include tobacco smoke, which increases the risk of lung cancer, and ultraviolet light from the sun. Long-term suppression of the immune system by disease (as in AIDS) or by drugs – for example, those given to prevent rejection of transplanted organs – also increases the risk of developing certain cancers. This demonstrates the importance of the immune system in removing abnormal cells with the potential to cause a tumour.

Overactivity of the immune system may also cause problems. It may respond excessively to an innocuous stimulus, as in hay fever (see Allergy, p.109), or may mount a reaction against normal tissues, leading to autoimmune diseases. These include rheumatoid arthritis, certain inflammatory skin disorders (for example, systemic lupus erythematosus), pernicious anemia, and some forms of hypothyroidism. Immune system activity can also be troublesome following an organ or tissue transplant, when it may lead to rejection of the foreign tissue. This shows the need for medication that can dampen the immune system and enable the body to accept the foreign tissue.

Why drugs are used

In cancer treatment, cytotoxic (cell-killing) drugs are used to eliminate abnormally dividing cells.

Types of cancer

Uncontrolled multiplication of cells leads to the formation of tumours that may be benign or malignant. Benign tumours do not spread to other tissues; however, malignant (cancerous) tumours do. Some of the main types of cancer are defined below.

Type of cancer	Tissues affected
Carcinoma	Skin and glandular tissue lining cells of internal organs
Sarcoma	Muscles, bones, and fibrous tissues and lining cells of blood vessels
Leukemia	White blood cells
Lymphoma	Lymph glands

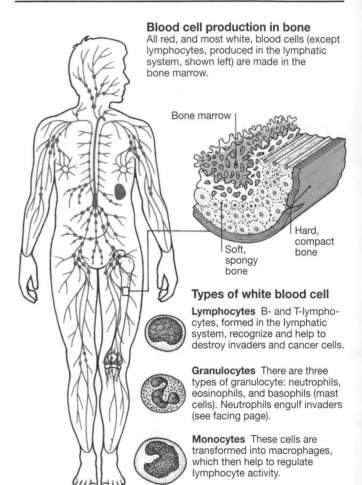

Blood cell production in bone

All red, and most white, blood cells (except lymphocytes, produced in the lymphatic system, shown left) are made in the bone marrow.

Bone marrow

Hard, compact bone

Soft, spongy bone

Types of white blood cell

Lymphocytes B- and T-lymphocytes, formed in the lymphatic system, recognize and help to destroy invaders and cancer cells.

Granulocytes There are three types of granulocyte: neutrophils, eosinophils, and basophils (mast cells). Neutrophils engulf invaders (see facing page).

Monocytes These cells are transformed into macrophages, which then help to regulate lymphocyte activity.

These slow the growth rate of tumours and sometimes lead to their complete disappearance. Because these drugs act against all rapidly dividing cells, they also reduce the number of normal cells, including blood cells, being produced from bone marrow. This can produce serious adverse effects, like *anemia* and neutropenia in cancer patients, but it can be useful in limiting white cell activity in autoimmune disorders. Some newer anticancer drugs are more selective in the cells they target.

Types of immune response

A specific response occurs when the immune system recognizes an invader. Two types of specific response, humoral and cellular, are described below. Phagocytosis, a non-specific response that does not depend on recognition of the invader, is also described.

Humoral response

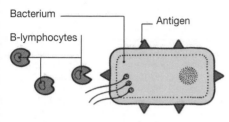

B-lymphocytes are activated by unfamiliar proteins (antigens) on the surface of the invading bacterium.

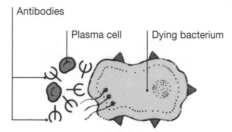

The activated B-lymphocytes form plasma cells, which release antibodies that bind to the invader and kill it.

Cellular response

T-lymphocytes recognize the antigens on abnormal or invading cells.

The T-lymphocytes bind to the abnormal cell and destroy it by altering chemical activity within the cell.

Engulfing invaders (phagocytosis)

Certain cells, such as neutrophils, are attracted by inflammatory chemicals to an area of bacterial infection.

The neutrophil flows around the bacterium, enclosing it within a fluid-filled space called a vacuole.

When the vacuole is formed, enzymes from areas called lysosomes in the neutrophil destroy the bacterium.

INTERFERONS

Interferons are natural proteins that limit viral infection by inhibiting viral replication within body cells. These substances also assist in the destruction of some types of cancer cells.

Effect on viral infection

Interferon binds to receptors on a virus-infected cell.

The presence of interferon triggers the release of enzymes that block viral replication. The virus is thus destroyed.

Effect on cancer cells

Interferon produced in response to a cancer cell activates T-lymphocytes.

T-lymphocytes attack and destroy the cancer cell.

Other drugs that have immunosuppressant effects include corticosteroids and cyclosporine, which are used following transplant surgery. No drugs are yet available that directly stimulate the entire immune system. However, growth factors may be used to increase the number and activity of some white blood cells, and antibody infusions may help those with deficient production or be used against specific targets in organ transplantation and cancer. For cervical cancer, there is a new preventive strategy. As a majority of cervical cancers are caused by a human papilloma virus (HPV) infection, vaccination against HPV in young women can reduce the risk of cervical cancer. HPV vaccine is recommended for females between the age of 9 and 26.

MAJOR DRUG GROUPS

Anticancer drugs
Immunosuppressant drugs
Drugs for immunodeficiency and AIDS

ANTICANCER DRUGS

Cancer is a general term that covers a wide range of disorders, ranging from the leukemias (blood cancers) to solid tumours of the lung, breast, and other organs. In all cancers, a group of cells escape from the normal controls on cell growth and multiplication. As a result, the malignant (cancerous) cells begin to crowd out the normal cells and a tumour develops. Cancerous cells are frequently unable to perform their usual functions, and this may lead to progressively impaired function of the organ or area concerned. Cancers may develop from cells of the blood, skin, muscle, or any other tissue.

Malignant tumours spread into nearby structures, blocking blood vessels and compressing nerves and other structures. Fragments of the tumour may become detached and carried in the bloodstream to other parts of the body, where they form secondary growths (metastases).

Many different factors, or a combination of them, can provoke cancerous changes in cells. These include an individual's genetic background, immune system failure, and exposure to cancer-causing agents (carcinogens). Known carcinogens include strong sunlight, tobacco smoke, radiation, certain chemicals, viruses, and dietary factors.

Treating cancer is a complicated process that depends on the type of cancer, its stage of development, and the patients' condition and wishes. Any of the following treatments may be used alone or in combination with the others: surgery, radiation treatment, and drug therapy.

Until recently, drug treatment of cancer relied heavily on hormonal drugs and cytotoxic agents (usually referred to as chemotherapy). Hormone treatments are suitable for only a few types of cancer, and cytotoxic drugs, although valuable, can have severe side effects because of the damage that they do to normal tissues. In recent years, as understanding of cancer biology has increased, new drugs have been developed. These include cytokines, such as interferon and interleukin-2, that stimulate the immune system to attack certain cancers, and monoclonal antibodies and growth-factor inhibitors that attack the cancer cells much more selectively.

Why they are used

Cytotoxic drugs can cure rapidly growing cancers and are the treatment of choice for leukemias, lymphomas, and certain cancers of the testis. They are less effective against slow-growing solid tumours, such as those of the breast and bowel, but they can relieve symptoms and prolong life when given as palliative chemotherapy (treatment that relieves symptoms but does not cure the disease). *Adjuvant* chemotherapy is increasingly being used after surgery, especially for breast and bowel tumours, to prevent regrowth of the cancer from cells left behind after surgery. Neoadjuvant, or primary, chemotherapy is sometimes used before surgery to reduce the size of the tumour. Hormone treatment is offered in cases of hormone-sensitive cancer, such as breast, uterine, and prostatic cancers, where they can be used to relieve disease symptoms or provide palliative treatment in advanced disease. Cytokines, monoclonal antibodies, and growth-factor inhibitors are used alone or alongside chemotherapy, sometimes with the aim of cure but more often to produce disease remission.

SUCCESSFUL CHEMOTHERAPY

Not all cancers respond to treatment with anticancer drugs. Some cancers can be cured by drug treatment. In others, drug treatment can slow or temporarily halt the progress of the disease. The table (right) summarizes the main cancers that fall into each of these two groups. In certain individual cases, drug treatment has no beneficial effect, but in some of these, other treatments, such as surgery, often produce significant benefits.

Successful drug treatment of cancer usually requires repeated courses of anticancer drugs because the treatment needs to be halted periodically to allow the blood-producing cells in the bone marrow to recover. The diagram below shows the number of cancer cells and normal blood cells before and after each course of treatment with cytotoxic anticancer drugs during successful chemotherapy. Both cancer cells and blood cells are reduced, but the blood cells recover quickly between courses of drug treatment. When treatment is effective, the number of cancer cells is reduced, so they no longer cause symptoms.

Response to chemotherapy

Cancers that can be cured by drugs
Some cancers of the lymphatic system (including Hodgkin's disease)
Acute leukemias (forms of blood cancer)
Choriocarcinoma (cancer of the placenta)
Germ cell tumours (cancers affecting sperm and egg cells)
Wilms' tumour (a rare form of kidney cancer that affects children)
Cancer of the testis

Cancers in which drugs produce worthwhile benefits
Breast cancer
Ovarian cancer
Some leukemias
Multiple myeloma (a bone marrow cancer)
Many types of lung cancer
Head and neck cancers
Cancer of the stomach
Cancer of the prostate
Some cancers of the lymphatic system
Bladder cancer
Endometrial cancer (cancer affecting the lining of the uterus)
Cancer of the large intestine
Cancer of the esophagus
Cancer of the pancreas
Cancer of the cervix

ACTION OF CYTOTOXIC ANTICANCER DRUGS

Each type of cytotoxic drug affects a separate stage of the cancer cell's development, and each type of drug kills the cell by a different mechanism of action. The action of some of the principal classes of cytotoxic drugs is described below.

Alkylating agents and cytotoxic antibiotics
These act within the cell's nucleus to damage the cell's genetic material, DNA. This prevents the cell from growing and dividing.

Nucleus
Cell DNA
Drug
Nutrients

Antimetabolites
These drugs prevent the cell from *metabolizing* (processing) nutrients and other substances that are necessary for normal activity in the cell.

Nucleus
Cell DNA
Drug
Nutrient

Most anticancer drug treatments, especially cytotoxic treatments, have side effects, sometimes severe, and so treatment decisions have to balance possible benefits against the risk of side effects. More aggressive treatments may be appropriate for patients who have curable cancers.

Often a combination of several drugs is used, either simultaneously or successively. Special regimes of different drugs used together and in succession have been devised to maximize their activity and minimize side effects.

Certain anticancer drugs are also used for their effect in suppressing immune system activity (see p.143).

How they work

Anticancer drugs work in many different ways. The main groups of drugs and how they work are described in this section.

Cytotoxic drugs

There are several classes of cytotoxic drugs, including the alkylating agents, antimetabolites, taxanes, and cytotoxic antibiotics. Each class has a different mechanism of action, but all act by interfering with basic processes of cell replication and division. They are particularly potent against rapidly dividing cells. These include cancer cells but also certain normal cells, especially those in the hair follicles, gut lining, and bone marrow. This explains their side effects (see below) and the need to schedule treatment carefully (see panel, p.140).

Hormone therapies

Hormone treatments act by counteracting the effects of the hormone that is encouraging growth of the cancer. For example, some breast cancers are stimulated by the female sex hormone estrogen; the action of estrogen is opposed by the drug tamoxifen. Other cancers are damaged by very high doses of a particular sex hormone. An example is medroxyprogesterone, a progesterone, that is often used to halt the spread of endometrial cancer.

Cytokines

The cytokines, interferon alfa and interleukin-2, stimulate the immune system to attack certain cancers. The mechanisms responsible for this action are not entirely understood.

Monoclonal antibodies

Antibodies are a fundamental building block of the immune system. They recognize and bind very specifically to "foreign" proteins on the surface of bacteria, viruses, and parasites, marking them out for destruction. Monoclonal antibodies are produced in tissue culture using cells genetically engineered to make antibodies against a particular target protein. If the target is carefully selected, the antibodies can be used to identify cancer cells for destruction by the immune system. If the target is found only on cancer cells, or on the cancer cells and the normal tissue from which it arose, the damage to healthy tissues during treatment is very limited. Once they have bound to a cell, antibodies interact with the immune system to kill cells in a variety of ways. They include attracting killer leukocytes and provoking a series of chemical reactions that dissolve the cell wall; this is called "complement fixation".

So far, two monoclonal antibodies are in routine use as cancer treatment: trastuzumab, which binds to a protein produced in particularly large quantities in about one-fifth of breast cancer cells, and rituximab. This antibody recognizes a protein found on most lymphatic cancer cells as well as some normal white blood cells. As these antibodies are so specific, they are useful only against particular cancers, in which they cause little of the toxicity of conventional chemotherapy. They do, however, often cause allergy-type reactions, especially at the beginning of treatment.

Growth-factor inhibitors

It has recently been discovered that the growth of cells, including cancer cells, is controlled by a complex network of growth factors that bind very specifically to receptor sites on the cell surface. This triggers a complex series of chemical reactions that transmit the "grow" message to the nucleus, triggering cell growth and replication. In many cancers, this system is faulty and there are either too many receptors on the cell surface or other abnormalities that result in the nucleus receiving inappropriate "grow" messages. The extra or abnormal cell surface receptors can be used as targets for monoclonal antibodies (see above).

Other defects in this system are being used as the basis for other new drugs. For example, imatinib very selectively interferes with an abnormal version of an enzyme that is found in certain leukemic cells. This abnormal enzyme results in the cell nucleus receiving a "grow" signal continuously, resulting in the uncontrolled growth of cancer. By stopping the enzyme working, it is possible to selectively "turn off" the growth of the abnormal cells. Imatinib is proving very successful in treating certain types of leukemia, with few serious side effects.

How they affect you

Cytotoxic drugs are generally associated with more side effects than other anticancer drugs. At the start of treatment, adverse effects of the drugs may be more noticeable than benefits. The most common side effect is nausea and vomiting, for which an anti-emetic drug (see p.74) will usually be prescribed. Effects on the blood are also common. Many cytotoxic drugs cause hair loss because of the effect of their activity on the hair follicle cells, but the hair usually starts to grow back after chemotherapy has been completed. Individual drugs may produce other side effects.

ACTION OF MONOCLONAL ANTIBODIES

Antibodies are a vital part of the body's immune system. They identify rogue cells, which are then destroyed in different ways by the action of the immune system; killer leukocytes are one type of immune response. Monoclonal antibodies are manufactured antibodies in the form of drugs that are designed to bind to proteins on the surface of specific cancer cells. The immune system is triggered into action and destroys the "tagged" cancer cells causing little or no harm to nearby normal cells.

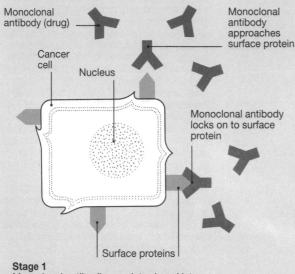

Monoclonal antibody (drug)

Cancer cell

Nucleus

Monoclonal antibody approaches surface protein

Monoclonal antibody locks on to surface protein

Surface proteins

Killer leukocyte is attracted to attached monoclonal antibody

Antibody-recognition sites

Nucleus

Cancer cell begins to disintegrate

Killer leukocyte is attached to cancer cell via monoclonal antibody

Stage 1
Monoclonal antibodies are introduced into the body. They are attracted to the surface proteins on a cancer cell and lock on to them. When sufficient antibodies have attached, the cell is recognized as rogue.

Stage 2
The "tagged" cancer cell becomes a target for destruction by killer leukocytes. Their antibody-recognition sites lock on to the monoclonal antibodies. This initiates destruction of the cell.

Cytotoxic drugs are, in most cases, administered in the highest doses that can be tolerated by the patient in order to kill as many cancer cells as quickly as possible.

The unpleasant side effects of intensive chemotherapy, combined with a delay of several weeks before any beneficial effects are seen, and the seriousness of the underlying disease often lead to depression in patients receiving anticancer drugs. Specialist counselling, support from family and friends, and, in some cases, treatment with anti-depressant drugs, may help.

Risks and special precautions

All cytotoxic anticancer drugs interfere with the activity of noncancerous cells and, for this reason, they often produce serious adverse effects during long-term treatment. In particular, these drugs often adversely affect rapidly dividing cells such as the blood-producing cells in the bone marrow. The numbers of red and white cells and the number of platelets (particles in the blood responsible for clotting) may all be reduced. In some cases, symptoms of *anemia* (weakness and fatigue) and an increased risk of abnormal or excessive bleeding may develop as a result of treatment with anticancer drugs. Reduction in the number of white blood cells may result in an increased susceptibility to infection.

A simple infection such as a sore throat may be a sign of depressed white cell production in a patient taking anticancer drugs, and it must be reported to the physician without delay. In addition, wounds may take longer to heal, and susceptible people can develop gout as a result of increased uric acid production due to cells being broken down.

Because of these problems, anticancer chemotherapy is often given in hospital, where the adverse effects can be closely monitored. Several short courses of drug treatment are usually given, thus allowing the bone marrow time to recover in the period between courses (see Successful chemotherapy, facing page). Blood tests are performed regularly. When necessary, blood transfusions, antibiotics, or other forms of treatment are used to overcome the adverse effects. When relevant, contraceptive advice is given early in treatment because most anticancer drugs can damage a developing baby.

In addition to these general effects, individual drugs may have adverse effects on particular organs. These are described under individual drug profiles in Part 4.

By contrast, other anticancer drugs, such as hormonal drugs, antibodies, and growth-factor inhibitors, are much more selective in their actions and generally have less serious side effects.

COMMON DRUGS

Alkylating agents
Chlorambucil
Cyclophosphamide ✱
Melphalan

Antimetabolites
Cytarabine
Fluorouracil
Mercaptopurine ✱
Methotrexate ✱

Cytotoxic antibiotics
Doxorubicin ✱
Epirubicin

Hormone treatments
Anastrozole ✱
Cyproterone acetate
Flutamide ✱
Goserelin ✱
Letrozole
Leuprolide
Medroxy-
    progesterone
    acetate ✱
Megestrol ✱
Tamoxifen ✱

Cytokines
Interferon alfa-2a ✱
Interferon alfa-2b ✱

Taxanes
Docetaxel
Paclitaxel

Monoclonal antibodies
Basiliximab
Bevacizumab
Daclizumab
Trastuzumab
Rituximab

Growth-factor inhibitors
Gefitinib
Imatinib

Vinca alkaloids and Analogs
Vinblastine
Vincristine
Vinorelbine

Other drugs
Carboplatin
Cisplatin ✱
Etoposide
Irinotecan

✱ See Part 4

IMMUNOSUPPRESSANT DRUGS

The body is protected against attack from bacteria, fungi, and viruses by the specialized cells and proteins in the blood and tissues that make up the immune system (see p.138). White blood cells known as lymphocytes either kill invading organisms directly or produce special proteins (*antibodies*) to destroy them. These mechanisms are also responsible for eliminating abnormal or unhealthy cells that could otherwise multiply and develop into a cancer.

In certain conditions it is medically necessary to dampen the activity of the immune system. These include a number of autoimmune disorders in which the immune system attacks normal body tissue. Autoimmune disorders may affect a single organ – for example, the kidneys in Goodpasture's syndrome or the thyroid gland in Hashimoto's disease – or they may result in widespread damage, for example, in rheumatoid arthritis or systemic lupus erythematosus.

Immune system activity may also need to be reduced following an organ transplant, when the body's defences would otherwise attack and reject the transplanted tissue.

Several types of drugs are used as immunosuppressants: anticancer drugs (p.140), corticosteroids (p.127), and cyclosporine (p.247).

Why they are used

Immunosuppressant drugs are given to treat autoimmune disorders, such as rheumatoid arthritis, when symptoms are severe and other treatments have not provided adequate relief. Corticosteroids are usually prescribed initially. The pronounced anti-inflammatory effect of these drugs, as well as their immunosuppressant action, helps to promote healing of tissue damaged by abnormal immune system activity. Anticancer drugs such as methotrexate may be used in addition to corticosteroids if these do not produce sufficient improvement or if their effect wanes (see also Antirheumatic drugs, p.103).

Immunosuppressant drugs are given before and after organ and other tissue transplants. Treatment may have to be continued indefinitely to prevent rejection. A number of drugs and drug combinations are used, depending on which organ is being transplanted and the underlying condition of the patient. However, cyclosporine, along with the related drug tacrolimus, is now the most widely used drug for preventing organ rejection. It is also increasingly used to treat autoimmune disorders. It is often used in combination with a corticosteroid or the more specific drug, mycophenolate mofetil.

Monoclonal antibodies which attack those parts of the immune system responsible for organ rejection are also used to aid transplantation.

How they work

Immunosuppressant drugs reduce the effectiveness of the immune system, either by depressing the production of lymphocytes or by altering their activity.

How they affect you

When immunosuppressants are given to treat an autoimmune disorder, they reduce the severity of the symptoms and may temporarily halt the progress of the disease. However, they cannot restore major tissue damage.

Immunosuppressant drugs can produce a variety of unwanted side effects. The side effects caused by corticosteroids are described in more detail on p.127. Anticancer drugs, when prescribed as immunosuppressants, are given in low doses that produce only mild side effects. They may cause nausea and vomiting, for which an anti-emetic drug (p.74) may be prescribed. Hair loss is rare and regrowth usually occurs when the drug treatment is discontinued. Cyclosporine may cause increased growth of facial hair, swelling of the gums, and tingling in the hands.

Risks and special precautions

All of these drugs may produce potentially serious adverse effects. By reducing the activity of the patient's immune system, immunosuppressant drugs can affect the body's ability to fight invading micro-organisms, thereby increasing the risk of serious infections. Because lymphocyte activity is also important for preventing the multiplication of abnormal cells, there is an increased risk of certain types of cancer. A major drawback of anticancer drugs is that, in addition to their effect on the production of lymphocytes, they interfere with the growth and division of other blood cells in the bone marrow. Reduced production of red blood cells can cause *anemia*; when the production of blood platelets is suppressed, blood clotting may be less efficient.

Although cyclosporine is more specific in its action than either corticosteroids or anticancer drugs, it can cause kidney damage and, in too high a dose, may affect the brain, causing hallucinations or fits. Cyclosporine also tends to raise blood pressure, and another drug may be required to counteract this effect (see Antihypertensive drugs, p.88).

ACTION OF IMMUNOSUPPRESSANTS

Before treatment
Many types of blood cell, each with a distinct role, form in the bone marrow. Lymphocytes respond to infection and foreign tissue. B-lymphocytes produce antibodies to attack invading organisms, whereas T-lymphocytes directly attack invading cells. Other blood cells help the action of the B- and T-cells.

Other blood cells

B-lymphocytes

T-lymphocytes

Antibodies

Anticancer drugs
These drugs slow the production of all cells in the bone marrow.

Corticosteroids
These drugs reduce the activity of both B- and T-lymphocytes.

Cyclosporine
This inhibits the activity of T-lymphocytes only, and not the activity of B-lymphocytes.

COMMON DRUGS

Anticancer drugs
Azathioprine ✳
Chlorambucil
Cyclophosphamide ✳
Methotrexate ✳
Mycophenolate
  mofetil

Other drugs
Cyclosporine ✳
Tacrolimus

Corticosteroids
(see p.127)

Antibodies
Lymphocyte immune globulin/
  anti-thymocyte globulin
Basiliximab
Daclizumab

✳ See Part 4

DRUGS FOR HIV AND AIDS

The disease AIDS (acquired immune deficiency syndrome) is caused by infection with the human immunodeficiency virus (HIV). This virus invades certain cells of the immune system, particularly the white blood cells called T-helper lymphocytes (or CD_4 cells), which normally activate other cells in the immune system to fight infection. Since HIV kills T-helper lymphocytes, the body cannot fight the virus or subsequent infections. Over the past few years the number of drugs available to treat HIV has increased considerably, as has the knowledge about how best to use the drugs in combination.

Why they are used

Drug treatments for HIV infection can be divided into the treatment of the initial infection and treatment of diseases and complications associated with AIDS.

Drugs that act directly against HIV are known as antiretrovirals and they can be divided into three groups. These work by interfering with enzymes vital for virus replication. The first group, which inhibit the reverse transcriptase enzyme, are divided by their chemical structure into nucleotide, nucleoside, and non-nucleoside inhibitors. The second group interfere with an enzyme called protease.

A challenge in the management of AIDS is the development of drug-resistant strains of HIV and some may not respond to a typical 3-drug regimen. Enfuvirtide, a new drug, appears to suppress the resistant strains and can be used in combination with the other drugs.

Treatment for HIV is usually started with two nucleoside transcriptase inhibitors and a non-nucleoside drug or a protease inhibitor. If combination therapy, called highly active antiretroviral therapy (HAART), is started before damage to the immune system is too great, it can reduce the level of HIV virus in the body and improve the outlook for HIV-infected individuals.

The mainstay of drug treatment for AIDS-related diseases are antimicrobial drugs for the bacterial, viral, fungal, and protozoal infections to which people with AIDS are particularly susceptible. These drugs include the antituberculous drugs (p.118), co-trimoxazole for the treatment of pneumocystis carinii pneumonia (PCP), and ganciclovir for the treatment of CMV (cytomegalovirus) infection.

COMMON DRUGS

Nucleoside reverse transcriptase inhibitors
Abacavir
Didanosine (ddl) ✱
Emtricitabine
Lamivudine (3TC)✱
Stavudine (d4T)
Zidovudine
  (AZT or ZDV) ✱

Nucleotide reverse transcriptase inhibitor
Tenofovir

Fusion inhibitor
Enfuvirtide
Maraviroc

Integrase inhibitor
Raltegravir

Non-nucleoside reverse transcriptase inhibitors
Delavirdine
Efavirenz ✱
Etravirine
Nevirapine

Protease inhibitors
Amprenavir
Atazanavir
Darunavir
Fosamprenavir
Indinavir
Lopinavir/ritonavir ✱
Nelfinavir
Saquinavir
Tipranavir

✱ See Part 4

HIV INFECTION AND POSSIBLE TREATMENTS

The illustrations below show how the human immunodeficiency virus (HIV) enters CD_4 cells and, once inside, replicates itself to produce new viruses. The action of already existing drugs, along with the possible action of future drugs is also shown.

Host cell
Nucleus
Receptor
HIV

Stage 1
The virus binds to a specialized site (receptor) on a body cell.

Stage 2
The virus enters the cell.

Possible drug intervention
Drugs such as enfuvirtide and maraviroc have been developed to block the entry of HIV into CD_4 cells.

Reverse transcriptase
Viral RNA

Stage 3
The virus loses its protective coat and releases RNA, its genetic material, and an enzyme known as reverse transcriptase.

Altered form of RNA

Drug intervention
The reverse transcriptase inhibitor drugs, such as zidovudine, efavirenz, and tenofovir, act here. Integrase inhibitors work by blocking the process here.

Stage 4
The enzyme reverse transcriptase converts viral RNA into a form that can enter the host cell's nucleus (DNA) and may become integrated with the cell's genetic material. This viral DNA is integrated into the DNA of the host cell by the enzyme integrase.

Protein
Viral RNA

Stage 5
The host cell starts to produce new viral RNA and protein from the viral material that has been incorporated into its nucleus.

New AIDS viruses
Dying host cell

Stage 6
The new viral RNA and proteins assemble to produce new viruses. These leave the host cell (which then dies) and are free to attack other cells in the body.

Drug intervention
The protease inhibitors prevent formation of viral proteins and viral assembly.

ANTIRETROVIRAL DRUGS

Drug name	Standard adult dose and cautions
Abacavir *Ziagen* (NRTI)	300mg twice daily. Can cause a severe allergic-type reaction.
Lamivudine, zidovudine (AZT) *Combivir* (NRTI)	1 tablet twice daily.
Didanosine (ddI) *Videx EC* (NRTI)	Adults over 60kg: 400mg daily in 1 or 2 divided doses. Adults under 60kg: 250mg in 1 or 2 divided doses.
Emtricitabine (FTC) *Emtriva* (NRTI). *Truvada*: emtricitabine and tenovir (NtRTI). *Atripla*: emtricitabine, tenovir (NtRTI), and efavirenz (NNRTI).	200mg once daily. May be taken with or without food.
Lamivudine (3TC) *Heptovir* (NRTI)	300mg in 1 or 2 divided doses. Can also be used to treat hepatitis B.
Stavudine (d4T) *Zerit* (NRTI)	Adults over 60kg: 40mg twice daily. Adults under 60kg: 30mg twice daily.
Lamivudine, zidovudine (AZT or ZDV), abacavir *Trizivir* (NRTI)	1 tablet twice daily. The abacavir contained within trizivir can cause a severe allergic-type reaction.
Zidovudine (AZT) *Retrovir* (NRTI)	500–600mg in 2–3 divided doses. Can cause anemia.
Tenofovir disoproxil *Viread* (NtRTI). Also see emtricitabine for combination products.	1 tablet once daily. Should be taken with food.
Nevirapine *Viramune* (NNRTI)	200mg daily for 2 weeks then, 200mg twice daily. Can cause a severe allergic-type reaction. Can cause psychiatric symptoms. Contraindicated in pregnancy.
Efavirenz *Sustiva* (NNRTI). Also see emtricitabine for combination products.	600mg once daily. Can cause a severe allergic-type rash.
Delavirdine (DLV) *Rescriptor* (NNRTI)	400mg three times daily. May be dissolved in water for easier swallowing.
Amprenavir *Agenerase* (PI)	Over 50kg in weight: tablets 1.2g twice daily. Capsules and solution are not interchangeable.

Drug name	Standard adult dose and cautions
Atazanavir *Reyataz* (PI)	300mg to 400mg once daily. Should be taken with food.
Darunavir (TMC-114) *Prezista* (PI)	Usually 600mg twice daily. Do not take this if you are allergic to ritonavir.
Tipranavir (TPV) *Aptivus* (PI)	Usually 500mg twice daily. Do not take this if you are allergic to ritonavir.
Fosamprenavir *Telzir* (PI)	Usually 1400mg twice daily (lower dose is used in PI-experienced patients). Tablets may be taken with or without food. Take solution on empty stomach.
Indinavir *Crixivan* (PI)	800mg every 8 hours. Should be taken with a low-fat meal or 1 hour before or 2 hours after any other meal.
Nelfinavir *Vircept* (PI)	1.25g twice daily or 750mg three times daily. Doses must be taken with a meal. Discuss risks with physician before initiating therapy.
Ritonavir *Norvir* (PI)	600mg every twice daily. Doses should be taken with food.
Lopinavir/ritonavir *Kaletra* (PI)	Three capsules twice daily. Doses should be taken with food.
Saquinavir *Fortovase, Invirase* (PI)	Invirase: 600mg every 8 hours; Fortovase: 1.2g every 8 hours. Doses should be taken within 2 hours of a full meal.
Enfuvirtide *Fuzeon* (FI)	90mg (1ml) twice daily. Injected subcutaneously. Reconstituted to be stored in refrigerator for no longer than 24 hours.
Maraviroc *Celsentri* (FI)	300mg twice daily; lower doses when given with certain drugs; higher doses given with some other drugs. Swallow tablets and do not chew them.
Raltegravir *Isentress* (II)	400mg twice daily.

KEY: NRTI = nucleoside reverse transcriptase inhibitor; NtRTI = nucleotide reverse transcriptase inhibitor; NNRTI = non-nucleoside reverse transcriptase inhibitor; PI = protease inhibitor; FI = fusion inhibitor; II = Integrase inhibitor.

REPRODUCTIVE & URINARY TRACTS

The reproductive systems of men and women consist of those organs that produce and release sperm (male), or store and release eggs, and then nurture a fertilized egg until it develops into a baby (female).

The urinary system filters wastes and water from the blood, producing urine, which is then expelled from the body. The reproductive and urinary systems of men are partially linked, but those of women form two physically close but functionally separate systems.

The female reproductive organs comprise the ovaries, fallopian tubes, and uterus (womb). The uterus opens via the cervix (neck of the uterus) into the vagina. The principal male reproductive organs are the two sperm-producing glands, the testes (testicles), which lie within the scrotum, and the penis. Other structures of the male reproductive tract include the prostate gland and several tubular structures – the tightly coiled epididymides, the vas deferens, the seminal vesicles and the urethra (see right).

The urinary organs in both sexes comprise the kidneys, which filter the blood and excrete urine (see also p.85), the ureters down which urine passes, and the bladder, where urine is stored until it is released from the body via the urethra.

What can go wrong

The reproductive and urinary tracts are both subject to infection. Such infections (apart from those transmitted by sexual activity) are relatively uncommon in men because the long male urethra prevents bacteria and other organisms passing easily to the bladder and upper urinary tract, and to the male sex organs. The shorter female urethra allows urinary tract infections, especially of the bladder (cystitis) and of the urethra (urethritis), to occur commonly. The female reproductive tract is also vulnerable to infection, which, in some cases, is sexually transmitted.

Reproductive function may also be disrupted by hormonal disturbances that lead to reduced fertility. Women may be troubled by symptoms arising from normal activity of the reproductive organs, including menstrual disorders as well as problems associated with childbirth.

The most common urinary problems apart from infection are those related to bladder function. Urine may be released involuntarily (incontinence) or it may be retained in the bladder. Such disorders are usually the result of abnormal nerve signals to the bladder or sphincter muscle. The filtering action of the kidneys may be affected by alteration

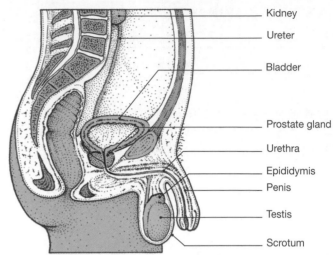

Male reproductive system
Sperm produced in each testis pass into the epididymis, a tightly coiled tube in which the sperm mature before passing along the vas deferens to the seminal vesicle. Sperm are stored in the seminal vesicle until they are ejaculated from the penis via the urethra, together with seminal fluid and secretions from the prostate gland.

Kidney
Ureter
Bladder
Prostate gland
Urethra
Epididymis
Penis
Testis
Scrotum

Epididymis
Seminiferous tubules
Tubule (enlarged)
Testis
Tubule wall
Sperm

How sperm are produced
Both testes contain tiny, coiled tubes (seminiferous tubules), where sperm are produced from the cells lining the walls. The sperm pass into the epididymides, where they mature for 2–4 weeks before passing into the seminal vesicles, where they are stored until ejaculation. Millions of sperm are produced daily and about 250 million are ejaculated at once.

of the composition of the blood or the hormones that regulate urine production, or by damage (from infection or inflammation) to the filtering units themselves.

Why drugs are used

Antibiotic drugs (p.114) are used to eliminate both urinary and reproductive tract infections (including sexually transmitted infections). Certain infections of the vagina are caused by fungi or yeasts and require antifungal drugs (p.124).

Hormone drugs are used both to reduce fertility deliberately (oral contraceptives) and to increase fertility in certain conditions in which it has not been

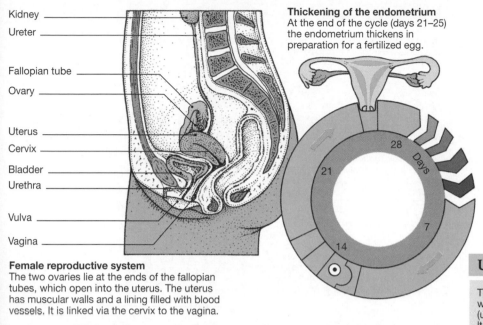

Kidney
Ureter
Fallopian tube
Ovary
Uterus
Cervix
Bladder
Urethra
Vulva
Vagina

Thickening of the endometrium
At the end of the cycle (days 21–25) the endometrium thickens in preparation for a fertilized egg.

Menstrual cycle
A monthly cycle of hormone interactions allows an egg to be released and, if it is fertilized, creates the correct environment for it to implant in the uterus. Major body changes occur, the most obvious being monthly vaginal bleeding (menstruation). The cycle usually starts between the ages of 11 and 14 years and continues until the menopause, which occurs at around 50. After the menopause, childbearing is no longer possible. The cycle is usually 28 days, but this varies with individuals.

Menstruation
If no egg is fertilized, the endometrium is shed (days 1–5).

Fertile period
Conception may take place in the two days after ovulation (days 14–16).

Female reproductive system
The two ovaries lie at the ends of the fallopian tubes, which open into the uterus. The uterus has muscular walls and a lining filled with blood vessels. It is linked via the cervix to the vagina.

Endometrium

The fertilized egg divides continually on the way down the fallopian tube.

One sperm fuses with the egg in the fallopian tube.

Ovarian follicle

Fallopian tube

Ovary

A fluid-filled cell cluster (follicle) nourishes the maturing egg. When the egg is ripe, it is released from the follicle.

The fertilized egg implants in the uterine wall and develops into an embryo.

Journey of the egg
Every month, hormone activity causes an egg within an ovarian follicle in one of the ovaries to ripen. It is then released (ovulation) and travels down the fallopian tube to the uterus.

URINARY SYSTEM

The kidneys extract waste and excess water from the blood. The waste liquid (urine) passes into the bladder, from which it is expelled via the urethra.

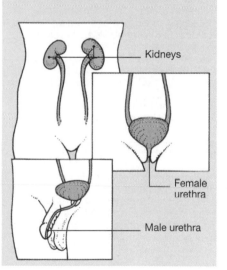

Kidneys

Female urethra

Male urethra

possible for a couple to conceive. Hormones may also be used to regulate menstruation when it is irregular or excessively painful or heavy. Analgesic drugs (p.64) are used to treat menstrual period pain and are also widely used for pain relief in labour. Other drugs used in labour include those that increase contraction of the muscles of the uterus and those that limit blood loss after the birth. Drugs may also be employed to halt premature labour.

Drugs that alter the transmission of nerve signals to the bladder muscles have an important role in the treatment of urinary incontinence and retention. Drugs that increase the kidneys' filtering action are commonly used to reduce blood pressure and fluid

retention (see Diuretics, p.85). Other drugs may alter the composition of the urine – for example, the uricosuric drugs that are used in the treatment of gout (p.105) increase the amount of uric acid.

MAJOR DRUG GROUPS

Drugs used to treat menstrual disorders
Oral contraceptives
Drugs for infertility
Drugs used in labour
Drugs used for urinary disorders

DRUGS USED TO TREAT MENSTRUAL DISORDERS

The menstrual cycle results from the actions of female sex hormones that cause ovulation (the release of an egg) and thickening of the endometrium (the lining of the uterus) each month in preparation for pregnancy. Unless the egg is fertilized, the endometrium will be shed about two weeks later during menstruation (see also p.147).

The main problems associated with menstruation that may require medical treatment are excessive blood loss (menorrhagia), pain during menstruation (dysmenorrhea), and distressing physical and psychological symptoms occurring prior to menstruation (premenstrual syndrome). The absence of periods (amenorrhea) is discussed under female sex hormones (p.133).

The drugs most commonly used to treat the menstrual disorders described above include estrogens, progestins, and analgesics.

Why they are used

Drug treatment for menstrual disorders is undertaken only when the physician has ruled out the possibility of an underlying gynecological disorder, such as a pelvic infection or fibroids. In some cases, especially in women over the age of 35, a D and C (dilatation and curettage) may be recommended. When no underlying reason for the problem is found, drug treatment aimed primarily at the relief of symptoms is usually prescribed.

Dysmenorrhea

Painful menstrual periods are usually treated initially with a simple analgesic (see p.64). Non-steroidal anti-inflammatory drugs (NSAIDs; see p.102), are often most effective because they counter the effects of prostaglandins, chemicals that are partly responsible for transmission of pain to the brain. Diclofenac and mefenamic acid are also used to reduce the excessive blood loss of menorrhagia (see below).

When these drugs are not sufficient to provide adequate pain relief, hormonal drug treatment may be recommended. If contraception is also required, treatment may involve an oral contraceptive pill containing both an estrogen and a progestin, or a progestin alone. However, non-contraceptive progestin preparations may also be prescribed. These are usually taken for only a few days during each month. The treatment of dysmenorrhea caused by endometriosis is described in the box above right.

Menorrhagia

Excessive blood loss during menstruation can sometimes be reduced by some NSAIDs. Tranexamic acid, an antifibrinolytic drug, is an effective treatment for menorrhagia. Alternatively, danazol, a drug that reduces production

ENDOMETRIOSIS

Endometriosis is a condition in which fragments of endometrial tissue (uterine lining) occur outside the uterus in the pelvic cavity. This disorder causes severe pain during menstruation, often causes pain during intercourse, and may sometimes lead to infertility.

Drugs used for this disorder are similar to those prescribed for heavy periods (menorrhagia). However, in this case the intention is to suppress endometrial development for an extended period so that the abnormal tissue eventually withers away. Progesterone supplements that suppress endometrial thickening may be prescribed throughout the menstrual cycle. Alternatively, danazol, which suppresses endometrial development by reducing estrogen production, may be prescribed. Any drug treatment usually needs to be continued for a minimum of six months.

When drug treatment is unsuccessful, surgical removal of the abnormal tissue is usually necessary.

Sites of endometriosis

Ovary — Wall of uterus — Fallopian tube

Bladder wall — Bowel wall

☐ Endometrial tissue

of the female sex hormone estrogen, may be prescribed to reduce blood loss.

Premenstrual syndrome

This is a collection of psychological and physical symptoms that affect many women to some degree in the days before menstruation. Psychological symptoms include mood changes such as increased irritability, depression, and anxiety. Principal physical symptoms are bloating, headache, and breast tenderness. Because some physicians believe that premenstrual syndrome is the result of a drop in progesterone levels in the last half of the menstrual cycle, non-contraceptive supplements of this hormone may be given in the week or so before menstruation. Oral contraceptives may be considered as an alternative. Other drugs sometimes used include pyridoxine (vitamin B_6), diuretics (p.85) if bloating due to fluid retention is a problem, and bromocriptine when breast tenderness is the major symptom. Anti-anxiety drugs (p.67) may be prescribed in rare cases where severe premenstrual psychological disturbance is experienced.

How they work

Drugs used in menstrual disorders act in a variety of ways. Hormonal treatments are aimed at suppressing the pattern of hormonal changes that is causing troublesome symptoms. Contraceptive preparations override the woman's normal menstrual cycle. Ovulation does not occur, and the endometrium does not

thicken normally. Bleeding that occurs at the end of a cycle is less likely to be abnormally heavy, to be accompanied by severe discomfort, or to be preceded by distressing symptoms. For further information on oral contraceptives, see facing page.

Non-contraceptive progestin such as medroxyprogesterone taken in the days before menstruation do not suppress ovulation. Increased progesterone during this time reduces premenstrual symptoms and prevents excessive thickening of the endometrium.

Danazol, a potent drug, prevents the thickening of the endometrium, thereby correcting excessively heavy periods. Blood loss is reduced, and in some cases menstruation ceases altogether during treatment.

COMMON DRUGS

Estrogens and progestins
(see p.133)

NSAID analgesics
ASA ✳
Diclofenac ✳
Diflunisal
Flurbiprofen
Ibuprofen ✳
Ketoprofen ✳
Mefenamic acid
Naproxen ✳

Diuretics
(see p.85)

Other drugs
Bromocriptine ✳
Buserelin
Danazol ✳
Goserelin ✳
Leuprolide
Nafarelin
Pyridoxine
Tranexamic acid
Triptorelin pamoate

☐ ✳ See Part 4

ORAL CONTRACEPTIVES

There are many different methods of ensuring that conception and pregnancy do not follow sexual intercourse, but for most women the oral contraceptive is the most effective method. It has the added advantage of being convenient and unobtrusive during lovemaking. Oral contraceptives are the method of choice for most young couples, especially teens, when combined with condoms, which are used for protection from sexually transmitted diseases.

Hormonal contraceptive formulations include oral tablets, vaginal ring, a patch applied on the skin, and an injection. Each vaginal ring and patch is left in/on for a period of 3 weeks; then a new package is used after a one-week homone-free interval (i.e. a new one used every 4 weeks). The ring and the patch contain a combination of an estrogen and a progestin hormone. The injection is administered every 3 months and contains only a progestin hormone. Oral contraceptives are available as a combined pill of estrogen and progestin or a progestin-only pill.

Why they are used
The combined pill
The combined pill is the most widely prescribed form of oral contraceptive and has the lowest failure rate in terms of unwanted pregnancies. It is referred to as the "pill" and is the type thought most suitable for young women who want to use a hormonal form of contraception. The combined pill is particularly suitable for those women who regularly experience exceptionally painful, heavy, or prolonged periods (see Drugs used to treat menstrual disorders, facing page).

COMPARISON OF RELIABILITY OF DIFFERENT METHODS OF CONTRACEPTION

The table indicates the number of pregnancies that occur with each method of contraception among 100 women using that method in a year. The wide variation that occurs with some methods takes into account pregnancies that occur as a result of incorrect use of the method.

Method	Pregnancies*
Combined and phased pills	2–3
Progestin-only pill	2.5–10
IUD (Intrauterine device)	up to 5
Condom	10–14
Diaphragm	10–14
Rhythm	25–30
Contraceptive sponge	10–14
Vaginal spermicide alone	2–30
Medoxy-progesterone depot	Less than 1
No contraception	80–85
"Morning after" pill	11–25

* Per 100 users per year.

There are many different products available containing a fixed dose of an estrogen and a progestin drug. They are usually divided into three groups according to their estrogen content (see Hormone content of common oral contraceptives, below). Low-dose products are chosen when possible to minimize the risk of adverse effects.

The combined pill is also available as "phased pills," where each pack is divided into two or three groups or phases. Each phase contains a different proportion of an estrogen and a progestin. The aim is to provide a hormonal balance that closely resembles the fluctuations of a normal menstrual cycle. Phased pills provide effective protection for many women who suffer side effects from other available forms of oral contraceptive.

Progestin-only pill
The progestin-only pill is often prescribed for women who react adversely to the estrogen in the combined pill or for whom the combined pill is considered unsuitable due to their age or medical history (see Risks and special precautions, p.150). It is also prescribed for women who are breast-feeding since it does not reduce milk production. The progestin pill has a higher failure rate than the combined pill and must be taken at precisely the same time each day for maximum contraceptive effect.

How they work
In a normal menstrual cycle, the ripening and release of an egg and the preparation of the uterus for implantation of the fertilized egg are the result of a complex interplay between the natural female sex hormones, estrogen and progesterone, and the pituitary hormones, follicle-stimulating hormone (FSH) and luteinizing hormone (LH) (see also p.133). The estrogen and progestins contained in oral contraceptives disrupt the normal menstrual cycle in such a way that conception is less likely.

With combined and phased pills, the increased levels of estrogen and progesterone produce similar effects to the hormonal changes of pregnancy. The actions of the hormones inhibit the production of FSH and LH, thereby preventing the egg from ripening in the ovary and from being released.

The progestin-only pill has a slightly different effect. It does not always prevent release of an egg; its main contraceptive action may be on the mucus that lines the cervix, which thickens so sperm cannot cross it. This effect occurs to some extent with combined pills and phased pills.

How they affect you
Each course of combined and phased pills lasts for 21 days, followed by a pill-free

HORMONE CONTENT OF COMMON ORAL CONTRACEPTIVES

The estrogen-containing forms are classified according to estrogen content as follows: Low: 20 micrograms; standard: 30–35 micrograms; high: 50 micrograms; phased pills: 30–40 micrograms.

Type of contraception (estrogen content)	Brand names
Combined (20mcg)	Alesse, Evra, Minestrin 1/20
(30–35mcg)	Brevicon 0.5/35, Brevicon 1/35, Cyclen Marvelon, Demulen 30, Diane-35, Loestrin 1.5/30, Min-Ovral, Ortho 0.5/35, Ortho 1/35, Ortho-Cept, Select 1/35, Yasmin
(50mcg)	Ovral
Phased (30–40mcg)	Linessa, Ortho7/7/7, Synphasic, Tri-cyclen, Tri-cyclen Lo, Triguilar, Triphasil
Progestin-only (no estrogen)	Micronor
Postcoital (morning after) (no estrogen)	Plan B

149

ORAL CONTRACEPTIVES continued

BALANCING THE RISKS AND BENEFITS OF ORAL CONTRACEPTIVES

Oral contraceptives are safe for the vast majority of young women. However, every woman considering oral contraception should discuss with her physician and pharmacist the risks and possible adverse effects of the drugs before deciding that a hormonal method is the most suitable in her case. A variety of factors must be taken into account, including the woman's age, her own medical history and that of her close relatives, and factors such as whether she is a smoker. The importance of such factors varies depending on the type of contraceptive. The table below gives the main advantages and disadvantages of estrogen-containing and progestin-only pills.

Type of oral contraceptive	Estrogen-containing combined and phased	Progestin-only
Advantages	● Very reliable ● Convenient/unobtrusive ● Regularizes menstruation ● Reduced menstrual pain and blood loss ● Reduced risk of: 　▼ benign breast disease 　▼ endometriosis 　▼ ectopic pregnancy 　▼ ovarian cysts 　▼ pelvic infection 　▼ ovarian and endometrial cancer	● Reasonably reliable ● Convenient/unobtrusive ● Suitable during breast-feeding ● Avoids estrogen-related side effects and risks ● Allows rapid return to fertility
Side effects	● Weight gain ● Depression ● Breast swelling ● Reduced sex drive ● Headaches ● Increased vaginal discharge ● Nausea	● Irregular menstruation ● Breast tenderness
Risks	● Thrombosis/embolism ● Heart disease ● High blood pressure ● Jaundice ● Cancer of the liver (rare) ● Gallstones	● Ectopic pregnancy ● Ovarian cysts
Factors that may prohibit use	● Previous thrombosis* ● Heart disease or high levels of lipid in blood ● Breast cancer ● Liver disease ● Blood disorders ● High blood pressure ● Unexplained vaginal bleeding ● Migraine with aura ● Otosclerosis ● Presence of several risk factors (below)	● Previous ectopic pregnancy ● Heart or circulatory disease ● Unexplained vaginal bleeding ● Breast cancer
Factors that increase risks	● Smoking* ● Obesity* ● Increasing age ● Diabetes mellitus ● Family history of heart or circulatory disease* ● Current treatment with other drugs	● As for estrogen-containing pills, but to a lesser degree

*Products containing desogestrel have a higher excess risk with these factors than other progestins.

How to minimize your health risks while taking the pill

▼ Give up smoking.
▼ Maintain a healthy weight and diet.
▼ Have regular blood pressure and blood lipid checks.
▼ Have regular cervical smear tests.

▼ Remind your physician that you are taking oral contraceptives before taking other prescription drugs.
▼ Stop taking estrogen-containing oral contraceptives four weeks before planned major surgery (use alternative contraception).

seven days (or sugar pills for the last seven days of a 28-day pack), during which time menstruation occurs. Some brands contain seven additional inactive pills (28-day pack). With these, the new course directly follows the last so the habit of taking the pill is not broken. Progestin-only pills are taken for 28 days each month. Menstruation usually occurs during the last few days of the menstrual cycle.

Women taking oral contraceptives, especially drugs that contain estrogen, usually find that their menstrual periods are lighter and relatively pain-free. Some women cease to menstruate altogether. This is not a cause for concern in itself, provided no pills have been missed, but it may make it difficult to determine if pregnancy has occurred. An apparently missed period probably indicates a light one, rather than pregnancy. However, if you have missed two consecutive periods and you feel that you may be pregnant, it is advisable to have a pregnancy test.

All forms of oral contraceptive may cause spotting of blood in mid-cycle ("breakthrough bleeding"), especially at first, but this can be a particular problem of the progestin-only pill.

Oral contraceptives that contain estrogen may produce any of a large number of mild side effects depending on the dose. Symptoms similar to those experienced early in pregnancy may occur, particularly in the first few months of pill use: some women complain of nausea and vomiting, weight gain, depression, altered libido, increased appetite, and cramps in the legs and abdomen. The pill

may also affect the circulation, producing minor headaches and dizziness. All these effects usually disappear within a few months, but if they persist, it may be advisable to change to a brand containing a lower dose of estrogen or to some other contraceptive method.

Risks and special precautions

All oral contraceptives need to be taken regularly for maximum protection against pregnancy. Contraceptive protection can be reduced by missing a pill (see What to do if you miss a pill, below). It may also be reduced by vomiting or diarrhea. If you suffer from either of these symptoms, it is advisable to act as if you had missed your last pill. Many drugs may also affect the action of oral contraceptives and it is essential to tell your physician and pharmacist that you are taking oral contraceptives before taking additional prescribed medications.

Oral contraceptives, particularly those containing an estrogen, have been found to carry a number of risks. These are summarized in the box on the facing page. One of the most serious potential adverse effects of estrogen-containing pills is development of a thrombus (blood clot) in a vein or artery. The thrombus may travel to the lungs or cause a stroke or heart attack. The risk of thrombus-formation increases with age and other factors, notably obesity, high blood pressure, and smoking. Physicians assess these risk factors for each person when prescribing oral contraceptives. A woman who is over 35 may be advised

POSTCOITAL CONTRACEPTION

Pregnancy following intercourse without contraception may be avoided by taking a short course of postcoital ("morning after") pills. The preparation used for this purpose contains a progestin and is usually taken in two doses 12 hours apart, within 72 hours following intercourse. These drugs postpone ovulation and act on the lining of the uterus to prevent implantation of the egg. However, the high doses required make them unsuitable for regular use. This method has a higher failure rate than the usual oral contraceptives.

against taking a combined pill, especially if she smokes or has an underlying medical condition such as diabetes mellitus. Concerns have been expressed about contraceptive pills containing the progestin desogestrel because several studies have found that preparations with this progestin carry a higher risk of thrombus formation than those containing other progestins. The drugs that contain desogestrel include Marvelon and Ortho-Cept. These preparations should be used only by those women who are intolerant of other contraceptive pills and are aware of the higher risk.

High blood pressure is a possible complication of oral contraceptives for some women. All women taking oral contraceptives should have their blood pressure measured before the pill is prescibed and monitored at six-month intervals thereafter.

Some very rare liver cancers have occurred in contraceptive pill-users, and breast cancer may be slightly more common. However, cancers of the ovaries and uterus are less common in women who take the contraceptive pill.

Although there is no evidence that oral contraceptives reduce a woman's fertility or that they damage the babies conceived after they are discontinued, physicians recommend that you wait for at least one normal menstrual period after stopping the pill before you attempt to become pregnant.

WHAT TO DO IF YOU MISS A PILL

Contraceptive protection may be reduced if blood levels of the hormones in the body fall as a result of missing a pill. It is particularly important to ensure that the progestogen-only pills are taken punctually. If you miss a pill, the action you should take depends on the degree of lateness and the type of pill being used (see below).

	Combined and phased pills	Progestin-only pills
3–12 hours late	Take the missed pill now. No additional precautions necessary.	Take the missed pill now. Take additional precautions for the next 7 days.
Over 12 hours late	Take the missed pill now and take the next pill on time (even if on the same day). If more than one pill has been missed, take the latest missed pill now and the next on time. Take additional precautions for the next 7 days. If the 7 days extends into the pill-free (or inactive pill) period, start the next pack without a break (or without taking inactive pills).	Take the missed pill now, and take the next on time. Take additional precautions for the next 7 days.

COMMON DRUGS

Progestins	Estrogens
Desogestrel	Ethinyl estradiol *
Drospirenone	Ethynodiol
Etonogestrel	diacetate
Levonorgestrel *	
Norelgestromin	
Norethindrone *	
Norgestimate	

* See Part 4

DRUGS FOR INFERTILITY

Conception and the establishment of pregnancy require a healthy reproductive system in both partners. The man must be able to produce sufficient numbers of healthy sperm; the woman must be able to produce a healthy egg that is able to pass freely down the fallopian tube to the uterus. The lining of the uterus must be in a condition that allows the implantation of the fertilized egg.

The cause of infertility may sometimes remain undiscovered, but in the majority of cases it is due to one of the following factors: intercourse taking place at the wrong time during the menstrual cycle; the man producing too few or unhealthy sperm; the woman either failing to ovulate (release an egg) or having blocked fallopian tubes perhaps as a result of previous pelvic infection. Alternatively, production of gonadotrophin hormones – follicle-stimulating hormone (FSH) and luteinizing hormone (LH) – needed for ovulation and implantation of the egg may be affected by illness or psychological stress.

If no simple explanation can be found, the man's semen will be analyzed. If these tests show that abnormally low numbers of sperm are being produced, or if a large proportion of the sperm produced are unhealthy, drug treatment may be tried.

If no abnormality of sperm production is discovered, the woman will be given a thorough medical examination. Ovulation is monitored and blood tests may be performed to assess hormone levels. If ovulation does not occur, the woman may be offered drug treatment.

Why they are used

In men, low sperm production may be treated with gonadotrophins (FSH or hCG) or a pituitary-stimulating drug (for example, clomifene) and unhealthy sperm may be controlled with corticosteroids.

In women, drugs are useful in helping to achieve pregnancy only when a hormone defect inhibiting ovulation has been diagnosed. Treatment may continue for months and does not always produce a pregnancy. Women in whom the pituitary gland produces some FSH and

ACTION OF FERTILITY DRUGS

Ovulation (release of an egg) and implantation are governed by hormones that are produced by the pituitary gland. FSH stimulates ripening of the egg follicle. LH triggers ovulation and ensures that progesterone is produced to prepare the uterus for the implantation of the egg. Drugs for female infertility boost the actions of these hormones.

FSH and hCG FSH adds to the action of the natural FSH early in the menstrual cycle. hCG mimics the action of natural LH at mid-cycle.

Clomiphene Normally, estrogen suppresses the output of FSH and LH by the pituitary gland. Clomiphene opposes the action of oestrogen so that FSH and LH continue to be produced.

Comparison of normal hormone fluctuation and timing of drug treatment

Days of menstrual cycle

LH may be given courses of clomiphene for several days during each month. Usually, up to three courses may be tried. An effective dose produces ovulation five to ten days after the last tablet is taken.

Clomiphene may thicken the cervical mucus, impeding the passage of sperm but the advantage of achieving ovulation outweighs the risk of this side effect. If treatment with clomiphene fails to produce ovulation, or if a disorder of the pituitary gland prevents the production of FSH and LH, treatment with FSH and gonadotrophin (human) chorionic may be given. FSH is given during the second week of the menstrual cycle, followed by an injection of gonadotrophin (human) chorionic.

How they work

Fertility drugs raise the chance of ovulation by boosting levels of LH and FSH. Clomiphene stimulates the pituitary gland to increase its output of these hormones. Artificially produced FSH and hCG mimic the action of naturally produced FSH and LH respectively. Both treatments, when successful, stimulate ovulation and implantation of the fertilized egg.

How they affect you

Clomiphene may produce hot flushes, nausea, headaches, and, rarely, ovarian cysts and visual disturbance, while hCG can cause tiredness, headaches, and mood changes. FSH can cause the ovaries to enlarge, producing abdominal discomfort. These drugs increase the likelihood of multiple births, usually twins.

DRUGS FOR IMPOTENCE

Impotence is a common male disorder and is defined as the inability to achieve or maintain an erection. The penis contains three cylinders of erectile tissue, the corpora cavernosa and the corpus spongiosum. Normally, when a man is sexually aroused, the arteries in the penis relax and widen, allowing more blood than usual to flow into the organ, filling the corpora cavernosa and the corpus spongiosum. As these tissues expand and harden, the veins that carry blood out of the penis become compressed, reducing outflow and resulting in an erection. In some forms of

impotence, this does not happen. In these situations, drugs that increase the blood flow into the penis to produce an erection can be used.

Drugs like Sildenafil (p.429) not only increase the blood flow into the penis but also prevent the muscle wall from relaxing, so the blood does not drain out of the blood vessels and the penis remains erect.

Alprostadil (p.183) is a prostaglandin drug that helps men achieve an erection by widening the blood vessels, but it must be injected directly into the penis, or applied into the urethra using a special syringe.

COMMON DRUGS

Buserelin	**Drugs for**
Clomiphene	**impotence**
Follitropin alpha	Alprostadil ✱
Follitropin beta	Sildenafil ✱
Ganirelix	Tadalafil
Gonadorelin	Vardenafil
Gonadotropin	
(human) chorionic ✱	
Goserelin ✱	
Menotropins	
Nafarelin	

✱ See Part 4

DRUGS USED IN LABOUR

Normal labour has three stages. In the first stage, the uterus begins to contract, initially irregularly and then gradually more regularly and powerfully, while the cervix dilates until it is fully stretched. During the second stage, powerful contractions of the uterus push the baby down the mother's birth canal and out of her body. The third stage involves the delivery of the placenta.

Drugs may be required during one or more stages of labour for any of the following reasons: to induce or augment labour; to delay premature labour (see Uterine muscle relaxants, below right); and to relieve pain. The administration of some drugs may be viewed as part of normal obstetric care; for example, the uterine stimulant ergometrine may be injected routinely before the third stage of labour. Other drugs are administered only when the condition of the mother or baby requires intervention. The possible adverse effects of the drug on both mother and baby are always carefully balanced against the benefits.

Drugs to induce or augment labour

Induction of labour may be advised when a physician considers it risky for the health of the mother or baby for the pregnancy to continue – for example, if natural labour does not occur within two weeks of the due date or when a woman has pre-eclampsia. Other common reasons for inducing labour include premature rupture of the membrane surrounding the baby (breaking of the waters), slow growth of the baby due to poor nourishment by the placenta, or death of the fetus in the uterus.

When labour needs to be induced, oxytocin, a uterine stimulant, may be administered intravenously. Alternatively, a prostaglandin vaginal suppository may be given to soften and dilate the cervix. If these methods are ineffective or cannot be used because of potential adverse effects (see Risks and special precautions, above right), a cesarean delivery may have to be performed.

DRUGS USED TO TERMINATE PREGNANCY

Drugs may be used in a hospital or in a clinic to terminate a pregnancy up to 20 weeks, or to empty the uterus after the death of the baby. A prostaglandin may be given first to dilate the cervix. Before 14 weeks of pregnancy, the fetus is then removed under anesthetic. After 14 weeks of pregnancy, labour is induced with a prostaglandin. These methods may be supplemented by oxytocin given by intravenous drip (see Drugs to induce or augment labour, above).

Oxytocin may also be used to strengthen the force of contractions in labour that has started spontaneously but has not continued normally.

A combination of oxytocin and another uterine stimulant, ergometrine, is given to most women as the baby is being born or immediately following birth to prevent excessive bleeding after the delivery of the placenta. This combination encourages the uterus to contract after delivery, which restricts the flow of blood.

Risks and special precautions
When oxytocin is used to induce labour, the dosage is carefully monitored throughout to prevent the possibility of excessively violent contractions. It is administered to women who have had surgery of the uterus only with careful monitoring. The drug is not known to affect the baby adversely. Ergometrine is not given to women who have suffered from high blood pressure during the course of pregnancy.

Drugs used for pain relief
Opioid analgesics
Meperidine, morphine, or other opioids may be given once active labour has been established (see Analgesics, p.64). Possible side effects for the mother include drowsiness, nausea, and vomiting. Opioid drugs may cause breathing difficulties for the new baby, but these problems may be reversed by the antidote naloxone.

Epidural anesthesia
This provides pain relief during labour and birth by numbing the nerves leading to the uterus and pelvic area. It is often used during a planned cesarean delivery, thus enabling the mother to be fully conscious for the birth.

An epidural involves the injection of a local anesthetic drug (see p.64) into the epidural space between the spinal cord and the vertebrae. An epidural may block the mother's urge to push during the second stage, and a forceps delivery may be necessary. Headaches may occasionally occur following epidural anesthesia.

Oxygen and nitrous oxide
These gases are combined to produce a mixture that reduces the pain caused by contractions. During the first and second stages of labour, gas is self-administered by inhalation through a mouthpiece or mask. If it is used over too long a period, it may produce nausea, confusion, and dehydration in the mother.

Local anesthetics
These drugs are injected inside the vagina or near the vaginal opening and are used to numb sensation during forceps delivery, before an episiotomy (an incision

WHEN DRUGS ARE USED IN LABOUR

The drugs used in each stage of labour are described below.

Before labour
Oxytocin
Prostaglandins

First stage
Epidural anesthetics
Morphine
Oxytocin
Meperidine

Second stage
Local anesthetics
Nitrous oxide
Oxytocin

Third stage
Ergometrine
Oxytocin

made to enlarge the vaginal opening), and when stitches are necessary. Side effects are rare.

Uterine muscle relaxants
When contractions of the uterus start before the 34th week of pregnancy, doctors usually advise bed rest and may also administer a drug that relaxes the muscles of the uterus and thus halts labour. Initially, the drug is given in hospital by injection, but it may be continued orally at home. These drugs work by stimulating the sympathetic nervous system (see Autonomic nervous system, p.63) and may cause palpitations and anxiety in the mother. They have not been shown to have adverse effects on the baby.

COMMON DRUGS

Prostaglandins
Dinoprostone

Pain relief
Fentanyl *
Morphine *
Meperidine

Uterine stimulants
Ergonovine
Oxytocin

Local anesthetics
Bupivacaine
Lidocaine

* See Part 4

DRUGS USED FOR URINARY DISORDERS

Urine is produced by the kidneys and stored in the bladder. As the urine accumulates, the bladder walls stretch and pressure within the bladder increases. Eventually, the stretching stimulates nerve endings that produce the urge to urinate. The ring of muscle (sphincter) around the bladder neck normally keeps the bladder closed until it is consciously relaxed, allowing urine to pass via the urethra out of the body.

A number of disorders can affect the urinary tract. The most common of these disorders are infection in the bladder (cystitis) or the urethra (urethritis), and loss of reliable control over urination (urinary incontinence). A less common problem is inability to expel urine (urinary retention). Drugs used to treat these problems include antibiotics and antibacterial drugs, analgesics, drugs to increase the acidity of the urine, and drugs that act on nerve control over the muscles of the bladder and sphincter.

Drugs for urinary infection

Nearly all infections of the bladder are caused by bacteria. Symptoms include a continual urge to urinate, although often nothing is passed; pain on urinating; and lower abdominal pain.

Many antibiotic and antibacterial drugs are used to treat urinary tract infections. Among the most widely used – because of their effectiveness – are cephalexin and norfloxacin (see Antibiotics, p.114, and Antibacterial drugs, p.117).

Measures are also sometimes taken to increase the acidity of the urine, thereby making it hostile to bacteria. Ascorbic acid (vitamin C) and acid fruit juices have this effect. Cranberry juice has also been tried

in preventing urinary infections. Once appropriate antibiotic treatment is started, symptoms are commonly relieved within a few hours.

For maximum effect, all drug treatments prescribed for urinary tract infections need to be accompanied by increased fluid intake.

Drugs for urinary incontinence

Urinary incontinence can occur for several reasons. A weak sphincter muscle allows the involuntary passage of urine when abdominal pressure is raised by coughing or physical exertion. This is known as stress incontinence and commonly affects women who have had children and post-menopausal women. Urgency – the sudden need to urinate – stems from oversensitivity of the bladder muscle; small quantities of urine stimulate the urge to urinate frequently.

Incontinence can also occur due to loss of nerve control in neurological disorders such as multiple sclerosis. In children, inability to control urination at night (nocturnal enuresis) is also a form of urinary incontinence.

Drug treatment is not necessary or appropriate for all forms of incontinence. In stress incontinence, exercises to strengthen the pelvic floor muscles or surgery to tighten stretched ligaments may be effective. In urgency, regular emptying of the bladder can often avoid the need for medical intervention. Incontinence caused by loss of nerve control is unlikely to be helped by drug treatment. Frequency of urination in urgency may be reduced by *anticholinergic* and *antispasmodic* drugs. These reduce nerve signals from the

muscles in the bladder, allowing greater volumes of urine to accumulate without stimulating the urge to pass urine. Tricyclic antidepressants, such as imipramine, have a strong anticholinergic action, and have been prescribed for nocturnal enuresis in children, but many doctors believe the risk of overdosage is unacceptable. Desmopressin, a synthetic derivative of antidiuretic hormone (see p.131), is also used for nocturnal enuresis.

Drugs for urinary retention

Urinary retention is the inability to empty the bladder. This usually results from the failure of the bladder muscle to contract sufficiently to expel accumulated urine. Possible causes include an enlarged prostate gland or tumour, or a long-standing neurological disorder. Some drugs can cause urinary retention.

Most cases of urinary retention need to be relieved by inserting a tube (catheter) into the urethra. Surgery may be needed to prevent a recurrence of the problem. Drugs that relax the sphincter or stimulate bladder contraction are now rarely used in the treatment of urinary retention, but two types of drug are used in the long-term management of prostatic enlargement. Finasteride prevents production of the male hormones that stimulate prostatic growth and alpha blockers, such as prazosin and terazosin, relax smooth muscle in the prostate gland and in the urethra, thereby improving urine outflow. Long-term drug treatment can relieve symptoms and delay the need for surgery.

COMMON DRUGS

Antibiotics and antibacterials
(see pp.114–117)

Anticholinergic/ antispasmodic
Darifenacin ✳
Desipramine
Flavoxate
Imipramine ✳
Oxybutynin ✳
Solifenacin
Tolterodine ✳
Trospium

Alpha blockers
Alfuzosin
Doxazosin ✳
Tamsulosin ✳
Terazosin

Other drugs
Desmopressin ✳
Dutasteride
Finasteride ✳
Vitamin C ✳

ACTION OF DRUGS ON URINATION

Normal bladder action
Urination occurs when the sphincter keeping the exit from the bladder into the urethra closed is consciously relaxed in response to signals from the bladder indicating that it is full. As the sphincter opens, the bladder wall contracts and urine is expelled.

Bladder

Sphincter muscle

Ureter

Openings of the ureters into bladder

Bladder wall

Urethra

How drugs act to improve bladder control

Anticholinergic drugs relax the bladder muscle by interfering with the passage of nerve impulses to the muscle.

Sympathomimetics act directly on the sphincter muscle, causing it to contract.

How drugs act to relieve urinary retention

Parasympathomimetics (cholinergics) stimulate contraction of the bladder wall.

Alpha blockers relax the muscle of the sphincter and urethra.

✳ See Part 4

EYES AND EARS

The eyes and ears are the two sense organs that provide us with the most information about the world around us. The eye is the organ of vision that converts light images into nerve signals, which are transmitted to the brain for interpretation. The ear not only provides the means by which sound is detected and communicated to the brain, but it also contains the organ of balance that tells the brain about the position and movement of the body. It is divided into three parts – outer, middle, and inner ear.

What can go wrong

The most common eye and ear disorders are infection and inflammation (sometimes caused by allergy). Many parts of the eye may be affected, notably the conjunctiva (the membrane that covers the front of the eye and lines the eyelids) and the iris. The middle and outer ear are more commonly affected by infection than the inner ear.

The eye may also be damaged by glaucoma, a disorder in which pressure of fluid within the eye builds up and may eventually threaten vision. Eye problems such as retinopathy (disease of the retina) or cataracts (clouding of the lens) may occur as a result of diabetes or for other reasons, but both are now treatable. Disorders for which no drug treatment is appropriate are beyond the scope of this book.

Other disorders affecting the ear include build-up of wax (cerumen) in the outer ear canal and disturbances to the balance mechanism (see Vertigo and Ménière's disease, p.74).

Why drugs are used

Doctors usually prescribe antibiotics (see p.114) to clear ear and eye infections. These may be given by mouth or *topically*. Topical eye and ear preparations may contain a corticosteroid (p.127) to reduce inflammation. When inflammation has been caused by allergy, antihistamines (p.110) may also be taken. Decongestant drugs (p.79) are often prescribed to help clear the eustachian tube in middle ear infections.

Various drugs are used to reduce fluid pressure in glaucoma. These include diuretics (p.85), beta blockers (p.83), and *miotics* to narrow the pupil. In other cases, the pupil may need to be widened by *mydriatic* drugs.

MAJOR DRUG GROUPS

Drugs for glaucoma	Drugs for ear disorders
Drugs affecting the pupil	

How the eye works
Light enters the eye through the cornea. The muscles of the iris control pupil size and thus the amount of light passing into the eye. In the eye, light hits the retina, which converts it to nerve signals that are carried by the optic nerve to the brain.

Retina
Conjunctiva
Iris
Lens
Cornea
Sclera
Optic nerve

Iris
Ciliary muscle
Lens
Cornea

The eye muscles
Both focusing and pupil size are governed by muscles controlled by the autonomic nervous system (p.63), which may be affected by many drugs. Disturbed vision is often a side effect of such drugs.

The ear
The outer ear canal is separated from the middle ear by the eardrum. Three bones in the middle ear connect it to the inner ear. This contains the cochlea (organ of hearing) and the labyrinth (organ of balance).

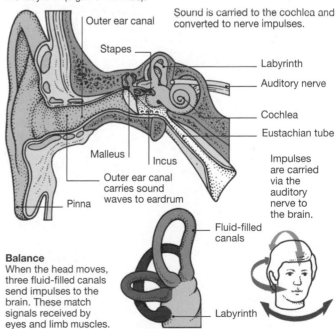

Outer ear canal
Sound is carried to the cochlea and converted to nerve impulses.
Stapes
Labyrinth
Auditory nerve
Cochlea
Eustachian tube
Impulses are carried via the auditory nerve to the brain.
Malleus
Incus
Outer ear canal carries sound waves to eardrum
Pinna
Fluid-filled canals

Balance
When the head moves, three fluid-filled canals send impulses to the brain. These match signals received by eyes and limb muscles.
Labyrinth

DRUGS FOR GLAUCOMA

Glaucoma is the name given to a group of conditions in which the pressure in the eye builds up to an abnormally high level. This compresses the blood vessels that supply the nerve connecting the eye to the brain (optic nerve) and may result in irreversible nerve damage and permanent loss of vision.

In the most common type of glaucoma, called chronic (or open-angle) glaucoma, reduced drainage of fluid from the eye causes pressure inside the eye to build up slowly. Progressive reduction in the peripheral field of vision may take months or years to be noticed. Acute (or closed-angle) glaucoma occurs when drainage of fluid is suddenly blocked by the iris. Fluid pressure usually builds up quite suddenly, blurring vision in the affected eye (see below). The eye becomes red and painful, accompanied by a headache and sometimes vomiting. The main attack is often preceded by milder warning attacks, such as seeing haloes around

lights in the previous weeks or months. Elderly, far-sighted people are particularly at risk of developing acute glaucoma. The angle may also narrow suddenly following injury or after taking certain drugs, for example, *anticholinergic* drugs. Closed-angle glaucoma may develop more slowly (chronic closed-angle glaucoma).

Drugs are used in the treatment of both types of glaucoma. These include miotics (see Drugs affecting the pupil, p.158) and beta blockers (p.83), as well as certain diuretics (carbonic anhydrase inhibitors and osmotics, p.85).

Why they are used
Chronic glaucoma
In this form of glaucoma, drugs are used to reduce pressure inside the eye. These drugs will prevent further deterioration of vision but cannot restore damage that has already been sustained, and therefore these drugs may be required lifelong. In most patients, treatment is begun with

eyedrops containing a beta blocker to reduce the production of fluid inside the eye. Miotic eyedrops to constrict the pupil and improve fluid drainage may be given. The prostaglandin, latanoprost, is also used to increase fluid outflow. If none of these drugs are effective, epinephrine, dipivefrine, or brimonidine may be tried to reduce secretion and help outflow. Sometimes a carbonic anhydrase inhibitor such as acetazolamide may be given by mouth to reduce fluid production. Laser treatment and surgery may also be used to improve fluid drainage from the eye.

Acute glaucoma
In acute glaucoma immediate medical treatment is required in order to prevent total loss of vision. Drugs are used initially to bring down the pressure within the eye. Laser treatment or surgery is then carried out to prevent a recurrence of the problem so that long-term drug treatment is seldom required.

WHAT HAPPENS IN GLAUCOMA

Normal eye
The ciliary body, situated at the root of the iris, continuously produces aqueous humour – a watery fluid that helps to maintain the normal shape of the eyeball. Aqueous humour drains via the angle between the cornea and iris through a mesh of fibres (the trabecular meshwork) into a channel in the sclera (white of the eye).

How vision is lost

In normal eye

In glaucoma

Pressure

Blood vessel

Compressed blood vessel

In glaucoma, rising pressure inside the eye compresses the blood vessels that supply the optic nerve.

The consequent reduction in blood supply causes damage to the optic nerve fibres and permanent loss of vision.

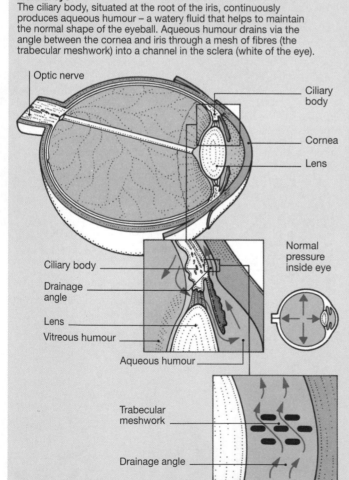

Optic nerve

Ciliary body

Cornea

Lens

Ciliary body

Drainage angle

Lens

Vitreous humour

Aqueous humour

Trabecular meshwork

Drainage angle

Normal pressure inside eye

Acute glaucoma
In acute glaucoma, the drainage angle between the cornea and the iris becomes completely closed, so the pressure inside the eye rises rapidly. This may cause permanent damage to the nerve fibres.

Iris

Drainage angle

Chronic glaucoma
In chronic glaucoma, the trabecular mesh-work through which the aqueous humour normally drains slowly closes off, so that fluid pressure builds up gradually and damages the optic nerve.

Trabecular meshwork

Drainage angle

Acetazolamide is often the first drug administered when the condition is diagnosed. This drug may be injected for rapid effect and thereafter administered by mouth. Frequent applications of eye drops containing pilocarpine or carbachol are given. An osmotic diuretic such as mannitol may be administered. This draws fluid out of all body tissues, including the eye, and reduces pressure within the eye.

How they work

The drugs used to treat glaucoma act in various ways to reduce the pressure of fluid in the eye. Miotics improve the drainage of the fluid out of the eye. In chronic glaucoma, this is achieved by increasing the outflow of aqueous humour through the drainage channel called the trabecular meshwork. In acute glaucoma, the pupil-constricting effect of miotics pulls the iris away from the drainage channel, allowing the aqueous humour to flow out in the normal way. Prostaglandin analogues act by increasing fluid flow from the eye. Beta blockers and carbonic anhydrase inhibitors act on the fluid-producing cells inside the eye to reduce the output of aqueous humour. Sympathomimetic drugs such as epinephrine, brimonidine, and apraclonidine are also thought to act partly in this way and partly by improving fluid drainage.

How they affect you

Drugs for acute glaucoma relieve pain and other symptoms within a few hours of their being used. The benefits of treatment in chronic glaucoma, however, may not be immediately apparent since treatment is only able to halt a further deterioration of vision.

People receiving miotic eye drops are likely to notice darkening of vision and difficulty seeing in the dark. Increased shortsightedness may be noticeable. Some miotics also cause irritation and redness of the eyes.

Beta blocker eye drops have few day-to-day side effects but carry risks for a few people (see right). Acetazolamide usually causes an increase in frequency of urination and thirst. Nausea and general malaise are also common.

ACTION OF DRUGS FOR GLAUCOMA

Miotics
These act on the circular muscle in the iris to reduce the size of the pupil. In acute glaucoma, this relieves any obstruction to the flow of aqueous humour by pulling the iris away from the cornea (right). In chronic glaucoma, miotic drugs act directly to increase the outflow of aqueous humour.

- Cornea
- Iris
- Lens
- Pupil

Beta blockers
The fluid-producing cells in the ciliary body are stimulated by signals passed through beta receptors. Beta blocking drugs prevent the transmission of signals through these receptors, thereby reducing the stimulus to produce fluid.

- Beta blocker
- Fluid-producing cell
- Aqueous humour

Before drug   **After drug**

- Fluid-producing cell
- Carbonic anhydrase
- Drug

Carbonic anhydrase inhibitors
These block carbonic anhydrase, an *enzyme* involved in the production of aqueous humour in the ciliary body.

Risks and special precautions

Miotics can cause alteration in vision. Beta blockers are absorbed into the body and can affect the lungs, heart, and circulation. As a result, a cardioselective beta blocker, such as betaxolol, may be prescribed with caution to people with asthma or certain circulatory disorders and, in some cases, such drugs are withheld altogether. The amount of the drug absorbed into the body can be reduced by applying the eye drops carefully, as described (left). Acetazolamide may cause troublesome adverse effects, including painful tingling of the hands and feet, the formation of kidney stones, and, rarely, kidney damage. People with existing kidney problems are not usually given this drug.

APPLYING EYE DROPS IN GLAUCOMA

To reduce the amount of drug absorbed into the blood via the lacrimal (tear) duct, apply eye drops as described. This also improves the effectiveness of the drug.

Lacrimal sac

Lacrimal duct

1 Press firmly on the lacrimal sac in the corner of the eye and apply the number of drops prescribed by your doctor.

2 Maintain pressure on the lacrimal sac for a few moments after applying the drops.

COMMON DRUGS

Miotics
Carbachol
Pilocarpine *

Carbonic anhydrase inhibitors
Acetazolamide
Brinzolamide
Dorzolamide *
Methazolamide

Prostaglandin analogues
Bimatoprost

Latanoprost *
Travoprost

Beta blockers
Betaxolol
Levobunolol
Timolol *

Sympathomimetics
Apraclonidine
Brimonidine
Epinephrine *

* See Part 4

DRUGS AFFECTING THE PUPIL

The pupil of the eye is the circular opening in the centre of the iris (the coloured part of the eye) through which light enters. It continually changes in size to adjust to variations in the intensity of light; in bright light it becomes quite small (constricts), but in dim light the pupil enlarges (dilates).

Eye drops containing drugs that act on the pupil are widely used by specialists. They are grouped into two categories: *mydriatics*, which dilate the pupil, and *miotics*, which constrict it.

Why they are used

Mydriatics are most often used to allow the physician to view the inside of the eye – particularly the retina, the optic nerve head, and the blood vessels that supply the retina. Many of these drugs cause a temporary paralysis of the eye's focusing mechanism, a state called cycloplegia. Cycloplegia is sometimes induced to help determine the presence of any focusing errors, especially in babies and young children. By producing cycloplegia, it is possible to determine the precise optical prescription required for a small child, especially in the case of a squint.

Dilation of the pupil is part of the treatment for uveitis, an inflammatory disease of the iris and focusing muscle. In uveitis, the inflamed iris may stick to the lens, and thus cause severe damage to the eye. This complication can be prevented by early dilation of the pupil so that the iris is no longer in contact with the lens.

Constriction of the pupil with miotic drugs is often required in the treatment of glaucoma (see p.157). Miotics can also be used to restore the pupil to a normal size after dilation is induced by mydriatics.

How they work

The size of the pupil is controlled by two separate sets of muscles in the iris, the circular muscle and the radial muscle. The two sets of muscles are governed by separate branches of the autonomic nervous system (see p.63): the radial muscle is controlled by the sympathetic nervous system, and the circular muscle is controlled by the parasympathetic nervous system.

Individual mydriatic and miotic drugs affect different branches of the autonomic nervous system, and cause the pupil to dilate or to contract, depending on the type of drug used (see above).

How they affect you

Mydriatic drugs – especially the long-acting types – impair the ability to focus the eye(s) for several hours after use. This interferes particularly with close activities such as reading. Bright light may cause discomfort. Miotics often interfere with night vision and may cause temporary short sight.

Normally, these eye drops produce few serious adverse effects. *Sympathomimetic* mydriatics may raise blood pressure and are used with caution in people with hypertension or heart disease. Miotics may irritate the eyes, but rarely cause generalized effects.

ACTION OF DRUGS AFFECTING THE PUPIL

The muscles of the iris
Pupil size is controlled by the coordinated action of the circular and radial muscles in the iris. The circular muscle forms a ring around the pupil; when this muscle contracts, the pupil becomes smaller. The radial muscle is composed of fibres that run from the pupil to the base of the iris like the spokes of a wheel. Contraction of these fibres causes the pupil to become larger.

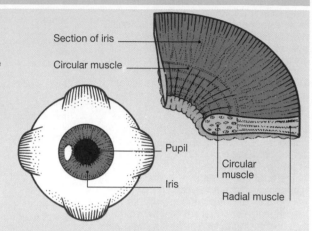

Section of iris
Circular muscle
Pupil
Circular muscle
Iris
Radial muscle

Radial muscle contracts
Circular muscle unable to contract

Circular muscle contracts

Mydriatics
Mydriatics enlarge the pupil in one of two ways. The *sympathomimetics* stimulate the radial muscle to contract. The *anticholinergics* prevent the circular muscle from contracting.

Miotics
Most miotics reduce the size of the pupil by stimulating the activity of the parasympathetic nervous system, which causes the circular muscle to contract.

ARTIFICIAL TEAR PREPARATIONS

Tears are continually produced to keep the front of the eye covered with a thin moist film. This is essential for clear vision and for keeping the front of the eye free from dirt and other irritants. In some conditions, known collectively as dry eye syndromes (for example, Sjögren's syndrome), inadequate tear production may make the eyes feel dry and sore. Sore eyes can also occur in disorders where the eyelids do not close properly, causing the eye to become dry.

Why they are used
Since prolonged deficiency of natural tears can damage the cornea, regular application of artificial tears in the form of eye drops is recommended for all of the conditions described above. Artificial tears may also be used to provide temporary relief from any feeling of discomfort and dryness in the eye caused by irritants, exposure to wind or sun, or following the initial wearing of contact lenses.

Although artificial tears are non-irritating, they often contain a preservative (for example, thimerosal or benzalkonium chloride) that may cause irritation. This risk of irritation is increased for wearers of soft contact lenses, who should ask their optician for advice before using any type of eye drops.

COMMON DRUGS

Sympathomimetic mydriatics
Epinephrine ✴
Phenylephrine

Miotics
Carbachol
Pilocarpine ✴

Anticholinergic mydriatics
Atropine ✴
Cyclopentolate
Homatropine
Tropicamide

✴ See Part 4

DRUGS FOR EAR DISORDERS

Inflammation and infection of the outer and middle ear are the most common ear disorders that are treated with drugs. Drug treatment for Ménière's disease, a condition that affects the inner ear, is described under Vertigo and Ménière's disease, p.74.

The type of drug treatment given for ear inflammation depends on the cause of the trouble and the site affected.

Inflammation of the outer ear

Inflammation of the external ear canal (otitis externa) can be caused by eczema or by a bacterial or fungal infection. The risk of inflammation is increased by swimming in dirty water, accumulation of wax in the ear, or scratching or poking too frequently at the ear.

Symptoms vary, but in many cases there is itching, pain (which may be severe if there is a boil in the ear canal), tenderness, and possibly some loss of hearing. If the ear is infected there will probably be a discharge.

Drug treatment
A corticosteroid (see p.127) in the form of ear drops may be used to treat inflammation of the outer ear when there is no infection. Aluminum acetate solution, as drops or applied on a piece of gauze, may also be used. Relief is usually obtained within a day or two. Prolonged use of corticosteroids is not advisable because they may reduce the ear's resistance to infection.

If there is both inflammation and infection, your physician may prescribe ear drops containing an antibiotic (see p.114) combined with a corticosteroid to relieve the inflammation. Usually, a combination of antibiotics is prescribed to make the treatment effective against a wide range of bacteria. Commonly used antibiotics include framycetin, neomycin, and polymyxin B. These antibiotics are not used if the eardrum is perforated.

EAR WAX REMOVAL

Ear wax (cerumen) is a natural secretion from the outer ear canal that keeps it free from dust and skin debris. Occasionally, wax may build up in the outer ear canal and become hard, leading to irritation and/or hearing loss.

A number of over-the-counter remedies are available to soften ear wax and hasten its expulsion. Such products may contain irritating substances that can cause inflammation. Some physicians advise application of olive or almond oil instead. A cotton plug should be inserted to retain the oil in the outer ear. When ear wax is not dislodged by such home treatment, a physician may syringe the ear with warm water. Do not use a stick or cotton swab.

Ear wax is produced in the outer ear canal.

Wax plug

Outer ear

Ear wax

Outer ear canal

Wax may build up and block the outer ear canal.

They are not usually applied for long periods because prolonged application can irritate the skin lining the ear canal.

Sometimes an antibiotic given in the form of drops is not effective, and another type of antibiotic may also have to be taken by mouth.

Infection of the middle ear

Infection of the middle ear (otitis media) often causes severe pain and hearing loss. It is particularly common in young children in whom infecting organisms are able to spread easily into the middle ear from the nose or throat via the eustachian tube.

Viral infections of the middle ear usually cure themselves and are less serious than those caused by bacteria, which are treated with antibiotics given by mouth or injection. Bacterial infections often cause the eustachian tube to swell and become blocked. When a blockage occurs, pus builds up in the middle ear and puts pressure on the eardrum, which may perforate as a result.

Drug treatment
Sometimes, an antibiotic is given by mouth to clear the infection.

Although antibiotics are not effective against viral infections, it is often difficult to distinguish between a viral and a bacterial infection of the middle ear, so your physician may prescribe an antibiotic as a precautionary measure. Acetaminophen or ibuprofen, an analgesic (see p.64), may be given to relieve pain.

HOW TO USE EAR DROPS

Ear drops for outer ear disorders are more easily and efficiently administered if you have someone to help you. Lie on your side while the other person drops the medication into the ear cavity, ensuring that the dropper does not touch the ear. If possible, it is advisable to remain lying in that position for a few minutes in order to allow the drops to bathe the ear canal. Ear drops should be discarded when the course of treatment has been completed.

Dropper

COMMON DRUGS

Antibiotic and antibacterial ear drops
Chloramphenicol *
Ciprofloxacin *
Clioquinol
Framycetin
Gentamicin *
Neomycin
Polymyxin B

Corticosteroids
Betamethasone *
Dexamethasone *
Flumethasone

Other drugs
Aluminum acetate

* See Part 4

SKIN

The skin waterproofs, cushions, and protects the rest of the body and is, in fact, its largest organ. It provides a barrier against innumerable infections and infestations, it helps the body to retain its vital fluids; it plays a major role in temperature control, and it houses the sensory nerves of touch.

The skin consists of two main layers: a thin, tough top layer, the epidermis, and below it a thicker layer, the dermis. The epidermis also has two layers: the skin surface, or stratum corneum (horny layer) consisting of dead cells, and below, a layer of active cells. The cells in the active layer divide and eventually die, maintaining the horny layer. Living cells produce keratin, which toughens the epidermis and is the basic substance of hair and nails. Some living cells in the epidermis produce melanin, a pigment released in increased amounts following exposure to sunlight.

The dermis contains different types of nerve ending for sensing pain, pressure, and temperature; sweat glands to cool the body; sebaceous glands that release an oil (sebum) that lubricates and waterproofs the skin; and white blood cells that help to keep the skin clear of infection.

What can go wrong

Most skin complaints are not serious, but they may be distressing if visible. They include infection, inflammation and irritation, infestation by skin parasites, and changes in skin structure and texture (for example, psoriasis, eczema, and acne).

Why drugs are used

Skin problems often resolve themselves without drug treatment. Over-the-counter preparations containing active ingredients are available, but physicians generally advise against their use without medical supervision because they could aggravate some skin conditions if used inappropriately. Drugs prescribed by physicians, however, are often highly effective, including antibiotics (p.114) for bacterial infections, antifungal drugs (p.124) for fungal infections, anti-infestation agents for skin parasites (p.164) and topical corticosteroids (p.162) for inflammatory conditions. Specialized drugs are available for conditions such as psoriasis and acne.

Although many drugs are *topical* medications, they must be used carefully because, like drugs taken orally, they can also cause adverse effects.

Structure of the skin
The epidermis contains keratin and melanin, while the dermis contains sweat glands, sebaceous glands, and nerve endings that sense pain, temperature, and pressure.

Epidermis
Active cell layer
Dermis
Sweat gland
Sebaceous gland
Hair follicle
Subcutaneous fat
Muscle

Hair shaft
Sweat pore
Stratum corneum
Nerve ending
Cold receptor
Heat receptor
Blood vessel

MAJOR DRUG GROUPS

Antipruritics	Drugs for psoriasis
Topical corticosteroids	Drugs for eczema
Anti-infective skin preparations	Drugs for dandruff
Drugs to treat skin parasites	Drugs for hair loss
Drugs used to treat acne	Sunscreens

SKIN

ANTIPRURITICS

Itching (irritation of the skin that creates the urge to scratch), also known as pruritus, most often occurs as a result of minor physical irritation or chemical changes in the skin caused by disease, allergy, inflammation, or exposure to irritant substances. People differ in their tolerance to itching, and an individual's threshold can be altered by stress and other psychological factors.

Itching is a common symptom of many skin disorders, including eczema and psoriasis and allergic conditions such as urticaria (hives). It is also sometimes caused by a localized fungal infection or parasitic infestation. Diseases such as chickenpox may also cause itching. Less commonly, itching may also occur as a symptom of diabetes mellitus, jaundice, and kidney failure.

In many cases, generalized itching is caused by dry skin. Itching in particular parts of the body is often caused by a specific problem. For example, itching around the anus (pruritus ani) may result from hemorrhoids or worm infestation, while genital itching in women (pruritus

vulvae) may be caused either by vaginal infection or, in older women, may be the result of a hormone deficiency.

Although scratching frequently provides temporary relief, it can often increase skin inflammation and make the condition worse. Continued scratching of an area of irritated skin may occasionally lead to a vicious circle of scratching and itching that continues long after the original cause of the trouble has been removed.

There are a number of different types of medicines used to relieve skin irritation. These products include soothing *topical* preparations applied to the affected skin and drugs that are taken by mouth. The main drugs used in antipruritic products include corticosteroids (see Topical corticosteroids, p.162), antihistamines (p.110), and local anesthetics (p.64). Simple *emollient* or cooling creams or ointments, which do not contain active ingredients, are often recommended.

Why they are used

For mild itching arising from sunburn, urticaria, or insect bites, a cooling lotion

such as calamine, perhaps containing menthol, phenol, or camphor, may be the most appropriate treatment. Local anesthetic creams are sometimes helpful for small areas of irritation, such as insect bites, but are unsuitable for widespread itching. The itching caused by dry skin is often soothed by a simple emollient. Avoiding excessive bathing and using moisturizing bath oils may also help.

Severe itching from eczema or other inflammatory skin conditions may be treated with a topical corticosteroid preparation. When the irritation prevents sleep, a physician may prescribe an antihistamine drug to be taken at night to promote sleep as well as to relieve itching (see also sleeping drugs, p.66). Antihistamines are also often included in topical preparations for the relief of skin irritation, but their effectiveness when administered in this way is doubtful. For the treatment of pruritus ani, see drugs for rectal and anal disorders (p.99). Post-menopausal pruritus vulvae may be helped by vaginal creams containing estrogen; for further information, see female sex hormones (p.133). Itching that is caused by an underlying illness cannot be helped by skin creams and requires treatment for the principal disorder.

Risks and special precautions

The main risk from any antipruritic, with the exception of simple emollient and soothing preparations, is skin irritation, and therefore aggravated itching, that is caused by prolonged or heavy use. Antihistamine and local anesthetic creams are especially likely to cause a reaction, and must be stopped if they do so. Antihistamines taken by mouth to relieve itching are likely to cause drowsiness. The special risks of topical corticosteroids are discussed on p.162.

Because itching can be a symptom of many underlying conditions, self-treatment should be continued for no longer than a week before seeking medical advice.

ACTION OF ANTIPRURITICS

Irritation of the skin causes the release of substances, such as histamine, that cause blood vessels to dilate and fluid to accumulate under the skin, which results in itching and inflammation. Antipruritic drugs act either by reducing inflammation, and therefore irritation, or by numbing the nerve impulses that transmit sensation to the brain.

Corticosteroids applied to the skin surface reduce itching caused by allergy within a few days, although the soothing effect of the cream may produce an immediate improvement. They pass into the underlying tissues and blood vessels and reduce the release of histamine, the chemical that causes itching and inflammation.

Antihistamines act within a few hours to reduce allergy-related skin inflammation. Applied to the skin, they pass into the underlying tissue and block the effects of histamine on the blood vessels beneath the skin. Taken by mouth, they also act on the brain to reduce the perception of irritation.

Local anesthetics absorbed through the skin may numb the transmission of signals from the nerves in the skin to the brain.

Soothing and emollient creams Calamine lotion and similar preparations applied to the skin surface reduce inflammation and itching by cooling the skin. Emollient creams lubricate the skin surface and prevent dryness.

Antihistamines by mouth
The action of these drugs on histamine in the brain reduces the response to signals from irritated skin.

Topical antipruritics
These antipruritics act locally to reduce itching.

Local anesthetics numb nerve endings.

Soothing creams act on the skin surface.

Corticosteroids reduce histamine release.

Histamine released into the tissues.

Antihistamines block the effects of histamine in the tissues.

Blood vessel

Nerve

COMMON DRUGS

Antihistamines
(see also p.110)
Diphenhydramine *
Hydroxyzine
Promethazine *

Corticosteroids
(see also p.127)
Hydrocortisone *

Local anesthetics
Benzocaine
Lidocaine
Tetracaine
Pramoxine

Emollient and cooling preparations
Aqueous cream
Calamine lotion
Cold cream
Emulsifying ointment

Other drugs
Crotamiton

* See Part 4

161

TOPICAL CORTICOSTEROIDS

Corticosteroid drugs (often simply called steroids) are related to the hormones produced by the adrenal glands. For a full description of these drugs, see p.127. *Topical* preparations containing a corticosteroid drug are often used to treat skin conditions in which inflammation is a prominent symptom.

Why they are used

Corticosteroid creams and ointments are most commonly given to relieve itching and inflammation associated with skin diseases such as eczema and dermatitis. These preparations may also be prescribed for psoriasis (see p.166). Corticosteroids do not affect the underlying cause of skin irritation, and the condition is therefore likely to recur unless the substance (allergen or irritant) that has provoked the irritation is removed, or the underlying condition is treated.

A physician might not prescribe a corticosteroid as the initial treatment, preferring to try a topical medicine that has fewer adverse effects (see Antipruritics, p.161). In most cases, treatment is started with a preparation containing a low concentration of a mild corticosteroid drug. A stronger preparation may be prescribed subsequently if the first product is ineffective.

How they affect you

Corticosteroids prevent the release of chemicals that trigger inflammation (see Action of corticosteroids on the skin, above right). Conditions treated with these drugs improve within a few days of starting the drug. Applied topically, corticosteroids rarely cause side effects, but the stronger drugs used in high concentrations have certain risks.

Risks and special precautions

Prolonged use of potent corticosteroids in high concentrations usually leads to

ACTION OF CORTICOSTEROIDS ON THE SKIN

Skin inflammation
Irritation of the skin, caused by allergens or irritant factors, provokes white blood cells to release substances that dilate the blood vessels. This makes the skin hot, red, and swollen.

Skin surface
Inflammation
Blood vessels
Fluid

Drug action
Applied to the skin surface, corticosteroids are absorbed into the underlying tissue. There they inhibit the action of the substances that cause inflammation, allowing the blood vessels to return to normal and reducing the swelling.

Drug
Inflammation reduced
Swelling reduced

permanent changes in the skin. The most common effect is thinning of the skin, sometimes resulting in permanent stretch marks. Fine blood vessels under the skin surface may become prominent (this condition is known as telangiectasia). Because the skin on the face is especially vulnerable to such damage, only weak corticosteroids should be prescribed for use on the face. Dark-skinned people sometimes suffer a temporary reduction in pigmentation at the site of application.

When corticosteroids have been used on the skin for a prolonged period, abrupt discontinuation can cause a reddening of the skin called rebound erythroderma. This effect may be avoided by a gradual reduction in dosage. Corticosteroids suppress the body's immune system (see p.143), thereby increasing the risk of infection. For this reason, they are never used alone to treat skin inflammation caused by bacterial or fungal infection. However, they are sometimes included in a topical preparation that also contains an antibiotic or antifungal agent (see Anti-infective skin preparations, facing page).

LONG-TERM EFFECTS OF TOPICAL CORTICOSTEROIDS

Prolonged use of topical corticosteroids causes drying and thinning of the epidermis, so that tiny blood vessels close to the skin surface become visible. In addition, long-term use of these drugs weakens the underlying connective tissue of the dermis, leading to an increased susceptibility to stretch marks.

Epidermis
Dermis

Normal skin

Stretch mark
Epidermis
Dermis
Weakened connective tissue

After prolonged use of topical corticosteroids

COMMON DRUGS

Very potent
Betamethasone
  dipropionate *
Clobetasol *
Halobetasol

Potent
Amcinonide
Betamethasone
  valerate *
Desoximetasone
Diflucortolone
Fluocinolone
Fluocinonide
Halcinonide
Mometasone *

Moderate
Clobetasone
Desonide
Flumethasone
Hydrocortisone
  valerate *
Prednicarbate
Triamcinolone

Mild
Hydrocortisone *

| * See Part 4 |

ANTI-INFECTIVE SKIN PREPARATIONS

The skin is the body's first line of defence against infection. Yet the skin can also become infected itself, especially if the outer layer (epidermis) is damaged by a burn, cut, scrape, insect bite, or an inflammatory skin condition – for example, eczema or dermatitis.

Several different types of organism may infect the skin, including bacteria, viruses, fungi, and yeasts. This page concentrates on drugs applied *topically* to treat bacterial skin infections. These drugs include antiseptics, antibiotics, and other antibacterial agents. Infection by other organisms is covered elsewhere (see Antiviral drugs, p.119, Antifungal drugs, p.124, and Drugs used to treat skin parasites, p.164).

Why they are used

Bacterial infection of a skin wound can usually be prevented by thorough cleansing of the damaged area and the application of antiseptic creams or lotions as described in the box (right). If infection does occur, the wound usually becomes inflamed and swollen, and pus may form. If you develop these signs, you should see your physician. The usual treatment for a wound infection is an antibiotic taken orally, although often an antibiotic cream is also prescribed.

An antibiotic or antibacterial skin cream may also be used to prevent infection when your physician considers this to be a particular risk – for example, in the case of severe burns.

Other skin disorders in which topical antibiotic treatment may be prescribed include impetigo and infected eczema, skin ulcers, bedsores, and nappy rash.

Often, a preparation containing two or more antibiotics is used in order to ensure that all bacteria are eradicated. The antibiotics selected for inclusion in topical preparations are usually drugs

ANTISEPTICS

Antiseptics (sometimes called germicides or skin disinfectants) are chemicals that kill or prevent the growth of microorganisms. They are weaker than household disinfectants, which are irritating to the skin.

Antiseptic lotions, creams, and solutions may be effective for preventing infection following wounds to the surface of the skin. Solutions can be added to water to clean wounds (if they are used undiluted, they may

cause inflammation and increase the risk of infection). Creams may be applied to wounds after cleansing.

Antiseptics are also included in some soaps and shampoos for the prevention of acne and dandruff, but their benefit in these disorders is doubtful. They are also included in some throat lozenges, but their effectiveness in curing throat infections is unproven.

Soaps, shampoos, throat lozenges and mouthwashes, skin lotions, creams, and ointments may contain antiseptic ingredients.

that are poorly absorbed through the skin (for example, the aminoglycosides). Thus the drug remains concentrated on the surface and in the skin's upper layers where it is intended to have its effect. However, if the infection is deep under the skin, or is causing fever and malaise, antibiotics may need to be given by mouth or injection.

Risks and special precautions

Any topical antibiotic product can irritate the skin or cause an allergic reaction.

Irritation is sometimes provoked by another ingredient of the preparation rather than the active drug, for example, a preservative contained in the product. An allergic reaction causing swelling and reddening of the skin is more likely to be caused by the antibiotic drug itself. Any adverse reaction of this kind should be reported to your physician, who may substitute another drug, or prescribe a different preparation.

Always follow your doctor's instructions on how long the treatment with antibiotics should be continued. Stopping too soon may cause the infection to flare up again.

Never use a skin preparation that has been prescribed for someone else since it may aggravate your condition. Always throw away any unused medication.

BASES FOR SKIN PREPARATIONS

Drugs that are applied to the skin are usually in a preparation known as a base (or vehicle), such as a cream, lotion, ointment, or paste. Many bases are beneficial on their own.

Creams These have an *emollient* effect. They are usually composed of an oil-in-water emulsion and are used in the treatment of dry skin disorders, such as psoriasis and dry eczema. They may contain other ingredients, such as camphor or menthol.

Barrier preparations These may be creams or ointments. They protect the skin against water and irritating substances. They may be used in the treatment of nappy rash and to protect the skin around an open sore. They may contain powders and water-repellent substances, such as silicones.

Lotions These thin, semi-liquid preparations are often used to cool and soothe inflamed skin. They are most suitable for use on large,

hairy areas. Preparations known as shake lotions contain fine powder that remains on the surface of the skin when the liquid has evaporated. They are used to encourage scabs to form.

Ointments These are usually greasy and are suitable for treating wet (weeping) eczema.

Pastes These are ointments containing large amounts of finely powdered solids such as starch or zinc oxide. Pastes protect the skin and absorb unwanted moisture. They are used for skin conditions that affect clearly defined areas, such as psoriasis.

Collodions These are preparations that, when applied to damaged areas of the skin such as ulcers and minor wounds, dry to form a protective film. They are sometimes used to keep a dissolved drug in contact with the skin.

COMMON DRUGS

Antibiotics	Antiseptics and other antibacterials
Bacitracin	
Framycetin	Chlorhexidine
Fusidic acid	Hexachlorophene
Gentamicin ✷	Metronidazole ✷
Mupirocin	Povidone iodine
Neomycin	Silver sulfadiazine
Polymyxin B	Triclosan

✷ See Part 4

DRUGS TO TREAT SKIN PARASITES

Mites and lice are the most common parasites that live on the skin. One common mite causes the skin disease scabies. The mite burrows into the skin and lays eggs, causing intense itching. Scratching the affected area results in bleeding and scab formation, as well as increasing the risk of infection.

There are three types of lice, each of which infests a different part of the human body: the head louse, the body (or clothes) louse, and the crab louse, which often infests the pubic areas but is also sometimes found on other hairy areas such as the eyebrows. All of these lice cause itching and lay eggs (nits) that look like white grains attached to hairs.

Both mites and lice are passed on by direct contact with an infected person (pubic lice are passed on during sexual intercourse) or, particularly in the case of body lice, by contact with infected bedding or clothing.

The drugs most often used to eliminate skin parasites are insecticides that kill both the adult insects and their eggs. The most effective drug for scabies is permethrin; lindane and precipitated sulfur in petrolatum are occasionally used. Very severe scabies may require oral ivermectin as well. For lice infestations, permethrin, pyrethrins with piperonyl butoxide, or lindane are used.

Why they are used

Skin parasites do not represent a serious threat to health, but they can cause severe irritation and spread rapidly if untreated. Prompt treatment of any parasite is essential. Drugs are used to eradicate the parasites from the body, but bedding and clothing may need to be disinfected to avoid the possibility of reinfestation.

How they are used

Lotions for the treatment of scabies (topical scabicides) should be applied to the entire body, including the face and scalp. It may be best to apply the lotion after showering and drying the skin thoroughly. After application of the scabicide, clothes can be worn. The lotion should be left on for 12 hours, then must be washed off.

One or two treatments are normally sufficient to remove the scabies mites. However, the itch associated with scabies may persist after the mite has been removed, so it may be necessary to use a soothing cream or medication containing an antipruritic drug (see p.161) to ease this. People who have direct skin-to-skin contact with a sufferer from scabies, such as family members and sexual partners, should also be treated with antiparasitic preparations at the same time.

Head and pubic lice infestations are usually treated by applying a preparation of one of the products and washing it off with water when and as instructed by the leaflet given with the preparation. If the skin has become infected as a result of scratching at the affected area, a *topical* antibiotic (see Anti-infective skin preparations, p.163) may also be prescribed.

Risks and special precautions

Lotions prescribed to control parasites can cause irritation and stinging that may be intense if the medication is allowed to come into contact with the eyes, mouth, or other moist membranes. Therefore, lotions and shampoos should be applied carefully, following the instructions of your physician or the manufacturer.

Because they are applied topically, antiparasitic drugs do not usually have generalized effects. Nevertheless, it is important not to apply these preparations more often than directed.

SITES AFFECTED BY SKIN PARASITES

Scabies
The female scabies mite burrows into the skin and lays its eggs under the skin surface. After hatching, larvae travel to the skin surface, where they mature for 10–17 days before starting the cycle again.

Skin surface | Eggs
Epidermis
Dermis

Scabies eggs in a burrow under the skin

Scabies mite

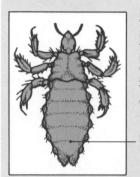
Head louse

Head lice
These tiny brown insects are transmitted from person to person (commonly among children). Their bites often cause itching.

Hair shaft
Nit

Nits
Head lice lay and attach their eggs near the base of the hair shaft, especially around the ears.

ELIMINATING PARASITES FROM BEDDING AND CLOTHING

Most skin parasites may also infest bedding and clothing that has been next to an infected person's skin. Therefore, to avoid reinfestation following removal of the parasites from the body, any insects and eggs lodged in the bedding or clothing must be eradicated.

Washing
Since all skin parasites are killed by heat, washing affected items of clothing and bedding in hot water and drying them in a hot dryer is an effective and convenient method of dealing with the problem.

Non-washable items
Items that cannot be washed should be isolated in plastic bags. The insects and their eggs cannot survive long without their human hosts and die within days. The length of time they can survive, and therefore the period of isolation, varies depending on the type of parasite (see the table below).

Parasite	Maximum survival time away from host Insects	Eggs	Isolation period
Scabies	2 days	0 days	2 days
Head lice	2 days	10 days	10 days
Crab lice	1 day	10 days	10 days
Body lice	10 days	30 days	30 days

COMMON DRUGS

Crotamiton
Lindane
Permethrin *
Piperonyl butoxide

Pyrethrins
Sulfur

* See Part 4

DRUGS USED TO TREAT ACNE

Acne, known medically as acne vulgaris, is a common condition caused by excess production of the skin's natural oil (sebum), leading to blockage of hair follicles (see What happens in acne, right). It chiefly affects adolescents but it may occur at any age, due to taking certain drugs, exposure to industrial chemicals, oily cosmetics, or hot, humid conditions.

Acne primarily affects the face, neck, back, and chest. The primary symptoms are blackheads, papules (inflamed spots), and pustules (raised pus-filled spots with a white centre). Mild acne may produce only blackheads and an occasional papule or pustule. Moderate cases are characterized by larger numbers of pustules and papules. In severe cases of acne, painful, inflamed cysts also develop. These can cause permanent pitting and scarring.

Medication for acne can be divided into two groups: *topical* preparations applied directly to the skin and *systemic* treatments taken by mouth.

Why they are used

Mild acne usually does not need medical treatment. It can be controlled by regular washing and by moderate exposure to sunlight or ultraviolet light. Over-the-counter antibacterial soaps and lotions are limited in use and may cause irritation.

When a physician or dermatologist thinks acne is severe enough to need medical treatment, he or she usually

CLEARING BLOCKED HAIR FOLLICLES

The most common treatment for acne is the application of keratolytic skin ointments. These encourage the layer of dead and hardened skin cells that form the skin surface to peel off. At the same time, this clears blackheads that block hair follicles and give rise to the formation of acne spots.

Blackhead
Trapped sebum

Blocked hair follicle
A hair follicle blocked by a plug of skin debris and sebum is ideal for acne spot formation.

Freed sebum

Cleared hair follicle
Once the follicle is unblocked, sebum can escape and air can enter, thereby limiting bacterial activity.

WHAT HAPPENS IN ACNE

In normal, healthy skin, sebum produced by a sebaceous gland attached to a hair follicle is able to flow out of the follicle along the hair. An acne spot forms when the flow of the sebum from the sebaceous gland is blocked by a plug of skin debris and hardened sebum, leading to an accumulation of sebum.

Hair
Skin surface
Sebaceous gland
Dermis
Hair follicle

Acne papules and pustules
Bacterial activity leads to the formation of pustules and papules. Irritant substances may leak into the surrounding skin, causing inflammation.

Sebum
Blackhead
Cyst

Cystic acne
When acne is severe, cysts may form in the inflamed dermis. These are pockets of pus enclosed within scar tissue.

recommends a topical preparation containing benzoyl peroxide or salicylic acid. If this does not produce improvement, an ointment containing tretinoin, a drug related to vitamin A or tetracycline, an antibiotic, may be prescribed.

If acne is severe or does not respond to topical treatments, a doctor may prescribe a course of antibiotics by mouth (usually tetracycline or minocycline). If these measures are unsuccessful, the more powerful vitamin A-like drug isotretinoin, taken by mouth, may be prescribed.

Estrogen drugs may have a beneficial effect on acne. A woman suffering from acne who also needs contraception may be given an estrogen-containing oral contraceptive (p.149). Alternatively, a preparation containing an estrogen and cyproterone (a drug that opposes male sex hormones) may be prescribed.

How they work

Drugs used to treat acne act in different ways. Some have a keratolytic effect – that is, they loosen the dead cells on the skin surface (see Clearing blocked hair follicles, left). Other drugs work by countering bacterial activity in the skin or reducing sebum production.

Topical preparations, such as benzoyl peroxide, salicylic acid, and tretinoin, have a keratolytic effect. Benzoyl peroxide also has an antibacterial effect. Topical or systemic tetracyclines reduce bacteria but may also have a direct anti-inflammatory effect on the skin. Isotretinoin reduces sebum production, soothes inflammation, and helps to unblock hair follicles.

How they affect you

Keratolytic preparations often cause soreness of the skin, especially at the

start of treatment. If this persists, a change to a milder preparation may be recommended. Day-to-day side effects are rare with antibiotics.

Treatment with isotretinoin often causes dry and scaly skin, particularly on the lips. The skin may become itchy and some hair loss may occur.

Risks and special precautions

Antibiotics in skin ointments may, in rare cases, provoke an allergic reaction requiring discontinuation of treatment. The tetracyclines, which are some of the most commonly used antibiotics for acne, have the advantage of being effective both topically and systemically. However, they are not suitable for use by mouth in pregnancy since they can affect the bones and teeth of the developing baby.

Isotretinoin sometimes increases levels of lipids in the blood. More seriously, the drug is known to damage the developing baby if taken during pregnancy. Women taking this drug need to make sure that they avoid conception during treatment.

COMMON DRUGS

Topical treatments	Oral and/or topical antibiotics
Adapalene	
Benzoyl peroxide *	Clindamycin *
Isotretinoin *	Doxycycline *
Salicylic acid	Erythromycin *
Tazarotene	Minocycline *
Tretinoin	Tetracycline *
Triclosan	

Other oral drugs
Cyproterone/
ethinyl estradiol
(women) *
Isotretinoin *
Levonorgestrel/
ethinyl estradiol
(women) *

* See Part 4

DRUGS FOR PSORIASIS

The skin is constantly being renewed; as fast as dead cells in the outermost layer (epidermis) are shed, they are replaced by cells from the base of the epidermis. Psoriasis occurs when the production of new cells increases while the shedding of old cells remains normal. As a result of increased cell production, the live skin cells accumulate and produce patches of inflamed, thickened skin covered by silvery scales. In some cases, the area of skin affected is extensive and causes severe embarrassment and physical discomfort. Psoriasis may occasionally be accompanied by arthritis, in which the joints become swollen and painful.

The underlying cause of psoriasis is not known. The disorder usually first occurs between the ages of 10 and 30, and it recurs throughout life. Outbreaks may be triggered by emotional stress, skin damage, drugs, and physical illness. Psoriasis can also occur as a consequence of the withdrawal of corticosteroid drugs.

There is no complete cure for psoriasis. Simple measures, including careful sunbathing or using an ultraviolet lamp, may help to clear mild psoriasis. An *emollient* cream (see Antipruritics, p.161) often soothes the irritation. When such measures fail to provide adequate relief, additional drug therapy is needed.

Why they are used

Drugs are used to decrease the size of affected skin areas and to reduce inflammation and scaling. Mild and moderate psoriasis are usually treated with a *topical* preparation. Coal tar preparations, available in the form of creams, pastes, or bath additives, are often helpful, although some people dislike the smell. Applied to the affected areas, the preparation is left for a few minutes or overnight (depending on which product is used), after which it is washed off. Coal tar can stain clothes and bed linen.

If this does not produce adequate benefit, ultraviolet light therapy in the form of regulated exposure to natural sunlight or to ultraviolet lamps (UVB) may be advised. Salicylic acid may be applied to help remove thick scale and crusts, especially from the scalp.

Topical corticosteroids (see p.162) may be used in difficult cases that do not respond to those treatments. They are particularly useful for the skinfold areas and may be given to counter irritation caused by dithranol.

If psoriasis is very severe and other treatments have not been effective, specialist treatment may include the use of more powerful drugs. These drugs include vitamin A derivatives (acitretin) taken by mouth in courses lasting approximately six months, and methotrexate, which is an anticancer drug.

PUVA

PUVA is the combined use of a psoralen drug (methoxsalen) and ultraviolet A light (UVA). The drug is applied *topically* or taken by mouth some hours before exposure to UVA, which enhances the effect of the drug on skin cells.

This therapy is given two to three times a week and produces an improvement in skin condition within about four to six weeks.

Possible adverse effects include nausea, itching, and painful reddening of the normal areas of skin. More seriously, there is a risk of the skin aging prematurely and a long-term risk of skin cancer, particularly in fair-skinned people. For these reasons, PUVA therapy is generally recommended only for severe psoriasis, when other treatments have failed.

In psoriasis
Skin cells form at the base of the epidermis faster than they can be shed from the skin surface. This causes the formation of patches of thickened, inflamed skin covered by a layer of flaking dead skin.

Normal skin

Skin in psoriasis

Epidermis

Rapidly dividing skin cells

Dermis

Skin cell

DNA

Drug

Psoralen drugs
In PUVA, psoralen drugs administered by mouth or as ointment penetrate the skin cells.

UVA rays

Drug

DNA restricted

Ultraviolet light
The drug is activated by exposure of the skin to ultraviolet light. It acts on the cell's genetic material (DNA) to regulate its rate of division.

Another form of specialist treatment, PUVA, is described in the box above.

How they work

Methotrexate slows down the rapid rate of cell division that causes thickening of the skin. Acitretin also reduces the production of keratin, the hard protein that forms in the outer layer of skin. Salicylic acid and coal tar remove the layers of dead skin cells. Corticosteroids reduce inflammation of underlying skin.

How they affect you

Appropriate treatment of psoriasis usually improves the appearance of the skin. However, since drugs cannot cure the underlying cause of the disorder, psoriasis tends to recur, even following successful treatment of an outbreak.

Individual drugs may cause side effects. Topical preparations can cause stinging and inflammation, especially if applied to normal skin. Coal tar increases the skin's sensitivity to sunlight; excessive sunbathing or overexposure to artificial ultraviolet light may damage skin and worsen the condition.

Acitretin and methotrexate can have several serious side effects, including gastrointestinal upsets. Acitretin can cause liver damage and methotrexate can cause bone marrow damage. Both are contraindicated in pregnancy, and women are advised not to become pregnant for two years after completing treatment with acitretin. Topical corticosteroids may cause rebound worsening of psoriasis when these drugs are stopped.

COMMON DRUGS

Acitretin
Calcipotriol ✳
Cyclosporine ✳
Coal tar
Dithranol

Methotrexate ✳
Methoxsalen
Salicylic acid
Tazarotene
Topical cortico-
steroids (see p.162)

✳ See Part 4

DRUGS AND OTHER TREATMENTS FOR ECZEMA

Eczema is a skin condition causing a dry, itchy rash that may be inflamed and blistered. There are several types, some of which are called dermatitis. Eczema can be triggered by allergy but often occurs for no known reason. In the long term, it can thicken the skin as a result of persistent scratching.

The most common type, atopic eczema, may appear in infancy, but many children grow out of it. There is often a family history of eczema, asthma, or allergic rhinitis. Atopic eczema commonly appears on the hands, due to their exposure to detergents, and the feet, due to the warm, moist conditions of enclosed footwear.

Contact dermatitis, another common form of eczema, is caused by chemicals, detergents, or soap. It may only appear after repeated exposure to the substance, but strong acids or alkalis can cause a reaction within minutes. It can also result from irritation of the skin by traces of detergent on clothes and bedding.

Allergic contact dermatitis can appear days or even years after initial contact has been made with triggers such as nickel, rubber, elastic, or drugs (such as antibiotics, antihistamines, antiseptics, or local anesthetics). Sunlight can also trigger contact dermatitis following use of aftershave or perfume.

Nummular eczema causes circular dry, scaly, itchy, patches to develop anywhere on the body, and bacteria are often found in these areas. The cause of nummular eczema is unknown.

Seborrhoeic dermatitis mainly affects the scalp and face (see Dandruff and hair loss p.168).

Why they are used
Emollients are used to soften and moisten the skin. Oral antihistamines (p.110) may be prescribed for a particularly itchy rash (*topical* antihistamines make the skin

COMMON SUBSTANCES THAT CAN CAUSE ECZEMA

Some substances produce an allergic reaction and some irritate the skin, causing eczema. The most common are listed below.

Allergens	Irritants
● Nickel, chromium	● Detergents
● Perfumes	● Soaps
● Plants	● Disinfectants
● Drugs	● Household cleaning products
● Rubber, elastic	● Paints
● Sticking plasters (especially zinc oxide ones)	● Glues and resins
● Cats and dogs	● Vegetable and fruit juices
● Tanning agents and dyes in leather and clothing	● Extremes of weather

PATCH TESTING

Low concentrations of the suspected substances are applied as spots to the skin of the back and held in place with non-absorbent adhesive tape. This method allows a number of potential allergens (substances that can cause an allergic reaction) to be tested at the same time.

After 48 hours, the adhesive tape is removed and the skin inspected for any redness, swelling, or blistering that has developed, which would indicate a positive reaction. The skin will be checked after a further 24 and 48 hours, in case the reaction has taken longer to develop.

Patches being applied

Patch containing allergen

Non-absorbent adhesive tape

Results of patch test

Normal skin

Blister

Reddened spot

Tape removed

more sensitive and should not be used). Coal tar or ichthammol may be used for chronic atopic eczema, but topical corticosteroids (p.162) may be needed to help control a flare up. Rarely, severe cases that are resistant to other treatments may need to be treated with the immuno-suppressant drug cyclosporine (p.243). Oral corticosteroids may be used to treat contact dermatitis. Nummular eczema usually requires corticosteroid treatment. If it is resistant, antibiotics (p.114) may be prescribed because infection is likely.

How they work
Emollients make the skin less dry and itchy. They are available as ointments, creams, lotions, soap substitutes, or bath oils. The effect is not long-lasting, so they need to be applied frequently. Emollients do not usually contain an active drug.

Antihistamines block the action of histamine (a chemical present in all cells). Histamine dilates the blood vessels in the skin, causing redness and swelling of the surrounding tissue due to fluid leaking from the circulation. Antihistamines also prevent histamine from irritating the nerve fibres, which causes itching.

Topical corticosteroids are absorbed into the tissues to relieve itching and inflammation. The least potent one that is effective is given. Hydrocortisone one per cent is often used in 1–2-week courses.

Oral or topical antibiotics destroy the bacteria sometimes present in broken, oozing, or blistered skin.

Cyclosporine blocks the action of white blood cells, which are involved in the immune response. The drug is given in short courses when the immune system responds inappropriately to an allergen.

Risks and special precautions
All types of eczema can become infected, and antibiotics may be needed. Herpes virus may infect atopic eczema, so direct contact with people who have a herpes infection, such as a cold sore, should be avoided. Emollients are generally well tolerated as are short-term topical mild corticosteroids. Cyclosporine, however, may produce some adverse effects.

Preventing eczema
Trigger substances can be identified using patch testing (see above) and avoided. PVC gloves should be worn to protect the hands from detergents. Cotton clothing should be worn next to the skin. Cosmetic moisturizers should be avoided because they usually contain perfumes and other sensitizers.

COMMON DRUGS

Emollient and cooling preparations
Aqueous cream
Cold cream
Emulsifying ointment
Calamine lotion

Antihistamines
(see also p.110)
Chlorpheniramine ✳
Diphenhydramine ✳
Hydroxyzine

Corticosteroids
(see also p.162)
Hydrocortisone ✳

Other drugs
Cyclosporine ✳
Coal tar
Tacrolimus

✳ See Part 4

DRUGS FOR DANDRUFF

Dandruff is an irritating, but harmless, condition that involves an acceleration in the normal shedding of skin cells from the scalp (see right). Extensive dandruff is considered to be a mild form of a type of dermatitis known as seborrhoeic dermatitis, which is caused by an overgrowth of a yeast organism that lives in the scalp. In severe cases, a rash and reddish yellow, scaly pimples appear along the hairline and on the face.

Why they are used

Frequent washing with a detergent shampoo usually keeps the scalp free of dandruff, but more persistent dandruff can be treated with shampoos medicated with zinc pyrithione or selenium sulfide (p.478), or with shampoos containing coal tar or salicylic acid. Severe cases of seborrhoeic dermatitis are best treated with shampoo containing the antifungal, ketoconazole (p.320). Ointments containing coal tar and salicylic acid are also available. Corticosteroid gels and lotions may be needed to treat an itchy rash, especially in cases of severe seborrhoeic dermatitis or psoriasis on the scalp (p.166).

How they work

Coal tar and salicylic acid preparations reduce the overproduction of new skin

WHAT HAPPENS IN DANDRUFF

All skin cells are replaced regularly as new cells grow from the epidermis. They gradually flatten as they die, and are shed on reaching the surface. Increased rate of production and sticking together of the cells produces dandruff. In children, dandruff may produce thick scaly flakes that can be 1–2cm across. In adults, smaller flakes are produced.

Normal shedding
- Normal scaling
- Epidermis
- Dermis

Dandruff
- Excessive scaling
- Thickened epidermis
- Dermis

cells and break down scales which are then washed off while shampooing. Antifungals (p.124) reduce the overgrowth of yeast on the scalp by altering the permeability of the fungal cell walls. Corticosteroids (p.127) help to relieve an itchy rash by reducing inflammation of the underlying skin.

COMMON DRUGS

Antifungals
Ketoconazole ✻
Zinc pyrithione

✻ See Part 4

Other drugs
Coal tar
Corticosteroids
Salicylic acid
Selenium sulfide ✻

DRUGS FOR HAIR LOSS

Hair loss (alopecia) is the result of greater than normal shedding of hairs, or reduced hair production. Hair loss can be caused by a skin condition such as scalp ringworm or scalp psoriasis.

Other forms of hair loss are due to a disorder of the follicles themselves and may be a response to illness, malnutrition, or a reaction to some drugs, such as anticancer drugs or anticoagulants. The hair loss may be diffuse or in a pattern, as in male-pattern baldness which is caused by oversensitivity to testosterone.

Why they are used

If the hair loss is caused by a skin disorder such as scalp ringworm, an antifungal will be used to kill the fungal growth. If male-pattern baldness is a response to the male hormone, testosterone, finasteride could be used to reduce the effect of the hormone. The antihypertensive drug minoxidil can be applied to the scalp to promote hair growth.

How they work

Hair loss can be reversed when the underlying illness is treated, or the drug treatment is stopped. Finasteride, taken by mouth, inhibits conversion of testosterone to its more active form and reduces sensitivity to androgens. The role of minoxidil (p.358) in hair growth is not fully understood, although it is thought to stimulate the hair follicles (see left).

Risks and special precautions

Finasteride can lead to loss of libido or impotence. Anyone with a history of heart disease or hypertension should consult their physician before using minoxidil, as the drug can be absorbed through skin.

HAIR REGROWTH IN MALE-PATTERN BALDNESS

Follicles on the scalp have periods of activity and rest. During the rest phase, the bottom of the hair detaches from the follicle and the hair falls out. Regular applications of minoxidil, the antihypertensive drug, stimulate follicles to produce new hair growth.

Normal hair growth
- Healthy hair
- Skin surface
- Follicle

Thinning hair
- Inactive hair follicle shrinks and no new hair is produced.

Hair regrowth
- Drug is applied to the surface of the scalp.
- Drug is absorbed and stimulates the hair follicle.
- New hair grows from the follicle.

COMMON DRUGS

Antifungals
Ketoconazole ✻
Terbinafine ✻

Other drugs
Minoxidil ✻
Finasteride ✻

✻ See Part 4

SUNSCREENS

Sunscreens and sunblocks are chemicals, usually formulated as creams or oils, that protect the skin from the damaging effects of ultraviolet radiation from the sun.

People vary in their sensitivity to sunlight. Fair-skinned people generally have the least tolerance and tend to burn easily when exposed to the sun, while those with darker skin, especially brown or black skin, can withstand exposure to the sun for longer periods.

In a few cases, the skin's sensitivity to sunlight is increased by a disease such as pellagra (see p.473) or herpes simplex infection. Some drugs, such as thiazide diuretics, phenothiazine antipsychotics, psoralens, sulfonamide antibacterials, tetracycline antibiotics, and nalidixic acid, can also increase the skin's sensitivity.

Apart from sunburn and premature ageing of the skin, the most serious effect from sunlight is skin cancer. Reducing the skin's exposure to sunlight can help to prevent skin cancers.

How they work

Sunlight consists of different wavelengths of radiation. Of these, ultraviolet (UV) radiation is particularly harmful to the skin. UV radiation ages the skin and causes burning. Excessive exposure to UV radiation also increases the risk of developing skin cancer. UV radiation is mainly composed of UVA and UVB rays, both of which age the skin. In addition, UVA rays cause tanning and UVB rays cause burning. Especially vulnerable are fair-skinned people and those being

ACTION OF SUNSCREENS

Fair skin unprotected by a sunscreen suffers damage as ultraviolet rays pass through to the layers beneath, causing pain and inflammation. Sunscreens act by blocking out some of these ultraviolet rays, while allowing a proportion of them to pass through the skin surface to the epidermis to stimulate the production of melanin, the pigment that gives the skin a tan and helps to protect it during further exposure to the sun.

Skin unprotected

- Ultraviolet rays
- Inflamed skin
- Epidermis
- Dermis
- Harmful rays penetrate the skin.

Skin protected by sunscreen

- Ultraviolet rays partly blocked by sunscreen.
- Fewer harmful rays penetrate the skin.

treated with immunosuppressant drugs. Sunscreens absorb some of the UVB radiation, ensuring that less of it reaches the skin. Sunscreens are graded using the Sun Protection Factor (SPF) (see below). Some preparations contain chemicals such as zinc oxide and titanium dioxide, which reflect both UVB and UVA rays; these are often called sunblocks.

A sunscreen is particularly advisable for visitors to tropical, subtropical, and mountainous areas, and for those who wish to sunbathe, because sunscreens can prevent burning while allowing the skin to tan. Sunscreens must be applied before exposure to the sun. People with fair skin should use a sunscreen with a higher SPF than people with darker skin.

Risks and special precautions

Sunscreens only form a physical barrier to the passage of UV radiation. They do not alter the skin to make it more resistant to sunlight. Sunscreen lotions must be applied frequently during exposure to the sun to maintain protection. People who are very fair skinned or are known to be very sensitive to sunlight should never expose their skin to direct sunlight, even if they are using a sunscreen, since not even sunscreens with high SPF values give complete protection.

Sunscreens can irritate the skin and some preparations may cause an allergic rash. People who are sensitive to some drugs, such as procaine and benzocaine and some hair dyes, might develop a rash after applying a sunscreen containing aminobenzoic acid or a benzophenone derivative such as oxybenzone.

SUN PROTECTION FACTORS

Sun protection factor (SPF) refers to the degree of protection given by a sunscreen against sunburn. It is a measure of the amount of UVB radiation a sunscreen absorbs. The higher the number, the greater the protection. The table below shows the major skin types and the minimum SPF recommended for each skin type.

This number only describes the protection against UVB radiation. Some sunscreens protect against UVA radiation as well and these are often called sunblocks. Some preparations carry a "star" classification for the UVA protection they give. The stars do not describe an absolute measure, but indicate a ratio of UVA to UVB protection. Four stars means that the product gives balanced protection against both UVA and UVB. Ratings of 1, 2, or 3 stars mean that the sunscreen has more protection again UVB than UVA.

Skin type	Type 1	Type 2	Type 3	Type 4	Type 5/6
Skin/hair tone	White or light skin, blue eyes, freckles	White or fair skin, fair hair	Medium white skin, brown hair	Olive skin, dark hair and eyes	Brown/ black skin, dark hair and eyes
Sun sensitivity	Always burns, never tans	Burns easily, tans eventually	Tans slowly, burns sometimes	Tans easily, burns occasionally	Very rarely burns
Minimum SPF	SPF 30 +	SPF 25 +	SPF 25	SPF 15 + SPF 25 for vulnerable areas	May not need; SPF 15 if at risk of burning

COMMON DRUGS

Ingredients in sunscreens and sunblocks
Aminobenzoic acid
Avobenzone
Benzophenones
Methyl anthranilate
Mexoryl Sx
Octocrylene
Octyl methoxy-cinnamate
Oxybenzone
Padimate-O
Titanium dioxide
Zinc oxide

4

A–Z
OF DRUGS

**A–Z OF MEDICAL DRUGS
A–Z OF VITAMINS, MINERALS,
AND SUPPLEMENTS
DRUGS OF ABUSE
ALTERNATIVE MEDICINE
DRUGS IN SPORT
MEDICINES AND TRAVEL**

A–Z OF MEDICAL DRUGS

The drug profiles in this section provide information and practical advice on 292 individual drugs. It is intended that the profiles should provide reference and guidance for non-medical readers taking drug treatment. However, it is impossible for this kind of book to take into account every variation in individual circumstances; readers should always follow their physician's or pharmacist's instructions in instances where these differ from the advice in this section.

The drugs have been selected in order to provide representative coverage of the principal classes of drugs in medical use today. For disorders for which a number of drugs are available, the most commonly used drugs have been selected.

Emphasis has also been placed on the drugs likely to be used in the home, although in a few cases drugs administered only in hospital have been included when the drug has been judged to be of sufficient general interest. At the end of this section, there are supplementary profiles on vitamins, minerals, and supplements (pp.468–482), drugs of abuse (pp.483–493), alternative medicine (pp.494–495), drugs in sport (p.496), and medicine and travel (pp.497–499).

Each drug profile is organized in the same way, using standard headings (see sample page, below). To help you make the most of the information provided, the terms used and the instructions given under each heading are discussed and explained on the following pages.

HOW TO UNDERSTAND THE PROFILES

For ease of reference, the information on each drug is arranged in a consistent format under standard headings.

Drug name
Tells you the drug's generic name, brand names under which the drug is marketed, and combined preparations that contain the drug.

General information
Gives you a brief summary of the drug's important characteristics.

Information for users
Practical information on how and when to take the drug, the usual recommended dosage, how soon it takes effect, how long it is active, and advice on diet, storage, and missed doses.

Possible adverse effects
Indicates adverse effects that you may experience with the drug.

Interactions
Tells you how the drug may interact with other drugs or substances taken at the same time.

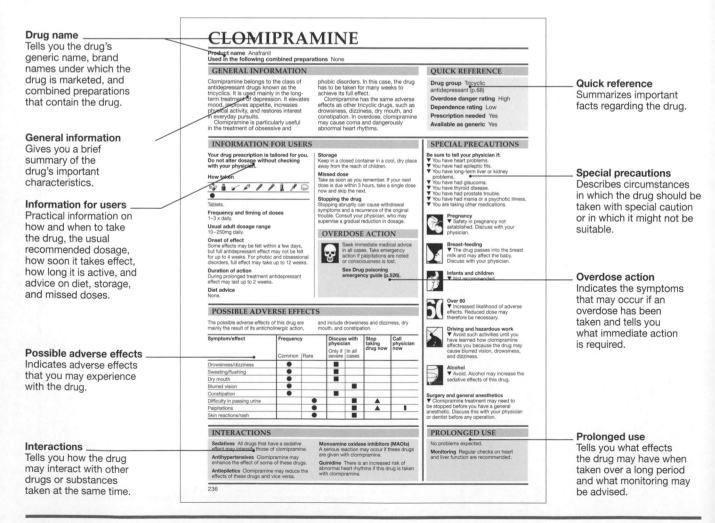

Quick reference
Summarizes important facts regarding the drug.

Special precautions
Describes circumstances in which the drug should be taken with special caution or in which it might not be suitable.

Overdose action
Indicates the symptoms that may occur if an overdose has been taken and tells you what immediate action is required.

Prolonged use
Tells you what effects the drug may have when taken over a long period and what monitoring may be advised.

Generic name

The main heading on the page is the drug's shortest generic name, unless the short name causes confusion with another drug, in which case the full generic name is given. For example, the antimalarial drug proguanil hydrochloride is listed as proguanil because there is no other generic drug of this name. However, magnesium hydroxide, an antacid, is listed under its full name to avoid confusing it with the mineral magnesium or other compounds, such as magnesium sulfate. If the drug has recently been renamed, the old name appears in brackets after the new one.

Brand names

Under the generic name are the brand names of products in which the drug is the major single active ingredient. If there are many different brand names of the drug, only the most commonly used ones are given because of limitations of space. The names of the principal preparations, if any, in which the drug is combined with other drugs, are also listed. For more information about brand names and generic names, see page 13.

AMILORIDE

Product name Midamor
Used in the following combined preparati

GENERAL INFORMATION

GENERAL INFORMATION

The information here gives an overall picture of the drug. It may include notes on the drug's history (for example, when it was first introduced) and the principal disorders for which it is prescribed. This section also discusses the drug's major advantages and disadvantages.

GENERAL INFORMATION

Cyclosporine is one of the immuno-suppressants, a group of drugs that suppress the body's natural defences against infection and foreign cells. This action is of particular use following organ transplants, when the recipient's

QUICK REFERENCE

The text in this box summarizes the important facts regarding your drug, and is organized under five headings, which are explained in detail below.

Drug group

This tells you which of the major groups the drug belongs to, and the page on which you can find out more about the drugs in the group and the various disorders or conditions they are used to treat. Where a drug belongs to more than one group, each group mentioned in the book is listed. For example, interferon is listed as an antiviral drug (p.119) and an anticancer drug (p.140).

Overdose danger rating

Gives an indication of the seriousness of the drug's effects if the dosage prescribed by your physician, or that recommended on the label of an over-the-counter drug, is exceeded. The ratings – low, medium, and high – are

QUICK REFERENCE

Drug group Immunosuppressant drug (p.143)

Overdose danger rating Medium

Dependence rating Low

Prescription needed Yes

explained to the left. The rating also determines the advice given under Exceeding the dose.

- **Low** Symptoms unlikely. Death unknown.
- **Medium** Medical advice needed. Death rare.
- **High** Medical attention needed urgently. Potentially fatal.

If you do exceed the dose, advice is given under Exceeding the dose.

Dependence rating

Drugs are rated low, medium, or high on the basis of the risk of dependence.

- **Low** Dependence unknown.
- **Medium** Rare possibility of dependence.
- **High** Dependence is likely in long-term use.

Prescription needed

This tells you whether or not you need a prescription to obtain the drug. Some drugs are currently having their status reviewed and may soon be available without prescription from the pharmacy counter. Certain other prescription drugs are subject to government regulations (see How drugs are classified, page 13).

Available as generic

Tells you if the drug is available as a generic product.

INFORMATION FOR USERS

This section contains information on the following: administration, i.e., the forms in which the drug is available, dosage frequency and amount, effects and actions, and advice on diet, storage, missed doses, stopping drug treatment, and overdose. All the information is generalized and should not be taken as a recommendation for an individual dosing schedule. Always follow your physician's instructions carefully when taking prescription drugs, and those of your pharmacist or the manufacturer when you buy over-the-counter medications.

How taken

The symbols in the box show how drugs can be administered. The dot below the symbol indicates the form in which a drug is available. This is a visual backup to the written information below the box.

Powder or granules

Liquid medication

Tablets/capsules, slow-release (SR) or modified-release (MR) tablets/ capsules, buccal tablets, dispersible tablets, pastilles, or wafers

Suppository, foam, enema, or bladder irrigation

Injection, implant injection, pen injection, or infusion pump

Cream, ointment, gel, lotion, solution, skin spray, shampoo, or scalp application

Inhaler, powder/capsules for inhaler, or inhalator

Eye, ear, or nose drops

Transdermal patch

INFORMATION FOR USERS continued

Frequency and timing of doses

This refers to the standard number of times each day that the drug should be taken and, where relevant, whether it should be taken with liquid, with meals, or on an empty stomach.

> **Frequency and timing of doses**
> *Relief of pain and fever* Every 4 hours as necessary, with food or milk. (SR-tablets, SR-capsules every 8–12 hours.)
> *Prevention of blood clots* Once daily.

> **Frequency and timing of doses**
> 1–3 x daily with meals.

Usual dosage range

This is generally given as the usual oral dosage range for an adult; dosages for injection are not usually given. In cases where the dosages for specific age groups vary significantly from the normal adult dosage, these will also be given. Where dosage varies according to use, the dosage for each is included.

The vast majority of drug dosages are expressed in metric units, usually milligrams (mg) or micrograms (mcg). In a few, dosage is given in units (u) or international units (IU). See also Weights and measures, facing page.

> **Usual adult dosage range**
> *Prevention of gout attacks* 0.6–1.2mg daily.
> *Relief of gout attacks* 1.0–1.2mg per dose initially, then 0.6mg every 2 hours, up to a maximum of 4–8mg daily until joint is better or gastrointestinal problems arise.

> **Usual dosage range**
> *Adults* 60–180ml daily (liquid); 1.5–9.5g daily (tablets).
> *Children over 6 years* Reduced dose according to age and weight.

Onset of effect

The onset of effect is the time it takes for the drug to become active in the body. This sometimes coincides with the onset of beneficial effects, but there may sometimes be an interval between the time when a drug is pharmacologically active and when you start to notice improvement in your symptoms or your underlying condition.

> **Onset of effect**
> In Parkinson's disease some benefits may be noticed within 1 hour, but full effect may not be felt for up to 2 weeks. In viral infections the severity and duration of symptoms is likely to be reduced during a 2-week course of treatment if the drug is begun within 48 ho

> **Onset of effect**
> 15–60 minutes.

Duration of action

The information given here refers to the length of time that one dose of the drug remains active in the body.

> **Duration of action**
> Up to 6 hours.

> **Duration of action**
> 6–8 hours (tablets, liquid, injection); 10–14 hours (SR-tablets).

Diet advice

With some drugs, it is important to avoid certain foods, either because they reduce the effect of the drug or because they interact adversely. This section of the profile tells you what, if any, dietary changes are necessary.

> **Diet advice**
> It is necessary to drink plenty of water during the 24 hours following treatment to reduce the risk of kidney damage.

Storage

Drugs will deteriorate and may become inactive if they are not stored under suitable conditions. The advice usually given is to store in a cool, dry place out of the reach of children. Some drugs must also be protected from light. Others, especially liquid medications, need to be kept in a refrigerator, but should not be frozen. For further advice on storing drugs, see p.29.

> **Storage**
> Keep in a closed container in a cool, dry place out of the reach of children. Protect from light.

Missed dose

This section gives advice on what to do if you forget a dose of your drug, so that the effectiveness and safety of your treatment is maintained as far as possible. If you forget to take several doses in succession, consult your physician. You can read more about missed doses on p.28.

> **Missed dose**
> Take as soon as your remember. If your next dose is due within 2 hours, take a single dose now and skip the next.

> **Missed dose**
> No cause for concern, but make up the missed dose or application as soon as you remember.

Stopping the drug

If you are taking a drug regularly you should know how and when you can safely stop taking it. Some drugs can be safely stopped as soon as you feel better, or as soon as your symptoms have disappeared. Others must not be stopped until the full course of treatment has been completed, or they must be gradually withdrawn under the supervision of a doctor. Failure to comply with instructions for stopping a drug may lead to adverse effects. It may also cause your condition to worsen or your symptoms to reappear. See also Ending drug treatment, p.28.

> **Stopping the drug**
> Can be safely stopped as soon as you no longer need it.

> **Stopping the drug**
> Do not stop the drug without consulting your physician; stopping the drug may lead to worsening of the underlying condition.

Exceeding the dose

The information in this section expands on that in the quick reference box on the drug's overdose danger rating. It explains possible consequences of exceeding the dose and what to do if an overdose is taken. Examples of wording used for low, medium, and high overdose ratings are:

Low

An occasional extra dose is unlikely to be a cause for concern. But if you notice any unusual symptoms, or if a large overdose has been taken, notify your physician.

Medium

An occasional extra dose is unlikely to cause problems. Large overdoses may cause [symptoms listed]. Notify your physician.

High

Seek immediate medical advice in all cases. Take emergency action if [relevant symptoms listed] occur.

> **Exceeding the dose**
> An occasional unintentional extra dose is unlikely to be a cause for concern. But if you notice any unusual symptoms, or if a large overdose has been taken, notify your physician.

> ### OVERDOSE ACTION
>
> Seek immediate medical advice in all cases. Take emergency action if palpitations are noted or consciousness is lost.
>
> **See Drug poisoning emergency guide (p.526).**

SPECIAL PRECAUTIONS

Many drugs need to be taken with care by people with a history of particular conditions. The profile lists conditions you should tell your physician about when you are prescribed a drug, or about which you should consult your physician or pharmacist before taking an over-the-counter drug. Certain groups of people (pregnant women, breast-feeding mothers, children, and the over 60s) may also be at special risk from drug treatment. Advice for each of these groups is given in every profile. Information is also included about driving, undertaking hazardous work, and drinking alcohol.

SPECIAL PRECAUTIONS

Cyclosporine is prescribed only under close medical supervision, taking account of your present condition and medical history.

Pregnancy
▼ Safety in pregnancy not established. Discuss with your physician.

Breast-feeding
▼ The drug passes into the breast milk and may affect the baby. Discuss with your physician.

Infants and children
▼ Not recommended.

Over 60
▼ No special problems.

Driving and hazardous work
▼ No special problems.

Alcohol
▼ Excessive intake of alcohol may irritate the stomach and increase the risk of bleeding.

WEIGHTS AND MEASURES

Metric equivalents of measurements used in this book:

1,000mcg (microgram) = 1mg (milligram)
1,000mg = 1g (gram)
1,000ml (millilitre) = 1l (litre)

Units or international units
Units (u) and international units (IU) are also used to express drug dosages. They represent the biological activity of a drug (its effect on the body). This ability cannot be measured in terms of weight or volume, but must be calculated in a laboratory.

POSSIBLE ADVERSE EFFECTS

The adverse effects discussed in the drug profile are symptoms or reactions that may arise when you take the drug. The emphasis is on symptoms that you, the patient, are likely to notice, rather than on the findings of laboratory tests that your physician may order. The bulk of the section is in the form of a table that lists the adverse effects and indicates how commonly they occur, when to tell your physician about them, and when to stop the drug. The headings in the table are explained below.

Frequency
Tells you whether the adverse effect is common or rare. Common effects are listed first.

Discuss with physician
The marker in this section indicates under what circumstances you need to inform your physician about an adverse effect you are experiencing.

Only if severe A marker in this column means that the symptom is unlikely to be serious, but that you should seek your physician's advice if it troubles you.
In all cases Adverse effects marked in this column require prompt, but not necessarily emergency, medical attention. (See also Call physician now, below.)

Stop taking drug now
In cases where certain unpleasant or dangerous adverse effects of a drug may override its beneficial effects, you are advised to stop taking the drug immediately, if necessary before seeing your physician.

Call physician now
Effects marked in this column require immediate medical help. They indicate a potentially dangerous response to the drug treatment, for which you should seek emergency medical attention.

Symptom/effect	Frequency		Discuss with physician		Stop taking drug now	Call physician now
	Common	Rare	Only if severe	In all cases		
Indigestion	●			■		
Weight gain		●		■		
Acne		●		■		
Muscle weakness		●		■		
Mood changes		●		■		
Bloody/black feces		●		■	▲	▮

INTERACTIONS

The interactions that are discussed here are those that may occur between the drug under discussion and other drugs. Information includes the name of the interacting drug or group of drugs and the effect of the interaction.

INTERACTIONS

General note Cyclosporine may interact with a large number of drugs. Check with your physician or pharmacist before taking

PROLONGED USE

The information given here concerns the adverse, and sometimes beneficial, effects of the drug that may occur during long-term use. These may differ from those listed under Possible adverse effects. This section of the profile also includes information on monitoring the effects of the drug during long-term treatment, explaining the tests you may be given if your physician thinks they are necessary.

PROLONGED USE

No problems expected from use of calcipotriol in low doses. If the effects of the skin preparation decline after several weeks, they may be regained by suspending use for a few weeks and then recommencing treatment.

Monitoring Regular checks on calcium levels in the blood or urine are required

ACARBOSE

Product name Glucobay
Used in the following combined preparations None

GENERAL INFORMATION

Acarbose is used in Type 2 Diabetes mellitus, usually in combination with other antidiabetic drugs. It inhibits an enzyme, alpha glucosidase, in the intestinal wall, which causes a delay in the breakdown of ingested carbohydrates and thereby reduces blood glucose levels after eating. As it works differently than other antidiabetic agents, it can be used with other antidiabetic drugs.

Acarbose should be taken with the first bite of a meal. To increase tolerability, it should be started once daily, then gradually increased up to three times daily. Common side effects with acarbose are flatulence, diarrhea, and abdominal discomfort. These effects can be minimized by starting with a small dose.

QUICK REFERENCE

Drug group Oral antidiabetic drug (p.128)

Overdose danger rating Medium

Dependence rating Low

Prescription needed Yes

Available as generic No

INFORMATION FOR USERS

Your drug prescription is tailored for you. Do not alter dosage without checking with your physician.

How taken

Tablets.

Frequency and timing of doses
1–3 x daily at mealtimes.

Usual adult dosage range
Starting dose: 25–50mg once daily.
Daily dose: 25–100mg.
Maximum dose: 300mg.

Onset of effect
Peak effect in 1 hour.

Duration of action
2–4 hours.

Diet advice
A diabetic diet will be recommended by your physician. Follow his or her advice.

Storage
Keep in a closed container in a cool, dry place out of the reach of children. Protect from light.

Missed dose
Skip the dose, and take the next dose with a meal. Acarbose should not be taken between meals. Do not take more doses each day than prescribed by your physician.

Stopping the drug
Do not stop the drug without consulting your physician; symptoms may recur.

Exceeding the dose
An occasional unintentional extra dose is unlikely to cause problems. Large overdoses may cause abdominal distension, flatulence, and diarrhea. Drinks and food containing carbohydrates should be avoided for 4–6 hours. If patient was also taking another drug, such as insulin for diabetes, overdose of this may cause low blood sugar. Should symptoms of low blood sugar occur, seek immediate medical advice.

SPECIAL PRECAUTIONS

Be sure to tell your physician if:
▼ You have had an allergic reaction to prandase.
▼ You have inflammation or ulceration of the bowel (Crohn's disease or ulcerative colitis).
▼ You have or have had a bowel obstruction.
▼ You have a kidney disorder.
▼ You have a large hernia.
▼ You are taking any digestive enzymes.
▼ You are taking other medications.

Pregnancy
▼ Safety not established. Discuss with your physician.

Breast-feeding
▼ Safety not established. Discuss with your physician.

Infants and children
▼ Not recommended.

Over 60
▼ Close monitoring may be required.

Driving and hazardous work
▼ Avoid such activities until you have learned how acarbose affects you.

Alcohol
▼ Avoid. Alcoholic drinks may upset diabetic control and increase the risk of hypoglycemia.

POSSIBLE ADVERSE EFFECTS

Adverse events associated with acarbose tend to be mild and transient in nature. The adverse events predominantly affect the skin and gastrointestinal tract.

Symptom/effect	Frequency		Discuss with physician		Stop taking drug now	Call physician now
	Common	Rare	Only if severe	In all cases		
Flatulence/bloating	●		■			
Diarrhea	●		■			
Nausea	●		■			
Abdominal pain/cramps	●			■		

INTERACTIONS

Diuretics, corticosteroids, estrogens, oral contraceptives, phenytoin, and sympathomimetics These drugs can increase blood glucose level and effect diabetic control.

Digestive enzymes These can decrease the effect of acarbose and should be avoided.

Chloestyramine This may enhance the effect of acarbose; monitor closely.

Digoxin Acarbose can effect digoxin absorption; dose adjustment of digoxin may be required.

PROLONGED USE

No problems expected.

Monitoring Regular testing of after-meal blood sugar levels is required.

ACETAMINOPHEN

Product names Abenol, Apo-Acetaminophen, Atasol, Tempra, Tylenol, and many others
Used in the following combined preparations Atasol-8, Dimetapp Nighttime Cold, Dristan, Exdol-15, Tylenol Cold, and others

GENERAL INFORMATION

Although acetaminophen has been known since the early 1900s, it was not widely used as an analgesic until the 1950s. One of a group of drugs known as the non-*opioid* analgesics, it is kept in the home to relieve occasional bouts of mild pain and to reduce fever. It is suitable for children as well as adults.

One of its primary advantages is that it does not cause stomach upset or bleeding problems. This makes it a useful alternative for people who suffer from peptic ulcers or those who cannot tolerate ASA. The drug is also safe for occasional use by those who are being treated with anticoagulants.

Although safe when used as directed, acetaminophen is dangerous when it is taken in overdose, and it is capable of causing serious damage to the liver and kidneys. Large doses of acetaminophen may also be *toxic* if you regularly drink even moderate amounts of alcohol or are malnourished.

INFORMATION FOR USERS

Follow instructions on the label. Call your physician if symptoms worsen.

How taken

Tablets, capsules, liquid, suppositories.

Frequency and timing of doses
Every 4–6 hours as necessary, but not more than 4 doses per 24 hours in children.

Usual dosage range
Adults 325mg–1g per dose up to 4g daily.
Children 60mg (2–3 months for fever after immunization; 2 doses only); 60–120mg per dose (3 months–1 year); 120–250mg per dose (1–5 years); 250–500mg per dose (6–12 years).

Onset of effect
Within 15–60 minutes.

Duration of action
Up to 6 hours.

Diet advice
None.

Storage
Keep in a closed container in a cool, dry place out of the reach of children.

Missed dose
Take as soon as you remember if required to relieve pain. Otherwise do not take the missed dose, and take a further dose only when you are in pain.

Stopping the drug
Can be safely stopped as soon as you no longer need it.

OVERDOSE ACTION

Seek immediate medical advice in all cases. Take emergency action if nausea, vomiting, or stomach pain occur.

See Drug poisoning emergency guide (p.526).

POSSIBLE ADVERSE EFFECTS

Acetaminophen has rarely been found to produce any side effects when taken as recommended. The drug should be stopped and your physician notified if a rash occurs.

Symptom/effect	Frequency		Discuss with physician		Stop taking drug now	Call physician now
	Common	Rare	Only if severe	In all cases		
Nausea	●		■			
Rash	●			■		▲

INTERACTIONS

Anticoagulants such as warfarin may need dosage adjustment if acetaminophen is taken regularly in high doses.

Cholestyramine reduces the absorption of acetaminophen and may reduce its effectiveness.

SPECIAL PRECAUTIONS

Be sure to consult your physician or pharmacist before using this drug if:
▼ You have long-term liver or kidney problems.
▼ You are taking other medications.

 Pregnancy
▼ No evidence of risk with occasional use.

 Breast-feeding
▼ No evidence of risk.

 Infants and children
▼ Infants aged 2–3 months on doctor's advice for post-immunization fever. Reduced dose necessary up to 12 years.

 Over 60
▼ No special problems.

 Driving and hazardous work
▼ No special problems.

 Alcohol
▼ Prolonged heavy intake of alcohol in combination with excess acetaminophen may substantially increase the risk of injury to the liver.

PROLONGED USE

You should not normally take this drug for longer than 48 hours except on the advice of your physician. However, there is no evidence of harm from long-term use.

ACYCLOVIR

Product names Zovirax and others
Used in the following combined preparations None

GENERAL INFORMATION

Acyclovir is an antiviral drug used in the treatment of herpes infections, which can cause cold sores and genital herpes. It is available as a cream, ointment, tablets, and injection. The cream is commonly used to treat cold sores and can be obtained without a prescription. It can speed up the healing of the lesions, provided application is started as soon as symptoms occur and before the lesions appear. Acyclovir tablets and injection are used to treat severe herpes infections, shingles, chickenpox, and genital herpes. The tablets can also be used to prevent the development of herpes infection in people who have reduced immunity.

INFORMATION FOR USERS

Your drug prescription is tailored for you. Do not alter dosage without checking with your physician.

How taken

Tablets, liquid, injection, cream, ointment.

Frequency and timing of doses
2–5 x daily. Start as soon as possible.

Usual adult dosage range
Tablets, liquid 1–4g daily (treatment); 600mg–1g daily (prevention).
Cream, ointment 5 x daily.

Onset of effect
Within 24 hours.

Duration of action
Up to 8 hours.

Diet advice
It is necessary to drink plenty of water when taking high doses by mouth or injection.

Storage
Keep in a closed container in a cool, dry place out of the reach of children. Protect from light.

Missed dose
Tablets/liquid Take as soon as you remember.
Cream, ointment Do not apply the missed dose. Apply your next dose as usual.

Stopping the drug
Complete the full course as directed.

Exceeding the dose
An occasional unintentional extra dose is unlikely to be a cause for concern. But if you notice any unusual symptoms, or if a large overdose has been taken, notify your physician.

SPECIAL PRECAUTIONS

Be sure to tell your physician if:
▼ You have a long-term kidney problem.
▼ You have reduced immunity.
▼ You are taking other medications.

Pregnancy
▼ Topical preparations carry no known risk, but oral and injectable forms are not usually prescribed, as the effects on the developing baby are unknown. Discuss with your physician.

Breast-feeding
▼ No evidence of risk with topical forms. The drug passes into the breast milk following injection or oral administration. Discuss with your physician.

Infants and children
▼ Reduced dose necessary in young children.

Over 60
▼ Reduced dose may be necessary.

Driving and hazardous work
▼ No known problems.

Alcohol
▼ No known problems.

POSSIBLE ADVERSE EFFECTS

Serious *adverse effects* are rare. The cream commonly causes discomfort at the site of application. Confusion and hallucinations occur rarely with injections.

Symptom/effect	Frequency		Discuss with physician		Stop taking drug now	Call physician now
	Common	Rare	Only if severe	In all cases		
Topical applications						
Burning/stinging/itching	●		■			
Rash		●		■	▲	
By mouth						
Nausea/vomiting		●	■			
Headache/dizziness/fatigue		●		■		
Rash		●		■	▲	
Injection						
Inflammation at injection site		●		■		
Confusion/hallucinations		●		■	▲	

PROLONGED USE

Acyclovir is usually given as a single course of treatment and is not given long term, except for people with reduced immunity.

INTERACTIONS (by mouth or injection only)

General note Any drug that affects the kidneys increases the risk of side effects with acyclovir.

Probenecid and cimetidine These drugs may increase the level of acyclovir in the blood.

Mycophenolate mofetil Acyclovir may increase the levels of this drug in the blood and vice versa.

ALENDRONATE

Product name Fosamax
Used in the following combined preparations Fosavance

GENERAL INFORMATION

Alendronate is used to treat osteoporosis in men and post-menopausal women. Alendronate tablets should be taken on getting up in the morning, and swallowed whole with a glass of tap water (mineral water or other drinks should not be used due to a possible negative effect on absorption of the drug). Following this, the individual should remain upright for at least 30 minutes to prevent the drug from staying in the esophagus, where it could cause irritation or, rarely, ulcers. Alendronate should be taken on an empty stomach. Calcium or vitamin D supplements, or other medications and food may be consumed 30 minutes (preferably longer) after taking alendronate.

QUICK REFERENCE

Drug group Drug for bone disorders (p.108)

Overdose danger rating Medium

Dependence rating Low

Prescription needed Yes

Available as generic Yes

INFORMATION FOR USERS

Your drug prescription is tailored for you. Do not alter dosage without checking with your physician.

How taken

Tablets.

Frequency and timing of doses
Once daily, first thing in the morning. Once weekly, first thing in the morning (post-menopausal women).

Usual adult dosage range
Treatment: men and postmenopausal women, 10mg; postmenopausal women may also use 70mg once weekly.
Prevention: 5mg (postmenopausal women).
Prevention and treatment of corticosteroid-induced osteoporosis: 5mg; postmenopausal women not taking HRT, 10mg.

Onset of effect
It may take months to notice an improvement.

Duration of action
Some effects may persist for months or years.

Diet advice
Absorption of alendronate is reduced by foods, especially those containing calcium (e.g. dairy products), so the drug should be taken on an empty stomach. The diet must contain adequate calcium and vitamin D; supplements may be given.

Storage
Keep in a closed container in a cool, dry place out of the reach of children.

Missed dose
Take the next dose at the usual time next morning.

Stopping the drug
Do not stop the drug without consulting your physician. Stopping the drug may lead to worsening of the underlying condition.

Exceeding the dose
An occasional unintentional extra dose is unlikely to cause problems. Large overdoses may cause stomach problems including heartburn, irritation, and ulcers. Notify your physician at once, and try to remain upright.

SPECIAL PRECAUTIONS

Be sure to tell your physician if:
▼ You have an abnormality of the esophagus.
▼ You have any unusual bone pain.
▼ You have stomach problems or a history of ulcers.
▼ You are unable to stand or sit upright for at least 30 minutes.
▼ You have hypocalcemia.
▼ You have kidney impairment.
▼ You are on any other medications.

Pregnancy
▼ Not recommended.

Breast-feeding
▼ Not recommended.

Infants and children
▼ Not recommended.

Over 60
▼ No special problems.

Driving and hazardous work
▼ No special problems.

Alcohol
▼ May cause further stomach irritation.

POSSIBLE ADVERSE EFFECTS

The most frequent adverse effect caused by alendronate is abdominal pain as a result of irritation to the esophagus, stomach, or the small intestine.

Symptom/effect	Frequency		Discuss with physician		Stop taking drug now	Call physician now
	Common	Rare	Only if severe	In all cases		
Abdominal pain/distension	●		■			
Diarrhea/constipation	●		■			
Muscle/bone pain	●			■		
Headache	●		■			
Nausea/vomiting		●	■			
Rash/photosensitivity		●		■		
Eye inflammation/discomfort		●		■		
Jaw pain		●		■	▲	▮

PROLONGED USE

Alendronate is usually prescribed indefinitely for osteoporosis without causing any problems.

Monitoring Blood and urine tests may be carried out at intervals.

INTERACTIONS

Antacids and calcium and iron salts reduce the absorption of alendronate.

ALGINATES/SODIUM ALGINATE

Product name Gaviscon
Used in the following combined preparations Gaviscon Heartburn Relief, Maalox HRF

GENERAL INFORMATION

"Alginates" is a group term that refers to a mixture of acidic compounds extracted from brown algae (seaweeds). When the powder extract is mixed with water, alginates become a thick viscous fluid or gel depending on the chemicals used. Alginates combined with antacids form a "raft" that floats on the surface of the stomach contents, which reduces reflux and protects the lining of the esophagus. Alginates are used to treat mild gastro-esophageal reflux disease. A number of indigestion remedies on sale to the public also contain alginates.

The properties of alginates are also used in wound dressings where, in the form of a woven pad, they absorb fluids from the surface of the wound, keeping it moist and allowing it to heal.

QUICK REFERENCE

Drug group Antacid (p.94)
Overdose danger rating Low
Dependence rating Low
Prescription needed No
Available as generic Yes

INFORMATION FOR USERS

Follow instructions on the label. Call your physician if symptoms worsen.

How taken

Tablets, liquid, powder.

Frequency and timing of doses
4 x daily after meals and at bedtime.

Usual adult dosage range
800-2000mg daily (tablets and liquid).

Onset of effect
10-20 minutes.

Duration of action
3-4 hours.

Diet advice
None.

Storage
Keep in a closed container in a cool, dry place out of the reach of children.

Missed dose
Take as soon as you remember, if you need it.

Stopping the drug
Alginates can be safely stopped as soon as you no longer need them.

Exceeding the dose
Overdose of alginates is likely to produce abdominal distension, without any other symptoms. Notify your physician if symptoms are severe.

POSSIBLE ADVERSE EFFECTS

The antacid salts used in combined oral preparations of alginates may cause abdominal discomfort and distension.

Symptom/effect	Frequency		Discuss with physician		Stop taking drug now	Call physician now
	Common	Rare	Only if severe	In all cases		
Stomach distension	●		■			
Nausea		●	■			

INTERACTIONS

Alginates combined with antacids could affect the absorption of some drugs.

SPECIAL PRECAUTIONS

Be sure to consult your physician or pharmacist before taking this drug if:
▼ You are on a salt-restricted diet.
▼ You are taking any other medications.

 Pregnancy
▼ No evidence of risk to developing baby. Some products can be used for heartburn in pregnancy.

 Breast-feeding
▼ No evidence of risk.

 Infants and children
▼ Reduced dose necessary.

 Over 60
▼ No special problems.

 Driving and hazardous work
▼ No known problems.

 Alcohol
▼ No known problems.

PROLONGED USE

No problems expected.

ALLOPURINOL

Product names Alloprin, Novo-Purol, Zyloprim
Used in the following combined preparations None

GENERAL INFORMATION

Allopurinol is used to prevent gout, which is caused by deposits of uric acid crystals in joints. Allopurinol blocks an enzyme called xanthine oxidase that is involved in forming uric acid. It is also used to lower high uric acid levels (hyperuricemia) caused by other drugs, such as anticancer drugs. Allopurinol should never be started until an acute attack is over because it may cause a further episode. Treatment with the drug should be continued indefinitely to prevent further attacks.

At the start of treatment, an acute attack may occur and colchicine or an anti-inflammatory drug may also be given, until uric acid levels are reduced. If an acute attack occurs while on allopurinol, treatment should continue along with an anti-inflammatory drug.

INFORMATION FOR USERS

Your drug prescription is tailored for you. Do not alter dosage without checking with your physician.

How taken

Tablets.

Frequency and timing of doses
1–3 x daily after food.

Usual adult dosage range
100–300mg daily.

Onset of effect
Within 24–48 hours. Full effect may not be felt for several weeks.

Duration of action
Up to 30 hours. Some effect may last for 1–2 weeks after the drug has been stopped.

Diet advice
A high fluid intake (2 litres of fluid daily) is recommended.

Storage
Keep in a closed container in a cool, dry place out of the reach of children.

Missed dose
If your next dose is not due for another 12 hours or more, take a dose as soon as you remember and take the next one as usual. Otherwise skip the missed dose and take your next dose on schedule.

Stopping the drug
Do not stop the drug without consulting your physician; symptoms may recur.

Exceeding the dose
An occasional unintentional extra dose is unlikely to cause problems. Large overdoses may cause nausea, vomiting, abdominal pain, diarrhea, and dizziness. Notify your physician.

POSSIBLE ADVERSE EFFECTS

Adverse effects of allopurinol are not very common. The most serious is an allergic rash that may require the drug to be stopped and an alternative treatment substituted. Nausea can be avoided by taking allopurinol after food.

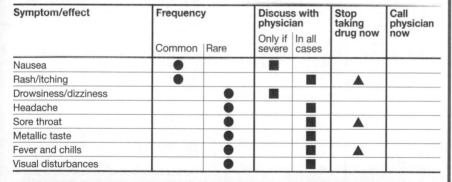

Symptom/effect	Frequency		Discuss with physician		Stop taking drug now	Call physician now
	Common	Rare	Only if severe	In all cases		
Nausea	●		■			
Rash/itching	●			■	▲	
Drowsiness/dizziness		●	■			
Headache		●		■		
Sore throat		●		■	▲	
Metallic taste		●		■		
Fever and chills		●		■	▲	
Visual disturbances		●		■		

INTERACTIONS

ACE inhibitors Allopurinol may increase the effects of these drugs.

ASA Large doses of ASA may reduce the effects of allopurinol.

Anticoagulant drugs Allopurinol may increase the effects of these drugs.

Theophylline Allopurinol may increase levels of this drug.

Mercaptopurine and azathioprine Allopurinol blocks the breakdown of these drugs, requiring a reduction in their dosage.

Chlorpropamide The hypoglycemic effects of chlorpropamide may be increased.

Cyclosporine Allopurinol may increase the effects of this drug.

SPECIAL PRECAUTIONS

Be sure to tell your physician if:
▼ You have long-term liver or kidney problems.
▼ You have had a previous sensitivity reaction to allopurinol.
▼ You have a current attack of gout.
▼ You are taking other medications.

Pregnancy
▼ Safety in pregnancy not established. Discuss with your physician.

Breast-feeding
▼ The drug passes into the breast milk and may affect the baby. Discuss with your physician.

Infants and children
▼ Reduced dose necessary.

Over 60
▼ Reduced dose may be necessary.

Driving and hazardous work
▼ Avoid such activities until you have learned how allopurinol affects you because the drug can cause drowsiness.

Alcohol
▼ Avoid. Alcohol may worsen gout.

PROLONGED USE

Apart from an increased risk of gout in the first weeks or months, no problems are expected.

Monitoring Periodic checks on uric acid levels in the blood and liver function tests are usually performed, and the dose of allopurinol adjusted if necessary.

ALPRAZOLAM

Product names Apo-Alpraz, Novo-Alprazol, Nu-Alpraz, Xanax
Used in the following combined preparations None

GENERAL INFORMATION

Alprazolam belongs to a group of drugs called the benzodiazepines. The actions and adverse effects of this group of drugs are described more fully under Anti-anxiety drugs (p.69).

Alprazolam is indicated for the short-term symptomatic relief of excessive anxiety. It is also used in the treatment of panic disorders and agrophobia (fear of open spaces), other phobias, and anxiety disorders of a general nature.

Panic disorders are characterized by recurrent panic attacks, which may present as periods of intense fear or discomfort.

Like other benzodiazepines, alprazolam can be habit-forming if taken regularly over a long period. Its effects may also grow weaker over time. For these reasons, treatment with alprazolam is reviewed by the physician at regular intervals.

QUICK REFERENCE

Drug group Benzodiazepine anti-anxiety drug (p.67)

Overdose danger rating Medium

Dependence rating High

Prescription needed Yes

Available as generic Yes

INFORMATION FOR USERS

Your drug prescription is tailored for you. Do not alter dosage without checking with your physician.

How taken

Tablets.

Frequency and timing of doses
2–3 x daily.

Usual dosage range
0.75–1.5mg daily. Occasionally, larger doses may be prescribed.

Onset of effect
1–2 hours.

Duration of action
Up to 24 hours.

Diet advice
None.

Storage
Keep in a tightly closed container in a cool, dry place away from reach of children. Protect from light.

Missed dose
No cause for concern, but take when you remember. If your next dose is due within 2 hours, take a single dose now and skip the next one.

Stopping the drug
If you have been taking the drug continuously for less than 2 weeks, it can be safely stopped as soon as you feel you no longer need it. However, if you have been taking it for longer, consult your physician, who may advise a gradual reduction in dosage. Stopping abruptly may lead to withdrawal symptoms.

Exceeding the dose
An occasional unintentional extra dose is unlikely to cause problems. Larger overdoses may cause unusual drowsiness, unsteadiness, or coma. Notify your physician.

SPECIAL PRECAUTIONS

Be sure to consult your physician or pharmacist before taking this drug if:
▼ You have impaired liver or kidney function.
▼ You have myasthenia gravis.
▼ You have glaucoma.
▼ You have had problems with alcohol or drug abuse.
▼ You are taking other medications.

Pregnancy
▼ Safety in pregnancy not established. Discuss with your physician.

Breast-feeding
▼ The drug passes into the breast milk. Its effects on the baby are not clearly known. Discuss with your physician.

Infants and children
▼ Not recommended in patients under 18 years.

Over 60
▼ Increased likelihood of adverse effects. Reduced dose may therefore be necessary.

Driving and hazardous work
▼ Avoid such activities until you have learned how the drug affects you: it can cause reduced alertness, blurred vision, and slowed reactions.

Alcohol
▼ Avoid. Alcohol may increase the sedative effects of this drug.

POSSIBLE ADVERSE EFFECTS

The principal adverse effects of this drug are related to its sedative and tranquilizing properties. These effects normally diminish after the first few days of treatment. If adverse effects persist, they can often be reduced by adjustment of dosage.

Symptom/effect	Frequency		Discuss with physician		Stop taking drug now	Call physician now
	Common	Rare	Only if severe	In all cases		
Drowsiness	●		■			
Dizziness/unsteadiness	●			■		
Blurred vision		●		■		
Forgetfulness/confusion		●		■		
Headache		●	■			
Rash		●		■		
Jaundice		●		■		

INTERACTIONS

Sedatives All drugs that have a sedative effect on the central nervous system are likely to increase the sedative properties of alprazolam. Such drugs include alcohol, sleeping drugs, antihistamines, antidepressants, narcotic analgesics, and antipsychotics.

PROLONGED USE

Regular use of this drug over several weeks can lead to a reduction in its effect as the body adapts. It may also be habit-forming when taken for extended periods, especially if larger-than-average doses are taken.

ALPROSTADIL

Product names Caverject, MUSE, Prostin VR
Used in the following combined preparations None

GENERAL INFORMATION

Alprostadil is a member of the prostaglandin group of drugs and is used to help impotent men to achieve an erection. It is either injected directly into the penis or applied as a gel into the urethra. The most common *side effect* of alprostadil is pain in the penis.

The first dose must be given by medically trained personnel, and self-administration may only be undertaken after proper training.

The drug Prostin VR is also used to treat patent ductus arteriosus, a congenital heart disorder in newborn babies. It works by keeping the ductus blood vessel (normally shut off at birth) open until it can be closed permanently by surgery. It is usually only administered to babies in hospital. Side effects such as heart and respiratory problems are common, and there is a risk of unusual bone growth, particularly after long use.

QUICK REFERENCE

Drug group Prostaglandin and drug for impotence (p.152)
Overdose danger rating Medium
Dependence rating Low
Prescription needed Yes
Available as generic No

INFORMATION FOR USERS

Your drug prescription is tailored for you. Do not alter dosage without checking with your physician.

How taken

Injection, gel.

Frequency and timing of doses
Caverjet up to 3 x per week. Not more than one dose in any 24 hour period.
MUSE no more than 2 doses in 24 hours.

Usual dosage range
Starts at 2.5mcg, individually adjusted by your physician to produce an erection lasting not more than 1 hour.

Onset of effect
Within a few minutes.

Duration of action
Erection should not last more than 1 hour.

Diet advice
None.

Storage
Store in a refrigerator, out of the reach of children. Do not freeze.

Missed dose
Take the next dose when needed. Use no more than one dose in any 24-hour period and no more than 3 doses per week.

Stopping the drug
Can be safely stopped as soon as you no longer need it.

Exceeding the dose
If an unintentional extra dose has been used close to the regular dose, notify your physician. If you notice any unusual symptoms or if a large overdose has been taken, notify your physician.

SPECIAL PRECAUTIONS

Be sure to tell your physician if:
▼ You are taking other medications for impotence.

Pregnancy
▼ Not prescribed.

Breast-feeding
▼ Not prescribed.

Infants and children
▼ Other than Prostin VR for newborn babies, not prescribed.

Over 60
▼ Doses are adjusted individually.

Driving and hazardous work
▼ No special problems.

Alcohol
▼ Excessive use of alcohol with alprostadil can contribute to erectile problems.

POSSIBLE ADVERSE EFFECTS

Breathing difficulties are a side effect of the drug in newborn babies. Less often, it may cause convulsions. In men, there is a risk of prolonged erection. You should report any erection lasting for more than 3 hours to your physician and stop taking the drug immediately.

Symptom/effect	Frequency		Discuss with physician		Stop taking drug now	Call physician now
	Common	Rare	Only if severe	In all cases		
Newborn babies						
Breathing difficulties		●		■		∣
Convulsions		●		■		∣
Men						
Penile pain	●		■			
Bruising/swelling	●			■		
Bleeding	●			■		
Prolonged erection	●			■	▲	∣
Testicular pain/swelling		●		■		
Dizziness/fainting		●		■		
Chest pain/palpitations		●		■		

PROLONGED USE

Prolonged use in newborn babies may cause abnormal bone development and weakening of some blood vessel walls.

Prolonged use for impotence may lead to development of fibrosis of the penis.

Monitoring Regular examinations for penile fibrosis are required.

INTERACTIONS

Antihypertensive and vasodilator drugs
The effects of these drugs may be increased by alprostadil.

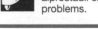

ALUMINUM HYDROXIDE

Product names Amphojel, Basaljel
Used in the following combined preparations Diovol, Gelusil, Maalox, Gaviscon Heartburn Relief Formula, Mucaine, and others

GENERAL INFORMATION

Aluminum hydroxide is a common ingredient of many over-the-counter remedies for indigestion and heartburn. Because the drug is constipating (it is sometimes used to treat diarrhea), it is usually combined with a magnesium-containing antacid with a balancing laxative effect.

The prolonged action of the drug makes it useful in preventing the pain of stomach and duodenal ulcers or heartburn. Aluminum hydroxide can also promote the healing of ulcers. The drug may be more effective as an antacid in liquid form rather than as tablets. Some antacid preparations include large amounts of sodium and these should be used with caution by those on low-sodium diets.

In the intestine, aluminum hydroxide binds with, and thereby reduces the absorption of, phosphate. This makes it helpful in treating high blood phosphate (hyperphosphatemia), which occurs in some people with impaired kidney function. However, prolonged heavy use can lead to phosphate deficiency and a consequent weakening of the bones.

QUICK REFERENCE

Drug group Antacid (p.94)
Overdose danger rating Low
Dependence rating Low
Prescription needed No
Available as generic Yes

INFORMATION FOR USERS

Follow instructions on the label. Call your physician if symptoms worsen.

How taken

Tablets, capsules, liquid (gel suspension). The tablets should be well chewed.

Frequency and timing of doses
As antacid 4–6 x daily as needed, or 1 hour before and after meals.
Peptic ulcer 6–7 x daily.
Hyperphosphatemia 3–4 x daily with meals.
Diarrhea 2–6 x daily.

Usual dosage range
Adults Up to 70ml daily (liquid), 2–10g daily (tablets or capsules).
Children over 6 years Reduced dose according to age and weight.

Onset of effect
Within 15 minutes.

Duration of action
2–4 hours.

Diet advice
For hyperphosphatemia, a low-phosphate diet may be advised in addition to aluminum hydroxide treatment.

Storage
Keep in a closed container in a cool, dry place out of the reach of children.

Missed dose
Do not take the missed dose. Take your next dose as usual.

Stopping the drug
Can be safely stopped as soon as you no longer need it (indigestion). When taken as ulcer treatment or for hyperphosphatemia resulting from kidney failure, do not stop without consulting your physician.

Exceeding the dose
An occasional unintentional extra dose is unlikely to be a cause for concern. But if you notice any unusual symptoms, or if a large overdose has been taken, notify your physician.

SPECIAL PRECAUTIONS

Be sure to consult your physician or pharmacist before taking this drug if:
▼ You have a long-term kidney problem.
▼ You have heart problems.
▼ You have high blood pressure.
▼ You suffer from constipation.
▼ You have a bone disease.
▼ You have porphyria.
▼ You are taking other medications.

 Pregnancy
▼ Safety in pregnancy not established. Discuss with your physician.

 Breast-feeding
▼ No evidence of risk.

 Infants and children
▼ Not recommended under 6 years except on the advice of a physician.

 Over 60
▼ Increased likelihood of adverse effects. Reduced dose may therefore be necessary.

 Driving and hazardous work
▼ No known problems.

 Alcohol
▼ No known problems.

POSSIBLE ADVERSE EFFECTS

Constipation is common with aluminum hydroxide; nausea and vomiting may occur due to the granular, powdery nature of the drug. Bone pain occurs only when large doses have been taken regularly for months or years.

Symptom/effect	Frequency		Discuss with physician		Stop taking drug now	Call physician now
	Common	Rare	Only if severe	In all cases		
Constipation	●		■			
Nausea		●	■			
Vomiting		●		■		

INTERACTIONS

General note Aluminum hydroxide may interfere with the absorption or excretion of many drugs, including oral anticoagulants, digoxin, many antibiotics, penicillamine, corticosteroids, antipsychotics, and phenytoin. It should only be taken at least 2 hours before or after other drugs.

***Enteric*-coated tablets** Aluminum hydroxide may lead to the break-up of the enteric coating of tablets (e.g., bisacodyl, or enteric-coated ASA) before they leave the stomach, leading to stomach irritation.

PROLONGED USE

Aluminum hydroxide should not be used for longer than 4 weeks without consulting your physician. Prolonged use in high doses may deplete blood phosphate and calcium levels, leading to weakening of the bones and fractures.

AMANTADINE

Product name Endantadine, Gen-Amantadine, Symmetrel
Used in the following combined preparations None

GENERAL INFORMATION

Amantadine was first used in the 1960s as an antiviral drug, originally for the prevention and treatment of influenza A. As a preventative against influenza A, it protects some 70 per cent of those not receiving vaccination. As treatment, it is effective in reducing the severity of symptoms when given within 48 hours of the onset of flu. It can also reduce pain following herpes zoster (shingles).

In 1969, amantadine was found to be helpful in *parkinsonism*, except when the condition is caused by drugs. Amantadine usually produces improvement of symptoms during the first few weeks, but its effectiveness wears off over six to eight weeks, requiring replacement by another drug. It is sometimes given with levodopa (see p.326), another drug for parkinsonism.

QUICK REFERENCE

Drug group Drug for parkinsonism (p.71) and antiviral drug (p.119)

Overdose danger rating Low

Dependence rating Low

Prescription needed Yes

Available as generic Yes

INFORMATION FOR USERS

Your drug prescription is tailored for you. Do not alter dosage without checking with your physician.

How taken

Capsules, liquid.

Frequency and timing of doses
1–2 x daily.

Usual dosage range
100–200mg daily.

Onset of effect
In parkinsonism the full effect may not be felt for up to 2 weeks. In viral infections the severity and duration of symptoms is likely to be reduced if the drug is begun within 48 hours of the onset of symptoms.

Duration of action
Up to 24 hours.

Diet advice
None.

Storage
Keep in a closed container in a cool, dry place out of the reach of children.

Missed dose
Take as soon as you remember. If your next dose is due within 2 hours, take a single dose now and skip the next dose.

Stopping the drug
Do not stop taking the drug without consulting your physician; symptoms may recur.

Exceeding the dose
An occasional unintentional extra dose is unlikely to cause problems. But if you notice any unusual symptoms, or if a large overdose has been taken, notify your physician.

SPECIAL PRECAUTIONS

Be sure to tell your physician if:
▼ You have long-term liver or kidney problems.
▼ You have a peptic ulcer.
▼ You have had epileptic fits.
▼ You have heart disease.
▼ You suffer from eczema.
▼ You are taking other medications.

Pregnancy
▼ Safety not established. Discuss with your physician.

Breast-feeding
▼ The drug passes into the breast milk and may affect the baby. Discuss with your physician.

Infants and children
▼ Not usually prescribed. Reduced dose necessary.

Over 60
▼ Increased likelihood of adverse effects. Reduced dose necessary.

Driving and hazardous work
▼ Avoid such activities until you have learned how amantadine affects you because the drug may cause blurred vision, dizziness, inability to concentrate, hallucinations, agaitation, and confusion.

Alcohol
▼ No known problems.

POSSIBLE ADVERSE EFFECTS

Adverse effects are uncommon and often wear off during continued treatment. They are rarely serious enough to require treatment to be stopped.

Symptom/effect	Frequency		Discuss with physician		Stop taking drug now	Call physician now
	Common	Rare	Only if severe	In all cases		
Nervousness/agitation	●		■			
Confusion/hallucinations	●			■		
Insomnia		●	■			
Dizziness		●		■		
Blurred vision		●		■		
Loss of appetite		●		■		
Ankle swelling		●		■		
Rash		●	■		▲	

INTERACTIONS

Anticholinergic drugs Amantadine may add to the effects of *anticholinergic* drugs. In that event your physician will probably reduce the dosage of the anticholinergic drugs.

PROLONGED USE

The beneficial effects of this drug usually diminish during continuous treatment for parkinsonism. When this occurs, another drug may be substituted for or given together with amantadine. Sometimes the effectiveness of amantadine can be restored if it is withdrawn by your physician for a few weeks and later reintroduced.

AMILORIDE

Product name Midamor
Used in the following combined preparations Moduret, Apo-Amilzide and others

GENERAL INFORMATION

Amiloride is a diuretic. It acts on the kidneys to increase the amount of urine that is passed. It is used in the treatment of edema (fluid retention), which can result from heart failure or liver disease and for hypertension (high blood pressure).

Amiloride's effect on urine flow may last for several hours. Preferably, it should be taken in the morning and no later than about 4 pm, otherwise you may need to pass urine during the night.

Amiloride causes the kidneys to conserve potassium (potassium-sparing diuretic) and should not be used when there is a high blood level of potassium. The drug is prescribed with caution in people taking potassium supplements or those with kidney disease. The drug is usually combined with other diuretics.

INFORMATION FOR USERS

Your drug prescription is tailored for you. Do not alter dosage without checking with your physician.

How taken

Tablets.

Frequency and timing of doses
Once daily, usually in the morning.

Usual adult dosage range
5–20mg daily.

Onset of effect
Within 2–4 hours.

Duration of action
12–24 hours.

Diet advice
Avoid foods that are high in potassium – for example, dried fruit, bananas, tomatoes, and salt substitutes.

Storage
Keep in a closed container in a cool, dry place out of the reach of children.

Missed dose
Take as soon as you remember. However, if it is late in the day, do not take the missed dose, or you may need to get up at night to pass urine. Take the next scheduled dose as usual.

Stopping the drug
Do not stop the drug without consulting your physician; symptoms may recur.

Exceeding the dose
An occasional unintentional extra dose is unlikely to be a cause for concern. But if you notice any unusual symptoms, or if a large overdose has been taken, notify your physician.

SPECIAL PRECAUTIONS

Be sure to tell your physician if:
▼ You have long-term liver or kidney problems.
▼ You have diabetes.
▼ You are taking other medications.

Pregnancy
▼ Not usually prescribed. May cause a reduction in the blood supply to the developing baby. Discuss with your physician.

Breast-feeding
▼ Not usually prescribed during breast-feeding. Discuss with your physician.

Infants and children
▼ Not recommended.

Over 60
▼ Increased likelihood of adverse effects. Reduced dose necessary.

Driving and hazardous work
▼ No known problems.

Alcohol
▼ No special problems.

POSSIBLE ADVERSE EFFECTS

Amiloride has few adverse effects; the main problem is the possibility that potassium may be retained by the body, causing muscle weakness and numbness.

Symptom/effect	Frequency		Discuss with physician		Stop taking drug now	Call physician now
	Common	Rare	Only if severe	In all cases		
Digestive disturbance		●	■			
Confusion		●		■		
Muscle weakness/cramps		●		■		
Rash		●		■	▲	
Dry mouth/thirst		●		■		
Dizziness		●		■		

PROLONGED USE

Monitoring Blood tests may be carried out to monitor levels of body salts.

INTERACTIONS

Lithium Amiloride may increase the blood levels of lithium, leading to an increased risk of lithium poisoning.

ACE inhibitors, cyclosporine, and NSAIDs These drugs may increase the risk of potassium retention if taken with amiloride.

AMIODARONE

Product names Apo-Amiodarone, Cordarone, Gen-Amiodarone, Novo-Amiodarone, and others
Used in the following combined preparations None

GENERAL INFORMATION

Introduced in the 1950s, amiodarone is used to treat a variety of abnormal heart rhythms (arrhythmias). It works by slowing nerve impulses in the heart muscle.

Amiodarone is given to prevent recurrent atrial and ventricular fibrillation and to treat ventricular and supraventricular tachycardias and Wolff-Parkinson-White Syndrome. Often the last choice when other treatments have failed, especially for long-term use, it has serious *adverse effects* including liver damage, thyroid problems, and eye and lung damage.

Treatment should be started only under specialist supervision or in hospital and the dosage carefully controlled in order to achieve the desired effect using the lowest possible dose.

QUICK REFERENCE

Drug group Anti-arrhythmic drug (p.86)

Overdose danger rating Medium

Dependence rating Low

Prescription needed Yes

Available as generic Yes

INFORMATION FOR USERS

Your drug prescription is tailored for you. Do not alter dosage without checking with your physician.

How taken

Tablets, injection.

Frequency and timing of doses
3 x daily or by injection initially, then 2 x daily, then 1x every 1 or 2 days (maintenance dose).

Usual adult dosage range
600–800mg daily, reduced gradually. Maintenance dose: 200–400mg

Onset of effect
By mouth, some effects may occur in 72 hours; full benefits may take some weeks to show. By injection, effects may occur within 30 minutes.

Duration of action
Up to 1 month.

Diet advice
None.

Storage
Keep in a closed container in a cool, dry place out of the reach of children. Protect from light.

Missed dose
Take as soon as you remember. If your next dose is due within 12 hours, do not take the missed dose. Take your next dose as usual.

Stopping the drug
Do not stop the drug without consulting your physician; symptoms may recur.

OVERDOSE ACTION

 Seek immediate medical advice in all cases. Take emergency action if palpitations are noted or consciousness is lost.

See Drug poisoning emergency guide (p.526).

POSSIBLE ADVERSE EFFECTS

Amiodarone may cause a greyish skin colour and increase the sensitivity of the skin to sunlight. Patients are advised to use sun block, wear a hat, and cover exposed skin.

Symptom/effect	Frequency		Discuss with physician		Stop taking drug now	Call physician now
	Common	Rare	Only if severe	In all cases		
Liver damage	●			■		
Photosensitivity	●			■		
Visual disturbances	●			■		
Thyroid problems		●		■		
Heart rate disturbances		●		■		
Numb, tingling extremities		●		■		
Shortness of breath/cough		●		■		
Headache/weakness/fatigue		●		■		
Grey skin colour		●		■		
Nausea/vomiting		●	■			

INTERACTIONS

General note Amiodarone can interact with many drugs. Consult your physician or pharmacist before taking other medications. Grapefruit juice can increase levels of oral amiodarone and should be avoided.

Diuretics These cause potassium loss that may increase amiodarone's *toxic* effects.

Other anti-arrhythmic drugs Amiodarone may increase the effects of drugs such as beta blockers, digoxin, diltiazem, or verapmil.

Warfarin Amiodarone may increase the anticoagulant effect of warfarin.

SPECIAL PRECAUTIONS

Be sure to tell your physician if:
▼ You have long-term liver or kidney problems.
▼ You have heart disease.
▼ You have eye disease.
▼ You have a lung disorder such as asthma or bronchitis.
▼ You have a thyroid disorder.
▼ You are sensitive to iodine.
▼ You are taking other medications.

 Pregnancy
▼ Not prescribed. Discuss with your physician.

 Breast-feeding
▼ The drug passes into the breast milk and may affect the baby. Discuss with your physician.

 Infants and children
▼ Not recommended.

 Over 60
▼ Increased likelihood of adverse effects. Reduced dose necessary.

 Driving and hazardous work
▼ Avoid these activities until you have learned how amiodarone affects you because the drug can cause the eyes to be dazzled by bright light.

 Alcohol
▼ No known problems.

PROLONGED USE

Prolonged use of this drug may cause a number of adverse effects on the eyes, lungs, thyroid gland, and liver.

Monitoring A chest X-ray may be taken before treatment starts. Blood tests are done before treatment starts and then every 6 months to check thyroid and liver function. Regular eye examinations are required.

AMITRIPTYLINE

Product name None
Used in the following combined preparation Triavil

GENERAL INFORMATION

Amitriptyline belongs to the tricyclic group of antidepressant drugs. The drug is used mainly for long-term depression. It elevates mood, increases physical activity, improves appetite, and restores interest in everyday activities.

More sedating than similar drugs, amitriptyline is useful when depression is accompanied by anxiety or insomnia.

Taken at night, the drug encourages sleep and helps to eliminate the need for additional sleeping drugs. This drug is sometimes used to treat nocturnal enuresis (bedwetting) in children. It may also be used to treat nerve pain such as postherpetic neuralgia after shingles.

In overdose, amitriptyline may cause coma, fits, and abnormal heart rhythms.

INFORMATION FOR USERS

Your drug prescription is tailored for you. Do not alter dosage without checking with your physician.

How taken

Tablets.

Frequency and timing of doses
1–4 x daily, usually as a single dose at night.

Usual adult dosage range
Depression: 50–200mg daily.
Neuropathic pain: 10–150mg daily.

Onset of effect
Sedation can appear within hours but full antidepressant effect may take 4 weeks.

Duration of action
Antidepressant effect may last for 6 weeks; common adverse effects, only a few days.

Diet advice
None.

Storage
Keep in a closed container in a cool, dry place out of the reach of children. Protect from light.

Missed dose
Take as soon as you remember. If your next dose is due within 3 hours, take a single dose now and skip the next.

Stopping the drug
An abrupt stop can cause withdrawal symptoms and a recurrence of the original trouble. Consult your physician, who may supervise a gradual reduction in dosage.

OVERDOSE ACTION

 Seek immediate medical advice in all cases. Take emergency action if palpitations are noted or consciousness is lost.

See Drug poisoning emergency guide (p.526).

SPECIAL PRECAUTIONS

Be sure to tell your physician if:
▼ You have heart problems.
▼ You have had epileptic fits.
▼ You have long-term liver or kidney problems.
▼ You have glaucoma.
▼ You have prostate trouble.
▼ You have thyroid disease.
▼ You have had mania or a psychotic illness.
▼ You are taking other medications.

 Pregnancy
▼ Safety in pregnancy not established. Discuss with your physician.

 Breast-feeding
▼ The drug passes into the breast milk and may affect the baby. Discuss with your physician.

 Infants and children
▼ Not recommended under 16 years for depression, or under 6 years for enuresis.

 Over 60
▼ Reduced dose may be necessary.

 Driving and hazardous work
▼ Avoid such activities until you have learned how amitriptyline affects you because the drug may cause blurred vision and reduced alertness.

 Alcohol
▼ Avoid. Alcohol may increase the sedative effects of this drug.

Surgery and general anesthetics
▼ Amitriptyline treatment may need to be stopped before you have a general anesthetic. Discuss this with your physician or dentist before any operation.

POSSIBLE ADVERSE EFFECTS

The possible adverse effects of this drug are mainly the result of its *anticholinergic* action and its blocking action on the transmission of signals through the heart.

Symptom/effect	Frequency		Discuss with physician		Stop taking drug now	Call physician now
	Common	Rare	Only if severe	In all cases		
Drowsiness	●		■			
Sweating	●		■			
Dry mouth/constipation	●		■			
Blurred vision	●			■		
Dizziness/fainting	●			■		
Difficulty passing urine		●		■	▲	
Sore throat		●		■	▲	
Palpitations		●		■	▲	■

INTERACTIONS

Monoamine oxidase inhibitors (MAOIs)
In the rare cases where these drugs are given with amitriptyline, there is a possibility of serious interactions.

Antiepileptics The effects of these drugs are reduced by amitriptyline as it lowers the fit threshold.

Sedatives All drugs that have *sedative* effects intensify those of amitriptyline.

Antiarrhythmic drugs There is an increased risk of abnormal heart rhythms when these drugs are taken with amitriptyline. Cimetidine, SSRIs, and beta blockers may increase amitriptyline levels.

PROLONGED USE

No problems expected.

AMLODIPINE

Product name Norvasc
Used in the following combined preparations Caduet

GENERAL INFORMATION

Amlodipine belongs to a group of drugs known as calcium channel blockers, which interfere with the conduction of signals in the muscles of the heart and blood vessels.

Amlodipine is used in the treatment of angina to help prevent attacks of chest pain. Unlike some other anti-angina drugs (such as beta blockers), it can be used safely by asthmatics and noninsulin-dependent diabetics.

Amlodipine is also used to reduce raised blood pressure (hypertension).

In common with other drugs of its class, amlodipine may cause blood pressure to fall too low at the start of treatment. In rare cases, angina may become worse at the start of amlodipine treatment. The drug may sometimes cause mild to moderate leg and ankle swelling.

QUICK REFERENCE

Drug group Anti-angina drug (p.87), antihypertensive drug (p.88)
Overdose danger rating Medium
Dependence rating Low
Prescription needed Yes
Available as generic No

INFORMATION FOR USERS

Your drug prescription is tailored for you. Do not alter dosage without checking with your physician.

How taken

Tablets.

Frequency and timing of doses
Once daily.

Usual adult dosage range
5–10mg daily.

Onset of effect
6–12 hours.

Duration of action
24 hours.

Diet advice
None.

Storage
Keep in a closed container in a cool, dry place out of the reach of children.

Missed dose
If you miss a dose and you remember it within 12 hours, take it as soon as you remember. However, if you do not remember until later, do not take the missed dose and do not double up the next one. Instead, go back to your regular schedule.

Stopping the drug
Do not stop taking the drug without consulting your physician; stopping the drug may lead to worsening of the underlying condition.

Exceeding the dose
An occasional unintentional extra dose is unlikely to cause problems. Large overdoses may cause a marked lowering of blood pressure. Notify your physician immediately.

SPECIAL PRECAUTIONS

Be sure to tell your physician if:
▼ You have long-term liver or kidney problems.
▼ You have heart failure.
▼ You have diabetes.
▼ You are taking other medications.

Pregnancy
▼ Safety in pregnancy not established. Discuss with your physician.

Breast-feeding
▼ It is not known if the drug passes into the breast milk. Discuss with your physician.

Infants and children
▼ Not recommended.

Over 60
▼ No special problems.

Driving and hazardous work
▼ Avoid such activities until you have learned how amlodipine affects you because the drug can cause dizziness owing to lowered blood pressure.

Alcohol
▼ Avoid. Alcohol may further reduce blood pressure, causing dizziness or other symptoms.

PROLONGED USE

No problems expected.

POSSIBLE ADVERSE EFFECTS

Amlodipine can cause a variety of minor adverse effects, including leg and ankle swelling, headache, dizziness, fatigue, and nausea. Dizziness, especially on rising, may be the result of an excessive reduction in blood pressure. The most serious effect is the rare possibility of angina becoming worse after starting amlodipine treatment. This should be reported to your physician.

Symptom/effect	Frequency		Discuss with physician		Stop taking drug now	Call physician now
	Common	Rare	Only if severe	In all cases		
Leg and ankle swelling	●			■		
Headache	●			■		
Dizziness/fatigue	●			■		
Flushing	●			■		
Nausea/abdominal pain		●		■		
Palpitations		●		■		
Worsening of angina		●		■	▲	■
Skin rash		●	■		▲	
Breathing difficulties		●		■	▲	

INTERACTIONS

Beta blockers Amlodipine may increase the effect of these drugs and vice versa.

AMOXICILLIN

Product names Apo-Amoxi, Gen-Amoxicillin, and others
Used in the following combined preparations Clavulin, Hp-PAC

GENERAL INFORMATION

Amoxicillin is a penicillin antibiotic. It is prescribed to treat a variety of infections, but is particularly useful for treating ear, nose, and throat infections, respiratory tract infections, cystitis, and uncomplicated gonorrhea. The drug is absorbed well by the body when taken orally.

Amoxicillin can cause minor stomach upsets and a skin rash. It can also provoke a severe allergic reaction with fever, swelling of the mouth and tongue, itching, and breathing difficulties. This suggests that the patient is allergic to penicillin antibiotics.

QUICK REFERENCE

Drug group Penicillin antibiotic (p.116)

Overdose danger rating Low

Dependence rating Low

Prescription needed Yes

Available as generic Yes

INFORMATION FOR USERS

Your drug prescription is tailored for you. Do not alter dosage without checking with your physician.

How taken

Tablets, capsules, powder (dissolved in water)

Frequency and timing of doses
Normally 3 x daily.

Usual dosage range
Adults 750mg–1.5g daily. In some cases a short course of up to 6g daily is given. A single dose of 3g may be given as a preventative.
Children Reduced dose according to age and weight.

Onset of effect
1–2 hours.

Duration of action
Up to 8 hours.

Diet advice
None.

Storage
Keep in a closed container in a cool, dry place out of the reach of children.

Missed dose
Take as soon as you remember. Take your next dose at the scheduled time.

Stopping the drug
Take the full course. Even if you feel better, the original infection may still be present and symptoms may recur if treatment is stopped too soon.

Exceeding the dose
An occasional unintentional extra dose is unlikely to be a cause for concern. But if you notice any unusual symptoms, or if a large overdose has been taken, notify your physician.

SPECIAL PRECAUTIONS

Be sure to tell your physician if:
▼ You have a long-term kidney problem.
▼ You have an allergy (for example, asthma, hay fever, or eczema).
▼ You have had a previous allergic reaction to a penicillin or cephalosporin antibiotic.
▼ You have ulcerative colitis.
▼ You have glandular fever.
▼ You have chronic leukemia.
▼ You are taking other medications.

Pregnancy
▼ No evidence of risk.

Breast-feeding
▼ The drug passes into the breast milk, but at normal doses adverse effects on the baby are unlikely. Discuss with your physician.

Infants and children
▼ Reduced dose necessary.

Over 60
▼ No known problems.

Driving and hazardous work
▼ No known problems.

Alcohol
▼ No known problems.

POSSIBLE ADVERSE EFFECTS

If you develop a rash, wheezing, itching, fever, or joint swelling, this may indicate an allergy. Call your physician, who may prescribe a different antibiotic.

Symptom/effect	Frequency		Discuss with physician		Stop taking drug now	Call physician now
	Common	Rare	Only if severe	In all cases		
Rash	●			■	▲	
Diarrhea	●			■		
Nausea/vomiting		●	■			
Wheezing		●		■	▲	▮
Itching		●		■	▲	▮
Swollen mouth/tongue		●		■	▲	▮

INTERACTIONS

Oral contraceptives Amoxicillin may reduce the effectiveness of the oral contraceptive pill and also increase the risk of breakthrough bleeding. Discuss with your physician.

Anticoagulant drugs Amoxicillin may alter the anticoagulant effect of these drugs so patients may have to be monitored more closely.

PROLONGED USE

Amoxicillin is usually given only for short courses of treatment.

AMPHOTERICIN

Product names Abelcet, AmBisome, Fungizone
Used in the following combined preparations None

GENERAL INFORMATION

Amphotericin is a highly effective and powerful antifungal drug. When given by injection, it is used to treat serious *systemic* fungal infections. It is also given by mouth to treat candida (thrush) infections of the mouth or intestines, but it is not used in vaginal candidiasis. Treatment administered by injection is carefully supervised, usually in hospital, because of potentially serious *adverse effects*. A test dose for allergy may be given before a full injection. The new, recently introduced formulations of this drug appear to be less toxic than the original injection. Adverse reactions to the oral forms are rare.

QUICK REFERENCE

Drug group Antifungal drug (p.124)
Overdose danger rating Low (oral)
Dependence rating Low
Prescription needed Yes
Available as generic No

INFORMATION FOR USERS

Your drug prescription is tailored for you. Do not alter dosage without checking with your physician.

How taken

Lozenges, liquid, injection.

Frequency and timing of doses
Every 6 hours (by mouth); daily, usually over a 6-hour period (injection).

Usual dosage range
400–800mg daily (tablets and liquid); 40–80mg daily (lozenges); the dosage for injection is determined individually.

Onset of effect
Improvement may be noticed after 2–4 days.

Duration of action
3–6 hours.

Diet advice
When given by injection, this drug may reduce the levels of potassium and magnesium in the blood. To correct this, mineral supplements may be recommended.

Storage
Keep in a closed container in a cool, dry place out of the reach of children. Some brands of injection should be stored in the fridge.

Missed dose
Take oral dose as soon as you remember. Take your next dose when scheduled.

Stopping the drug
Take the full course as prescribed. Even if symptoms improve, the original infection may still be present and symptoms may recur if treatment is stopped too soon.

Exceeding the dose
An occasional unintentional extra oral dose is unlikely to be a cause for concern. But if you notice unusual symptoms, notify your physician.

SPECIAL PRECAUTIONS

Be sure to tell your physician if:
▼ You have a long-term kidney problem.
▼ You have previously had an allergic reaction to amphotericin.
▼ You are taking other medications.

Pregnancy
▼ There is no evidence of risk from the oral forms of the drug. Injections are given only when the infection is very serious.

Breast-feeding
▼ No evidence of risk from oral forms of the drug. It is not known whether the drug passes into the breast milk when given by injection. Discuss with your physician.

Infants and children
▼ Reduced dose may be necessary.

Over 60
▼ No special problems.

Driving and hazardous work
▼ No known problems.

Alcohol
▼ No known problems.

POSSIBLE ADVERSE EFFECTS

Amphotericin is given by injection only under close medical supervision. Adverse effects are thus carefully monitored and promptly treated. Adverse effects from oral administration are rare.

Symptom/effect	Frequency		Discuss with physician		Stop taking drug now	Call physician now
	Common	Rare	Only if severe	In all cases		
Injection						
Pain at injection site	●			■		
Nausea/vomiting	●			■		
Headache/fever	●			■		
Unusual bleeding		●		■		
Muscle and joint pain		●		■		
Indigestion/abdominal pain		●		■		

INTERACTIONS (INJECTION ONLY)

Digoxin Amphotericin may increase the *toxicity* of digoxin.

Diuretics Amphotericin increases the risk of low potassium levels with diuretics.

Aminoglycoside antibiotics Taken with amphotericin, these drugs increase the likelihood of kidney damage.

Corticosteroids may increase loss of potassium from the body caused by amphotericin.

Cyclosporine increases the likelihood of kidney damage.

PROLONGED USE

Given by injection, the drug may cause a reduction in blood levels of potassium and magnesium. It may also damage the kidneys and cause blood disorders.

Monitoring Regular blood tests to monitor liver and kidney function, blood cell counts, and potassium and magnesium levels are advised during treatment by injection.

ANAKINRA

Product name Kineret
Used in the following combined preparations None

GENERAL INFORMATION

Anakinra may be used alone, or with other medications, to decrease the pain and swelling associated with moderate to severe rheumatoid arthritis (RA). This class of medications, called biologic response modifiers, works by blocking receptors for interleukins, which are mediators released in the body and can cause inflammation.

Anakinra is administered by subcutaneous injection, usually in the outer thigh, back of arms, stomach, or buttocks. It can be self-administered. The syringes should not be shaken prior to use and should not used if there is any discoloration. While on anakinra, patients should consult their physician before receiving any vaccinations such as the flu shot.

INFORMATION FOR USERS

Your drug prescription is tailored for you. Do not alter dosage without checking with your physician.

How taken

Parenteral (subcutaneous injection).

Frequency and timing of doses
Once daily.

Usual adult dosage range
100mg daily.

Onset of effect
Several weeks to see full benefit.

Duration of action
Up to 24 hours.

Diet advice
None.

Storage
Store in refrigerator, but do not freeze. Keep away from light. Keep in a closed container and out of the reach of children.

Missed dose
If you miss a dose, take it as soon as you remember. If it is near the time of the next dose, skip the missed dose and resume your usual dosing schedule. Do not double up to catch up on a missed dose.

Stopping the drug
Do not stop the drug without consulting your physician. Stopping the drug may lead to worsening of the underlying condition.

Exceeding the dose
Overdosage is unlikely since treatment is monitored closely. If an extra dose is administered, notify your physician immediately.

SPECIAL PRECAUTIONS

Be sure to tell your physician if:
▼ You have infections, asthma, HIV, or kidney disease.
▼ You are considering getting vaccinations, such as the flu shot.
▼ You have allergy to proteins from bacterial cells (E-coli) or latex.
▼ You are taking other medications.

 Pregnancy
▼ Not usually prescribed. Discuss with your physician.

 Breast-feeding
▼ Safety not established. Discuss with your physician.

 Infants and children
▼ Safety not established.

 Over 60
▼ A reduced dose may be needed depending on kidney function.

 Driving and hazardous work
▼ No special problems.

 Alcohol
▼ No special problems.

POSSIBLE ADVERSE EFFECTS

Common side effects relate to redness and pain at the site of injection. If you develop a fever or sore throat while on this medication, contact your physician right away.

Symptom/effect	Common	Rare	Only if severe	In all cases	Stop taking drug now	Call physician now
Redness, swelling, pain at injection site	●		■			
Headache	●		■			
Upset stomach	●		■			
Diarrhea	●		■			
Runny nose	●		■			
Infection		●		■	▲	■
Stomach pain		●	■			
Flu-like symptoms		●		■		■
Rash		●		■		■
Fever, sore throat, chills		●		■		■
Coughing, wheezing, chest pain		●		■		■

INTERACTIONS

Etanercept, adalimumab, infliximab
Anakinra should not be used with these types of agents, due to a greater risk of infection.

Vaccinations Vaccinations may not be effective if patient is on anakinra. Discuss with physician prior to receiving any vaccinations.

PROLONGED USE

This medication should be reassessed periodically.

ANASTROZOLE

Product name Arimidex
Used in the following combined preparations None

GENERAL INFORMATION

Anastrozole is a potent non-steroidal inhibitor of the enzymes that manufacture estradiol (natural estrogen) in the body. It can reduce production of estradiol by more than 80 per cent. Anastrozole is used in the treatment of breast cancer in post-menopausal women. It has not been proved to have any effect in cancers that do not have estrogen receptors. It is not used in premenopausal women and is contraindicated in pregnancy and breast-feeding.

Anastrozole is generally well tolerated; adverse effects are mainly gastrointestinal or gynecological, and are generally similar to menopausal symptoms. If there is any doubt about whether the woman to be treated is post-menopausal, a biochemical test will be performed.

QUICK REFERENCE

Drug group Anticancer drug (p.140)
Overdose danger rating Low
Dependence rating Low
Prescription needed Yes
Available as generic No

INFORMATION FOR USERS

Your drug prescription is tailored for you. Do not alter dosage without checking with your physician.

How taken

Tablets.

Frequency and timing of doses
Once daily.

Usual adult dosage range
1mg.

Onset of effect
30 minutes.

Duration of action
24 hours.

Diet advice
None.

Storage
Keep in a closed container in a cool, dry place out of the reach of children.

Missed dose
Take as soon as you remember. If your next dose is due within 2 hours, take a single dose now and skip the next.

Stopping the drug
Do not stop the drug without consulting your physician. Stopping the drug may lead to worsening of the underlying condition.

Exceeding the dose
An occasional unintentional extra dose is unlikely to be a cause for concern. But if you notice any unusual symptoms, or a large overdose has been taken, notify your physician.

POSSIBLE ADVERSE EFFECTS

Anastrozole is usually well tolerated, and any side effects are relatively minor.

Symptom/effect	Frequency		Discuss with physician		Stop taking drug now	Call physician now
	Common	Rare	Only if severe	In all cases		
Hot flushes	●		■			
Headache/fatigue/dizziness	●		■			
Joint pain/stiffness		●	■			
Vaginal dryness		●	■			
Rash/hair thinning		●	■			
Nausea/constipation		●	■			

INTERACTIONS

Tamoxifen and estrogens may oppose the effects of anastrozole.

SPECIAL PRECAUTIONS

Be sure to tell your physician if:
▼ You are premenopausal.
▼ You have kidney or liver problems.
▼ You are allergic to anastrozole.
▼ You are taking other medications.

Pregnancy
▼ Not prescribed in pregnancy.

Breast-feeding
▼ Not prescribed when breast-feeding.

Infants and children
▼ Not recommended.

Over 60
▼ No special problems.

Driving and hazardous work
▼ Do not drive until you know how the drug affects you. It can cause drowsiness.

Alcohol
▼ No known problems.

PROLONGED USE

No known problems.

Monitoring Women with osteoporosis or at risk of osteoporosis will have their bone mineral density assessed at the start of treatment and at regular intervals.

ASA (ACETYLSALICYLIC ACID)

Product names Aspirin, Coated Aspirin, Entrophen, Novasen
Used in the following combined preparations Fiorinal, Midol, 222 Tablets, Norgesic, Robaxisal, Percodan, and others

GENERAL INFORMATION

In use for over 80 years, ASA relieves pain, reduces fever, and alleviates the symptoms of arthritis. In low doses, it helps to prevent blood clots, particularly in atherosclerosis or angina due to coronary artery disease, and it reduces the risk of heart attacks and strokes.

It is present in many medicines for colds, flu, headaches, menstrual period pains, and joint or muscular aches.

ASA may irritate the stomach and cause stomach ulcers or bleeding. Coated ASA can minimize stomach upsets.

ASA can also provoke asthma attacks, and, in children, can cause Reye's syndrome, a rare but serious brain and liver disorder. For this reason, ASA should not be given to children under the age of 16 years, except on the advice of a physician.

INFORMATION FOR USERS

Follow instructions on the label. Call your physician if symptoms worsen.

How taken

Tablets, suppositories.

Frequency and timing of doses
Relief of pain or fever Every 4–6 hours, as necessary, with or after food or milk.
Prevention of blood clots Once daily.

Usual adult dosage range
Relief of pain or fever 300–900mg per dose.
Prevention of blood clots 75–300mg daily.

Onset of effect
30–60 minutes (regular aspirin); 1½–8 hours (coated tablets or SR-capsules).

Duration of action
Up to 12 hours. Effect persists for several days when used to prevent blood clotting.

Diet advice
Take with or immediately after food.

Storage
Keep in a closed container in a cool, dry place out of the reach of children.

Missed dose
Take as soon as you remember. If your next dose is due within 2 hours, take a single dose now and skip the next.

Stopping the drug
If you have been prescribed ASA by your physician for a long-term condition, you should seek medical advice before stopping the drug. Otherwise it can be safely stopped.

OVERDOSE ACTION

Seek immediate medical advice in all cases. Take emergency action if there is restlessness, stomach pain, ringing noises in the ears, blurred vision, or vomiting.

See Drug poisoning emergency guide (p.526).

POSSIBLE ADVERSE EFFECTS

Adverse effects are more likely to occur with high doses of ASA, but may be reduced by taking the drug with food or in buffered or enteric coated forms.

Symptom/effect	Frequency		Discuss with physician		Stop taking drug now	Call physician now
	Common	Rare	Only if severe	In all cases		
Indigestion	●		■		▲	
Nausea/vomiting		●		■		
Rash		●		■	▲	
Breathlessness/wheezing		●		■	▲	
Blood in vomit/black feces		●		■	▲	▮
Ringing in the ears/dizziness		●	■		▲	▮

INTERACTIONS

Anticoagulants ASA may add to the anticoagulant effect of such drugs, leading to an increased risk of abnormal bleeding.

Drugs for gout ASA may reduce the effect of these drugs.

Corticosteroids These drugs may increase the risk of stomach bleeding with ASA.

NSAIDs These drugs may increase the likelihood of stomach irritation with ASA.

Methotrexate ASA may increase the *toxicity* of this drug.

Oral antidiabetic drugs ASA may increase the effect of these drugs.

SPECIAL PRECAUTIONS

Be sure to consult your physician or pharmacist before taking this drug if:
▼ You have long-term liver or kidney problems.
▼ You have asthma.
▼ You are allergic to ASA.
▼ You have a blood clotting disorder.
▼ You have had a stomach ulcer.
▼ You are taking other medications.

Pregnancy
▼ Not usually recommended. An alternative drug may be safer. Discuss with your physician.

Breast-feeding
▼ The drug passes into the breast milk. Discuss with your physician.

Infants and children
▼ Do not give to children under 16 years, except on a physician's advice.

Over 60
▼ Adverse effects more likely.

Driving and hazardous work
▼ No special problems.

Alcohol
▼ Avoid. Alcohol increases the likelihood of stomach irritation with this drug.

Surgery and general anesthetics
▼ Regular treatment with ASA may need to be stopped about one week before surgery. Discuss with your physician or dentist before any operation.

PROLONGED USE

Except for low doses to help prevent blood clotting, ASA should not be taken for longer than 2 days except on your physician's advice. Prolonged use of ASA may lead to bleeding in the stomach and to stomach ulcers.

ATENOLOL

Product names Apo-Atenol, Tenormin, Novo-Atenol, and others
Used in the following combined preparations Tenoretic

GENERAL INFORMATION

Atenolol belongs to the group of drugs known as beta blockers. It prevents the heart from beating too quickly and is used mainly to treat chest pain (angina), and high blood pressure (hypertension).

Atenolol is a cardioselective beta blocker (see p.83) and is less likely to provoke breathing difficulties, but it should still be used with caution by people with asthma, bronchitis, or other forms of respiratory disease. Atenolol is sometimes prescribed with a diuretic for high blood pressure, and may also be given after a heart attack to protect the heart from further damage.

Atenolol does not cure heart disease, it only controls the symptoms, so it usually has to be taken long term.

QUICK REFERENCE

Drug group Beta blocker (p.83)
Overdose danger rating Medium
Dependence rating Low
Prescription needed Yes
Available as generic Yes

INFORMATION FOR USERS

Your drug prescription is tailored for you. Do not alter dosage without checking with your physician.

How taken

Tablets.

Frequency and timing of doses
Once daily.

Usual adult dosage range
25–100mg daily.

Onset of effect
2–4 hours.

Duration of action
20–30 hours.

Diet advice
None.

Storage
Keep in a tightly closed container in a cool, dry place out of the reach of children. Protect from light.

Missed dose
Take as soon as you remember. If your next dose is due within 6 hours, do not take the missed dose but take the next scheduled dose as usual.

Stopping the drug
Do not stop taking the drug without consulting your physician; sudden withdrawal may lead to dangerous worsening of the underlying condition. It should be withdrawn gradually.

Exceeding the dose
An occasional unintentional extra dose is unlikely to be a cause for concern. But if you notice any unusual symptoms, or if a large overdose has been taken, notify your physician.

SPECIAL PRECAUTIONS

Be sure to tell your physician if:
▼ You have any other heart condition.
▼ You have a long-term kidney problem.
▼ You have diabetes.
▼ You have a lung disorder such as asthma or bronchitis.
▼ You are taking other medications.

Pregnancy
▼ Safety in pregnancy not established. Discuss with your physician.

Breast-feeding
▼ The drug passes into the breast milk. Discuss with your physician.

Infants and children
▼ Not recommended.

Over 60
▼ No special problems. Reduced dose may be necessary if there is impaired kidney function.

Driving and hazardous work
▼ Avoid such activities until you have learned how atenolol affects you because the drug can cause dizziness.

Alcohol
▼ No special problems with small intake.

Surgery and general anesthetics
▼ Atenolol may need to be stopped before you have a general anesthetic. Discuss this with your physician or dentist before any surgery.

POSSIBLE ADVERSE EFFECTS

Atenolol has adverse effects that are common to most beta blockers. Symptoms are usually temporary and tend to diminish with long-term use.

Symptom/effect	Frequency		Discuss with physician		Stop taking drug now	Call physician now
	Common	Rare	Only if severe	In all cases		
Muscle ache	●		■			
Fatigue/dry eyes	●			■		
Cold hands and feet		●	■			
Nightmares/sleeplessness		●	■			
Headache		●		■		
Rash		●		■	▲	
Breathing difficulties		●		■	▲	■
Dizziness		●		■		

INTERACTIONS

Anti-arrhythmic drugs When used together with atenolol they may increase the risk of adverse effects on the heart.

Antidiabetic drugs including insulin used with atenolol may increase the risk and/or mask many symptoms of low blood sugar.

Decongestants used with atenolol may increase blood pressure and heart rate.

Calcium channel blockers Taken with atenolol, some of these drugs may further decrease blood pressure and/or heart rate. They may also reduce the force of the heart's pumping action.

Non-steroidal anti-inflammatory drugs (NSAIDs) may reduce the antihypertensive effect of atenolol.

PROLONGED USE

No special problems expected.

ATOMOXETINE

Product name Strattera
Used in the following combined preparations None

GENERAL INFORMATION

Atomoxetine is a drug prescribed for adolescents and adults with attention-deficit hyperactivity disorder (ADHD). It can also be used in children 6 years of age or older. Studies indicate that after 6–12 weeks of treatment this drug can decrease some of the symptoms of ADHD in about 70% of cases. It is not a stimulant and may be an option in those who have not responded to, or are not able to tolerate, the stimulant class of drugs. Dosing in children is based on the individual's weight. The starting dose may be gradually increased as appropriate. It may take 3–4 weeks of regular use to start to see a benefit. It should be used cautiously in those with heart problems, high blood pressure, or uncontrolled overactive thyroid. It may also affect a child's growth and weight. Benefits and risks should be discussed with a physician prior to starting therapy.

QUICK REFERENCE

Drug group Drug used in attention-deficit hyperactivity disorder (ADHD) (for other drugs for ADHD, see p.72)
Overdose danger rating High
Dependence rating Low
Prescription needed Yes
Available as generic No

INFORMATION FOR USERS

Your drug prescription is tailored for you. Do not alter dosage without checking with your physician.

How taken

Capsules.

Frequency and timing of doses
Usually once or twice daily.

Usual adult dosage range
Initial dose: 40mg daily to start; may increase gradually as appropriate; maximum 100mg/day.

Onset of effect
3–4 weeks; full beneficial effects take 6–12 weeks.

Duration of action
Up to 24 hours.

Diet advice
None.

Storage
Keep in a closed container in a cool, dry place out of the reach of children.

Missed dose
If you miss a dose, take it as soon as you remember. If it is near the time of the next dose, skip the missed dose and resume your usual dosing schedule. Do not take more than the total daily dose.

Stopping the drug
Do not stop the drug without consulting your physician. Stopping the drug may lead to worsening of the underlying condition.

OVERDOSE ACTION

Seek immediate medical advice in all cases. Take emergency action if loss of consciousness occurs.

See Drug poisoning emergency guide (p.526).

SPECIAL PRECAUTIONS

Be sure to tell your physician if:
▼ You have liver problems.
▼ You have tics.
▼ You or anyone else in your family has depression or bipolar disorder.
▼ You have had seizures.
▼ You have a history of glaucoma.
▼ You have any heart conditions or heart rhythm problems.
▼ You have thyroid disease.
▼ You have high blood pressure.
▼ You are involved in strenuous activities.
▼ You have a family history of sudden death related to a heart condition.
▼ You are taking other medications.

Pregnancy
▼ Safety in pregnancy not established. Discuss with your physician.

Breast-feeding
▼ Safety not established. Discuss with your physician.

Infants and children
▼ Not recommended in those less than 6 years of age. Discuss with your physician.

Over 60
▼ Safety and efficacy not established in older individuals.

Driving and hazardous work
▼ May cause drowsiness or dizziness. Do not drive a car or operate machinery until you feel you are mentally alert.

Alcohol
▼ Avoid. Alcohol may increase the risk of drowsiness caused by this drug.

POSSIBLE ADVERSE EFFECTS

The most common are upset stomach, nausea, headaches, sedation, decrease in appetite, small changes in heart rate or blood pressure. Rarely, this drug may cause liver problems.

Symptom/effect	Frequency		Discuss with physician		Stop taking drug now	Call physician now
	Common	Rare	Only if severe	In all cases		
Headache	●		■			
Dizziness/fatigue	●		■			
Abdominal discomfort/pain	●		■			
Nausea/vomiting		●	■			
Appetite changes	●		■		▲	
Jaundice		●		■		▮
Irregular heartbeat		●		■		▮
Skin rash/hives		●		■		▮
Emotional changes		●			▲	▮
Flu-like symptoms		●		■		▮

INTERACTIONS

Fluoxetine, Paroxetine, Quinidine These medications may decrease the breakdown of atomoxetine and increase its effects.

Salbutamol If used at the same time, may increase heart rate.

Phenelzine, tranylcypromine, selegiline Atomoxetine should not be taken with, or within 14 days of stopping, these drugs.

PROLONGED USE

Prolonged treatment can adversely affect liver function.

Monitoring Regular blood tests to check liver function are recommended. Tests of muscle function may be carried out if problems are suspected.

ATORVASTATIN

Product name Lipitor
Used in the following combined preparations Caduet

GENERAL INFORMATION

Atorvastatin is a member of the statin group of lipid-lowering drugs. It is used to treat hypercholesterolemia (high blood cholesterol levels) in patients who have not responded to other treatments, such as a special diet, and are at risk of developing heart disease.

Atorvastatin blocks the action, in the liver, of an enzyme that is needed for the manufacture of cholesterol. As a result, blood levels of cholesterol are lowered, which can help to prevent coronary heart disease.

Rarely, atorvastatin can cause muscle pain, inflammation, and muscle damage. The risk is increased if the drug is given with a fibrate (another kind of lipid-lowering drug).

INFORMATION FOR USERS

Your drug prescription is tailored for you. Do not alter dosage without checking with your physician.

How taken

Tablets.

Frequency and timing of doses
Once daily.

Usual adult dosage range
10–40mg; up to 80mg (inherited hypercholesterolemia).

Onset of effect
Within 2 weeks. Full beneficial effects may not be seen for 4–6 weeks.

Duration of action
20–30 hours.

Diet advice
A low-fat diet is usually recommended.

Storage
Keep in a closed container in a cool, dry place out of the reach of children.

Missed dose
Take as soon as you remember. If your next dose is due within 8 hours, do not take the missed dose, but take the next one on schedule.

Stopping the drug
Do not stop taking the drug without consulting your physician. Stopping the drug may lead to a recurrence of the original condition.

Exceeding the dose
An occasional unintentional extra dose is unlikely to cause problems. Large overdoses may cause liver problems. Notify your physician.

SPECIAL PRECAUTIONS

Be sure to tell your physician if:
▼ You have had liver problems.
▼ You are a heavy drinker.
▼ You are taking other medications.
▼ You are allergic to statins or atorvastatin.
▼ You have had kidney problems.
▼ You have thyroid problems.
▼ You have a family history of muscular disorders.
▼ You are diabetic.

Pregnancy
▼ Not usually prescribed. Safety not established. Discuss with your physician.

Breast-feeding
▼ Safety not established. Discuss with your physician.

Infants and children
▼ Not recommended.

Over 60
▼ No special problems.

Driving and hazardous work
▼ No special problems.

Alcohol
▼ Avoid excessive amounts. Alcohol may increase the risk of developing liver problems with atorvastatin.

POSSIBLE ADVERSE EFFECTS

Adverse effects of atorvastatin are usually mild and transient. Muscle damage is a rare side effect and muscle aching or weakness should be reported to your physician at once.

Symptom/effect	Frequency		Discuss with physician		Stop taking drug now	Call physician now
	Common	Rare	Only if severe	In all cases		
Nausea	●		■			
Headache	●		■			
Skin rash		●		■	▲	
Muscle pain/weakness		●		■	▲	▮
Jaundice		●		■	▲	▮
Insomnia		●	■			
Urine discolouration		●		■	▲	▮
Change in cognition		●				▮

INTERACTIONS

Anticoagulant drugs Atorvastatin may increase the effect of anticoagulants.

Antifungal drugs Itraconazole, ketoconazole, and possibly other antifungals, may increase the risk of muscle damage with atorvastatin. Clarithromycin and erythromycin may also increase the level of atorvastatin.

Grapefruit juice may increase the level of atorvastatin in the blood.

Other lipid-lowering drugs Taken with atorvastatin, these drugs may increase the risk of muscle damage.

Cyclosporine and other immuno-suppressant drugs Atorvastatin is not usually prescribed with these drugs because of the increased risk of muscle damage. However, if using the drugs together is unavoidable, close monitoring is advised.

PROLONGED USE

Long-term use of atorvastatin can affect liver function.

Monitoring Regular blood tests to check liver function are needed. Tests of muscle function may be carried out if problems are suspected.

ATROPINE

Product names Isopto Atropine, Minims Atropine, and others
Used in the following combined preparation Lomotil

GENERAL INFORMATION

Atropine is an *anticholinergic* drug. Because of its *antispasmodic* action, which relaxes the muscle wall of the intestine, the drug has been used to relieve abdominal cramps in irritable bowel syndrome. Atropine may also be prescribed in combination with diphenoxylate, an antidiarrheal drug. However, this combination can be dangerous in overdosage, particularly in young children.

Atropine eye drops, used to enlarge the pupil during eye examinations, are part of the treatment for uveitis.

Atropine may be used as part of the *premedication* before a general anesthetic. It is occasionally injected to restore normal heart beat in heart block (p.86).

Atropine must be used with caution in children and the elderly due to their sensitivity to the drug's effects.

QUICK REFERENCE

Drug group Anticholinergic drug for irritable bowel syndrome (p.98) and mydriatic drug (p.158)

Overdose danger rating High

Dependence rating Low

Prescription needed Yes (except powder)

Available as generic Yes

INFORMATION FOR USERS

Your drug prescription is tailored for you. Do not alter dosage without checking with your physician.

How taken

Tablets, injection, eye ointment, eye drops.

Frequency and timing of doses
Once only, or up to 4 times daily according to condition (eye drops); as directed (other forms).

Usual adult dosage range
1–2 drops as directed (eye drops); as directed (other forms).

Onset of effect
Varies according to method of administration. 30 minutes (eye drops).

Duration of action
7 days or longer (eye drops); several hours (other forms).

Diet advice
None.

Storage
Keep in a closed container in a cool, dry place out of the reach of children. Protect from light.

Missed dose
Take as soon as you remember. If your next dose is due within 2 hours, take a single dose now and skip the next.

Stopping the drug
Do not stop the drug without consulting your physician.

OVERDOSE ACTION

 Seek immediate medical advice in all cases. Take emergency action if palpitations, tremor, delirium, fits, or loss of consciousness occur.

See Drug poisoning emergency guide (p.526).

SPECIAL PRECAUTIONS

Be sure to tell your physician if:
▼ You have long-term liver or kidney problems.
▼ You have prostate problems.
▼ You have gastro-esophageal reflux.
▼ You have glaucoma.
▼ You have urinary difficulties.
▼ You have myasthenia gravis.
▼ You have ulcerative colitis.
▼ You wear contact lenses (eye drops).
▼ You have heart problems or high blood pressure.
▼ You are taking other medications.

Pregnancy
▼ Safety in pregnancy not established. Discuss with your physician.

Breast-feeding
▼ The drug passes into the breast milk and may affect the baby. Discuss with your physician.

Infants and children
▼ Combination with diphenoxylate not recommended under 4 years; reduced dose necessary in older children.

Over 60
▼ Increased likelihood of adverse effects.

Driving and hazardous work
▼ Avoid such activities until you have learned how atropine affects you because the drug can cause blurred vision and may impair concentration.

Alcohol
▼ Avoid. Alcohol increases the likelihood of confusion when taken with atropine.

POSSIBLE ADVERSE EFFECTS

The use of this drug is limited by the frequency of anticholinergic effects.

In addition to these effects, atropine eye drops may cause stinging.

Symptom/effect	Frequency		Discuss with physician		Stop taking drug now	Call physician now
	Common	Rare	Only if severe	In all cases		
Blurred vision/dry mouth/thirst	●		■			
Constipation	●		■			
Flushing/dry skin	●			■		
Difficulty in passing urine		●		■		
Eye pain and irritation		●		■	▲	■
Palpitations/confusion		●		■	▲	■
Contact rash		●		■	▲	
Nausea/vomiting		●	■			
Dizziness		●	■			

INTERACTIONS

Anticholinergic drugs Atropine increases the risk of *side effects* from drugs that also have anticholinergic effects.

Ketoconazole Atropine reduces the absorption of this drug from the digestive tract. Increased dose may be necessary.

PROLONGED USE

Usually used for short duration of therapy.

ATTAPULGITE

Product names Fowler's Antidiarrheal tablets, Kaopectate
Used in the following combined preparations None

GENERAL INFORMATION

Attapulgite is used in the treatment of diarrhea. It decreases diarrhea by absorbing fluid in the intestine. This medication is usually taken after each loose bowel movement. In cases where diarrhea lasts for longer than 2 days, or there is blood in the stool, or the person has a fever, a physician should be consulted. Attapulgite is usually only used for a few days. With diarrhea, it is important to maintain an adequate fluid intake to prevent dehydration. Young children and the elderly are more susceptible to dehydration from diarrhea.

QUICK REFERENCE

Drug group Antidiarrheal drugs (p.96)

Overdose danger rating Low

Dependence rating Low

Prescription needed No

Available as generic Yes

INFORMATION FOR USERS

Follow instructions on the label. Call your physician if symptoms worsen.

How taken

Tablets, liquid.

Frequency and timing of doses
Taken as needed after each bowel movement.

Usual dosage range
Adults 600–750mg per dose; take 2 tablets to start with, then 2 tablets following each loose bowel movement to a maximum of 6 doses in 24 hours.
Children 6 to 12 years, 600mg per dose; take 1 tablet to start with, then 1 tablet following each bowel movement to a maximum of 6 doses in 24 hours; < 6 years, consult with your physician.

Onset of effect
30 minutes to 1 hour.

Duration of action
24 hours.

Diet advice
Ensure adequate fluid, sugar, and salt intake during a diarrheal illness.

Storage
Keep in a closed container in a cool, dry place out of the reach of children.

Missed dose
If you miss a dose, take it as soon as you remember. If it is near the time of the next dose, skip the missed dose and resume your using dosing schedule. Do not double up to catch up on a missed dose.

Stopping the drug
Can be safely stopped as soon as you no longer need it.

Exceeding the dose
An occasional unintentional extra dose is unlikely to be a cause for concern. Large overdoses may cause constipation and cramping. Notify your physician.

SPECIAL PRECAUTIONS

Be sure to consult your physician or pharmacist before taking this drug if:
▼ You have heart disease.
▼ You have bowel problems.
▼ You are taking other medications.

 Pregnancy
▼ No evidence of risk. Discuss with your physician prior to use.

 Breast-feeding
▼ No evidence of risk. Discuss with your physician.

 Infants and children
▼ Dosage is reduced. Children are more susceptible to dehydration with diarrhea.

 Over 60
▼ No special problems expected. The elderly are more susceptible to dehydration with diarrhea.

 Driving and hazardous work
▼ No known problems.

 Alcohol
▼ No known problems.

POSSIBLE ADVERSE EFFECTS

Generally well tolerated. Common adverse effect may be stomach upset.

Symptom/effect	Frequency		Discuss with physician		Stop taking drug now	Call physician now
	Common	Rare	Only if severe	In all cases		
Stomach upset	●		■			
Abdominal pain		●		■		

INTERACTIONS

Recommended not to administer attapulgite at the same time as other medications and to space them apart.

PROLONGED USE

Usually only used for a few days.

AZATHIOPRINE

Product names Apo-Azathioprine, Imuran, Novo-Azathioprine
Used in the following combined preparations None

GENERAL INFORMATION

Azathioprine is an immunosuppressant drug used to prevent immune system rejection of transplanted organs. The drug is also given for severe rheumatoid arthritis that has failed to respond to conventional drug therapy.

Autoimmune and collagen diseases (including polymyositis, systemic lupus erythematosus, myasthenia gravis, and dermatomyositis) may be treated with azathioprine, usually when corticosteroids have not been effective.

Azathioprine is administered only under close supervision because of the risk of serious *adverse effects*. These include suppression of the production of white blood cells, thereby increasing the risk of infection as well as the risk of excessive or prolonged bleeding.

QUICK REFERENCE

Drug group Antirheumatic drug (p.103) and immunosuppressant drug (p.143)

Overdose danger rating Medium

Dependence rating Low

Prescription needed Yes

Available as generic Yes

INFORMATION FOR USERS

Your drug prescription is tailored for you. Do not alter dosage without checking with your physician.

How taken

Tablets, injection.

Frequency and timing of doses
Usually once daily with or after food.

Usual dosage range
Initially according to body weight and the condition being treated and then adjusted according to response.

Onset of effect
2–4 weeks. Antirheumatic effect may not be felt for 8 weeks or more.

Duration of action
Immunosuppressant effects may last for several weeks after the drug is stopped.

Diet advice
None.

Storage
Keep in a closed container in a cool, dry place out of the reach of children. Protect from light.

Missed dose
Take as soon as you remember, then return to your normal schedule. If more than 2 doses are missed, consult your physician.

Stopping the drug
Do not stop the drug without consulting your physician. If taken to prevent graft transplant rejection, stopping treatment could provoke the rejection of the transplant.

Exceeding the dose
An occasional unintentional extra dose is unlikely to cause problems. Large overdoses may cause nausea, vomiting, abdominal pains, and diarrhea. Notify your physician.

POSSIBLE ADVERSE EFFECTS

Digestive disturbances and adverse effects on the blood which could lead to sore throat, fever, and weakness are common with azathioprine. Unusual bleeding or bruising while taking this drug may be a sign of reduced levels of platelets in the blood.

Symptom/effect	Frequency		Discuss with physician		Stop taking drug now	Call physician now
	Common	Rare	Only if severe	In all cases		
Nausea/vomiting	●		■			
Hair loss	●		■			
Loss of appetite	●			■		
Weakness/fatigue		●		■		
Unusual bleeding/bruising		●		■		▮
Jaundice		●		■		▮
Rash		●		■		▮
Fever/chills		●		■		▮
Pain in the side/urinary difficulty		●		■		▮

INTERACTIONS

ACE inhibitors could increase risk of blood cell changes if taken with azathioprine.

Allopurinol increases effects and *toxicity* of azathioprine; dosage of azathioprine will need to be reduced.

Warfarin Azathioprine may reduce its effect.

Co-trimoxazole and trimethoprim may increase the risk of blood problems if taken with azathioprine.

Corticosteroids may increase infection risk.

SPECIAL PRECAUTIONS

Be sure to tell your physician if:
▼ You have long-term liver or kidney problems.
▼ You have had a previous allergic reaction to azathioprine or 6-mercaptopurine.
▼ You have recently had shingles or chickenpox.
▼ You have an infection.
▼ You have a blood disorder.
▼ You are taking other medications.

Pregnancy
▼ Azathioprine has been taken in pregnancy without problems. Discuss with your physician.

Breast-feeding
▼ A small amount of the drug passes into the breast milk. Discuss with your physician.

Infants and children
▼ No special problems.

Over 60
▼ Increased likelihood of adverse effects. Reduced dose necessary.

Driving and hazardous work
▼ Avoid such activities until you have learned how azathioprine affects you because the drug can cause dizziness.

Alcohol
▼ No known problems.

PROLONGED USE

There may be a slightly increased risk of some cancers with long-term use of azathioprine. Blood changes may also occur. Avoidance of exposure to sunlight may help to prevent adverse skin effects.

Monitoring Regular checks on blood composition are usually carried out.

AZITHROMYCIN

Product names Apo-Azithromycin, CO Azithromycin, Novo-Azithromycin, PMS-Azithromycin, Zithromax, Z-PAK
Used in the following combined preparations None

GENERAL INFORMATION

Azithromycin is a marcolide antibiotic similar to erythromycin (p.270) from which it is derived. It has similar actions and uses to erythromycin. It is used for upper respiratory tract infections, such as middle ear infections, pharyngitis and tonsilitis, and lower respiratory tract infections, such as bacterial exacerbation of chronic obstructive lung disease, bronchitis, and pneumonia, as well as for skin and soft tissue infections, including gonorrhoea.

Prolonged use with azithromycin is usually not necessary.

INFORMATION FOR USERS

Your drug prescription is tailored for you. Do not alter dosage without checking with your physician.

How taken

Tablets, liquid (reconstituted from powder), injection.

Frequency and timing of doses
Once daily.

Usual dosage range
250mg–1.5g daily.

Onset of effect
1–3 hours.

Duration of action
Up to 24 hours.

Diet advice
None.

Storage
Keep in a closed container in a cool, dry place out of the reach of children.
Store the reconstituted solution between 5 and 30°C and discard any unused portion after 10 days.

Missed dose
If you miss a dose, take it as soon as you remember. If it is near the time of the next dose, skip the missed dose and resume your usual dosing schedule. Do not double up to catch up on a missed dose.

Stopping the drug
Take the full course. Even if you feel better, the infection may still be present and symptoms may recur if treatment is stopped too soon.

Exceeding the dose
An occasional unintentional extra dose is unlikely to be a cause for concern. But if you notice any unusual symptoms, or if a large overdose has been taken, notify your physician.

POSSIBLE ADVERSE EFFECTS

Azithromycin is usually well tolerated. Nausea and diarrhea may occur.

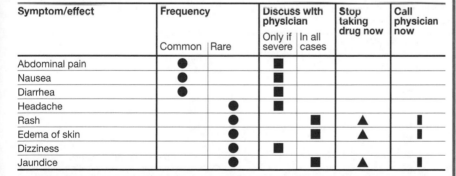

Symptom/effect	Frequency		Discuss with physician		Stop taking drug now	Call physician now
	Common	Rare	Only if severe	In all cases		
Abdominal pain	●		■			
Nausea	●		■			
Diarrhea	●		■			
Headache		●	■			
Rash		●		■	▲	▮
Edema of skin		●		■	▲	▮
Dizziness		●	■			
Jaundice		●		■	▲	▮

INTERACTIONS

Antacids Aluminum- and magnesium-containing antacids can affect azithromycin's peak effect. Do not take at the same time as azithromycin.

Cyclosporine, digoxin, triazolam, disopyramide Azithromycin may increase the effect of these drugs.

SPECIAL PRECAUTIONS

Be sure to tell your physician if:
▼ You have liver or kidney problems.
▼ You have had an allergic reaction to erythromycin, clarithromycin, or azithromycin.
▼ You have a heart problem.
▼ You have porphyria.
▼ You are taking other medications.

 Pregnancy
▼ Safety has not been established. Discuss with your physician.

 Breast-feeding
▼ Safety in breast-feeding not established. Discuss with your physician.

 Infants and children
▼ Reduced dose necessary.

 Over 60
▼ No special problems.

 Driving and hazardous work
▼ No special problems.

 Alcohol
▼ No known problems.

PROLONGED USE

Usually not used for prolonged periods. During prolonged therapy, periodic liver function tests may be done.

Monitoring Regular blood tests to check liver function are recommended.

BACLOFEN

Product name Lioresal
Used in the following combined preparations None

GENERAL INFORMATION

Baclofen is a muscle-relaxant drug that acts on the central nervous system, including the spinal cord. The drug relieves the spasms, cramping, and rigidity of muscles caused by a variety of disorders, including multiple sclerosis and spinal cord injury. Baclofen is also used to treat the spasticity that results from brain injury, cerebral palsy, or stroke. Although this drug does not cure any of these disorders, it increases mobility, allowing other treatment, such as physiotherapy, to be carried out.

Baclofen is less likely to cause muscle weakness than similar drugs, and its *side effects*, such as dizziness or drowsiness, are usually temporary. Elderly people are more susceptible to side effects, especially during early stages of treatment.

INFORMATION FOR USERS

Your drug prescription is tailored for you. Do not alter dosage without checking with your physician.

How taken

Tablets, injection (specialist use).

Frequency and timing of doses
3 x daily with food or milk.

Usual adult dosage range
15mg daily (starting dose). Daily dose may be increased by 15mg every 3 days as necessary. Maximum daily dose: 80mg.

Onset of effect
Some benefits may appear after 1–3 hours, but full beneficial effects may not be felt for several weeks. A dose 1 hour before a specific task will improve mobility.

Duration of action
Up to 8 hours.

Diet advice
None.

Storage
Keep in a closed container in a cool, dry place out of the reach of children. Protect liquid from light.

Missed dose
Take as soon as you remember. If your next dose is due within 2 hours, take a single dose now and skip the next.

Stopping the drug
Do not stop taking the drug without consulting your physician who will supervise a gradual reduction in dosage. Abrupt cessation may cause hallucinations, fits, and worsening spasticity.

Exceeding the dose
An occasional unintentional extra dose is unlikely to cause problems. Large overdoses may cause weakness, vomiting, and severe drowsiness. Notify your physician.

SPECIAL PRECAUTIONS

Be sure to tell your physician if:
▼ You have long-term liver or kidney problems.
▼ You have difficulty in passing urine.
▼ You have had a peptic ulcer.
▼ You have had epileptic fits.
▼ You have diabetes.
▼ You suffer with breathing problems.
▼ You are taking other medications.

Pregnancy
▼ Safety in pregnancy not established. Discuss with your physician.

Breast-feeding
▼ The drug passes into the breast milk. Discuss with your physician.

Infants and children
▼ Reduced dose necessary.

Over 60
▼ Increased likelihood of adverse effects. Reduced dose may therefore be necessary.

Driving and hazardous work
▼ Avoid such activities until you have learned how baclofen affects you because the drug can cause drowsiness.

Alcohol
▼ Avoid. Alcohol may increase the sedative effects of this drug.

Surgery and general anesthetics
▼ Be sure to inform your physician or dentist that you are taking baclofen before you have a general anesthetic.

POSSIBLE ADVERSE EFFECTS

The common *adverse effects* are related to the sedative effects of the drug. Such effects are minimized by starting with a low dose that is gradually increased.

Symptom/effect	Frequency		Discuss with physician		Stop taking drug now	Call physician now
	Common	Rare	Only if severe	In all cases		
Dizziness	●		■			
Drowsiness	●		■			
Nausea	●		■			
Muscle fatigue/weakness	●		■			
Difficulty in passing urine	●		■			
Constipation/diarrhea		●	■			
Headache		●	■			
Confusion		●		■		

INTERACTIONS

Antihypertensive and diuretic drugs The effect of such drugs may be increased.

Drugs for *parkinsonism* Some of these drugs may cause confusion or hallucinations if taken with baclofen.

Antidiabetic drugs or insulin Dosage may need adjusting, as baclofen may increase blood glucose levels.

Sedatives These drugs may increase the sedative properties of baclofen.

Tricyclic antidepressants may increase baclofen's effects, causing muscle weakness.

PROLONGED USE

No problems expected.

BECLOMETHASONE

Product names Alti-Beclamethasone, Qvar, Rivanase AQ
Used in the following combined preparation Ventide

GENERAL INFORMATION

Beclomethasone is a corticosteroid drug prescribed to relieve the symptoms of allergic rhinitis (as a nasal spray) and to control asthma (as an inhalant). It controls nasal symptoms by reducing inflammation and mucus production in the nose. It also helps to reduce chest symptoms, such as wheezing and coughing. Asthma sufferers may take it regularly to reduce the severity and frequency of attacks. However, once an attack has started, the drug does not relieve symptoms.

Beclomethasone is given primarily to people whose asthma has not responded to bronchodilators alone (p.78). Beclomethasone is also used as the main ingredient in some skin creams and ointments to treat inflammatory conditions, particularly eczema. As it is potent it is not usually used on the face.

There are few serious *adverse effects* associated with beclomethasone as it is given *topically* by nasal spray or inhaler. Fungal infections causing irritation of the mouth and throat are a possible *side effect* of inhaling beclomethasone. These can be avoided to some degree by rinsing the mouth and gargling with water after each inhalation.

INFORMATION FOR USERS

Your drug prescription is tailored for you. Do not alter dosage without checking with your physician.

How taken

Cream, inhaler, nasal spray.

Frequency and timing of doses
2–4 x daily.

Usual dosage range
Adults 1–2 puffs 2–4 x daily according to preparation used (asthma); 1–2 sprays in each nostril 2–4 x daily (allergic rhinitis); as directed but usually 1–2 x daily (skin conditions). *Children* Reduced dose according to age and weight.

Onset of effect
Within 1 week (asthma); 1–3 days (allergic rhinitis). Full benefit may not be felt for up to 4 weeks.

Duration of action
Several days after stopping the drug.

Diet advice
None.

Storage
Keep in a closed container in a cool, dry place out of the reach of children. Protect from light.

Missed dose
Take as soon as you remember. If your next dose is due within 2 hours, take a single dose now and skip the next.

Stopping the drug
Do not stop the drug without consulting your physician; symptoms may recur. Sometimes a gradual reduction in dosage is recommended.

Exceeding the dose
An occasional unintentional extra dose is unlikely to cause problems. But if you notice any unusual symptoms, or if a large overdose has been taken, notify your physician. Adverse effects may occur if the recommended dose is regularly exceeded over a prolonged period.

SPECIAL PRECAUTIONS

Be sure to tell your physician if:
▼ You have had tuberculosis or another nasal or respiratory infection.
▼ You have a skin infection (cream/ointment).
▼ You have varicose ulcers (cream/ointment).

Pregnancy
▼ No evidence of risk with inhaler or topical product.

Breast-feeding
▼ No evidence of risk with inhaler or topical product.

Infants and children
▼ Reduced dose necessary. Avoid prolonged use of ointment in infants and children.

Over 60
▼ No known problems.

Driving and hazardous work
▼ No known problems.

Alcohol
▼ No known problems.

POSSIBLE ADVERSE EFFECTS

The main side effects of the nasal spray and inhaler are irritation of the nasal passages and fungal infection of the throat and mouth. More serious side effects, such as permanent skin changes, may be seen with the ointment, which should not normally be used on the face.

Symptom/effect	Frequency		Discuss with physician		Stop taking drug now	Call physician now
	Common	Rare	Only if severe	In all cases		
Inhaler/nasal spray						
Nasal discomfort/irritation	●		■			
Cough	●		■			
Sore throat/hoarseness	●			■		
Nosebleed	●			■		
Cream/ointment						
Skin changes		●		■		

INTERACTIONS

None.

PROLONGED USE

No problems expected when used for asthma or rhinitis, but high doses of nasal spray can give systemic effects. Prolonged use of cream or ointment should be avoided where possible because it can cause permanent skin changes, especially on the face, and high doses can suppress the body's own corticosteroid production.

Monitoring Periodic checks to ensure that the adrenal glands are functioning healthily may be required if large doses are being used.

BENZOYL PEROXIDE

Product names Acetoxyl, Benoxyl, Benzac, Benzagel, Oxyderm, Panoxyl
Used in the following combined preparation Benzamycin

GENERAL INFORMATION

Benzoyl peroxide is used in a variety of *topical* preparations for the treatment of acne. Available over the counter, it comes in concentrations of varying strengths for moderate acne.

Benzoyl peroxide works by removing the top layer of skin and unblocking the sebaceous glands. It can also reduce inflammation of blocked hair follicles by killing the bacteria that infect them.

Benzoyl peroxide may cause irritation due to its drying effect on the skin, but this generally diminishes with time. The drug should be applied to the affected areas as directed on the label. Washing the area prior to application greatly enhances the drug's beneficial effects. *Side effects* are less likely if treatment is started with a preparation containing a low concentration of benzoyl peroxide, and changed to a stronger preparation only if necessary. Marked dryness and peeling of the skin, which may occur, can usually be controlled by reducing the frequency of application. Care should be taken to avoid contact of the drug with the eyes, mouth, and mucous membranes. It is also advisble to avoid excessive exposure to sunlight. Preparations of benzoyl peroxide may bleach clothing.

INFORMATION FOR USERS

Your drug prescription is tailored for you. Do not alter dosage without checking with your physician.

How taken

Lotion, gel, bar, facial cleanser.

Frequency and timing of doses
1–2 x daily.

Usual dosage range
Apply sparingly to affected skin, as instructed on the label.

Onset of effect
Reduces oiliness of skin immediately. Acne usually improves within 4–6 weeks.

Duration of action
24–48 hours.

Diet advice
None.

Storage
Keep in a closed container in a cool, dry place out of the reach of children.

Missed dose
Apply as soon as you remember.

Stopping the drug
Can be safely stopped as soon as you no longer need it.

Exceeding the dose
A single extra application is unlikely to cause problems. Regular overuse may result in extensive irritation, peeling, redness, and swelling of the skin.

POSSIBLE ADVERSE EFFECTS

Application of benzoyl peroxide may cause temporary burning or stinging of the skin. Redness, peeling, and swelling may result from excessive drying of the skin and usually clears up if the treatment is stopped or used less frequently. If severe burning, blistering, or crusting occur, stop using benzoyl peroxide and consult your physician.

Symptom/effect	Frequency		Discuss with physician		Stop taking drug now	Call physician now
	Common	Rare	Only if severe	In all cases		
Skin irritation	●		■			
Dryness/peeling	●		■			
Stinging/redness	●		■			
Blistering/crusting/swelling		●		■	▲	

INTERACTIONS

Skin-drying preparations Medicated cosmetics, soaps, toiletries, and other anti-acne preparations increase the likelihood of dryness and irritation of the skin with benzoyl peroxide.

SPECIAL PRECAUTIONS

Be sure to consult your physician or pharmacist before taking this drug if:
▼ You have eczema.
▼ You have sunburn.
▼ You have had a previous allergic reaction to benzoyl peroxide.
▼ You are taking other medications.

Pregnancy
▼ No evidence of risk.

Breast-feeding
▼ No evidence of risk.

Infants and children
▼ Not usually recommended under 12 years except under medical supervision.

Over 60
▼ Not usually required.

Driving and hazardous work
▼ No known problems.

Alcohol
▼ No known problems.

PROLONGED USE

Benzoyl peroxide usually takes 4–6 weeks to produce an effect. Continuation beyond this time should be on the advice of your physician.

BETAHISTINE

Product name Serc
Used in the following combined preparations None

GENERAL INFORMATION

Betahistine, a drug that resembles the naturally occurring substance histamine in some of its effects, was introduced in the 1970s as a treatment for Ménière's disease, which is caused by the pressure of excess fluid in the inner ear.

Taken regularly, betahistine reduces both the frequency and the severity of the nausea and vertigo attacks that characterize this condition. It is also effective in treating tinnitus (ringing in the ears). Betahistine is thought to work by reducing pressure in the inner ear, possibly by improving blood flow in the small blood vessels. Drug treatment is not successful in all cases, however, and surgery may be needed.

QUICK REFERENCE

Drug group Drug for Ménière's disease (p.74)

Overdose danger rating High

Dependence rating Low

Prescription needed Yes

Available as generic No

INFORMATION FOR USERS

Your drug prescription is tailored for you. Do not alter dosage without checking with your physician.

How taken

Tablets.

Frequency and timing of doses
3 x daily after food.

Usual adult dosage range
24–48mg daily.

Onset of effect
Within 1 hour.

Duration of action
6–12 hours.

Diet advice
None.

Storage
Keep in a closed container in a cool, dry place out of the reach of children.

Missed dose
Take as soon as you remember. If your next dose is due within 2 hours, take a single dose now and skip the next.

Stopping the drug
Do not stop the drug without consulting your physician; symptoms may recur.

OVERDOSE ACTION

 Seek immediate medical advice in all cases. Large overdoses may cause collapse requiring emergency action.

POSSIBLE ADVERSE EFFECTS

Adverse effects from betahistine are minor and rarely cause problems.

Symptom/effect	Frequency		Discuss with physician		Stop taking drug now	Call physician now
	Common	Rare	Only if severe	In all cases		
Nausea	●		■			
Indigestion	●		■			
Headache		●	■			
Rash		●		■		

INTERACTIONS

Antihistamines Although unproven, there is a possibility that betahistine may reduce the effects of these drugs.

SPECIAL PRECAUTIONS

Be sure to tell your physician if:
▼ You have asthma.
▼ You have a peptic ulcer.
▼ You have pheochromocytoma.
▼ You are taking other medications.

 Pregnancy
▼ Safety in pregnancy not established. Discuss with your physician.

 Breast-feeding
▼ The drug passes into the breast milk, but at normal doses adverse effects on the baby are unlikely. Discuss with your physician.

 Infants and children
▼ Not recommended.

 Over 60
No special problems.

 Driving and hazardous work
▼ No special problems.

 Alcohol
▼ No special problems.

PROLONGED USE

No special problems.

BETAMETHASONE

Product names Betaderm, Betaject, Betnesol, Celestone, Diprosone, Prevex B, Valisone
Used in the following combined preparations Dovobet, Lotriderm, Diprosalic, Garasone, Valisone-G

GENERAL INFORMATION

Betamethasone is a corticosteroid drug used to treat a variety of conditions. It is available as different esters such as dipropionate and valerate, with variable potency. When injected directly into the joints it relieves joint inflammation and the pain and stiffness of rheumatoid arthritis. It is also used *topically* to treat skin complaints, such as eczema and psoriasis. When taken for short periods, low or moderate doses of this drug rarely cause serious *side effects*. High dosages or prolonged use can lead to many symptoms (see below).

INFORMATION FOR USERS

Your drug prescription is tailored for you. Do not alter dosage without checking with your physician.

How taken

Injection, cream, ointment, rectal enema, scalp solution, eye ointment, eye/ear drops.

Frequency and timing of doses
Usually once daily in the morning (*systemic*). Otherwise varies according to disorder being treated.

Usual dosage range
Varies; follow your physician's instructions.

Onset of effect
Within 30 minutes (injection); within 48 hours (other forms).

Duration of action
Up to 24 hours.

Diet advice
None

Storage
Keep in a closed container in a cool, dry place out of the reach of children. Protect from light.

Missed dose
Take as soon as you remember. If your next dose is due within 2 hours, take a single dose now and skip the next.

Stopping the drug
Can be safely stopped as soon as you no longer need it.

Exceeding the dose
An occasional unintentional extra dose is unlikely to cause problems. But if you notice any unusual symptoms, notify your physician.

POSSIBLE ADVERSE EFFECTS

Serious adverse effects occur only when high doses are taken by mouth for long periods.

Topical preparations are unlikely to cause adverse effects unless overused.

Symptom/effect	Frequency		Discuss with physician		Stop taking drug now	Call physician now
	Common	Rare	Only if severe	In all cases		
Indigestion	●			■		
Weight gain		●		■		
Acne		●		■		
Muscle weakness		●		■		
Mood changes		●		■		
Bloody/black feces		●		■	▲	▮

INTERACTIONS

Insulin, antidiabetic drugs, and oral anticoagulant drugs Betamethasone may alter insulin requirements and the effects of these drugs.

Vaccines Serious reactions can occur when certain vaccinations are given during betamethasone treatment.

Antihypertensive drugs and drugs used in myasthenia gravis Betamethasone may reduce the effects of these drugs.

Anticonvulsants These drugs may reduce the effects of betamethasone.

SPECIAL PRECAUTIONS

Be sure to tell your physician if:
▼ You suffer from a mental disorder.
▼ You have a heart condition.
▼ You have glaucoma.
▼ You have high blood pressure.
▼ You have a history of epilepsy.
▼ You have had a peptic ulcer.
▼ You have had tuberculosis.
▼ You have any infection.
▼ You have diabetes.
▼ You have liver or kidney problems.
▼ You are taking other medications.

Avoid exposure to chickenpox, measles, or shingles if you are on systemic treatment.

Pregnancy
▼ No evidence of risk with topical preparations. Discuss with your physician.

Breast-feeding
▼ No risk with topical preparations. Discuss with your physician.

Infants and children
▼ Reduced dose necessary.

Over 60
▼ Reduced dose may be necessary.

Driving and hazardous work
▼ No known problems.

Alcohol
▼ Keep consumption low. Betamethasone tablets increase the risk of peptic ulcers.

PROLONGED USE

Prolonged use of topical treatment may lead to skin thinning. This drug can also retard growth in children.

BEZAFIBRATE

Product names Benzalip-SR, PMS-Bezafibrate
Used in the following combined preparations None

GENERAL INFORMATION

Bezafibrate belongs to a group of drugs, usually called fibrates, that lower lipid levels in the blood. Fibrates are particularly effective in decreasing levels of triglycerides in the blood. They also reduce blood levels of cholesterol. Raised levels of lipids (fats) in the blood are associated with atherosclerosis (deposition of fat in blood vessel walls).

This can lead to coronary heart disease (for example, angina and heart attacks) and cerebrovascular disease (for example, stroke). When bezafibrate is taken with a diet low in saturated fats, there is some evidence that the risk of coronary heart disease is reduced.

INFORMATION FOR USERS

Your drug prescription is tailored for you. Do not alter dosage without checking with your physician.

How taken

Tablets.

Frequency and timing of doses
1–3 x daily with a little liquid after a meal; SR: with evening meal

Usual adult dosage range
400–600mg daily.

Onset of effect
A beneficial effect on blood fat levels may not be produced for weeks, and it takes months or years for fat deposits in the arteries to be reduced. Treatment should be stopped if no adequate response is obtained in 3–4 months.

Duration of action
About 6–24 hours. This may vary according to the individual.

Diet advice
A low-fat diet will have been recommended. Follow the advice of your physician.

Storage
Keep in a closed container in a cool, dry place out of the reach of children.

Missed dose
Take as soon as you remember. If your next dose is due within 4 hours (and you take it once daily), take a single dose now and skip the next. If you take 2–3 times daily, take the next dose as normal.

Stopping the drug
Do not stop the drug without consulting your physician.

Exceeding the dose
An occasional unintentional extra dose is unlikely to be a cause for concern. But if you notice unusual symptoms, notify your physician.

SPECIAL PRECAUTIONS

Be sure to tell your physician if:
▼ You have long-term liver or kidney problems.
▼ You have a history of gallbladder disease.
▼ You are taking other medications.

Pregnancy
▼ Safety in pregnancy not established. Discuss with your physician.

Breast-feeding
▼ The drug may pass into the breast milk and may affect the baby. Discuss with your physician.

Infants and children
▼ Not usually prescribed.

Over 60
▼ No special problems expected.

Driving and hazardous work
▼ No special problems.

Alcohol
▼ No special problems.

POSSIBLE ADVERSE EFFECTS

The most common *adverse effects* are those on the gastrointestinal tract, such as loss of appetite and nausea. These effects normally diminish as treatment continues.

Symptom/effect	Frequency		Discuss with physician		Stop taking drug now	Call physician now
	Common	Rare	Only if severe	In all cases		
Nausea	●		■			
Loss of appetite	●		■			
Abdominal pain	●		■			
Skin rash		●		■		
Headache		●		■		
Muscular pain/cramp		●		■		
Dizziness/fatigue		●		■		

INTERACTIONS

Anticoagulants Bezafibrate may increase the effect of anticoagulants such as warfarin. Your physician will reduce the dosage of your anticoagulant when starting bezafibrate.

Monoamine oxidase inhibitors (MAOIs) There is a risk of liver damage when bezafibrate is taken with an MAOI.

Antidiabetic drugs Bezafibrate may interact with these drugs to lower blood sugar levels.

Pravastatin, simvastatin, and other lipid-lowering drugs whose names end in 'statin' There is an increased risk of muscle damage if bezafibrate is taken with these drugs.

PROLONGED USE

No problems expected, but patients with kidney disease will need special care as there is a high risk of muscle problems developing.

Monitoring Blood tests will be performed occasionally to monitor the effect of the drug on lipids in the blood, and to periodically measure kidney and liver function.

BISACODYL

Product names Apo-Bisacodyl, Correctol, Dulcolax, Feen-A-Mint, Gentlax, Laxcodyl, PMS-Bisacodyl, Soflax Ex
Used in the following combined preparations Bicholate Lilas, Fruitatives, Gentlax S

GENERAL INFORMATION

Bisacodyl is recommended for the treatment of occasional constipation. It may also be given in preparation for diagnostic procedures. Bisacodyl is a stimulant laxative that is thought to work by acting on the nerve endings on the wall of the bowel, which triggers contraction of the intestinal muscles and speeds up the process of fecal matter moving through the bowel. With regular use for more than a week, the bowel can become dependent on laxatives for its normal function; long-term use with bisacodyl is not recommended.

Bisacodyl, as with other laxatives, should not be used in someone who is experiencing abdominal pain, nausea, vomiting, or fever. Bisacodyl tablets should be swallowed whole and not taken with milk or antacids.

QUICK REFERENCE

Drug group Laxatives (p.97)
Overdose danger rating Medium
Dependence rating Low
Prescription needed No
Available as generic Yes

INFORMATION FOR USERS

Follow instructions on the label. Call your physician if symptoms worsen.

How taken

Tablets, suppositories, enema.

Frequency and timing of doses
Once daily on an occasional basis.

Usual adult dosage range
Oral tablets 5–15mg.
Suppository 10mg.
Micro-enema Contents of one enema.

Onset of effect
Tablets within 6–8 hours.
Suppository and micro-enema: within 30 minutes.

Duration of action
Up to 24 hours.

Diet advice
Maintaining adequate fluid and fiber intake is important in preventing constipation.

Storage
Keep in a closed container in a cool, dry place out of the reach of children.

Missed dose
If you miss a dose, take it as soon as you remember. Resume normal dose thereafter. Do not double up on a dose.

Stopping the drug
Can be safely stopped as soon as you no longer need it.

Exceeding the dose
An occasional unintentional extra dose is unlikely to be a cause for concern. Large doses can cause watery stools, abdominal cramps, and loss of electrolytes. Notify your physician.

SPECIAL PRECAUTIONS

Be sure to consult your physician or pharmacist before taking this drug if:
▼ You have severe constipation, and/or nausea, vomiting, or abdominal pain.
▼ You have unexplained rectal bleeding.
▼ You have difficulty swallowing.
▼ You have a known narrowing of the bowel.
▼ You have any obstruction of the bowel.
▼ You have an acute appendicitis or inflammatory bowel disease.
▼ You are sensitive or allergic to triarylmethane products.
▼ You are taking other medications.

Pregnancy
▼ Safety not established. Discuss with your physician.

Breast-feeding
▼ No evidence of risk. Discuss with your physician.

Infants and children
▼ Not recommended in children under 6 years of age without medical advice.

Over 60
▼ No special problems expected.

Driving and hazardous work
▼ No known problems.

Alcohol
▼ No known problems.

POSSIBLE ADVERSE EFFECTS

Generally well tolerated.

Symptom/effect	Frequency		Discuss with physician		Stop taking drug now	Call physician now
	Common	Rare	Only if severe	In all cases		
Abdominal pain/discomfort		●		■		
Dizziness		●		■		
Diarrhea		●		■		
Muscle weakness		●		■		
Suppositories and enema:						
Local irritation	●		■			
Painful sensation		●		■		

INTERACTIONS

Diuretics Prolonged use of bisacodyl can affect electrolyte balance, which can be potentiated further with diuretic use.

Digoxin Changes in electrolytes with bisacodyl could increase the effect of digoxin.

PROLONGED USE

Prolonged use of the oral preparation can make the bowel dependent on laxatives. For regular use, consult your physician or pharmacist.

BOTULINUM TOXIN

Product names Botox, Botox Cosmetic
Used in the following combined preparations None

GENERAL INFORMATION

Botulinum toxin is a neurotoxin (nerve poison) produced naturally by the bacterium *Clostridium botulinum*. The toxin causes botulism, a rare but serious form of food poisoning,

Research has found that there are several slightly different components in the toxin. Two are used medically: botulinum A toxin and botulinum B toxin. They are used therapeutically to treat conditions in which there are painful muscle spasms, for example spastic foot deformity, blepharospasm (spasm of the eyelids, causing them

almost to close), hemifacial spasm, and spasmodic torticollis (spasms of the neck muscles, causing the head to jerk). Toxin A is also used to treat very resistant and distressing cases of hyperhidrosis (excessive sweating). The effects produced by the toxins may last for 2-3 months, until new nerve endings have formed.

Botulinum toxin is used cosmetically to remove facial wrinkles by paralysing the muscles under the skin.

INFORMATION FOR USERS

This drug is given only under medical supervision and is not for self-administration.

How taken

Injection.

Frequency and timing of doses
Every 2–3 months, depending on response.

Usual adult dosage range
Dose depends on the particular condition being treated. Individual injections may range from 1.25 units to 50 units. The number of injection sites depends on the size and number of the muscles to be paralysed. Specialist judgement is necessary.

Onset of effect
Within 3 days to 2 weeks. The maximum

benefit of the drug will be seen around 6 weeks after treatment.

Duration of action
2–3 months.

Diet advice
None.

Storage
Not applicable as the drug is not normally kept in the home.

Missed dose
Attend for treatment at the next possible time.

Stopping the drug
Discuss with your physician whether you should stop receiving the drug.

Exceeding the dose
Overdose is unlikely since treatment is carefully monitored, and the drug is given by injection only under close supervision.

SPECIAL PRECAUTIONS

Be sure to tell your physician if:
▼ You have any disorder of muscle activity such as myasthenia gravis.
▼ You are taking an anticoagulant drug or have a bleeding disorder.
▼ You are allergic to botulinum toxin.

 Pregnancy
▼ Not prescribed.

 Breast-feeding
▼ Not prescribed.

 Infants and children
▼ Reduced dose necessary.

 Over 60
▼ No special problems.

 Driving and hazardous work
▼ Do not drive until you know how botulinum toxin affects you; the drug may impair ability.

 Alcohol
▼ No known problems.

POSSIBLE ADVERSE EFFECTS

Some of the adverse effects depend on the site of injection. Misplaced injections may

paralyse unintended muscle groups. All paralyses are likely to be long lasting.

Symptom/effect	Frequency		Discuss with physician		Stop taking drug now	Call physician now
	Common	Rare	Only if severe	In all cases		
Reduced blinking/dry eye	●			■		
Painful swallowing	●			■		▮
Pain at site	●			■		
Glaucoma/painful eye		●		■		
Neck weakness/head tremor		●		■		▮
Weakness (local or general)	●			■		
Hypersensitivity reactions		●		■		

PROLONGED USE

To maintain the desired effects, the drug may have to be administered at regular intervals.

INTERACTIONS

None.

BROMOCRIPTINE

Product name Parlodel
Used in the following combined preparations None

GENERAL INFORMATION

By inhibiting secretion of the hormone prolactin from the pituitary gland, bromocriptine is used in the treatment of conditions associated with excessive prolactin production. Such conditions include some types of female infertility and occasionally male infertility and impotence. It is effective in treating some benign breast conditions and other symptoms of menstrual disorders. Bromocriptine may also be used to suppress lactation in women who do not wish to breast-feed.

Bromocriptine is also effective for relieving the symptoms of *parkinsonism*. The drug is widely used to treat people with advanced parkinsonism when other drugs have failed or are unsuitable.

Bromocriptine reduces the release of growth hormone, and is therefore used to treat acromegaly (see p.133).

Serious *adverse effects* are rare with low doses. Nausea and vomiting can be minimized by taking bromocriptine with meals. Bromocriptine may in rare cases cause ulceration of the stomach.

QUICK REFERENCE

Drug group Drug for parkinsonism (p.71) and pituitary agent (p.131)

Overdose danger rating Low

Dependence rating Low

Prescription needed Yes

Available as generic Yes

INFORMATION FOR USERS

Your drug prescription is tailored for you. Do not alter dosage without checking with your physician.

How taken

Tablets, capsules.

Frequency and timing of doses
1–4 x daily with food.

Usual adult dosage range
The dose given depends on the condition being treated and your response. In most cases treatment starts with a daily dose of 1–1.25mg. This is gradually increased until a satisfactory response is achieved.

Onset of effect
Variable depending on the condition.

Duration of action
About 8 hours.

Diet advice
None.

Storage
Keep in a closed container in a cool, dry place out of the reach of children. Protect from light.

Missed dose
Take as soon as you remember. If your next dose is due within 2 hours, take a single dose now and skip the next.

Stopping the drug
Do not stop the drug without consulting your physician; symptoms may recur.

Exceeding the dose
An occasional unintentional extra dose is unlikely to be a cause for concern. If you notice any unusual symptoms, or if a large overdose has been taken, notify your physician.

SPECIAL PRECAUTIONS

Be sure to tell your physician if:
▼ You have poor circulation.
▼ You have a stomach ulcer.
▼ You have a history of psychiatric disorders.
▼ You have high blood pressure.
▼ You have porphyria.
▼ You have a history of lung disease.
▼ You are allergic to ergot alkaloids.
▼ You are taking other medications.

Pregnancy
▼ Safety in pregnancy not established. Discuss with your physician.

Breast-feeding
▼ The drug suppresses milk production, and prevents it completely if given within 12 hours of delivery. If you wish to breast-feed, consult your physician.

Infants and children
▼ Not usually prescribed under 15 years.

Over 60
▼ Reduced dose may be necessary.

Driving and hazardous work
▼ Avoid such activities until you have learned how bromocriptine affects you because the drug may cause dizziness and drowsiness.

Alcohol
▼ Avoid. Alcohol increases the likelihood of confusion and reduces *tolerance* to bromocriptine.

POSSIBLE ADVERSE EFFECTS

Common adverse effects include headache, lightheadedness, dizziness, and nausea/vomiting. May cause abnormal movements when used for parkinsonism.

Symptom/effect	Frequency		Discuss with physician		Stop taking drug now	Call physician now
	Common	Rare	Only if severe	In all cases		
Confusion/dizziness	●			■		
Circulatory problems	●			■		
Nausea/vomiting	●		■			
Severe headache		●		■	▲	▮
Constipation		●	■			
Abnormal movements		●		■		
Drowsiness		●		■	▲	▮
Hypertension		●		■	▲	▮

INTERACTIONS

Antipsychotic drugs These drugs oppose the action of bromocriptine and increase the risk of parkinsonism.

Ephedrine, pseudoephedrine, and phenothiazines These drugs are found in some over-the-counter cough and cold remedies. Use of these with bromocriptine may lead to severe adverse effects.

Erythromycin and other macrolide antibiotics These drugs may lead to increased levels of bromocriptine and the risk of adverse effects.

Domperidone and metoclopramide These drugs may reduce some of the effects of bromocriptine.

PROLONGED USE

No special problems.

Monitoring Periodic blood tests may be performed to check hormone levels. Gynecological tests may be carried out annually (or every six months in post-menopausal women). Monitoring for other, rare, adverse effects (e.g., peptic ulcer in acromegaly) may also be carried out.

BUDESONIDE

Product names Entocort, Pulmicort, Rhinocort Aqua
Used in the following combined preparation Symbicort

GENERAL INFORMATION

Budesonide is a corticosteroid drug used in the form of slow-release capsules to relieve the symptoms of Crohn's disease and as an enema to treat ulcerative colitis. It is also used as an inhaler to prevent attacks of asthma but will not stop an existing attack. Like other corticosteroids, budesonide is used by people whose asthma is not controlled by bronchodilators (p.76) alone. It is also used as a nasal spray to relieve the symptoms of allergic rhinitis and for nasal polyps.

Budesonide controls symptoms by reducing inflammation, whether it is in the nose, lungs, or intestine.

There are fewer, usually less serious, *side effects* when budesonide is taken by inhaler or nasal spray because the drug is absorbed by the body in much smaller quantities than when it is taken by mouth.

QUICK REFERENCE

Drug group Corticosteroid (p.127)
Overdose danger rating Low
Dependence rating Low
Prescription needed Yes
Available as generic Yes

INFORMATION FOR USERS

Your drug prescription is tailored for you. Do not alter dosage without checking with your physician.

How taken

SR-capsules, enema, inhaler, powder for inhalation, nasal spray.

Frequency and timing of doses
Once daily in morning before meal (capsules); once daily at bedtime (enema); twice daily (inhaler); once or twice daily (nasal spray).

Usual dosage range
3–9mg (capsules); 2mg (enema); 200mcg–1,600mcg (inhaler), 100–200mcg (nasal spray).

Onset of effect
Asthma Within 1 week.
Other conditions 1–3 days.

Duration of action
12–24 hours.

Diet advice
None.

Storage
Keep in a closed container in a cool, dry place out of the reach of children.

Missed dose
Take as soon as you remember. If your next dose is due within 2 hours, take a single dose now and skip the next.

Stopping the drug
Do not stop taking the drug without consulting your physician; symptoms may recur. The SR-capsules used in Crohn's disease should be withdrawn gradually.

Exceeding the dose
An occasional extra dose is unlikely to be a cause for concern. But if you notice any unusual symptoms, or if a large overdose has been taken, notify your physician.

SPECIAL PRECAUTIONS

Be sure to tell your physician if:
▼ You have had tuberculosis or another respiratory infection.
▼ You are taking other medications.

 Pregnancy
▼ Discuss with physician, especially if used for Crohn's disease.

 Breast-feeding
▼ Discuss with physician, especially if used for Crohn's disease.

 Infants and children
▼ Reduced dose necessary.

 Over 60
▼ No special problems.

 Driving and hazardous work
▼ No special problems.

 Alcohol
▼ No special problems.

POSSIBLE ADVERSE EFFECTS

The main side effects of inhalers and nasal spray are confined to the nasal passages and mouth. Capsules and enemas can cause gastrointestinal disturbances and rashes.

High doses of budesonide by any route can cause weight gain and other long-term side effects associated with corticosteroids.

Symptom/effect	Frequency		Discuss with physician		Stop taking drug now	Call physician now
	Common	Rare	Only if severe	In all cases		
Inhalers and nasal spray						
Nasal irritation	●		■			
Cough	●		■			
Sore throat/hoarseness	●			■		
Nosebleed		●		■		
Capsules and enema						
Diarrhea/constipation	●		■			
Rash/itching		●		■		
Mood disorders		●		■		
All preparations						
Weight gain		●		■		
Pain in the eye		●		■	▲	■

PROLONGED USE

Asthma prevention is the condition for which prolonged use may be required. There may be a small risk of glaucoma, cataracts, and effects on bone with high doses inhaled for a prolonged period. Patients taking budesonide long term are advised to carry a steroid card or wear a Medic-alert bracelet.

Monitoring If budesonide is being taken in large doses, periodic checks may be needed to make sure that the adrenal glands are working properly. Children using inhalers may have their growth (height) monitored regularly.

INTERACTIONS

Ketoconazole/other azole antifungals Can increase the blood level of oral budesonide.

BUMETANIDE

Product name Burinex
Used in the following combined preparations None

GENERAL INFORMATION

Bumetanide is a powerful, short-acting loop diuretic used to treat edema (accumulation of fluid in tissue spaces) resulting from heart failure, nephrotic syndrome, and cirrhosis of the liver. Bumetanide is particularly useful in treating people with impaired kidney function who do not respond well to thiazide diuretics. Because it is fast-acting, it is often injected in an emergency to relieve pulmonary edema (fluid in the lungs).

Bumetanide increases potassium loss in the urine, which can result in a wide variety of symptoms (see p.85). For this reason, potassium supplements or a potassium-sparing diuretic are often given with the drug.

INFORMATION FOR USERS

Your drug prescription is tailored for you. Do not alter dosage without checking with your physician.

How taken

Tablets.

Frequency and timing of doses
Usually once daily in the morning. In some cases, twice daily.

Usual dosage range
0.5–5mg daily. Dose may be increased if kidney function is impaired.

Onset of effect
Within 30 minutes by mouth.

Duration of action
2–4 hours.

Diet advice
Use of this drug may reduce potassium in the body. Eat plenty of fresh fruit and vegetables, such as bananas and tomatoes.

Storage
Keep in a closed container in a cool, dry place out of the reach of children. Protect from light.

Missed dose
No cause for concern, but take as soon as you remember. However, if it is late in the day do not take the missed dose, or you may need to get up during the night to pass urine. Take the next scheduled dose as usual.

Stopping the drug
Do not stop the drug without consulting your physician; symptoms may recur.

Exceeding the dose
An occasional unintentional extra dose is unlikely to be a cause for concern. But if you notice any unusual symptoms, or if a large overdose has been taken, notify your physician.

SPECIAL PRECAUTIONS

Be sure to tell your physician if:
▼ You have long-term liver or kidney problems.
▼ You have diabetes.
▼ You have prostate trouble.
▼ You have gout.
▼ You are taking other medications.

Pregnancy
▼ Not usually prescribed. May cause a reduction in blood supply to the developing baby. Discuss with your physician.

Breast-feeding
▼ This drug may reduce your milk supply. Discuss with your physician.

Infants and children
▼ Not usually prescribed. Reduced dose necessary.

Over 60
▼ Dosage is often reduced.

Driving and hazardous work
▼ Avoid such activities until you have learned how bumetanide affects you because the drug may cause dizziness and faintness.

Alcohol
▼ Keep consumption low. The drug increases the likelihood of dehydration and hangovers after drinking alcohol.

POSSIBLE ADVERSE EFFECTS

Adverse effects are caused mainly by the rapid fluid loss produced by bumetanide. These diminish as the body adjusts to the drug. Bumetanide may precipitate gout in susceptible individuals and can affect the control of diabetes.

Symptom/effect	Frequency		Discuss with physician		Stop taking drug now	Call physician now
	Common	Rare	Only if severe	In all cases		
Dizziness/fainting	●		■			
Lethargy/fatigue		●	■			
Muscle cramps		●	■			
Rash/photosensitivity		●		■		
Nausea/vomiting		●		■		
Pain in joints		●		■		

INTERACTIONS

Anti-arrhythmic drugs Low potassium levels may increase these drugs' toxicity.

Antibacterials Bumetanide can increase the ear damage that is caused by some antibiotics.

Digoxin Excessive potassium loss may increase the adverse effects of digoxin.

Non-steroidal anti-inflammatory drugs (NSAIDs) These drugs may reduce the diuretic effect of bumetanide.

Lithium Bumetanide may increase the blood levels of lithium, leading to an increased risk of lithium *toxicity*.

Pimozide Low potassium levels increase the risk of abnormal heart rhythms with this antipsychotic drug.

PROLONGED USE

Serious problems are unlikely, but the levels of certain salts in the body may occasionally become abnormal during prolonged use.

Monitoring Regular blood tests may be performed to check on kidney function and levels of body salts.

BUPROPION

Product names Wellbutrin SR, Zyban
Used in the following combined preparations None

GENERAL INFORMATION

Bupropion is an antidepressant; chemically it is unrelated to other antidepressant drugs. Although it has been used to treat depression, it is generally used as an aid for people who are trying to give up tobacco smoking. The person being treated must commit in advance to a stop date. Treatment is started while the patient is still smoking and the "target stop date" decided on within the first two weeks of treatment. Bupropion will be stopped after 7 weeks if the smoker has not made significant progress in giving up smoking by then. Although the drug can be an effective aid, nicotine replacement therapy is more popular.

Bupropion should not be prescribed for people with a history of seizures or eating disorders, or who are withdrawing from benzodiazepine or alcohol. Neither should the drug be used by people with manic depression or psychosis because there is a risk of mania developing.

QUICK REFERENCE

Drug group Nicotine withdrawal aid (pp.24, 367)

Overdose danger rating High

Dependence rating Low

Prescription needed Yes

Available as generic Yes

INFORMATION FOR USERS

Your drug prescription is tailored for you. Do not alter dosage without checking with your physician.

How taken

SR-tablets.

Frequency and timing of doses
1–2 x daily.

Usual adult dosage range
150–300mg (maximum dose).

Onset of effect
Up to 4 weeks for full effect.

Duration of action
12 hours.

Diet advice
None.

Storage
Keep in original closed container in a cool, dry place out of the reach of children.

Missed dose
Take as soon as you remember. If your next dose is due within 2 hours, take a single dose now and skip the next dose.

Stopping the drug
Do not stop the drug without consulting your physician. The physician may want to taper the dose.

OVERDOSE ACTION

 Seek immediate medical advice in all cases. Take emergency action if consciousness is lost.

See Drug poisoning emergency guide (p.526)

POSSIBLE ADVERSE EFFECTS

Some effects, for example agitation, tremor, sweating, and insomnia, may be due to the withdrawal of nicotine rather than to the effects of bupropion itself.

Symptom/effect	Frequency		Discuss with physician		Stop taking drug now	Call physician now
	Common	Rare	Only if severe	In all cases		
Insomnia/poor concentration	●		■			
Headache/dizziness/tremor	●		■			
Nausea/vomiting	●		■			
Rash/fever	●			■		
Palpitations/fainting		●		■		
Confusion/anxiety		●		■		
Seizures		●		■	▲	▮
Dry mouth	●		■			
Depression	●			■		

INTERACTIONS

General note A wide range of drugs increases the likelihood of seizures when taken with bupropion. Check with your physician if you are on other medications.

Ritonavir, amantadine, and levodopa may all increase the risk of side effects with bupropion.

Antiepileptics Phenytoin and carbamazepine may reduce the blood levels and effects of bupropion. Valproate may increase its blood levels and effects.

SPECIAL PRECAUTIONS

Be sure to tell your physician if:
▼ You have a head injury or history of seizures.
▼ You have an eating disorder.
▼ You have cancer of the nervous system.
▼ You have diabetes.
▼ You have manic depression or a psychosis.
▼ You have kidney or liver problems.
▼ You are withdrawing from alcohol or benzodiazepine dependence.
▼ You are taking other medications.

 Pregnancy
▼ Safety in pregnancy is not established. Try to give up smoking without using drugs.

 Breast-feeding
▼ Safety not established. The drug passes into the breast milk and may affect the baby.

 Infants and children
▼ Not recommended.

 Over 60
▼ Increased sensitivity to drug's effects. Reduced dose may therefore be necessary.

 Driving and hazardous work
▼ Avoid until you have learned how bupropion affects you. The drug may cause impaired concentration and dizziness.

 Alcohol
▼ Avoid. Alcohol will increase any sedative effects.

PROLONGED USE

Bupropion is used for up to 9 weeks for cessation of smoking.

Monitoring Progress will be reviewed after about 3–4 weeks, and the drug continued only if it is having some effect.

BUSPIRONE

Product names Apo-Buspirone, BuSpar, Novo-Buspirone, and others
Used in the following combined preparations None

GENERAL INFORMATION

Buspirone is an anti-anxiety drug that is used for the treatment of anxiety disorders marked by persistent, unrealistic, and excessive worry and anxiety. It is used in conjunction with counselling. It is thought to act by increasing 5-HT (serotonin) and dopamine levels in the brain.

Buspirone is as effective as benzodiazepine drugs (see p.67), but has a far lesser sedating effect. It may take one to two weeks to see an effect, and up to four weeks for the maximum benefit of the drug to be achieved.

see p.67

QUICK REFERENCE

Drug group Anti-anxiety (p.67)
Overdose danger rating Medium
Dependence rating Low
Prescription needed Yes
Available as generic Yes

(p.67)

INFORMATION FOR USERS

Your drug prescription is tailored for you. Do not alter dosage without checking with your physician.

How taken

Tablets.

Frequency and timing of doses
2–3 x daily.

Usual dosage range
5–30 mg daily.

Onset of effect
40–90 minutes.

Duration of action
Variable; up to 11 hours.

Diet advice
None.

Storage
Keep in a closed container in a cool, dry place away from the reach of children.

Missed dose
No cause for concern, but take when you next feel you need the drug. If your next dose is due within 2 hours, take a single dose now and skip the next dose.

Stopping the drug
If you have been taking the drug continuously for less than 2 weeks, it can be safely stopped if you no longer need it. However, if you have been taking it for a longer period of time, consult your physician. Stopping abruptly may lead to withdrawal symptoms.

Exceeding the dose
An occasional, unintentional extra dose is unlikely to cause problems. Larger overdoses may cause unusual drowsiness. Notify your physician.

SPECIAL PRECAUTIONS

Be sure to tell your physician if:
▼ You have impaired kidney or liver function.
▼ You have any form of epilepsy or any other convulsive disorder.
▼ You have a problem with alcohol or drug abuse.
▼ You are taking other medications.

Pregnancy
▼ Safety in pregnancy not established. Discuss with your physician.

Breast-feeding
▼ Safety in breast-feeding not established. Discuss with your physician.

Infants and children
▼ Not recommended for patients under 18 years of age.

Over 60
▼ Increased chance of adverse effects. Reduced dosage, therefore, may be necessary.

Driving and hazardous work
▼ Avoid such activities until you have learned how the drug affects you; it can cause reduced alertness and slowed reactions.

Alcohol
▼ Avoid. Alcohol may increase the sedative effects of this drug.

POSSIBLE ADVERSE EFFECTS

The most common adverse reactions encountered with buspirone are dizziness, headache, drowsiness, and nausea. They normally diminish after the first few days and if troublesome, they can usually be reduced by adjustment of dosage.

Symptom/effect	Frequency		Discuss with physician		Stop taking drug now	Call physician now
	Common	Rare	Only if severe	In all cases		
Dizziness/lightheadedness	●		■			
Headache	●			■		
Daytime drowsiness	●			■		
Nausea	●		■			
Skin rash		●		■	▲	▮
Sore throat		●		■	▲	▮

INTERACTIONS

Sedatives All drugs, including alcohol, that have a sedating effect on the central nervous system are likely to increase the sedative effects of buspirone.

Cyclosporine and haloperidol Buspirone may increase blood levels of these drugs.

Verapamil, diltiazem, itraconazole, and erythromycin may increase blood levels of buspirone.

Monamine oxidase inhibitors (MAOIs) Phenelzine, tranylcypromine, and moclobemide taken with buspirone may cause increased blood pressure; therefore, they should not be used together.

Grapefruit juice Regular intake of grapefruit juice can increase buspirone levels; avoid.

PROLONGED USE

If buspirone is taken for longer than 3–4 weeks, the need for continued therapy should be reassessed regularly.

CALCIPOTRIOL

Product name Dovonex
Used in the following combined preparations Dovobet

GENERAL INFORMATION

Calcipotriol is used in the treatment of psoriasis affecting up to 40 per cent of the patient's skin area, and also for scalp psoriasis.

Calcipotriol is similar to vitamin D. It is thought to work by reducing production of the skin cells that cause skin thickening and scaling, which are the most common symptoms of psoriasis. Because this drug is related to vitamin D, excessive use (more than 100g per week) can lead to a rise in calcium levels in the body; otherwise calcipotriol is unlikely to cause any serious *adverse effects*.

The drug is applied to the affected areas in the form of cream, ointment, or scalp solution. It should not be used on the face, and it is important that the hands are washed following application of this ointment to avoid accidental transfer to unaffected areas. Local irritation may occur during the early stages of treatment.

QUICK REFERENCE

Drug group Drug for psoriasis (p.166)

Overdose danger rating Low

Dependence rating Low

Prescription needed Yes

Available as generic No

INFORMATION FOR USERS

Your drug prescription is tailored for you. Do not alter dosage without checking with your physician.

How taken

Cream, ointment, scalp solution.

Frequency and timing of doses
1–2 x daily.

Usual adult dosage range
Maximum 100g each week. Scalp solution, maximum 60ml each week. Less if both preparations are used together.

Onset of effect
Improvement is seen within 2 weeks.

Duration of action
One application lasts up to 12 hours. Beneficial effects are longer lasting.

Diet advice
None.

Storage
Store at room temperature out of the reach of children.

Missed dose
Apply the next dose at the scheduled time.

Stopping the drug
Do not stop taking the drug without consulting your physician; symptoms may recur.

Exceeding the dose
Excessive prolonged use may lead to an increase in blood calcium levels, which can cause nausea, constipation, thirst, and frequent urination. Notify your physician.

POSSIBLE ADVERSE EFFECTS

Temporary local irritation may occur when treatment is started. The other effects are usually due to heavy or prolonged use, leading to high calcium levels in the blood.

Symptom/effect	Frequency		Discuss with physician		Stop taking drug now	Call physician now
	Common	Rare	Only if severe	In all cases		
Local irritation	●		■			
Rash on face/mouth		●		■		
Thirst/frequent urination		●		■		
Nausea/constipation		●		■		
Light sensitive rash		●		■		

INTERACTIONS

None known.

SPECIAL PRECAUTIONS

Be sure to tell your physician if:
▼ You have a metabolic disorder.
▼ You have previously had a hypersensitivity reaction to the drug.
▼ You are taking other medications.

 Pregnancy
▼ Safety in pregnancy not established. Discuss with your physician.

 Breast-feeding
▼ Not known if excreted into breast milk. Discuss with your physician.

 Infants and children
▼ Not recommended under 6 years. Lower dose recommended in children under 14 years.

 Over 60
▼ No problems expected.

 Driving and hazardous work
▼ No problems expected.

 Alcohol
▼ No problems expected.

PROLONGED USE

No problems expected from use of calcipotriol in low doses. If the effects of the skin preparation decline after several weeks, they may be regained by suspending use for a few weeks and then recommencing treatment.

Monitoring Regular checks on calcium levels in the blood or urine are required during prolonged or heavy use.

CAPTOPRIL

Product names Apo-Capto, Capoten, Gen-Captopril, and others
Used in the following combined preparations None

GENERAL INFORMATION

Captopril belongs to the class of drugs called ACE inhibitors, used to treat high blood pressure and heart failure. The drug works by relaxing the muscles around blood vessels, allowing them to dilate and thereby easing blood flow.

Captopril lowers blood pressure rapidly but may require several weeks to achieve full effect. People with heart failure may be given captopril in addition to diuretics. It can achieve dramatic results, relaxing muscle in blood vessel walls and reducing the heart's workload.

The first dose is usually very small and taken while lying down as there is a risk of a sudden fall in blood pressure. Diuretics are often given at the same time.

A variety of minor *side effects* may occur. Some people experience loss of taste, while others get a persistent dry cough. A reduction in dose may help minimize these effects.

QUICK REFERENCE

Drug group ACE inhibitor (p.84)
Overdose danger rating Medium
Dependence rating Low
Prescription needed Yes
Available as generic Yes

INFORMATION FOR USERS

Your drug prescription is tailored for you. Do not alter dosage without checking with your physician.

How taken

Tablets.

Frequency and timing of doses
2–3 x daily.

Usual adult dosage range
12.5–25mg daily initially, gradually increased to 50–150mg daily. Starting doses of 6.25mg may be used.

Onset of effect
30–60 minutes.

Duration of action
6–8 hours.

Diet advice
None.

Storage
Keep in a closed container in a cool, dry place out of the reach of children.

Missed dose
Take as soon as you remember. If your next dose is due within 2 hours, take a single dose now and skip the next.

Stopping the drug
Do not stop the drug without consulting your physician; stopping the drug may lead to worsening of the underlying condition.

Exceeding the dose
An occasional unintentional extra dose is unlikely to cause problems. Large overdoses may cause dizziness or fainting. Notify your physician.

SPECIAL PRECAUTIONS

Be sure to tell your physician if:
▼ You have long-term kidney problems.
▼ You have coronary artery disease.
▼ You are on a low sodium diet.
▼ You are allergic to ACE inhibitors.
▼ You are taking other medications.

Pregnancy
▼ Not usually prescribed. There is evidence of harm to the developing fetus. Discuss with your physician.

Breast-feeding
▼ The drug passes into the breast milk, but at normal doses adverse effects on the baby are unlikely. Discuss with your physician.

Infants and children
▼ Not usually prescribed. Reduced dose necessary.

Over 60
▼ Reduced dose may be necessary.

Driving and hazardous work
▼ Avoid such activities until you have learned how captopril affects you because the drug can cause dizziness and fainting.

Alcohol
▼ Avoid. Alcohol may increase the blood-pressure lowering and adverse effects of the drug.

Surgery and general anesthetics
▼ Captopril may need to be stopped before you have a general anesthetic. Discuss with your physician or dentist before any operation.

POSSIBLE ADVERSE EFFECTS

Captopril causes a variety of minor adverse effects, primarily rashes and gastrointestinal symptoms. These usually disappear soon after treatment has started.

Symptom/effect	Frequency		Discuss with physician		Stop taking drug now	Call physician now
	Common	Rare	Only if severe	In all cases		
Loss of taste	●		■			
Rash	●			■		
Persistent dry cough	●			■		
Mouth ulcers/sore mouth		●		■		
Dizziness/fainting		●		■		
Sore throat/fever		●		■		
Swelling of mouth/lips		●		■	▲	■

INTERACTIONS

Non-steroidal anti-inflammatory drugs (NSAIDs) may reduce the effectiveness of captopril. There is also a risk of kidney damage when they are taken with captopril.

Lithium Blood levels of lithium may be raised by captopril.

Vasodilators (e.g., nitrates) These drugs may reduce blood pressure even further.

Potassium supplements and potassium-sparing diuretics increase the risk of high potassium levels when taken with captopril.

Cyclosporine This drug increases the risk of high potassium levels in the blood when taken with captopril.

Diuretics Taking captopril with these drugs can cause a rapid fall in blood pressure.

PROLONGED USE

Rarely, prolonged use can lead to changes in the blood count or kidney function.

Monitoring Periodic checks on potassium levels, white blood cell count, kidney function, and urine are usually performed.

CARBAMAZEPINE

Product names Apo-Carbamazepine, Novo-Carbamaz, Tegretol, and others
Used in the following combined preparations None

GENERAL INFORMATION

Carbamazepine is used to treat some forms of epilepsy as it reduces the likelihood of fits caused by abnormal nerve signals in the brain.

Carbamazepine is also prescribed to relieve the intermittent severe pain caused by damage to the cranial nerves in trigeminal neuralgia. Carbamazepine is also occasionally prescribed to treat manic depression and diabetes insipidus and is used for pain relief in diabetic neuropathy.

In order to avoid *side effects*, carbamazepine therapy is usually commenced at a low dose and is gradually increased. It is recommended that patients stick to the brand of carbamazepine prescribed.

INFORMATION FOR USERS

Your drug prescription is tailored for you. Do not alter dosage without checking with your physician.

How taken

CR (controlled release) tablets, tablets chewable tablets, liquid, suppositories.

Frequency and timing of doses
1–2 x daily.

Usual adult dosage range
Epilepsy 100–2,000mg daily (low starting dose that is slowly increased every 2 weeks).
Pain relief 100–1,600mg daily.
Psychiatric disorders 400–1,600mg daily.

Onset of effect
Within 4 hours.

Duration of action
12–24 hours.

Diet advice
None.

Storage
Keep in a closed container in a cool, dry place out of the reach of children.

Missed dose
Take as soon as you remember. If your next dose is due within 2 hours, take a single dose now and skip the next.

Stopping the drug
Do not stop the drug without consulting your physician; symptoms may recur.

Exceeding the dose
An occasional unintentional extra dose is unlikely to cause problems. Large overdoses may cause tremor, convulsions, and coma. Notify your physician.

SPECIAL PRECAUTIONS

Be sure to tell your physician if:
▼ You have long-term liver or kidney problems.
▼ You have heart problems.
▼ You have had blood problems with other drugs or porphyria.
▼ You are taking other medications.

Pregnancy
▼ May be associated with abnormalities in the unborn baby. Folic acid supplements should be taken before and during pregnancy. Discuss with your physician.

Breast-feeding
▼ The drug passes into the breast milk, but at normal doses adverse effects on the baby are unlikely. Discuss with your physician.

Infants and children
▼ Reduced dose necessary.

Over 60
▼ May cause confused or agitated behaviour in the elderly. Reduced dose may be necessary.

Driving and hazardous work
▼ Discuss with your physician. Your underlying condition, as well as the possibility of reduced alertness while taking carbamazepine, may make such activities inadvisable.

Alcohol
▼ Avoid. Alcohol may increase the sedative effects of this drug.

POSSIBLE ADVERSE EFFECTS

Most people experience very few adverse effects with this drug, but when blood levels get too high, adverse effects are common and the dose may need to be reduced.

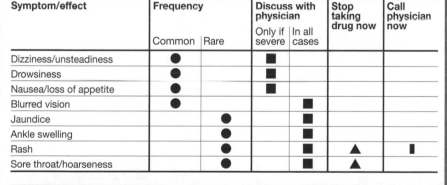

Symptom/effect	Frequency		Discuss with physician		Stop taking drug now	Call physician now
	Common	Rare	Only if severe	In all cases		
Dizziness/unsteadiness	●		■			
Drowsiness	●		■			
Nausea/loss of appetite	●		■			
Blurred vision	●			■		
Jaundice		●		■		
Ankle swelling		●		■		
Rash		●		■	▲	▮
Sore throat/hoarseness		●		■	▲	

INTERACTIONS

General note Many drugs may increase or reduce the effects of carbamazepine. Discuss with your physician or pharmacist before taking other medications.

Other antiepileptic drugs Complex and variable interactions can occur between these drugs and carbamazepine.

Grapefruit juice May increase carbamazepine blood levels; avoid.

Oral contraceptives Carbamazepine may affect the blood level of oral contraceptives

PROLONGED USE

There is a slight risk of changes in liver function or of skin or blood abnormalities occurring during prolonged use.

Monitoring Periodic blood tests are usually performed to monitor levels of the drug, blood cell counts, and liver and kidney function.

CEFUROXIME

Product names Apo-Cefuroxime, Ceftin, Ratio-Cefuroxime
Used in the following combined preparations None

GENERAL INFORMATION

Cefuroxime is a cephalosporin antibiotic that is prescribed for a variety of mild to moderately severe infections. It is used for upper respiratory tract infections such as pharyngitis, tonsillitis, ear infections, and sinus infections. It is also used in lower respiratory tract infections such as pneumonia and bronchitis. Cefuroxime may be used in some skin and soft tissue infections, urinary tract infections, and for gonorrhea. The injectable form can be used to treat meningitis.

Cefuroxime axetil is an orally active drug of cefuroxime. Absorption of the oral formulation is better when administered with food. The liquid suspension should be shaken well before use.

Patients who are allergic to penicillins have a higher chance of being allergic to a cephalosporin antibiotic and cefuroxime should be used cautiously in these individuals.

INFORMATION FOR USERS

Your drug prescription is tailored for you. Do not alter dosage without checking with your physician.

How taken

Tablets, liquid, injection.

Frequency and timing of doses
1–2 times daily. Take oral dose with food.

Usual dosage range
Adults 500mg–1g daily.
Children 3 months to < 12 years Dose based on body weight.

Onset of effect
Within 1 hour.

Duration of action
6–12 hours.

Diet advice
None.

Storage
Keep tablets in a closed container in a cool, dry place out of the reach of children. The solution should be stored between 2 and 25°C, preferably in the refrigerator. Any leftover solution should be discarded after 10 days.

Missed dose
Take as soon as you remember, then continue with your regular dosing regiment.

Stopping the drug
Take the full course. Even if you feel better, the original infection may still be present and may recur if treatment is stopped too soon.

Exceeding the dose
An occasional unintentional extra dose is unlikely to cause problems. But if you notice any unusual symptoms, or if a large overdose has been taken, notify your physician.

SPECIAL PRECAUTIONS

Be sure to tell your physician if:
▼ You have a long-term kidney problem.
▼ You have had a previous allergic reaction to a penicillin or a cephalosporin.
▼ You have a history of blood disorders.
▼ You have a gastrointestinal disease such as colitis.
▼ You are taking other medications.

Pregnancy
▼ Safety not established. Discuss with your physician.

Breast-feeding
▼ Safety not established. Discuss with your physician.

Infants and children
▼ May be used in children older than 3 months.

Over 60
▼ May require a reduced dose.

Driving and hazardous work
▼ No known problems.

Alcohol
▼ No known problems.

POSSIBLE ADVERSE EFFECTS

Diarrhea can occur but is usually mild. A physician should be consulted for ongoing or worsening diarrhea or diarrhea occurring after finishing the antibiotic course.

Symptom/effect	Frequency		Discuss with physician		Stop taking drug now	Call physician now
	Common	Rare	Only if severe	In all cases		
Diarrhea	●		■			
Headache/dizziness	●		■			
Nausea/vomiting	●		■			
Rash		●		■	▲	▌
Itching/swelling/wheezing		●		■	▲	▌
Jaundice/tiredness		●		■		▌

INTERACTIONS

Aminoglycosides When administered with cefuroxime, increase risk of kidney problems. Monitor closely.

Probenecid May increase the level of cefuroxime. Monitor closely.

PROLONGED USE

Cefuroxime is usually given only for short courses of treatment. Use of large doses or prolonged therapy requires close monitoring.

CELECOXIB

Product name Celebrex
Used in the following combined preparations None

GENERAL INFORMATION

Celecoxib is one of a subgroup of NSAIDs called cyclo-oxygenase-2 (COX-2) selective inhibitors; these drugs have a lower risk of causing irritation and ulceration to the upper gastrointestinal tract than other NSAIDs. It is useful for people who need an NSAID but who have had problems, such as stomach ulcers, with other drugs. It is also given to groups at high risk of developing gastro-intestinal problems, such as the elderly.

Celecoxib reduces pain, stiffness, and inflammation and is used to relieve the symptoms of both rheumatoid arthritis and osteoarthritis.

Elderly patients and those with kidney problems may be more sensitive to the drug's effects; they are usually prescribed a low dose to begin with.

Celecoxib does not protect against coronary heart disease as is the case with aspirin and some other NSAIDs.

QUICK REFERENCE

Drug group Analgesic (p.64) and non steroidal anti-inflammatory drug (p.102)
Overdose danger rating Medium
Dependence rating Low
Prescription needed Yes
Available as generic No

INFORMATION FOR USERS

Your drug prescription is tailored for you. Do not alter dosage without checking with your physician.

How taken

Capsules.

Frequency and timing of doses
1–2 x daily.

Usual adult dosage range
200–400mg daily.

Onset of effect
1 hour.

Duration of action
8–12 hours.

Diet advice
None.

Storage
Keep in a cool, dry place out of the reach of children.

Missed dose
Take as soon as you remember. If your next dose is due within 4 hours, take a single dose now and skip the next.

Stopping the drug
If being used short term, the drug can safely be stopped as soon as you no longer need it. If prescribed for long-term use, you should not stop taking the drug without consulting your physician.

Exceeding the dose
An occasional unintentional extra dose is unlikely to cause problems. Large overdoses can cause stomach and intestinal pain and damage. Notify your physician.

SPECIAL PRECAUTIONS

Be sure to tell your physician if:
▼ You have asthma.
▼ You have angina/coronary heart disease.
▼ You are allergic to ASA or celecoxib.
▼ You are allergic to sulfonamides.
▼ You have a peptic ulcer or gastrointestinal bleeding.
▼ You have inflammatory bowel disease.
▼ You have congestive heart failure.
▼ You are taking other medicines.

Pregnancy
▼ Not prescribed.

Breast-feeding
▼ Not prescribed.

Infants and children
▼ Not recommended.

Over 60
▼ Elderly people may be more sensitive to the drug's effects. Lower doses may be necessary.

Driving and hazardous work
▼ Avoid until you know how the drug affects you. It can cause dizziness, vertigo, and sleepiness.

Alcohol
▼ Alcohol may increase drowsiness and the risk of stomach irritation.

POSSIBLE ADVERSE EFFECTS

Gastrointestinal, nervous, and respiratory symptoms are the most likely adverse effects.

Symptom/effect	Frequency		Discuss with physician		Stop taking drug now	Call physician now
	Common	Rare	Only if severe	In all cases		
Indigestion/abdominal pain	●		■			
Diarrhea/flatulence	●		■			
Dizziness/insomnia	●		■			
Rash	●			■		
Swollen ankles	●			■		
Palpitations/difficulty breathing		●		■		▮
Black/bloody vomit/feces		●		■	▲	▮

INTERACTIONS

Anticoagulants The effecs of warfarin are increased by celecoxib.

ACE inhibitors increase the risk of renal failure.

Antihypertensives and diuretics Blood pressure-lowering effects may be reduced by celecoxib.

Lithium levels and effects are increased when taken with celecoxib.

Cyclosporine and tacrolimus may increase the risk of renal toxicity if taken with celecoxib.

Methotrexate Excretion of this drug is slowed by NSAIDs (possibly including celecoxib) causing increased toxicity.

Carbamazepine, fluconazole, rifampin, and barbiturates reduce the effects of celecoxib.

PROLONGED USE

There is a smaller risk of peptic ulcers compared to other NSAIDs when used long-term.

Monitoring Periodic tests of kidney function may be performed.

CEPHALEXIN

Product names Apo-Cephalex, Novo-Lexin, and others
Used in the following combined preparations None

GENERAL INFORMATION

Cephalexin is a cephalosporin antibiotic that is prescribed for a variety of mild to moderate infections. Cephalexin does not have such a wide range of uses as some other antibiotics, but it is helpful in treating bronchitis, cystitis, and certain skin and soft tissue infections. In some cases it is prescribed as follow-up treatment for severe infections after a more powerful cephalosporin has been given by injection.

Diarrhea is the most common *side effect* of cephalexin, although it tends to be less severe than with other cephalosporin antibiotics. In addition, some people may find that they are allergic to this drug, especially if they are sensitive to penicillin.

INFORMATION FOR USERS

Your drug prescription is tailored for you. Do not alter dosage without checking with your physician.

How taken

Tablets, capsules, liquid.

Frequency and timing of doses
Usually 4 x daily. May take with food.

Usual dosage range
Adults 1–2g daily, up to a maximum of 4g.
Children Reduced dose according to age and weight.

Onset of effect
Within 1 hour.

Duration of action
6–12 hours.

Diet advice
None.

Storage
Keep tablets and capsules in a closed container in a cool, dry place out of the reach of children. Refrigerate liquid, but do not freeze, and keep for no longer than 10 days. Protect from light.

Missed dose
Take as soon as you remember. If your next dose is due at this time, take both doses now.

Stopping the drug
Take the full course. Even if you feel better, the original infection may still be present and may recur if treatment is stopped too soon.

Exceeding the dose
An occasional unintentional extra dose is unlikely to be a cause for concern. But if you notice any unusual symptoms, or if a large overdose has been taken, notify your physician.

SPECIAL PRECAUTIONS

Be sure to tell your physician if:
▼ You have a long-term kidney problem.
▼ You have had a previous allergic reaction to a penicillin or cephalosporin antibiotic.
▼ You have a history of blood disorders.
▼ You are taking other medications.

Pregnancy
▼ No evidence of risk to the developing baby.

Breast-feeding
▼ The drug passes into the breast milk but at normal doses adverse effects on the baby are unlikely. Discuss with your physician.

Infants and children
▼ Reduced dose necessary.

Over 60
▼ No special problems.

Driving and hazardous work
▼ No known problems.

Alcohol
▼ No known problems.

POSSIBLE ADVERSE EFFECTS

Most people do not suffer serious adverse effects while taking cephalexin. Diarrhea is common but it tends not to be severe. The rarer adverse effects are usually due to an allergic reaction and may necessitate stopping the drug.

Symptom/effect	Frequency		Discuss with physician		Stop taking drug now	Call physician now
	Common	Rare	Only if severe	In all cases		
Diarrhea	●		■			
Nausea/vomiting	●		■			
Abdominal pain		●		■		
Rash		●		■	▲	∎
Itching/swelling/wheezing		●		■	▲	∎

INTERACTIONS

Probenecid This drug increases the level of cephalexin in the blood. The dosage of cephalexin may need to be adjusted accordingly.

Oral contraceptives Cephalexin may reduce the contraceptive effect of these drugs. Discuss with your physician.

PROLONGED USE

Cephalexin is usually given only for short courses of treatment. Use of large doses or prolonged therapy requires close monitoring.

CETIRIZINE

Product names Reactine, Apo-Cetrizine
Used in the following combined preparations None

GENERAL INFORMATION

Cetirizine is a long-acting antihistamine. Its main use is in the treatment of allergic rhinitis, particularly hay fever. It is also used to treat a number of allergic skin conditions, such as urticaria (hives).

The principal difference between cetirizine and traditional antihistamines such as chlorpheniramine is that this has a less *sedative* effect on the central nervous system and may therefore be suitable for people when they need to avoid sleepiness – for example, when driving or at work. However, because these drugs can cause drowsiness in some people, you should learn how cetirizine affects you before you undertake any activities that require concentration.

INFORMATION FOR USERS

Your drug prescription is tailored for you. Do not alter dosage without checking with your physician.

How taken

Tablets, liquid.

Frequency and timing of doses
1–2 x daily.

Usual adult dosage range
5–10mg daily. Maximum dose: 20mg.

Onset of effect
1–3 hours. Some effects may not be felt for 1–2 days.

Duration of action
Up to 24 hours.

Diet advice
None.

Storage
Keep in a closed container in a cool, dry place out of the reach of children.

Missed dose
No cause for concern, but take as soon as you remember. If your next dose is due within 8 hours, take a single dose now and skip the next.

Stopping the drug
Can be safely stopped as soon as you no longer need it.

Exceeding the dose
An occasional unintentional extra dose is unlikely to cause problems. Large overdoses may cause nausea or drowsiness and have adverse effects on the heart. Notify your physician.

POSSIBLE ADVERSE EFFECTS

The most common adverse effects are drowsiness, dry mouth, and fatigue.

Side effects may be reduced if the dose of cetirizine is taken as 5mg twice a day.

Symptom/effect	Frequency		Discuss with physician		Stop taking drug now	Call physician now
	Common	Rare	Only if severe	In all cases		
Drowsiness/fatigue		●	■			
Dry mouth		●	■			

INTERACTIONS

Anticholinergic drugs The *anticholinergic* effects of cetirizine may be increased by all drugs that have anticholinergic effects, including anti-psychotics and tricyclic antidepressants.

Sedatives Cetirizine may increase the *sedative* effects of anti-anxiety drugs, sleeping drugs, antidepressants, and antipsychotic drugs.

Allergy tests Antihistamines should be discontinued approximately 2–4 days before allergy skin testing.

SPECIAL PRECAUTIONS

Be sure to consult your physician if:
▼ You have long-term liver or kidney problems.
▼ You have glaucoma.
▼ You are allergic to hydroxyzine.
▼ You are taking other medications.

Pregnancy
▼ Safety in pregnancy not established. Discuss with your physician.

Breast-feeding
▼ The drug passes into the breast milk. Discuss with your physician.

Infants and children
▼ Not recommended under 2 years, but may be prescribed for special use under 6 years.

Over 60
▼ No problems expected.

Driving and hazardous work
▼ Avoid such activities until you have learned how cetirizine affects you because the drug can cause drowsiness in some people.

Alcohol
▼ Keep consumption low.

PROLONGED USE

No problems expected.

CHLORAMPHENICOL

Product names Chloromycetin, Pentamycetin
Used in the following combined preparation Pentamycetin/HC

GENERAL INFORMATION

Chloramphenicol is an antibiotic used *topically* to treat eye and ear infections. Given by mouth or injection, it is used in the treatment of meningitis and brain abscesses. It is also effective in acute infections such as typhoid, pneumonia, epiglottitis, or meningitis caused by bacteria resistant to other antibiotics.

Although most people experience few *adverse effects*, chloramphenicol occasionally causes serious or even fatal blood disorders. For this reason, chloramphenicol by mouth or injection is normally only given to treat life-threatening infections that do not respond to safer drugs.

INFORMATION FOR USERS

Your drug prescription is tailored for you. Do not alter dosage without checking with your physician.

How taken

Capsules, injection, cream, eye and ear drops, eye and ear ointment.

Frequency and timing of doses
Every 6 hours (by mouth or injection); every 3–6 hours (eye preparations); 3–4 x daily (ear drops).

Usual adult dosage range
Varies according to preparation and condition. Follow your doctor's instructions.

Onset of effect
1–3 days, depending on the condition and preparation.

Duration of action
6–8 hours.

Diet advice
None.

Storage
Keep in a closed container in a cool, dry place out of the reach of children. Protect from light.

Missed dose
Take as soon as you remember (if by mouth). If your next dose is due, double the dose to make up the missed dose. For skin, eye, and ear preparations, apply as soon as you remember.

Stopping the drug
Take the full course. Even if you feel better the infection may still be present and may recur if treatment is stopped too soon.

Exceeding the dose
An occasional unintentional extra dose is unlikely to be a cause for concern. But if you notice any unusual symptoms, or if a large overdose has been taken, notify your physician.

POSSIBLE ADVERSE EFFECTS

Transient irritation may occur with eye or ear drops. Sore throat, fever, and unusual tiredness with any form of chloramphenicol may be signs of blood abnormalities and should be reported to your physician without delay, even if treatment has been stopped.

Symptom/effect	Frequency		Discuss with physician		Stop taking drug now	Call physician now
	Common	Rare	Only if severe	In all cases		
Burning/stinging (drops)		●	■			
Nausea/vomiting/diarrhea		●	■			
Numb/tingling hands/feet		●		■		
Rash/itching		●		■		
Impaired vision		●		■	▲	▮
Sore throat		●		■	▲	▮
Fever/weakness		●		■	▲	▮
Painful mouth/tongue		●		■	▲	▮

INTERACTIONS

General note Chloramphenicol may increase the effect of certain other drugs, including phenytoin, oral anticoagulants, and oral antidiabetics. Phenobarbital or rifampin may reduce the effect of chloramphenicol.

Antidiabetic drugs Chloramphenicol may increase the effect of antidiabetic drugs.

Cyclosporine, tacrolimus, and sirolimus The blood levels of these drugs may rise if given at the same time as chloramphenicol capsules or injection.

SPECIAL PRECAUTIONS

Be sure to tell your physician if:
▼ You have long-term liver or kidney problems.
▼ You have a blood disorder.
▼ You are taking other medications.

Pregnancy
▼ No evidence of risk with eye or ear preparations. Safety in pregnancy, of other methods of administration, not established. Discuss with your physician.

Breast-feeding
▼ No evidence of risk with eye or ear preparations. Taken by mouth, the drug passes into the breast milk and may increase the risk of blood disorders in the baby. Discuss with your physician.

Infants and children
▼ Reduced dose necessary.

Over 60
▼ No problems expected.

Driving and hazardous work
▼ No known problems.

Alcohol
▼ No known problems.

PROLONGED USE

Prolonged or repeated use of this drug may increase the risk of serious blood disorders and eye damage.

Monitoring Periodic blood cell counts and eye tests may be performed. Blood levels of the drug are usually monitored in infants given chloramphenicol by mouth or injection.

CHLORDIAZEPOXIDE

Product name Apo-Chlordiazepoxide
Used in the following combined preparations Apo-Chlorax, Librax

GENERAL INFORMATION

Chlordiazepoxide was introduced in the mid-1960s and belongs to the group of anti-anxiety drugs known as the benzodiazepines. These drugs are used to help relieve tension and nervousness, relax muscles, and encourage sleep. The actions and the *adverse effects* of this drug group are described more fully on page 67.

Prescribed primarily to treat anxiety, chlordiazepoxide has also been used to relieve symptoms of alcohol withdrawal.
Chlordiazepoxide may lead to mild dependence and withdrawal symptoms if taken regularly over a long period, and it may also lose effectiveness with time. For these reasons, courses of treatment are usually limited to two to four weeks.

QUICK REFERENCE

Drug group Benzodiazepine anti-anxiety drug (p.67)

Overdose danger rating Medium

Dependence rating Medium

Prescription needed Yes

Available as generic Yes

INFORMATION FOR USERS

Your drug prescription is tailored for you. Do not alter dosage without checking with your physician.

How taken

Tablets, capsules.

Frequency and timing of doses
1–3 x daily.

Usual adult dosage range
10–100mg daily. The dosage varies considerably from person to person.

Onset of effect
1–2 hours.

Duration of action
12–24 hours, but some effect may last up to 4 days.

Diet advice
None.

Storage
Keep in a closed container in a cool, dry place out of the reach of children.

Missed dose
No cause for concern, but take when you remember. If your next dose is due within 2 hours, take a single dose now and skip the next.

Stopping the drug
If you have been taking the drug for less than 2 weeks, it can be safely stopped as soon as you feel you no longer need it. However, if you have been taking the drug for longer, consult your physician, who may supervise a gradual reduction in dosage. Stopping abruptly may lead to withdrawal symptoms.

Exceeding the dose
An occasional unintentional extra dose is unlikely to cause problems. Large overdoses may cause excessive drowsiness or coma. Notify your physician.

POSSIBLE ADVERSE EFFECTS

The principal adverse effects of this drug are related to its *sedative* properties. These effects normally diminish after the first few days of treatment.

Symptom/effect	Frequency		Discuss with physician		Stop taking drug now	Call physician now
	Common	Rare	Only if severe	In all cases		
Daytime drowsiness	●		■			
Dizziness/unsteadiness	●			■		
Forgetfulness/confusion		●		■		
Headache		●	■			
Blurred vision		●		■		
Rash		●		■	▲	

INTERACTIONS

Sedatives All drugs that have a *sedative* effect are likely to increase the sedative properties of chlordiazepoxide. Such drugs include anti-anxiety and sleeping drugs, antihistamines, opioid analgesics, antidepressants, and antipsychotics.

Anticonvulsant drugs Chlordiazepoxide may increase or decrease the effects of some anticonvulsant drugs.

SPECIAL PRECAUTIONS

Be sure to tell your physician if:
▼ You have long-term liver or kidney problems.
▼ You have a history of breathing problems.
▼ You have had problems with alcohol or drug abuse.
▼ You are taking other medications.

Pregnancy
▼ Safety in pregnancy not established. Discuss with your physician.

Breast-feeding
▼ The drug passes into the breast milk and may affect the baby. Discuss with your physician.

Infants and children
▼ Not recommended.

Over 60
▼ Reduced dose may be necessary.

Driving and hazardous work
▼ Avoid such activities until you have learned how chlordiazepoxide affects you because the drug can cause reduced alertness and slowed reactions.

Alcohol
▼ Avoid. Alcohol may increase the sedative effects of this drug.

PROLONGED USE

Regular use of this drug over several weeks can lead to a reduction in its effect as the body adapts. It may also be habit-forming when taken for extended periods, especially if it is taken in doses that are larger than average.

CHLOROQUINE

Product name Novo-Chloroquine
Used in the following combined preparation None

GENERAL INFORMATION

Chloroquine is used for the prevention and treatment of malaria. It usually clears an attack in three days. Injections may be given for a severe attack. To prevent malaria, a low dose is given once weekly, starting one week before visiting a high-risk area and continuing through four weeks after leaving. Chloroquine is not suitable for use in all parts of the world as resistance to the drug has developed in some areas. The other use is in the treatment of amebiasis (a parasitic disease).

Common *side effects* include nausea, headache, diarrhea, and abdominal cramps. Occasionally a rash develops. Chloroquine can damage the retina during prolonged treatment, causing blurred vision that may progress to blindness. Regular eye examinations are performed to detect early changes.

QUICK REFERENCE

Drug group Antimalarial drug (p.123) and antirheumatic drug (p.103)

Overdose danger rating High

Dependence rating Low

Prescription needed Yes

Available as generic Yes

INFORMATION FOR USERS

Your drug prescription is tailored for you. Do not alter dosage without checking with your physician.

How taken

Tablets.

Frequency and timing of doses
By mouth 1 x weekly (prevention of malaria); 1–4 x daily (treatment of malaria).

Usual adult dosage range
Prevention of malaria 300mg (2 tablets) as a single dose on the same day each week. Start 1 week before entering endemic area, and continue for 4 weeks after leaving.
Treatment of malaria Initial dose 600mg (4 tablets) and following doses 300mg.

Onset of effect
2–3 days.

Duration of action
Up to 1 week.

Diet advice
None.

Storage
Keep in a closed container in a cool, dry, place out of the reach of children. Protect from light.

Missed dose
Take as soon as you remember but if your next dose is due within 24 hours (1 x weekly schedule), or 6 hours (1–2 x daily schedule), take a single dose now and skip the next.

Stopping the drug
Do not stop the drug without consulting your physician.

OVERDOSE ACTION

 Seek immediate medical advice in all cases. Take emergency action if breathing difficulties, fits, or loss of consciousness occur.

See Drug poisoning emergency guide (p.526).

POSSIBLE ADVERSE EFFECTS

Side effects such as nausea, diarrhea, and abdominal pain might be avoided by taking the drug with food. Changes in vision should be reported promptly.

Symptom/effect	Frequency		Discuss with physician		Stop taking drug now	Call physician now
	Common	Rare	Only if severe	In all cases		
Nausea	●		■			
Diarrhea/abdominal pain	●		■			
Headache/dizziness		●		■		
Hearing disorders		●		■		
Mood changes		●		■		
Rash		●		■	▲	▮
Sore throat		●		■		
Blurred vision		●		■	▲	▮

INTERACTIONS

Antiepileptic drugs Chloroquine may reduce the effect of these drugs.

Amiodarone Chloroquine may increase the risk of abnormal heart rhythms if taken with this drug.

Digoxin The level of digoxin in the blood may be increased by chloroquine.

Cyclosporine Chloroquine increases the blood level of cyclosporine.

SPECIAL PRECAUTIONS

Be sure to tell your physician if:
▼ You have liver or kidney problems.
▼ You have glucose-6-phosphate dehydrogenase (G6PD) deficiency.
▼ You have eye or vision problems.
▼ You have psoriasis.
▼ You have a history of epilepsy.
▼ You suffer from porphyria.
▼ You are taking other medications.

 Pregnancy
▼ No evidence of risk with low doses. High doses may affect the baby. Discuss with your physician.

 Breast-feeding
▼ The drug may pass into breast milk in small amounts. At normal doses effects on the baby are unlikely. Discuss with your physician.

 Infants and children
▼ Reduced dose necessary.

 Over 60
▼ No special problems, except that it may be difficult to tell between changes in eyesight due to aging, and those that are drug-induced.

 Driving and hazardous work
▼ Avoid such activities until you have learned how chloroquine affects you because the drug may cause dizziness.

 Alcohol
▼ Keep consumption low.

PROLONGED USE

Prolonged use may cause eye damage and blood disorders.

Monitoring Periodic eye tests and blood counts must be carried out.

CHLORPHENIRAMINE

Product name Chlor-Tripolon
Used in the following combined preparations Dristan, Omni-Tuss, Sinutab with Codeine, Tylenol Cold and Flu, and others

GENERAL INFORMATION

Chlorpheniramine has been used for over 30 years to treat allergies such as hay fever, allergic conjunctivitis, urticaria (hives), insect bites and stings, and angioedema (allergic swellings). It is included in several over-the-counter cold remedies (see p.80).

Like other antihistamines, it relieves allergic skin symptoms such as itching, swelling, and redness. It also reduces sneezing and the runny nose and itching eyes of hay fever. Chlorpheniramine also has a mild *anticholinergic* action, which suppresses mucus secretion.

Chlorpheniramine may also be used to prevent or treat allergic reactions to blood transfusions or X-ray contrast material.

QUICK REFERENCE

Drug group Antihistamine (p.110)
Overdose danger rating Medium
Dependence rating Low
Prescription needed No (tablets and liquid); yes (injection)
Available as generic Yes

INFORMATION FOR USERS

Follow instructions on the label. Call your physician if symptoms worsen.

How taken

Tablets, repetabs, liquid, injection.

Frequency and timing of doses
1–6 x daily (tablets, liquid); 2 x daily (repetabs).

Usual dosage range
Adults 12–24mg daily.
Children Reduced dose according to age and weight.

Onset of effect
Within 60 minutes.

Duration of action
4–6 hours (tablets, liquid).

Diet advice
None.

Storage
Keep in a closed container in a cool, dry place out of the reach of children.

Missed dose
Take as soon as you remember. If your next dose is due within 2 hours, take a single dose now and skip the next.

Stopping the drug
Can be safely stopped as soon as you no longer need it.

Exceeding the dose
An occasional unintentional extra dose is unlikely to cause problems. Large overdoses may cause drowsiness or agitation. Notify your physician.

SPECIAL PRECAUTIONS

Be sure to consult your physician or pharmacist before taking this drug if:
▼ You have a long-term liver problem.
▼ You have had epileptic fits.
▼ You have glaucoma.
▼ You have urinary difficulties.
▼ You are taking other medications.

 Pregnancy
▼ Safety in pregnancy not established. Discuss with your physician.

 Breast-feeding
▼ The drug passes into the breast milk, but at normal doses adverse effects on the baby are unlikely. Discuss with your physician.

 Infants and children
▼ Reduced dose necessary.

 Over 60
▼ Reduced dose may be necessary. Increased likelihood of adverse effects.

 Driving and hazardous work
▼ Avoid such activities until you have learned how chlorpheniramine affects you because the drug can cause drowsiness, dizziness, and blurred vision.

 Alcohol
▼ Avoid. Alcohol may increase the sedative effects of this drug.

POSSIBLE ADVERSE EFFECTS

Drowsiness is the most common adverse effect of chlorpheniramine; other *side effects* are rare. Some of these, such as dryness of the mouth, blurred vision, and difficulty passing urine, are due to its *anticholinergic* effects. Gastrointestinal irritation may be reduced by taking the tablets or liquid with food or drink.

Symptom/effect	Frequency		Discuss with physician		Stop taking drug now	Call physician now
	Common	Rare	Only if severe	In all cases		
Drowsiness/dizziness	●			■		
Digestive disturbances		●		■		
Difficulty in passing urine		●		■		
Dry mouth		●		■		
Blurred vision		●			■	
Excitation (children)		●			■	▲
Rash		●		■		▲

INTERACTIONS

Anticholinergic drugs All drugs, including some drugs for *parkinsonism*, that have an anticholinergic effect are likely to increase the anticholinergic effect of chlorpheniramine.

Phenytoin The effects of phenytoin may be enhanced by chlorpheniramine.

Monoamine oxidase inhibitors (MAOIs) and tricyclic antidepressants These drugs may increase the side effects of chlorpheniramine.

Sedatives All drugs with a *sedative* effect are likely to increase the sedative properties of chlorpheniramine.

PROLONGED USE

The effect of the drug may become weaker with prolonged use over a period of weeks or months as the body adapts. Transfer to a different antihistamine may be recommended.

CHLORPROMAZINE

Product names Apo-Chlorpromazine, Novo-Chlorpromazine
Used in the following combined preparations None

GENERAL INFORMATION

Chlorpromazine was the first anti-psychotic drug to be marketed. It has a tranquillizing effect that is useful in the short-term treatment of anxiety, agitation, and aggressive behaviour.

Chlorpromazine is prescribed for the treatment of schizophrenia, mania, and other disorders where confused, aggressive, or abnormal behaviour may occur and a degree of sedation is required. Other uses of this drug include the treatment of nausea and vomiting, especially when caused by drug or radiation treatment; and treating severe, prolonged hiccoughs.

The drug can produce a number of adverse effects, some of which may be serious. After continuous use of chlorpromazine over several years, eye changes and skin discoloration may occur, particularly in women.

INFORMATION FOR USERS

Your drug prescription is tailored for you. Do not alter dosage without checking with your physician.

How taken

Tablets, liquid, injection, suppositories.

Frequency and timing of doses
1–4 x daily.

Usual adult oral dosage range
Mental illness 75–300mg daily; dose is started low and gradually increased. Some patients may need higher doses.
Nausea and vomiting 40–150mg daily.

Onset of effect
30–60 minutes (by mouth); 15–20 minutes (injection); up to 30 minutes (suppository).

Duration of action
8–12 hours (by mouth or injection); 3–4 hours (suppository). Some effect may persist for up to 3 weeks when stopping the drug after regular use.

Diet advice
None.

Storage
Keep in a closed container in a cool, dry place out of the reach of children. Protect from light.

Missed dose
Take as soon as you remember. If your next dose is due within 2 hours, do not take the missed dose. Take your next scheduled dose as usual.

Stopping the drug
Do not stop taking the drug without consulting your physician; symptoms may recur.

Exceeding the dose
An occasional unintentional extra dose is unlikely to cause problems. Larger overdoses may cause unusual drowsiness, fainting, abnormal heart rhythms, muscle rigidity, and agitation. Notify your physician.

SPECIAL PRECAUTIONS

Be sure to tell your physician if:
▼ You have long-term liver or kidney problems.
▼ You have had heart problems.
▼ You have had epileptic fits.
▼ You have thyroid disease.
▼ You have Parkinson's disease.
▼ You have glaucoma.
▼ You are taking other medications.

Pregnancy
▼ Not usually prescribed. Taken near the time of delivery it can prolong labour and may cause drowsiness in the newborn baby. Discuss with your physician.

Breast-feeding
▼ The drug passes into the breast milk and may affect the baby. Discuss with your physician.

Infants and children
▼ Not recommended for infants under 1 year. Reduced dose necessary for older children.

Over 60
▼ Initial dosage is low; it may be increased if there are no adverse reactions, such as abnormal limb movements or low blood pressure.

Driving and hazardous work
▼ Avoid such activities until you have learned how chlorpromazine affects you as the drug can cause drowsiness and slowed reactions.

Alcohol
▼ Avoid. Alcohol may increase the sedative effects of this drug.

Surgery and general anesthetics
▼ Chlorpromazine treatment may need to be stopped before you have a general anesthetic. Discuss this with your physician or dentist before any operation.

POSSIBLE ADVERSE EFFECTS

Chlorpromazine commonly causes mild drowsiness and has an *anticholinergic* effect, which can cause symptoms. The most significant adverse effect is *parkinsonism*.

Symptom/effect	Frequency		Discuss with physician		Stop taking drug now	Call physician now
	Common	Rare	Only if severe	In all cases		
Drowsiness/lethargy	●		■			
Weight gain	●		■			
Tremor/parkinsonism	●			■		
Blurred vision	●			■		
Dizziness/fainting	●			■		
Infrequent periods		●		■		
Light sensitive rash		●		■	▲	
Jaundice		●		■	▲	

INTERACTIONS

Drugs for parkinsonism Chlorpromazine may reduce the effect of these drugs.

Anticholinergic drugs These drugs may intensify the *anticholinergic* properties of chlorpromazine.

Sedatives All drugs that have a *sedative* effect on the central nervous system are likely to increase the sedative properties of chlorpromazine.

PROLONGED USE

If used for more than a few months, chlorpromazine may cause movement disorders. Occasionally, *jaundice* may occur due to an allergic effect of the drug.

CHOLESTYRAMINE

Product names Novo-Cholamine, PHL-Cholestyramine Light
Used in the following combined preparations None

GENERAL INFORMATION

Cholestyramine is a resin that binds bile acids in the intestine, preventing their reabsorption. Cholesterol in the body is normally converted to bile acids. Therefore, cholestyramine reduces cholesterol levels in the blood. This action on bile acids makes bowel movements bulkier, creating an antidiarrheal effect. Cholestyramine is used to treat hyperlipidemia (high levels of cholesterol in the blood) in people who have not responded to dietary changes.

In liver disorders, such as primary biliary cirrhosis, bile salts sometimes accumulate in the bloodstream, and cholestyramine may be prescribed to alleviate any accompanying itching.

Taken in large doses, cholestyramine often causes bloating, mild nausea, and constipation. It may also interfere with the body's ability to absorb fat and certain fat-soluble vitamins, causing pale, bulky, foul-smelling feces.

INFORMATION FOR USERS

Your drug prescription is tailored for you. Do not alter dosage without checking with your physician.

How taken

Powder mixed with water, juice, or apple sauce.

Frequency and timing of doses
1–4 x daily before meals and at bedtime.

Usual dosage range
4–24g daily.

Onset of effect
May take several weeks to achieve full beneficial effects.

Duration of action
12–24 hours.

Diet advice
A low-fat, low-calorie diet may be advised for patients who are overweight. Use of this drug may deplete levels of certain vitamins. Supplements may be advised.

Storage
Keep in a closed container in a cool, dry place out of the reach of children.

Missed dose
Take as soon as you remember.

Stopping the drug
Do not stop taking the drug without consulting your physician.

Exceeding the dose
An occasional unintentional extra dose is unlikely to cause problems. But if you notice any unusual symptoms, or if a large overdose has been taken, notify your physician.

SPECIAL PRECAUTIONS

Be sure to tell your physician if:
▼ You have jaundice.
▼ You have a peptic ulcer.
▼ You suffer from hemorrhoids.
▼ You are taking other medications.

Pregnancy
▼ Safety in pregnancy not established. Discuss with your physician.

Breast feeding
▼ Safety not established. The drug binds fat-soluble vitamins long-term and may cause vitamin deficiency in the baby. Discuss with your physician.

Infants and children
▼ Not recommended under 6 years. Reduced dose necessary in older children.

Over 60
▼ Increased likelihood of adverse effects.

Driving and hazardous work
▼ No special problems.

Alcohol
▼ Although this drug does not interact with alcohol, your underlying condition may make it inadvisable to take alcohol.

POSSIBLE ADVERSE EFFECTS

Adverse effects are more likely if large doses are taken by people over 60. Minor side effects such as indigestion and abdominal discomfort are rarely a cause for concern. More serious adverse effects are usually the result of vitamin deficiency.

Symptom/effect	Frequency		Discuss with physician		Stop taking drug now	Call physician now
	Common	Rare	Only if severe	In all cases		
Indigestion	●			■		
Abdominal discomfort	●			■		
Nausea/vomiting	●			■		
Constipation	●			■		
Bruising/increased bleeding		●		■	■	
Diarrhea (high doses)		●		■		

INTERACTIONS

General note Cholestyramine reduces the body's ability to absorb other drugs. If you are taking other medicines, you should tell either your physician or pharmacist so that they can discuss with you the best way to take all your drugs. To avoid any problems, take other drugs at least 1 hour before, or 4–6 hours after, cholestyramine. The dosage of other drugs you take may need to be adjusted.

PROLONGED USE

As this drug reduces vitamin absorption, supplements of vitamins A, D, and K and folic acid may be advised.

Monitoring Periodic blood checks are usually required to monitor the level of cholesterol in the blood.

CIMETIDINE

Product names Apo-Cimetidine, Gen-Cimetidine, and others
Used in the following combined preparations None

GENERAL INFORMATION

Introduced in the 1970s, cimetidine was the first of a new group of anti-ulcer drugs. Cimetidine reduces the secretion of gastric acid and of pepsin, an enzyme that helps in the digestion of protein. By reducing levels of acid and pepsin, it promotes healing of ulcers in the stomach and duodenum (see p.95). It is also used for reflux esophagitis, in which acid stomach contents may flow up the esophagus. Treatment is usually given in four- to eight-week courses, with further short courses if symptoms recur.

Cimetidine also affects the actions of certain enzymes in the liver, where many drugs are broken down. It is therefore prescribed with caution to people who are receiving other drugs, particularly anticoagulants and anticonvulsants, whose levels need to be carefully controlled. Since cimetidine promotes healing of the stomach lining, it may mask the symptoms of stomach cancer and delay diagnosis. It is therefore prescribed with caution if symptoms persist.

INFORMATION FOR USERS

Follow instructions on the label. Call your physician if symptoms worsen.

How taken

Tablets, liquid.

Frequency and timing of doses
1–4 x daily (after meals and at bedtime).

Usual adult dosage range
800–1,600mg daily.

Onset of effect
Within 90 minutes.

Duration of action
2–6 hours.

Diet advice
None.

Storage
Keep in a closed container in a cool, dry place away from the reach of children. Protect from light.

Missed dose
Do not take the missed dose. Take your next dose as usual.

Stopping the drug
If prescribed by your physician, do not stop taking the drug without consulting him or her because symptoms may recur.

Exceeding the dose
An occasional unintentional extra dose is unlikely to be a cause for concern. But if you notice any unusual symptoms, or if a large overdose has been taken, notify your physician.

SPECIAL PRECAUTIONS

Be sure to consult your physician or pharmacist before taking this drug if:
▼ You have long-term liver or kidney problems.
▼ You are taking other medications.

 Pregnancy
▼ Safety in pregnancy not established. Discuss with your physician.

 Breast-feeding
▼ The drug passes into the breast milk, but at normal doses adverse effects on the baby are unlikely. Discuss with your physician.

 Infants and children
▼ Reduced dose necessary.

 Over 60
▼ No special problems unless kidney function is reduced. Risk of stomach cancer is higher in the elderly and it must be excluded before cimetidine is prescribed.

 Driving and hazardous work
▼ Avoid such activities until you have learned how cimetidine affects you because the drug may cause dizziness and confusion.

 Alcohol
▼ Avoid. Alcohol may aggravate the underlying condition and counter the beneficial effects of cimetidine.

POSSIBLE ADVERSE EFFECTS

Adverse effects of cimetidine are uncommon. They are usually related to dosage level and almost always disappear when the drug is stopped.

Symptom/effect	Frequency		Discuss with physician		Stop taking drug now	Call physician now
	Common	Rare	Only if severe	In all cases		
Diarrhea	●		■			
Dizziness/confusion/tiredness	●			■		
Muscle pain		●		■		
Breast enlargement (men)		●		■		
Impotence		●		■		
Rash		●		■	▲	

INTERACTIONS

Benzodiazepines Cimetidine may increase the blood levels of some of these drugs, increasing the risk of adverse effects.

Theophylline/aminophylline Cimetidine may increase the blood levels of these drugs. Their dose may need to be reduced.

Sildenafil and oral contraceptives Cimetidine may increase the blood level of these drugs.

Beta blockers and antiarrhythmic drugs Cimetidine may increase the blood levels of these drugs.

Anticoagulant drugs Cimetidine may increase their effect.

Ketoconazole Cimetidine may affect its absorption.

PROLONGED USE

Courses of longer than 8 weeks are not usually necessary.

CIPROFLOXACIN

Product names Cipro, Ciloxan
Used in the following combined preparations Cipro HC

GENERAL INFORMATION

Ciprofloxacin, a quinolone antibacterial, is used to treat several types of bacteria resistant to other commonly used antibiotics. It is especially useful for some types of chest infections, and skin, intestinal, and urinary tract infections. It can also be used to treat gonorrhea.

When taken by mouth, ciprofloxacin is well absorbed by the body and works quickly and effectively. In more severe systemic bacterial infections the drug may need to be administered by injection.

Ciprofloxacin has a long duration of action and needs to be taken only once or twice daily. Its most common *side effect* is gastrointestinal disturbance.

INFORMATION FOR USERS

Your drug prescription is tailored for you. Do not alter dosage without checking with your physician.

How taken

Tablets, liquid, injection, eye ointment and drops, ear drops.

Frequency and timing of doses
2 x daily with plenty of fluids.

Usual adult dosage range
500mg–1.5g daily (tablets); 200–400mg daily (injection).

Onset of effect
The drug begins to work within a few hours, although full beneficial effect may not be felt for several days.

Duration of action
About 12 hours.

Diet advice
Do not get dehydrated; ensure that you drink fluids regularly.

Storage
Keep in a closed container in a cool, dry place out of the reach of children. The injection must be protected from light.

Missed dose
Take as soon as you remember, and take your next dose as usual.

Stopping the drug
Take the full course. Even if you feel better the original infection may still be present, and symptoms may recur if treatment is stopped too soon.

Exceeding the dose
An occasional unintentional extra dose is unlikely to cause problems. Large overdoses may cause mental disturbance and fits. Notify your physician.

SPECIAL PRECAUTIONS

Be sure to tell your physician if:
▼ You have long-term liver or kidney problems.
▼ You have had epileptic fits.
▼ You have glucose-6-phosphate dehydrogenase (G6PD) deficiency.
▼ You are taking other medications.

Pregnancy
▼ Safety in pregnancy not established. Discuss with your physician.

Breast-feeding
▼ The drug passes into the breast milk and may affect the baby adversely. Discuss with your physician.

Infants and children
▼ Not usually recommended.

Over 60
▼ The drug may make the elderly more susceptible to tendinitis.

Driving and hazardous work
▼ Avoid such activities until you have learned how ciprofloxacin affects you because the drug can cause dizziness.

Alcohol
▼ Avoid. Alcohol may increase the sedative effects of this drug.

Sunlight
▼ Avoid excessive exposure.

PROLONGED USE

No problems expected.

Monitoring Blood tests may be necessary to monitor kidney and liver function.

POSSIBLE ADVERSE EFFECTS

Ciprofloxacin commonly causes nausea and vomiting; other side effects are less common, except when very high doses are given. Painful and inflamed tendons should be reported to your physician at once, treatment should be discontinued, and the affected limbs rested.

Symptom/effect	Frequency		Discuss with physician		Stop taking drug now	Call physician now
	Common	Rare	Only if severe	In all cases		
Nausea/vomiting	●		■			
Abdominal pain/diarrhea	●		■			
Rash/itching	●			■		
Dizziness/headache		●	■			
Joint pain		●	■			
Sleep disturbance		●	■			
Photosensitivity		●		■		
Jaundice		●		■		
Confusion/convulsions		●		■	▲	▎
Painful, inflamed tendons		●		■	▲	▎

INTERACTIONS

Oral iron preparations and antacids containing magnesium or aluminum hydroxide interfere with absorption of ciprofloxacin. Do not take antacids within 2 hours of taking ciprofloxacin tablets.

Anticoagulants and oral antidiabetics Blood levels of these drugs may be increased; their dosage may need adjusting.

Theophylline Ciprofloxacin may increase blood levels of this drug; its dose may need adjusting and its blood levels monitored.

Phenytoin Ciprofloxacin may increase the blood levels of this drug.

Non-steroidal anti-inflammatory drugs These drugs increase the risk of epileptic fits.

CISPLATIN

Product name None
Used in the following combined preparations None

GENERAL INFORMATION

Cisplatin is one of the most effective drugs available to treat a wide variety of cancers including those of the ovaries, testes, head, neck, bladder, cervix, and lung. It is also used in treating certain children's cancers and some cancers of the blood. It is usually given along with other anticancer drugs.

The most common and serious *adverse effect* of cisplatin is impaired kidney function. To reduce the risk of permanent kidney damage, the drug is usually given only once every three weeks, allowing the kidneys time to recover between courses of treatment. Plenty of fluid must be taken to dilute the drug in the kidneys. Nausea and vomiting may occur after administration of cisplatin. These symptoms usually start within an hour and last for up to 24 hours, in some case persisting for up to a week. Because they may be quite severe, anti-emetic drugs are given.

Damage to hearing is common and may be more severe in children. Use of cisplatin may also increase the risk of anemia, blood clotting disorders, and infection during treatment.

QUICK REFERENCE

Drug group Anticancer drug (p.140)
Overdose danger rating High
Dependence rating Low
Prescription needed Yes
Available as generic Yes

INFORMATION FOR USERS

This drug is given only under medical supervision and is not for self-administration.

How taken

Injection.

Frequency and timing of doses
Every 3 weeks for up to 5 days; it may be given alone or in combination with other anticancer drugs.

Usual adult dosage range
Dosage is determined individually according to body height, weight, and response.

Onset of effect
Some adverse effects, such as nausea and vomiting, may appear within 1 hour of starting treatment.

Duration of action
Some adverse effects may last for up to 1 week after treatment has stopped.

Diet advice
Prior to treatment it is important that the body is well hydrated. Therefore, 1–2 litres of fluid are usually given by infusion over 8–12 hours.

Storage
Not applicable. The drug is not normally kept in the home.

Missed dose
Not applicable. The drug is given only in hospital under medical supervision.

Stopping the drug
Not applicable. The drug will be stopped under medical supervision.

Exceeding the dose
Overdosage is unlikely since treatment is carefully monitored, and the drug is given intravenously only under close supervision.

POSSIBLE ADVERSE EFFECTS

Most adverse effects appear within a few hours of injection and are carefully monitored in hospital after each dose. Some effects wear off within 24 hours. Nausea and loss of appetite may last for up to a week.

Symptom/effect	Frequency		Discuss with physician		Stop taking drug now	Call physician now
	Common	Rare	Only if severe	In all cases		
Loss of appetite/taste	●		■			
Nausea/vomiting	●			■		
Ringing in the ears/hearing loss	●			■		
Breathing difficulties		●		■		▌
Abnormal sensations		●		■		▌
Wheezing		●		■		▌
Swollen face/rash		●		■		▌

INTERACTIONS

General note A number of drugs (e.g., antibacterials such as gentamicin) increase the adverse effects of cisplatin. Because cisplatin is given only under close medical supervision, these interactions are carefully monitored and the dosage is adjusted accordingly.

SPECIAL PRECAUTIONS

Cisplatin is prescribed only under close medical supervision, taking account of your present condition and your medical history.

Pregnancy
▼ Not usually prescribed. Cisplatin may cause birth defects or premature birth. Discuss with your physician.

Breast-feeding
▼ Not advised. The drug passes into the breast milk and may affect the baby adversely. Discuss with your physician.

Infants and children
▼ The risk of hearing loss is increased. Reduced dose used.

Over 60
▼ Reduced dose may be necessary. Increased likelihood of adverse effects.

Driving and hazardous work
▼ No known problems.

Alcohol
▼ No known problems.

PROLONGED USE

Prolonged use of this drug increases the risk of damage to the kidneys, nerves, and bone marrow, and to hearing.

Monitoring Hearing tests and blood checks to monitor kidney function and bone marrow activity are carried out regularly.

CITALOPRAM

Products name Apo-Citalopram, Celexa
Used in the following combined preparations None

GENERAL INFORMATION

Citalopram is a member of the selective serotonin re-uptake inhibitor (SSRI) group of antidepressant drugs. It is used for depressive illness and panic disorder. Citalopram gradually improves the patient's mood, increases physical activity, and restores interest in everyday pursuits.

Citalopram is generally well tolerated, and any gastrointestinal *adverse effects*, such as nausea, vomiting, or diarrhea, are dose related and usually diminish with continued use of the drug.

Like other SSRIs, citalopram causes fewer *anticholinergic side effects* and is less sedating than the tricyclic antidepressants. It is also less likely to be harmful if taken in overdose. It can, however, cause drowsiness and impair performance of tasks such as driving.

INFORMATION FOR USERS

Your drug prescription is tailored for you. Do not alter dosage without checking with your physician.

How taken

Tablets.

Frequency and timing of doses
Once daily in the morning or evening.

Usual adult dosage range
Depressive illness 20–60mg.
Panic attacks 10mg (starting dose); 20–30mg (usual range).

Onset of effect
Full benefits may not be felt for 2–4 weeks.

Duration of action
Antidepressant effect may persist for some weeks following prolonged treatment.

Diet advice
None.

Storage
Keep in a closed container in a cool, dry place out of the reach of children.

Missed dose
Take as soon as you remember. If your next dose is due within 8 hours, take a single dose now and skip the next.

Stopping the drug
Do not stop taking the drug without consulting your physician. Stopping abruptly can cause withdrawal symptoms.

Exceeding the dose
An occasional unintentional extra dose is unlikely to be a cause for concern. If you notice any unusual symptoms, or if a large overdose has been taken, notify your physician.

POSSIBLE ADVERSE EFFECTS

Common adverse effects such as nausea, indigestion, and diarrhea usually diminish with reduction in dosage. If convulsions or a rash occur, consult your physician immediately.

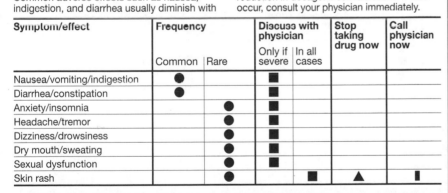

Symptom/effect	Frequency		Discuss with physician		Stop taking drug now	Call physician now
	Common	Rare	Only if severe	In all cases		
Nausea/vomiting/indigestion	●		■			
Diarrhea/constipation	●		■			
Anxiety/insomnia		●	■			
Headache/tremor		●	■			
Dizziness/drowsiness		●	■			
Dry mouth/sweating		●	■			
Sexual dysfunction		●	■			
Skin rash		●		■	▲	▮

INTERACTIONS

General note Any drug that affects the breakdown of others in the liver may alter blood levels of citalopram, and vice versa.

Sumatriptan and other 5HT1 agonists and lithium There is an increased risk of adverse effects when citalopram is taken with these drugs.

Monoamine oxidase inhibitors (MAOIs) These drugs may cause a severe reaction if they are taken with citalopram. Avoid taking citalopram if MAOIs have been taken in the last 14 days.

Anticoagulants The effect of these drugs may be increased by citalopram.

SPECIAL PRECAUTIONS

Be sure to tell your physician if:
▼ You have epilepsy.
▼ You have liver or kidney problems.
▼ You have had a manic-depressive illness.
▼ You have had heart problems.
▼ You have been taking monoamine oxidase inhibitors (MAOIs) or other antidepressants.
▼ You are taking other medications.

 Pregnancy
▼ Safety in pregnancy not established. Discuss with your physician.

 Breast-feeding
▼ The drug may pass into breast milk and may affect the baby. Discuss with your physician.

 Infants and children
▼ Not recommended.

 Over 60
▼ Reduced dose necessary.

 Driving and hazardous work
▼ Avoid such activities until you have learned how citalopram affects you because the drug can cause drowsiness.

 Alcohol
▼ No special problems.

PROLONGED USE

No problems expected. However, mild withdrawal symptoms may occur if the drug is not stopped gradually.

CLARITHROMYCIN

Product names Biaxin, Biaxin BID, Biaxin XL
Used in the following combined preparations Hp-PAC

GENERAL INFORMATION

Clarithromycin is a macrolide antibiotic similar to erythromycin (p.274) from which it is derived. It has similar actions and uses to erythromycin, but is slightly more active in certain situations. It is used for upper respiratory tract infections, such as middle ear infections, sinusitis, and pharyngitis, and lower respiratory tract infections, including whooping cough,

bronchitis, and pneumonia, as well as for skin and soft tissue infections, including gonorrhoea. Given with anti-ulcer drugs (p.95) and other antibiotics, clarithromycin is used to eradicate *Helicobacter pylori*, the bacterium that causes many peptic ulcers.

Prolonged use of clarithromycin is not usually necessary.

INFORMATION FOR USERS

Your drug prescription is tailored for you. Do not alter dosage without checking with your physician.

How taken

Tablets, liquid, extended release tablets.

Frequency and timing of doses
2 x daily, up to 14 days.

Usual adult dosage range
500mg–1g daily.

Onset of effect
1–4 hours.

Duration of action
1–12 hours.

Diet advice
None.

Storage
Keep in a closed container in a cool, dry place out of the reach of children. Protect from light.

Missed dose
Take as soon as you remember. If your next dose is due within 2 hours, take a single dose now and skip the next.

Stopping the drug
Take the full course. Even if you feel better, the infection may still be present and symptoms may recur if treatment is stopped too soon.

Exceeding the dose
An occasional unintentional extra dose is unlikely to be a cause for concern. But if you notice any unusual symptoms, or if a large overdose has been taken, notify your physician.

SPECIAL PRECAUTIONS

Be sure to tell your physician if:
▼ You have liver or kidney problems.
▼ You have had an allergic reaction to erythromycin or clarithromycin.
▼ You have a heart problem.
▼ You have porphyria.
▼ You are taking other medications.

Pregnancy
▼ Safety has not been established. Discuss with your physician.

Breast-feeding
▼ Clarithromycin passes into the breast milk and may affect the baby. Discuss with your physician.

Infants and children
▼ Reduced dose necessary.

Over 60
▼ No special problems.

Driving and hazardous work
▼ No known problems.

Alcohol
▼ No known problems.

POSSIBLE ADVERSE EFFECTS

Clarithromycin is generally well tolerated. Gastrointestinal disturbances are the most common problems encountered. Hearing loss is a rare possibility, but it is usually reversible on stopping the drug.

Symptom/effect	Frequency		Discuss with physician		Stop taking drug now	Call physician now
	Common	Rare	Only if severe	In all cases		
Nausea/vomiting/diarrhea	●		■			
Indigestion	●		■			
Headache	●		■			
Joint/muscle pain	●		■			
Rash	●			■		
Altered sense of taste/smell		●		■		
Anxiety/insomnia		●		■		
Confusion/hallucinations		●		■		
Jaundice		●		■	▲	

INTERACTIONS

Digoxin, warfarin, triazolam, midazolam, disopyramide, lovastatin, rifabutin, phenytoin, cyclosporine, and tacrolimus Blood levels and effects of these drugs are increased by clarithromycin.

Carbamazepine, theophylline, and digoxin Blood levels and toxicity of these drugs are increased by clarithromycin.

Zidovudine Blood levels are reduced if this drug is taken at the same time as clarithromycin.

Ergot derivatives There is an increased risk of ergot toxicity if these drugs are taken with clarithromycin.

Pimozide may cause cardiac arrhythmias if taken with clarithromycin.

Lipid-lowering drugs whose names end in 'statin' If these drugs are taken with clarithromycin, there is a risk of rhabdomyolysis (muscle damage).

PROLONGED USE

In courses of over 14 days, there is a risk of developing antibiotic-resistant infections.

CLINDAMYCIN

Product names Apo-Clindamycin, Clinda-T, Clindets, Dalacin C, Gen-Clindamycin, Novo-Clindamycin, Ratio-Clindamycin
Used in the following combined preparations Benzaclin topical gel, Clindoxyl gel

GENERAL INFORMATION

Clindamycin is an antibiotic that is prescribed for a variety of mild to moderate infections. It is used to treat infections of the skin, the respiratory tract, vagina, and abdomen. It may also be used prior to certain surgical procedures. It is also available as a topical product, which is prescribed for moderate acne. When taken by mouth, clindamycin is usually given every 6–8 hours. It should be taken with a full glass of water. Diarrhea can sometimes occur. If significant diarrhea occurs, the physician should be called.

A vaginal cream is also available to treat bacterial infection; this is usually used intravaginally for 7 nights.

QUICK REFERENCE

Drug group Antibiotics (p.116)
Overdose danger rating Low
Dependence rating Low
Prescription needed Yes
Available as generic Yes

INFORMATION FOR USERS

Your drug prescription is tailored for you. Do not alter dosage without checking with your physician.

How taken

Capsules, oral solution, parenteral injection (IM, IV), topical gel, topical cream, topical pad, topical solution, vaginal cream.

Frequency and timing of doses
Orally: every 6–8 hours; topically: twice daily.

Usual adult dosage range
Oral dose: 600–1800mg daily; maximum 1800mg daily.

Onset of effect
Within 48 hours; for acne, may take several days to see effect.

Duration of action
6–8 hours.

Diet advice
None

Storage
Keep in a closed container in a cool, dry place out of the reach of children. Reconstituted oral solution should not be refrigerated and is kept at room temperature for 14 days. Discard any unused medication; talk to your pharmacist about proper disposal.

Missed dose
If you miss a dose, take it as soon as you remember. If it is near the time of the next dose, skip the missed dose and resume your usual dosing schedule. Do not double up to catch up on a missed dose.

Stopping the drug
Do not stop the drug without consulting your physician. Stopping the drug may lead to worsening of the underlying condition.

Exceeding the dose
An occasional unintentional extra dose is unlikely to cause problems. With large overdoses, seek help right away and notify your physician.

SPECIAL PRECAUTIONS

Be sure to tell your physician if:
▼ You are allergic to any antibiotics or tartrazine (a yellow dye used in foods).
▼ You have kidney disease.
▼ You have gastrointestinal disease.
▼ You have liver problems.
▼ You are taking other medications.

 Pregnancy
▼ Safety in pregnancy not established. Discuss with your physician.

 Breast-feeding
▼ Safety not established. Discuss with your physician.

 Infants and children
▼ Not recommended.

 Over 60
▼ When diarrhea occurs, requires more close monitoring and follow-up.

 Driving and hazardous work
▼ No special problems.

 Alcohol
▼ No known problems.

POSSIBLE ADVERSE EFFECTS

Clindamycin is usually well tolerated.
Some may experience an upset stomach.

Symptom/effect	Frequency		Discuss with physician		Stop taking drug now	Call physician now
	Common	Rare	Only if severe	In all cases		
Skin rash		●			▲	▮
Diarrhea	●			■		
Vomiting	●		■			
Upset stomach	●		■			
When used topically or vaginally						
Redness/irritation	●		■			
Burning	●		■			

INTERACTIONS

Tubocurarine, pancuronium These drugs should be used with caution and close monitoring is required when used with clindamycin.

Erythromycin Usually not used with clindamycin as it may effect the efficacy of both agents.

PROLONGED USE

Clindamycin, when used by injection, orally, or vaginally, is usually given only for short courses of treatment. When used topically, continued use should be regularly reassessed.

CLOBETASOL

Product names Clobex Lotion, Clobex Shampoo, Dermovate
Used in the following combined preparation None

GENERAL INFORMATION

Clobetasol is a corticosteroid drug (p.127) used for short-term treatment of severe skin conditions such as discoid lupus erythematosus, lichen planus and lichen simplex, eczema, and psoriasis. It is the strongest *topical* corticosteroid and is used only when the disorder has not responded to treatment with another topical corticosteroid.

It is important to apply clobetasol thinly and sparingly to affected areas because it can cause *systemic adverse*

effects such as suppression of the pituitary and adrenal glands and Cushing's syndrome. Other side effects include irreversible changes to the structure of the skin in the areas that have been treated. Also, clobetasol can exacerbate eczema infected with a virus such as herpes simplex.

Treatment of psoriasis with clobetasol must only be carried out with specialist care and supervision.

QUICK REFERENCE

Drug group Topical corticosteroid (p.162)

Overdose danger rating Low

Dependence rating Low

Prescription needed Yes

Available as generic Yes

INFORMATION FOR USERS

Your drug prescription is tailored for you. Do not alter dosage without checking with your physician.

How taken

Cream, ointment, solution, scalp application.

Frequency and timing of doses
1 x 2 times daily. If treating the face, use for no more than 5 days.

Usual dosage range
No more than 50g weekly.

Onset of effect
12 hours. Full beneficial effect after 48 hours.

Duration of action
Up to 24 hours.

Diet advice
None.

Storage
Keep in a closed container, in a cool, dry place out of the reach of children.

Missed dose
Use as soon as you remember. If your next application is due within 8 hours, apply the usual amount now and skip the next application.

Stopping the drug
Do not stop using the drug without consulting your physician; symptoms may recur.

Exceeding the dose
An occasional unintentional extra application is unlikely to cause problems. But if you notice any unusual symptoms, notify your physician.

POSSIBLE ADVERSE EFFECTS

Most people who use clobetasol as directed do not have problems. Adverse effects mainly affect the skin. Some of these effects cannot be reversed.

Symptom/effect	Frequency		Discuss with physician		Stop taking drug now	Call physician now
	Common	Rare	Only if severe	In all cases		
Thinning of the skin	●			■		
Stretch marks	●			■		
Increased capillary size in skin	●			■		
Acne/dermatitis around mouth	●			■		
Loss of skin pigment	●		■			
Mood changes		●		■		
Weight gain		●		■		

INTERACTIONS

None.

SPECIAL PRECAUTIONS

Be sure to tell your physician if:
▼ You have a cold sore or chickenpox.
▼ You have any other infection.
▼ You have psoriasis.
▼ You have acne or rosacea.
▼ You are taking other medications.

Pregnancy
▼ Safety in pregnancy not established. Discuss with your physician.

Breast-feeding
▼ The drug passes into the breast milk and may affect the baby. Discuss with your physician.

Infants and children
▼ Not recommended for infants under 1 year. Used only with great caution for short periods in older children because overuse can slow growth.

Over 60
▼ No special problems.

Driving and hazardous work
▼ No special problems.

Alcohol
▼ No special problems.

PROLONGED USE

Clobetasol is not normally used for more than 4 weeks. If the condition has not improved in 2 to 4 weeks, you should notify your physician.

CLOMIPHENE

Product names Clomid, Serophene
Used in the following combined preparations None

GENERAL INFORMATION

Clomiphene increases the output of hormones by the pituitary gland, thereby stimulating ovulation (egg release) in women. If hormone levels in the blood fail to rise after the drug is taken, the gland is not working as it should.

For female infertility, tablets are taken within about five days of the onset of each menstrual cycle. This stimulates ovulation. If clomiphene does not stimulate ovulation after several months, other drugs may be prescribed.

Multiple pregnancies (usually twins) occur more commonly in women treated with clomiphene than in those who have not been treated. Adverse effects include an increased risk of ovarian cysts and ectopic pregnancy.

QUICK REFERENCE

Drug group Drug for infertility (p.152)

Overdose danger rating Low

Dependence rating Low

Prescription needed Yes

Available as generic Yes

INFORMATION FOR USERS

Your drug prescription is tailored for you. Do not alter dosage without checking with your physician.

How taken

Tablets.

Frequency and timing of doses
Once daily for 5 days during each menstrual cycle.

Dosage range
50mg daily initially; dose may be increased up to 100mg daily.

Onset of effect
Ovulation occurs 4–10 days after the last dose in any cycle. However, ovulation may not occur for several months.

Duration of action
5 days.

Diet advice
None.

Storage
Keep in a closed container in a cool, dry place away from the reach of children. Protect from light.

Missed dose
Take as soon as you remember. If your next dose is due at this time, take the missed dose and the next scheduled dose together.

Stopping the drug
Take as directed by your physician. Stopping the drug will reduce the chances of conception.

Exceeding the dose
An occasional unintentional extra dose is unlikely to be a cause for concern. But if you notice any unusual symptoms, or if a large overdose has been taken, notify your physician.

SPECIAL PRECAUTIONS

Be sure to tell your physician if:
▼ You have a long-term liver problem.
▼ You are taking other medications.

 Pregnancy
▼ Not prescribed. The drug is stopped as soon as pregnancy occurs.

 Breast-feeding
▼ Not prescribed.

 Infants and children
▼ Not prescribed.

 Over 60
▼ Not prescribed.

 Driving and hazardous work
▼ Avoid such activities until you have learned how clomiphene affects you because the drug can cause blurred vision.

 Alcohol
▼ Keep consumption low.

POSSIBLE ADVERSE EFFECTS

Most *side effects* are related to the dose taken. Ovarian enlargement and cyst formation can occur. If this happens the problem usually resolves within a few weeks of stopping the drug.

Symptom/effect	Frequency		Discuss with physician		Stop taking drug now	Call physician now
	Common	Rare	Only if severe	In all cases		
Hot flushes	●		■			
Nausea/vomiting	●		■			
"Breakthrough" bleeding	●		■			
Abdominal discomfort/bloating	●			■		
Impaired vision		●		■	▲	
Severe pain in chest/abdomen		●		■	▲	▮
Breast tenderness		●		■		
Dry skin/hair loss/rash		●		■		
Convulsions		●		■	▲	▮
Dizziness		●		■		

PROLONGED USE

Prolonged use of clomiphene may cause visual impairment. Also, no more than 6 courses of treatment are recommended since this may lead to an increased risk of ovarian cancer.

Monitoring Eye tests may be recommended if symptoms of visual impairment are noticed. Monitoring of body temperature and blood or urine hormone levels is performed to detect signs of ovulation and pregnancy.

INTERACTIONS

None.

CLOMIPRAMINE

Product name Anafranil
Used in the following combined preparations None

GENERAL INFORMATION

Clomipramine belongs to the class of antidepressant drugs known as the tricyclics. It is used mainly in the long-term treatment of depression. It elevates mood, improves appetite, increases physical activity, and restores interest in everyday pursuits.

Clomipramine is particularly useful in the treatment of obsessive and phobic disorders. In this case, the drug has to be taken for many weeks to achieve its full effect.

Clomipramine has the same adverse effects as other tricyclic drugs, such as drowsiness, dizziness, dry mouth, and constipation. In overdose, clomipramine may cause coma and dangerously abnormal heart rhythms.

QUICK REFERENCE

Drug group Tricyclic antidepressant (p.68)

Overdose danger rating High

Dependence rating Low

Prescription needed Yes

Available as generic Yes

INFORMATION FOR USERS

Your drug prescription is tailored for you. Do not alter dosage without checking with your physician.

How taken

Tablets.

Frequency and timing of doses
1–3 x daily.

Usual adult dosage range
10–250mg daily.

Onset of effect
Some effects may be felt within a few days, but full antidepressant effect may not be felt for up to 4 weeks. For phobic and obsessional disorders, full effect may take up to 12 weeks.

Duration of action
During prolonged treatment antidepressant effect may last up to 2 weeks.

Diet advice
None.

Storage
Keep in a closed container in a cool, dry place away from the reach of children.

Missed dose
Take as soon as you remember. If your next dose is due within 3 hours, take a single dose now and skip the next.

Stopping the drug
Stopping abruptly can cause withdrawal symptoms and a recurrence of the original trouble. Consult your physician, who may supervise a gradual reduction in dosage.

OVERDOSE ACTION

 Seek immediate medical advice in all cases. Take emergency action if palpitations are noted or consciousness is lost.

See Drug poisoning emergency guide (p.526).

SPECIAL PRECAUTIONS

Be sure to tell your physician if:
▼ You have heart problems.
▼ You have had epileptic fits.
▼ You have long-term liver or kidney problems.
▼ You have had glaucoma.
▼ You have thyroid disease.
▼ You have had prostate trouble.
▼ You have had mania or a psychotic illness.
▼ You are taking other medications.

 Pregnancy
▼ Safety in pregnancy not established. Discuss with your physician.

 Breast-feeding
▼ The drug passes into the breast milk and may affect the baby. Discuss with your physician.

 Infants and children
▼ Not recommended.

 Over 60
▼ Increased likelihood of adverse effects. Reduced dose may therefore be necessary.

 Driving and hazardous work
▼ Avoid such activities until you have learned how clomipramine affects you because the drug may cause blurred vision, drowsiness, and dizziness.

 Alcohol
▼ Avoid. Alcohol may increase the sedative effects of this drug.

Surgery and general anesthetics
▼ Clomipramine treatment may need to be stopped before you have a general anesthetic. Discuss this with your physician or dentist before any operation.

POSSIBLE ADVERSE EFFECTS

The possible *adverse effects* of this drug are mainly the result of its *anticholinergic* action, and include drowsiness and dizziness, dry mouth, and constipation.

Symptom/effect	Frequency		Discuss with physician		Stop taking drug now	Call physician now
	Common	Rare	Only if severe	In all cases		
Drowsiness/dizziness	●		■			
Sweating/flushing	●		■			
Dry mouth	●		■			
Blurred vision	●			■		
Constipation	●		■			
Difficulty in passing urine		●		■	▲	
Palpitations		●		■	▲	■
Skin reactions/rash		●		■		

INTERACTIONS

Sedatives All drugs that have a *sedative* effect may intensify those of clomipramine.

Antihypertensives Clomipramine may enhance the effect of some of these drugs.

Antiepiletics Clomipramine may reduce the effects of these drugs and vice versa.

Monoamine oxidase inhibitors (MAOIs) A serious reaction may occur if these drugs are given with clomipramine.

Quinidine There is an increased risk of abnormal heart rhythms if this drug is taken with clomipramine.

PROLONGED USE

No problems expected.

Monitoring Regular checks on heart and liver function are recommended.

CLONAZEPAM

Product names Apo-Clonazepam, Novo-Clonazepam, Rivotril, and others
Used in the following combined preparations None

GENERAL INFORMATION

Clonazepam belongs to a group of drugs known as the benzodiazepines, which are mainly used in the treatment of anxiety and insomnia (see p.67). However, clonazepam is used almost exclusively as an anticonvulsant to prevent and treat epileptic fits. It is particularly useful for the prevention of brief muscle spasms (myoclonus) and absence seizures (petit mal) in children but other forms of epilepsy, such as sudden flaccidity or fits induced by flashing lights, also respond to clonazepam treatment. Being a benzodiazepine, the drug also has tranquillizing and sedative effects.

Clonazepam is used either alone or together with other anticonvulsant drugs. Its anticonvulsant effect may begin to wear off after some months.

QUICK REFERENCE

Drug group Benzodiazepine anticonvulsant drug (p.70)

Overdose danger rating Medium

Dependence rating Medium

Prescription needed Yes

Available as generic Yes

INFORMATION FOR USERS

Your drug prescription is tailored for you. Do not alter dosage without checking with your physician.

How taken

Tablets.

Frequency and timing of doses
1–3 x daily.

Usual dosage range
Adults 0.5mg daily at night (starting dose), increased gradually to 4–8mg daily (maintenance dose).
Children Reduced dose according to age and weight.

Onset of effect
1–4 hours.

Duration of action
Approximately 6–12 hours.

Diet advice
None.

Storage
Keep in a closed container in a cool, dry place away from the reach of children.

Missed dose
No cause for concern, but take as soon as you remember. Take your next dose when it is due.

Stopping the drug
Do not stop the drug without consulting your physician because symptoms may recur.

Exceeding the dose
An occasional unintentional extra dose is unlikely to cause problems. Larger overdoses may cause excessive drowsiness and confusion. Notify your physician.

SPECIAL PRECAUTIONS

Be sure to tell your physician if:
▼ You have severe respiratory disease.
▼ You have long-term liver or kidney problems.
▼ You are taking other medications.
▼ You have had problems with drug or alcohol abuse.

 Pregnancy
▼ Safety in pregnancy not established. Discuss with your physician.

 Breast-feeding
▼ The drug passes into the breast milk and may affect the baby adversely. Discuss with your physician.

 Infants and children
▼ Reduced dose necessary.

 Over 60
▼ Reduced dose may be necessary.

 Driving and hazardous work
▼ Your underlying condition, as well as the possibility of drowsiness while taking clonazepam, may make such activities inadvisable. Discuss with your physician.

 Alcohol
▼ Avoid. Alcohol may increase the sedative effects of this drug.

POSSIBLE ADVERSE EFFECTS

The principal *adverse effects* of this drug are related to its sedative and tranquillizing properties. These effects normally diminish after the first few days of treatment and can often be reduced by medically supervised adjustment of dosage.

Symptom/effect	Frequency		Discuss with physician		Stop taking drug now	Call physician now
	Common	Rare	Only if severe	In all cases		
Daytime drowsiness	●		■			
Dizziness/unsteadiness	●		■			
Increased salivation	●		■			
Altered behaviour	●			■		
Forgetfulness/confusion		●		■		
Muscle weakness		●		■		

INTERACTIONS

Sedatives All drugs that have a *sedative* effect on the central nervous system are likely to increase the sedative properties of clonazepam. Such drugs include anti-anxiety and sleeping drugs, antihistamines, opioid analgesics, antidepressants, and antipsychotics.

Other anticonvulsants Clonazepam may alter the effects of other anticonvulsants you are taking, or they may alter its effect. Adjustment of dosage or change of drug may be necessary.

PROLONGED USE

Both beneficial and adverse effects of clonazepam may become less marked during prolonged treatment as the body adapts.

CLOPIDOGREL

Product name Plavix
Used in the following combined preparations None

GENERAL INFORMATION

Clopidogrel is an antiplatelet drug that is used to prevent blood clots from forming. It is prescribed to patients who have a tendency to form clots in the fast-flowing blood of the arteries and heart, or those who have had a stroke or a heart attack.

The drug may be suitable for people who cannot take ASA for its antiplatelet effects. It reduces the tendency of platelets to stick together when blood flow is disrupted. However, this can lead to abnormal bleeding. You should, report any unusual bleeding to your physician at once, and, if you require dental treatment, you should tell your dentist that you are taking the drug.

Adverse effects are common with clopidogrel and are usually associated with bleeding.

INFORMATION FOR USERS

Your drug prescription is tailored for you. Do not alter dosage without checking with your physician.

How taken

Tablets.

Frequency and timing of doses
Once daily.

Usual dosage range
75mg.

Onset of effect
1 hour.

Duration of action
24 hours.

Diet advice
None.

Storage
Keep in a closed container in a cool, dry place out of the reach of children.

Missed dose
Take as soon as you remember. If your next dose is due within 4 hours, take a single dose now and skip the next.

Stopping the drug
Do not stop taking the drug without consulting your physician. Stopping the drug may lead to a recurrence of the original condition.

Exceeding the dose
An occasional unintentional extra dose is unlikely to be a cause for concern. But if you notice any unusual symptoms, or if a large overdose has been taken, notify your physician.

SPECIAL PRECAUTIONS

Be sure to tell your physician if:
▼ You have liver or kidney problems.
▼ You have a condition, such as a peptic ulcer, that makes you more likely to bleed.
▼ You are taking other medications.

Pregnancy
▼ Safety in pregnancy not established. Discuss with your physician.

Breast-feeding
▼ The drug passes into the breast milk and may affect the baby. Discuss with your physician.

Infants and children
▼ Not recommended.

Over 60
▼ No special problems.

Driving and hazardous work
▼ No special problems.

Alcohol
▼ Excessive intake of alcohol may irritate the stomach and increase the risk of bleeding.

Surgery and general anesthetics
▼ Clopidogrel may need to be stopped a week before surgery. Discuss this with your physician or dentist.

POSSIBLE ADVERSE EFFECTS

The most frequent adverse effects of clopidogrel are bleeding and bruising. Nausea and diarrhea are less common.

Symptom/effect	Frequency		Discuss with physician		Stop taking drug now	Call physician now
	Common	Rare	Only if severe	In all cases		
Gastrointestinal bleeding/ulcers		●		■		
Bruising/nosebleeds	●			■		
Blood in urine		●		■		
Nausea/vomiting		●	■			
Diarrhea/abdominal pain		●	■			
Headache/dizziness		●	■			
Rash/itching		●		■		
Sore throat		●		■		■

INTERACTIONS

ASA and other non-steroidal anti-inflammatory drugs (NSAIDs) Clopidogrel increases the effect of ASA on platelets. The risk of gastrointestinal bleeding is increased when clopidogrel is used with these drugs.

Anticoagulant drugs (e.g., warfarin) The anticoagulant effect of these drugs is increased if they are taken with clopidogrel.

PROLONGED USE

No special problems.

CLOTRIMAZOLE

Product names Canesten, Clotrimaderm
Used in the following combined preparations Lotriderm

GENERAL INFORMATION

Clotrimazole is an antifungal drug that is commonly used to treat fungal and yeast infections. It is used for treating tinea (ringworm) infections of the skin, and candida (thrush) infections of the vagina or penis. The drug is applied in the form of a cream to the affected area, and inserted as vaginal suppositories or applied as cream for vaginal conditions such as candida.

Adverse effects from clotrimazole are very rare, although some people may experience burning and irritation on the skin surface in the area where the drug has been applied.

QUICK REFERENCE

Drug group Antifungal drug (p.124)
Overdose danger rating Low
Dependence rating Low
Prescription needed Yes (for combined preparations)
Available as generic Yes

INFORMATION FOR USERS

Your drug prescription is tailored for you. Do not alter dosage without checking with your physician.

How taken

Suppositories, vaginal cream, topical cream.

Frequency and timing of doses
2–3 x daily (skin cream);
once daily at bedtime (vaginal suppositories);
1–2 x daily (vaginal cream).

Usual dosage range
Vaginal infections One applicatorful (5g) per dose (vaginal cream); 100–500mg per dose (vaginal suppositories).
Skin infections (skin cream) as directed.

Onset of effect
Within 2–3 days.

Duration of action
Up to 12 hours.

Diet advice
None.

Storage
Keep in a closed container in a cool, dry place away from the reach of children.

Missed dose
No cause for concern, but make up the missed dose or application as soon as you remember.

Stopping the drug
Apply the full course. Even if symptoms disappear, the original infection may still be present and symptoms may recur if treatment is stopped too soon.

Exceeding the dose
An occasional unintentional extra dose is unlikely to cause problems. But if you notice unusual symptoms or if a large amount has been swallowed, notify your physician.

POSSIBLE ADVERSE EFFECTS

Clotrimazole rarely causes adverse effects. Skin preparations and vaginal applications may occasionally cause localized burning and irritation.

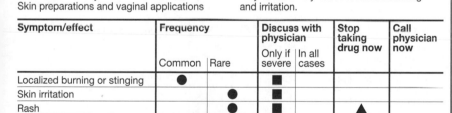

Symptom/effect	Frequency		Discuss with physician		Stop taking drug now	Call physician now
	Common	Rare	Only if severe	In all cases		
Localized burning or stinging	●		■			
Skin irritation		●	■			
Rash		●	■		▲	

INTERACTIONS

None known.

SPECIAL PRECAUTIONS

Be sure to tell your physician if:
▼ You are taking other medications.

 Pregnancy
▼ No evidence of risk to developing baby, but only use with the advice of your physician.

 Breast-feeding
▼ No evidence of risk.

 Infants and children
▼ No special problems, but use of vaginal suppositories not advised.

 Over 60
▼ No special problems.

 Driving and hazardous work
▼ No known problems.

Alcohol
▼ No known problems.

PROLONGED USE

No problems expected.

CLOXACILLIN

Product names Apo-Cloxi, Novo-Cloxin, Nu-Cloxi
Used in the following combined preparations None

GENERAL INFORMATION

Cloxacillin, a penicillin antibiotic first available in 1963, is prescribed to treat staphylococcal infections. These are usually resistant to treatment with other forms of penicillin because the bacteria produce an enzyme that breaks down the antibiotic. Cloxacillin, however, is not affected by the enzyme. Common sites where staphylococcal infection may occur include the skin and the soft tissues.

For maximum effect, cloxacillin needs to be taken on an empty stomach, because food interferes with absorption of the drug from the digestive tract.

Diarrhea is the most common side effect. As with other penicillin antibiotics, there is a risk of an allergic reaction – rash and possibly fever, itching, swelling of the mouth and tongue, and breathing difficulty.

INFORMATION FOR USERS

Your drug prescription is tailored for you. Do not alter dosage without checking with your physician.

How taken

● ● ●

Capsules, oral liquid, injection.

Frequency and timing of doses
4 x daily at least 1 hour before, or 2 hours after eating.

Dosage range
Adults 1–2g daily (by mouth).
Children Reduced dose according to age and weight.

Onset of effect
Symptoms usually improve within 1–3 days, depending on the condition.

Duration of action
Up to 6 hours.

Diet advice
None.

Storage
Keep in a closed container in a cool, dry place away from the reach of children. Refrigerate liquid, but do not freeze, and do not keep for longer than 14 days.

Missed dose
Take as soon as you remember. If your next dose is due at this time, take both doses now.

Stopping the drug
Take the full course. Even if you feel better, the original infection may still be present and symptoms may recur if treatment is stopped too soon.

Exceeding the dose
An occasional unintentional extra dose is unlikely to cause problems. But if you notice unusual symptoms, or if a large overdose has been taken, notify your physician.

SPECIAL PRECAUTIONS

Be sure to tell your physician if:
▼ You have an allergy (for example, asthma, hay fever, eczema, or hives).
▼ You have ulcerative colitis.
▼ You have had a rash after taking a penicillin or cephalosporin antibiotic.
▼ You are taking other medications.

Pregnancy
▼ Is prescribed during pregnancy, but risks to baby have not been fully established. Discuss with your physician.

Breast-feeding
▼ The drug passes into the breast milk and may affect the baby adversely. Discuss with your physician.

Infants and children
▼ Safety in premature and newborn infants not established. Reduced dose necessary for children.

Over 60
▼ Reduced dose necessary.

Driving and hazardous work
▼ No known problems.

Alcohol
▼ No known problems.

POSSIBLE ADVERSE EFFECTS

If you develop a rash, wheezing, itching, fever, or joint swelling, this may indicate an allergy to cloxacillin, making it necessary to take a different antibiotic.

Symptom/effect	Frequency		Discuss with physician		Stop taking drug now	Call physician now
	Common	Rare	Only if severe	In all cases		
Rash	●			■		
Nausea/vomiting		●	■			
Unusual thirst		●	■			
Tiredness/weakness		●	■			
Diarrhea		●		■		
Wheezing/breathlessness		●		■	▲	▮
Itching		●		■	▲	▮
Swollen mouth/tongue		●		■	▲	▮

PROLONGED USE

Cloxacillin is usually given only for short courses of treatment.

INTERACTIONS

Probenecid This drug can increase blood levels of cloxacillin.

CLOZAPINE

Product names Apo-Clozapine, Clozaril
Used in the following combined preparations None

GENERAL INFORMATION

Clozapine is an atypical antipsychotic drug for schizophrenia. It is given to patients who have not responded to other treatments or who have experienced intolerable *side effects* with other drugs. Clozapine helps control severe resistant schizophrenia, helping the patient to re-establish a more normal lifestyle. The improvement is gradual, and relief of severe symptoms can take more than three weeks. All treatment is usually started and supervised by a hospital and all patients must be registered with the Clozaril Support and Assistance Network (CSAN). The drug can cause a very serious side effect: agranulocytosis (a large decrease in white blood cells). Blood tests are done before and during treatment; the drug is supplied only if results are normal. Clozapine is less likely than other antipsychotics to cause *parkinsonism*.

INFORMATION FOR USERS

This drug is given only under strict medical supervision and continual monitoring.

How taken

Tablets.

Frequency and timing of doses
1–3 x daily; a larger dose may be given at night.

Usual adult dosage range
2.5–900mg daily.

Onset of effect
Gradual. Some effect may appear within 3–5 days, but the full beneficial effect may not be felt for over 3 weeks.

Duration of action
Up to 16 hours.

Diet advice
None.

Storage
Keep in a closed container in a cool, dry place away from the reach of children.

Missed dose
Take as soon as you remember. If your next dose is due within 2 hours, take a single dose now and skip the next. If you miss more than 2 days of tablets, notify your physician because you may need to restart at a lower dose.

Stopping the drug
Do not stop the drug without consulting your physician because symptoms may recur.

Exceeding the dose
An occasional unintentional extra dose is unlikely to cause problems. Large overdoses may cause unusual drowsiness, fits, and agitation. Notify your physician.

SPECIAL PRECAUTIONS

Be sure to tell your physician if:
▼ You have long-term liver or kidney problems.
▼ You have a history of blood disorders.
▼ You have had epileptic fits.
▼ You have heart problems.
▼ You have colon problems or have had bowel surgery.
▼ You have diabetes.
▼ You have glaucoma.
▼ You have prostate problems.
▼ You are taking other medications.

 Pregnancy
▼ Not usually prescribed. Safety not established. Discuss with your physician.

 Breast-feeding
▼ The drug passes into the breast milk and may affect the baby. Discuss with your physician.

 Infants and children
▼ Not prescribed.

 Over 60
▼ Adverse effects are more likely. Initial dose is low and is slowly increased.

 Driving and hazardous work
▼ Avoid such activities until you know how clozapine affects you because the drug can cause blurred vision, drowsiness, and dizziness.

 Alcohol
▼ Avoid. Alcohol may increase the sedative effects of this drug.

POSSIBLE ADVERSE EFFECTS

Clozapine is less likely to cause parkinsonian side effects (tremor and stiffness), which occur with the use of other anti-psychotic drugs. The most serious side effect is agranulocytosis, and strict monitoring is necessary.

Symptom/effect	Frequency		Discuss with physician		Stop taking drug now	Call physician now
	Common	Rare	Only if severe	In all cases		
Drowsiness/tiredness	●		■			
Excess saliva	●		■			
Dry mouth	●		■			
Weight gain	●		■			
Fast heartbeat	●			■		
Dizziness/fainting	●			■		
Constipation	●			■		
Blurred vision		●		■		
Tremor/muscle rigidity		●		■		
Urinary difficulties		●		■		
Fever/sore throat		●		■		▮
Fits or seizures		●		■		▮

INTERACTIONS

General note A number of drugs increase the risk of adverse effects on the blood. Do not take other medication without checking with your physician or pharmacist.

Sedatives All drugs that have a *sedative* effect on the central nervous system are likely to increase the sedative properties of clozapine.

PROLONGED USE

Agranulocytosis may occur, and occasionally liver function may be upset. Significant weight gain may also occur.

Monitoring Blood tests are carried out weekly for 18 weeks, fortnightly until the end of the first year, and, if blood counts are stable, every 4 weeks thereafter. Liver function tests may also be performed.

CODEINE

Product Name Codeine Contin
Used in the following combined preparations Atasol-8, Exdol-15, Fiorinal-C1/4, Novo-Gesic C15, and many others

GENERAL INFORMATION

Codeine is a mild *opioid* analgesic that is similar to, but weaker than, morphine. It has been in common medical use since the beginning of this century.

Codeine is prescribed primarily to relieve mild to moderate pain, and is often combined with a non-opioid analgesic such as acetaminophen. It is also an effective cough suppressant and, for this reason, is included as an ingredient in many non-prescription cough syrups and cold relief preparations.

Like the other opioid drugs, codeine is constipating, a characteristic that sometimes makes it useful in the short-term control of diarrhea.

Although codeine is habit-forming, addiction seldom occurs if the drug is used for a limited period of time and the recommended dosage is followed.

Constipation is common with codeine. Other, rare, *adverse effects* include breathing difficulties, which should be reported to your physician without delay.

QUICK REFERENCE

Drug group Opioid analgesic (p.64), antidiarrheal drug (p.96), and cough suppressant (p.80)

Overdose danger rating High

Dependence rating Medium

Prescription needed Yes (some preparations)

Available as generic Yes

INFORMATION FOR USERS

Your drug prescription is tailored for you. Do not alter dosage without checking with your physician.

How taken

Tablets, liquid, injection.

Frequency and timing of doses
4–6 x daily (pain); 3–4 x daily when necessary (cough); every 4–6 hours when necessary (diarrhea).

Usual adult dosage range
120–240mg daily (pain); 45–120mg daily (cough); 30–180mg daily (diarrhoea).

Onset of effect
30–60 minutes.

Duration of action
4–6 hours.

Diet advice
None.

Storage
Keep in a closed container in a cool, dry place out of the reach of children. Protect from light.

Missed dose
Take as soon as you remember if needed for relief of symptoms. If not needed, do not take the missed dose, and return to your normal dose schedule when necessary.

Stopping the drug
Can be safely stopped as soon as you no longer need it.

OVERDOSE ACTION

 Seek immediate medical advice in all cases. Take emergency action if there are symptoms such as slow or irregular breathing, severe drowsiness, or loss of consciousness.

See Drug poisoning emergency guide (p.526).

SPECIAL PRECAUTIONS

Be sure to tell your physician if:
▼ You have long-term liver or kidney problems.
▼ You have a lung disorder such as asthma or bronchitis.
▼ You are taking other medications.

 Pregnancy
▼ No evidence of risk, but may adversely affect the baby's breathing if taken during labour.

 Breast-feeding
▼ The drug passes into the breast milk, but at normal doses adverse effects on the baby are unlikely. Discuss with your physician.

 Infants and children
▼ Reduced dose necessary.

 Over 60
▼ Reduced dose may be necessary.

 Driving and hazardous work
▼ Avoid such activities until you have learned how codeine affects you because the drug may cause dizziness and drowsiness.

 Alcohol
▼ Avoid. Alcohol may increase the sedative effects of this drug.

PROLONGED USE

Codeine is normally used only for short-term relief of symptoms. It can be habit-forming if taken for extended periods, especially if higher-than-average doses are taken.

POSSIBLE ADVERSE EFFECTS

Serious adverse effects are rare with codeine. Constipation occurs especially with prolonged use, but other side effects, such as nausea, vomiting, and drowsiness, are not usually troublesome at recommended doses, and usually disappear if the dose is reduced.

Symptom/effect	Frequency		Discuss with physician		Stop taking drug now	Call physician now
	Common	Rare	Only if severe	In all cases		
Constipation	●		■			
Nausea/vomiting		●		■		
Drowsiness		●		■		
Dizziness		●		■		
Agitation/restlessness		●		■	▲	
Rash/hives		●		■	▲	▮
Wheezing/breathlessness		●		■	▲	▮

INTERACTIONS

Sedatives All drugs, including alcohol, that have a *sedative* effect on the central nervous system are likely to increase sedation with codeine. Such drugs include sleeping drugs, antidepressant drugs, and antihistamines.

COLCHICINE

Product name None
Used in the following combined preparations None

GENERAL INFORMATION

Colchicine, a drug originally extracted from the autumn crocus flower and later synthesized, has been used since the 18th century for gout. Although it has now, to some extent, been superseded by newer drugs, it is still often used to relieve joint pain and inflammation in flare-ups of gout. Colchicine is most effective when taken at the first sign of symptoms, and almost always produces an improvement. The drug may also be given during the first few months of treatment with allopurinol or probenecid (other drugs used for treating gout), because these may at first increase the frequency of gout attacks.

Colchicine is occasionally prescribed for the relief of the symptoms of familial Mediterranean fever (a rare congenital condition).

QUICK REFERENCE

Drug group Drug for gout (p.105)
Overdose danger rating High
Dependence rating Low
Prescription needed Yes
Available as generic Yes

INFORMATION FOR USERS

Your drug prescription is tailored for you. Do not alter dosage without checking with your physician.

How taken

Tablets.

Frequency and timing of doses
Prevention of gout attacks 2–3 x daily.
Relief of gout attacks Every 2–3 hours.

Usual adult dosage range
Prevention of gout attacks 0.5mg 1–4 x weekly to 1.8mg daily.
Relief of gout attacks 1mg initially, followed by 0.5 or 0.6mg every 2–3 hours, until relief of pain, vomiting, or diarrhea occurs, or until a total dose of 8mg is reached. This course must not be repeated within 3 days.

Onset of effect
Relief of symptoms in an attack may be felt in 6–24 hours. Full effect in gout prevention may not be felt for several days.

Duration of action
Up to 2 hours. Some effect may last longer.

Diet advice
Certain foods are known to make gout worse. Discuss with your physician.

Storage
Keep in a closed container in a cool, dry place out of the reach of children. Protect from light.

Missed dose
Take as soon as you remember. If your next dose is due within 30 minutes, take a single dose now and skip the next.

Stopping the drug
When taking colchicine frequently during an acute attack of gout, stop if diarrhea or abdominal pain develop. In other cases, do not stop without consulting your physician.

OVERDOSE ACTION

 Seek immediate medical advice in all cases; some reactions can be fatal. Take emergency action if severe nausea, vomiting, bloody diarrhea, severe abdominal pain, or loss of consciousness occur.

See Drug poisoning emergency guide (p.526).

SPECIAL PRECAUTIONS

Be sure to tell your physician if:
▼ You have long-term liver or kidney problems.
▼ You have heart problems.
▼ You have a blood disorder.
▼ You have stomach ulcers.
▼ You have chronic inflammation of the bowel.
▼ You are taking other medications.

 Pregnancy
▼ Not usually prescribed. May cause defects in the unborn baby. Discuss with your physician.

 Breast-feeding
▼ The drug passes into the breast milk and may affect the baby. Discuss with your physician.

 Infants and children
▼ Not recommended.

 Over 60
▼ Increased likelihood of adverse effects.

 Driving and hazardous work
▼ No special problems.

 Alcohol
▼ Avoid. Alcohol may increase stomach irritation caused by colchicine.

PROLONGED USE

Prolonged use of this drug may lead to hair loss, rashes, tingling in the hands and feet, muscle pain and weakness, and blood disorders.

Monitoring Periodic blood checks are usually required.

POSSIBLE ADVERSE EFFECTS

The appearance of any symptom that may be an *adverse effect* of the drug is a sign that you should stop the drug until you have received further medical advice.

Symptom/effect	Frequency		Discuss with physician		Stop taking drug now	Call physician now
	Common	Rare	Only if severe	In all cases		
Nausea/vomiting	●			■	▲	
Diarrhea/abdominal pain	●			■	▲	
Numbness and tingling		●		■	▲	
Unusual bleeding/bruising		●		■	▲	
Rash		●		■	▲	

INTERACTIONS

Cyclosporine Taking cyclosporine with colchicine may lead to adverse effects on the kidneys.

CONJUGATED ESTROGENS

Product names C.E.S., Congest, Premarin
Used in the following combined preparations Premplus

GENERAL INFORMATION

Preparations of conjugated estrogens consist of naturally occurring estrogens similar to those found in the urine of pregnant mares. Given by mouth, they are used to relieve symptoms of menopause such as hot flushes. They can also help prevent post-menopausal osteoporosis (bone loss), although they are not used to treat osteoporosis.

As replacement therapy, conjugated estrogens are usually taken on a cyclic dosing schedule, often in conjunction with a progestin, to simulate hormonal changes that occur in a normal menstrual cycle. Conjugated estrogens are also available as a vaginal cream to relieve pain and dryness of the vagina or vulva after the menopause.

Conjugated estrogens do not provide contraception. A woman can still get pregnant for 2 years after her last period (if she is under 50 years) or for 1 year after the end of menstruation (if she is over 50 years). Conjugated estrogens on their own are not recommended for women who have a "working" uterus.

QUICK REFERENCE

Drug group Female sex hormone (p.133) and drug for bone disorders (p.108)

Overdose danger rating Low

Dependence rating Low

Prescription needed Yes

Available as generic Yes

INFORMATION FOR USERS

Your drug prescription is tailored for you. Do not alter dosage without checking with your physician.

How taken

Tablets, cream.

Frequency and timing of doses
Once daily (tablets).
Once daily (cream).

Usual adult dosage range
0.3–1.25mg daily (tablets); 1–2g daily (cream).

Onset of effect
5–20 days.

Duration of action
1–2 days.

Diet advice
None.

Storage
Keep in a closed container in a cool, dry place out of the reach of children.

Missed dose
Take as soon as you remember.

Stopping the drug
Do not stop the drug without consulting your physician because symptoms may recur.

Exceeding the dose
An occasional unintentional extra dose is unlikely to be a cause for concern. But if you notice any unusual symptoms, or if a large overdose has been taken, notify your physician.

SPECIAL PRECAUTIONS

Be sure to tell your physician or pharmacist if:
▼ You have heart failure or high blood pressure.
▼ You have had blood clots or a stroke.
▼ You have a history of breast disease.
▼ You have had fibroids in the uterus.
▼ You suffer from migraine or epilepsy.
▼ You are taking other medications.
▼ You have long-term liver or kidney problems.

 Pregnancy
▼ Not prescribed. May affect the baby adversely. Discuss with your physician.

 Breast-feeding
▼ Not prescribed. The drug passes into the breast milk and may inhibit its flow. Discuss with your physician.

 Infants and children
▼ Not prescribed.

 Over 60
▼ No special problems.

 Driving and hazardous work
▼ No known problems.

 Alcohol
▼ No known problems.

Surgery and general anesthetics
▼ Conjugated estrogens may need to be stopped several weeks before you have surgery. Discuss with your physician.

POSSIBLE ADVERSE EFFECTS

The most common *adverse effects* of conjugated estrogens are similar to symptoms that occur in the early stages of pregnancy, and generally diminish or disappear after 2–3 months of treatment. Women on a cyclic schedule will have a menstrual bleed towards the end of each cycle. Sudden, sharp pain in the chest, groin, or legs may indicate an abnormal blood clot that requires urgent medical attention.

Symptom/effect	Frequency		Discuss with physician		Stop taking drug now	Call physician now
	Common	Rare	Only if severe	In all cases		
Nausea/vomiting	●		■			
Breast swelling/tenderness	●		■			
Increase or decrease in weight	●		■			
Reduced sex drive		●	■			
Depression		●		■		
Vaginal bleeding		●		■		
Pain in chest/groin/legs		●		■		■

INTERACTIONS

Tobacco smoking Smoking increases the risk of serious adverse effects on the heart and circulation with conjugated estrogens.

Oral anticoagulant drugs Conjugated estrogens reduce the *anticoagulant* effect of these drugs.

PROLONGED USE

There is a higher risk of breast cancer, cancer of the uterus, gallbladder disease, and abnormal blood clots in some people.

Monitoring Regular physical examinations (e.g., mammograms) and blood pressure checks are advised.

CO-TRIMOXAZOLE

Product name Septra
Used in the following combined preparations (Co-trimoxazole is a combination of two drugs)

GENERAL INFORMATION

Co-trimoxazole is a mixture of two antibacterial drugs: trimethoprim and sulfamethoxazole. It is prescribed for prevention and treatment of urinary tract infections and treatment of skin, ear, and gastrointestinal infections. Co-trimoxazole is also used to treat pneumocystis pneumonia, toxoplasmosis, and the bacterial infection nocardiasis.

Although co-trimoxazole was widely prescribed in the past, its use has declined in recent years with the introduction of new, more effective, and safer drugs.

Rare but serious adverse effects of co-trimoxazole may occur and these include skin rashes, blood disorders, and liver or kidney damage.

QUICK REFERENCE

Drug group Antibacterial drug (p.117)

Overdose danger rating Medium

Dependence rating Low

Prescription needed Yes

Available as generic Yes

INFORMATION FOR USERS

Your drug prescription is tailored for you. Do not alter dosage without checking with your physician.

How taken

Tablets, tablets double strength (DS), liquid, injection.

Frequency and timing of doses
Normally 2 x daily, preferably with food.

Usual adult dosage range
Usually 4 tablets daily (each standard tablet is 80mg trimethroprim and 400mg sulfamethox-azole) or 2 DS daily. Higher doses may be used for the treatment of pneumocystis pneumonia, toxoplasmosis, and nocardiasis.

Onset of effect
1–4 hours.

Duration of action
12 hours.

Diet advice
Drink plenty of fluids, particularly in warm weather.

Storage
Keep in a closed container in a cool, dry place out of the reach of children. Protect from light.

Missed dose
Take as soon as you remember. If your normal dose is 80/400mg, double this; if it is more than 80/400mg, take one dose only.

Stopping the drug
Take the full course. Even if you feel better, the original infection may still be present and symptoms may recur if treatment is stopped too soon.

Exceeding the dose
An occasional unintentional extra dose is unlikely to be a cause for concern. Large overdoses may cause nausea, vomiting, dizziness, and confusion. Notify your physician.

SPECIAL PRECAUTIONS

Be sure to tell your physician if:
▼ You have long-term liver or kidney problems.
▼ You have a blood disorder.
▼ You have glucose-6-phosphate dehydrogenase (G6PD) deficiency.
▼ You are allergic to sulfonamide drugs.
▼ You suffer from porphyria.
▼ You are taking other medications.

Pregnancy
▼ Not usually prescribed. May cause defects in the baby. Discuss with your physician.

Breast-feeding
▼ The drug passes into the breast milk, but at normal levels adverse effects on the baby are unlikely. Discuss with your physician.

Infants and children
▼ Not recommended in infants under 6 weeks old. Reduced dose necessary in older children.

Over 60
▼ Side effects are more likely. Used only when necessary, and often in reduced dosage.

Driving and hazardous work
▼ No known problems.

Alcohol
▼ No known problems.

POSSIBLE ADVERSE EFFECTS

The most common problems are nausea and rash, and itching. Other less common reactions include vomiting, diarrhea, sore tongue, and headache.

Symptom/effect	Frequency		Discuss with physician		Stop taking drug now	Call physician now
	Common	Rare	Only if severe	In all cases		
Rash/itching	●			■	▲	▮
Nausea/vomiting		●		■		
Diarrhea		●	■			
Sore tongue		●		■		
Headache		●		■		
Jaundice		●		■		▮

INTERACTIONS

Warfarin Co-trimoxazole may increase its *anticoagulant* effect; the dose of warfarin may have to be reduced. Blood-clotting status may have to be checked.

Cyclosporine Taking cyclosporine with co-trimoxazole can impair kidney function.

Phenytoin Co-trimoxazole may cause a build-up of phenytoin in the body; the dose of phenytoin may have to be reduced.

Oral antidiabetic drugs Co-trimoxazole may increase the blood sugar lowering effect of these drugs.

PROLONGED USE

Long-term use of this drug may lead to folic acid deficiency, which can cause anemia. Folic acid supplements may be needed.

Monitoring Regular blood tests are recommended.

CYCLOPHOSPHAMIDE

Product names Cytoxan, Procytox
Used in the following combined preparations None

GENERAL INFORMATION

Cyclophosphamide belongs to a group of anticancer drugs known as alkylating agents. It is used for a wide range of cancers, including lymphomas (lymph gland cancers), leukemias, and solid tumours, particularly of the breast and lung. It is commonly given together with radiotherapy or other drugs. Cyclophosphamide has also been used for autoimmune diseases.

Cyclophosphamide causes nausea, vomiting, and hair loss, and can affect the heart, lungs, and liver. It can also cause bladder damage in susceptible people because it produces a toxic substance called acrolein. To reduce *toxicity*, people considered to be at risk may be given a drug called mesna before and after each dose of cyclophosphamide. Also, because the drug often reduces production of blood cells, it may lead to abnormal bleeding, increased risk of infection, and reduced fertility in men.

INFORMATION FOR USERS

Your drug prescription is tailored for you. Do not alter dosage without checking with your physician.

How taken

Tablets, injection.

Frequency and timing of doses
Varies from once daily to every 3 weeks, depending on the condition being treated.

Usual dosage range
Dosage is determined individually according to the nature of the condition, body weight, and response.

Onset of effect
Some effects may appear within hours of starting treatment. Full beneficial effects may not be felt for many weeks.

Duration of action
Several weeks.

Diet advice
High fluid intake with frequent bladder emptying is recommended. This will usually prevent the drug causing bladder irritation.

Storage
Keep in a closed container in a cool, dry place out of the reach of children. Protect from light.

Missed dose
Injections are given only in hospital. If you are taking tablets, take the missed dose as soon as you remember. If your next dose is due within 6 hours, take a single dose now and skip the next. Tell your physician that you missed a dose.

Stopping the drug
The drug will be stopped under medical supervision (injection). Do not stop taking the drug without consulting your physician (tablets); stopping the drug may lead to worsening of the underlying condition.

Exceeding the dose
An occasional unintentional extra dose is unlikely to cause problems. Large overdoses may cause nausea, vomiting, and bladder damage. Notify your physician.

SPECIAL PRECAUTIONS

Cyclophosphamide is prescribed only under close medical supervision, taking account of your present condition and medical history.

Pregnancy
▼ Not usually prescribed. May cause birth defects. Discuss with your physician.

Breast-feeding
▼ Not advised. The drug passes into the breast milk and may affect the baby adversely. Discuss with your physician.

Infants and children
▼ Reduced dose necessary.

Over 60
▼ No special problems.

Driving and hazardous work
▼ No known problems.

Alcohol
▼ No problems expected, but avoid excessive amounts.

Surgery and general anesthetics
Infom your anesthesiologist that you are taking the drug prior to surgery.

PROLONGED USE

Prolonged use of this drug may reduce the production of blood cells.

Monitoring Periodic checks on blood composition and on all effects of the drug are usually required.

POSSIBLE ADVERSE EFFECTS

Cyclophosphamide often causes nausea and vomiting, which usually diminish as your body adjusts. Also, women often experience irregular periods. Blood in the urine may be a sign of bladder damage and requires prompt medical attention. Those thought to be at risk of bladder damage may be given mesna before and after doses of cyclophosphamide.

Symptom/effect	Frequency		Discuss with physician		Stop taking drug now	Call physician now
	Common	Rare	Only if severe	In all cases		
Nausea/vomiting	●		■			
Hair loss	●		■			
Irregular menstruation	●			■		
Mouth ulcers		●		■		
Bloodstained urine		●		■		■

INTERACTIONS

Phenytoin Can increase the breakdown of cyclophosphamide.

Allopurinol and phenothiazines Can inhibit breakdown of cyclophosphamide.

CYCLOSPORINE

Product names Neoral, Sandimmune
Used in the following combined preparations None

GENERAL INFORMATION

Cyclosporine is one of the immuno-suppressants, a group of drugs that suppress the body's natural defences against infection and foreign cells. This action is of particular use following organ transplants, when the recipient's immune system may reject the transplanted organ unless the immune system is controlled.

Cyclosporine is widely used after many types of transplant, such as heart, bone marrow, kidney, liver, and pancreas; its use has considerably reduced the risk of rejection. It is sometimes used to treat rheumatoid arthritis, severe psoriasis, and in nephrotic syndrome, when other treatments have failed.

Because cyclosporine reduces the effectiveness of the immune system, people being treated with this drug are more susceptible than usual to infections. Cyclosporine can also cause kidney damage.

Different brands of cyclosporine may reach different levels in your blood. It is important to know which brand you are taking. Do not try to make dose changes on your own. Ask your pharmacist for a patient information leaflet on the product you are taking.

QUICK REFERENCE

Drug group Immunosuppressant drug (p.143)

Overdose danger rating Medium

Dependence rating Low

Prescription needed Yes

Available as generic Yes

INFORMATION FOR USERS

Your drug prescription is tailored for you. Do not alter dosage without checking with your physician.

How taken

Capsules, liquid, injection.

Frequency and timing of doses
1–2 x daily. The liquid can be mixed with water, apple juice, or orange juice just before taking. Do not mix with grapefruit juice.

Usual dosage range
Dosage is calculated on an individual basis according to age and weight.

Onset of effect
Within 12 hours.

Duration of action
Up to 3 days.

Diet advice
Avoid high-potassium foods, such as bananas and tomatoes, and potassium supplements. Avoid grapefruit juice.

Storage
Capsules should be left in the blister pack until required. Keep in a closed container in a cool, dry place out of the reach of children. Do not refrigerate liquid.

Missed dose
Take as soon as you remember. If your dose is more than 36 hours late, consult your physician.

Stopping the drug
Do not stop taking the drug without consulting your physician; stopping the drug may lead to transplant rejection.

Exceeding the dose
An occasional unintentional extra dose is unlikely to cause problems. Large overdoses may cause vomiting and diarrhea and may affect kidney function. Notify your physician.

SPECIAL PRECAUTIONS

Cyclosporine is prescribed only under close medical supervision, taking account of your present condition and medical history.

Pregnancy
▼ Not usually prescribed. Safety in pregnancy not established. Discuss with your physician.

Breast-feeding
▼ Not recommended. The drug passes into the breast milk and safety has not been established. Discuss with your physician.

Infants and children
▼ Safety not established; used only with great caution.

Over 60
▼ Reduced dose may be necessary.

Driving and hazardous work
▼ No known problems.

Alcohol
▼ No known problems.

Sunlight
▼ Avoid prolonged, unprotected exposure.

POSSIBLE ADVERSE EFFECTS

The most common *adverse effects* are gum swelling, excessive hair growth, nausea and vomiting, and tremor. Headache and muscle cramps may also occur. Less common effects are diarrhea, facial swelling, flushing, "pins and needles" sensations, rash, and itching.

Symptom/effect	Frequency		Discuss with physician		Stop taking drug now	Call physician now
	Common	Rare	Only if severe	In all cases		
Increased body hair	●		■			
Nausea/vomiting	●			■		
Tremor	●			■		
Headache	●			■		
Sore throat/chills		●		■		
Swelling of gums	●			■		
High blood pressure	●			■		■

INTERACTIONS

General note Cyclosporine may interact with a large number of drugs. Check with your physician or pharmacist before taking any new prescription or over-the-counter medications.

Grapefuit juice can increase blood levels of cyclosporine. Avoid grapefruit juice.

PROLONGED USE

Long-term use, especially in high doses, can affect kidney and/or liver function. It may reduce numbers of white blood cells, thus increasing susceptibility to infection.

Monitoring Regular blood tests should be carried out as well as tests for liver and kidney function. Cyclosporine blood levels and blood pressure should also be checked regularly.

DANAZOL

Product name Cyclomen
Used in the following combined preparations None

GENERAL INFORMATION

Danazol is a synthetic steroid hormone that inhibits hormones called pituitary gonadotrophins.

It is used in a range of conditions, including endometriosis (fragments of endometrial tissue growing outside the uterus), menorrhagia, and, in men, to reduce gynecomastia (breast swelling). Danazol has also been used, long term, to treat hereditary angioedema (a rare allergic disorder that causes facial swelling).

Danazol is also used to relieve pain, tenderness, and lumpiness in the breasts caused by fibrocystic disease. Treatment commonly disrupts normal menstrual periods and in some cases periods may stop altogether. Women taking high doses may notice unusual hair growth and deepening of the voice.

INFORMATION FOR USERS

Your drug prescription is tailored for you. Do not alter dosage without checking with your physician.

How taken

Capsules.

Frequency and timing of doses
2–4 x daily.

Usual adult dosage range
200–800mg daily, depending on the condition being treated, its severity, and the response to the drug.

Onset of effect
Some effects occur after a few days. Full beneficial effects may take some months.

Duration of action
1–2 days.

Diet advice
None.

Storage
Keep in a closed container in a cool, dry place out of the reach of children.

Missed dose
Take as soon as you remember. If your next dose is due within 2 hours, take a single dose now and skip the next.

Stopping the drug
Do not stop the drug without consulting your physician; symptoms may recur.

Exceeding the dose
An occasional unintentional extra dose is unlikely to cause problems. But if you notice any unusual symptoms, or if a large overdose has been taken, notify your physician.

SPECIAL PRECAUTIONS

Be sure to tell your physician if:
▼ You have long-term liver or kidney problems.
▼ You have heart disease.
▼ You have had epileptic fits.
▼ You suffer from migraine.
▼ You suffer from unexplained vaginal bleeding.
▼ You have diabetes mellitus.
▼ You are taking other medications.

Pregnancy
▼ Not prescribed. May cause masculine characteristics in a female baby. Non-hormonal methods of contraception should be used for women of childbearing age; and pregnancy should be avoided for 3 months after the end of treatment.

Breast-feeding
▼ The drug passes into the breast milk and may affect the baby. Discuss with your physician.

Infants and children
▼ Not recommended.

Over 60
▼ Unlikely to be required.

Driving and hazardous work
▼ No known problems.

Alcohol
▼ No known problems.

POSSIBLE ADVERSE EFFECTS

Danazol rarely causes *adverse effects* in low doses. Adverse effects from higher doses, including acne, weight gain, and nausea, are the result of hormonal changes. Voice changes and unusual hair growth in women are largely reversed after treatment.

Symptom/effect	Frequency		Discuss with physician		Stop taking drug now	Call physician now
	Common	Rare	Only if severe	In all cases		
Swollen feet/ankles	●		■			
Weight gain	●		■			
Nausea/dizziness	●		■			
Acne/oily skin	●		■			
Backache/cramps	●		■			
Women only						
Unusual hair growth and loss	●			■		
Reduced breast size		●	■			
Voice changes		●		■		
Menstrual disturbances	●			■		

INTERACTIONS

Oral anticoagulant drugs Danazol may increase the effects of these drugs.

Anticonvulsant drugs Danazol may increase the effects of carbamazepine, and possibly other antiepileptic drugs.

Immunosuppressants Danazol may increase the effects of cyclosporine and tacrolimus.

Oral antidiabetic drugs Danazol may reduce the effects of these drugs.

PROLONGED USE

The drug is normally taken for 3–9 months depending on the condition being treated. There is a slight risk of liver damage. See also Possible adverse effects, left.

Monitoring Periodic liver function tests may be carried out.

DARIFENACIN

Product name Enablex
Used in the following combined preparations None

GENERAL INFORMATION

Darifenacin is used to treat an overactive bladder, and can help minimize symptoms of frequent urination and the urgency to urinate. It works by relaxing the bladder muscle. Darifenacin is available as an extended-release tablet and is taken once daily. The tablets should be swallowed whole and should not be chewed, split, or crushed. It is best to take it at the same time every day. As darifenacin can decrease sweating, precautions should be taken in hot environments to prevent heat prostration.

QUICK REFERENCE

Drug group Drug for urinary disorders (p.154)

Overdose danger rating Medium

Dependence rating Low

Prescription needed Yes

Available as generic No

INFORMATION FOR USERS

Your drug prescription is tailored for you. Do not alter dosage without checking with your physician.

How taken

Extended-release tablets.

Frequency and timing of doses
Usually once daily.

Usual adult dosage range
7.5–15mg daily.

Onset of effect
May take 1–2 weeks to see full benefit.

Duration of action
Up to 24 hours.

Diet advice
None.

Storage
Keep in a closed container in a cool, dry place out of the reach of children.

Missed dose
If you miss a dose, skip the missed dose and continue your usual dosing schedule. Do not double up to catch up on a missed dose.

Stopping the drug
Do not stop the drug without consulting your physician. Stopping the drug may lead to worsening of the underlying condition.

Exceeding the dose
An occasional unintentional extra dose is unlikely to cause problems. With large overdoses, seek help right away and notify your physician.

SPECIAL PRECAUTIONS

Be sure to tell your physician if:
▼ You are allergic to darifenacin or other medications.
▼ You have had difficulty passing urine.
▼ You have or have had prostate enlargement.
▼ You have had severe constipation.
▼ You have or have had liver disease.
▼ You have or have had glaucoma.
▼ You have or have had any disorders of the nervous system.
▼ You are taking other medications.

 Pregnancy
▼ Not usually prescribed. Safety in pregnancy not established. Discuss with your physician.

 Breast-feeding
▼ Safety not established. Discuss with your physician.

 Infants and children
▼ Not recommended.

 Over 60
▼ No special problems.

 Driving and hazardous work
▼ May cause blurred vision or dizziness. Do not drive a car or operate machinery until you know how this medication affects you.

 Alcohol
▼ No special problems

POSSIBLE ADVERSE EFFECTS

Common side effects include dry mouth, constipation, and an upset stomach.

Additional side effects are associated with higher doses.

Symptom/effect	Frequency		Discuss with physician		Stop taking drug now	Call physician now
	Common	Rare	Only if severe	In all cases		
Dry mouth	●			■		
Constipation	●			■		
Upset stomach	●			■		
Dry eyes	●			■		
Diarrhea		●		■		
Difficulty urinating		●				∎
Burning pain during urination		●				∎
Rash		●				∎
Itching		●				∎

INTERACTIONS

Flavoxate, oxybutynin, tolterodine, solifenacin These drugs also affect the bladder muscle. These are not usually used at the same time as darifenacin.

Flecainide Darifenacin can increase levels of flecainide, leading to possible adverse effects.

Ketoconazole, telithromycin, clarithromycin, erythromycin Some antifungals and antibiotics increase the level of darifenacin. May require dose adjustment.

Anticholinergics Drugs with anticholinergic properties can affect urination and should generally not be used with darifenacin. Examples include diphenhydramine, amitriptyline, clozapine, benztropine, and scopolamine.

Donepezil, galantamine, rivastigmine, tacrine Taking darifenacin with these medications can make both drugs less effective. Patients on both should be closely monitored.

PROLONGED USE

No problems expected.

DESMOPRESSIN

Product names DDAVP, Minirin, Octostim
Used in the following combined preparations None

GENERAL INFORMATION

Desmopressin is a synthetic form of the hormone vasopressin. Low levels of vasopressin in the body can lead to diabetes insipidus, which causes frequent urination and continual thirst.

Desmopressin can be used to correct the deficiency of vasopressin. It is also used to test for diabetes insipidus, to check kidney function, and to treat nocturnal enuresis (bedwetting) in both children and adults. When given by injection, it helps to boost clotting factors in hemophilia.

Side effects of the drug include low blood sodium and fluid retention (which sometimes requires monitoring of body weight and blood pressure to check the body's water balance).

Desmopressin should not be taken during an episode of vomiting and diarrhea because the body's fluid balance may be upset.

QUICK REFERENCE

Drug group Drug for diabetes insipidus (p.128)

Overdose danger rating Medium

Dependence rating Low

Prescription needed Yes

Available as generic Yes

INFORMATION FOR USERS

Your drug prescription is tailored for you. Do not alter dosage without checking with your physician.

How taken

Tablets, injection, nasal solution, nasal spray.

Frequency and timing of doses
Diabetes insipidus 3 x daily (tablets); 1–2 x daily (nasal spray/solution).
Nocturnal enuresis At bedtime (tablets, nasal spray/solution). Avoid fluids from 1 hour before bedtime to 8 hours afterwards.

Usual dosage range
Diabetes insipidus: *Adults* 300–600mcg daily (tablets); 1–4 puffs (nasal spray); 10–40mcg daily (nasal solution).
Children 300–600mcg daily (tablets); up to 2 puffs (nasal spray); 20mcg (nasal solution). Nocturnal enuresis: 200–400mcg for children over 5 years only (tablets); 20–40mcg (nasal solution); 2–4 puffs (nasal spray).

Onset of effect
Begins within a few minutes with full effects in a few hours (injection, nasal solution, and nasal spray); 30–90 minutes (tablets).

Duration of action
Tablets 8 hours; injection and nasal solutions 8–12 hours; nasal spray 10–12 hours.

Diet advice
Your physician may advise you to monitor your fluid intake.

Storage
Keep in a cool, dry place (tablets) or in a refrigerator, without freezing (nasal solution and nasal spray), out of the reach of children. Protect from light.

Missed dose
Take as soon as you remember. If your next dose is due within 2 hours, take a single dose now and skip the next.

Stopping the drug
Do not stop the drug without consulting your physician; symptoms of diabetes insipidus may recur.

Exceeding the dose
An occasional unintentional extra dose is unlikely to cause problems. Large overdoses may prevent the kidneys from eliminating fluid, with ensuing problems including convulsions. Notify your physician immediately.

SPECIAL PRECAUTIONS

Be sure to tell your physician if:
▼ You have heart problems.
▼ You have high blood pressure.
▼ You have kidney problems.
▼ You have cystic fibrosis.
▼ You have asthma or allergic rhinitis.
▼ You have epilepsy.
▼ You are taking other medications.

Pregnancy
▼ Used with caution in pregnancy.

Breast-feeding
▼ The drug passes into breast milk, in small amounts, but adverse effects on the baby are unlikely.

Infants and children
▼ No special problems in children; infants may need monitoring to ensure that fluid balance is correct.

Over 60
▼ May need monitoring to ensure that fluid balance is correct.

Driving and hazardous work
▼ No known problems.

Alcohol
▼ Your physician may advise on fluid intake.

PROLONGED USE

Diabetes insipidus: no problems expected.

Nocturnal enuresis: the drug will be withdrawn for at least a week after 3 months for assessment of the need to continue treatment.

POSSIBLE ADVERSE EFFECTS

Desmopressin can cause fluid retention and low blood sodium (in serious cases with convulsions). Headache, nausea, vomiting, and epistaxis (nosebleeds) may also occur.

Symptom/effect	Frequency		Discuss with physician		Stop taking drug now	Call physician now
	Common	Rare	Only if severe	In all cases		
Headache		●	■			
Nausea/vomiting		●	■			
Nasal congestion		●	■			
Nosebleeds		●	■			
Increased body weight		●		■		
Stomach pain		●		■		
Convulsions		●		■	▲	▮

INTERACTIONS

Antidepressants, chlorpropamide, and carbamazepine These drugs may increase the effects of desmopressin.

Indomethacin This anti-inflammatory drug may increase the body's response to desmopressin.

DEXAMETHASONE

Product name Maxidex
Used in the following combined preparations Sofracort, Maxitrol, Tobradex

GENERAL INFORMATION

Dexamethasone is a long-acting corticosteroid drug that is prescribed to suppress inflammatory and allergic disorders, such as rheumatoid arthritis, shock, and brain swelling (due to injury or tumour).

It is also used in conjunction with other drugs to alleviate the nausea and vomiting associated with chemotherapy.

Dexamethasone is available in different forms, including tablets, oral solution, injection, and eye and ear drops.

Low doses of dexamethasone taken for short periods rarely cause serious *side effects*. However, as with other corticosteroids, long-term treatment with high doses can cause unpleasant or dangerous side effects.

QUICK REFERENCE

Drug group Corticosteroid (p.127)
Overdose danger rating Low
Dependence rating Low
Prescription needed Yes
Available as generic Yes

INFORMATION FOR USERS

Your drug prescription is tailored for you. Do not alter dosage without checking with your physician.

How taken

Tablets, liquid, injection, eye ointment, eye/ear drops.

Frequency and timing of doses
1–4 x daily (with food when taken by mouth); 1–6 hourly (eye drops); 1–4 x daily (ear drops); 1–2 x daily (eye ointment).

Usual dosage range
0.5–10mg daily (by mouth).

Onset of effect
1–4 days.

Duration of action
Some effects may last several days.

Diet advice
None.

Storage
Keep in a closed container in a cool, dry place out of the reach of children. Protect from light.

Missed dose
Take as soon as you remember. If your next dose is due within 2 hours, take a single dose now and skip the next.

Stopping the drug
Do not stop taking the drug without consulting your physician. It may be necessary to withdraw the drug gradually.

Exceeding the dose
An occasional unintentional extra dose is unlikely to be a cause for concern. But if you notice any unusual symptoms, or if a large overdose has been taken, notify your physician.

SPECIAL PRECAUTIONS

Be sure to tell your physician if:
▼ You have had a peptic ulcer.
▼ You have glaucoma.
▼ You have had tuberculosis.
▼ You have suffered from depression or mental illness.
▼ You have a herpes infection.
▼ You are taking an NSAID regularly.
▼ You are taking other medications.

Avoid exposure to chickenpox or shingles if you are on *systemic* treatment.

Pregnancy
▼ Safety in pregnancy not established. Discuss with your physician.

Breast-feeding
▼ The drug passes into the breast milk, but at normal doses adverse effects on the baby are unlikely. Discuss with your physician.

Infants and children
▼ Reduced dose necessary.

Over 60
▼ No known problems.

Driving and hazardous work
▼ No known problems.

Alcohol
▼ Avoid. Alcohol may increase the risk of peptic ulcer with this drug.

POSSIBLE ADVERSE EFFECTS

The more serious adverse effects only occur when dexamethasone is taken in high doses for long periods of time. These are carefully monitored during prolonged treatment.

Symptom/effect	Frequency		Discuss with physician		Stop taking drug now	Call physician now
	Common	Rare	Only if severe	In all cases		
Indigestion	●		■			
Weight gain		●	■			
Acne and other skin effects		●	■			
Fluid retention		●		■		
Muscle weakness		●		■		
Mood changes		●		■		

INTERACTIONS

Antidiabetic drugs Dexamethasone reduces the action of these drugs. Dosage may need to be adjusted accordingly to prevent abnormally high blood sugar.

Barbiturates, phenytoin, rifampin, and carbamazepine These drugs may reduce the effectiveness of dexamethasone. The dosage may need to be adjusted accordingly.

Oral anticoagulant drugs Dexamethasone may increase the effects of these drugs.

Non-steroidal anti-inflammatory drugs These drugs may increase the likelihood of indigestion from dexamethasone.

Antacids These drugs may reduce the effectiveness of, and should be taken at least 2 hours apart from, dexamethasone.

Vaccines Dexamethasone can interact with some vaccines. Discuss with your physician before having any vaccinations.

PROLONGED USE

Prolonged use of this drug can lead to weight gain, glaucoma, cataracts, diabetes, mental disturbances, muscle wasting, fragile bones, and thin skin, and can retard growth in children. People receiving long-term treatment with this drug are advised to carry a 'steroid treatment' card.

DEXTROMETHORPHAN

Product names Balminil DM, Benylin DM, Koffex DM, Robitussin Children's, and many others
Used in the following combined preparations Tylenol Cough, Triaminic Cold, Cough and Fever, Neocitran DM, and others

GENERAL INFORMATION

Dextromethorphan is a cough suppressant available over-the-counter in a large number of cough and cold remedies. It is useful for suppressing persistent, dry coughing, especially if the cough is causing disturbed sleep.

Dextromethorphan has little general *sedative* effect. Additionally, unlike the stronger opioid cough suppressants, its use is unlikely to lead to dependence when it is taken as recommended.

Like other cough suppressants, dextromethorphan should not be used to treat phlegm-producing coughs. This is because its use may prolong a chest infection by preventing the normal elimination of sputum through coughing.

Although dextromethorphan is less sedating than many similar cough suppressants, its principal adverse effect is drowsiness. However, side effects from this drug are rare when it is taken in recommended doses.

QUICK REFERENCE

Drug group Cough suppressant (p.80)

Overdose danger rating Medium

Dependence rating Medium

Prescription needed No

Available as generic Yes

INFORMATION FOR USERS

Follow instructions on the label. Call your physician if symptoms worsen.

How taken

Tablets, SR-tablets, capsules, liquid, powder for solution.

Frequency and timing of doses
Up to 4 x daily as required. SR products 1–2 x daily.

Usual adult dosage range
Adults 12 years and older, 15–30mg per dose, up to a maximum of 120mg/24 hours. *Children* 6–11 years, 15mg per dose up to a maximum of 60mg/24 hours; 2–5 years, 7.5mg per dose up to a maximum of 30mg/24 hours.

Onset of effect
Within 30 minutes.

Duration of action
4–8 hours.

Diet advice
None.

Storage
Keep in a closed container in a cool, dry place out of the reach of children.

Missed dose
Take as soon as you remember if needed to relieve coughing. If you are using a sustained release product, and if your next dose is less than 4 hours away, take a dose now and skip the next dose.

Stopping the drug
Can be safely stopped as soon as you no longer need it.

Exceeding the dose
An occasional unintentional extra dose is unlikely to cause problems. Larger overdoses may cause nausea, vomiting, stomach pain, dizziness, drowsiness, and breathing problems. Notify your physician.

SPECIAL PRECAUTIONS

Be sure to consult your physician or pharmacist before taking this drug if:
▼ You have a liver disorder.
▼ You suffer from asthma or another serious respiratory problem.
▼ You are taking other medications.

Pregnancy
▼ No evidence of risk to the developing baby when normal doses are used for short periods Discuss with your physician.

Breast-feeding
▼ The drug passes into the breast milk, but at normal doses adverse effects on the baby are unlikely. Discuss with your physician.

Infants and children
▼ Not recommended for children under 2 years of age. Consult with your physician or pharmacist before using this medication in children.

Over 60
▼ Reduced dose necessary.

Driving and hazardous work
▼ Avoid such activities until you have learned how the drug affects you; it may reduce alertness.

Alcohol
▼ Avoid. Alcohol may increase the sedative effects of this drug.

POSSIBLE ADVERSE EFFECTS

The principal adverse effects of this drug are related to its sedative properties. The effects normally diminish after a few days and can often be reduced by adjustment of dosage.

Symptom/effect	Frequency		Discuss with physician		Stop taking drug now	Call physician now
	Common	Rare	Only if severe	In all cases		
Dizziness/drowsiness		●		■		
Constipation		●		■		
Nausea/vomiting		●		■		
Abdominal pain		●		■		

PROLONGED USE

Dextromethorphan should not be taken for longer than 1 week except on the advice of a physician.

INTERACTIONS

Sedatives All drugs, including alcohol, that have a *sedative* effect on the central nervous system can increase the sedative properties of dextromethorphan. Such drugs include anti-anxiety and sleeping drugs, antihistamines, opioid analgesics, antidepressants, and antipsychotics.

Monoamine oxidase inhibitors (MAOIs) These drugs may interact dangerously with dextromethorphan to cause excitation and fever.

Fluoxetine, quinidine, paroxetine, rizatriptan and similar drugs can increase dextromethorphan levels.

DIAZEPAM

Product names Apo-Diazepam, Diastat, Diazemuls, Valium Roche Oral
Used in the following combined preparations None

GENERAL INFORMATION

Introduced in the early 1960s, diazepam is the best known and most widely used of the benzodiazepine group of drugs. The benzodiazepines help relieve tension and nervousness, relax muscles, and encourage sleep. Their actions and *adverse effects* are described more fully on page 67.

Diazepam has a wide range of uses. Besides being commonly used in the treatment of anxiety and anxiety-related insomnia, it is prescribed as a muscle relaxant, in the treatment of alcohol withdrawal, and for the relief of epileptic fits. Given intravenously, it is used to sedate people undergoing certain uncomfortable medical procedures.

Diazepam can be habit-forming if taken regularly over a long period. Its effects may also diminish with time. For these reasons, courses of treatment with diazepam are limited to two weeks whenever possible.

QUICK REFERENCE

Drug group Benzodiazepine anti-anxiety drug (p.67), muscle relaxant (p.106), and anticonvulsant (p.70)

Overdose danger rating Medium

Dependence rating High

Prescription needed Yes

Available as generic Yes

INFORMATION FOR USERS

Your drug prescription is tailored for you. Do not alter dosage without checking with your physician.

How taken

Tablets, injection, rectal solution.

Frequency and timing of doses
1–4 x daily.

Usual adult dosage range
Anxiety 6–30mg daily.
Muscle spasm 2–60mg daily.

Onset of effect
Immediate effect (injection); 30 minutes–2 hours (other methods of administration).

Duration of action
Up to 24 hours. Some effect may last up to 4 days.

Diet advice
None.

Storage
Keep in a closed container in a cool, dry place out of the reach of children.

Missed dose
Take as soon as you remember. If your next dose is due within 2 hours, take a single dose now and skip the next.

Stopping the drug
If you have been taking the drug continuously for less than 2 weeks, it can be safely stopped as soon as you no longer need it. However, if you have been taking it for longer, consult your physician, who will supervise a gradual reduction in dosage. Stopping abruptly may lead to withdrawal symptoms (see p.63).

Exceeding the dose
An occasional unintentional extra dose is unlikely to cause problems. Larger overdoses may cause excessive drowsiness. Notify your physician.

SPECIAL PRECAUTIONS

Be sure to tell your physician if:
▼ You have severe respiratory disease.
▼ You have long-term liver or kidney problems.
▼ You have had problems with alcohol or drug abuse.
▼ You are taking other medications.

Pregnancy
▼ Safety in pregnancy not established. Discuss with your physician.

Breast-feeding
▼ The drug passes into the breast milk and may affect the baby. Discuss with your physician.

Infants and children
▼ Reduced dose necessary.

Over 60
▼ Increased likelihood of adverse effects. Reduced dose may therefore be necessary.

Driving and hazardous work
▼ Avoid such activities until you have learned how diazepam affects you because the drug can cause reduced alertness, slowed reactions, and increased aggression.

Alcohol
▼ Avoid. Alcohol may increase the sedative effects of this drug.

POSSIBLE ADVERSE EFFECTS

The principal adverse effects of this drug are related to its sedative properties. The effects normally diminish after a few days and can often be reduced by adjustment of dosage.

Symptom/effect	Frequency		Discuss with physician		Stop taking drug now	Call physician now
	Common	Rare	Only if severe	In all cases		
Daytime drowsiness	●		■			
Dizziness/unsteadiness	●			■		
Headache		●	■			
Blurred vision		●		■		
Forgetfulness/confusion		●		■		
Rash		●		■	▲	

INTERACTIONS

Sedatives All drugs that have a *sedative* effect on the central nervous system can increase the sedative properties of diazepam.

Grapefruit juice may increase diazepam level.

Cimetidine, fluconazole, fluoxetine, erythromycin, clarithromycin, ciprofloxacin, isoniazid, ritonavir, and indinavir These drugs may inhibit the breakdown of diazepam leading to increased levels in the blood and risk of adverse effects.

PROLONGED USE

Regular use of this drug over several weeks can lead to a reduction in its effect as the body adapts. It may also be habit-forming when taken for extended periods, and severe withdrawal reactions can occur.

DICLOFENAC

Product names Apo-Diclo, Novo-Difenac, Nu-Diclo, Voltaren, Voltaren Rapide, and others
Used in the following combined preparation Arthrotec

GENERAL INFORMATION

Taken as a single dose, diclofenac has analgesic properties similar to those of acetaminophen. It is taken to relieve mild to moderate headache, menstrual pain, and pain following minor surgery. When diclofenac is given regularly over a long period, it exerts an anti-inflammatory effect and is used to relieve the pain and stiffness associated with rheumatoid arthritis and advanced osteoarthritis. Diclofenac may also be prescribed to treat acute attacks of gout.

The combined preparation, Arthrotec, contains diclofenac and misoprostol (see p.374). Misoprostol helps prevent gastroduodenal ulceration, which is sometimes caused by diclofenac, and may be particularly useful in patients at risk of developing this problem.

INFORMATION FOR USERS

Your drug prescription is tailored for you. Do not alter dosage without checking with your physician.

How taken

Tablets, extended-release tablets, topical solution, ophthalmic solution, rectal suppository.

Frequency and timing of doses
1–3 x daily with food.

Usual adult dosage range
75–150mg daily.

Onset of effect
Around 1 hour (pain relief); full anti-inflammatory effect may take 2 weeks.

Duration of action
Up to 12 hours; up to 24 hours (SR-preparations).

Diet advice
None.

Storage
Keep in a closed container in a cool, dry place out of the reach of children.

Missed dose
Take as soon as you remember. If your next dose is due within 2 hours, take a single dose now and skip the next.

Stopping the drug
When taken for short-term pain relief, diclofenac can be safely stopped as soon as you no longer need it. If prescribed for long-term treatment (e.g., for arthritis), speak to your physician before stopping the drug.

Exceeding the dose
An occasional unintentional extra dose is unlikely to be a cause for concern. But if you notice any unusual symptoms or if a large overdose has been taken, notify your physician.

SPECIAL PRECAUTIONS

Be sure to tell your physician if:
▼ You have long-term liver or kidney problems.
▼ You have a bleeding disorder.
▼ You have had a peptic ulcer or esophagitis.
▼ You have porphyria.
▼ You suffer from indigestion.
▼ You are allergic to ASA.
▼ You suffer from asthma.
▼ You have heart problems or high blood pressure.
▼ You are taking other medications.

Pregnancy
▼ Not usually prescribed in the last 3 months of pregnancy as it may increase the risk of adverse effects on the baby's heart and may prolong labour. Discuss with your physician.

Breast-feeding
▼ Small amounts of the drug pass into the breast milk, but adverse effects on the baby are unlikely. Discuss with your physician.

Infants and children
▼ Reduced dose necessary.

Over 60
▼ Increased risk of adverse effects. Reduced dose may therefore be necessary.

Driving and hazardous work
▼ No problems expected.

Alcohol
▼ Keep consumption low. Alcohol may increase the risk of stomach irritation.

Surgery and general anesthetics
▼ Discuss with your physician or dentist before any surgery.

POSSIBLE ADVERSE EFFECTS

The most common adverse effects are gastrointestinal disturbances. Black or bloodstained vomit or feces should be reported to your physician without delay.

Symptom/effect	Frequency		Discuss with physician		Stop taking drug now	Call physician now
	Common	Rare	Only if severe	In all cases		
Gastrointestinal disorders	●		■			
Headache/dizziness		●	■			
Drowsiness		●	■			
Swollen feet/ankles		●		■		
Rash		●		■	▲	
Wheezing/breathlessness		●		■	▲	▐
Black/bloodstained feces/vomit		●		■	▲	▐

INTERACTIONS

General note Interacts with other NSAIDs, oral anticoagulants, and corticosteroids to increase the risk of bleeding and/or ulcers.

Antihypertensive drugs and diuretics The beneficial effects of these drugs may be reduced with diclofenac.

Cyclosporine Diclofenac may increase the risk of kidney problems.

Lithium, digoxin, and methotrexate Diclofenac may increase the blood levels of these drugs to an undesirable extent.

Indigestion remedies These should not be taken at the same time of day as *enteric* coated diclofenac preparations as they disrupt this coating.

PROLONGED USE

There is an increased risk of bleeding from peptic ulcers and in the bowel with prolonged use of diclofenac.

DICYCLOMINE

Product names Bentylol, Lomine
Used in the following combined preparation None

GENERAL INFORMATION

Dicyclomine is a mild *anticholinergic* antispasmodic drug that relieves painful abdominal cramps occurring in the gastrointestinal tract. It can be used to treat irritable bowel syndrome, indigestion not associated with ulcers, and colicky conditions in babies (only over 6 months).

Because the drug has anticholinergic properties, it is also included in some combined preparations used to treat flatulence, indigestion, and diarrhea. Dicyclomine relieves symptoms but does not cure the underlying condition. Additional treatment with other drugs and self-help measures, such as dietary changes, may be recommended by your physician.

Side effects with dicyclomine are rare, but they include headaches, constipation, urinary difficulties, and palpitations.

INFORMATION FOR USERS

Your drug prescription is tailored for you. Do not alter dosage without checking with your physician.

How taken

Tablets, liquid.

Frequency and timing of doses
3–4 x daily before or after meals.

Usual dosage range
Adults 30–80mg daily.
Children Reduced dose according to age and weight.

Onset of effect
Within 1–2 hours.

Duration of action
4–6 hours.

Diet advice
None.

Storage
Keep in a closed container in a cool, dry place out of the reach of children. Protect from light.

Missed dose
Take as soon as you remember. If your next dose is due within 2 hours, take a single dose now and skip the next.

Stopping the drug
The drug can be stopped without causing problems when it is no longer needed.

Exceeding the dose
An occasional unintentional extra dose is unlikely to cause problems. Large overdoses may cause drowsiness, dizziness, and difficulty in swallowing. Notify your physician.

POSSIBLE ADVERSE EFFECTS

Most people do not notice any *adverse effects* when taking dicyclomine. Those that do occur are related to its anticholinergic properties and include drowsiness and dry mouth. Such symptoms may be overcome by adjusting the dosage, or they may disappear after a few days of usage as your body adjusts to the drug.

Symptom/effect	Frequency		Discuss with physician		Stop taking drug now	Call physician now
	Common	Rare	Only if severe	In all cases		
Dry mouth		●	■			
Headache		●	■			
Blurred vision		●	■			
Constipation		●	■			
Drowsiness/dizziness		●	■			
Difficulty in passing urine		●		■		
Palpitations		●		■		

INTERACTIONS

Sedatives All drugs that have a *sedative* effect on the central nervous system may increase the sedative properties of dicyclomine.

Anticholinergic drugs These drug may increase the adverse effects of dicyclomine.

SPECIAL PRECAUTIONS

Be sure to tell your physician if:
▼ You have glaucoma.
▼ You have urinary problems.
▼ You have hiatus hernia.
▼ You are taking other medications.

Pregnancy
▼ No evidence of risk.

Breast-feeding
▼ The drug passes into the breast milk, but at normal doses adverse effects on the baby are unlikely. Discuss with your physician.

Infants and children
▼ Reduced dose necessary. Not recommended in infants under 6 months.

Over 60
▼ Reduced dose necessary. The elderly are more susceptible to anticholinergic side effects.

Driving and hazardous work
▼ Avoid such activities until you have learned how dicyclomine affects you because the drug can cause drowsiness and blurred vision.

Alcohol
▼ Avoid. Alcohol may increase the sedative effects of this drug.

PROLONGED USE

No problems expected.

DIGOXIN

Product name Lanoxin
Used in the following combined preparations None

GENERAL INFORMATION

Digoxin is the most widely used extract of digitalis, a compound obtained from the leaves of the foxglove plant. It is sometimes given in the treatment of congestive heart failure and certain alterations of heart rhythm.

Digoxin increases the force of the heartbeat making it more effective in pumping blood around the body. This in turn helps to control breathlessness, fluid retention, and tiredness.

The effective dose of digoxin can be close to the toxic dose and, therefore, treatment needs careful monitoring to prevent toxic doses being reached. A number of *adverse effects* (see below) may indicate that the toxic level is close and should be reported to your physician.

QUICK REFERENCE

Drug group Digitalis drug (p.82)
Overdose danger rating High
Dependence rating Low
Prescription needed Yes
Available as generic Yes

INFORMATION FOR USERS

Your drug prescription is tailored for you. Do not alter dosage without checking with your physician.

How taken

Tablets, liquid, injection.

Frequency and timing of doses
Usually once daily. Starting dose may be given up to 3 x daily.

Usual adult dosage range
0.0625–0.25mg daily (by mouth).

Onset of effect
Within a few minutes (injection); within 1–2 hours (by mouth).

Duration of action
Up to 4 days.

Diet advice
This drug may be more toxic if potassium levels are depleted, so you should include potassium-rich fruit and vegetables, such as bananas and tomatoes, in your diet.

Storage
Keep in a closed container in a cool, dry place out of the reach of children. Protect from light.

Missed dose
Take as soon as you remember. If your next dose is due within 8 hours, take a dose now and skip the next.

Stopping the drug
Do not stop the drug without consulting your physician; stopping the drug may lead to worsening of the underlying condition.

OVERDOSE ACTION

 Seek immediate medical advice in all cases. Take emergency action if palpitations, severe weakness, chest pain, or loss of consciousness occur.

See Drug poisoning emergency guide (p.526).

SPECIAL PRECAUTIONS

Be sure to tell your physician if:
▼ You have a long-term liver problem.
▼ You have thyroid trouble.
▼ You are taking other medications.

 Pregnancy
▼ No evidence of risk, but adjustment in dose may be necessary.

 Breast-feeding
▼ The drug passes into breast milk, but at normal doses adverse effects on the baby are unlikely. Discuss with your physician.

 Infants and children
▼ Reduced dose necessary.

 Over 60
▼ Increased likelihood of adverse effects. Reduced dose may therefore be necessary.

 Driving and hazardous work
▼ Special problems are unlikely, but do not undertake these activities until you know how digoxin affects you.

 Alcohol
▼ No special problems.

POSSIBLE ADVERSE EFFECTS

The possible adverse effects of digoxin are usually due to increased levels of the drug in the blood. Any symptoms should be reported to your physician without delay.

Symptom/effect	Frequency		Discuss with physician		Stop taking drug now	Call physician now
	Common	Rare	Only if severe	In all cases		
Tiredness	●		■			
Nausea/loss of appetite	●			■		
Confusion		●		■		
Visual disturbance		●		■	▲	▮
Palpitations		●		■	▲	▮

INTERACTIONS

General note Many drugs interact with digoxin. Do not take any medication without the advice of your physician or pharmacist.

Diuretics may increase the risk of adverse effects from digoxin.

Antacids may reduce the effects of digoxin. The effect of digoxin may increase when such drugs are stopped.

Anti-arrhythmic drugs may increase blood levels of digoxin.

PROLONGED USE

No problems expected.

Monitoring Periodic checks on blood levels of digoxin and body salts may be advised.

DILTIAZEM

Product names Cardizem, Cardizem CD, Tiazac
Used in the following combined preparations None

GENERAL INFORMATION

Diltiazem belongs to the group of drugs known as calcium channel blockers (p.87). These drugs interfere with the conduction of signals in the muscles of the heart and blood vessels.

Diltiazem is used in the treatment of angina and longer acting formulations are used to treat high blood pressure. When this drug is taken regularly, it reduces the frequency of angina attacks but does not work quickly enough to reduce the pain of an angina attack that is already in progress.

Diltiazem does not adversely affect breathing and is valuable for people who suffer from asthma, for whom other anti-angina drugs may not be suitable.

Different brands of diltiazem may not be equivalent so you should always take the same brand.

QUICK REFERENCE

Drug group Calcium channel blocker (p.87) and antihypertensive drug (p.88)

Overdose danger rating Medium

Dependence rating Low

Prescription needed Yes

Available as generic Yes

INFORMATION FOR USERS

Your drug prescription is tailored for you. Do not alter dosage without checking with your physician.

How taken

Tablets, SR-capsules, CD-capsules.

Frequency and timing of doses
3 x daily (tablets); 2 x daily (SR-capsules), 1 x daily (CD capsules).

Usual adult dosage range
180–360mg daily.

Onset of effect
2–3 hours.

Duration of action
6–8 hours.

Diet advice
None.

Storage
Keep in a closed container in a cool, dry place out of the reach of children.

Missed dose
Take as soon as you remember. If your next dose is due within 2 hours, take a single dose now and skip the next.

Stopping the drug
Do not stop taking the drug without consulting your physician; symptoms may recur. Stopping suddenly may worsen angina.

Exceeding the dose
An occasional unintentional extra dose is unlikely to cause problems. Large overdoses may cause dizziness or collapse. Notify your physician urgently.

SPECIAL PRECAUTIONS

Be sure to tell your physician if:
▼ You have long-term liver or kidney problems.
▼ You have heart failure.
▼ You are taking other medications.

Pregnancy
▼ Not usually prescribed. Discuss with your physician.

Breast-feeding
▼ The drug passes into the breast milk and may affect the baby. Discuss with your physician.

Infants and children
▼ Not recommended.

Over 60
▼ Increased likelihood of adverse effects. Reduced dose may therefore be necessary.

Driving and hazardous work
▼ Avoid such activities until you have learned how diltiazem affects you because the drug can cause dizziness due to lowered blood pressure.

Alcohol
▼ Avoid. Alcohol may lower blood pressure, causing dizziness.

POSSIBLE ADVERSE EFFECTS

Diltiazem can cause various minor symptoms that are common to other calcium channel blockers as well. These include headache and nausea. The most serious effect is the possibility of a slowed heart beat, which may cause tiredness or dizziness. These effects can sometimes be controlled by an adjustment in dosage.

Symptom/effect	Frequency		Discuss with physician		Stop taking drug now	Call physician now
	Common	Rare	Only if severe	In all cases		
Headache	●		■			
Nausea	●		■			
Dry mouth	●		■			
Leg and ankle swelling	●			■		
Tiredness		●		■		
Dizziness		●		■		
Rash		●		■	▲	

INTERACTIONS

Antihypertensive drugs Diltiazem increases the effects of these drugs, leading to a further reduction in blood pressure.

Anticonvulsant drugs Levels of these drugs may be altered by diltiazem.

Anti-arrhythmic drugs There is a risk of side effects on the heart if these are taken with diltiazem.

Digoxin Blood levels and adverse effects of this drug may be increased if it is taken with diltiazem. The dosage of digoxin may need to be reduced.

Theophylline/aminophylline Diltiazem may increase the levels of this drug.

Beta blockers increase the risk of the heart slowing.

PROLONGED USE

No problems expected.

DIMENHYDRINATE

Product names Apo-Dimenhydrinate, Gravol, Novo-Dimenate, PMS Dimenhydrinate, Travel Tabs
Used in the following combined preparations None

GENERAL INFORMATION

Dimenhydrinate is an antihistamine that is mainly used as an anti-emetic drug. It is especially effective for treating the nausea and vomiting that occur with vertigo. It is also prescribed to relieve the symptoms of inner ear disorders such as Meniere's disease and to prevent and treat motion sickness. Dimenhydrinate is often effective in treating other forms of nausea and vomiting, including those caused by drugs and radiation treatments for cancer.

Like other antihistamines, dimenhydrinate has a sedative effect that can cause problems if you need to drive or operate machinery.

INFORMATION FOR USERS

Follow instructions on the label. Call your physician if symptoms worsen.

How taken

Tablets, slow-release (SR) capsules, oral liquid, injection, rectal suppositories, chewable tablets.

Frequency and timing of doses
Adults Every 4 hours
Children Every 6–8 hours. To prevent motion sickness the first dose should be taken 30 minutes before travel.

Usual oral dosage range
Adults 50–100mg per dose (maximum 400mg/24 hours)
Children 2–6 years, 15–25mg per dose (maximum 75mg/24 hours); 6–12 years, 25–50mg per dose (maximum 150mg/24 hours); 12 years and over, 50mg per dose (maximum 300mg/24 hours).

Onset of effect
Within 30 minutes.

Duration of action
6–8 hours

Diet advice
None.

Storage
Keep in a closed container in a cool, dry place away from reach of children.

Missed dose
Take when you remember. Adjust the timing of your next dose accordingly.

Stopping the drug
Can be safely stopped as soon as you no longer need it.

Exceeding the dose
An occasional unintentional extra dose is unlikely to cause problems. Larger overdoses may cause unusual drowsiness. Notify your physician.

POSSIBLE ADVERSE EFFECTS

The principal adverse effects of this drug are related to its anticholinergic properties and, if troublesome, can sometimes be reduced by adjustment of dosage.

Symptom/effect	Frequency		Discuss with physician		Stop taking drug now	Call physician now
	Common	Rare	Only if severe	In all cases		
Drowsiness	●		■			
Dry mouth	●		■			
Blurred vision	●			■		
Confusion/nervousness		●		■		

INTERACTIONS

Alcohol and other sedatives All drugs that have a sedative effect on the central nervous system are likely to increase the sedative properties of dimenhydrinate. Such drugs include alcohol, anti-anxiety and sleeping drugs, antidepressants, opioid analgesics, and antipsychotics.

SPECIAL PRECAUTIONS

Be sure to consult your physician or pharmacist before taking this drug if:
▼ You have impaired liver or kidney function.
▼ You have chronic lung disease.
▼ You have had glaucoma.
▼ You have prostate trouble.
▼ You have had seizures/fits.
▼ You are taking other medications.

Pregnancy
▼ While there is no evidence of risk to the developing baby, absolute safety in pregnancy has not been established. Discuss with your physician.

Breast-feeding
▼ The drug passes into the breast milk. Its effects on the baby are not clearly known. Discuss with your physician.

Infants and children
▼ Only as prescribed by your physician in children under 2 years. Reduced dose necessary in older children.

Over 60
▼ No special problems.

Driving and hazardous work
▼ Because of the possibility of drowsiness, avoid such activities until you have learned how the drug affects you .

Alcohol
▼ Avoid. Alcohol may increase the sedative effects of this drug.

PROLONGED USE

No special problems, but this drug should not be used for more than a few days except on medical advice.

Anti-emetics may mask the presence of underlying organic abnormalities or the toxic effects of other drugs.

Antihistamines should be discontinued approximately 48 hours prior to allergy skin testing.

DIPHENHYDRAMINE

Product names Allerdryl, Benadryl, Nytol, Simply Sleep, Unisom, and others
Used in the following combined preparations Balminil Night-Time, Contac Cough, Sinutab Nighttime, and others

GENERAL INFORMATION

Diphenhydramine, one of the oldest antihistamines, is used for treating allergies such as allergic rhinitis and urticaria (hives). Injected diphenhydramine is also used in the treatment of anaphylaxis and hypersensitivity reactions to food, drugs, or insect stings.

Because it has anticholinergic properties, it is useful in the treatment of parkinsonism and movement disorders caused by antipsychotic drugs (p.69). It is also an effective anti-emetic, used to prevent and treat vertigo and motion sickness.

Diphenhydramine has a marked sedative action and often causes drowsiness. It is included in several over-the-counter sleeping preparations.

QUICK REFERENCE

Drug group Antihistamine (p.110), anti-emetic drug (p.74), and sleeping drug (p.66)

Overdose danger rating Medium

Dependence rating Low

Prescription needed No

Available as generic No

INFORMATION FOR USERS

Follow instructions on the label. Call your physician if symptoms worsen.

How taken

Tablets, chewable tablets, capsules, oral liquid, injection, cream.

Frequency and timing of doses
By mouth 3–4 x daily (allergic conditions); 30 minutes before travelling and before meals (motion sickness); 30 minutes before bedtime (insomnia).
Injection Every 2–3 hours (adults).
Cream As directed.

Usual dosage range
Adults 25–200mg daily (by mouth); up to 400mg daily (by injection).
Children Reduced dose necessary according to age and weight.

Onset of effect
Within 1 hour (by mouth); within 20 minutes (injection).

Duration of action
4–6 hours.

Diet advice
None.

Storage
Keep in a closed container in a cool, dry place away from reach of children. Do not freeze.

Missed dose
Take as soon as you remember. If your next dose is due within 2 hours, take a single dose now and skip the next.

Stopping the drug
Can be safely stopped as soon as you no longer need it.

Exceeding the dose
An occasional, unintentional extra dose is unlikely to cause problems. Large overdoses may cause drowsiness or agitation. Notify your physician.

SPECIAL PRECAUTIONS

Be sure to consult your physician or pharmacist before taking this drug if
▼ You have impaired liver function.
▼ You have chronic lung disease.
▼ You have had epileptic seizures.
▼ You have glaucoma.
▼ You have urinary difficulties.
▼ You are taking other medications.

Pregnancy
▼ No evidence of risk to the developing baby when normal doses are used for short periods. Discuss with your physician.

Breast-feeding
▼ The drug passes into the breast milk and may make the baby drowsy or irritable. It may also inhibit milk secretion. Discuss with your physician.

Infants and children
▼ Not recommended for newborn or premature infants. Reduced dose necessary for older children.

Over 60
▼ Reduced dose may be necessary. Discuss with your physician.

Driving and hazardous work
▼ Avoid such activities until you have learned how the drug affects you; it can cause drowsiness.

Alcohol
▼ Avoid. Alcohol may increase the sedative effects of this drug.

POSSIBLE ADVERSE EFFECTS

Drowsiness is the most common adverse effect of diphenhydramine. Other side effects, such as dry mouth and blurred vision, are due to its anticholinergic action.

Symptom/effect	Frequency		Discuss with physician		Stop taking drug now	Call physician now
	Common	Rare	Only if severe	In all cases		
Drowsiness	●		■			
Dry mouth		●	■			
Nausea/abdominal pain		●	■			
Blurred vision		●		■		
Urinary difficulties		●		■		
Disorientation/excitation		●		■		

INTERACTIONS

Sedatives All sedatives, including alcohol, are likely to enhance the sedative effect of this drug.

Anticholinergic drugs are likely to increase the anticholinergic effects of diphenhydramine.

PROLONGED USE

The effect of this drug may become weaker with prolonged use over a period of weeks or months as the body adapts. Transfer to a different antihistamine may be recommended.

Antihistamines should be discontinued approximately 48 hours prior to allergy skin testing.

DIPHENOXYLATE

Product name None
Used in the following combined preparations Lomotil

GENERAL INFORMATION

Diphenoxylate is an antidiarrheal drug that is chemically related to the opioid analgesics. It reduces bowel contractions and, therefore, the fluidity and frequency of bowel movements. Available in tablet form, it is prescribed for the relief of sudden or recurrent bouts of diarrhea.

The drug is not suitable for diarrhea that is caused by infection, poisons, or antibiotics as it may delay recovery by slowing expulsion of harmful substances from the bowel. Diphenoxylate can cause toxic

megacolon, a dangerous dilation of the bowel that shuts off blood supply to the wall of the bowel and increases the risk of perforation.

At recommended doses, serious adverse effects are rare. To guard against addiction, atropine is added to diphenoxylate tablets. If these are taken in excessive amounts, the atropine will cause highly unpleasant anticholinergic effects. Diphenoxylate is especially dangerous for young children; be sure to store the drug out of their reach.

QUICK REFERENCE

Drug group Opioid antidiarrheal drug (p.96)

Overdose danger rating Medium

Dependence rating Medium

Prescription needed Yes

Available as generic No

INFORMATION FOR USERS

Your drug prescription is tailored for you. Do not alter dosage without checking with your physician.

How taken

Tablets.

Frequency and timing of doses
3–4 x daily.

Usual dosage range
Adults 5mg initially, followed by doses of 2.5–5mg. Maximum dose: 20mg in 24 hours.
Children Reduced dose necessary according to age and weight.

Onset of effect
Within 1 hour. Control of diarrhea may take some hours.

Duration of action
Up to 24 hours.

Diet advice
Ensure adequate fluid intake during an attack of diarrhea.

Storage
Keep in a closed container in a cool, dry place out of the reach of children. Protect from light.

Missed dose
Take as soon as you remember. If your next dose is due within 3 hours, take a single dose now and skip the next.

Stopping the drug
Can be safely stopped as soon as you no longer need it.

Exceeding the dose
An occasional, unintentional extra dose is unlikely to cause problems. Large overdoses may cause unusual drowsiness, dryness of the mouth and skin, restlessness, and in extreme cases, loss of consciousness. Symptoms of overdose may be delayed. Notify your physician.

SPECIAL PRECAUTIONS

Be sure to tell your physician if
▼ You have a long-term liver problem.
▼ You have severe abdominal pain.
▼ You have bloodstained diarrhea.
▼ You have ulcerative colitis.
▼ You have recently taken antibiotics.
▼ You have recently travelled abroad.
▼ You are taking other medications.

Pregnancy
▼ Safety in pregnancy not established. Discuss with your physician.

Breast-feeding
▼ The drug passes into the breast milk and may cause drowsiness in the baby. Discuss with your physician.

Infants and children
▼ Not recommended under 4 years. Reduced dose necessary for older children.

Over 60
▼ Reduced dose may be necessary.

Driving and hazardous work
▼ Avoid such activities until you have learned how diphenoxylate affects you because the drug may cause drowsiness and dizziness.

Alcohol
▼ Avoid. Alcohol may increase the sedative effects of this drug.

PROLONGED USE

Not usually recommended.

POSSIBLE ADVERSE EFFECTS

Side effects occur infrequently with diphenoxylate. If abdominal pain or distension, nausea or vomiting occur, notify your physician.

Symptom/effect	Frequency		Discuss with physician		Stop taking drug now	Call physician now
	Common	Rare	Only if severe	In all cases		
Drowsiness	●		■			
Restlessness		●	■			
Headache		●	■			
Skin rash/itching		●		■		
Dizziness		●		■		
Nausea/vomiting		●		■	▲	▌
Abdominal discomfort		●		■	▲	▌

INTERACTIONS

Sedatives All drugs that have a sedative effect on the central nervous system may increase the sedative effect of diphenoxylate.

Monoamine oxidase inhibitors (MAOIs) There is a risk of a dangerous rise in blood pressure if MAOIs are taken together with diphenoxylate.

DIPYRIDAMOLE

Product name Persantine
Used in the following combined preparation Aggrenox

GENERAL INFORMATION

Dipyridamole was introduced in the late 1970s as an anti-angina drug; its purpose was to improve the capability of people with angina to exercise. Although more effective drugs are now available to help with this problem, dipyridamole is still prescribed as an antiplatelet drug. It acts by "thinning" the blood, which reduces the likelihood of clots forming in the bloodstream. This is especially important in people who have had a stroke or have undergone heart valve replacement surgery.

Dipyridamole is usually given together with other drugs such as warfarin or ASA. The drug can also be given by injection during certain types of diagnostic test on the heart.

Side effects may occur, especially during the early days of treatment. If they persist, your physician may advise a reduction in dosage.

INFORMATION FOR USERS

Your drug prescription is tailored for you. Do not alter dosage without checking with your physician.

How taken

Tablets, capsules, injection (for diagnostic tests only).

Frequency and timing of doses
4 x daily (tablets).
2 x daily (Aggrenox capsules).

Usual adult dosage range
300–400mg daily.

Onset of effect
Within 1 hour. Full therapeutic effect may not be reached for 2–3 weeks.

Duration of action
Up to 8 hours.

Diet advice
None.

Storage
Keep in a closed container in a cool, dry place out of the reach of children. Protect from light.

Missed dose
Take as soon as you remember. If your next dose is due within 2 hours, take a single dose now and skip the next.

Stopping the drug
Do not stop taking the drug without consulting your physician; withdrawal of the drug could lead to abnormal blood clotting.

Exceeding the dose
An occasional unintentional extra dose is unlikely to be a cause for concern. Large overdoses may cause dizziness or vomiting. Notify your physician.

SPECIAL PRECAUTIONS

Be sure to tell your physician if:
▼ You have low blood pressure.
▼ Your suffer from migraine.
▼ You have angina.
▼ You have had a recent heart attack.
▼ You are taking other medications.

Pregnancy
▼ Safety in pregnancy not established. Discuss with your physician.

Breast-feeding
▼ The drug passes into the breast milk but at normal doses adverse effects on the baby are unlikely. Discuss with your physician.

Infants and children
▼ Reduced dose necessary.

Over 60
▼ No special problems.

Driving and hazardous work
▼ Avoid such activities until you have learned how dipyridamole affects you because the drug may cause dizziness and faintness.

Alcohol
▼ No known problems.

POSSIBLE ADVERSE EFFECTS

Adverse effects are rare. Possible symptoms include dizziness, headache, fainting, stomach upsets including nausea, and rash. In rare cases, the drug may aggravate angina.

Symptom/effect	Frequency		Discuss with physician		Stop taking drug now	Call physician now
	Common	Rare	Only if severe	In all cases		
Stomach upset/nausea	●		■			
Headache	●			■		
Diarrhea		●	■			
Dizziness/fainting		●		■		
Rash		●		■	▲	

INTERACTIONS

Anticoagulant drugs The effect of these drugs may be increased by dipyridamole, thereby increasing the risk of uncontrolled bleeding. The dosage of the anticoagulant should be reduced accordingly.

Antacids may reduce the effectiveness of dipyridamole.

PROLONGED USE

No known problems.

DOCUSATE SODIUM

Product names Colace, Correctol Stool Softener, Novo-Docusate Sodium, Selax, Soflax
Used in the following combined preparations Gentlax S, Fruitatives, Senokot-S

GENERAL INFORMATION

Docusate is a stool softener and is used in the management of constipation due to hard stools. Taking it regularly makes the stools softer and easier to pass. Docusate may be recommended to be used by those with heart conditions to ease the passage of stools and to avoid straining on defecation.

Laxatives, including docusate, should not be used in those experiencing vomiting, abdominal pain, or fever.

INFORMATION FOR USERS

Follow instructions on the label. Call your physician if symptoms worsen.

How taken

Capsules, liquid, drops.

Frequency and timing of doses
Once to twice daily.

Usual adult dosage range
100–200mg.

Onset of effect
Within 1–2 days.

Duration of action
Up to 24 hours.

Diet advice
None.

Storage
Keep in a closed container in a cool, dry place out of the reach of children.

Missed dose
If you miss a dose, take it as soon as you remember. Resume normal dose thereafter.

Stopping the drug
Can be safely stopped as soon as you no longer need it.

Exceeding the dose
An occasional unintentional extra dose is unlikely to be a cause for concern. But if you notice unusual symptoms, or if a large overdose has been taken, notify your physician. Large overdoses may cause constipation and cramping. Notify your physician.

SPECIAL PRECAUTIONS

Be sure to consult your physician or pharmacist before taking this drug if:
▼ You have severe constipation, and/or nausea, vomiting, or abdominal pain.
▼ You have unexplained rectal bleeding.
▼ You have difficulty swallowing.
▼ You have a known narrowing of the bowel.
▼ You are taking other medications.

Pregnancy
▼ Safety in pregnancy not established. Discuss with your physician.

Breast-feeding
▼ Safety in breast-feeding not established. Discuss with your physician.

Infants and children
▼ Reduced dose recommended in children.

Over 60
▼ No special problems expected.

Driving and hazardous work
▼ No known problems.

Alcohol
▼ No known problems.

POSSIBLE ADVERSE EFFECTS

Generally well tolerated.

Symptom/effect	Frequency		Discuss with physician		Stop taking drug now	Call physician now
	Common	Rare	Only if severe	In all cases		
Abdominal pain		●		■		
Cramping		●		■		
Rash		●		■		

INTERACTIONS

Mineral oil Docusate should not be administered with mineral oil as this may increase the absorption of the oil.

All medications Generally recommended that docusate not be administered within 2 hours of other medications.

PROLONGED USE

No problems expected.

DOMPERIDONE

Product names Apo-Domperidone, Novo-Domperidone, and others
Used in the following combined preparation None

GENERAL INFORMATION

Domperidone, which increases gastric motility, is particularly effective for treating nausea and vomiting caused by gastroenteritis, chemotherapy or radiotherapy. It is not effective for treating motion sickness or nausea caused by inner ear disorders such as Ménière's disease.

The main advantage of domperidone over other anti-emetic drugs is that it does not usually cause drowsiness or other *adverse effects* such as abnormal movement. Domperidone is not suitable, however, for the long-term treatment of gastrointestinal disorders, for which an alternative drug treatment is often prescribed.

Domperidone may also be used to relieve dyspepsia (indigestion and heartburn); and, in combination with acetaminophen, it is sometimes used to treat acute attacks of migraine.

QUICK REFERENCE

Drug group Anti-emetic drug (p.74)
Overdose danger rating Medium
Dependence rating Low
Prescription needed No
Available as generic Yes

INFORMATION FOR USERS

Your drug prescription is tailored for you. Do not alter dosage without checking with your physician.

How taken

Tablets, liquid, suppositories.

Frequency and timing of doses
Nausea/vomiting Every 4–8 hours as required.
Dyspepsia 3 x daily with water before meals and at night (tablets only).

Usual adult dosage range
Nausea/vomiting 10–20mg (by mouth); 30–60mg (rectally).

Onset of effect
Within 1 hour. The effects of the drug may be delayed if taken after the onset of nausea.

Duration of action
Approximately 6 hours.

Diet advice
None.

Storage
Keep in a closed container in a cool, dry place out of the reach of children. Protect from light.

Missed dose
Take as soon as you remember for dyspepsia. If your next dose is due within 4 hours, take a single dose now and skip the next. Then return to your normal dose schedule.

Stopping the drug
Can be stopped when you no longer need it.

Exceeding the dose
An occasional unintentional extra dose is unlikely to cause problems. Large overdoses may cause dizziness. Notify your physician.

POSSIBLE ADVERSE EFFECTS

Adverse effects from this drug are rare.

Symptom/effect	Frequency		Discuss with physician		Stop taking drug now	Call physician now
	Common	Rare	Only if severe	In all cases		
Breast enlargement		●		■		
Milk secretion from breast		●		■		
Muscle spasms/tremors		●		■		
Reduced libido		●		■		
Rash		●		■		

INTERACTIONS

Anticholinergic **drugs** These may reduce the beneficial effects of domperidone.

Opioid **analgesics** These may reduce the beneficial effects of domperidone.

Bromocriptine and cabergoline Domperidone may reduce the effects of these drugs in some people.

Ketoconazole, erythromycin, azithromycin, SSRIs These drugs can increase the level of domperidone, resulting in adverse effects.

Grapefruit juice Can potentially increase the effect of domperidone.

SPECIAL PRECAUTIONS

Be sure to tell your physician if:
▼ You have a long-term kidney problem.
▼ You have thyroid disease.
▼ You are taking other medications.

Pregnancy
▼ Safety in pregnancy not established. Discuss with your physician.

Breast-feeding
▼ The drug may pass into the breast milk, but at normal doses adverse effects on the baby are unlikely. Discuss with your physician.

Infants and children
▼ Prescribed only to treat nausea and vomiting caused by anticancer drugs or radiation therapy. Reduced dose necessary.

Over 60
▼ No special problems.

Driving and hazardous work
▼ No special problems.

Alcohol
▼ No special problems, but alcohol is best avoided in cases of nausea and vomiting.

PROLONGED USE

Not prescribed for longer than 12 weeks.

DONEPEZIL

Product name Aricept
Used in the following combined preparations None

GENERAL INFORMATION

Donepezil is an inhibitor of the enzyme acetylcholinesterase. This enzyme breaks down the natural *neurotransmitter* acetylcholine to limit its effects. Blocking the enzyme raises the levels of acetylcholine which, in the brain, increases alertness. Donepezil has been found to improve the symptoms of dementia in Alzheimer's disease and is used to diminish deterioration in that disease. It is not currently recommended for dementia due to other causes. It is usual to assess anyone being treated with donepezil after about three months to decide whether the drug is helping and whether it is worth continuing treatment.

Side effects may include bladder outflow obstruction and psychiatric problems, such as agitation and aggression, which might be thought due to the disease.

QUICK REFERENCE

Drug group Drug for dementia (p.71)

Overdose danger rating Medium

Dependence rating Low

Prescription needed Yes

Available as generic No

INFORMATION FOR USERS

Your drug prescription is tailored for you. Do not alter dosage without checking with your physician.

How taken

Tablets.

Frequency and timing of doses
Once daily in the evening.

Usual adult dosage range
5–10mg.

Onset of effect
1 hour. Full effects might take up to 3 months.

Duration of action
1–2 days.

Diet advice
None.

Storage
Keep in a closed container in a cool, dry place out of the reach of children.

Missed dose
Take as soon as you remember. A carer should ensure that the maximum dose taken in 24 hours does not exceed 10mg.

Stopping the drug
Do not stop taking the drug without consulting your physician; symptoms may recur.

Exceeding the dose
An occasional unintentional extra dose is unlikely to be a cause for concern. But if you notice any unusual symptoms, or if a large overdose has been taken, notify your physician.

SPECIAL PRECAUTIONS

Be sure to tell your physician if:
▼ You have a heart problem.
▼ You have asthma or respiratory problems.
▼ You have had a gastric or duodenal ulcer.
▼ You are taking an NSAID regularly.
▼ You are taking other medications.

Pregnancy
▼ Safety in pregnancy not established.

Breast-feeding
▼ Not recommended.

Infants and children
▼ Not recommended.

Over 60
▼ No special problems.

Driving and hazardous work
▼ Your underlying condition may make such activities inadvisable. Discuss with your physician.

Alcohol
▼ Avoid. Alcohol may reduce the effect of donepezil.

Surgery and general anesthetics
▼ Treatment with donepezil may need to be stopped before you have a general anesthetic. Discuss this with your physician or dentist before any operation.

POSSIBLE ADVERSE EFFECTS

Adverse effects include such problems as accidents, which are common in this group of people even when not treated.

Symptom/effect	Frequency		Discuss with physician		Stop taking drug now	Call physician now
	Common	Rare	Only if severe	In all cases		
Nausea/vomiting	●		■			
Diarrhea	●		■			
Fatigue/insomnia	●		■			
Muscle cramps	●		■			
Headache		●	■			
Fainting/dizziness		●		■		
Palpitations		●		■		
Difficulty in passing urine		●		■		

INTERACTIONS

General note This drug is relatively new and interactions with other drugs are not fully established. If changes to the effect of donepezil are noticed when other drugs are taken or removed, discuss with your physician.

Paroxetine, erythromycin, and grapefruit juice Could increase donepezil levels in the blood and possibly its side effects.

Muscle relaxants used in surgery Donepezil may increase the effect of some muscle relaxants, but it may also block some others.

Carbamazepine, phenytoin, and rifampin These drugs can all decrease the effectiveness of donepezil.

PROLONGED USE

May be continued for as long as there is benefit. Stopping the drug leads to a gradual loss of the improvements.

Monitoring Periodic checks may be performed to test whether the drug is still providing some benefit.

DORZOLAMIDE

Product name Trusopt
Used in the following combined preparation Cosopt

GENERAL INFORMATION

Dorzolamide is a carbonic anhydrase inhibitor (a kind of diuretic) that is used, in the form of eye drops only, to treat glaucoma. It is also used for ocular hypertension (high blood pressure inside the eye). The drug relieves the pressure by reducing production of aqueous humour, the fluid in the front chamber of the eye.

Dorzolamide may be used alone or combined with a beta blocker by people resistant to the effects of beta blockers or for whom beta blockers are not suitable.

Most *side effects* of dorzolamide are local to the eye, but *systemic* effects may occur if enough of the drug is absorbed by the body.

INFORMATION FOR USERS

Your drug prescription is tailored for you. Do not alter dosage without checking with your physician.

How taken

Eye drops.

Frequency and timing of doses
3 x daily (on its own); 2 x daily (combined preparation).

Usual adult dosage range
1 drop in the affected eye(s) or as directed.

Onset of effect
15–30 minutes.

Duration of action
4–8 hours.

Diet advice
None.

Storage
Keep in a closed container in a cool, dry place out of the reach of children. Protect from light. Discard eye drops 4 weeks after opening.

Missed dose
Use as soon as you remember. If your next dose is due, skip the missed dose and then go back to your normal dosing schedule.

Stopping the drug
Do not stop the drug without consulting your physician; symptoms may recur.

Exceeding the dose
An occasional unintentional extra application is unlikely to cause problems. Excessive use may provoke side effects as described below.

SPECIAL PRECAUTIONS

Be sure to tell your physician if:
▼ You have liver or kidney problems.
▼ You are allergic to sulfonamide drugs.
▼ You are allergic to benzalkonium chloride.
▼ You are taking other medications.

 Pregnancy
▼ Not prescribed. Discuss with your physician.

 Breast-feeding
▼ Not recommended. Discuss with your physician.

 Infants and children
▼ Not recommended.

 Over 60
▼ No special problems.

 Driving and hazardous work
▼ Avoid such activities until you have learned how dorzolamide affects you because the drug can cause dizziness and blurred vision.

 Alcohol
▼ No special problems.

POSSIBLE ADVERSE EFFECTS

Local side effects of dorzolamide include conjunctivitis and keratitis (inflammation of the cornea, the transparent part of the eye). *Systemic* side effects such as nausea and headache may also occur. If you develop a rash or breathing difficulties, you should consult your physician urgently.

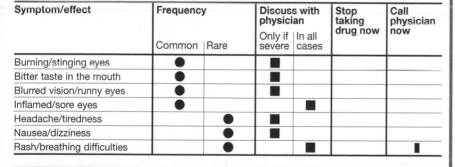

Symptom/effect	Frequency		Discuss with physician		Stop taking drug now	Call physician now
	Common	Rare	Only if severe	In all cases		
Burning/stinging eyes	●		■			
Bitter taste in the mouth	●		■			
Blurred vision/runny eyes	●		■			
Inflamed/sore eyes	●			■		
Headache/tiredness		●	■			
Nausea/dizziness		●	■			
Rash/breathing difficulties		●		■		■

PROLONGED USE

No special problems.

INTERACTIONS

General note Dorzolamide may interact with the following drugs, but there do not appear to be any published reports of problems. Consult your physician.

Thiazide diuretics Excessive loss of potassium may occur when these drugs are taken with dorzolamide.

ASA this drug may increase the levels of dorzolamide and increase the risk of adverse effects.

Lithium Dorzolamide may reduce blood levels of lithium.

DOXAZOSIN

Product names Cardura-1, Cardura-2, Cardura-4
Used in the following combined preparations None

GENERAL INFORMATION

Doxazosin is an antihypertensive vaso-dilator drug that relieves hypertension (high blood pressure) by relaxing the muscles in the blood vessel walls, which, in turn, enables more blood to pass through. As doxazosin is removed slowly from the body, it is usually given only once daily. It may be administered together with other antihypertensive drugs, including beta blockers, since its effects on blood pressure are increased when it is combined with most other antihypertensives.

Doxazosin can also be given to patients with an enlarged prostate gland. It relaxes the muscles around the bladder exit and prostate gland allowing urine to flow out more easily.

Dizziness and fainting may occur at the onset of treatment with doxazosin, because the first dose may cause a marked fall in blood pressure. For this reason, the initial dose is usually low. It should be taken at home, preferably just before bedtime.

QUICK REFERENCE

Drug group A vasodilator (p.84), antihypertensive drug (p.88), and drug for urinary disorders (p.154)

Overdose danger rating Medium

Dependence rating Low

Prescription needed Yes

Available as generic Yes

INFORMATION FOR USERS

Your drug prescription is tailored for you. Do not alter dosage without checking with your physician.

How taken

Tablets.

Frequency and timing of doses
Once daily, at the same time each day.

Usual adult dosage range
Hypertension 1mg (starting dose), increased gradually as necessary up to 16mg.
Enlarged prostate 1mg (starting dose), increased gradually at 1–2-week intervals up to 8mg.

Onset of effect
Within 2 hours.

Duration of action
24 hours.

Diet advice
None.

Storage
Keep in a closed container in a cool, dry place out of the reach of children.

Missed dose
If you forget to take a tablet, skip that dose completely but carry on as normal the following day.

Stopping the drug
Do not stop taking the drug without consulting your physician; stopping the drug may lead to a rise in blood pressure.

Exceeding the dose
An occasional unintentional extra dose is unlikely to be a cause for concern. Larger overdoses may cause dizziness or fainting. Notify your physician.

SPECIAL PRECAUTIONS

Be sure to tell your physician if:
▼ You have long-term liver or kidney problems.
▼ You have had an allergic reaction to doxazosin in the past.
▼ You are due to have an operation.
▼ You are taking other medications.

 Pregnancy
▼ Safety in pregnancy not established. Discuss with your physician.

 Breast-feeding
▼ The drug passes into the breast milk. Discuss with your physician.

 Infants and children
▼ Not recommended.

 Over 60
▼ Reduced dose may be necessary. Take extra care when standing up until you have learned how the drug affects you.

 Driving and hazardous work
▼ Avoid such activities until you have learned how doxazosin affects you because the drug can cause drowsiness, dizziness, and fainting.

Alcohol
▼ Avoid excessive amounts. Alcohol may increase some of the *adverse effects* of this drug, such as dizziness, drowsiness, and fainting.

Surgery and general anesthetics
▼ A general anesthetic may increase the low blood pressure effect of doxazosin.

POSSIBLE ADVERSE EFFECTS

Nausea, headache, and weakness are common with doxazosin, but the main problem is that it may cause dizziness or fainting when you stand up.

Symptom/effect	Frequency		Discuss with physician		Stop taking drug now	Call physician now
	Common	Rare	Only if severe	In all cases		
Nausea	●		■			
Weakness/drowsiness	●		■			
Headache	●		■			
Dizziness/fainting		●	■			
Stuffy/runny nose		●	■			
Palpitations/chest pain		●		■		■
Rash		●		■		

INTERACTIONS

Hypotensive drugs Any drugs that can reduce blood pressure are likely to have an increased effect when taken with doxazosin. These include diuretics, beta blockers, ACE inhibitors, nitrates, calcium channel blockers, and some antipsychotics and antidepressants.

PROLONGED USE

No known problems.

DOXORUBICIN

Product names Adriamycin PFS, Caelyx, Myocet
Used in the following combined preparations None

GENERAL INFORMATION

Doxorubicin is one of the most effective anticancer drugs. It is prescribed to treat a wide variety of cancers, usually in conjunction with other anticancer drugs. It is used in cancer of the lymph nodes (Hodgkin's disease), lung, breast, bladder, stomach, thyroid, and reproductive organs. It is also used to treat Kaposi's sarcoma in AIDS patients.

Nausea and vomiting after injection are the most common *side effects* of doxorubicin. Although these symptoms are unpleasant, they tend to be less severe as the body adjusts to treatment. The drug may stain the urine bright red, but this is not harmful. More seriously,

because doxorubicin interferes with the production of blood cells, blood clotting disorders, *anemia*, and infections may occur. Therefore, effects on the blood are carefully monitored. Hair loss is also a common side effect. Rarely, heart rhythm disturbance and heart failure are dose-dependent side effects that may also occur.

The brand-name drugs Caelyx and Myocet are special formulations in which the doxorubicin is enclosed in fatty spheres. This makes the drug more suitable for treating certain types of cancers, for example AIDS-related Kaposi's sarcoma.

INFORMATION FOR USERS

This drug is given only under medical supervision and is not for self-administration.

How taken

Injection, *bladder instillation*.

Frequency and timing of doses
Every 1–3 weeks.

Usual adult dosage range
Dosage is determined individually according to body height, weight, and response.

Onset of effect
Some adverse effects may appear within one hour of starting treatment, but full beneficial effects may not be felt for up to 4 weeks.

Duration of action
Adverse effects can persist for up to 2 weeks after stopping treatment.

Diet advice
None.

Storage
Not applicable. The drug is not normally kept in the home.

Missed dose
The drug is administered in hospital under close medical supervision. If for some reason you skip your dose, contact your physician as soon as you can.

Stopping the drug
Discuss with your physician. Stopping the drug prematurely may lead to a worsening of the underlying condition.

Exceeding the dose
Overdosage is unlikely since treatment is carefully monitored and supervised.

SPECIAL PRECAUTIONS

Doxorubicin is prescribed only under close medical supervision, taking account of your present condition and medical history.

Pregnancy
▼ Not usually prescribed. Doxorubicin may cause birth defects or premature birth. Discuss with your physician.

Breast-feeding
▼ Not advised. The drug passes into the breast milk and may affect the baby adversely. Discuss with your physician.

Infants and children
▼ Reduced dose necessary.

Over 60
▼ Increased risk of adverse effects. Reduced dose may be necessary.

Driving and hazardous work
▼ No known problems.

Alcohol
▼ No known problems.

POSSIBLE ADVERSE EFFECTS

Nausea and vomiting generally occur within an hour of injection. Many people also experience hair loss and loss of appetite. Palpitations may indicate an adverse effect of the drug on the heart. Since treatment is closely supervised in hospital, all adverse effects are monitored.

Symptom/effect	Frequency		Discuss with physician		Stop taking drug now	Call physician now
	Common	Rare	Only if severe	In all cases		
Nausea/vomiting	●			■		
Loss of appetite	●			■		
Hair loss	●			■		
Diarrhea		●		■		
Mouth ulcers		●		■		
Skin irritation/ulcers		●		■		
Palpitations		●		■		■

INTERACTIONS

Cyclosporine Treatment with cyclosporine while receiving doxorubicin can lead to adverse effects on the nervous system.

PROLONGED USE

Prolonged use of doxorubicin may reduce the activity of the bone marrow, leading to reduced production of all types of blood cell. It may also affect the heart adversely.

Monitoring Periodic checks on blood composition are usually required. Regular heart examinations are also carried out.

DOXYCYCLINE

Product names Vibramycin, Vibra-Tabs
Used in the following combined preparations None

GENERAL INFORMATION

Doxycycline is a tetracycline antibiotic. It is used to treat infections of the urinary, respiratory, and gastrointestinal tracts. It is also prescribed for treatment of some sexually transmitted diseases, skin, eye, and prostate infections, acne, and malaria prevention (in some parts of the world, see p.123).

Doxycycline is less likely to cause diarrhea than other tetracyclines, and its absorption is not significantly impaired by milk and food. It can therefore be taken with meals to reduce *side effects* such as nausea or indigestion. It is also safer than most other tetracyclines for people with impaired kidney function. Like other tetracyclines, it can stain developing teeth and may affect development of bone; it is therefore usually avoided in children under 12 years old and pregnant women.

INFORMATION FOR USERS

Your drug prescription is tailored for you. Do not alter dosage without checking with your physician.

How taken

Tablets, capsules.

Frequency and timing of doses
1–2 x daily with water, or with or after food, in a sitting or standing position, and well before going to bed to avoid risk of throat irritation.

Usual dosage range
100–200mg daily.

Onset of effect
1–12 hours; several weeks (acne).

Duration of action
Up to 24 hours; several weeks (acne).

Diet advice
None.

Storage
Keep in closed container in a cool, dry place out of the reach of children.

Missed dose
Take as soon as you remember. If your next dose is due within 6 hours, take a single dose now and skip the next.

Stopping the drug
Take the full course. Even if you feel better, the original infection may still be present and symptoms may recur if treatment is stopped too soon.

Exceeding the dose
An occasional unintentional extra dose is unlikely to be a cause for concern. But if you notice any unusual symptoms, or if a large overdose has been taken, notify your physician.

POSSIBLE ADVERSE EFFECTS

Adverse effects from doxycycline are rare, although nausea, vomiting, or diarrhea may occur. Rash, itching, and photosensitivity of the skin are other possible adverse effects.

Symptom/effect	Frequency		Discuss with physician		Stop taking drug now	Call physician now
	Common	Rare	Only if severe	In all cases		
Nausea/vomiting		●	■			
Mouth ulcers		●	■			
Diarrhea		●	■			
Rash/itching		●		■	▲	
Photosensitivity		●		■	▲	
Headache/visual disturbances		●		■	▲	■

INTERACTIONS

Penicillin antibiotics Doxycycline interferes with the antibacterial action of these drugs.

Barbiturates, carbamazepine, and phenytoin All these drugs reduce the effectiveness of doxycycline. Doxycycline dosage may need to be increased.

Oral contraceptives There is a slight risk of doxycycline reducing the effectiveness of oral contraceptives. Discuss with your physician.

Oral anticoagulant drugs Doxycycline may increase the anticoagulant action of these drugs.

Antacids and preparations containing iron, calcium, or magnesium may impair absorption of this drug. Do not take within 2–3 hours of doxycycline.

Cyclosporine, digoxin, and lithium Doxycycline may increase the blood levels of these drugs.

SPECIAL PRECAUTIONS

Be sure to tell your physician if:
▼ You have a long-term liver problem.
▼ You have previously suffered an allergic reaction to a tetracycline antibiotic.
▼ You have porphyria.
▼ You have systemic lupus erythematosus.
▼ You have myasthenia gravis.
▼ You are taking other medications.

Pregnancy
▼ Not used in pregnancy. May discolour the teeth of the developing baby.

Breast-feeding
▼ The drug passes into the breast milk and may lead to discoloration of the baby's teeth and may also have other adverse effects. Discuss with your physician.

Infants and children
▼ Not recommended under 12 years. Reduced dose necessary for older children.

Over 60
▼ No special problems. Ensure that medication is taken in upright position to minimize esophageal irritation or ulceration.

Driving and hazardous work
▼ No known problems.

Alcohol
▼ Excessive amounts may decrease the effectiveness of doxycycline.

Surgery and general anesthetics
▼ Nofity your physician or dentist that you are taking doxycycline.

PROLONGED USE

Not usually prescribed long term, except for acne.

EFAVIRENZ

Product name Sustiva
Used in the following combined preparations Atripla

GENERAL INFORMATION

Efavirenz is a non-nucleoside reverse transcriptase inhibitor, which is a type of antiretroviral drug that is used to treat HIV infection. It is used together with other antiretrovirals, for example, two nucleoside analogues, as combination therapy to slow down the production of the virus. The aim of this treatment is to reduce the damage done to the immune system by the virus. Combination antiretroviral therapy is not a cure for HIV. If the drugs are taken regularly on a long-term basis, they can reduce the level of the virus in the body and improve the outlook for the HIV patient. However, the patient will remain infectious, and will suffer a relapse if treatment is stopped.

INFORMATION FOR USERS

Your drug prescription is tailored for you. Do not alter dosage without checking with your physician.

How taken

Capsules.

Frequency and timing of doses
Once daily, usually at night to minimize adverse effects.

Usual adult dosage range
600mg, but may be reduced according to body weight.

Onset of effect
1 hour.

Duration of action
24 hours.

Diet advice
None.

Storage
Keep in the original container in a cool, dry place out of the reach of children.

Missed dose
Take as soon as you remember. If your next dose is due within 2 hours, take a single dose now and skip the next. It is very important not to miss doses on a regular basis as this can lead to the development of drug-resistant HIV.

Stopping the drug
Do not stop taking the drug without consulting your physician. It may be necessary to withdraw all your drugs gradually, starting with efavirenz.

Exceeding the dose
An occasional unintentional extra dose is unlikely to cause problems. But if you notice any unusual symptoms, or if a large overdose has been taken, notify your physician.

POSSIBLE ADVERSE EFFECTS

Gastrointestinal upset and rash are the most common adverse effects. Efavirenz can cause vivid dreams and changes in sleep patterns, but these tend to wear off with time.

Symptom/effect	Frequency		Discuss with physician		Stop taking drug now	Call physician now
	Common	Rare	Only if severe	In all cases		
Nausea/vomiting	●		■			
Diarrhea	●		■			
Vivid dreams	●		■			
Rash	●			■		▮
Mood changes	●			■		▮

INTERACTIONS

General note A wide range of drugs may interact with efavirenz, causing either an increase in adverse effects or a reduction in the effect of the antiretroviral drugs. Check with your physician or pharmacist before taking any new drugs, including those from the dentist and supermarket, and herbal medicines.

SPECIAL PRECAUTIONS

Be sure to tell your physician if:
▼ You have liver or kidney problems.
▼ You have an infection such as hepatitis B or C.
▼ You are pregnant or planning pregnancy.
▼ You are taking other medications.

Pregnancy
▼ Should not be used during pregnancy. Pregnancy should be avoided when taking efavirenz by using barrier methods of contraception in addition to other methods. Discuss with your physician.

Breast-feeding
▼ Safety in breast-feeding not established. Breast-feeding is not recommended for HIV-positive mothers as the virus may be passed to the baby.

Infants and children
▼ Not prescribed to children under 3 years. Reduced dose necessary in older children.

Over 60
▼ Reduced dose may be necessary to minimize adverse effects.

Driving and hazardous work
▼ Avoid such activities until you have learned how efavirenz affects you because the drug can cause dizziness.

Alcohol
▼ No known problems, although some people may find the effects of alcohol are more pronounced while taking efavirenz.

PROLONGED USE

No known problems.

Monitoring Your physician will take regular blood samples to check the drug's effects on the virus. Blood will also be checked for changes in lipid, cholesterol, and sugar levels.

ENALAPRIL/ENALAPRILAT

Product name Vasotec
Used in the following combined preparation Vaseretic

GENERAL INFORMATION

Enalapril belongs to the ACE inhibitor group of *vasodilator* drugs, which are used to treat hypertension (high blood pressure) and heart failure (inability of the heart to cope with its workload). It is also given to patients following a heart attack.

The first dose of enalapril may cause a sudden drop in blood pressure. For this reason, you should be resting at the time and be able to lie down for 2 to 3 hours afterwards.

The more common *adverse effects* of enalapril, such as dizziness and headache, usually diminish with long-term treatment. Rashes can also occur but usually disappear when the drug is stopped. In some cases, they clear up on their own despite continued treatment with enalapril.

QUICK REFERENCE

Drug group ACE inhibitor (p.84) and antihypertensive drug (p.88)

Overdose danger rating Medium

Dependence rating Low

Prescription needed Yes

Available as generic Yes

INFORMATION FOR USERS

Your drug prescription is tailored for you. Do not alter dosage without checking with your physician.

How taken

Tablets, injection.

Frequency and timing of doses
1–2 x daily.

Usual adult dosage range
2.5–5mg daily (starting dose), increased to 10–40mg daily (maintenance dose).

Onset of effect
Within 1 hour.

Duration of action
24 hours.

Diet advice
None.

Storage
Keep in a closed container in a dry place below 25°C out of the reach of children. Protect from light.

Missed dose
Take as soon as you remember. If your next dose is due within 8 hours, take a single dose now and skip the next.

Stopping the drug
Do not stop the drug without consulting your physician; stopping the drug may lead to worsening of the underlying condition.

Exceeding the dose
An occasional unintentional extra dose is unlikely to be a cause for concern. Large overdoses may cause dizziness or fainting. Notify your physician.

SPECIAL PRECAUTIONS

Be sure to tell your physician if:
▼ You have a long-term kidney problem.
▼ You have a heart problem.
▼ You have angioedema.
▼ You have had a previous allergic reaction to an ACE inhibitor drug.
▼ You have porphyria.
▼ You are taking other medications.

Pregnancy
▼ Not normally prescribed. May cause abnormalities in the fetus. Discuss with your physician.

Breast-feeding
▼ The drug passes into the breast milk, but at normal doses adverse effects on the baby are unlikely. Discuss with your physician.

Infants and children
▼ Not recommended.

Over 60
▼ Reduced dose may be necessary.

Driving and hazardous work
▼ Avoid such activities until you have learned how enalapril affects you because the drug can cause dizziness and fainting.

Alcohol
▼ Avoid. Alcohol increases the likelihood of an excessive drop in blood pressure that may cause dizziness.

Surgery and general anesthetics
▼ Discuss with your physician or dentist before any operation.

POSSIBLE ADVERSE EFFECTS

Common adverse effects such as dizziness and headache usually diminish with long-term treatment. Less common problems may also diminish wtih time but dose adjustment may be necessary. Rashes may occur, but usually disappear when the drug is stopped.

Symptom/effect	Frequency		Discuss with physician		Stop taking drug now	Call physician now
	Common	Rare	Only if severe	In all cases		
Dizziness	●		■			
Headache	●		■			
Persistent dry cough	●			■		
Nausea/loss of appetite		●	■			
Diarrhea		●	■			
Fainting		●		■		
Rash/urticaria		●		■		
Muscle cramps		●		■		
Wheezing/swelling		●		■	▲	■

INTERACTIONS

Antihypertensive drugs and NSAIDs These drugs are likely to enhance the blood pressure-lowering effect of enalapril.

Lithium Enalapril increases the levels of lithium in the blood, and serious adverse effects from lithium excess may occur.

Cyclosporine Taken with enalapril, this drug may increase blood levels of potassium.

Potassium supplements and potassium-sparing diuretics Enalapril may enhance the effect of these drugs, leading to raised levels of potassium in the blood.

Non-steroidal anti-inflammatory drugs (NSAIDs) Some of these drugs may reduce the effectiveness of enalapril. There is also risk of kidney damage when they are taken with enalapril.

PROLONGED USE

No problems expected.

Monitoring Periodic tests on blood and urine should be performed.

EPHEDRINE

Product names Ephedra, Ephedrine sulfate
Used in the following combined preparations None

GENERAL INFORMATION

In use for more than 50 years, ephedrine promotes the release of norephedrine, a *neurotransmitter*. It was once widely prescribed as a bronchodilator to relax the muscles surrounding the airways, easing breathing difficulty caused by asthma, bronchitis, and emphysema. More effective drugs have largely replaced ephedrine for these uses. Its main use now is as a decongestant in cough preparations. Ephedrine injections may be used as a method of restoring normal blood pressure after anaesthetic procedures.

Adverse effects of ephedrine include stimulation of the heart and the central nervous system, causing palpitations and anxiety. It is not recommended for the elderly, or those with heart problems, high blood pressure, thyroid disease, diabetes, or an enlarged prostate.

QUICK REFERENCE

Drug group Bronchodilator (p.76) and decongestant (p.79)

Overdose danger rating Medium

Dependence rating Low

Prescription needed No

Available as generic Yes

INFORMATION FOR USERS

Follow instructions on the label. Call your physician if symptoms worsen.

How taken

Tablets, injection.

Frequency and timing of doses
By mouth 3 x daily.

Usual dosage range
Adults 15–30mg daily (by mouth);
3–6mg every 3–4 minutes to a maximum of 30mg (injection).
Children Reduced dose according to age and weight.

Onset of effect
Within 15–60 minutes.

Duration of action
3–6 hours.

Diet advice
None.

Storage
Keep in a closed container in a cool, dry place out of the reach of children. Protect from light.

Missed dose
Do not take the missed dose. Take your next dose as usual.

Stopping the drug
Can be safely stopped as soon as you no longer need it.

Exceeding the dose
An occasional unintentional extra dose is unlikely to cause problems. Large overdoses may cause shortness of breath, high fever, fits, or loss of consciousness. Notify your physician immediately.

SPECIAL PRECAUTIONS

Be sure to consult your physician or pharmacist before taking this drug if:
▼ You have a long-term kidney problem.
▼ You have heart disease.
▼ You have high blood pressure.
▼ You have diabetes.
▼ You have an overactive thyroid gland.
▼ You have had glaucoma.
▼ You have urinary difficulties.
▼ You are taking other medications.

 Pregnancy
▼ Safety in pregnancy not established. Discuss with your physician.

 Breast-feeding
▼ The drug passes into the breast milk and may affect the baby. Discuss with your physician.

 Infants and children
▼ For children in general, but especially for those under 2 years of age, consult your health care provider. Reduced dose necessary for all children.

 Over 60
▼ Not usually prescribed.

 Driving and hazardous work
▼ Avoid such activities until you have learned how ephedrine affects you.

 Alcohol
▼ No special problems.

Surgery and general anesthetics
▼ Ephedrine may need to be stopped before you have a general anesthetic. Discuss this with your physician or dentist before surgery.

POSSIBLE ADVERSE EFFECTS

When taken by mouth, the drug may have adverse effects on the central nervous system (for example, insomnia and anxiety) and the cardiovascular system (palpitations). Taking the last dose before 4 pm may help to prevent insomnia.

Symptom/effect	Frequency		Discuss with physician		Stop taking drug now	Call physician now
	Common	Rare	Only if severe	In all cases		
Anxiety/restlessness	●		■			
Insomnia	●		■			
Cold extremities		●	■			
Dry mouth		●	■			
Tremor		●	■			
Urinary difficulties		●		■		
Palpitations/chest pain		●		■	▲	■

INTERACTIONS

Monoamine oxidase inhibitors (MAOIs) Ephedrine may interact with these drugs to cause a dangerous rise in blood pressure.

Beta blockers Ephedrine may interact with these drugs to cause a dangerous rise in blood pressure.

Antihypertensive drugs Ephedrine may counteract the effects of some antihypertensive drugs.

PROLONGED USE

Prolonged use is not recommended except on medical advice. Please consult with your physician or pharmacist before using ephedrine.

EPINEPHRINE (ADRENALINE)

Product name Epipen
Used in the following combined preparations Sensorcaine with epinephrine, Xylocaine with epinephrine

GENERAL INFORMATION

Epinephrine is a *neurotransmitter* that is produced in the centre (medulla) of the adrenal glands. Synthetic epinephrine has been made since 1900. The drug is given in an emergency to stimulate heart activity and raise low blood pressure. It also narrows blood vessels in the skin and intestine.

Epinephrine is injected to counteract cardiac arrest, or to relieve severe allergic reactions (anaphylaxis) to drugs, food, or insect stings. For patients who are at risk of anaphylaxis, it is provided as a pre-filled syringe for immediate self-injection at the start of an attack.

Because it constricts blood vessels, epinephrine is used to control bleeding and to slow the dispersal, and thereby prolong the effect, of local *anesthetics*.

QUICK REFERENCE

Drug group Drug for glaucoma (p.156), cardiac resuscitation, and anaphylaxis

Overdose danger rating High

Dependence rating Low

Prescription needed Yes

Available as generic Yes

INFORMATION FOR USERS

Your drug prescription is tailored for you. Do not alter dosage without checking with your physician.

How taken

Injection, eye drops, intranasal solution.

Frequency and timing of doses
As directed according to method of administration and underlying disorder.

Usual dosage range
As directed according to method of administration and underlying disorder.

Onset of effect
Within 5 minutes (injection); within 1 hour (eye drops).

Duration of action
Up to 4 hours (injection); up to 24 hours (eye drops).

Diet advice
None.

Storage
Keep in a closed container in a cool, dry place out of the reach of children. Protect from light.

Missed dose
Do not take the missed dose. Take the next dose as usual.

Stopping the drug
Do not stop using the drug without consulting your physician; stopping may lead to worsening of the underlying condition.

OVERDOSE ACTION

Seek immediate medical advice in all cases. Take emergency action if palpitations, breathing difficulties, or loss of consciousness occur.

See Drug poisoning emergency guide (p.526).

SPECIAL PRECAUTIONS

Be sure to tell your physician if:
▼ You have a heart problem.
▼ You have diabetes.
▼ You have an overactive thyroid gland.
▼ You have a nervous system problem.
▼ You have high blood pressure.
▼ You are taking other medications.

Pregnancy
▼ Not usually prescribed. May cause defects in the fetus and prolong labour. Discuss with your physician.

Breast-feeding
▼ Adverse effects on the baby are unlikely. Discuss with your physician.

Infants and children
▼ Reduced dose necessary.

Over 60
▼ Increased likelihood of adverse effects. Reduced dose may therefore be necessary.

Driving and hazardous work
▼ No known problems.

Alcohol
▼ No known problems.

Surgery and general anesthetics
▼ Epinephrine may need to be stopped before you have a general anesthetic. Discuss this with your physician or dentist before surgery.

POSSIBLE ADVERSE EFFECTS

The principal *adverse effects* of this drug are related to its stimulant action on the heart and central nervous system.

Symptom/effect	Frequency		Discuss with physician		Stop taking drug now	Call physician now
	Common	Rare	Only if severe	In all cases		
Dry mouth	●		■			
Nervousness/restlessness	●		■			
Nausea/vomiting	●		■			
Cold extremities	●		■			
Palpitations	●				■	
Headache/blurred vision	●				■	

INTERACTIONS

General note A variety of drugs interact with epinephrine to increase the risk of palpitations and/or high blood pressure. Such drugs include monoamine oxidase inhibitors (MAOIs) and tricyclic antidepressants, such as amitriptyline.

Beta blockers Epinephrine can produce a dangerous rise in blood pressure with certain beta blockers, such as propranolol.

Antidiabetic drugs Epinephrine may reduce the effectiveness of these drugs.

PROLONGED USE

Long-term use of epinephrine eye drops is not recommended.

ERGOTAMINE

Product name None
Used in the following combined preparations Bellergal Spacetabs, Cafergot, Ergodryl

GENERAL INFORMATION

Ergotamine is used to treat migraine but its use has largely been superseded by newer agents with fewer adverse effects. Ergotamine may also be used in the prevention of cluster headaches. Its use in migraine should be restricted to when other analgesics are ineffective. It should be taken at the first sign of migraine (the "aura"). Later use may be ineffective and cause stomach upset.

Ergotamine causes temporary narrowing of blood vessels and, therefore should not be used by people with poor circulation. If taken too frequently, the drug can dangerously reduce circulation to the hands and feet; it should never be taken regularly.

Frequent migraine attacks may indicate the need for a different drug to prevent migraine.

INFORMATION FOR USERS

Your drug prescription is tailored for you. Do not alter dosage without checking with your physician.

How taken

Capsules, tablets, suppositories, nasal spray.

Frequency and timing of doses
Once at the onset, repeated if needed after 30 minutes (tablets) up to the maximum dose (see below).

Usual adult dosage range
Varies according to product. Generally, 1–2mg per dose. Take no more than 4mg in 24 hours or 8mg in 1 week. Treatment should not be repeated within 4 days or more than twice a month.

Onset of effect
15–30 minutes.

Duration of action
Up to 24 hours.

Diet advice
Changes in diet are unlikely to affect the action of this drug, but certain foods may provoke migraine attacks in some people.

Storage
Keep in a closed container in a cool, dry place out of the reach of children. Protect from light.

Missed dose
Regular doses of this drug are not necessary and may be dangerous. Take only when you have symptoms of migraine.

Stopping the drug
Can be safely stopped as soon as you no longer need it.

Exceeding the dose
An occasional unintentional extra dose is unlikely to cause problems. Large overdoses may cause vomiting, dizziness, fits, or coma. Notify your physician immediately.

SPECIAL PRECAUTIONS

Be sure to tell your physician if:
▼ You have long-term liver or kidney problems.
▼ You have heart problems.
▼ You have poor circulation.
▼ You have high blood pressure.
▼ You have had a recent stroke.
▼ You have an overactive thyroid gland.
▼ You are taking other medications.

Pregnancy
▼ Not usually prescribed. Ergotamine can cause contractions of the uterus.

Breast-feeding
▼ Not recommended. The drug passes into the milk and may have adverse effects on the baby. It may also reduce your milk supply.

Infants and children
▼ Not usually prescribed.

Over 60
▼ Not recommended. May aggravate existing heart or circulatory problems.

Driving and hazardous work
▼ Avoid such activities until you have learned how ergotamine affects you because the drug can cause vertigo.

Alcohol
▼ No special problems, but some spirits may provoke migraine in some people.

Surgery and general anesthetics
▼ Notify your physician if you have used ergotamine within 48 hours prior to surgery.

POSSIBLE ADVERSE EFFECTS

Digestive disturbances and nausea (for which an anti-emetic may be given) are common with ergotamine treatment. Rare but serious *adverse effects* may result from arterial spasm.

Symptom/effect	Frequency		Discuss with physician		Stop taking drug now	Call physician now
	Common	Rare	Only if severe	In all cases		
Nausea/vomiting	●		■			
Abdominal pain	●		■			
Muscle cramps	●		■			
Diarrhea		●	■			
Dizziness		●		■		
Muscle pain/stiffness		●		■		
Chest pain		●		■	▲	▌
Leg/groin pain		●		■	▲	▌
Cold/numb fingers/toes		●		■	▲	▌

INTERACTIONS

Beta blockers These drugs may increase circulatory problems with ergotamine.

Sumatriptan and related drugs There is an increased risk of adverse effects on the blood circulation if ergotamine is used with these drugs.

Erythromycin and related antibiotics and antivirals taken with ergotamine increase the likelihood of adverse effects.

Oral contraceptives There is an increased risk of blood clotting in women taking these drugs with ergotamine.

PROLONGED USE

Reduced circulation to the hands and feet may result if doses near to the maximum are taken for too long. The recommended dosage and length of treatment should not be exceeded. Rebound headache may occur if it is taken too frequently.

ERYTHROMYCIN

Product names EES 200, EryC
Used in the following combined preparation Benzamycin, Erysol, Pediazole

GENERAL INFORMATION

One of the safest and most widely used antibiotics, erythromycin is effective against many bacteria. It is commonly used as an alternative in people allergic to penicillin and related antibiotics.

Erythromycin is used to treat throat, middle ear, and chest infections (including some rare types of pneumonia such as Legionnaires' disease). It is also used for sexually transmitted diseases such as chlamydial infections, and in some forms of gastroenteritis.

Erythromycin may also be included as part of the treatment for diphtheria and is sometimes given to treat, and reduce the likelihood of infecting others with, pertussis (whooping cough).

When taken by mouth, erythromycin may sometimes cause nausea and vomiting. Other possible *adverse effects* include rash as well as a rare risk of liver disorders. Oral administration or topical application of the drug is sometimes helpful in treating acne.

INFORMATION FOR USERS

Your drug prescription is tailored for you. Do not alter dosage without consulting your physician.

How taken

Tablets, capsules, liquid, injection, topical solution, eye ointment.

Frequency and timing of doses
Every 6–12 hours before or with meals.

Usual dosage range
1–4g daily.

Onset of effect
1–4 hours.

Duration of action
6–12 hours.

Diet advice
None.

Storage
Keep in a closed container in a cool, dry place out of the reach of children.

Missed dose
Take as soon as you remember. If your next dose is due within 2 hours, take a single dose now and skip the next.

Stopping the drug
Take the full course. Even if you feel better, the original infection may still be present and symptoms may recur if treatment is stopped too soon.

Exceeding the dose
An occasional unintentional extra dose is unlikely to be a cause for concern. But if you notice any unusual symptoms, or if a large overdose has been taken, notify your physician.

SPECIAL PRECAUTIONS

Be sure to tell your physician if:
▼ You have a long-term liver problem.
▼ You have had a previous allergic reaction to erythromycin.
▼ You have porphyria.
▼ You are taking other medications.

Pregnancy
▼ No evidence of risk to the developing fetus.

Breast-feeding
▼ The drug passes into the breast milk, but at normal doses adverse effects on the baby are unlikely. Discuss with your physician.

Infants and children
▼ Reduced dose necessary.

Over 60
▼ No special problems.

Driving and hazardous work
▼ No known problems.

Alcohol
▼ No known problems.

POSSIBLE ADVERSE EFFECTS

Nausea and vomiting are common and most likely with large doses taken by mouth. Fever, rash, and *jaundice* may be signs of a liver disorder; inform your physician.

Symptom/effect	Frequency		Discuss with physician		Stop taking drug now	Call physician now
	Common	Rare	Only if severe	In all cases		
Nausea/vomiting	●		■			
Diarrhea	●		■			
Rash/itching	●			■	▲	
Deafness		●		■		▮
Jaundice		●		■	▲	▮
Unexplained fever		●		■	▲	▮
Skin blisters/ulcers		●		■	▲	▮

INTERACTIONS

General note Erythromycin interacts with a number of other drugs, particularly:

Warfarin Erythromycin increases the risk of bleeding with warfarin.

Ergotamine Erythromycin increases the risk of side effects with this drug.

Carbamazepine, digoxin, and some immunosuppressants Erythromycin may increase blood levels of these drugs.

Theophylline/aminophylline Erythromycin increases the risk of adverse effects with these drugs.

Lipid-lowering drugs ending in -statin Erythromycin may increase the risk of muscular aches and pains with statins.

PROLONGED USE

Courses of longer than 14 days may increase the risk of liver damage.

ERYTHROPOIESIS STIMULATORS

Product names Aranesp, Eprex
Used in the following combined preparations None

GENERAL INFORMATION

Epoetin alfa (erythropoietin) and darbepoetin are both erythropoiesis-stimulating agents (ESA). Erythropoietin is a hormone naturally produced by the kidneys; it stimulates the body to produce red blood cells. Epoetin and darbepoetin are manufactured forms of erythropoetin that are used to treat anemia associated with chronic kidney disease.

ESA are also used to treat anemia caused by certain cancer treatments. They are also used to boost the level of red blood cells before surgery. Patients donate blood before surgery and this is then used during or after the surgery. Epoetin may also be used as an alternative to blood transfusions in major orthopedic (bone) surgery.

Darbepoetin is a derivative of epoetin and it has a longer duration of action. It can, therefore, be given less frequently.

The doses of these drugs are titrated gradually, with close monitoring of the hemoglobin level.

QUICK REFERENCE

Drug group Kidney hormone (p.126)
Overdose danger rating Low
Dependence rating Low
Prescription needed Yes
Available as generic No

INFORMATION FOR USERS

Your drug prescription is tailored for you. Do not alter dosage without checking with your physician.

How taken

Injection.

Frequency and timing of doses
1–3 x weekly, depending on the product and condition being treated.

Usual dosage range
Dosage is calculated on an individual basis according to body weight. The dosage also varies depending on the product and condition being treated.

Onset of effect
Active inside the body within 4 hours, but effects may not be noted for 2–3 months.

Duration of action
Some effects may persist for several days.

Diet advice
None. However, if you have kidney failure, you may have to follow a special diet.

Storage
Store at 2–8°C, out of the reach of children. Do not freeze or shake. Protect from light.

Missed dose
Do not make up any missed doses.

Stopping the drug
Discuss with your physician.

Exceeding the dose
A single excessive dose is unlikely to be a cause for concern. Too high a dose over a long period can increase the likelihood of adverse effects.

SPECIAL PRECAUTIONS

Be sure to tell your physician if:
▼ You have high blood pressure.
▼ You have a long-term liver problem.
▼ You have previously suffered allergic reactions to any drugs.
▼ You have peripheral vascular disease.
▼ You have had epileptic fits.
▼ You are taking other medications.

Pregnancy
▼ Not usually prescribed. Safety in pregnancy not established. Discuss with your physician.

Breast-feeding
▼ Safety not established. Discuss with your physician.

Infants and children
▼ Reduced dose necessary.

Over 60
▼ No known problems.

Driving and hazardous work
▼ Not applicable.

Alcohol
▼ Follow your physician's advice regarding alcohol.

POSSIBLE ADVERSE EFFECTS

The most common effects are increased blood pressure and problems at the site of the injection; all unusual symptoms should be discussed with your physician immediately.

Symptom/effect	Frequency		Discuss with physician		Stop taking drug now	Call physician now
	Common	Rare	Only if severe	In all cases		
Increased blood pressure	●			■		
Problems at injection site	●			■		
Flu symptoms/bone pain		●		■		
Epileptic fits		●		■		▮
Skin reactions		●		■		
Headache (stabbing pain)		●		■		▮
Chest pain, difficulty breathing		●				▮
Blurred vision, changes in speech		●				▮

PROLONGED USE

The long-term effects of the drug are still under investigation, but problems are unlikely if treatment is carefully monitored.

Monitoring Regular blood tests to monitor blood composition and blood pressure monitoring are required.

INTERACTIONS

ACE inhibitor drugs These drugs may increase the level of potassium in the blood and epoetin may enhance their blood pressure-lowering effect.

Iron supplements These may increase the effect of epoetin if you have a low level of iron in your blood.

ESTRADIOL

Product names Climara, Estrace, Estraderm, Estring, Estrogel
Used in the following combined preparations Estalis, Estracomb

GENERAL INFORMATION

Estradiol is a naturally occurring estrogen (a female sex hormone). It is mainly used as hormone replacement therapy (HRT) to treat menopausal and post-menopausal symptoms such as hot flushes, night sweats, and vaginal atrophy. It is also used in contraceptive products with a progestin (another female sex hormone 133). HRT also helps prevent the loss of bone tissue that occurs in osteoporosis. Estradiol is often given with a progestin, either as separate drugs or as a combined product. Estradiol is not recommended on its own for women with a "working" uterus.

Use of estradiol may increase the risk of developing a blood clot (thrombosis) particularly in the veins of the legs. Women with a history of these conditions should discuss this with their physician.

Estradiol is available in a variety of forms, including topical gels and skin patches. Skin patches of the drug may cause local rash and itching.

QUICK REFERENCE

Drug group Female sex hormone (p.133)

Overdose danger rating Low

Dependence rating Low

Prescription needed Yes

Available as generic No

INFORMATION FOR USERS

Your drug prescription is tailored for you. Do not alter dosage without checking with your physician.

How taken

Tablets, vaginal tablets, vaginal rings, skin gel, patches.

Frequency and timing of doses
Once daily (tablets, gel); every 1–7 days (skin patches); daily to twice weekly (vaginal tablets); every 3 months (vaginal ring).

Usual adult dosage range
1–2mg daily (tablets); 2–4 measures daily (skin gel); 25–100mcg daily (skin patches); 25mcg per dose (vaginal tablets); 7.5mcg daily (vaginal ring).

Onset of effect
10–20 days.

Duration of action
Up to 24 hours; some effects may be longer lasting.

Diet advice
None.

Storage
Keep in a closed container in a cool, dry place out of the reach of children.

Missed dose
Take as soon as you remember. If your next daily treatment is due within 4 hours, take a single dose now and skip the next.

Stopping the drug
Do not stop the drug without consulting your physician; symptoms may recur.

Exceeding the dose
An occasional unintentional extra dose is unlikely to be a cause for concern. But if you notice any unusual symptoms, or if a large overdose has been taken, notify your physician.

SPECIAL PRECAUTIONS

Be sure to tell your physician if:
▼ You have a long-term liver problem.
▼ You have heart or circulation problems.
▼ You have porphyria.
▼ You have had blood clots or a stroke.
▼ You have diabetes.
▼ You are a smoker.
▼ You suffer from migraine or epilepsy.
▼ You are taking other medications.

Pregnancy
▼ Not prescribed.

Breast-feeding
▼ Not prescribed. The drug passes into breast milk and may inhibit its flow. Discuss with your physician.

Infants and children
▼ Not usually prescribed.

Over 60
▼ No special problems.

Driving and hazardous work
▼ No problems expected.

Alcohol
▼ No known problems.

Surgery and general anesthetics
▼ You may need to stop taking estradiol several weeks before having major surgery.

POSSIBLE ADVERSE EFFECTS

The most common *adverse effects* are similar to symptoms of early pregnancy, and generally diminish with time. Sudden sharp pain in the chest, groin, or legs may indicate a blood clot.

Symptom/effect	Frequency		Discuss with physician		Stop taking drug now	Call physician now
	Common	Rare	Only if severe	In all cases		
Nausea/vomiting	●		■			
Breast swelling/tenderness	●			■		
Weight gain	●		■			
Headache		●	■			
Depression		●		■		
Pain in chest/groin/legs		●		■	▲	▮

INTERACTIONS

Anticoagulant drugs The effects of these drugs are reduced by estradiol.

St John's wort May reduce the effect of estradiol.

Rifampin This drug may reduce the effects of estradiol.

Tobacco smoking This increases the risk of serious adverse effects on the heart and circulation with estradiol.

Anticonvulsants The effects of estradiol are reduced by carbamazepine, phenytoin, and phenobarbital.

PROLONGED USE

In some circumstances, prolonged use of estradiol may slightly increase the risk of cancer of the uterus and breast. The risk of gallstones may also be higher.

Monitoring Blood pressure checks and physical examinations, including regular mammograms, may be performed.

ETHAMBUTOL

Product name Etibi
Used in the following combined preparations None

GENERAL INFORMATION

Ethambutol is an antibiotic used in the treatment of tuberculosis. It is combined with other antituberculous drugs to enhance its effect and reduce the risk of the infection becoming drug resistant. Ethambutol is not used in all cases of tuberculosis. It is more likely to be used in people with a history of tuberculosis; those with a low immune status; and in those in whom the infection may be caused by a resistant organism.

Although the drug has few common *adverse effects*, it may occasionally cause optic neuritis, a type of eye damage leading to blurring and fading of vision. As a result, ethambutol is not usually prescribed for children under six years of age or for other patients who are unable to communicate their symptoms adequately. Before starting treatment, a full ophthalmic examination is recommended.

INFORMATION FOR USERS

Your drug prescription is tailored for you. Do not alter dosage without checking with your physician.

How taken

Tablets.

Frequency and timing of doses
Once daily.

Usual adult dosage range
According to body weight.

Onset of effect
It may take several days for symptoms to improve.

Duration of action
Up to 24 hours.

Diet advice
None.

Storage
Keep in a closed container in a cool, dry, place out of the reach of children.

Missed dose
Take as soon as you remember. If your next dose is due within 6 hours, take a single dose now and skip the next.

Stopping the drug
Take the full course. Even if you feel better the original infection may still be present and may recur if treatment is stopped too soon.

Exceeding the dose
An occasional unintentional extra dose is unlikely to cause problems. Large overdoses may cause headache and abdominal pain. Notify your physician.

SPECIAL PRECAUTIONS

Be sure to tell your physician if:
▼ You have a kidney problem.
▼ You have cataracts or other eye problems.
▼ You have gout.
▼ You have had a previous allergic reaction to this drug.
▼ You are taking other medications.

Pregnancy
▼ Safety in pregnancy not established. Discuss with your physician.

Breast-feeding
▼ The drug passes into the breast milk, but at normal doses adverse effects on the baby are unlikely. Discuss with your physician.

Infants and children
▼ Not generally prescribed under 6 years, and often not under 13 years.

Over 60
▼ Increased likelihood of adverse effects. Reduced dose may therefore be necessary.

Driving and hazardous work
▼ Avoid such activities until you have learned how ethambutol affects you because the drug may cause dizziness.

Alcohol
▼ No known problems.

POSSIBLE ADVERSE EFFECTS

Side effects are uncommon with this drug but are more likely after prolonged treatment at high doses. Blurred vision or eye pain require prompt medical attention.

Symptom/effect	Frequency		Discuss with physician		Stop taking drug now	Call physician now
	Common	Rare	Only if severe	In all cases		
Nausea/vomiting		●	■			
Dizziness		●	■			
Numb/tingling hands/feet		●		■		
Blurred vision		●		■	▲	▌
Eye pain		●		■	▲	▌
Loss of colour vision		●		■	▲	▌
Rash/itching		●		■	▲	

INTERACTIONS

Antacids Those containing aluminium salts may decrease levels of ethambutol, and should be taken at least 2 hours before or after ethambutol.

PROLONGED USE

Prolonged use may increase the risk of eye damage.

Monitoring Periodic eye tests are usually necessary.

ETHINYL ESTRADIOL

Used in the following combined preparations Combined oral contraceptives (e.g. Diane-35, Marvelon, Ortho-Cept, Demulen 30, Alesse, Min-Ovral, Triphasil)

GENERAL INFORMATION

Ethinyl estradiol is a synthetic estrogen similar to estradiol, a natural female sex hormone. It is widely used in oral contraceptives, in combination with a synthetic progestin. The drug is also very occasionally used (often with a progestin) to supplement estrogen during the menopause.

Ethinyl estradiol is sometimes given to control heavy bleeding from the uterus and to treat delayed female sexual development (hypogonadism). Certain breast and prostate cancers respond to ethinyl estradiol. With cyproterone, it is used to treat severe acne in women.

Women taking an oral contraceptive pill containing ethinyl estradiol have an increased risk of developing thrombosis (a blood clot). This risk increases in overweight women and smokers.

QUICK REFERENCE

Drug group Female sex hormone (p.133) and oral contraceptive (p.149)

Overdose danger rating Low

Dependence rating Low

Prescription needed Yes

Available as generic Yes

INFORMATION FOR USERS

Your drug prescription is tailored for you. Do not alter dosage without checking with your physician.

How taken

Tablets.

Frequency and timing of doses
Once daily. Often at certain times of the menstrual cycle.

Usual adult dosage range
Menopausal symptoms 10–20mcg daily.
Hormone deficiency 10–50mcg daily.
Combined contraceptive pills 20–40mcg daily depending on preparation.
Acne 35mcg daily.
Breast cancer 1–3mg daily.

Onset of effect
10–20 days. Contraceptive protection is effective after 7 days in most cases.

Duration of action
1–2 days.

Diet advice
None.

Storage
Keep in a closed container in a cool, dry place out of the reach of children.

Missed dose
Take as soon as you remember. If your next dose is due within 4 hours, take a single dose now and skip the next. If you are taking the drug for contraceptive purposes, see What to do if you miss a pill (p.151).

Stopping the drug
Do not stop the drug without consulting your physician. Contraceptive protection is lost unless an alternative is used.

Exceeding the dose
An occasional unintentional extra dose is unlikely to be a cause for concern. If you notice any unusual symptoms, or if a large overdose has been taken, notify your physician.

SPECIAL PRECAUTIONS

Be sure to tell your physician or pharmacist before taking this drug if:
▼ You have heart failure or high blood pressure.
▼ You or a close relative have had blood clots or a stroke.
▼ You have a long-term liver problem.
▼ You have had breast or endometrial cancer.
▼ You have sickle cell anemia.
▼ You have porphyria.
▼ You are a smoker.
▼ You have diabetes.
▼ You suffer from migraine or epilepsy.
▼ You are taking other medications.

Pregnancy
▼ Not prescribed. High doses may adversely affect the baby. Discuss with your physician.

Breast-feeding
▼ The drug passes into the breast milk; it may also inhibit milk flow. Discuss with your physician.

Infants and children
▼ Not usually prescribed.

Over 60
▼ No special problems.

Driving and hazardous work
▼ No known problems.

Alcohol
▼ No known problems.

Surgery and general anesthetics
▼ Ethinyl estradiol may need to be stopped several weeks before you have major surgery. Discuss this with your physician.

POSSIBLE ADVERSE EFFECTS

The most common *adverse effects* with ethinyl estradiol are similar to symptoms in the early stages of pregnancy and generally diminish with time. Sudden, sharp pain in the chest, groin, or legs may indicate an abnormal blood clot and requires urgent attention.

Symptom/effect	Frequency Common	Frequency Rare	Discuss with physician Only if severe	Discuss with physician In all cases	Stop taking drug now	Call physician now
Nausea/vomiting	●		■			
Breast swelling/tenderness	●		■			
Weight gain	●		■			
Bleeding between periods	●		■			
Headache		●	■			
Depression		●		■		
Pain in chest/groin/legs		●		■	▲	▋
Sudden breathlessness		●		■	▲	▋
Itching/jaundice		●		■	▲	▋

INTERACTIONS

Tobacco smoking This increases the risk of serious adverse effects on the heart and circulation with ethinyl estradiol.

Rifampin and anticonvulsant drugs These drugs significantly reduce the effectiveness of oral contraceptives containing ethinyl estradiol.

Antihypertensive drugs and diuretics Ethinyl estradiol may reduce the effectiveness of these drugs.

Antibiotics and St John's wort May reduce the effectiveness of oral contraceptives containing ethinyl estradiol. Discuss with your physician or pharmacist.

PROLONGED USE

Prolonged use of ethinyl estradiol without a progestin slightly increases the risk of postmenopausal cancer of the uterus. There may also be an increased risk of gallstones and breast cancer.

Monitoring Physical examinations and blood pressure checks may be performed.

ETIDRONATE

Product name Didronel
Used in the following combined preparation Didrocal

GENERAL INFORMATION

Etidronate is given for the treatment of bone disorders such as Paget's disease. It acts only on the bones, reducing the activity of the bone cells and thereby stopping the progress of the disease. This action also stops calcium from being released from the bones into the bloodstream, so it reduces the amount of calcium in the blood. Etidronate is also used together with calcium tablets to treat osteoporosis in post-menopausal women and to prevent steroid-induced osteoporosis. The drug's *side effects* are usually mild. The most common is diarrhea. If taken at high doses (20mg/kg body weight daily), the drug can lead to thinning of the bones and fractures. The effect is reversed on stopping the drug. When used for osteoporosis, the drug is taken for 14 days, followed by a gap of 76 days before the next 14 day cycle. In Didrocel, calcium carbonate tablets are included, to be taken for the 76 days.

INFORMATION FOR USERS

Your drug prescription is tailored for you. Do not alter dosage without checking with your physician.

How taken

Tablets.

Frequency and timing of doses
Once daily on an empty stomach, 2 hours before or after food.

Usual dosage range
Paget's disease 5–20mg/kg body weight daily for a maximum of 3–6 months. Courses may be repeated after a break of at least 3 months. *Osteoporosis* 400mg daily for 2 weeks, repeated every 3 months.

Onset of effect
Paget's disease/osteoporosis Beneficial effects may not be felt for several months.

Duration of action
Some effects may persist for several weeks or months.

Diet advice
Absorption of etidronate is reduced by foods, especially those containing calcium (e.g., dairy products), so the drug should be taken on an empty stomach. The diet must contain adequate calcium, and vitamin D; supplements may be given.

Storage
Keep in a closed container in a dry place below 30°C out of the reach of children. Protect from light.

Missed dose
Take as soon as you remember. If your next dose is due within 6 hours, take a single dose now and skip the next.

Stopping the drug
Do not stop the drug without consulting your physician. Stopping the drug may lead to worsening of the underlying condition.

Exceeding the dose
An occasional unintentional extra dose is unlikely to cause problems. Large overdoses may cause numbness and muscle spasm. Notify your physician.

SPECIAL PRECAUTIONS

Be sure to tell your physician if:
▼ You have a long-term kidney problem
▼ You have osteomalacia.
▼ You have unusual bone pain.
▼ You have had a previous allergic reaction to etidronate or other bisphosphonates.
▼ You have an overactive parathyroid gland.
▼ You have a high concentration of calcium in your blood or urine.
▼ You have colitis.
▼ You are taking other medications.

 Pregnancy
▼ Safety in pregnancy not established. Discuss with your physician.

 Breast-feeding
▼ Safety in breast-feeding not established. Discuss with your physician.

 Infants and children
▼ Not recommended.

 Over 60
▼ No special problems.

 Driving and hazardous work
▼ No special problems.

 Alcohol
▼ No special problems.

POSSIBLE ADVERSE EFFECTS

The most common side effect, diarrhea, is more likely if the dose is increased above 5mg/kg daily. In some patients with Paget's disease, bone pain may be increased initially, but this symptom usually disappears with further treatment.

Symptom/effect	Frequency Common	Frequency Rare	Discuss with physician Only if severe	Discuss with physician In all cases	Stop taking drug now	Call physician now
Diarrhea	●		■			
Nausea	●		■			
Constipation/abdominal pain	●		■			
Headache		●	■			
Rash/itching		●		■		
Bone pain/bruising		●		■		▮
Fever/sore throat		●		■		▮
Eye inflammation/vision change		●		■		

INTERACTIONS

Antacids and products containing calcium, magnesium, or iron These products should be given at least 2 hours before or after etidronate to minimize the risk of reduced absorption of etidronate.

PROLONGED USE

When used in bone disorders such as Paget's disease, courses of treatment longer than 3 to 6 months are not usually prescribed, but repeat courses may be required. This drug can be used long term for osteoporosis.

Monitoring Blood and urine tests may be carried out.

EZETIMIBE

Product name Ezetrol
Used in the following combined preparations None

GENERAL INFORMATION

Ezetimibe is in a new class of lipid-lowering drug that is used in the treatment of high cholesterol. It lowers blood cholesterol by blocking the absorption of cholesterol, including dietary cholesterol, from the intestines. It is usually used in addition to another lipid-lowering medication, a statin (p.89). Ezetimibe can be taken at any time, once daily, and preferably taken at the same time.

QUICK REFERENCE

Drug group Lipid-lowering drugs (p.89)

Overdose danger rating Low

Dependence rating Low

Prescription needed Yes

Available as generic No

INFORMATION FOR USERS

Your drug prescription is tailored for you. Do not alter dosage without checking with your physician.

How taken

Tablets.

Frequency and timing of doses
Once daily.

Usual adult dosage range
10mg daily.

Onset of effect
1–4 hours.

Duration of action
Up to 24 hours.

Diet advice
Patients should be on a cholesterol-lowering diet.

Storage
Keep in a closed container in a cool, dry place out of the reach of children.

Missed dose
If you miss a dose, take it as soon as you remember. If it is near the time of the next dose, skip the missed dose and resume your using dosing schedule.

Stopping the drug
Do not stop the drug without consulting your physician. Stopping the drug may lead to worsening of the underlying condition.

Exceeding the dose
An occasional unintentional extra dose is unlikely to cause problems. However, if you notice any unusual symptoms, or if a large overdose has been taken, notify your physician.

SPECIAL PRECAUTIONS

Be sure to tell your physician if:
▼ You have ever had an allergic reaction to ezetimibe.
▼ You have liver problems or liver disease.
▼ You have kidney problems or kidney disease.
▼ You are on any other medications.

Pregnancy
▼ Safety in pregnancy not established. Discuss with your physician.

Breast-feeding
▼ Safety in breast-feeding has not established. Discuss use with your physician.

Infants and children
▼ Not recommended in children less than 10 years of age.

Over 60
▼ No special problems.

Driving and hazardous work
▼ No known problems.

Alcohol
▼ No known problems.

POSSIBLE ADVERSE EFFECTS

Ezetimibe is usually well tolerated and serious side effects are rare.

Symptom/effect	Frequency		Discuss with physician		Stop taking drug now	Call physician now
	Common	Rare	Only if severe	In all cases		
Abdominal pain		●	■			
Dizziness		●	■			
Diarrhea	●			■		
Headache	●		■			
Sinusitis		●		■		
Muscle ache		●		■		

INTERACTIONS

Antacids May decrease the rate of absorption of ezetimibe, although these do not significantly affect the total amount of ezetimibe absorbed.

Cholestyramine May decrease absorption of ezetimibe, when taken at the same time.

Fibrates Ezetimibe is not recommended to be used with fibrates (p.89) which also decrease cholesterol.

Cyclosporine May increase levels of ezetimibe; close monitoring recommended.

PROLONGED USE

No known problems.

Monitoring If administered with a statin, certain blood tests will be done periodically.

FAMCICLOVIR

Product name Famvir
Used in the following combined preparations None

GENERAL INFORMATION

Famciclovir is an antiviral drug used in the treatment of shingles (herpes zoster) and genital herpes.

Early treatment in shingles can decrease symptoms. Treatment should be initiated within 72 hours of the appearance of rash. Famciclovir is also beneficial in those with shingles who are over 50 years of age or those who are experiencing severe pain with shingles.

In genital herpes, it may be used to treat an acute episode or to suppress recurrent episodes in those who have had 6 or more episodes in a year. Famciclovir should be started in the prodrome stage or as soon as lesions appear.

INFORMATION FOR USERS

Your drug prescription is tailored for you. Do not alter dosage without checking with your physician.

How taken

Tablets.

Frequency and timing of doses
Herpes zoster: 3 times daily.
Suppression of recurrent genital herpes: twice daily.

Usual adult dosage range
250–1500mg daily.

Onset of effect
Within 24 hours.

Duration of action
Up to 8–12 hours.

Diet advice
None.

Storage
Keep in a closed container in a cool, dry place out of the reach of children.

Missed dose
If you miss a dose, take it as soon as you remember. If it is near the time of the next dose, skip the missed dose and resume your using dosing schedule. Do not double up to catch up on a missed dose.

Stopping the drug
Complete the full course as directed.

Exceeding the drug
An occasional unintentional extra dose is unlikely to cause problems. However, if you notice any unusual symptoms, or if a large overdose has been taken, notify your physician.

SPECIAL PRECAUTIONS

Be sure to tell your physician if:
▼ You have ever had an allergic reaction to famciclovir or another antiviral drug.
▼ You have impaired liver or kidney function or disease.
▼ You have reduced immunity.
▼ You are on any other medications.

 Pregnancy
▼ Safety in pregnancy not established. Discuss with your physician.

 Breast-feeding
▼ Safety in breast-feeding has not established. Discuss use with your physician.

 Infants and children
▼ Not recommended.

 Over 60
▼ No special problems.

 Driving and hazardous work
▼ No known problems.

Alcohol
▼ No known problems.

POSSIBLE ADVERSE EFFECTS

Common side effects include headache, nausea, and diarrhea. These effects are generally not bothersome after the first few days.

Symptom/effect	Frequency		Discuss with physician		Stop taking drug now	Call physician now
	Common	Rare	Only if severe	In all cases		
Headache	●		■			
Nausea	●		■			
Diarrhea	●		■			
Vomiting		●		■		
Dizziness		●		■		
Rash		●		■		▮

INTERACTIONS

Probenecid Drugs such as probenecid, which are eliminated by the kidneys, may decrease the elimination of famciclovir, resulting in its effects being increased.

PROLONGED USE

Famciclovir is usually given for 5 or 7 days. It may be used up to a year in prevention of genital herpes.

Monitoring When used for longer than a few days, periodic monitoring of liver and kidney function may be done.

FAMOTIDINE

Product names Apo-Famotidine, Famotidine Omega, Gen-Famotidine, Maalox H$_2$ Acid Controller, Novo-Famotidine, Nu-Famotidine, Pepcid, Pepcid AC, Peptic Guard **Used in the following combined preparation** Pepcid Complete

GENERAL INFORMATION

Famotidine is prescribed in the treatment of stomach and duodenal ulcers. It is also used to protect against duodenal ulcers in people taking NSAIDs (p.102), who may be prone to ulcers. This drug reduces the discomfort and ulceration of reflux esophagitis, and may prevent stress ulceration and gastric bleeding in severely ill patients. Famotidine reduces the amount of stomach acid produced, allowing ulcers to heal. It is usually given in courses lasting four to eight weeks, with further courses if symptoms recur. Unlike the similar drug cimetidine, famotidine does not increase blood levels of other drugs

such as anticoagulants and anti-convulsants, which might reduce the effectiveness of treatment. It is available in smaller doses over-the-counter for self-management of the discomfort of acid indigestion.

Most people experience no serious effects during famotidine treatment. As it promotes healing of the stomach lining, there is a risk that famotidine may mask stomach cancer, delaying diagnosis. It is therefore usually prescribed only when the possibility of stomach cancer has been ruled out.

QUICK REFERENCE

Drug group Anti-ulcer drug (p.95)

Overdose danger rating Low

Dependence rating Low

Prescription needed Yes, for most doses

Available as generic Yes

INFORMATION FOR USERS

Your drug prescription is tailored for you. Do not alter dosage without checking with your physician.

How taken

Tablets, chewable tablets, injection.

Frequency and timing of doses
Once to twice daily. For prevention of acid-related symptoms associated with food intake, take 15 minutes before eating.

Usual dosage range
10–40mg daily.

Onset of effect
1 hour

Duration of action
Up to 12 hours.

Diet advice
None.

Storage
Keep in a closed container in a cool, dry place out of the reach of children. Protect from light.

Missed dose
If you miss a dose, take it as soon as you remember. If your next dose is within 3 hours, take a single dose now and skip the next.

Stopping the drug
Do not stop the drug without consulting your physician; symptoms may recur.

Exceeding the dose
An occasional unintentional extra dose is unlikely to be a cause for concern. But if you notice any unusual symptoms, or if a large overdose has been taken, notify your physician.

SPECIAL PRECAUTIONS

Be sure to tell your physician if:
▼ You have liver or kidney problems.
▼ You have porphyria.
▼ You have had an allergic reaction to famotidine or another H$_2$ blocker.
▼ You are taking other medications.

Pregnancy
▼ Safety in pregnancy not established. Discuss with your physician.

Breast-feeding
▼ The drug passes into the breast milk and may affect the baby. Discuss with your physician.

Infants and children
▼ Not recommended.

Over 60
▼ No special problems.

Driving and hazardous work
▼ No known problems. Dizziness may occur in a very small proportion of patients.

Alcohol
▼ Avoid. Alcohol may aggravate your underlying condition and reduce the beneficial effects of this drug.

PROLONGED USE

No problems expected.

POSSIBLE ADVERSE EFFECTS

Adverse effects such as headache is usually related to dosage level and almost always disappear when treatment finishes.

Symptom/effect	Frequency		Discuss with physician		Stop taking drug now	Call physician now
	Common	Rare	Only if severe	In all cases		
Headache	●		■			
Diarrhea		●	■			
Dizziness		●	■			
Drowsiness		●	■			
Constipation		●	■			
Jaundice		●		■		
Mental problems		●		■		

INTERACTIONS

Ketoconazole Famotidine may reduce the absorption of ketoconazole.

FENTANYL

Product names Duragesic, Fentanyl citrate
Used in the following combined preparations None

GENERAL INFORMATION

Fentanyl is an opioid analgesic indicated in the management of persistent, moderate to severe, chronic pain in individuals already requiring continous opioid medication. It is available as a patch or an injection. The patch provides a more constant management of pain.

It is recommended that the patches not be cut or divided as this may lead to uncontrolled release of the drug. The patch should be applied to non-irritated skin on a flat surface such as the chest, back, flank, or upper arm. When applying a new patch, ensure that the old patch is removed and disposed of safely by folding it so that the adhesive side sticks to itself and flushing it down the toilet. Fentanyl injection may be used to help with anesthesia.

Individuals at risk of serious side effects include those with a fever, those whose patch area is exposed to sources of heat such as heating pads and hot water bottles, and those using drugs that may interact with this medication. The elderly are more susceptible to adverse effects.

QUICK REFERENCE

Drug group Opioid analgesic (p.64)

Overdose danger rating High

Dependence rating High

Prescription needed Yes

Available as generic Yes

Factors that increase the risk of life-threatening hypoventilation include fever, exposure to external heat sources, and drug interactions.

INFORMATION FOR USERS

Your drug prescription is tailored for you. Do not alter dosage without checking with your physician.

How taken

Injection, patch.

Frequency and timing of doses
One patch every 72 hours (3 days.)

Usual adult dosage range
Variable and based on previous opioid dose. Patch available in 4 different strengths.

Onset of effect
The peak effect from a patch usually occurs around 12 hours.

Duration of action
Up to 72 hours.

Diet advice
To relieve constipation, increase intake of fluids and high fiber foods.

Storage
Keep in a closed container in a cool, dry place out of the reach of children before and after use.

Missed dose
If you miss a dose, apply the patch when you remember; the next patch should be used at the appropriate interval of 72 hours. Do not double up a dose.

Stopping the drug
Always discuss with your physician. When stopping opioid medications, a gradual downward titration is recommended.

OVERDOSE ACTION

 Seek immediate medical advice. Take emergency action in cases of slow, shallow, or irregular breathing, severe drowsiness, inability to think, or slow pulse.

See Drug poisoning emergency guide (p.526).

SPECIAL PRECAUTIONS

Be sure to tell your physician if:
▼ You have impaired liver or kidney function.
▼ You have heart or circulatory problems.
▼ You have a lung disorder such as asthma, bronchitis, or emphysema.
▼ You have sleep apnea.
▼ You have thyroid disease.
▼ You are taking other medications.

Pregnancy
▼ Safety in pregnancy not established. Taken near the time of delivery, the drug may cause breathing difficulties in the newborn baby. Discuss with your physician.

Breast-feeding
▼ Low levels of the drug have been detected in human milk. Safety in breast-feeding not established. Discuss with your physician.

Infants and children
▼ Not recommended.

Over 60
▼ Increased likelihood of adverse effects. Reduced dose necessary.

Driving and hazardous work
▼ Patients receiving fentanyl are unlikely to be well enough to undertake such activities.

Alcohol
▼ Avoid. Alcohol increases the sedative effects of fentanyl.

POSSIBLE ADVERSE EFFECTS

As with other opioids, fentanyl may produce nausea, vomiting, dizziness, loss of appetite, and constipation. Dosage adjustments may lessen some effects.

Symptom/effect	Frequency		Discuss with physician		Stop taking drug now	Call physician now
	Common	Rare	Only if severe	In all cases		
Sedation	●		■			
Constipation	●		■			
Nausea/vomiting	●			■		
Dizziness/light headedness	●			■		
Wheezing/difficulty breathing		●		■	▲	▮
Confusion/vivid dreams		●		■		

INTERACTIONS

CNS depressants Fentanyl increases the sedative properties of all drugs that have a sedative effect.

Ritonavir, ketoconazole, itraconazole, troleandomycin, clarithromycin, nelfinavir These drugs increase the effect of fentanyl, leading to serious effects on breathing. If any of these drugs is used with fentanyl, very close monitoring is required.

Monoamine oxidase inhibitors These may produce a severe rise in blood pressure when taken with fentanyl.

PROLONGED USE

The effects of fentanyl usually become weaker during prolonged use as the body adapts. This is known as tolerance. Other effects of long-term use include physical and psychological dependence.

FILGRASTIM

Product name Neupogen
Used in the following combined preparations None

GENERAL INFORMATION

Filgrastim is a synthetic form of G-CSF (granulocyte-colony stimulating factor), a naturally occurring protein responsible for the manufacture of white blood cells, which fight infection. Deficiency of G-CSF, therefore, increases the risk of infection. The drug works by stimulating bone marrow to produce white blood cells. It also causes bone marrow cells to move into the bloodstream, where they can be collected for use in the treatment of bone marrow disease, or to replace bone marrow lost during intensive cancer treatment.

Filgrastim is used to treat patients with congenital neutropenia (deficiency of G-CSF from birth), some AIDS patients, and those who have recently received high doses of chemo- or radiotherapy during bone-marrow transplantation or cancer treatment. Such patients are prone to frequent and severe infections.

Bone pain is a common *adverse effect* but it can be controlled using painkillers. There is an increased risk of leukemia (cancer of white blood cells) if filgrastim is given to patients with certain rare blood disorders.

QUICK REFERENCE

Drug group Blood stimulant
Overdose danger rating Medium
Dependence rating High
Prescription needed Yes
Available as generic No

INFORMATION FOR USERS

Your drug prescription is tailored for you. Do not alter dosage without checking with your physician.

How taken

Injection.

Frequency and timing of doses
Once daily.

Usual adult dosage range
0.5mcg/kg body weight–12mcg/kg body weight per day, depending upon condition being treated and response to treatment.

Onset of effect
24 hours (increase in numbers of white blood cells); several weeks (recovery of normal numbers of white blood cells).

Duration of action
Approximately 2 days.

Diet advice
None.

Storage
Store in a refrigerator out of the reach of children.

Missed dose
Take as soon as you remember. If your next dose is due within 6 hours, do not take the missed dose. Take the next scheduled dose as usual.

Stopping the drug
Do not stop taking the drug without consulting your physician; stopping the drug may lead to worsening of the underlying condition.

Exceeding the dose
An occasional unintentional extra dose is unlikely to cause problems. But if you notice any unusual symptoms or if a large overdose has been taken, notify your physician.

SPECIAL PRECAUTIONS

Be sure to tell your physician if:
▼ You suffer from any blood disorders.
▼ You are taking other medications.

Pregnancy
▼ Safety in pregnancy not established. Discuss with your physician.

Breast-feeding
▼ Safety in breast-feeding not established. Discuss with your physician.

Infants and children
▼ No special problems.

Over 60
▼ No special problems.

Driving and hazardous work
▼ No known problems.

Alcohol
▼ No known problems.

POSSIBLE ADVERSE EFFECTS

Adverse effects resulting from short courses of filgrastim are unusual. Most common is bone pain, which is probably linked to the stimulant effect of the drug on bone marrow.

Symptom/effect	Frequency		Discuss with physician		Stop taking drug now	Call physician now
	Common	Rare	Only if severe	In all cases		
Bone/muscle pain	●		■			
Difficulty/pain on urination		●		■		
Skin rash		●		■		

INTERACTIONS

***Cytotoxic* chemotherapy or radiotherapy** should not be administered within 24 hours of taking filgrastim because of the risk of increasing the damage these treatments inflict on the bone marrow.

PROLONGED USE

Prolonged use may lead to a slightly increased risk of certain leukemias. Cutaneous vasculitis (inflammation of blood vessels of the skin), osteoporosis (weakening of the bones), hair thinning, enlargement of the spleen and liver, and bleeding due to reduction in platelet numbers may also occur.

Monitoring Blood checks and regular physical examinations are performed, as well as X-rays or bone scans to check for bone thinning.

FINASTERIDE

Product names Propecia, Proscar
Used in the following combined preparations None

GENERAL INFORMATION

Finasteride is an an anti-androgen drug (see Male sex hormones, p.132) used to treat benign prostatic hyperplasia (BPH), in which the prostate gland, which surrounds the urethra, increases in size, making urination difficult. The drug works by gradually shrinking the prostate gland, which improves urine flow and other obstructive symptoms such as difficulty in starting urination.

Because finasteride is excreted in semen and can feminize a male fetus, you should use a condom if your sexual partner may be, or is likely to become, pregnant. Also, women of childbearing age should not handle broken or crushed tablets because small quantities of the drug are absorbed through the skin.

The symptoms of BPH are similar to those of prostate cancer and so the drug is used only when the possibility of cancer has been ruled out.

Finasteride is also used in men, at a lower dose, to reverse male-pattern baldness by preventing the hair follicles from becoming inactive. Noticeable improvements may take about three months but will disappear within a year of treatment being stopped.

QUICK REFERENCE

Drug group Drug used for urinary disorders, p.154
Overdose danger rating Low
Dependence rating Low
Prescription needed Yes
Available as generic No

INFORMATION FOR USERS

Your drug prescription is tailored for you. Do not alter dosage without checking with your physician.

How taken

Tablets.

Frequency and timing of doses
Once daily.

Usual adult dosage range
Prostate disease 5mg.
Male-pattern baldness 1mg.

Onset of effect
Within 1 hour, but beneficial effects may take several months.

Duration of action
24 hours.

Diet advice
None.

Storage
Keep in a closed container, in a cool, dry place out of the reach of children. Protect from light.

Missed dose
Do not take the missed dose, but take your next scheduled dose as usual.

Stopping the drug
Do not stop taking the drug without consulting your physician; stopping the drug may lead to worsening of the underlying condition.

Exceeding the dose
An occasional unintentional extra dose is unlikely to cause problems. But if you notice any unusual symptoms, or if a large overdose has been taken, notify your physician.

SPECIAL PRECAUTIONS

Be sure to tell your physician if:
▼ You are taking other medications.

Pregnancy
▼ Not prescribed.

Breast-feeding
▼ Not prescribed.

Infants and children
▼ Not prescribed.

Over 60
▼ No special problems.

Driving and hazardous work
▼ No special problems.

Alcohol
▼ No special problems.

POSSIBLE ADVERSE EFFECTS

Most people experience very few adverse effects when taking finasteride.

Symptom/effect	Frequency		Discuss with physician		Stop taking drug now	Call physician now
	Common	Rare	Only if severe	In all cases		
Impotence/decreased libido	●		■			
Reduced ejaculate volume	●		■			
Breast swelling or tenderness		●	■			
Rash/lip swelling/wheezing		●		■	▲	▮

INTERACTIONS

None.

PROLONGED USE

Treatment with finasteride for benign prostatic hyperplasia and male-pattern baldness is reviewed after about six months to see if it has been effective.

FLUCONAZOLE

Product names Diflucan, Diflucan-150
Used in the following combined preparations None

GENERAL INFORMATION

Fluconazole is an antifungal drug that is used to treat local candida infections ("thrush") affecting the vagina, mouth, and skin as well as *systemic* or more widespread candida infections. The drug is also used to treat some more unusual fungal infections, including cryptococcal meningitis. It may also be used to prevent fungal infections in patients with defective immunity. The dosage and length of course will depend on the condition being treated.

The drug is generally well tolerated, although *side effects* such as nausea and vomiting, diarrhea, and abdominal discomfort are common.

QUICK REFERENCE

Drug group Antifungal drug (p.124)
Overdose danger rating Medium
Dependence rating Low
Prescription needed Yes
Available as generic Yes

INFORMATION FOR USERS

Your drug prescription is tailored for you. Do not alter dosage without checking with your physician.

How taken

Tablets, liquid, injection.

Frequency and timing of doses
Once daily; single 150mg dose for vaginal candidiasis.

Usual adult dosage range
50–400mg daily.

Onset of effect
Within a few hours, but full beneficial effects may take several days.

Duration of action
Up to 24 hours.

Diet advice
None.

Storage
Keep in a closed container in a cool, dry place out of the reach of children. Store liquid in a refrigerator (do not freeze) for no longer than 14 days.

Missed dose
Take as soon as you remember. If your next dose is due within 6 hours, take a single dose now and skip the next.

Stopping the drug
Take the full course. Even if you feel better, the original infection may still be present and may recur if treatment is stopped too soon.

Exceeding the dose
An occasional unintentional extra dose is unlikely to be a cause for concern. But if you notice any unusual symptoms, or a large overdose has been taken, notify your physician.

SPECIAL PRECAUTIONS

Be sure to tell your physician if:
▼ You have long-term liver or kidney problems.
▼ You have previously had an allergic reaction to antifungal drugs.
▼ You are taking other medications.

Pregnancy
▼ Safety in pregnancy not established. Discuss with your physician.

Breast-feeding
▼ Not recommended. The drug passes into the breast milk. Discuss with your physician.

Infants and children
▼ Reduced dose necessary.

Over 60
▼ Normal dose used as long as kidney function is not impaired.

Driving and hazardous work
▼ No known problems.

Alcohol
▼ No known problems.

POSSIBLE ADVERSE EFFECTS

Fluconazole is generally well tolerated. Most side effects affect the gastrointestinal tract.

Rarely, a rash may occur and should be reported to your physician.

Symptom/effect	Frequency		Discuss with physician		Stop taking drug now	Call physician now
	Common	Rare	Only if severe	In all cases		
Nausea/vomiting	●		■			
Abdominal discomfort	●		■			
Diarrhea	●		■			
Flatulence	●		■			
Rash		●		■		▲

INTERACTIONS

General note Most interactions with other drugs relate to multiple doses of fluconazole. The relevance of a single dose of fluconazole is not established.

Rifampin The effect of fluconazole may be reduced by rifampin.

Oral antidiabetic drugs Fluconazole may increase the risk of hypoglycemia with oral sulfonylureas, such as gliclazide, glibencglyburide, chlorpropamide, and tolbutamide.

Phenytoin, theophylline/aminophylline, cyclosporine, tacrolimus, and zidovudine Fluconazole may increase the blood levels of these drugs.

Anticoagulant drugs Fluconazole may increase the effect of oral anticoagulants such as warfarin.

PROLONGED USE

Fluconazole is usually given for short courses of treatment. However, for prevention of relapse of cryptococcal meningitis in patients with defective immunity, it may be administered indefinitely.

FLUOXETINE

Product name Prozac
Used in the following combined preparations None

GENERAL INFORMATION

Fluoxetine belongs to the group of antidepressants called selective serotonin re-uptake inhibitors (SSRIs). These drugs tend to cause less sedation and have different *side effects* to older antidepressants. Fluoxetine elevates mood, increases physical activity, and restores interest in everyday pursuits.

Fluoxetine is broken down slowly and remains in the body for several weeks after treatment is stopped. It is used to treat depression, to reduce binge eating and purging activity (bulimia nervosa), and to treat obsessive-compulsive disorder.

QUICK REFERENCE

Drug group Antidepressant (p.68)
Overdose danger rating Medium
Dependence rating Low
Prescription needed Yes
Available as generic Yes

INFORMATION FOR USERS

Your drug prescription is tailored for you. Do not alter dosage without checking with your physician.

How taken

Capsules, liquid.

Frequency and timing of doses
Once daily in the morning.

Usual adult dosage range
20–60mg daily.

Onset of effect
The full benefits of fluoxetine may not be felt for 4 weeks or more.

Duration of action
Beneficial effects may last for up to 6 weeks following prolonged treatment. Adverse effects may wear off within a few days.

Diet advice
None.

Storage
Keep in a closed container in a cool, dry place out of the reach of children.

Missed dose
Take as soon as you remember. If your next dose is due within 8 hours, take a single dose now and skip the next.

Stopping the drug
Do not stop the drug without consulting your physician, who may supervise a gradual reduction in dosage.

Exceeding the dose
An occasional unintentional extra dose is unlikely to cause problems. Large overdoses may cause adverse effects. Notify your physician.

SPECIAL PRECAUTIONS

Be sure to tell your physician if:
▼ You have long-term liver or kidney problems.
▼ You have heart problems.
▼ You have diabetes.
▼ You have had epileptic fits.
▼ You have previously had an allergic reaction to fluoxetine or other SSRIs.
▼ You are taking other medications.

 Pregnancy
▼ Safety in pregnancy not established. Discuss with your physician.

 Breast-feeding
▼ The drug passes into the breast milk. Discuss with your physician.

 Infants and children
▼ Safety and effectiveness not established. Discuss with your physician.

 Over 60
▼ A reduced dose may be necessary.

 Driving and hazardous work
▼ Avoid such activities until you have learned how fluoxetine affects you because the drug can cause drowsiness and can affect your judgment and coordination.

 Alcohol
▼ No special problems.

POSSIBLE ADVERSE EFFECTS

The most common adverse effects of this drug are restlessness, insomnia, and intestinal irregularities. Fluoxetine produces fewer *anticholinergic* side effects than the tricyclics.

Symptom/effect	Frequency		Discuss with physician		Stop taking drug now	Call physician now
	Common	Rare	Only if severe	In all cases		
Headache/nervousness	●		■			
Insomnia/anxiety	●			■		
Nausea/diarrhea	●			■		
Weight loss	●			■		
Drowsiness		●	■			
Sexual dysfunction		●	■			
Rash		●		■	▲	▮

INTERACTIONS

General note: Any drug that affects the breakdown of other drugs in the liver may alter blood levels of fluoxetine.

Sedatives All drugs having a *sedative* effect may increase the sedative effects of fluoxetine.

Monoamine oxidase inhibitors (MAOIs) Fluoxetine should not be started less than 14 days after stopping an MAOI (except moclobemide) as serious adverse effects can occur. An MAOI should not be started less than 5 weeks after stopping fluoxetine.

Tricyclic antidepressants Fluoxetine reduces the breakdown of tricyclics and may increase the toxicity of these drugs.

Lithium Fluoxetine increases blood levels and *toxicity* of lithium.

Tryptophan Taken together, tryptophan and fluoxetine may produce agitation, restlessness, and gastric distress.

Anticoagulants Fluoxetine can increase the effect of warfarin so dose may need adjustment.

PROLONGED USE

No problems expected. Side effects tend to decrease with time.

FLUPENTIXOL

Product name Fluanxol
Used in the following combined preparations None

GENERAL INFORMATION

Flupentixol is an antipsychotic drug that is prescribed to treat schizophrenia and similar illnesses. Flupentixol's *side effects* are similar to those of phenothiazines, but it is less sedating. The drug is not suitable for any patients who suffer from mania because it may worsen the symptoms.

The drug has fewer *anticholinergic* effects than the phenothiazines but is more likely to cause side effects such as *parkinsonism*. Control of severe symptoms can take six months; a lower maintenance dose is then prescribed.

QUICK REFERENCE

Drug group Antipsychotic drug (p.69)
Overdose danger rating Medium
Dependence rating Low
Prescription needed Yes
Available as generic No

INFORMATION FOR USERS

Your drug prescription is tailored for you. Do not alter dosage without checking with your physician.

How taken

Tablets, injection.

Frequency and timing of doses
1–3 x daily no later than 4 pm (tablets); every 2–4 weeks (injection).

Usual adult dosage range
Schizophrenia and other psychoses 3–12mg daily (tablets); from 20–40mg every 4 weeks (injection).

Onset of effect
10 days (side effects may appear much sooner).

Duration of action
Up to 12 hours (by mouth); 2–4 weeks (by injection).

Diet advice
None.

Storage
Store at room temperature out of the reach of children. Protect injections from light.

Missed dose
Take as soon as you remember. If your next dose is due within 2 hours, do not take the missed dose, but take your next scheduled dose as usual.

Stopping the drug
Do not stop taking the drug without consulting your physician, who will supervise a gradual reduction in dosage. Abrupt cessation of the drug may cause withdrawal symptoms and a recurrence of the original problem.

Exceeding the dose
An occasional unintentional extra dose is unlikely to cause problems. Larger overdoses may cause severe drowsiness, fits, low blood pressure, high or low body temperature, or shock. Notify your physician.

SPECIAL PRECAUTIONS

Be sure to tell your physician if:
▼ You have long-term liver or kidney problems.
▼ You have heart problems.
▼ You have porphyria.
▼ You have had epileptic fits.
▼ You have thyroid disease.
▼ You have Parkinson's disease.
▼ You have glaucoma.
▼ You are taking other medications.

Pregnancy
▼ Not usually prescribed. May cause lethargy in the baby during labour. Discuss with your physician.

Breast-feeding
▼ The drug passes into the breast milk and may affect the baby. Discuss with your physician.

Infants and children
▼ Not recommended.

Over 60
▼ Reduced dose necessary. Increased risk of late-appearing movement disorders or confusion.

Driving and hazardous work
▼ Avoid such activities until you have learned how flupentixol affects you because the drug can cause drowsiness and slowed reactions.

Alcohol
▼ Avoid. Flupentixol enhances the sedative effect of alcohol.

Surgery and general anesthetics
▼ Treatment may need to be stopped before you have any surgery. Discuss this with your physician or dentist.

POSSIBLE ADVERSE EFFECTS

The possible adverse effects of this drug are mainly the result of its anticholinergic action and its blocking action on the transmission of signals through the heart.

Symptom/effect	Frequency		Discuss with physician		Stop taking drug now	Call physician now
	Common	Rare	Only if severe	In all cases		
Blurred vision	●			■		
Weight gain	●		■			
Nausea	●		■			
Drowsiness	●		■			
Rapid heartbeat/palpitations	●			■		▮
Dizziness/fainting/confusion	●			■		▮
Parkinsonism/tremor	●			■		
Epileptic fits		●		■	▲	▮
Rash		●		■	▲	
Persistent infection/sore throat		●		■		
Jaundice		●		■	▲	

INTERACTIONS

Antiarrhythmic drugs Taken with these drugs, flupentixol may increase the risk of arrhythmias.

Anticholinergic drugs Flupentixol may increase the effects of these drugs.

Anticonvulsant drugs Flupentixol may reduce the effects of these drugs.

Sedatives Flupentixol enhances the effect of all sedative drugs.

PROLONGED USE

The risk of late-appearing movement disorders increases as treatment with flupentixol continues. Blood disorders, as well as *jaundice* and other liver disorders, are occasionally seen.

Monitoring Blood tests may be performed, particularly if there is persistent infection.

FLUTAMIDE

Product name Euflex
Used in the following combined preparations None

GENERAL INFORMATION

Flutamide is an anti-androgen drug used in the treatment of advanced prostate cancer, often in combination with drugs such as goserelin that control the production of the male sex hormones (androgens). Both drugs are effective because the cancer is dependent on androgens for its continued development. Treatment with goserelin-type drugs causes an initial increase in release of the hormone testosterone, leading to a growth spurt of the cancer ("tumour flare"), which

flutamide is prescribed to stop. Flutamide treatment is begun in combination with the goserelin-type drug. Flutamide is also used to treat prostate cancer when goserelin-type drugs are not prescribed.

Flutamide may discolour the urine amber or yellow-green, but this is harmless. However, you should always notify your physician straight away if your urine becomes dark coloured, because this may be an indication of liver damage.

INFORMATION FOR USERS

Your drug prescription is tailored for you. Do not alter dosage without checking with your physician.

How taken

Tablets.

Frequency and timing of doses
3 x daily, starting 3 days before the goserelin-type drug and continuing for 3 weeks.

Usual adult dosage range
250mg.

Onset of effect
1 hour.

Duration of action
8 hours.

Diet advice
None.

Storage
Keep in a closed container in a cool, dry place out of the reach of children.

Missed dose
Take as soon as you remember. If your next dose is due within 2 hours, take a single dose now and skip the next.

Stopping the drug
Do not stop taking the drug without consulting your physician because the condition may worsen rapidly.

Exceeding the dose
An occasional unintentional extra dose is unlikely to be a cause for concern. But if you notice any unusual symptoms, or if a large overdose has been taken, notify your physician.

SPECIAL PRECAUTIONS

Be sure to tell your physician if:
▼ You have heart problems.
▼ You have liver problems.
▼ You are taking other medications.

Pregnancy
▼ Not prescribed.

Breast-feeding
▼ Not prescribed.

Infants and children
▼ Not prescribed.

Over 60
▼ No special problems.

Driving and hazardous work
▼ Do not undertake such activities until you have learned how flutamide affects you because the drug can cause blurred vision and dizziness.

Alcohol
▼ No special problems, but excessive consumption should be avoided.

POSSIBLE ADVERSE EFFECTS

Nausea and tiredness are common. Breast swelling also occurs when the drug is given in an effective dose; this is usually reversible when treatment stops or dosage is reduced.

Symptom/effect	Frequency		Discuss with physician		Stop taking drug now	Call physician now
	Common	Rare	Only if severe	In all cases		
Breast swelling/tenderness	●		■			
Nausea/vomiting/diarrhea	●		■			
Insomnia/tiredness/headache	●		■			
Dizziness/blurred vision		●	■			
Skin reactions		●		■		
Jaundice/dark urine		●		■	▲	■

INTERACTIONS

Warfarin Flutamide increases the effect of this drug.

PROLONGED USE

Prolonged use of flutamide may cause liver damage. Because it is an anti-androgen, the drug also reduces sperm count.

Monitoring Periodic liver-function tests are usually performed.

FLUTICASONE

Product names Avamys, Flonase, Flovent
Used in the following combined preparation Advair

GENERAL INFORMATION

Fluticasone is a corticosteroid drug used to control inflammation in asthma and allergic rhinitis. Fluticasone does not produce relief immediately, so it is important to take the drug regularly. For allergic rhinitis, treatment with the nasal spray needs to begin two to three weeks before the hay fever season commences. People who suffer from asthma should take fluticasone regularly by inhaler in order to prevent attacks. Proper instruction is essential to ensure that the inhaler is used correctly.

There are few serious *adverse effects* associated with fluticasone because it is administered directly into the lungs (by the inhaler) or nasal mucosa (by the nasal spray). Fungal infection causing irritation of the mouth and throat is a possible side effect of the inhaled form but can be minimized by thoroughly rinsing the mouth and gargling with water after each inhalation.

QUICK REFERENCE

Drug group Corticosteroid (p.127)
Overdose danger rating Low
Dependence rating Low
Prescription needed Yes
Available as generic Yes

INFORMATION FOR USERS

Your drug prescription is tailored for you. Do not alter dosage without checking with your physician.

How taken

Inhaler, nasal spray.

Frequency and timing of doses
Allergic rhinitis 1–2 x daily; *asthma* 2 x daily.

Usual adult dosage range
Allergic rhinitis 2 sprays into each nostril; *asthma* 200–500mcg per day.

Onset of effect
4–7 days (asthma); 3–4 days (allergic rhinitis).

Duration of action
The effects can last for several days after stopping the drug.

Diet advice
None.

Storage
Keep in a cool, dry place out of the reach of children.

Missed dose
Take as soon as you remember.

Stopping the drug
Do not stop the drug without consulting your physician; symptoms may recur.

Exceeding the dose
An occasional unintentional extra dose is unlikely to be a cause for concern. Adverse effects may occur if the recommended dose is regularly exceeded over a prolonged period.

SPECIAL PRECAUTIONS

Be sure to tell your physician if:
▼ You have chronic sinusitis.
▼ You have had nasal ulcers or surgery.
▼ You have had tuberculosis or another respiratory infection.
▼ You are taking other medications.

Pregnancy
▼ Safety in pregnancy not established. Discuss with your physician.

Breast-feeding
▼ Safety in breast-feeding not established. However, fluticasone is unlikely to pass into breast milk. Discuss with your physician.

Infants and children
▼ Not recommended under 4 years. Reduced dose necessary in older children. For use in children 12 years and older, discuss with their physician.

Over 60
▼ No known problems.

Driving and hazardous work
▼ No known problems.

Alcohol
▼ No known problems.

POSSIBLE ADVERSE EFFECTS

Adverse effects are unlikely to occur. The main side effect is fungal infection of the throat and mouth (inhaler). This can be minimized by thoroughly rinsing the mouth, brushing the teeth, or gargling with water.

Symptom/effect	Frequency		Discuss with physician		Stop taking drug now	Call physician now
	Common	Rare	Only if severe	In all cases		
Nasal irritation	●		■			
Sore throat/mouth/hoarseness	●			■		
Taste/smell disturbances		●	■			
Nosebleeds		●		■		
Breathing difficulties		●		■		▮
Rash/facial swelling		●		■		▮

INTERACTIONS

None.

PROLONGED USE

Long-term use of high doses may, rarely, lead to suppression of adrenal gland function. Patients on long-term fluticasone should carry a steroid card or wear a Medic-alert bracelet.

Monitoring Periodic checks on adrenal gland function may be required if large doses are being taken.

FLUVOXAMINE

Product names Apo-Fluvoxamine, Dom-Fluvoxamine, Luvox, and others
Used in the following combined preparation None

GENERAL INFORMATION

Fluvoxamine belongs to the group of antidepressants called selective serotonin re-uptake inhibitors (SSRIs). These drugs tend to cause less sedation than older antidepressants such as amitriptyline (tricyclic antidepressants).

Fluvoxamine is indicated in the management of depression and obsessive-compulsive disorder. Like other SSRIs, it elevates mood, increases physical activity, and restores interest in the individual's usual activities.

QUICK REFERENCE

Drug group Antidepressant (p.68)
Overdose danger rating Medium
Dependence rating Low
Prescription needed Yes
Available as generic Yes

INFORMATION FOR USERS

Your drug prescription is tailored for you. Do not alter dosage without checking with your physician.

How taken

Tablets.

Frequency and timing of doses
Once daily.

Usual adult dosage range
Initial dose: 50mg at bedtime; may increase gradually as appropriate; maximum 300mg/day.

Onset of effect
The full benefits of fluvoxamine may not be felt for 4 weeks or more.

Duration of action
Up to 24 hours.

Diet advice
None.

Storage
Keep in a closed container in a cool, dry place out of the reach of children.

Missed dose
If you miss a dose, take it as soon as you remember. If it is near the time of the next dose, skip the missed dose and resume your usual dosing schedule. Do not take more than the total daily prescribed dose in a day.

Stopping the drug
Do not stop the drug without consulting your physician. This drug needs to be withdrawn gradually over several weeks to minimize the potential for withdrawal effects.

Exceeding the does
An occasional unintentional extra dose is unlikely to cause problems. For overdoses seek immediate medical advice and contact your physician right away. Take emergency action if seizures or loss of consciousness occurs. **See Drug poisoning emergency guide (p.526)**.

SPECIAL PRECAUTIONS

Be sure to tell your physician if:
▼ You have diabetes.
▼ You have seizure disorders or epilepsy.
▼ You or anyone else in your family has depression or obsessive compulsive disorder.
▼ You have a history of mania or hypomania.
▼ You have had seizures.
▼ You have liver or kidney disease.
▼ You have high blood pressure.
▼ You are taking medications that can affect bleeding.
▼ You are taking other medications.

Pregnancy
▼ Safety in pregnancy not established. Discuss with your physician.

Breast-feeding
▼ Safety not established. Discuss with your physician.

Infants and children
▼ Safety not established. Discuss risks and benefits with your physician.

Over 60
▼ A reduced dose may be necessary.

Driving and hazardous work
▼ Avoid such activities until you have learned how fluvoxamine affects you because the drug can cause drowsiness and can affect your judgment and coordination.

Alcohol
▼ No special problems.

POSSIBLE ADVERSE EFFECTS

The most common are nausea, headaches, upset stomach, sedation, small changes in heart rate or blood pressure, decrease in appetite. Rarely, may cause liver problems.

Symptom/effect	Frequency		Discuss with physician		Stop taking drug now	Call physician now
	Common	Rare	Only if severe	In all cases		
Tiredness	●		■			
Drowsiness	●		■			
Nausea	●		■			
Diarrhea		●		■		
Insomnia		●	■			
Tremor/agitation		●		■		
Constipation	●		■			
Headache	●		■			
Changes in sexual performance		●		■		
Mental/mood changes		●		■		■

INTERACTIONS

Grapefruit juice Can increase the level of fluvoxamine.

Tizanidine and Monoamine Oxidase Inhibitors (MAOIs) Fluvoxamine should not be used with these drugs. Fluvoxamine and MAOIs should not be used within 2 weeks of each other.

St. John's Wort, lithium, tryptophan Use with caution with fluvoxamine as there is a potential for interaction.

Anticoagulants Fluvoxamine can increase the effect of warfarin; may require dose adjustment.

PROLONGED USE

No problems expected.

FORMOTEROL

Product names Foradil, Oxeze Turbuhaler
Used in the following combined preparation Symbicort Turbuhaler

GENERAL INFORMATION

Formoterol is a long-acting sympathomimetic bronchodilator that relaxes the muscle surrounding the bronchioles (airways in the lungs).

This drug is used in the maintenance therapy (as a "preventer") of asthma, chronic bronchitis, and emphysema. A shorter-acting bronchodilator may be used for relief of acute symptoms. However, in those over 12 years of age, Oxeze can be used as a reliever for acute symptoms and for exercise-induced asthma.

Formoterol is used by inhalation and is very effective because the drug is delivered directly to the bronchioles, allowing for smaller doses and causing fewer side effects. The most common side effect is fine tremor of the hands. Anxiety, tension, and restlessness may also occur.

INFORMATION FOR USERS

Your drug prescription is tailored for you. Do not alter dosage without checking with your physician.

How taken

Powder in capsule for inhalation, metered dose inhaler.

Frequency and timing of doses
2 x daily.

Usual dosage range
Adults 1 puff or inhaled capsule (6mcg or 12mcg); daily maximum 48mcg.
Children 6–16 years 1 puff or inhaled capsule (6mcg or 12mcg); daily maximum 24mcg. Not recommended in children less than 6 years.

Onset of effect
1–3 minutes; peak at about 15 minutes.

Duration of action
12 hours.

Diet advice
None.

Storage
Keep in a cool, dry place out of the reach of children. Protect from light. Do not puncture or burn inhalers.

Missed dose
If you remember within 6 hours of the missed dose, take your usual dose as soon as possible, then go back to your regular schedule. If it is longer than 6 hours, just take your next dose on time.

Stopping the drug
Do not stop the drug without consulting your physician; symptoms may recur.

Exceeding the dose
An occasional unintentional extra dose is unlikely to be a cause for concern. But if you notice any unusual symptoms, or if a large overdose has been taken, notify your physician immediately.

SPECIAL PRECAUTIONS

Be sure to tell your physician if:
▼ You have heart problems.
▼ You have high blood pressure.
▼ You have had an overactive thyroid gland.
▼ You have diabetes.
▼ You are taking other medications.

 Pregnancy
▼ Safety in pregnancy not established. Discuss with your physician.

 Breast-feeding
▼ Safety in breast-feeding not established. Discuss with your physician.

 Infants and children
▼ Not recommended under 6 years.

 Over 60
▼ Increased likelihood of adverse effects. Reduced dose may therefore be necessary.

 Driving and hazardous work
▼ Avoid such activities until you have learned how formoterol affects you because the drug can cause some dizziness and tremors.

 Alcohol
▼ No known problems.

POSSIBLE ADVERSE EFFECTS

Muscle tremor, which particularly affects the hands, anxiety, and restlessness are the most common adverse effects. Palpitations and headaches are rare; should these occur, see your physician.

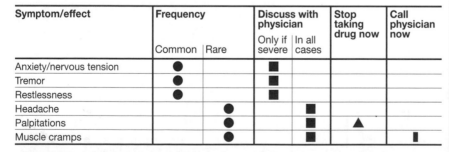

Symptom/effect	Frequency		Discuss with physician		Stop taking drug now	Call physician now
	Common	Rare	Only if severe	In all cases		
Anxiety/nervous tension	●		■			
Tremor	●		■			
Restlessness	●		■			
Headache		●		■		
Palpitations		●		■	▲	
Muscle cramps		●		■		▮

PROLONGED USE

No problems expected. However, you should contact your physician if you need to use higher doses than prescribed, or require 48mcg for 3 or more days, or if you feel that your short-acting bronchodilator is not as effective.

Monitoring Periodic blood tests for potassium may be needed in people on high-dose treatment with formoterol combined with other asthma drugs.

INTERACTIONS

Theophylline When taken with formoterol, there is a risk of low blood potassium level.

Other sympathomimetic drugs Increase the effects of formoterol, thereby also increasing the risk of adverse effects.

Beta blockers Drugs in this group may reduce the action of formoterol.

Monoamine Oxidase Inhibitors (MAOIs) Tranylcypromine, moclobemide, and phenelzine can interact with formoterol to cause a dangerous rise in blood pressure.

FUROSEMIDE

Product name Lasix
Used in the following combined preparations None

GENERAL INFORMATION

Furosemide is a powerful, short-acting loop diuretic that has been in use for over 20 years. Like other diuretics, it is used to treat edema (accumulation of fluid in tissue spaces) caused by heart failure, and certain lung, liver, and kidney disorders.

Because it is fast acting, furosemide is often used in emergencies to relieve pulmonary edema (fluid in the lungs).

Furosemide is particularly useful for people who have impaired kidney function because they do not respond well to thiazide diuretics (see p.85).

Furosemide increases potassium loss, which can produce a wide variety of symptoms. For this reason, potassium supplements or a potassium-sparing diuretic are often given with the drug.

QUICK REFERENCE

Drug group Loop diuretic (p.85) and antihypertensive drug (p.88)

Overdose danger rating Low

Dependence rating Low

Prescription needed Yes

Available as generic Yes

INFORMATION FOR USERS

Your drug prescription is tailored for you. Do not alter dosage without checking with your physician.

How taken

Tablets, liquid, injection.

Frequency and timing of doses
Once daily, usually in the morning; 4–6 x hourly (high dose therapy).

Usual adult dosage range
20–80mg daily. Dose may be increased to a maximum of 2g daily if kidney function is impaired.

Onset of effect
Within 1 hour (by mouth); within 5 minutes (by injection).

Duration of action
Up to 6 hours.

Diet advice
Use of this drug may reduce potassium in the body. Eat plenty of potassium-rich fresh fruits and vegetables, such as bananas and tomatoes.

Storage
Keep in a closed container in a cool, dry place out of the reach of children. Protect from light.

Missed dose
No cause for concern, but take as soon as you remember. However, if it is late in the day do not take the missed dose, or you may need to get up during the night to pass urine. Take the next scheduled dose as usual.

Stopping the drug
Do not stop the drug without consulting your physician; symptoms may recur.

Exceeding the dose
An occasional unintentional extra dose is unlikely to be a cause for concern. But if you notice any unusual symptoms, or if a large overdose has been taken, notify your physician.

POSSIBLE ADVERSE EFFECTS

Adverse effects are caused mainly by the rapid fluid loss produced by furosemide. These tend to diminish as the body adjusts to taking the drug. The disturbance in body salts and water balance can result in muscle cramps, headaches, and dizziness.

Symptom/effect	Frequency		Discuss with physician		Stop taking drug now	Call physician now
	Common	Rare	Only if severe	In all cases		
Dizziness/nausea	●		■			
Lethargy		●	■			
Noise in ears (high dose)		●	■			
Muscle cramps		●		■		
Rash/photosensitivity		●		■	▲	
Palpitations		●		■	▲	■

INTERACTIONS

Non-steroidal anti-inflammatory drugs (NSAIDs) Some of these drugs may reduce the diuretic effect of furosemide.

Lithium Furosemide may increase blood levels of lithium, leading to an increased risk of lithium poisoning.

Digoxin Loss of potassium may lead to digoxin *toxicity* when furosemide is taken with this drug.

Aminoglycoside antibiotics The risk of hearing and kidney problems may be increased when these drugs are taken with furosemide.

Angiotensin-converting enzyme inhibitors There is a risk of low blood pressure when these drugs are taken with furosemide.

SPECIAL PRECAUTIONS

Be sure to tell your physician if:
▼ You have long-term liver problems.
▼ You have gout.
▼ You have diabetes.
▼ You have previously had an allergic reaction to furosemide or sulfonamides.
▼ You have prostate trouble.
▼ If you are taking laxatives.
▼ You are taking other medications.

Pregnancy
▼ Safety in pregnancy not established. Discuss with your physician.

Breast-feeding
▼ The drug may reduce milk supply, but the amount in the milk is unlikely to affect the baby. Discuss with your physician.

Infants and children
▼ Reduced dose necessary.

Over 60
▼ Reduced dose may be necessary.

Driving and hazardous work
▼ Avoid such activities until you have learned how furosemide affects you because the drug may reduce mental alertness and cause dizziness.

Alcohol
▼ Keep consumption low. Furosemide increases the likelihood of dehydration and hangovers after the consumption of alcohol.

PROLONGED USE

Serious problems are unlikely, but levels of salts, such as potassium, sodium, and calcium, may become depleted. Low blood pressure, palpitations, headaches, problems passing urine, or muscle cramps may develop, particularly in the elderly.

Monitoring Periodic tests may be performed to check kidney function and levels of body salts.

GABAPENTIN

Product name Neurontin
Used in the following combined preparations None

GENERAL INFORMATION

Gabapentin is an antiepileptic drug (see Anticonvulsant drugs, p.70) used to treat partial seizures, and is often prescribed in combination with other drugs when a patient's epilepsy is not being satisfactorily controlled with the other drugs alone. Unlike some of the other antiepileptics, gabapentin does not require blood level monitoring. In addition, it does not have any interactions with the other anticonvulsant drugs.

Gabapentin has also been studied in relieving neuropathic pain, such as the pain suffered after shingles.

Patients with impaired kidney function should be given smaller doses, and diabetic patients taking gabapentin may notice fluctuations in their blood sugar levels.

INFORMATION FOR USERS

Your drug prescription is tailored for you. Do not alter dosage without checking with your physician.

How taken

Tablets, capsules.

Frequency and timing of doses
Twice daily initially, increasing to three times daily as maintenance treatment. No more than 12 hours should elapse between doses.

Usual adult dosage range
Epilepsy 900–1800mg daily; maintenance dose reached gradually over a few days. *Neuropathic pain* Maximum of 1800mg daily, reached gradually over a few days.

Onset of effect
The full antiepileptic effect may not be seen for 48 hours.

Duration of action
6–8 hours.

Diet advice
None.

Storage
Keep in a cool, dry place out of the reach of children.

Missed dose
Take as soon as you remember. If your next dose is due within 4 hours, take a dose now and skip the next.

Stopping the drug
Gabapentin should not be stopped abruptly. Gradual withdrawal over at least 7 days, in consultation with a physician, is advised to reduce the risk of seizures in epileptics.

Exceeding the dose
An occasional unintentional extra dose is unlikely to be a cause for concern. Large overdoses may cause dizziness, double vision, and slurred speech. Notify your physician.

SPECIAL PRECAUTIONS

Be sure to tell your physician if:
▼ You have a kidney problem.
▼ You have diabetes.
▼ You have a history of psychiatric illness.
▼ You are taking any other medications.

Pregnancy
▼ The drug is likely to reach the fetus and its effects are unknown. Discuss with your physician.

Breast-feeding
▼ The drug passes into the breast milk, and the effects on the baby are unknown. Discuss with your physician.

Infants and children
▼ Not recommended in children uner 6 years. Reduced doses based on body weight are required in children under 12 years.

Over 60
▼ Doses may have to be adjusted to allow for decreased kidney function.

Driving and hazardous work
▼ Avoid driving or hazardous work until you have learned how the drug affects you. Gabapentin may produce drowsiness or dizziness.

Alcohol
▼ Alcohol may increase the sedative effects of gabapentin.

POSSIBLE ADVERSE EFFECTS

The most common adverse effects of gabapentin are sleepiness and dizziness. Vision difficulties are less common, as are indigestion and weight gain. The most unusual adverse effect are mood changes and rash.

Symptom/effect	Frequency		Discuss with physician		Stop taking drug now	Call physician now
	Common	Rare	Only if severe	In all cases		
Drowsiness/dizziness/fatigue	●		■			
Muscle tremor	●			■		
Vision disturbances		●		■		
Indigestion		●		■		
Weight gain		●		■		
Mood changes/hallucinations		●		■		▮
Rash		●		■		▮

INTERACTIONS

Antacids containing aluminum or magnesium These may reduce the effect of gabapentin. The drug should not be taken within 2 hours of antacid preparations.

Urinary protein tests for diabetics
False-positive readings have been recorded with some tests. Special procedures are required for diabetics taking gabapentin.

PROLONGED USE

No problems expected.

GALANTAMINE

Product names Reminyl, Reminyl ER
Used in the following combined preparations None

GENERAL INFORMATION

Galantamine is an inhibitor of the enzyme cholinesterase, which breaks down the naturally occurring neurotransmitter acetylcholine to limit its effect. Blocking this raises the level of acetylcholine which, in the brain, increases alertness. Galantamine can improve the symptoms of mild to moderate dementia in Alzheimer's disease, and may slow the rate of deterioration. It is not currently recommended for dementia due to other causes. It is usual to assess those on the drug after three months to decide whether it is helping and if it should be continued. As the disease progresses, the benefit obtained may diminish.

Common side effects include change in appetite, drowsiness, agitation, and confusion, which can appear to be similar to Alzheimer's disease.

The starting dose in usually 8mg; this can then be gradually increased up to 24mg daily. Caregiver should be overseeing the taking of tablet(s).

QUICK REFERENCE

Drug group Drug for dementia (p.71)

Overdose danger rating Medium

Dependence rating Low

Prescription needed Yes

Available as generic No

INFORMATION FOR USERS

Your drug prescription is tailored for you. Do not alter dosage without checking with your physician.

How taken

Tablets, capsules.

Frequency and timing of doses
Twice daily (regular release tablets — RR); once daily (extended release capsules — ER).

Usual adult dosage range
Maintenance dose 16–24mg.

Onset of effect
1–3 hours (regular).

Duration of action
8–12 hours (RR tablets).

Up to 24 hours (ER capsules).

Diet advice
None.

Storage
Keep in a closed container in a cool, dry place out of the reach of children.

Missed dose
Take as soon as you remember. If your next regular tablet dose is within 4 hours, take a dose now and skip the next.

Stopping the drug
Do not stop taking the drug without consulting your physician; symptoms may recur.

Exceeding the dose
An occasional unintentional extra dose is unlikely to be a problem. Large overdoses may cause vomiting, diarrhea, and a low heart rate. Notify your physician.

SPECIAL PRECAUTIONS

Be sure to tell your physician if:
▼ You have a heart problem.
▼ You have liver or kidney problems.
▼ You have asthma or respiratory problems.
▼ You have had a gastric or duodenal ulcer.
▼ You have urinary incontinence or bladder problem.
▼ You are taking other medications.

Pregnancy
▼ Safety in pregnancy not established.

Breast-feeding
▼ Not recommended.

Infants and children
▼ Not recommended.

Over 60
▼ No special problems expected.

Driving and hazardous work
▼ Your underlying condition may make such activities inadvisable. Discuss with your physician.

Alcohol
▼ Avoid. Alcohol increases the sedative effects of galantamine.

POSSIBLE ADVERSE EFFECTS

Adverse effects include mental changes and intestinal problems. Although these are common, they are usually mild. However, women may be more susceptible to nausea, vomiting, and weight loss.

Symptom/effect	Frequency		Discuss with physician		Stop taking drug now	Call physician now
	Common	Rare	Only if severe	In all cases		
Nausea/vomiting	●			■		
Reduced appetite/ weight loss	●			■		
Tiredness	●		■			
Diarrhea		●		■		
Dizziness/drowsiness	●			■		
Headache	●		■			
Agitation/confusion/depression	●			■		
Low heart rate		●		■		
Convulsions		●		■		

INTERACTIONS

Anticholinergic medications
Cholinesterase inhibitors such as galantamine or rivastigmine may interfere with the activity of these anticholinergic agents, such as benztropine.

Ketoconazole, erythromycin, paroxetine, grapefruit juice These may increase the effect of galantamine and the dose of galantamine may need to be adjusted.

Muscle relaxants used in surgery
Galantamine may increase the effects of some muscle relaxants, but it may also block the effects of some others.

PROLONGED USE

May be continued for as long as there is benefit. Stopping the drug leads to a gradual loss of the improvements.

Monitoring Periodic checks may be performed to test whether the drug is still providing some benefit.

GATIFLOXACIN

Product name Zymar
Used in the following combined preparations None

GENERAL INFORMATION

Gatifloxacin, a quinolone antibiotic, is available as eye drops and is used in the treatment of bacterial conjunctivitis. To use the drops, wash your hands first, then tilt the head back and pull down the lower eyelid to form a pouch. Place a drop of the medication in the pouch. Close your eyes gently for about 30 seconds, without blinking. Do not touch the applicator tip to the eyelid as this can contaminate it.

Use the antibiotic for the full treatment period recommended by your physician, even if your eye starts to feel better. Do not wear contact lenses when you have a bacterial eye infection, until it is resolved.

INFORMATION FOR USERS

Your drug prescription is tailored for you. Do not alter dosage without checking with your physician.

How taken

Eye drops.

Frequency and timing of doses
4–8 times daily.

Usual adult dosage range
Usually for days 1 and 2, one drop every 2 hours while awake, up to 8 times daily. On days 3 to 7, one drop four times daily, spaced evenly apart.

Onset of effect
Within 48 hours.

Duration of action
2–4 hours.

Diet advice
None.

Storage
Store between 15°C and 25°C. Do not freeze. Discard container 28 days after opening.

Missed dose
If you miss a dose, apply it as soon as you remember. If it is near the time of the next dose, skip the missed dose and resume your usual dosing schedule.

Stopping the drug
Take the full course. Even if you feel better, the original infection may still be present, and symptoms may recur if treatment is stopped too soon.

Exceeding the dose
An occasional unintentional extra dose is unlikely to be a cause for concern. If too many drops are used accidentally, the eye can be flushed with warm water. If you notice any unusual symptoms, notify your physician.

SPECIAL PRECAUTIONS

Be sure to tell your physician if:
▼ You have allergy to quinolone antibiotics or any other medications.
▼ You wear contact lenses.
▼ You are using any other eye drops.
▼ You are taking other medications.

Pregnancy
▼ Safety in pregnancy not established. Discuss with your physician.

Breast-feeding
▼ Safety not established. Discuss with your physician.

Infants and children
▼ Not recommended in children less than one year of age. Limited experience in children.

Over 60
▼ No specific problems.

Driving and hazardous work
▼ Avoid such activities until you have learned how the eye drops affect your vision.

Alcohol
▼ No special problems.

POSSIBLE ADVERSE EFFECTS

The most frequently reported symptoms include eye irritation and dry eyes.

Symptom/effect	Frequency		Discuss with physician		Stop taking drug now	Call physician now
	Common	Rare	Only if severe	In all cases		
Eye irritation/dryness	●		■			
Increased tearing	●		■			
Changes in vision		●		■		▮
Swelling or redness of eye		●		■		
Redness of the skin or hives		●			▲	▮
Unusual aftertaste	●		■			
Runny nose		●	■			
Sore throat		●	■			
Headache		●		■		
Eye pain		●		■		

INTERACTIONS

Specific interactions with gatifloxacin eye drops have not been studied.

PROLONGED USE

This medication is usually applied for a short duration of therapy.

GEMFIBROZIL

Product names Apo-Gemfibrozil, Lopid, Novo-Gemfibrozil, Nu-Gemfibrozil, and others
Used in the following combined preparations None

GENERAL INFORMATION

Gemfibrozil belongs to a group of drugs, usually called fibrates, that lower lipid levels in the blood. Fibrates are particularly effective in decreasing triglyceride levels in the blood. They also reduce blood levels of cholesterol. Raised levels of lipids (fats) in the blood are associated with atherosclerosis (deposition of fat in blood vessel walls).

This can lead to coronary heart disease (for example, angina and heart attacks) and cerebrovascular disease (for example, stroke). When gemfibrozil is taken with a diet low in saturated fats, there is some evidence that the risk of coronary heart disease is reduced.

INFORMATION FOR USERS

Your drug prescription is tailored for you. Do not alter dosage without checking with your physician.

How taken

Tablets, capsules.

Frequency and timing of doses
Twice daily, 30 minutes before morning and evening meals.

Usual adult dosage range
1200mg.

Onset of effect
See onset of effect in 2–5 days; may take up to 4 weeks to see maximum benefit.

Duration of action
3–6 hours.

Diet advice
A low-fat diet is usually recommended.

Storage
Keep in a closed container in a cool, dry place out of the reach of children.

Missed dose
If you miss a dose, take it as soon as you remember. If it is near the time of the next dose, skip the missed dose and resume your usual dosing schedule. Do not double up to catch up on a missed dose.

Stopping the drug
Do not stop the drug without consulting your physician. Stopping the drug may lead to worsening of the underlying condition.

Exceeding the dose
An occasional unintentional extra dose is unlikely to cause problems. Large overdoses may cause liver problems. Notify your physician and seek medical assistance right away.

SPECIAL PRECAUTIONS

Be sure to tell your physician if:
▼ You have liver or kidney problems.
▼ You have muscle weakness.
▼ You have angina or other heart disease.
▼ You have high blood pressure.
▼ You are taking other medications.

 Pregnancy
▼ Safety not established. Discuss with your physician.

 Breast-feeding
▼ Safety not established. Discuss with your physician.

 Infants and children
▼ Not usually prescribed.

 Over 60
▼ No special problems expected.

 Driving and hazardous work
▼ No known problems.

 Alcohol
▼ No known problems.

POSSIBLE ADVERSE EFFECTS

The common adverse effects are those on the gastrointestinal tract, such as loss of appetite and nausea. These effects normally diminish as treatment continues.

Symptom/effect	Frequency		Discuss with physician		Stop taking drug now	Call physician now
	Common	Rare	Only if severe	In all cases		
Nausea	●		■			
Vomiting		●		■		
Loss of appetite	●		■			
Abdominal pain	●		■			
Epigastric pain	●		■			
Headache		●		■		
Skin rash		●		■		
Muscle pain/cramp		●		■		
Dizziness/fatigue		●		■		

PROLONGED USE

No problems expected, but patients with kidney disease will need special care as there is a high risk of developing muscle problems.

Monitoring Blood tests will be performed occasionally to monitor the effect of the drug on lipids in the blood, and to periodically measure kidney and liver function.

INTERACTIONS

Anticoagulants Gemfibrozil may increase the effect of anticoagulants such as warfarin. Dosage adjustment may be needed.

Pravastatin, atorvastatin, simvastatin, and other lipid-lowering drugs belonging to 'statins' There is an increased risk of muscle damage if gemfibrozil is taken with these drugs.

Cholestyramine, colestipol May decrease absorption of gemfibrozil. Take two hours apart.

Repaglinide Gemfibrozil can increase the effect of repaglinide.

Amlodipine, verapamil, carvedilol, losartan, phenytoin, diazepam, tolbutamide Gemfibrozil may increase the effect of these drugs.

GENTAMICIN

Product name Garamycin
Used in the following combined preparations Garasone, Valisone-G

GENERAL INFORMATION

Gentamicin is one of the aminoglycoside antibiotics. The injectable form is usually reserved for hospital treatment of serious infections. These include lung, urinary tract, bone, joint, and wound infections, as well as peritonitis, septicemia, and meningitis. This form is also used together with a penicillin for prevention and treatment of heart valve infections (endocarditis).

In the form of drops, gentamicin is used to treat eye and ear infections.

Gentamicin given by injection can have serious *adverse effects* on the ears and the kidneys. Damage to the ears may lead to deafness and problems with the balance mechanism in the inner ear. Courses of treatment are, therefore, limited to seven days when this is possible. Treatment is monitored with particular care when high doses are needed or kidney function is poor.

QUICK REFERENCE

Drug group Aminoglycoside antibiotic (p.114)
Overdose danger rating Low
Dependence rating Low
Prescription needed Yes
Available as generic Yes

INFORMATION FOR USERS

Your drug prescription is tailored for you. Do not alter dosage without checking with your physician.

How taken

Injection, eye and ear drops.

Frequency and timing of doses
1–3 x daily (injection); 3–4 x daily or as directed (ear drops); every 2 hours or as directed (eye drops).

Usual adult dosage range
According to condition and response (injection); according to your physician's instructions (eye and ear drops).

Onset of effect
Within 1–2 hours.

Duration of action
8–12 hours.

Diet advice
None.

Storage
Keep in closed container in a cool, dry place out of the reach of children.

Missed dose
Apply eye and ear preparations as soon as you remember.

Stopping the drug
Complete the course. Even if you feel better, the original infection may still be present and may recur if treatment is stopped too soon.

Exceeding the dose
Although overdose by injection is dangerous, it is unlikely because treatment is carefully monitored. For other preparations of the drug, an occasional unintentional extra dose is unlikely to cause concern. But if you notice any unusual symptoms, notify your physician.

SPECIAL PRECAUTIONS

Be sure to tell your physician if:
▼ You have a long-term kidney problem.
▼ You have a hearing disorder.
▼ You have myasthenia gravis.
▼ You have Parkinson's disease.
▼ You have previously had an allergic reaction to aminoglycosides.
▼ You are taking other medications.

Pregnancy
▼ No evidence of risk with eye or ear drops. Injections are not prescribed, as they may cause hearing defects in the baby. Discuss with your physician.

Breast-feeding
▼ No evidence of risk with eye or ear preparations. Given by injection, the drug may pass into the breast milk. Discuss with your physician.

Infants and children
▼ Reduced dose necessary for injections.

Over 60
▼ Increased likelihood of adverse effects. Reduced dose may therefore be necessary.

Driving and hazardous work
▼ No known problems from preparations for the eye or ear.

Alcohol
▼ No known problems.

POSSIBLE ADVERSE EFFECTS

Adverse effects are rare but those that occur with the injectable form of gentamicin may be serious. Dizziness, loss of balance (vertigo), impaired hearing, and changes in the urine should be reported promptly. Allergic reactions, including rash and itching, may occur with all preparations that contain gentamicin. Blurred vision or eye irritation may occur with the eye preparations and should be reported to your physician.

Symptom/effect	Frequency		Discuss with physician		Stop taking drug now	Call physician now
	Common	Rare	Only if severe	In all cases		
Nausea/vomiting		●	■			
Dizziness/vertigo		●		■	▲	❘
Rash/itching		●		■	▲	❘
Ringing in the ears		●		■	▲	❘
Loss of hearing		●		■	▲	❘
Bloody/cloudy urine		●		■	▲	❘

INTERACTIONS

General note A range of drugs, including furosemide, vancomycin, amphotericin B, and cephalosporins, increase the risk of hearing loss and/or kidney failure with gentamicin given by injection.

PROLONGED USE

Not usually given for longer than seven days. When given by injection, there is a risk of adverse effects on hearing and balance.

Monitoring Blood levels of the drug are usually checked if it is given by injection. Tests on kidney function are also usually carried out.

GLICLAZIDE

Product names Apo-Gliclazide, Diamicron, Diamicron MR, Novo-Gliclazide
Used in the following combined preparations None

GENERAL INFORMATION

Gliclazide is an oral antidiabetic drug belonging to the sulfonylurea group. It stimulates the production and secretion of insulin from the islet cells in the pancreas. This promotes the uptake of sugar into body cells thereby lowering the level of sugar in the blood.

The drug is used to treat adult (maturity-onset) diabetes mellitus, in conjunction with a diabetic diet low in carbohydrates and fats

In conditions of severe illness, injury, stress, or surgery, the drug may lose its effectiveness necessitating the use of insulin injections. *Adverse effects* of gliclazide are generally mild. However, symptoms of poor diabetic control will occur if the dosage is not appropriate.

QUICK REFERENCE

Drug group Oral antidiabetic drug (p.128)

Overdose danger rating High

Dependence rating Low

Prescription needed Yes

Available as generic Yes

INFORMATION FOR USERS

Your drug prescription is tailored for you. Do not alter dosage without checking with your physician.

How taken

Tablets, MR-tablets.

Frequency and timing of doses
1–2 x daily (in the morning and evening with a meal).

Usual dosage range
40–320mg daily (doses above 160mg are divided into two doses).

Onset of effect
Within 1 hour.

Duration of action
12–24 hours.

Diet advice
An individual low-fat, low-carbohydrate diet must be maintained for the drug to be fully effective. Follow the advice of your physician.

Storage
Keep in a closed container in a cool, dry place out of the reach of children.

Missed dose
Take with next meal; do not double the dose to account for missed dose.

Stopping the drug
Do not stop the drug without consulting your physician; stopping the drug may lead to worsening of the underlying condition.

OVERDOSE ACTION

 Seek immediate medical advice in all cases. If early warning symptoms of excessively low blood sugar such as fainting, sweating, trembling, confusion, or headache occur, eat or drink something sugary at once. Take emergency action if fits or loss of consciousness occur.

See Drug poisoning emergency guide (p.526).

SPECIAL PRECAUTIONS

Be sure to tell your physician if:
▼ You have long-term liver or kidney problems.
▼ You are allergic to sulfonylurea drugs.
▼ You have thyroid problems.
▼ You have porphyria.
▼ You have ever had problems with your adrenal glands.
▼ You are taking other medications.

 Pregnancy
▼ Not recommended. May cause abnormally low blood sugar in the newborn baby. Insulin is generally substituted in pregnancy because it gives better diabetic control.

 Breast-feeding
▼ The drug passes into the breast milk. Discuss with your physician.

 Infants and children
▼ Not prescribed.

 Over 60
▼ Signs of low blood sugar may be more difficult to recognize. Reduced dose may be necessary.

 Driving and hazardous work
▼ Avoid such activities until you have learned how gliclazide affects you because it can cause dizziness, drowsiness, and confusion. Avoid these activities if you have warning signs of low blood pressure.

 Alcohol
▼ Avoid. Alcoholic drinks may upset diabetic control increasing the risk of hypoglycemia.

Surgery and general anesthetics
▼ Notify your physician or dentist that you are diabetic before undergoing any type of surgery.

POSSIBLE ADVERSE EFFECTS

Serious adverse effects are rare. Dizziness, confusion, tremors, sweating, and weakness may be signs of low blood sugar due to lack of food or too high a dose of gliclazide.

Symptom/effect	Frequency		Discuss with physician		Stop taking drug now	Call physician now
	Common	Rare	Only if severe	In all cases		
Faintness/confusion	●			■		
Weakness/tremor	●			■		
Sweating	●			■		
Constipation/diarrhea	●		■			
Nausea/vomiting		●		■		
Rash/itching		●		■		
Jaundice		●		■		■
Weight changes		●				

INTERACTIONS

General note A variety of drugs may reduce the effect of gliclazide and so may raise blood sugar levels. These include corticosteroids, estrogens, diuretics, and rifampin. Other drugs increase the risk of low blood sugar. These include warfarin, sulfonamides and other antibacterials, ASA, beta blockers, ACE inhibitors, and antifungals, particularly miconazole.

PROLONGED USE

No problems expected.

Monitoring Regular testing of sugar levels in the blood and urine is required. Periodic assessment of the eyes, heart, and kidneys may also be advised.

GLIMEPIRIDE

Product names Amaryl, Apo-Glimepiride, Co-Glimepiride, Novo-Glimepiride, Ratio-Glimepiride, Sandoz Glimepiride
Used in the following combined preparations Avandaryl (rosiglitazone + glimepiride)

GENERAL INFORMATION

Glimepiride is an oral antidiabetic drug belonging to the sulfonylurea class. Like other drugs in this class, glimepiride stimulates insulin secretion from the islets cells in the pancreas. This allows for the uptake of glucose (sugar) into the cells of the body, thereby lowering blood glucose. This drug is used in Type 2 or typically maturity-onset diabetes mellitus, in conjunction with a diabetic diet low in carbohydrates and fats. Glimepiride is a long-acting drug, which can be administered once daily.

QUICK REFERENCE

Drug group Oral antidiabetic (p.129)
Overdose danger rating High
Dependence rating Low
Prescription needed Yes
Available as generic Yes

INFORMATION FOR USERS

Your drug prescription is tailored for you. Do not alter dosage without checking with your physician.

How taken

Tablets.

Frequency and timing of doses
Once daily.

Usual adult dosage range
1–8mg daily.

Onset of effect
1–3 hours.

Duration of action
24 hours.

Diet advice
A low carbohydrate, low fat diet. Follow the advice of your physician.

Storage
Keep in a closed container in a cool, dry place out of the reach of children.

Missed dose
If you miss a dose, take it as soon as you remember it. If it is time for a snack, take the medication with the snack. If it is near the time for the next dose, skip the missed dose and resume your usual dosing schedule. Do not double up to catch up on a missed dose.

Stopping the drug
Do not stop the drug without consulting your physician. Stopping the drug may lead to worsening of the underlying condition.

OVERDOSE ACTION

Seek immediate medical advice in all cases. If any early warning symptoms of excessively low blood sugar occur, eat or drink something containing sugar, e.g., 1tbsp of sugar dissolved in water or ¾ cup of juice or regular (not diet) soft drink. Take emergency action and dial 911 if seizures (fits) or loss of consciousness occur.

See Drug poisoning emergency guide (p.526).

SPECIAL PRECAUTIONS

Be sure to tell your physician if:
▼ You have liver disease.
▼ You had or have had kidney disease.
▼ You had or have had ketoacidosis.
▼ You have had problems with alcohol abuse.
▼ You are taking other medications.

Pregnancy
▼ Safety in pregnancy not established. Discuss with your physician.

Breast-feeding
▼ Not recommended. Discuss with your physician.

Infants and children
▼ Not prescribed.

Over 60
▼ No special problems.

Driving and hazardous work
▼ Usually no problems. Avoid these activities if you have warning signs of low blood sugar.

Alcohol
▼ Avoid. Alcoholic drinks may upset diabetic control, increasing the risk of hypoglycemia.

PROLONGED USE

No problems expected.

Monitoring Regular monitoring of blood glucose in blood and urine is needed. Periodic assessment of the eyes, heart, and kidneys is also advised.

POSSIBLE ADVERSE EFFECTS

This drug is generally well tolerated. The most common adverse effects include weight gain and the risk of hypoglycemia. The risk for these is lower than with other drugs in this class.

Symptom/effect	Frequency		Discuss with physician		Stop taking drug now	Call physician now
	Common	Rare	Only if severe	In all cases		
Weight gain	●		■			
Light headedness/confusion		●		■		▮
Headache/dizziness	●		■			
Weakness/tremor		●		■		▮
Sweating		●		■		▮
Constipation or diarrhea	●		■			
Nausea	●		■			
Rash/itching		●		■		
Jaundice		●		■		▮

INTERACTIONS

General note A variety of drugs may reduce the effect of glimepiride and may raise blood glucose levels. These include corticosteroids, estrogens, diuretics, and rifampin. Other drugs, including sulfonamides and other antibacterials, antifungals, ASA, warfarin, ACE inhibitors, and beta-blockers, increase the risk of low blood glucose.

GLYBURIDE

Product names Diabeta, Euglucon, Gen Glybe, Med Glybe, Penta-Glyburide, Riva-Glyburide, Rhoxal-Glyburide, and others
Used in the following combined preparations None

GENERAL INFORMATION

Glyburide is an oral antidiabetic drug belonging to the sulfonylurea class. Like other drugs of this type, glyburide stimulates the production and secretion of insulin from the islet cells in the pancreas. This promotes the uptake of sugar into body cells, thereby lowering the level of sugar in the blood.

This drug is used in the treatment of adult (maturity-onset) diabetes mellitus, in conjunction with a diabetic diet low in carbohydrates and fats.

In conditions of severe illness, injury, or stress, glyburide may lose its effectiveness, making insulin injections necessary. *Adverse effects* are generally mild. Symptoms of poor diabetic control will occur if the dosage of glyburide is not appropriate.

QUICK REFERENCE

Drug group Oral antidiabetic drug (p.128)

Overdose danger rating High

Dependence rating Low

Prescription needed Yes

Available as generic Yes

INFORMATION FOR USERS

Your drug prescription is tailored for you. Do not alter dosage without checking with your physician.

How taken

Tablets.

Frequency and timing of doses
Once daily in the morning with breakfast.

Usual adult dosage range
5–15mg daily.

Onset of effect
Within 3 hours.

Duration of action
10–15 hours.

Diet advice
A low-carbohydrate, low-fat diet must be maintained in order for the drug to be fully effective. Follow the advice of your physician.

Storage
Keep in a closed container in a cool, dry place out of the reach of children. Protect from light.

Missed dose
Take with next meal; do not double the dose to account for missed dose.

Stopping the drug
Do not stop the drug without consulting your physician; stopping the drug may lead to worsening of your diabetes.

OVERDOSE ACTION

Seek immediate medical advice in all cases. If any early warning symptoms of excessively low blood sugar (such as fainting, sweating, trembling, confusion, or headache) occur, eat or drink something sugary. Take emergency action if fits or loss of consciousness occur.

See Drug poisoning emergency guide (p.526).

POSSIBLE ADVERSE EFFECTS

Serious adverse effects are rare. More common symptoms, often accompanied by hunger, may be signs of low blood sugar due to lack of food or too high a dose of the drug.

Symptom/effect	Frequency		Discuss with physician		Stop taking drug now	Call physician now
	Common	Rare	Only if severe	In all cases		
Faintness/confusion		●		■		●
Weakness/tremor	●			■		
Sweating	●			■		
Constipation/diarrhea	●		■			
Nausea/vomiting		●		■		
Rash/itching		●		■		
Jaundice		●		■		■
Weight changes		●		■		

INTERACTIONS

General note A variety of drugs may reduce the effect of glyburide and so may raise blood sugar levels. These include corticosteroids, estrogens, diuretics, and rifampin. Other drugs increase the risk of low blood sugar. These include warfarin, sulfonamides and other antibacterials, antifungals, ASA, beta blockers, and ACE inhibitors.

SPECIAL PRECAUTIONS

Be sure to tell your physician if:
▼ You have long-term liver or kidney problems.
▼ You are allergic to sulfonylurea drugs.
▼ You have thyroid problems.
▼ You have porphyria.
▼ You have ever had problems with your adrenal glands.
▼ You are taking other medications.

 Pregnancy
▼ Not usually prescribed. Insulin is generally substituted in pregnancy because it gives better diabetic control.

 Breast-feeding
▼ The drug passes into the breast milk. Discuss with your physician.

 Infants and children
▼ Not prescribed.

 Over 60
▼ Reduced dose may be necessary. Greater likelihood of low blood sugar exists when glyburide is used.

 Driving and hazardous work
▼ Usually no problems. Avoid these activities if you have warning signs of low blood sugar.

 Alcohol
▼ Avoid. Alcoholic drinks may upset diabetic control increasing the risk of hypoglycemia.

Surgery and general anesthetics
▼ Notify your physician or dentist that you are diabetic before undergoing any type of surgery.

PROLONGED USE

No problems expected.

Monitoring Regular monitoring of levels of sugar in the blood and urine is needed. Periodic assessment of the eyes, heart, and kidneys may also be advised.

GONADOTROPIN CHORIONIC

Product names Pregnyl, Profasi HP
Used in the following combined preparations None

GENERAL INFORMATION

Produced by the placenta, human chorionic gonadotropin (hCG) is a hormone that stimulates the ovaries to produce two other hormones, estrogen and progesterone, that are essential to the conception and early growth of the fetus. The hormone is extracted from the urine of pregnant women and has several medical purposes.

Its principal value is in the treatment of female infertility. Given by injection, usually with another hormone, hCG encourages the ovaries to release an egg (known as ovulation) so that it can be fertilized. Ovulation usually occurs 18 hours after injection, and intercourse should follow within 48 hours. The likelihood of multiple births increases because several eggs may be released by the ovaries at once.

In rare cases chorionic gonadotropin is also given to young boys to treat undescended testes.

The drug is occasionally given to men to improve sperm production; treatment may take as long as six to nine months.

QUICK REFERENCE

Drug group Drug for infertility (p.152)

Overdose danger rating Low

Dependence rating Low

Prescription needed Yes

Available as generic No

INFORMATION FOR USERS

This drug is given only under medical supervision and is not for self-administration.

How taken

Injection.

Frequency and timing of doses
1–3 x per week.

Usual dosage range
Dosage varies from person to person, and may need adjustment during treatment.

Onset of effect
1–8 days (female infertility); 6–9 months (male infertility).

Duration of action
2–3 days.

Diet advice
None.

Storage
Not applicable. This drug is not kept in the home.

Missed dose
Arrange to receive the missed dose as soon as possible. Delay of more than 24 hours may reduce the chance of conception.

Stopping the drug
Complete the course of treatment as directed. Stopping the drug prematurely will reduce the chance of conception.

Exceeding the dose
The drug is always injected under close medical supervision. Overdose is unlikely.

SPECIAL PRECAUTIONS

Be sure to tell your physician if:
▼ You have a long-term kidney problem.
▼ You have asthma.
▼ You have had epileptic fits.
▼ You suffer from migraine.
▼ You have a heart disorder.
▼ You have had a previous allergic reaction to this drug.
▼ You have prostate trouble.
▼ You are taking other medications.

Pregnancy
▼ Not prescribed.

Breast feeding
▼ Not prescribed.

Infants and children
▼ hCG is safely prescribed to treat undescended testes in boys.

Over 60
▼ Not usually required.

Driving and hazardous work
▼ Avoid such activities until you have learned how hCG affects you because the drug can cause tiredness.

Alcohol
▼ Avoid excessive amounts. Alcohol increases tiredness and, if taken in excess, may reduce fertility.

POSSIBLE ADVERSE EFFECTS

When taken for fertility problems, the more common *adverse effects* of hCG are rarely severe and tend to diminish with time.

Women who take large doses of the drug may experience abdominal pain or swelling due to overstimulation of the ovaries.

Symptom/effect	Frequency		Discuss with physician		Stop taking drug now	Call physician now
	Common	Rare	Only if severe	In all cases		
Headache/tiredness	●		■			
Pain at injection site	●		■			
Mood changes	●			■		
Women only						
Abdominal pain		●		■		
Men only						
Enlarged breasts		●		■	▲	
Swollen feet/ankles		●		■		

INTERACTIONS

None.

PROLONGED USE

No special problems.

Monitoring Women taking hCG to improve fertility usually have regular pelvic examinations and checks on cervical mucus to confirm that ovulation is taking place. Men are given regular sperm counts.

GOSERELIN

Product names Zoladex, Zoladex LA
Used in the following combined preparations None

GENERAL INFORMATION

Goserelin is a synthetic drug chemically related to the hormone gonadorelin. Like gonadorelin, it stimulates the release of other hormones from the pituitary gland, which in turn control production of the sex hormones.

Goserelin is used to suppress the production of sex hormones in breast and prostate cancer. At the start of treatment for prostate cancer, it is often given with an anti-androgen drug (see p.132) to control an initial growth spurt of the tumour – known as 'tumour flare'.

The drug is also used in the management of fibroids, infertility, and endometriosis. The first dose is normally given during menstruation to avoid the possibility that the patient may be pregnant. It is advisable for women of childbearing age to use barrier methods of contraception during treatment.

Loss of bone density is an important *side effect* in women.Therefore, repeat courses of of the drug are given only for cancerous conditions.

INFORMATION FOR USERS

Your drug prescription is tailored for you. Do not alter dosage without checking with your physician.

How taken

Implant injection, long-acting implant injection.

Frequency and timing of doses
Endometriosis Every 28 days, maximum of a single 6-month treatment course only (implant).
Fibroids Implant every 28 days, maximum 3 months' treatment.
Breast and prostate cancer Every 28 days.
Prostate cancer Every 12 weeks (LA implant).

Usual adult dosage range
3.6mg every 28 days (endometriosis/fibroids/breast cancer); 10.8mg every 3 months (prostate).

Onset of effect
Within 24 hours (endometriosis/fibroids/breast cancer);
1–2 weeks after tumour flare (prostate).

Duration of action
28 days (implant); 12 weeks (long-acting implant).

Diet advice
None.

Storage
Not applicable. The drug is not kept in the home.

Missed dose
No cause for concern. Treatment can be resumed when possible.

Stopping the drug
Do not stop treatment without consulting your physician.

Exceeding the dose
Overdosage is unlikely since treatment is not self-administered.

SPECIAL PRECAUTIONS

Be sure to tell your physician if:
▼ You have osteoporosis.
▼ You have previously been treated with goserelin (or another gonadorelin analogue) for endometriosis or fibroids.
▼ You have polycystic ovarian disease.
▼ You are allergic to gonadorelin analogues.
▼ You are taking other medications.

Pregnancy
▼ Not prescribed.

Breast-feeding
▼ Not recommended. Discuss with your physician.

Infants and children
▼ Not recommended.

Over 60
▼ No special problems.

Driving and hazardous work
▼ No special problems.

Alcohol
▼ No special problems.

POSSIBLE ADVERSE EFFECTS

Symptoms similar to those of the menopause, such as hot flushes and changes in breast size are common. Rare adverse effects should be reported to your physician straight away.

Symptom/effect	Frequency		Discuss with physician		Stop taking drug now	Call physician now
	Common	Rare	Only if severe	In all cases		
Hot flushes	●		■			
Headache	●		■			
Bleeding on stopping drug	●		■			
Rash/wheezing		●		■		▮
Reaction at injection site		●		■		
Ovarian cysts		●		■		
Dizziness/fainting		●		■		

INTERACTIONS

None.

PROLONGED USE

Goserelin is only used in the long term for treatment of prostate or breast cancer. Bone density is lost over time in women taking the drug, but this may be partly recoverable once treatment stops.

Monitoring Women are usually monitored for changes in bone density.

HALOPERIDOL

Product names Apo-Haloperidol, Novo-Peridol, and others
Used in the following combined preparations None

GENERAL INFORMATION

First introduced in the 1960s, haloperidol is used to reduce the violent, aggressive manifestations of mental illnesses such as schizophrenia, mania, dementia, and other disorders in which hallucinations are experienced. It does not cure the underlying mental disorder but is used to relieve the distressing symptoms.

Haloperidol is also used in the control of Tourette's syndrome and may be of benefit in children who have severe behavioural problems for which other drugs are ineffective.

The main drawback of haloperidol is that it produces the disturbing *side effect* of abnormal, involuntary movements and stiffness of the face and limbs.

QUICK REFERENCE

Drug group Butyrophenone antipsychotic drug (p.69)

Overdose danger rating Medium

Dependence rating Low

Prescription needed Yes

Available as generic Yes

INFORMATION FOR USERS

Your drug prescription is tailored for you. Do not alter dosage without checking with your physician.

How taken

Tablets, liquid, injection, *depot* injection.

Frequency and timing of doses
1–3 x daily.

Usual adult dosage range
Schizophrenia 1.5–3mg daily initially, up to a maximum of 20mg daily.

Onset of effect
2–3 hours (by mouth); 20–30 minutes (by injection).

Duration of action
6–24 hours (by mouth); 2–4 hours (injection); up to 4 weeks (depot injection).

Diet advice
None.

Storage
Keep in a closed container in a cool, dry place out of the reach of children.

Missed dose
Take as soon as you remember. If your next dose is due within 3 hours, take a single dose now and skip the next.

Stopping the drug
Do not stop the drug without consulting your physician; symptoms may recur.

Exceeding the dose
An occasional unintentional extra dose is unlikely to cause problems. Larger overdoses may cause unusual drowsiness, muscle weakness or rigidity, and/or faintness. Notify your physician.

SPECIAL PRECAUTIONS

Be sure to tell your physician if:
▼ You have long-term liver or kidney problems.
▼ You have heart or circulation problems.
▼ You have had epileptic fits.
▼ You have an overactive thyroid gland.
▼ You have Parkinson's disease.
▼ You have had glaucoma.
▼ You have asthma, bronchitis, or another lung disorder.
▼ You have ever had pheochromocytoma.
▼ You are taking other medications.

Pregnancy
▼ Safety in pregnancy not established. Discuss with your physician.

Breast-feeding
▼ The drug passes into the breast milk and may affect the baby. Discuss with your physician.

Infants and children
▼ Rarely required. Reduced dose necessary.

Over 60
▼ Reduced dose may be necessary.

Driving and hazardous work
▼ Avoid such activities until you have learned how haloperidol affects you because the drug may cause drowsiness and slowed reactions.

Alcohol
▼ Avoid. Alcohol may increase the sedative effect of this drug.

POSSIBLE ADVERSE EFFECTS

Haloperidol can cause a variety of minor *anticholinergic* symptoms that often become less marked with time. The most significant adverse effect, abnormal movements of the face and limbs (parkinsonism), may be controlled by dosage adjustment.

Symptom/effect	Frequency		Discuss with physician		Stop taking drug now	Call physician now
	Common	Rare	Only if severe	In all cases		
Drowsiness/lethargy	●		■			
Loss of appetite	●		■			
Parkinsonism	●			■		
Dizziness/fainting		●		■		
Rash		●		■	▲	
High fever/confusion		●		■	▲	▮

INTERACTIONS

Sedatives *Sedatives* are likely to increase the sedative properties of haloperidol.

Rifampin and anticonvulsant drugs These drugs may reduce the effects of haloperidol, the dosage of which may need to be increased.

Lithium This drug may increase the risk of parkinsonism and effects on the nerves.

Methyldopa This drug may increase the risk of parkinsonism and low blood pressure.

Anticholinergic drugs Haloperidol may increase the side effects of these drugs.

PROLONGED USE

Use of this drug for more than a few months may lead to *tardive dyskinesia* (abnormal, involuntary movements of the eyes, face, and tongue). Occasionally, *jaundice* may occur.

HEPARIN/LMWH

Product names Hepalean, Heparin-Leo; [LMWH] Fragmin, Fraxiparine, Innohep, Lovenox
Used in the following combined preparations None

GENERAL INFORMATION

Heparin is an anticoagulant drug used to prevent the formation of, and aid in the dispersion of, blood clots. As the drug acts quickly, it is useful in emergencies, for instance, to prevent further clotting when a clot has already reached the lungs or the brain. People undergoing open heart surgery or kidney dialysis are also given heparin to prevent clotting. A low dose is sometimes given after surgery to prevent the development of deep vein thromboses (clots forming in the leg veins). Heparin is often given with other slower-acting anticoagulants, such as warfarin. It is also used to treat unstable angina. Low molecular weight heparins are fragments of heparin and include dalteparin, enoxaparin, nadroparin, and tinzaparin. Their advantage is that they act longer and do not require close blood monitoring as heparin does.

The most serious *adverse effect* of heparin is the risk of excessive bleeding, so the ability of the blood to clot is monitored carefully.

INFORMATION FOR USERS

Your drug prescription is tailored for you. Do not alter dosage without checking with your physician.

How taken

Injection.

Frequency and timing of doses
Every 8–12 hours or continuous intravenous infusion; once daily (LMWH).

Usual dosage range
Dosage is determined by the nature of the condition being treated or prevented.

Onset of effect
Within 15 minutes.

Duration of action
4–12 hours after treatment is stopped; 24 hours after end of treatment (LMWH).

Diet advice
None.

Storage
Keep in a cool, dry place out of the reach of children.

Missed dose
Notify your physician.

Stopping the drug
Do not stop taking the drug without consulting your physician. Stopping the drug may lead to clotting of blood.

OVERDOSE ACTION

 Seek immediate medical advice in all cases. Take emergency action if bleeding, severe headache, or loss of consciousness occur. Overdose can be reversed under medical supervision by a drug called protamine.

See Drug poisoning emergency guide (p.526).

POSSIBLE ADVERSE EFFECTS

As with all anticoagulants, bleeding is the most common adverse effect of heparin.

The less common effects may occur during long-term treatment.

Symptom/effect	Frequency		Discuss with physician		Stop taking drug now	Call physician now
	Common	Rare	Only if severe	In all cases		
Bleeding/bruising	●			■		▮
Alopecia		●		■		
Aching bones		●		■		
Rash		●		■	▲	▮
Breathing difficulties		●		■		▮
Jaundice/vomiting blood		●		■		▮

INTERACTIONS

Clopidogrel, ticlopidine, and dipyridamole The anticoagulant effect of heparin may be increased when it is taken with these drugs. The dosage of heparin may need to be adjusted accordingly.

ASA Do not take ASA, which may increase the anticoagulant effect of this drug and the risk of bleeding in the intestines or joints. Discuss with your physician.

SPECIAL PRECAUTIONS

Be sure to tell your physician if:
▼ You have long-term liver or kidney problems.
▼ You have high blood pressure.
▼ You bleed easily.
▼ You have any allergies.
▼ You have stomach ulcers.
▼ You are taking other medications.

 Pregnancy
▼ Careful monitoring is necessary as it may cause the mother to bleed excessively if taken near delivery. Discuss with your physician.

 Breast-feeding
▼ No evidence of risk.

 Infants and children
▼ Reduced dose necessary according to age and weight.

 Over 60
▼ No special problems.

 Driving and hazardous work
▼ Avoid risk of injury, since excessive bruising and bleeding may occur.

  Alcohol
▼ No special problems.

Surgery and general anesthetics
▼ Heparin may need to be stopped. Discuss this with your physician or dentist before having any surgery.

PROLONGED USE

Osteoporosis and hair loss may occur very rarely; tolerance to heparin may develop.

Monitoring Periodic blood and liver function tests will be required.

HYDROCHLOROTHIAZIDE

Product name Apo-Hydro
Used in the following combined preparations Moduret, Atacand Plus, Inhibace Plus, Vaseretic, Avalide, Hyzaar, and others

GENERAL INFORMATION

Hydrochlorothiazide belongs to the thiazide group of diuretic drugs, which remove excess water from the body and reduce edema (fluid retention) in people with congestive heart failure, kidney disorders, and cirrhosis of the liver. This drug is used to treat high blood pressure (see Antihypertensive drugs, p.88).

Hydrochlorothiazide increases the loss of potassium in the urine, which can cause a variety of symptoms (see p.83), and increases the likelihood of irregular heart rhythms, particularly in patients who are taking drugs such as digoxin. For this reason, potassium supplements are often given with hydrochlorothiazide.

QUICK REFERENCE

Drug group Thiazide diuretic (p.85)
Overdose danger rating Low
Dependence rating Low
Prescription needed Yes
Available as generic Yes

INFORMATION FOR USERS

Your drug prescription is tailored for you. Do not alter dosage without checking with your physician.

How taken

Tablets.

Frequency and timing of doses
Once daily, or every 2 days, early in the day.

Usual adult dosage range
12.5–50mg daily.

Onset of effect
Within 2 hours.

Duration of action
6–12 hours.

Diet advice
Use of this drug may reduce potassium in the body. Eat plenty of fresh fruit and vegetables. Discuss with your physician the advisability of reducing your salt intake.

Storage
Keep in a closed container in a cool, dry place out of the reach of children. Protect from light.

Missed dose
No cause for concern, but take as soon as you remember. However, if it is late in the day do not take the missed dose, or you may have to get up during the night to pass urine. Take the next scheduled dose as usual.

Stopping the drug
Do not stop the drug without consulting your physician; symptoms may recur.

Exceeding the dose
An occasional unintentional extra dose is unlikely to be a cause for concern. But if you notice any unusual symptoms, or if a large overdose has been taken, notify your physician.

SPECIAL PRECAUTIONS

Be sure to tell your physician if:
▼ You have long-term liver or kidney problems.
▼ You have had gout.
▼ You have diabetes.
▼ You have porphyria.
▼ You have Addison's disease or systemic lupus erythematosus.
▼ You are taking other medications.

Pregnancy
▼ Not usually prescribed. May cause *jaundice* in the newborn baby. Discuss with your physician.

Breast-feeding
▼ The drug passes into the breast milk, but at normal doses adverse effects on the baby are unlikely. Discuss with your physician.

Infants and children
▼ Not usually prescribed. Reduced dose necessary.

Over 60
▼ Increased likelihood of adverse effects.

Driving and hazardous work
▼ Avoid such activities until you have learned how hydrochlorothiazide affects you because the drug may reduce mental alertness and cause dizziness.

Alcohol
▼ Keep consumption low. Hydrochlorothiazide increases the likelihood of dehydration and hangovers after consumption of alcohol.

POSSIBLE ADVERSE EFFECTS

Most effects are caused by excessive loss of potassium. This can usually be put right by taking a potassium supplement. In rare cases, gout may occur in susceptible people, and certain forms of diabetes may become more difficult to control.

Symptom/effect	Frequency		Discuss with physician		Stop taking drug now	Call physician now
	Common	Rare	Only if severe	In all cases		
Muscle cramps	●			■		
Lethargy		●	■			
Dizziness		●		■		
Digestive disturbance		●	■			
Temporary impotence		●	■			
Rash		●		■	▲	

INTERACTIONS

Non-steroidal anti-inflammatory drugs (NSAIDs) Some NSAIDs may reduce the diuretic effect of hydrochlorothiazide, whose dosage may need to be adjusted.

Digoxin Adverse effects may be increased if excessive potassium is lost.

Corticosteroids These drugs further increase loss of potassium from the body when taken with hydrochlorothiazide.

Lithium Hydrochlorothiazide may increase lithium levels in the blood, leading to a risk of serious *adverse effects*.

PROLONGED USE

Excessive loss of potassium and imbalances of other salts may result, especially in the elderly.

Monitoring Blood tests may be performed periodically to check kidney function and levels of potassium and other salts.

HYDROCODONE

Product name Hycodan
Used in the following combined preparations Hycomine, Dimetane Expectorant-DC

GENERAL INFORMATION

Hydrocodone is a opioid antitussive (cough suppressant) drug with a pronounced sedative effect. It is used on its own or in a combined preparation with other drugs (for example, decongestants and antihistamines) to suppress troublesome dry coughs when non-opioid cough suppressants have not been effective.

Like other opioid drugs, hydrocodone can be constipating.

It may also depress breathing, and is therefore unsuitable for people with asthma or emphysema.

Hydrocodone may produce euphoria and has the potential to cause psychological and physical dependence if used in larger-than-recommended amounts over an extended period of time. It is therefore recommended to be used only for short-term treatment.

QUICK REFERENCE

Drug group Opioid cough suppressant (p.80)
Overdose danger rating High
Dependence rating Medium
Prescription needed Yes
Available as generic Yes

INFORMATION FOR USERS

Your drug prescription is tailored for you. Do not alter dosage without checking with your physician.

How taken

Tablets, oral liquid.

Frequency and timing of doses
3–4 x daily with food or milk.

Usual adult dosage range
5–15mg, not to exceed 30mg daily. Maximum single dose: 15mg.

Onset of effect
15–30 minutes.

Duration of action
4 hours.

Diet advice
None.

Storage
Keep in a closed container in a cool, dry place away from reach of children. Protect from light.

Missed dose
Take as soon as you remember. Adjust the timing of subsequent doses accordingly

Stopping the drug
Can be safely stopped following short-term treatment.

OVERDOSE ACTION

 Seek immediate medical advice in all cases. Take emergency action if there are symptoms such as slow or irregular breathing, severe drowsiness, or loss of consciousness.

See Drug poisoning emergency guide (p.526).

POSSIBLE ADVERSE EFFECTS

All opioid drugs can produce a variety of adverse effects; these are more frequent in children and older persons.

Symptom/effect	Frequency		Discuss with physician		Stop taking drug now	Call physician now
	Common	Rare	Only if severe	In all cases		
Constipation	●		■			
Drowsiness/dizziness	●		■			
Nausea/vomiting		●		■		
Slow respiration		●		■	▲	▐
Slow heartbeat		●		■	▲	▐
Confusion		●		■	▲	

INTERACTIONS

Sedatives All drugs, including alcohol, that have a sedative effect on the central nervous system are likely to increase sedation with hydrocodone. Such drugs include antidepressants, antipsychotics, sleeping drugs, and antihistamines.

Monoamine oxidase inhibitors (MAOIs) Hydrocodone may interact with these drugs to cause a dangerous rise in blood pressure.

SPECIAL PRECAUTIONS

Be sure to tell your physician if:
▼ You have impaired liver or kidney function.
▼ You have a heart or circulatory disorder.
▼ You have a lung disorder such as asthma, bronchitis, or emphysema.
▼ You have thyroid disease.
▼ You are taking other medications.

 Pregnancy
▼ Safety in pregnancy not established. Discuss with your physician.

 Breast-feeding
▼ The drug passes into the breast milk and may affect the baby. Discuss with your physician.

 Infants and children
▼ Reduced dose necessary.

 Over 60
▼ Increase likelihood of adverse effects. Reduced dose necessary.

 Driving and hazardous work
▼ Avoid such activities until you have learned how the drug affects you; it can cause dizziness, drowsiness, or blurred vision.

 Alcohol
▼ Avoid. Alcohol may increase the sedative effects of hydrocodone.

PROLONGED USE

If hydrocodone has been taken in large doses and/or over a long period of time, withdrawal symptoms are likely to occur upon stopping the drug abruptly.

HYDROCORTISONE

Product names Cortate, Cortef, Cortifoam, Cortoderm, Westcort
Used in the following combined preparations Fucidin H, Pentamycetin HC, Proctofoam-HC, Rectogel HC, and others

GENERAL INFORMATION

Hydrocortisone is chemically identical to the hormone cortisol, which is produced by the adrenal glands. For this reason, the drug is prescribed to replace natural hormones in adrenal insufficiency (Addison's disease).

The main use of hydrocortisone is in the treatment of a variety of allergic and inflammatory conditions. Used in *topical* preparations, it provides prompt relief from inflammation of the skin, eye, and outer ear. Hydrocortisone is used in oral form to relieve inflammatory bowel disease. Injected directly into the joints, the drug relieves pain and stiffness (see p.104). Injections may also be given to relieve severe attacks of asthma.

Overuse of skin preparations with hydrocortisone can lead to permanent thinning of the skin. Long-term treatment with high doses may cause serious *side effects*.

QUICK REFERENCE

Drug group Corticosteroid (p.127)

Overdose danger rating Low

Dependence rating Low

Prescription needed Yes (except for some topical preparations)

Available as generic Yes

INFORMATION FOR USERS

Your drug prescription is tailored for you. Do not alter dosage without checking with your physician.

How taken

Topical (cream, ointment, lotion), injection, rectal suppositories, rectal enema, eye ointment, ear solution, oral tablets.

Frequency and timing of doses
Varies according to condition.

Usual dosage range
Varies according to condition.

Onset of effect
Within 1–4 days.

Duration of action
Up to 12 hours.

Diet advice
Salt intake may need to be restricted when the drug is taken by mouth. It may also be necessary to take potassium supplements.

Storage
Keep in a closed container in a cool, dry place out of the reach of children.

Missed dose
Take as soon as you remember. If your next dose is due within 2 hours, take a single dose now and skip the next.

Stopping the drug
Do not stop taking the drug without consulting your physician. A gradual reduction in dosage is required following prolonged treatment with oral hydrocortisone.

Exceeding the dose
An occasional unintentional extra dose is unlikely to be a cause for concern. But if you notice any unusual symptoms, or if a large overdose has been taken, notify your physician.

SPECIAL PRECAUTIONS

Be sure to tell your physician if:
▼ You have liver or kidney problems.
▼ You have had a peptic ulcer.
▼ You have had a mental illness or epilepsy.
▼ You have glaucoma.
▼ You have had tuberculosis.
▼ You have diabetes or heart problems.
▼ You are taking other medications.

Avoid exposure to chickenpox, shingles, or measles if you are on systemic treatment.

Pregnancy
▼ No evidence of risk with topical preparations. Oral doses may adversely affect the developing baby. Discuss with your physician.

Breast-feeding
▼ The drug passes into the breast milk and may affect the baby. Discuss with your physician.

Infants and children
▼ Reduced dose necessary.

Over 60
▼ Reduced dose may be necessary.

Driving and hazardous work
▼ No special problems.

Alcohol
▼ Avoid. Alcohol may increase the risk of peptic ulcers when this drug is taken by mouth.

POSSIBLE ADVERSE EFFECTS

The most serious adverse effects only occur when hydrocortisone is taken by mouth in high doses for long periods of time. These are carefully monitored during treatment.

Symptom/effect	Frequency		Discuss with physician		Stop taking drug now	Call physician now
	Common	Rare	Only if severe	In all cases		
Indigestion	●		■			
Weight gain	●		■			
Acne	●		■			
Fluid retention		●		■		
Muscle weakness		●		■		
Mood changes		●		■		

INTERACTIONS (by mouth only)

Barbiturates, anticonvulsants, and rifampin These drugs reduce the effectiveness of hydrocortisone.

Antidiabetic drugs Hydrocortisone reduces the action of these drugs.

Antihypertensive drugs Hydrocortisone reduces the effects of these drugs.

Vaccines Severe reactions can occur if certain vaccines are given while taking hydrocortisone.

PROLONGED USE

Depending on method of administration, prolonged high dosage may cause diabetes, glaucoma, fragile bones, and thin skin, and may retard growth in children. People on long-term treatment are advised to carry a treatment card.

Monitoring Periodic checks on blood pressure are usually required when the drug is taken by mouth.

HYDROMORPHONE

Product names Dilaudid, Hydromorphone HP, Hydromorph Contin
Used in the following combined preparations None

GENERAL INFORMATION

Hydromorphone is chemically related to morphine. Small doses produce effective relief of acute and chronic pain. The onset of relief is faster after injection than after oral doses. Hydromorphone is used to relieve severe pain and anxiety following surgery, heart attacks, severe injuries, and in painful diseases such as cancer. The drug causes some drowsiness, although this is usually not pronounced. It is habit forming: physical and psychological dependence can occur with repeated use. However, this is usually less likely to occur when used to control chronic pain, such as that associated with cancer. When used for short periods of time for acute pain, most patients can stop taking the drug without difficulty.

QUICK REFERENCE

Drug group Opioid analgesic (p.64)
Overdose danger rating High
Dependence rating High
Prescription needed Yes (no repeats)
Available as generic Yes

INFORMATION FOR USERS

Your drug prescription is tailored for you. Do not alter dosage without checking with your physician.

How taken

Tablets, SR tablets, injection, rectal suppositories, liquid.

Frequency and timing of doses
Every 4–6 hours (tablets, SR tablets, injection). Doses by rectal suppository are required less frequently.

Usual adult dosage range
2–4mg per dose (tablets); 3 mg per dose (rectal suppository). Dosage by injection varies considerably between individuals.

Onset of effect
Within 30 minutes (tablets); within 15 minutes (injection).

Duration of action
4–6 hours.

Diet advice
To relieve constipation, increase intake of fluids and high fiber foods.

Storage
Keep in a closed container in a cool, dry place that is well secured and away from reach of children.

Missed dose
Take as soon as you remember. Return to your normal dosing schedule as soon as possible.

Stopping the drug
If the reason for taking the drug no longer exists, you may stop taking the drug after discussing it with your physician.

OVERDOSE ACTION

Seek immediate medical advice in all cases. Take emergency action if there are symptoms such as slow or irregular breathing, severe drowsiness, loss of consciousness, or slow or irregular pulse.

See Drug poisoning emergency guide (p.526).

POSSIBLE ADVERSE EFFECTS

As with other opioids, hydromorphone may produce nausea, vomiting, dizziness, loss of appetite, and constipation. Dosage adjustments may lessen some effects.

Symptom/effect	Frequency		Discuss with physician		Stop taking drug now	Call physician now
	Common	Rare	Only if severe	In all cases		
Sedation	●		■			
Constipation	●		■			
Nausea/vomiting	●			■		
Dizziness/lightheadedness	●			■		
Wheezing/difficult breathing		●		■	▲	▮
Confusion/vivid dreams		●		■		

INTERACTIONS

Sedatives Hydromorphone increases the sedative properties of all drugs that have a sedative effect. Such drugs include alcohol, antidepressants, antipsychotics, sleeping drugs, and antihistamines.

Monoamine oxidase inhibitors (MAOIs) May produce a severe rise in blood pressure when taken with hydromorphone.

SPECIAL PRECAUTIONS

Be sure to tell your physician if:
▼ You have impaired liver or kidney function.
▼ You have heart or circulatory problems .
▼ You have a lung disorder such as asthma, bronchitis, or emphysema.
▼ You have thyroid disease.
▼ You are taking other medications.

Pregnancy
▼ Not recommended. Taken near the time of delivery, the drug may cause breathing difficulties in the newborn baby. Discuss with your physician.

Breast-feeding
▼ Low levels of opioid analgesics have been detected in human milk, and may affect the baby adversely. Discuss with your physician.

Infants and children
▼ Not recommended.

Over 60
▼ Increased likelihood of adverse effects. Reduced dose may therefore be necessary.

Driving and hazardous work
▼ Persons receiving hydromorphone are unlikely to be well enough to undertake such acitivities.

Alcohol
▼ Avoid. Alcohol increases the sedative effect of hydromorphone.

PROLONGED USE

The effects of hydromorphone usually become weaker during prolonged use as the body adapts. This is known as *tolerance*. Other effects of long-term use include physical and psychological dependence, sexual impotence, and loss of sexual desire.

IBUPROFEN

Product names Advil, Apo-ibuprofen, Motrin, Novo-Profen, Nu-Ibuprofen
Used in the following combined preparation Advil Cold and Sinus, Dristan Decongestant, Sudafed Sinus Advance, and others

GENERAL INFORMATION

Ibuprofen is a non-steroidal anti-inflammatory drug (NSAID) which, like other drugs in this group, reduces pain, stiffness, and inflammation. It is an effective treatment for the symptoms of osteoarthritis, rheumatoid arthritis, and gout. In the treatment of rheumatoid arthritis, ibuprofen may be prescribed with slower-acting drugs. Other uses of the drug include the relief of mild to moderate headache, menstrual and dental pain, pain resulting from soft tissue injuries, or the pain that may follow an operation.

Ibuprofen has fewer *side effects* than many of the other NSAIDs. Unlike ASA, it has the benefit of rarely causing bleeding in the stomach.

Ibuprofen in a smaller dosage form is available over-the-counter.

QUICK REFERENCE

Drug group Analgesic (p.64) and non-steroidal anti-inflammatory drug (p.102)

Overdose danger rating Low

Dependence rating Low

Prescription needed No (some preparations)

Available as generic Yes

INFORMATION FOR USERS

Follow instructions on the label. Call your physician if symptoms worsen.

How taken

Tablets, chewable tablets, gel caps, liquid.

Frequency and timing of doses
4–6 x daily (general pain relief); 3–4 x daily with food (arthritis).

Usual adult dosage range
General pain relief 600mg–1.8g daily.
Arthritis 1.2–2.4g daily.

Onset of effect
Pain relief begins in 1–2 hours. The full anti-inflammatory effect in arthritic conditions may not be felt for up to 2 weeks.

Duration of action
5–10 hours.

Diet advice
None.

Storage
Keep in a closed container in a cool, dry place out of the reach of children.

Missed dose
Take as soon as you remember. If your next dose is due within 2 hours, take a single dose now and skip the next.

Stopping the drug
When taken for short-term pain relief, the drug can be safely stopped as soon as you no longer need it. If prescribed for the long-term treatment of arthritis, however, you should seek medical advice before stopping the drug.

Exceeding the dose
An occasional unintentional extra dose is unlikely to be a cause for concern. But if you notice any unusual symptoms, or if a large overdose has been taken, notify your physician.

POSSIBLE ADVERSE EFFECTS

The most common adverse effects are the result of gastrointestinal disturbances. Black or bloodstained feces should be reported to your physician without delay.

Symptom/effect	Frequency		Discuss with physician		Stop taking drug now	Call physician now
	Common	Rare	Only if severe	In all cases		
Heartburn/indigestion	●		■			
Nausea/vomiting		●	■			
Rash/fever		●		■	▲	▌
Wheezing/breathlessness		●		■	▲	▌
Black/bloodstained feces		●		■	▲	▌
Swollen feet and ankles		●		■		
Ringing in the ears		●		■		
Changes in vision		●		■		▌

INTERACTIONS

General note Ibuprofen interacts with a wide range of drugs to increase the risk of bleeding and/or peptic ulcers. Such drugs include other non-steroidal anti-inflammatory drugs (NSAIDs), ASA, oral anticoagulants, and corticosteroids.

Ciprofloxacin The risk of seizures with this drug and related antibiotics may be increased by ibuprofen.

Antihypertensive drugs and diuretics The beneficial effects of these drugs may be reduced by ibuprofen.

Lithium, digoxin, and methotrexate Ibuprofen may increase the blood levels of these drugs to an undesirable extent.

SPECIAL PRECAUTIONS

Be sure to consult your physician or pharmacist before taking this drug if:
▼ You have a long-term kidney problem.
▼ You have a long-term liver problem.
▼ You have high blood pressure.
▼ You have had a peptic ulcer, esophagitis, or acid indigestion.
▼ You are allergic to ASA.
▼ You have asthma.
▼ You are taking other medications.

Pregnancy
▼ Not usually prescribed. May affect the unborn baby and may prolong labour. Discuss with your physician.

Breast-feeding
▼ The drug passes into the breast milk, but at normal doses adverse effects on the baby are unlikely. Discuss with your physician.

Infants and children
▼ Reduced dose necessary.

Over 60
▼ Reduced dose may be necessary.

Driving and hazardous work
▼ No problems expected.

Alcohol
▼ Avoid. Alcohol may increase the risk of stomach disorders with ibuprofen.

Surgery and general anesthetics
▼ Ibuprofen may prolong bleeding. Discuss the possibility of stopping treatment temporarily with your physician or dentist.

PROLONGED USE

There is an increased risk of bleeding from peptic ulcers and in the bowel with prolonged use of ibuprofen.

IMIPRAMINE

Product name Tofranil
Used in the following combined preparations None

GENERAL INFORMATION

Imipramine belongs to the tricyclic class of antidepressant drugs. The drug is used mainly in the long-term treatment of depression to elevate mood, improve appetite, increase physical activity, and restore interest in everyday life. Because imipramine is less sedating than other tricyclic antidepressants, it is particularly useful when a depressed person is withdrawn or apathetic, although it can aggravate insomnia if it is taken in the evening.

Imipramine is also prescribed to treat night-time enuresis (bedwetting) in children, although proof of its benefit is not conclusive. Imipramine can cause a variety of *side effects*. In overdose, the drug may cause coma and dangerous heart rhythms.

QUICK REFERENCE

Drug group Tricyclic anti-depressant (p.84) and drug for urinary disorders (p.170)

Overdose danger rating High

Dependence rating Low

Prescription needed Yes

Available as generic Yes

INFORMATION FOR USERS

Your drug prescription is tailored for you. Do not alter dosage without checking with your physician.

How taken

Tablets.

Frequency and timing of doses
1–3 x daily.

Usual dosage range
Adults Usually 75–200mg daily (up to a maximum of 300mg in hospital patients). *Children* Reduced dose according to age and weight.

Onset of effect
Some benefits and effects may appear within hours, but full antidepressant effect may not be felt for 4 weeks.

Duration of action
Following prolonged treatment, antidepressant effect may persist for up to 6 weeks. Any adverse effects may wear off within days.

Diet advice
None.

Storage
Keep in a closed container in a cool, dry place out of the reach of children.

Missed dose
Take as soon as you remember. If your next dose is due within 3 hours, take a single dose now and skip the next.

Stopping the drug
Do not stop taking the drug without consulting your physician, who will supervise a gradual reduction in dosage. Stopping abruptly may cause withdrawal symptoms.

OVERDOSE ACTION

Seek immediate medical advice in all cases. Take emergency action if consciousness is lost.

See Drug poisoning emergency guide (p.526).

POSSIBLE ADVERSE EFFECTS

The possible adverse effects of this drug are mainly the result of its *anticholinergic* action and its effect on the normal rhythm of the heart.

Symptom/effect	Frequency		Discuss with physician		Stop taking drug now	Call physician now
	Common	Rare	Only if severe	In all cases		
Sweating/flushing	●		■			
Dry mouth/constipation	●		■			
Blurred vision	●			■		
Dizziness/drowsiness		●		■		
Rash		●		■	▲	
Palpitations		●		■	▲	▮
Weight gain	●		■			

INTERACTIONS

Monoamine oxidase inhibitors (MAOIs) There is a possibility of a serious interaction. Such drugs are prescribed with imipramine only under strict supervision.

Amiodarone, and sotalol These drugs may increase the risk of abnormal heart rhythms.

Sedatives Imipramine may increase the effects of sedative drugs.

Antihypertensive drugs Imipramine may reduce the effectiveness of these drugs.

Phenytoin Imipramine may increase levels of phenytoin.

SPECIAL PRECAUTIONS

Be sure to tell your physician if:
▼ You have had heart problems.
▼ You have long-term liver or kidney problems.
▼ You have had epileptic fits.
▼ You have porphyria.
▼ You have had glaucoma.
▼ You have prostate trouble.
▼ You have had mania or a psychotic illness.
▼ You are taking other medications.

Pregnancy
▼ Safety in pregnancy not established. Discuss with your physician.

Breast-feeding
▼ The drug passes into the breast milk, but at normal doses adverse effects on the baby are unlikely. Discuss with your physician.

Infants and children
▼ Not recommended under 7 years. Reduced dose necessary in older children.

Over 60
▼ Increased likelihood of adverse effects. Reduced dose may therefore be necessary.

Driving and hazardous work
▼ Avoid such activities until you have learned how imipramine affects you because the drug can cause reduced alertness and blurred vision.

Alcohol
▼ Avoid. Alcohol may increase the sedative effect of imipramine.

Surgery and general anesthetics
▼ Imipramine treatment may need to be stopped before you have a general anesthetic. Discuss this with your physician or dentist before any operation.

PROLONGED USE

No problems expected. Imipramine is not usually prescribed for children as a treatment for bedwetting for longer than three months.

INDAPAMIDE

Product names Apo-Indapamide, Dom-Indapamide, Gen-Indapamide, Lozide, PMS-Indapamide
Used in the following combined preparation Coversyl Plus

GENERAL INFORMATION

Indapamide is a drug related in its effects and uses to the thiazide diuretic group of drugs, and is used to treat hypertension (high blood pressure).

The drug prevents the hormone norepinephrine (noradrenaline) from constricting blood vessels, thereby allowing them to dilate. It also acts on the kidneys to increase excretion of sodium.

Indapamide is sometimes combined with other antihypertensive drugs but not with other diuretics. Indapamide's diuretic effects are slight at low doses, but susceptible people need to have their blood levels of potassium and uric acid monitored. These include the elderly, those taking digoxin, or those with gout or hyperaldosteronism (overproduction of the hormone aldosterone). Unlike the thiazides, indapamide does not affect control of diabetes.

QUICK REFERENCE

Drug group Diuretic (p.85)
Overdose danger rating Low
Dependence rating Low
Prescription needed Yes
Available as generic Yes

INFORMATION FOR USERS

Your drug prescription is tailored for you. Do not alter dosage without checking with your physician.

How taken

Tablets.

Frequency and timing of doses
Once daily in the morning.

Usual adult dosage range
1.5–2.5mg.

Onset of effect
1–2 hours, but the full effect may not be felt for several months.

Duration of action
12–24 hours.

Diet advice
None.

Storage
Keep in a closed container in a cool, dry place out of the reach of children.

Missed dose
Take as soon as you remember. If your next dose is due within 4 hours, take a single dose now and skip the next.

Stopping the drug
Do not stop taking the drug without consulting your physician; high blood pressure may return.

Exceeding the dose
An occasional unintentional extra dose is unlikely to cause problems. But if you notice any unusual symptoms, or if a large overdose has been taken, notify your physician.

SPECIAL PRECAUTIONS

Be sure to tell your physician if:
▼ You have had a stroke.
▼ You have liver or kidney problems.
▼ You have gout.
▼ You have hyperaldosteronism or hyperparathyroidism.
▼ You are allergic to sulfonamide drugs.
▼ You are taking digoxin.
▼ You are taking other medications.

 Pregnancy
▼ Safety not established. Discuss with your physician.

 Breast-feeding
▼ Safety not established. Discuss with your physician.

 Infants and children
▼ Not prescribed.

 Over 60
▼ No special problems.

 Driving and hazardous work
▼ No special problems.

 Alcohol
▼ No special problems.

POSSIBLE ADVERSE EFFECTS

Headaches and muscle cramps are common, but other symptoms rarely cause problems.

Symptom/effect	Frequency		Discuss with physician		Stop taking drug now	Call physician now
	Common	Rare	Only if severe	In all cases		
Headache/dizziness	●		■			
Fatigue/muscle cramps	●		■			
Diarrhea/constipation		●	■			
Skin rash		●		■		
Palpitations/fainting		●		■		
Jaundice		●		■		
Sore throat		●		■		
Tingling/"pins and needles"		●		■		
Impotence		●		■		

INTERACTIONS

Diuretics There is a risk of imbalance of salts in the blood if these drugs are taken with indapamide.

Digoxin Loss of potassium may lead to *toxicity* of this drug with indapamide.

Lithium Blood levels of lithium are increased when it is taken with indapamide.

Antiarrhythmic drugs Loss of potassium may make these drugs less effective if they are taken with indapamide.

PROLONGED USE

Long-term use of indapamide may lead to potassium loss, especially in the elderly.

Monitoring Blood potassium and uric acid levels may be checked periodically.

INSULIN

Product names Humulin, Novolin, Humalog, Innovo
Used in the following combined preparations None

GENERAL INFORMATION

Insulin is a hormone manufactured by the pancreas and vital to the body's ability to use sugar. It is given by injection to supplement or replace natural insulin in the treatment of diabetes mellitus. It is the only effective treatment in juvenile (insulin-dependent or Type 1) diabetes and may also be prescribed in adult (maturity-onset or Type 2) diabetes.

Insulin should be used with a carefully controlled diet. Illness, vomiting, or alterations in diet or in exercise levels may require dosage adjustment.

Insulin is available in a wide variety of preparations – short-, medium-, or long-acting. Combinations of types are often given. People receiving insulin should carry a warning card or tag.

QUICK REFERENCE

Drug group Drug for diabetes (p.128)

Overdose danger rating High

Dependence rating Low

Prescription needed Yes

Available as generic No

INFORMATION FOR USERS

Your drug prescription is tailored for you. Do not alter dosage without checking with your physician.

How taken

Injection, infusion pump, pen injection.

Frequency and timing of doses
1–4 x daily. Short-acting insulin is usually given 15–30 minutes before meals. Some newer forms can be given directly before or after eating. However, the exact timing of injections and longer-acting preparations will be tailored to your individual needs; follow the instructions you are given.

Usual dosage range
The dose (and type) of insulin is determined according to the needs of the individual.

Onset of effect
15–60 minutes (short-acting); 1–2 hours (medium- and long-acting).

Duration of action
6–8 hours (short-acting); 18–26 hours (medium-acting); 28–36 hours (long-acting).

Diet advice
A low-carbohydrate diet is necessary. Follow your physician's advice.

Storage
Refrigerate but once opened may be stored at room temperature for 1 month. Do not freeze. Follow the instructions on the container.

Missed dose
Discuss with your physician. Appropriate action depends on dose and type of insulin.

Stopping the drug
Do not stop taking the drug without consulting your physician; confusion and coma may occur.

OVERDOSE ACTION

 Seek immediate medical advice. You may notice symptoms of low blood sugar, such as faintness, hunger, sweating, trembling. Eat or drink something sugary. Take emergency action if fits or loss of consciousness occur.

See Drug poisoning emergency guide (p.526).

POSSIBLE ADVERSE EFFECTS

Symptoms such as dizziness, sweating, weakness, and confusion indicate low blood sugar. Serious allergic reactions (rash, swelling, and shortness of breath) are rare.

Symptom/effect	Frequency		Discuss with physician		Stop taking drug now	Call physician now
	Common	Rare	Only if severe	In all cases		
Injection-site irritation	●			■		
Weakness/sweating	●			■		
Dimpling at injection site		●		■		
Eyesight problems		●		■		
Rash/facial swelling		●		■		▮
Shortness of breath		●		■		▮

SPECIAL PRECAUTIONS

Be sure to tell your physician if:
▼ You have had a previous allergic reaction to insulin.
▼ You are taking other medications, or your other drug treatment is changed.

 Pregnancy
▼ No evidence of risk to the developing baby from insulin, but poor control of diabetes increases the risk of birth defects. Careful monitoring is required.

 Breast-feeding
▼ No evidence of risk. Adjustment in dose may be necessary while breast-feeding.

 Infants and children
▼ Reduced dose necessary.

 Over 60
▼ No special problems.

 Driving and hazardous work
▼ Usually no problem, but strenuous exercise alters your insulin and sugar requirements. Avoid these activities if you have warning signs of low blood sugar.

 Alcohol
▼ Avoid. Alcoholic drinks upset diabetic control.

Surgery and general anesthetics
▼ Insulin requirements may increase during surgery, and blood glucose levels will need to be monitored during and after an operation. Notify your physician or dentist that you are diabetic before any surgery.

INTERACTIONS

General note 1 Many drugs, including some antibiotics, monoamine oxidase inhibitors (MAOIs), and oral antidiabetic drugs, increase the risk of low blood sugar.

Corticosteroids and diuretics may oppose the effect of insulin.

General note 2 Check with your physician or pharmacist before taking any medicines; some contain sugar and may upset control of diabetes.

Beta blockers may affect insulin needs and mask signs of low blood sugar.

PROLONGED USE

No problems expected.

Monitoring Regular monitoring of levels of sugar in the blood and/or urine is required.

INTERFERON

Product names Avonex, Betaseron, Intron A, Rebif
Used in the following combined preparations None

GENERAL INFORMATION

Interferons are a group of substances normally produced in human and animal cells that have been infected with viruses or stimulated by other substances. They are thought to promote resistance to several types of viral infection (see p.113). Three main types of interferon (alpha, beta, and gamma) are used to treat a range of diseases. Interferon alpha is used for leukemias, other cancers, and chronic hepatitis B and C. Peginterferon alfa-2a and 2b are indicated in the management of hepatic C; 2a is also indicated in hepatitis B. Interferon beta reduces the frequency and severity of relapses in multiple sclerosis. Interferon gamma is prescribed in conjunction with antibiotics for patients suffering from chronic granulomatous disease.

Interferons can cause severe *adverse effects* (see below).

INFORMATION FOR USERS

This drug is given only under medical supervision and is not for self-administration.

How taken

Injection.

Frequency and timing of doses
Once daily or once weekly depending on product and condition being treated.

Usual adult dosage range
The dosage is calculated taking account of the body surface area of the patient and the condition being treated.

Onset of effect
Active inside the body within 1 hour, but effects may not be noted for 1–2 months.

Duration of action
Immediate effects last for about 12 hours.

Diet advice
None.

Storage
Store in a refrigerator at 2–8°C (36–46°F). Do not let it freeze, and protect from light. Keep out of the reach of children.

Missed dose
Not applicable. This drug is usually given only in hospital under close medical supervision.

Stopping the drug
Discuss with your physician.

Exceeding the dose
Overdosage is unlikely since treatment is carefully monitored.

SPECIAL PRECAUTIONS

Interferon is prescribed only under close medical supervision, taking account of your present condition and medical history. However, be sure to tell your physician if:
▼ You have long-term liver or kidney problems.
▼ You have heart disease.
▼ You have had epileptic fits.
▼ You have previously suffered allergic reactions to any drugs.
▼ You have had asthma or eczema.
▼ You suffer from depression.
▼ You are taking other medications.

 Pregnancy
▼ Not usually prescribed. Safety in pregnancy not established. Discuss with your physician.

 Breast-feeding
▼ It is not known whether the drug passes into the breast milk. Discuss with your physician.

 Infants and children
▼ Not usually used.

 Over 60
▼ Increased likelihood of adverse effects. Reduced dose may be necessary.

 Driving and hazardous work
▼ Not applicable.

 Alcohol
▼ Avoid. Alcohol may increase the sedative effects of this drug.

POSSIBLE ADVERSE EFFECTS

The symptoms listed below are the most common problems. All unusual symptoms should be brought to your physician's attention without delay. Some of these symptoms are dose-related, and a reduction in dosage may be necessary to eliminate them.

Symptom/effect	Frequency		Discuss with physician		Stop taking drug now	Call physician now
	Common	Rare	Only if severe	In all cases		
Headache	●		■			
Lethargy/depression	●			■		
Dizziness/drowsiness	●			■		
Digestive disturbances	●			■		
Chills, fever, muscle-ache	●			■		
Poor appetite and weight loss	●			■		
Hair loss		●		■		
Mood changes		●		■		■

INTERACTIONS

General note A number of drugs increase the risk of adverse effects on the blood, heart, or nervous system. This is taken into account when prescribing an interferon with other drugs.

Sedatives All drugs that have a sedative effect on the central nervous system are likely to increase the sedative properties of interferon. Such drugs include *opioid* analgesics, anti-anxiety and sleeping drugs, antihistamines, antidepressants, and antipsychotics.

Vaccines Interferon may reduce the effectiveness of vaccines.

Theophylline/aminophylline The effects of this drug may be increased by interferon.

PROLONGED USE

There may be an increased risk of liver damage. Blood cell production in the bone marrow may be reduced. Repeated large doses are associated with lethargy, fatigue, collapse, and coma.

Monitoring Frequent blood tests are required to monitor blood composition and liver function.

IPRATROPIUM BROMIDE

Product name Atrovent
Used in the following combined preparations Combivent, Duovent

GENERAL INFORMATION

Ipratropium bromide is an *anticholinergic* bronchodilator that relaxes the muscles surrounding the bronchioles (airways in the lung). It is used primarily in the maintenance treatment of reversible airway disorders, particularly chronic bronchitis. It is given only by inhaler or via a nebulizer for these conditions. Although its effect lasts longer, the drug has a slower onset of action than the *sympathomimetic* bronchodilators. For this reason, it is not as effective in treating acute attacks of wheezing, or

in the emergency treatment of asthma, and it is usually used together with the faster-acting drugs. Ipratropium bromide is also prescribed as a nasal spray for the treatment of a continually runny nose due to allergy.

Unlike other anticholinergic drugs, *side effects* are rare. It is not likely to affect the heart, eyes, bowel, or bladder. Ipratropium bromide must be used with caution by people with glaucoma, but problems are unlikely at normal doses and if inhalers are used correctly.

QUICK REFERENCE

Drug group Bronchodilator (p.76)
Overdose danger rating Low
Dependence rating Low
Prescription needed Yes
Available as generic Yes

INFORMATION FOR USERS

Your drug prescription is tailored for you. Do not alter dosage without checking with your physician.

How taken

Inhaler, nasal spray, liquid for nebulizer.

Frequency and timing of doses
3–4 x daily.

Usual adult dosage range
80–320mcg daily (inhaler); 125–500mcg per dose (nebulizer); 1–2 puffs to the affected nostril 2–3 x daily (nasal spray).

Onset of effect
5–15 minutes.

Duration of action
Up to 8 hours.

Diet advice
None.

Storage
Keep in a cool, dry place out of the reach of children. Do not puncture or burn containers.

Missed dose
Take as soon as you remember. If your next dose is due within 2 hours, take a single dose now and skip the next.

Stopping the drug
Do not stop taking the drug without consulting your physician; symptoms may recur.

Exceeding the dose
An occasional unintentional extra dose is unlikely to be a cause for concern. But if you notice any unusual symptoms, or if a large overdose has been taken, notify your physician.

SPECIAL PRECAUTIONS

Be sure to tell your physician if:
▼ You have glaucoma.
▼ You have prostate problems.
▼ You have difficulty in passing urine.
▼ You are taking other medications.

Pregnancy
▼ No evidence of risk, but discuss with your physician before using in the first 3 months of pregnancy.

Breast-feeding
▼ No evidence of risk, but discuss with your physician.

Infants and children
▼ Reduced dose necessary.

Over 60
▼ No special problems.

Driving and hazardous work
▼ No special problems.

Alcohol
▼ No known problems.

POSSIBLE ADVERSE EFFECTS

Side effects are rare. The most common is dry mouth or throat.

Symptom/effect	Frequency		Discuss with physician		Stop taking drug now	Call physician now
	Common	Rare	Only if severe	In all cases		
Dry mouth/throat	●		■			
Constipation		●	■			
Urinary hesitancy		●	■			

INTERACTIONS

Anticholinergic drugs Although absorption is minimal from the inhaler/spray, additive anticholinergic effects could occur.

PROLONGED USE

No special problems.

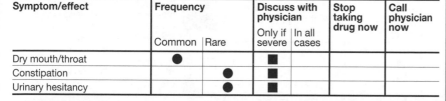

IRBESARTAN

Product name Avapro
Used in the following combined preparations Avalide

GENERAL INFORMATION

Irbesartan is a member of the group of vasodilator drugs called angiotensin-II blockers. Used to treat hypertension, the drug works by blocking the action of angiotensin-II (a naturally occurring substance that constricts blood vessels). This action causes the blood vessel walls to relax, thereby lowering blood pressure.

Unlike ACE inhibitors, irbesartan does not cause a persistent dry cough. Along with other angiotensin-II blockers,

it is being evaluated for the treatment of some of the other conditions, such as heart failure, for which ACE inhibitors are used. Irbesartan is also available in combination with a diuretic.

Irbesartan is prescribed with caution to people with stenosis (narrowing) of the arteries to the kidneys because the initial dose causes a sudden drop in blood pressure. It is important to notify your physician if you know that you have this condition.

QUICK REFERENCE

Drug group Vasodilator (p.84) and antihypertensive drug (p.88)

Overdose danger rating Medium

Dependence rating Low

Prescription needed Yes

Available as generic No

INFORMATION FOR USERS

Your drug prescription is tailored for you. Do not alter dosage without checking with your physician.

How taken

Tablets.

Frequency and timing of doses
Once daily.

Usual adult dosage range
150–300mg, but 75mg may be used in people over 75 years or with liver problems.

Onset of effect
Within 1 hour. Blood pressure is lowered within 1–2 weeks, and maximum beneficial effect is felt 4–6 weeks from start of treatment.

Duration of action
24 hours.

Diet advice
None.

Storage
Keep in a closed container in a cool, dry place out of the reach of children.

Missed dose
Take as soon as you remember. If your next dose is due within 8 hours, take a single dose now and skip the next.

Stopping the drug
Do not stop the drug without consulting your physician. Stopping the drug may lead to worsening of the high blood pressure.

Exceeding the dose
An occasional unintentional extra dose is unlikely to be a cause for concern. Large overdoses may cause dizziness and fainting. Notify your physician.

SPECIAL PRECAUTIONS

Be sure to tell your physician if:
▼ You have kidney problems or renal artery stenosis.
▼ You have heart problems.
▼ You have congestive heart failure.
▼ You have primary aldosteronism.
▼ You are taking other medications.

 Pregnancy
▼ Not prescribed.

 Breast-feeding
▼ Safety not established. Discuss with your physician.

 Infants and children
▼ Not prescribed.

 Over 60
▼ Reduced dose may be necessary in people over 75 years.

 Driving and hazardous work
▼ Avoid such activities until you have learned how irbesartan affects you because the drug can cause dizziness and fatigue.

 Alcohol
▼ Avoid. Regular intake of alcohol may raise the blood pressure and reduce the effectiveness of irbesartan. Alcohol may also increase the likelihood of an excessive fall in blood pressure.

POSSIBLE ADVERSE EFFECTS

Adverse effects are usually mild.

Symptom/effect	Frequency		Discuss with physician		Stop taking drug now	Call physician now
	Common	Rare	Only if severe	In all cases		
Dizziness/fatigue	●			■		
Flushing	●		■			
Headache		●	■			
Rash		●		■		

INTERACTIONS

Diuretics There is a risk of a sudden fall in blood pressure if these drugs are being taken when irbesartan treatment is started.

Potassium supplements, potassium-sparing diuretics, and cyclosporine Irbesartan enhances the effect of these drugs, leading to raised levels of potassium in the blood.

Lithium Irbesartan increases the blood levels and *toxicity* of lithium.

NSAIDs Certain of these drugs may reduce the blood-pressure lowering effects of irbesartan.

PROLONGED USE

No special problems.

Monitoring
Periodic checks on blood potassium levels may be performed.

ISONIAZID

Product name Isotamine
Used in the following combined preparations Rifater

GENERAL INFORMATION

Isoniazid (also known as INH) has been in use for over 30 years and remains an effective drug for tuberculosis. It is given alone to prevent tuberculosis and in combination with other drugs for the treatment of the disease. Treatment usually lasts for six months. However, courses lasting nine months or a year may sometimes be prescribed.

One of the *side effects* of isoniazid is the increased loss of pyridoxine (vitamin B_6) from the body. This effect, which is more likely with high doses, is rare in children but common among people with poor nutrition. Since pyridoxine deficiency can lead to irreversible nerve damage, supplements are usually given.

QUICK REFERENCE

Drug group Antituberculous drug (p.118)

Overdose danger rating High

Dependence rating Low

Prescription needed Yes

Available as generic Yes

INFORMATION FOR USERS

Your drug prescription is tailored for you. Do not alter dosage without checking with your physician.

How taken

Tablets, liquid, injection.

Frequency and timing of doses
Normally once daily.

Usual dosage range
Adults 300mg daily. Can be given 2 or 3 x weekly in some cases.
Children According to age and weight.

Onset of effect
Over 2–3 days.

Duration of action
Up to 24 hours.

Diet advice
Isoniazid may deplete pyridoxine (vitamin B_6) levels, so supplements are usually prescribed.

Storage
Keep in a closed container in a cool, dry place out of the reach of children. Protect from light.

Missed dose
Take as soon as you remember. If your next dose is scheduled within 8 hours, take a single dose now and skip the next.

Stopping the drug
Take the full course. Even if you feel better, the infection may still be present and may recur if treatment is stopped too soon.

OVERDOSE ACTION

 Seek immediate medical advice in all cases. Take emergency action if breathing difficulties, fits, or loss of consciousness occur.

See Drug poisoning emergency guide (p.526).

SPECIAL PRECAUTIONS

Be sure to tell your physician if:
▼ You have long-term liver or kidney problems.
▼ You have had liver damage following isoniazid treatment in the past.
▼ If you have problems with drugs or alcohol abuse.
▼ You have diabetes.
▼ You have porphyria.
▼ You have HIV infection.
▼ You have had epileptic fits.
▼ You are taking other medications.

 Pregnancy
▼ Not known to be harmful to the fetus. Discuss with your physician.

 Breast-feeding
▼ The drug passes into the breast milk and may affect the baby. The infant should be monitored for signs of toxic effects. Discuss with your physician.

 Infants and children
▼ Reduced dose necessary.

 Over 60
▼ Increased likelihood of adverse effects.

 Driving and hazardous work
▼ No special problems.

 Alcohol
▼ Avoid excessive amounts.

POSSIBLE ADVERSE EFFECTS

Although serious problems are uncommon, all adverse effects of this drug should receive prompt medical attention because of the possibility of nerve or liver damage.

Symptom/effect	Frequency		Discuss with physician		Stop taking drug now	Call physician now
	Common	Rare	Only if severe	In all cases		
Nausea/vomiting		●	■			
Fatigue/weakness		●		■		
Numbness/tingling		●		■		
Rash		●		■		
Mood changes		●		■		
Blurred vision		●		■	▲	
Jaundice		●		■	▲	▍
Twitching/muscle weakness		●		■	▲	▍

INTERACTIONS

Alcohol and rifampin Large quantities of alcohol may reduce the effectiveness of isoniazid. If alcohol and isoniazid are taken together, the likelihood of liver damage is increased; if, in addition, rifampin is being taken, the risk of liver damage is increased even further.

Antiepileptics The effects of these drugs may be increased with isoniazid.

Antacids These drugs may reduce the absorption of isoniazid.

Ketoconazole Isoniazid reduces the blood concentration of ketoconazole.

PROLONGED USE

Pyridoxine (vitamin B_6) deficiency may occur with prolonged use and lead to nerve damage. Supplements are usually prescribed. There is also a risk of serious liver damage.

Monitoring Periodic blood tests are usually performed to monitor liver function.

ISOSORBIDE DINITRATE/MONONITRATE

Product names [Dinitrate] Apo-ISDN, Cedocard SR [Mononitrate] Imdur
Used in the following combined preparation None

GENERAL INFORMATION

Isosorbide dinitrate and mononitrate are vasodilator drugs similar to nitroglycerin. They are usually used to treat patients suffering from angina, and are also used in some cases of heart failure.

Unlike nitroglycerin, however, both isosorbide dintrate and isosorbide mononitrate are stable and can be stored for long periods without losing their effectiveness.

Headaches, flushing, and dizziness are common *side effects* during the early stages of treatment; gradual increase in dose can minimize these symptoms. As tolerance can develop with round-the-clock use, an appropriate dosing schedule will include a nitrate-free interval of 10–12 hours each day. This should be discussed with your physician or pharmacist.

QUICK REFERENCE

Drug group Nitrate vasodilator (p.84) and anti-angina drug (p.87)
Overdose danger rating Medium
Dependence rating Low
Prescription needed No
Available as generic Yes (dinitrate)

INFORMATION FOR USERS

Your drug prescription is tailored for you. Do not alter dosage without checking with your physician.

How taken

Dinitrate Sublingual tablets (held under the tongue), SR-tablets, tablets.
Mononitrate SR-tablets.

Frequency and timing of doses
Relief of angina attacks Tablets (dinitrate) sublingual under the tongue as needed.
Prevention of angina 2–4 x daily; 1 x daily (SR-tablets).

Usual adult dosage range
Relief of angina attacks 5–10mg per dose.
Prevention of angina 30–120mg daily (mononitrate).

Onset of effect
2–3 minutes when chewed or held under the tongue (certain preparations only); 30 minutes when swallowed.

Duration of action
Up to 2 hours (chewed); up to 5 hours (swallowed); up to 10 hours (SR-tablets).

Diet advice
None.

Storage
Keep in a closed container in a cool, dry place out of the reach of children. Protect from light.

Missed dose
Take as soon as you remember. If your next dose is due within 2 hours, take a single dose now and skip the next.

Stopping the drug
Do not stop taking the drug without consulting your physician; stopping the drug may lead to worsening of the underlying condition.

Exceeding the dose
An occasional unintentional extra dose is unlikely to cause problems. Large overdoses may cause dizziness and headache. Notify your physician.

SPECIAL PRECAUTIONS

Be sure to tell your physician if:
▼ You have long-term liver or kidney problems.
▼ You have any blood disorders or anemia.
▼ You have had glaucoma.
▼ You have low blood pressure.
▼ You have ever had a heart attack.
▼ You have an underactive thyroid.
▼ You are taking other medications.

Pregnancy
▼ Safety in pregnancy not established. Discuss with your physician.

Breast-feeding
▼ Safety not established. Discuss with your physician.

Infants and children
▼ Not usually prescribed.

Over 60
▼ No special problems.

Driving and hazardous work
▼ Avoid such activities until you have learned how isosorbide dinitrate or mononitrate affect you because these drugs can cause dizziness.

Alcohol
▼ Avoid. Alcohol may further lower blood pressure, depressing the heart and causing dizziness and fainting.

POSSIBLE ADVERSE EFFECTS

The most serious adverse effect is excessively lowered blood pressure, and this may need to be monitored on a regular basis. Other adverse effects of both forms of the drug usually improve after regular use; dose adjustment may help.

Symptom/effect	Frequency		Discuss with physician		Stop taking drug now	Call physician now
	Common	Rare	Only if severe	In all cases		
Headache	●		■			
Flushing	●		■			
Dizziness	●			■		
Fainting/weakness		●		■		

INTERACTIONS

Sildenafil The blood-pressure lowering effect of nitrate drugs is significantly enhanced by sildenafil and the two drugs should not be used together.

Antihypertensives A further lowering of blood pressure occurs when such drugs are taken with isosorbide dinitrate.

PROLONGED USE

The initial adverse effects may disappear with continued use. To prevent tolerance, an appropriate dosing schedule will include a 10–12 hour nitrate-free period during each day. Discuss this with your physician or pharmacist.

ISOTRETINOIN

Product names Accutane, Clarus
Used in the following combined preparation None

GENERAL INFORMATION

Isotretinoin, a drug that is chemically related to vitamin A, is prescribed for the treatment of severe acne that has failed to respond to other treatments.

The drug reduces production of the skin's natural oils (sebum) and of the horny protein (keratin) in the outer layers of the skin, making it useful in conditions such as ichthyosis, in which the skin thickens abnormally, causing scaling.

A 12–16-week course of treatment often clears the acne. The skin may be very dry, flaky, and itchy at first, but this usually improves as treatment continues. Serious *adverse effects* include liver damage and bowel inflammation.

QUICK REFERENCE

Drug group Drug for acne (p.165)
Overdose danger rating Medium
Dependence rating Low
Prescription needed Yes
Available as generic Yes

INFORMATION FOR USERS

Your drug prescription is tailored for you. Do not alter dosage without checking with your physician.

How taken

Capsules.

Frequency and timing of doses
1–2 x daily (take capsules with food or milk).

Usual adult dosage range
Dosage is determined individually.

Onset of effect
2–4 weeks. Acne may worsen during the first few weeks of treatment in some people.

Duration of action
Effects persist for several weeks after the drug has been stopped. Acne is usually completely cleared.

Diet advice
None.

Storage
Keep in a closed container in a cool, dry place out of the reach of children. Protect from light.

Missed dose
Take as soon as you remember. If your next dose is due within 4 hours, take a single dose now and skip the next.

Stopping the drug
Can be safely stopped as soon as you no longer need it, but best results are achieved when the course of treatment is completed as prescribed.

Exceeding the dose
An occasional unintentional extra dose is unlikely to cause problems. Large overdoses may cause headaches, vomiting, abdominal pain, facial flushing, incoordination, and dizziness. Notify your physician.

SPECIAL PRECAUTIONS

Do not donate blood during, or for at least a month after, taking oral isotretinoin. Be sure to tell your physician or pharmacist before taking this drug if:
▼ You have long-term liver or kidney problems.
▼ You suffer from arthritis.
▼ You have diabetes.
▼ You have high blood fat levels.
▼ You wear contact lenses.
▼ You suffer from gout.
▼ You are taking other medications.

Pregnancy
▼ Must not be prescribed. The drug is known to cause abnormalities in the developing baby. Effective contraception must be used during treatment and for at least a month before and after.

Breast-feeding
▼ The drug passes into the breast milk and may affect the baby. Discuss with your physician.

Infants and children
▼ Not prescribed.

Over 60
▼ Not usually prescribed.

Driving and hazardous work
▼ Avoid such activities until you have learned how the drug affects you because it can cause vision problems in dim light or darkness.

Alcohol
▼ Regular heavy drinking may raise blood fat levels with isotretinoin.

Sunlight
▼ Avoid exposure to the sun and sunlamps.

POSSIBLE ADVERSE EFFECTS

Dryness of the nose, mouth, and eyes, inflammation of the lips, and flaking of the skin occur in most cases. Temporary loss or increase of hair may also occur. If headache accompanied by symptoms such as nausea and vomiting, abdominal pain with diarrhea, blood in the feces, or visual impairment occur, consult your physician promptly.

Symptom/effect	Frequency		Discuss with physician		Stop taking drug now	Call physician now
	Common	Rare	Only if severe	In all cases		
Dry skin/nosebleeds	●		■			
Muscle/joint pain	●		■			
Lip/eye dryness/inflammation	●			■		
Headache		●		■		
Impaired vision		●		■		
Nausea/vomiting		●		■		
Abdominal pain/diarrhea		●		■	▲	▮
Mood changes		●	■			

INTERACTIONS

Tetracycline antibiotics These may increase the risk of high pressure in the skull, leading to headaches, nausea, and vomiting.

Skin-drying preparations Medicated cosmetics, soaps, toiletries, and anti-acne preparations increase the likelihood of dryness and irritation of the skin with isotretinoin.

Vitamin A Supplements of this vitamin increase the risk of adverse effects from isotretinoin.

PROLONGED USE

Treatment rarely exceeds 16 weeks. Prolonged use may raise blood fat levels, and increase the risk of heart and blood vessel disease. Bone changes may occur.

Monitoring Liver function tests and checks on blood fat levels are performed.

KETOCONAZOLE

Product names Ketoderm, Nizoral
Used in the following combined preparations None

GENERAL INFORMATION

Ketoconazole is prescribed for severe, internal *systemic* fungal infections. It is also given to treat serious infections of the skin and mucous membranes caused by the *Candida* yeast. People with rare fungal diseases (for example, paracoccidioidomycosis, histoplasmosis, and coccidioidomycosis) may also be given this antifungal drug.

Ketoconazole is applied as a cream to treat fungal skin infections, and as a shampoo for the treatment of scalp infections and seborrhoeic dermatitis.

The most common *side effect* of ketoconazole is nausea, which can be reduced by taking the drug at bedtime or with meals. Ketoconazole may also cause liver damage.

QUICK REFERENCE

Drug group Antifungal drug (p.124)

Overdose danger rating Medium

Dependence rating Low

Prescription needed Yes (except for some shampoos)

Available as generic Yes (oral)

INFORMATION FOR USERS

Your drug prescription is tailored for you. Do not alter dosage without checking with your physician.

How taken

Tablets, cream, shampoo.

Frequency and timing of doses
Once daily with food (by mouth); 1–2 x daily (cream); 1–2 times weekly (shampoo used for seborrhoeic dermatitis).

Usual dosage range
Adults 200–400mg daily (by mouth).
Children Reduced dose according to age and weight.

Onset of effect
The drug begins to work within a few hours; full beneficial effect may take several days.

Duration of action
Up to 24 hours.

Diet advice
None.

Storage
Keep in a closed container in a cool, dry place out of the reach of children.

Missed dose (oral)
Take as soon as you remember. If your next dose is due within 6 hours, take a single dose now and skip the next.

Stopping the drug
Take the full course. Even if you feel better, the infection may still be present; symptoms may recur if treatment is stopped too soon.

Exceeding the dose
An occasional unintentional extra dose is unlikely to be a cause for concern. Large overdoses may cause gastric problems. Notify your physician.

SPECIAL PRECAUTIONS

Be sure to tell your physician if:
▼ You have long-term liver or kidney problems.
▼ You have porphyria.
▼ You have previously had an allergic reaction to antifungal drugs.
▼ You are taking other medications.

Pregnancy
▼ Not usually prescribed. May cause defects in the developing baby. Discuss with your physician.

Breast-feeding
▼ The drug passes into the breast milk and may affect the baby. Discuss with your physician.

Infants and children
▼ Reduced dose necessary.

Over 60
▼ No special problems.

Driving and hazardous work
▼ No special problems.

Alcohol
▼ Avoid. Alcohol may interact with this drug to cause flushing and nausea.

POSSIBLE ADVERSE EFFECTS

Nausea is the most common side effect of ketoconazole; liver damage is a rare but serious adverse effect causing *jaundice* that may necessitate stopping the drug.

Symptom/effect	Frequency		Discuss with physician		Stop taking drug now	Call physician now
	Common	Rare	Only if severe	In all cases		
Nausea/vomiting	●		■			
Headache		●	■			
Abdominal pain		●	■			
Itching/rash		●		■	▲	
Painful breasts (men)		●		■	▲	
Jaundice		●		■	▲	▮

INTERACTIONS (administration by mouth only)

Antacids, cimetidine, and ranitidine These drugs may reduce the effectiveness of ketoconazole if they are taken within 2 hours before or after ketoconazole.

Rifampin and phenytoin These drugs may reduce the effect of ketoconazole.

Sedatives, warfarin, cyclosporine, tacrolimus, sirolimus, theophylline, and sildenafil Ketoconazole increases the effects of these drugs.

Eletriptan Use of this drug with ketoconazole is not recommended.

Antiviral drugs Adjustments in doses of these drugs may be necessary if used with ketoconazole.

Antimalarials The use of artemether with lumefantrine should be avoided when taking ketoconazole.

Simvastatin Ketoconazole may increase the risk of muscle damage if simvastatin or other statins are taken with it.

PROLONGED USE

The risk of liver damage increases with use for more than 14 days.

Monitoring Periodic blood tests are usually performed to check the effect of the drug on the liver.

KETOPROFEN

Product names Apo-Keto, and others
Used in the following combined preparations None

GENERAL INFORMATION

Ketoprofen is a non-steroidal anti-inflammatory (NSAID) drug which, like other NSAIDs, relieves pain and reduces inflammation and stiffness in rheumatoid arthritis, osteoarthritis, and ankylosing spondylitis. The drug does not cure the underlying disease, however.

Ketoprofen is also given to relieve mild to moderate pain of menstruation and soft tissue injuries, and the pain that occurs following operations.

The most common *adverse reactions* to ketoprofen, as with all NSAIDs, are gastrointestinal disturbances such as nausea and indigestion. Switching to another NSAID may be recommended by your physician if unwanted effects are persistent or troublesome.

QUICK REFERENCE

Drug group Non-steroidal anti-inflammatory drug (p.102)
Overdose danger rating Medium
Dependence rating Low
Prescription needed Yes
Available as generic Yes

INFORMATION FOR USERS

Your drug prescription is tailored for you. Do not alter dosage without checking with your physician.

How taken

Tablets, SR-tablets, capsules, SR-capsules, suppositories.

Frequency and timing of doses
Once daily (SR-tablets/capsules) or 2 x daily (tablets/capsules) with food; 2 x daily (suppositories).

Usual adult dosage range
100–200mg daily.

Onset of effect
Pain relief may be felt in 30 minutes to 2 hours. Full anti-inflammatory effect may not be felt for up to 2 weeks.

Duration of action
Up to 8–12 hours.

Diet advice
None.

Storage
Keep in a closed container in a cool, dry place out of the reach of children.

Missed dose
Take as soon as you remember. If your next dose is due within 4 hours, take a single dose now and skip the next.

Stopping the drug
Seek medical advice before stopping the drug.

Exceeding the dose
An occasional unintentional extra dose is unlikely to be a cause for concern. Large overdoses may cause vomiting, confusion, or irritability. Notify your physician.

SPECIAL PRECAUTIONS

Be sure to tell your physician if:
▼ You have long-term liver or kidney problems.
▼ You have heart problems.
▼ You have high blood pressure.
▼ You have asthma.
▼ You have had a peptic ulcer, esophagitis, or acid indigestion.
▼ You have bleeding problems.
▼ You are allergic to ASA or other NSAIDs.
▼ You are taking other medications.

Pregnancy
▼ Safety in pregnancy not established. Discuss with your physician.

Breast-feeding
▼ The drug passes into the breast milk and may affect the baby. Discuss with your physician.

Infants and children
▼ Not recommended for children under 12 years.

Over 60
▼ Increased likelihood of adverse effects. Reduced dose may therefore be necessary.

Driving and hazardous work
▼ Avoid such activities until you have learned how ketoprofen affects you because the drug can cause dizziness and drowsiness.

Alcohol
▼ Avoid. Alcohol may increase the risk of stomach disorders with ketoprofen.

Surgery and general anesthetics
▼ Ketoprofen may prolong bleeding. Discuss this with your physician or dentist before having any surgery.

POSSIBLE ADVERSE EFFECTS

Gastrointestinal disturbances, such as nausea, abdominal pain, and indigestion, commonly occur with ketoprofen when taken by mouth.

Suppositories may cause rectal irritation. Black or bloodstained feces should be reported promptly.

Symptom/effect	Frequency		Discuss with physician		Stop taking drug now	Call physician now
	Common	Rare	Only if severe	In all cases		
Nausea/vomiting	●			■		
Abdominal pain	●			■		
Heartburn	●		■			
Headache		●	■			
Dizziness/drowsiness		●	■			
Swollen feet or legs		●	■			
Weight gain		●	■			
Rash/itching		●		■	▲	▮
Wheezing/breathlessness		●		■	▲	▮
Black/bloodstained feces		●		■	▲	▮

INTERACTIONS

General note Ketoprofen interacts with a wide range of drugs, such as other NSAIDs including ASA, oral anticoagulants, and corticosteroids, to increase the risk of bleeding and/or stomach ulcers.

Lithium, digoxin, and methotrexate Ketoprofen may raise blood levels of these drugs to an undesirable extent.

Phenytoin Ketoprofen may enhance the effects of phenytoin.

Quinolone antibiotics Ketoprofen may increase the risk of seizures if taken with these drugs.

Antihypertensive drugs Ketoprofen may reduce the beneficial effects of these drugs.

PROLONGED USE

There is an increased risk of bleeding from peptic ulcers and in the bowel with prolonged use of ketoprofen.

LACTULOSE

Product names Apo-lactulose, PMS-lactulose
Used in the following combined preparations None

GENERAL INFORMATION

Lactulose is an effective laxative that softens feces by increasing the amount of water in the large intestine. It is used for the relief of constipation and fecal impaction, especially in the elderly. This drug is less likely than some of the other laxatives to disrupt normal bowel action.

Lactulose is also used for preventing and treating brain disturbance associated with liver failure, known as hepatic encephalopathy.

Because lactulose acts locally in the large intestine and is not absorbed into the body, it is safer than many other laxatives. However, the drug can cause stomach cramps and flatulence especially at the start of treatment.

INFORMATION FOR USERS

Follow instructions on the label. Call your physician if symptoms worsen.

How taken

Liquid.

Frequency and timing of doses
2 x daily (chronic constipation);
3–4 x daily (liver failure).

Usual adult dosage range
15–30ml daily (chronic constipation);
30–120ml daily (liver failure). May dilute drug with water or juice.

Onset of effect
24–48 hours.

Duration of action
6–18 hours.

Diet advice
Maintaining adequate fluid intake is important.

Storage
Keep in a closed container in a cool, dry place out of the reach of children. Do not store after diluting.

Missed dose
Take as soon as you remember. If your next dose is due within 3 hours, take a single dose now and skip the next.

Stopping the drug
In the treatment of constipation, the drug can be safely stopped as soon as you no longer need it.

Exceeding the dose
An occasional unintentional extra dose is unlikely to be a cause for concern. But if you notice any unusual symptoms, or if a large overdose has been taken, notify your physician.

SPECIAL PRECAUTIONS

Be sure to consult your physician or pharmacist before taking this drug if:
▼ You have severe abdominal pain.
▼ You suffer from lactose intolerance or galactosemia.
▼ You are taking other medications.

Pregnancy
▼ No evidence of risk. Discuss with your physician.

Breast-feeding
▼ No evidence of risk.

Infants and children
▼ Reduced dose necessary.

Over 60
▼ No special problems.

Driving and hazardous work
▼ No known problems.

Alcohol
▼ No known problems.

POSSIBLE ADVERSE EFFECTS

Adverse effects are rarely serious and often disappear when your body adjusts to the medicine. Diarrhea may indicate that the dosage of lactulose is too high.

Symptom/effect	Frequency		Discuss with physician		Stop taking drug now	Call physician now
	Common	Rare	Only if severe	In all cases		
Flatulence/belching	●		■			
Stomach cramps	●		■			
Nausea		●	■			
Abdominal distension		●		■		
Diarrhea		●		■		

INTERACTIONS

Mesalazine Lactulose may reduce the release of mesalazine at the site of action.

PROLONGED USE

In children, prolonged use may contribute to the development of dental caries.

LAMOTRIGINE

Product name Lamictal
Used in the following combined preparations None

GENERAL INFORMATION

Lamotrigine is an anticonvulsant drug that is prescribed, either alone or in combination with other anticonvulsants, for the treatment of epilepsy. The drug acts by restoring the balance between excitatory and inhibitory *neurotransmitters* in the brain. Lamotrigine may be less sedating than older anticonvulsants, and there is no need for blood tests to determine the level of the drug in the blood.

Lamotrigine may cause a number of minor *adverse effects* (see below), most of which will respond to an adjustment in dosage. Unlike many of the older anticonvulsant drugs, lamotrigine does not interfere with the action of the oral contraceptive pill.

INFORMATION FOR USERS

Your drug prescription is tailored for you. Do not alter dosage without checking with your physician.

How taken

Tablets, dispersible/chewable tablets.

Frequency and timing of doses
1 – 2 x daily.

Usual adult dosage range
100–500mg daily (maintenance) (100–200mg with valproic acid). Smaller doses are used at start of treatment. Dose may vary if other anticonvulsant drugs are being taken.

Onset of effect
Approximately 5 days at a constant dose.

Duration of action
Up to 24 hours.

Diet advice
None.

Storage
Keep in a closed container in a cool, dry place out of the reach of children.

Missed dose
Take as soon as you remember. If your next dose is due within 2 hours, take a single dose now and skip the next.

Stopping the drug
Do not stop taking the drug without consulting your physician, who will supervise a gradual reduction in dosage over a period of about two weeks. Abrupt cessation increases the risk of rebound fits.

Exceeding the dose
An occasional unintentional extra dose is unlikely to be a cause for concern. Large overdoses may cause sedation, double vision, loss of muscular coordination, nausea, and vomiting. Contact your physician immediately.

POSSIBLE ADVERSE EFFECTS

Serious adverse effects are rare. The most common side effects are skin rash, nausea, headache, tiredness, insomnia, blurred or double vision, dizziness, agitation, confusion, and poor muscle coordination. Although common, a rash may indicate a serious hypersenstivity reaction; call your physician immediately. If sore throat, flu-like symptoms, or persistent or unusual bruising occur, call your physician immediately.

Symptom/effect	Frequency		Discuss with physician		Stop taking drug now	Call physician now
	Common	Rare	Only if severe	In all cases		
Headache	●		■			
Rash	●			■		▮
Blurred vision/double vision	●			■		
Tremor/incoordination	●			■		
Nausea		●	■			
Flu-like symptoms		●		■		▮
Sore throat/bruising		●		▮		▮
Swelling around the face		●		■		▮

INTERACTIONS

Valproic acid increases and prolongs the effectiveness of lamotrigine. A reduced dose of lamotrigine will be used.

Antidepressants, antipsychotics, mefloquine, and chloroquine may counteract the anticonvulsant effect of lamotrigine.

Carbamazepine may reduce lamotrigine blood levels, but lamotrigine may increase the side effects of carbamazepine.

Phenytoin and phenobarbital may decrease blood levels of lamotrigine so a higher dose of lamotrigine may be needed.

SPECIAL PRECAUTIONS

Be sure to tell your physician if:
▼ You have long-term liver or kidney problems.
▼ You suffer from thalassemia.
▼ You have a heart condition.
▼ You are taking other medications.

Pregnancy
▼ Safety in pregnancy not established. Discuss with your physician.

Breast-feeding
▼ The drug passes into the breast milk and may affect the baby. Discuss with your physician.

Infants and children
▼ Not recommended under 2 years. Not recommended as a single therapy under 12 years. Doses may be relatively higher than adult doses due to increased metabolism.

Over 60s
▼ No special problems.

Driving and hazardous work
▼ Your underlying condition, in addition to the possibility of sedation, dizziness, and vision disturbances while taking lamotrigine, may make such activities inadvisable. Discuss with your physician.

Alcohol
▼ Alcohol may increase the adverse effects of this drug.

PROLONGED USE

No special problems.

LANSOPRAZOLE

Product name Prevacid
Used in the following combined preparations Hp-PAC

GENERAL INFORMATION

Lansoprazole is an anti-ulcer drug belonging to the group called proton pump inhibitors (p.95). It is used to treat peptic ulcers, gastro-esophageal reflux (in which the stomach acid rises into and irritates the esophagus), and Zollinger-Ellison syndrome (in which large quantities of stomach acid are produced, leading to ulceration).

Lansoprazole may be used alone or, for peptic ulcers, with two antibiotics, as part of a seven-day regimen to eradicate *Helicobacter pylori* bacteria, the main cause of such ulcers.

Because lansoprazole may mask the symptoms of stomach cancer, it is prescribed only when the possibility of this disease has been ruled out.

QUICK REFERENCE

Drug group Anti-ulcer drug (p.95)
Overdose danger rating Low
Dependence rating Low
Prescription needed Yes
Available as generic No

INFORMATION FOR USERS

Your drug prescription is tailored for you. Do not alter dosage without checking with your physician.

How taken

Capsules, oral suspension.

Frequency and timing of doses
1–2 x daily in the morning.

Usual adult dosage range
Benign gastric ulcer 15–30mg daily in the morning.
NSAID-associated gastric ulcer 15–30mg daily in the morning.
Duodenal ulcer 15mg daily in the morning.
H. pylori-associated ulcer 30mg daily with appropriate antibiotics.

Onset of effect
1–2 hours.

Duration of action
24 hours.

Diet advice
None, although spicy foods and alcohol may exacerbate the condition being treated.

Storage
Keep in a closed container in a cool, dry place out of the reach of children.

Missed dose
Take as soon as you remember. If your next dose is due within 8 hours, take a single dose now and skip the next.

Stopping the drug
Do not stop taking the drug without consulting your physician; symptoms may recur.

Exceeding the dose
An occasional unintentional extra dose is unlikely to be a cause for concern. But if you notice any unusual symptoms, or if a large overdose has been taken, notify your physician.

SPECIAL PRECAUTIONS

Be sure to tell your physician if:
▼ You have liver problems.
▼ You are taking other medications.

Pregnancy
▼ Safety not established. Discuss with your physician.

Breast-feeding
▼ Safety not established. Discuss with your physician.

Infants and children
▼ Not recommended.

Over 60
▼ No special problems.

Driving and hazardous work
▼ No special problems.

Alcohol
▼ Avoid. Alcohol may aggravate your condition and reduce the beneficial effects of lansoprazole.

PROLONGED USE

No problems expected.

POSSIBLE ADVERSE EFFECTS

Common *side effects* include headache, indigestion, and diarrhea. A sore throat or breathlessness are rare but should be reported to your physician at once.

Symptom/effect	Frequency		Discuss with physician		Stop taking drug now	Call physician now
	Common	Rare	Only if severe	In all cases		
Headache/dizziness	●		■			
Diarrhea/constipation	●		■			
Flatulence/abdominal pain	●		■			
Fatigue/malaise		●	■			
Muscle/joint pain		●		■		
Bruising/swollen extremities		●		■		
Rash/itching		●		■	▲	
Sore throat		●		■	▲	▮
Wheeziness/breathing difficulty		●		■	▲	▮

INTERACTIONS

Oral contraceptives, phenytoin, carbamazepine, warfarin, and theophylline Lansoprazole may reduce the effect of these drugs.

Antacids and sucralfate These drugs may reduce the absorption of, and should not be taken within an hour of, lansoprazole.

LATANOPROST

Product name Xalatan
Used in the following combined preparation Xalacom

GENERAL INFORMATION

Latanoprost is a synthetic derivative of the prostaglandin dinoprost, which constricts the smooth muscle in the blood vessels and bronchi. Latanoprost is used as eye drops to reduce pressure inside the eye in open angle (chronic) glaucoma (p.156) by constricting the pupils. The drug is used when patients have not responded to or cannot tolerate the drug of first choice, usually a beta blocker (for example timolol, p.449). Sometimes, combined eye drops of latanoprost and timolol may be prescribed when timolol alone is not adequately controlling the pressure.

Latanoprost eye drops can gradually increase the amount of brown pigment in the eye, darkening the iris (because of increased amounts of melanin). This will be particularly noticeable if only one eye needs treatment. Irises of mixed coloration are especially susceptible; pure blue eyes do not seem to be affected. Latanoprost has also been reported to cause darkening, thickening, and lengthening of eyelashes.

QUICK REFERENCE

Drug group Drug for glaucoma (p.156)

Overdose danger rating Medium

Dependence rating Low

Prescription needed Yes

Available as generic No

INFORMATION FOR USERS

Your drug prescription is tailored for you. Do not alter dosage without checking with your physician.

How taken

Eye drops.

Frequency and timing of doses
1x daily, in the evening.

Usual adult dosage range
1 drop per eye, daily.

Onset of effect
15-30 minutes.

Duration of action
24 hours.

Diet advice
None.

Storage
Keep the eyedrops in the outer cardboard package to protect from light. Store in a refrigerator between 2°C and 8°C, out of the reach of children.

Missed dose
Use the next dose as normal.

Stopping the drug
Do not stop the drug without consulting your physician. Symptoms may recur.

Exceeding the dose
An occasional unintentional extra application is unlikely to cause problems. Excessive use may irritate the eye and produce adverse effects in other parts of the body. Notify your physician.

POSSIBLE ADVERSE EFFECTS

Darkening of the iris is very common. Changes to the eyelashes occur almost as often. Irritation of the eye is also a very common adverse effect.

Symptom/effect	Frequency		Discuss with physician		Stop taking drug now	Call physician now
	Common	Rare	Only if severe	In all cases		
Darkening of iris	●		■			
Eye irritation	●		■			
Eyelash changes	●		■			
Eye pain	●			■		
Bloodshot eye	●			■		
Inflamed eyelids	●			■		
Eye/facial swelling		●		■		
Chest pains		●		■	▲	
Wheezing/breathing difficulty		●		■	▲	

INTERACTIONS

Thiomersal-containing eye drops should not be used within 5 minutes of using latanoprost (thiomersal is a preservative used in some eye drops).

SPECIAL PRECAUTIONS

Be sure to consult your physician or pharmacist before taking this drug if:
▼ You wear contact lenses.
▼ You are allergic to benzalkonium chloride or latanoprost.
▼ You have asthma.
▼ You are taking other medications.

Pregnancy
▼ Safety not established. Prostaglandins may affect the fetus.

Breast-feeding
▼ The drug may pass into the breast milk and may affect the baby. Discuss with your physician.

Infants and children
▼ Not recommended.

Over 60
▼ No special problems.

Driving and hazardous work
▼ No known problems.

Alcohol
▼ No known problems.

PROLONGED USE

No known problems apart from changes to iris pigment and eyelash colour.

Monitoring Although there should be no problems with long-term use, your physician will continue to monitor eye pigmentation as well as control of the glaucoma.

LEVODOPA

Product name None
Used in the following combined preparations Prolopa, Sinemet, Sinemet CR

GENERAL INFORMATION

The treatment of Parkinson's disease underwent dramatic change in the 1960s with the introduction of levodopa. Since the body can transform levodopa into dopamine, a chemical messenger in the brain the absence or shortage of which causes Parkinson's disease (see p.71), rapid improvements in control were obtained. These improvements were not a cure of the disease but a marked relief of symptoms.

However, it was found that, while levodopa was effective, it produced severe *side effects*, such as nausea, dizziness, and palpitations. Even when treatment was initiated gradually, it was difficult to balance the benefits against the *adverse reactions*.

Today the drug is combined with carbidopa or benserazide, both of which enhance the effects of levodopa in the brain and also help to reduce the side effects of levodopa.

INFORMATION FOR USERS

Your drug prescription is tailored for you. Do not alter dosage without checking with your physician.

How taken

Tablets, controlled-release tablets, capsules.

Frequency and timing of doses
3–6 x daily with food or milk.

Usual adult dosage range
125–500mg initially, increased until benefits and side effects are balanced.

Onset of effect
Within 1 hour.

Duration of action
2–12 hours.

Diet advice
None.

Storage
Keep in a closed container in a cool, dry place out of the reach of children. Protect from light.

Missed dose
Take as soon as you remember. If your next dose is due within 2 hours, take a single dose now and skip the next.

Stopping the drug
Do not stop taking the drug without consulting your physician; stopping the drug may lead to severe worsening of the underlying condition.

Exceeding the dose
An occasional unintentional extra dose is unlikely to cause problems. Larger overdoses may cause vomiting or drowsiness. Notify your physician.

POSSIBLE ADVERSE EFFECTS

Adverse effects of levodopa are related to dosage levels. At the start of treatment, on a low dosage, unwanted effects are likely to be mild. Such effects may increase in severity as dosage is increased. All adverse effects should be discussed with your physician.

Symptom/effect	Frequency		Discuss with physician		Stop taking drug now	Call physician now
	Common	Rare	Only if severe	In all cases		
Digestive disturbance	●			■		
Abnormal movement	●			■		
Nervousness/agitation	●			■		
Dark urine	●		■			
Dizziness/fainting		●		■		
Confusion/vivid dreams		●		■		
Palpitations		●		■	▲	▮

INTERACTIONS

Antidepressant drugs Levodopa may interact with monoamine oxidase inhibitors (MAOIs) to cause a dangerous rise in blood pressure. It may also interact with tricyclic antidepressants.

Pyridoxine (vitamin B$_6$) Excessive intake of this vitamin may reduce the effect of levodopa if levodopa is used on its own.

Iron Absorption of levodopa may be reduced by iron.

Antipsychotic drugs Some of these drugs may reduce the effect of levodopa.

Bupropion The side effects of levodopa will be increased if used with this drug.

SPECIAL PRECAUTIONS

Be sure to tell your physician if:
▼ You have heart problems.
▼ You have long-term liver or kidney problems.
▼ You have a lung disorder, such as asthma or bronchitis.
▼ You have an overactive thyroid gland.
▼ You have had glaucoma.
▼ You have a peptic ulcer.
▼ You have diabetes.
▼ You have any serious mental illness.
▼ You have ever had malignant melanoma.
▼ You are taking other medications.

Pregnancy
▼ Unlikely to be required.

Breast-feeding
▼ Unlikely to be required.

Infants and children
▼ Not normally used in children (and rarely given to patients under 25 years).

Over 60
▼ No special problems.

Driving and hazardous work
▼ Your underlying condition, as well as the possibility of levodopa causing fainting and dizziness, may make such activities inadvisable. Discuss with your physician.

Alcohol
▼ No known problems.

PROLONGED USE

Effectiveness usually declines in time, necessitating increased dosage and/or addition of other medications. The adverse effects may become so severe that ultimately the drug must be stopped.

LEVOFLOXACIN

Product name Levaquin
Used in the following combined preparations None

GENERAL INFORMATION

Levofloxacin is a quinolone antibacterial drug used for soft-tissue and respiratory and urinary tract infections that have not responded to other antibiotics.

The drug is usually prescribed in the form of tablets, but it is administered by intravenous *infusion* to people with serious *systemic* infections or to those who cannot take drugs by mouth.

Like other quinolones, levofloxacin may occasionally cause tendon inflammation and damage, especially in the elderly or in people taking corticosteroids. You should, therefore, report tendon pain or inflammation to your physician straight away and stop taking the drug. The affected limb or limbs should be rested until the symptoms have subsided.

INFORMATION FOR USERS

Your drug prescription is tailored for you. Do not alter dosage without checking with your physician.

How taken

Tablets, injection.

Frequency and timing of doses
1 x 2 times daily for 7–14 days depending on infection (tablets).

Usual adult dosage range
250–1,000mg daily.

Onset of effect
1 hour.

Duration of action
12–24 hours.

Diet advice
None.

Storage
Keep in a closed container in a cool, dry place out of the reach of children.

Missed dose
Take as soon as you remember, then take your next dose when it is due.

Stopping the drug
Take the full course. Even if you feel better, the original infection may still be present, and symptoms may recur if treatment is stopped too soon.

Exceeding the dose
An occasional unintentional extra dose is unlikely to cause problems. Larger overdoses may cause mental disturbances and fits. Notify your physician.

POSSIBLE ADVERSE EFFECTS

Given by injection, levofloxacin may cause palpitations and a fall in blood pressure.

Nausea and vomiting are the most common *side effects* of the drug taken by mouth.

Symptom/effect	Frequency		Discuss with physician		Stop taking drug now	Call physician now
	Common	Rare	Only if severe	In all cases		
Nausea/vomiting	●		■			
Diarrhea/abdominal pain	●		■			
Headache/dizziness		●	■			
Skin rash/itching		●	■			
Drowsiness/restlessness		●	■			
Jaundice		●		■	▲	
Confusion/hallucinations		●		■	▲	
Fever/allergic reaction		●		■	▲	
Painful or inflamed tendons		●		■	▲	■

INTERACTIONS

Non-steroidal anti-inflammatory drugs (NSAIDs) and theophylline There is an increased risk of convulsions when these drugs are taken with levofloxacin.

Anticoagulants The effect of these drugs may be increased by levofloxacin.

Antacids, adsorbents, sucralfate, iron, and zinc These drugs may reduce the absorption of levofloxacin.

Cyclosporine There is an increased risk of kidney damage if cyclosporine is taken with levofloxacin.

SPECIAL PRECAUTIONS

Be sure to tell your physician if:
▼ You have kidney problems.
▼ You suffer from epilepsy.
▼ You have glucose-6-phosphate dehydrogenase (G6PD) deficiency.
▼ You have porphyria.
▼ You have diabetes.
▼ You are taking ASA or another NSAID.
▼ You have had a previous allergic reaction to a quinolone antibacterial.
▼ You have had a previous tendon problem with a quinolone.
▼ You are taking other medications.

Pregnancy
▼ Safety not established. Discuss with your physician.

Breast-feeding
▼ Safety not established. Discuss with your physician.

Infants and children
▼ Not recommended.

Over 60
▼ No special problems, except that tendon damage is more likely over the age of 60.

Driving and hazardous work
▼ Avoid such activities until you have learned how levofloxacin affects you because the drug can cause dizziness, drowsiness, visual disturbances, and hallucinations.

Alcohol
▼ Avoid. Alcohol may increase the sedative effects of levofloxacin.

Sunlight
▼ Avoid exposure to strong sunlight or artificial ultraviolet rays because photosensitization may occur.

PROLONGED USE

Levofloxacin is not usually prescribed for long-term use.

LEVONORGESTREL

Product names Plan B, Mirena
Used in the following combined preparations Alesse, Min-Ovral, Triphasil

---

GENERAL INFORMATION

Levonorgestrel is a synthetic hormone similar to progesterone, a natural female sex hormone. The drug's primary use is as an ingredient in oral contraceptives. It performs this function by thickening the mucus at the neck of the uterus (cervix), thereby making it difficult for sperm to enter the uterus.

Levonorgestrel is available both in combined oral contraceptives with an estrogen drug and in progestin-only preparations.

It is given for emergency, post-coital contraception. (It is also given in combination with an estrogen drug in hormone replacement therapy to treat menopausal symptoms.)

Levonorgestrel rarely causes serious *adverse effects*. When it is used without an estrogen, menstrual irregularities, especially mid-cycle, or "breakthrough", bleeding are common.

INFORMATION FOR USERS

Your drug prescription is tailored for you. Do not alter dosage without checking with your physician.

How taken

Tablets, intrauterine device (IUD).

Frequency and timing of doses
Once daily, at the same time each day.

Usual adult dosage range
Oral contraceptive 0.5–1mg with estrogen.
Post-coital contraceptive 750mcg; two doses 12 hours apart.

Onset of effect
Levonorgestrel starts to act within 4 hours, but contraceptive protection may not be fully effective for 14 days, depending on which day of the cycle the tablets are started.

Duration of action
24 hours. Some effects, not including contraception, may persist for up to 3 months after levonorgestrel is stopped.

Diet advice
None.

Storage
Keep in a closed container in a cool, dry place out of the reach of children.

Missed dose
If a tablet is delayed by 3 hours or more, regard it as a missed dose. See What to do if you miss a pill (p.151).

Stopping the drug
The drug can be safely stopped as soon as contraceptive protection is no longer required. For treatment of menopausal symptoms, consult your physician before stopping the drug.

Exceeding the dose
An occasional unintentional extra dose is unlikely to be a cause for concern. But if you notice any unusual symptoms, or if a large overdose has been taken, notify your physician.

SPECIAL PRECAUTIONS

Be sure to consult your physician or pharmacist before taking this drug if:
▼ You have a liver problem.
▼ You have heart failure or high blood pressure.
▼ You have diabetes.
▼ You have unexplained abnormal vaginal bleeding.
▼ You have had blood clots or a stroke.
▼ You have ever had migraines or severe headaches.
▼ You are taking other medications.

Pregnancy
▼ Not prescribed. May cause abnormalities in the developing baby. Discuss with your physician.

Breast-feeding
▼ The drug passes into the breast milk, but at normal doses adverse effects on the baby are unlikely. Discuss with your physician.

Infants and children
▼ Not prescribed.

Over 60
▼ Not prescribed.

Driving and hazardous work
▼ No known problems.

Alcohol
▼ No known problems.

POSSIBLE ADVERSE EFFECTS

Menstrual irregularities (blood spotting between menstrual periods or absence of menstruation) are the most common side effects of levonorgestrel alone.

Symptom/effect	Frequency		Discuss with physician		Stop taking drug now	Call physician now
	Common	Rare	Only if severe	In all cases		
Swollen feet/ankles	●		■			
Weight gain	●		■			
Irregular vaginal bleeding	●			■		
Nausea/vomiting		●	■			
Breast tenderness		●	■			
Depression		●		■		
Headache		●		■		

INTERACTIONS

General note The beneficial effects of many drugs, including bromocriptine, oral anticoagulants, anticonvulsants, and antihypertensive and antidiabetic drugs, may be affected by levonorgestrel. Many other drugs may reduce contraceptive protection. These include anticonvulsants, antituberculous drugs, and antibiotics. Inform your physician before taking any additional prescribed medication.

PROLONGED USE

Problems are rare.

LEVOTHYROXINE

Product names Eltroxin, Synthroid
Used in the following combined preparations None

GENERAL INFORMATION

Levothyroxine is the major hormone produced by the thyroid gland. A deficiency of the natural hormone causes hypothyroidism and may sometimes lead to myxedema, a condition characterized by slowing of body functions and facial puffiness. A synthetic preparation is used to replace the natural hormone when it is deficient.

Certain types of goitre (an enlarged thyroid gland) are helped by levothyroxine, and it may be prescribed to prevent the development of goitre during treatment with antithyroid drugs. Levothyroxine is also prescribed for some forms of thyroid cancer.

Adults who have a severe thyroid deficiency are sensitive to thyroid hormones, so treatment is introduced gradually, and increased slowly, to prevent *adverse effects*. Particular care is required in patients with heart problems such as angina.

INFORMATION FOR USERS

Your drug prescription is tailored for you. Do not alter dosage without checking with your physician.

How taken

Tablets.

Frequency and timing of doses
Once daily.

Usual dosage range
Adults Doses of 50–100mcg daily, increased at 3–4-week intervals as required. The maximum dose is 200mcg daily.

Onset of effect
Within 48 hours. Full beneficial effects may not be felt for several weeks.

Duration of action
1–3 weeks.

Diet advice
None.

Storage
Keep in a closed container in a cool, dry place out of the reach of children. Protect from light.

Missed dose
Take as soon as you remember. If your next dose is due within 8 hours, take a single dose now and skip the next.

Stopping the drug
Do not stop the drug without consulting your physician; symptoms may recur.

Exceeding the dose
An occasional unintentional extra dose is unlikely to cause problems. Large overdoses may cause palpitations during the next few days. Notify your physician.

SPECIAL PRECAUTIONS

Be sure to tell your physician if:
▼ You have high blood pressure.
▼ You have heart problems.
▼ You have diabetes.
▼ You are taking other medications.

Pregnancy
▼ No evidence of risk, but dosage adjustment may be necessary.

Breast-feeding
▼ The drug passes into the breast milk, but at normal doses adverse effects on the baby are unlikely. Discuss with your physician.

Infants and children
▼ Dosage depends on age and weight.

Over 60
▼ Reduced dose usually necessary.

Driving and hazardous work
▼ No known problems.

Alcohol
▼ No known problems.

POSSIBLE ADVERSE EFFECTS

Adverse effects are rare with levothyroxine and are usually the result of overdosage causing thyroid overactivity. These effects diminish as the dose is lowered. Too low a dose of levothyroxine may cause signs of thyroid underactivity.

Symptom/effect	Frequency		Discuss with physician		Stop taking drug now	Call physician now
	Common	Rare	Only if severe	In all cases		
Anxiety/nervousness		●		■		
Diarrhea		●		■		
Weight loss		●		■		
Sweating/flushing		●		■		
Muscle cramps/tremor		●		■		
Insomnia		●		■		
Palpitations/chest pain		●		■		■

PROLONGED USE

No special problems.

Monitoring Periodic tests of thyroid function are usually required.

INTERACTIONS

Oral anticoagulants Levothyroxine may increase the effect of these drugs.

Antidiabetic agents The doses of these drugs may need increasing once levothyroxine treatment is started.

Cholestyramine and sucralfate may both reduce absorption of levothyroxine.

Amiodarone may affect thyroid activity and levothyroxine dosage may need adjustment.

Antiepileptic drugs These drugs may reduce the effect of levothyroxine.

LISINOPRIL

Product names Prinivil, Zestril
Used in the following combined preparations Zestoretic, Prinzide

GENERAL INFORMATION

Lisinopril is an ACE inhibitor drug used in the treatment of high blood pressure (including that caused by diabetic kidney problems), heart failure, and following a heart attack. It works by relaxing the muscles in blood vessel walls, allowing them to dilate (widen), thereby easing blood flow.

Lisinopril can initially cause a rapid fall in blood pressure, especially when taken with a diuretic drug. Therefore, treatment for heart failure is usually started under close medical supervision, in hospital in severe cases. The first dose is usually very small, and should be taken while lying down, preferably at bedtime.

QUICK REFERENCE

Drug group ACE inhibitor (p.84)
Overdose danger rating Medium
Dependence rating Low
Prescription needed Yes
Available as generic Yes

INFORMATION FOR USERS

Your drug prescription is tailored for you. Do not alter dosage without checking with your physician.

How taken

Tablets.

Frequency and timing of doses
Once daily.

Usual adult dosage range
Hypertension 2.5mg (starting dose) up to 40mg.
Heart failure/diabetic nephropathy 2.5mg (starting dose) up to 20mg.
Prevention of further heart attacks 2.5–5mg (starting dose) up to 10mg.

Onset of effect
1–2 hours; full beneficial effect may take several weeks.

Duration of action
12–24 hours.

Diet advice
None.

Storage
Keep in a closed container in a cool, dry place out of the reach of children.

Missed dose
Take as soon as you remember. If your next dose is due within 8 hours, take a single dose now and skip the next.

Stopping the drug
Do not stop taking the drug without consulting your physician. Stopping the drug may lead to worsening of the underlying condition.

Exceeding the dose
An occasional unintentional extra dose is unlikely to be a cause for concern. Larger overdoses may cause dizziness or fainting. Notify your physician.

POSSIBLE ADVERSE EFFECTS

Common but unusual *side effects* of lisinopril are persistent dry cough and an altered sense of taste. A reduction of dosage may minimize these effects.

Symptom/effect	Frequency		Discuss with physician		Stop taking drug now	Call physician now
	Common	Rare	Only if severe	In all cases		
Nausea/vomiting	●		■			
Rash/itching		●	■			
Chest pain/palpitations		●		■		
Dry cough/altered sense of taste	●			■		
Dizziness/fainting		●		■		
Runny nose/sore throat		●		■		
Confusion/mood changes		●		■		
Jaundice		●		■		
Facial swelling		●		■	▲	■

INTERACTIONS

Potassium supplements, potassium-sparing diuretics, and cyclosporine Taken with lisinopril, these drugs increase the risk of high blood potassium levels.

Non-steroidal anti-inflammatory drugs (NSAIDs) Some of these drugs may reduce the effect of lisinopril, and the risk of kidney damage is increased.

Vasodilators, diuretics, and other drugs for hypertension These drugs may increase the effect of lisinopril.

Lithium Blood levels of lithium may be increased by lisinopril.

Insulin and antidiabetic drugs Lisinopril may increase the effect of these drugs.

SPECIAL PRECAUTIONS

Be sure to tell your physician if:
▼ You are allergic to other ACE inhibitors.
▼ You have a history of angioedema.
▼ You have kidney problems or are on dialysis.
▼ You are taking a diuretic drug.
▼ You are on a low sodium diet.
▼ You are taking other medications.

Pregnancy
▼ Not prescribed. May harm the developing baby.

Breast-feeding
▼ Safety not established. Discuss with your physician.

Infants and children
▼ Not recommended.

Over 60
▼ No special problems.

Driving and hazardous work
▼ Avoid such activities until you have learned how lisinopril affects you because the drug can cause dizziness and fainting.

Alcohol
▼ Avoid. Alcohol may increase the blood-pressure lowering and adverse effects of this drug.

PROLONGED USE

Rarely, prolonged use of lisinopril can lead to changes in blood count or kidney function.

Monitoring Periodic checks on potassium levels, white blood cell counts and urine are usually performed.

LITHIUM

Product names Carbolith, Duralith, Lithane
Used in the following combined preparation None

GENERAL INFORMATION

Lithium, the lightest known metal, has been used since the 1940s to treat manic depression or bipolar affective disorder. Lithium decreases the intensity and frequency of the swings from extreme excitement to deep depression that characterize the disorder.

It is sometimes used along with an antidepressant drug for depression that has not responded to an antidepressant alone. Treatment with lithium may be started in hospital for the seriously ill.

Careful monitoring is required because high levels of lithium can cause serious *adverse effects*. It may take two to three weeks for any apparent benefit, so an antipsychotic drug is often given with lithium until it becomes effective.

INFORMATION FOR USERS

Your drug prescription is tailored for you. Do not alter dosage without checking with your physician.

How taken

Capsules, tablets, SR-tablets, liquid.

Frequency and timing of doses
1–3 x daily with meals. Always take the same brand of lithium to ensure a consistent effect; change of brand must be closely supervised.

Usual adult dosage range
0.3–1.2g daily. Dosage may vary according to individual response.

Onset of effect
Some effects may be noticed in 3–5 days, but full benefits may not be felt for 3 weeks.

Duration of action
18–36 hours. Some effect may last for several days.

Diet advice
Lithium levels in the blood are affected by the amount of salt in the body, so do not suddenly alter the amount of salt in your diet. Be sure to drink plenty of fluids, especially in hot weather.

Storage
Keep in a closed container in a cool, dry place out of the reach of children.

Missed dose
Take as soon as you remember. If your next dose is due within 4 hours, take a single dose now and skip the next.

Stopping the drug
Do not stop the drug without consulting your physician; symptoms may recur.

OVERDOSE ACTION

Seek immediate medical advice in all cases. Take emergency action if convulsions or loss of consciousness occur.

See Drug poisoning emergency guide (p.526).

POSSIBLE ADVERSE EFFECTS

Many of the symptoms below are signs of a high lithium level in the blood. Stop taking the drug and seek medical advice promptly if you notice any of these symptoms.

Symptom/effect	Frequency		Discuss with physician		Stop taking drug now	Call physician now
	Common	Rare	Only if severe	In all cases		
Nausea/vomiting/diarrhea	●			■	▲	
Tremor	●			■		
Weight gain		●	■			
Drowsiness/lethargy		●		■	▲	
Blurred vision		●		■	▲	
Rash		●		■	▲	
Muscle weakness		●		■		
Increase in urine/thirst		●		■		

INTERACTIONS

General note Many drugs interact with lithium. Do not take any over-the-counter or prescription drugs without consulting your physician or pharmacist. Acetaminophen should be used in preference to other analgesics for everyday pain relief.

SPECIAL PRECAUTIONS

Be sure to tell your physician if:
▼ You have long-term liver or kidney problems.
▼ You have heart or circulation problems.
▼ You have an overactive thyroid gland.
▼ You have myasthenia gravis.
▼ You have Addison's disease.
▼ You are taking other medications.

Pregnancy
▼ Not usually prescribed. May cause defects in the unborn baby. Discuss with your physician.

Breast-feeding
▼ The drug passes into the breast milk and may affect the baby. Discuss with your physician.

Infants and children
▼ Not recommended.

Over 60
▼ Increased likelihood of adverse effects. Reduced dose may therefore be necessary.

Driving and hazardous work
▼ Avoid such activities until you have learned how lithium affects you because the drug can cause reduced alertness.

Alcohol
▼ Avoid. Alcohol may increase the sedative effects of this drug.

PROLONGED USE

Prolonged use may lead to kidney problems. Treatment for periods of longer than 5 years is not normally advised unless the benefits are significant and tests show no sign of reduced kidney function.

Monitoring Once stabilized, lithium levels should be checked every 3 months. Thyroid function should be checked every 6–12 months. Kidney function should also be monitored regularly.

LOPERAMIDE

Product name Imodium
Used in the following combined preparation Imodium Advanced

GENERAL INFORMATION

Loperamide is an antidiarrheal drug available in tablet, capsule, or liquid form. It reduces the loss of water and salts from the bowel and slows bowel activity, resulting in the passage of firmer bowel movements at less frequent intervals.

A fast-acting drug, loperamide is widely prescribed for both sudden and recurrent bouts of diarrhea. However, it is not generally recommended for diarrhea caused by infection because it may delay the expulsion of harmful substances from the bowel. Loperamide is often prescribed for people who have had a colostomy or an ileostomy, to reduce fluid loss from the stoma (outlet).

Adverse effects from this drug are rare. It can be purchased over-the-counter in a pharmacy.

QUICK REFERENCE

Drug group Antidiarrheal drug (p.96)

Overdose danger rating Medium

Dependence rating Low

Prescription needed No (most preparations)

Available as generic Yes

INFORMATION FOR USERS

Follow instructions on the label. Call your physician if symptoms worsen.

How taken

Tablets, caplets, quick dissolve tablets, chewable tablets, liquid.

Frequency and timing of doses
Acute diarrhea Take a double dose at start of treatment, then a single dose after each loose feces, up to the maximum daily dose.
Chronic diarrhea 2 x daily.

Usual dosage range
Acute diarrhea 4mg (starting dose), then 2mg after each loose bowel movement (up to 16mg daily); usual dose 6–8mg daily. Use for up to 5 days only (3 days only for children 4–8 years), then consult your physician.
Chronic diarrhea 4–8mg daily (up to 16mg daily).

Onset of effect
Within 1–2 hours.

Duration of action
6–18 hours.

Diet advice
Ensure adequate fluid, sugar, and salt intake during a diarrheal illness.

Storage
Keep in a closed container in a cool, dry place out of the reach of children.

Missed dose
Do not take the missed dose. Take your next dose if needed.

Stopping the drug
Can be safely stopped as soon as you no longer need it.

Exceeding the dose
An occasional unintentional extra dose is unlikely to be a cause for concern. Large overdoses may cause constipation, vomiting, or drowsiness, and affect breathing. Notify your physician.

SPECIAL PRECAUTIONS

Be sure to consult your physician or pharmacist before taking this drug if:
▼ You have long-term liver or kidney problems.
▼ You have had recent abdominal surgery.
▼ You have an infection or blockage in the intestine, pseudomembranous colitis, or ulcerative colitis.
▼ You are taking other medications.

Pregnancy
▼ Safety in pregnancy not established. Discuss with your physician.

Breast-feeding
▼ The drug passes into the breast milk and may affect the baby. Discuss with your physician.

Infants and children
▼ Not to be given to children under 4 years. Reduced dose necessary in older children. Children can be very sensitive to the effects of this drug so care should be taken.

Over 60
▼ No special problems.

Driving and hazardous work
▼ No known problems.

Alcohol
▼ No known problems.

POSSIBLE ADVERSE EFFECTS

Adverse effects are rare with loperamide and often difficult to distinguish from the effects of the diarrhea it is used to treat. If symptoms such as bloating, abdominal pain, or fever persist or worsen during treatment with loperamide, consult your physician.

Symptom/effect	Frequency		Discuss with physician		Stop taking drug now	Call physician now
	Common	Rare	Only if severe	In all cases		
Constipation		●	■		▲	
Bloating		●	■			
Abdominal pain		●	■			
Dry mouth		●	■			
Drowsiness or dizziness		●	■			
Itching skin		●		■		
Rash		●		■	▲	

INTERACTIONS

Opioid analgesics may cause severe constipation; avoid using them with loperamide.

PROLONGED USE

Although this drug is not usually taken for prolonged periods (except by persons with a medically diagnosed long-term gastrointestinal condition), special problems are not expected during long-term use.

LOPINAVIR/RITONAVIR

Product name Kaletra
Used in the following combined preparations None

GENERAL INFORMATION

Lopinavir and ritonavir are both antiretroviral drugs from the same class of drugs, known as protease inhibitors. Combined together as a single drug, they are used in the treatment of HIV infection. The drugs work by interfering with an enzyme used by the virus to produce genetic material.

The combination drug is prescribed with other antiretroviral drugs, usually two nucleoside analogues, which together slow down the production of HIV. The aim of this combination therapy is to reduce the damage done to the immune system by the virus.

Combination antiretroviral therapy is not a cure for HIV. Taken regularly on a long-term basis, it can reduce the level of the virus in the body and improve the outlook for the HIV patient. However, the patient will remain infectious, and will suffer a relapse if the treatment is stopped.

QUICK REFERENCE

Drug group Drug for HIV and immune deficiency (p.144)

Overdose danger rating Medium

Dependence rating Low

Prescription needed Yes

Available as generic No

INFORMATION FOR USERS

Your drug prescription is tailored for you. Do not alter dosage without checking with your physician.

How taken

Capsules, liquid.

Frequency and timing of doses
Every 12 hours, with food.

Usual adult dosage range
3 capsules or 5ml liquid.

Onset of effect
Within 1 hour.

Duration of action
12 hours.

Diet advice
None.

Storage
Keep in the fridge in the original container out of the reach of children.

Missed dose
Take as soon as you remember. If your next dose is due within 2 hours, take a single dose now and skip the next. It is very important not to miss doses on a regular basis as this can lead to the development of drug-restant HIV.

Stopping the drug
Do not stop taking the drug without consulting your physician.

Exceeding the dose
An occasional unintentional extra dose is unlikely to cause problems. But if you notice any unusual symptoms, or if a large overdose has been taken, notify your physician.

SPECIAL PRECAUTIONS

Be sure to tell your physician if:
▼ You have long-term liver or kidney problems.
▼ You take recreational drugs.
▼ You are taking other medications.

Pregnancy
▼ Safety in pregnancy not established. Discuss with your physician.

Breast-feeding
▼ Safety in breast-feeding not established. Breast-feeding is not recommended for HIV-positive mothers as the virus may be passed to the baby.

Infants and children
▼ Not recommended in children under 2 years. Reduced dose recommended in children over 2 years.

Over 60
▼ Reduced dose may be necessary to minimize adverse effects.

Driving and hazardous work
▼ No known problems.

Alcohol
▼ The liquid form of the drug contains a small amount of alcohol, so care should be taken if alcoholic drinks are consumed as well.

POSSIBLE ADVERSE EFFECTS

Gastrointestinal upset is the most common adverse effect. Other problems, which are more likely to occur with prolonged use, include changes in body shape, and should be discussed with your physician.

Symptom/effect	Frequency		Discuss with physician		Stop taking drug now	Call physician now
	Common	Rare	Only if severe	In all cases		
Nausea/vomiting/diarrhea	●			■		
Loss of appetite	●			■		
Fatigue	●			■		
Body shape changes		●		■		
Severe abdominal pain		●			■	▮

INTERACTIONS

General note A wide range of drugs may interact with lopinavir and ritonavir, causing either an increase in adverse effects or a reduction in the effect of the antiretroviral drugs. Check with your physician or pharmacist before taking any new drugs, including those from the dentist and supermarket, and herbal medicines. Ritonavir is known to interact with some recreational drugs, including ecstasy, and it is essential that you discuss the use of such drugs with your physician or pharmacist.

PROLONGED USE

Changes in body shape may occur.

Monitoring Your physician will take regular blood samples to check the effect of the drugs on the virus. Blood will also be checked for changes in lipids, cholesterol, and sugar levels.

LORATADINE/DESLORATADINE

Product names Aerius, Claritin, Claritin Kids
Used in the following combined preparations Chlor-Tripolon ND, Claritin Extra, Claritin Liberator

GENERAL INFORMATION

Loratadine, a long-acting antihistamine drug, is used for the relief of symptoms associated with allergic rhinitis, such as sneezing, nasal discharge, and itching and burning of the eyes. Symptoms are normally relieved within an hour of oral administration. Loratadine is also used to treat allergic skin conditions such as chronic urticaria (itching). An advantage of loratadine over older antihistamines, such as chlorpheniramine, is that it

has fewer sedative and *anticholinergic* effects, so this drug is less likely to cause drowsiness.

Desloratadine is an active breakdown product of loratadine. It is available as a separate product (Aerius).

Loratadine and desloratadine should be discontinued about four days prior to skin testing for allergy as they may decrease or prevent the detection of positive results.

INFORMATION FOR USERS

Follow instructions on the label. Call your physician if symptoms worsen.

How taken

Tablets, liquid, rapid-dissolve tablets (loratadine).

Frequency and timing of doses
Once daily.

Usual adult dosage range
10mg daily (loratadine); 5mg daily (desloratadine).

Onset of effect
Usually within 1 hour.

Duration of action
Up to 24 hours.

Diet advice
None.

Storage
Keep in a closed container in a cool, dry place out of the reach of children.

Missed dose
Take as soon as you remember. If your next dose is due within 6 hours, take a single dose now and skip the next.

Stopping the drug
Can be safely stopped as soon as you no longer need it.

Exceeding the dose
An occasional unintentional extra dose is unlikely to be a cause for concern. But if you notice any unusual symptoms, or if a large overdose has been taken, notify your physician.

SPECIAL PRECAUTIONS

Be sure to consult your physician or pharmacist before taking this drug if:
▼ You are taking other medications.

Pregnancy
▼ Safety in pregnancy not established. Discuss with your physician.

Breast-feeding
▼ The drug passes into the breast milk. Discuss with your physician.

Infants and children
▼ Not recommended for children under 2 years. Reduced dose necessary for older children.

Over 60
▼ No problems expected.

Driving and hazardous work
▼ Problems are unlikely, but be aware of how the drug affects you before driving or carrying out hazardous work.

Alcohol
▼ No known problems, but avoid excessive amounts.

POSSIBLE ADVERSE EFFECTS

The incidence of adverse effects with loratadine/desloratadine is low.

Symptom/effect	Frequency		Discuss with physician		Stop taking drug now	Call physician now
	Common	Rare	Only if severe	In all cases		
Fatigue		●	■			
Nausea		●	■			
Headache		●	■			
Palpitations		●		■		
Fainting		●		■		

INTERACTIONS

Cimetidine, clarithromycin, erythromycin, ketoconazole, fluoxetine, fluconazole, and quinidine These drugs may increase the blood levels and effects of loratadine, but this has not been found to cause problems.

PROLONGED USE

No problems expected.

LORAZEPAM

Product names Apo-Lorazepam, Ativan, Novo-Lorazem, Nu-Loraz
Used in the following combined preparation None

GENERAL INFORMATION

Lorazepam belongs to a group of drugs known as the benzodiazepines, which help to relieve anxiety and encourage sleep. The actions and adverse effects of this group of drugs are described more fully on page 67.

Lorazepam is used for the short-term treatment of excessive anxiety. In those with anxiety and insomnia, taking a dose at bedtime can help with sleep. The injectable form of the drug may be used as an anticonvulsant for the control of status epilepticus (see p.70). Lorazepam is less likely than some of the other benzodiazepines to accumulate in the body.

In common with other benzodiazepines, lorazepam can be habit-forming if taken regularly over a long period of time. Its effects may also diminish with time. For those reasons, treatment should be reviewed regularly.

(see p.70)

QUICK REFERENCE

Drug group Benzodiazepine anti-anxiety drug (p.67)

Overdose danger rating Medium

Dependence rating High

Prescription needed Yes

Available as generic Yes

INFORMATION FOR USERS

Your drug prescription is tailored for you. Do not alter dosage without checking with your physician.

How taken

Tablets, sublingual tablets, injection.

Frequency and timing of doses
1–4 x daily.

Usual adult dosage range
1–6mg daily (by mouth); varies with condition under treatment (injection) and age.

Onset of effect
30–60 minutes (oral tablets); 5–10 minutes (intravenous injection); less than 30 minutes (intramuscular injection, sublingual tablets).

Duration of action
Up to 12 hours.

Diet advice
None.

Storage
Keep in a closed container in a cool, dry place out of the reach of children. Protect from light.

Missed dose
If you are taking the drug once daily for insomnia, a missed dose is no cause for concern. Return to your normal dose schedule the following night, if necessary. On a daytime schedule, take the missed dose when you remember. If your next dose is due within 2 hours, take a single dose now and skip the next.

Stopping the drug
If you have been taking the drug continuously for less than 2 weeks, it can be safely stopped as soon as you feel you no longer need it. However, if you have been taking the drug for longer, consult your physician, who will supervise a gradual reduction in dosage. Stopping abruptly may lead to withdrawal symptoms (see p.66)

Exceeding the dose
An occasional unintentional extra dose is unlikely to cause problems. Larger overdoses may cause unusual drowsiness. Notify your physician.

(see p.66)

SPECIAL PRECAUTIONS

Be sure to tell your physician if:
▼ You have severe respiratory disease.
▼ You have impaired liver or kidney function.
▼ You have myasthenia gravis.
▼ You have glaucoma.
▼ You have or have had any problems with alcohol or drug abuse.
▼ You are taking other medications.

Pregnancy
▼ Safety in pregnancy not established. Discuss with your physician.

Breast-feeding
▼ The drug passes into the breast milk. Its effects on the baby are not clearly known. Discuss with your physician.

Infants and children
▼ Not recommended for those under 18 years.

Over 60
▼ Increased likelihood of adverse effects. Reduced dose may be therefore be necessary.

Driving and hazardous work
▼ Do not undertake such activities until you have learned how the drug affects you; it can cause reduced alertness and slowed reactions.

Alcohol
▼ Avoid. Alcohol increases the sedative effects of this drug.

POSSIBLE ADVERSE EFFECTS

The principal adverse effects of this drug are related to its sedative and tranquilizing properties and normally diminish after the first few days of treatment.

Symptom/effect	Frequency		Discuss with physician		Stop taking drug now	Call physician now
	Common	Rare	Only if severe	In all cases		
Daytime drowsiness	●		■			
Dizziness/unsteadiness		●		■		
Headache		●		■		
Nausea/vomiting		●		■		
Amnesia		●		■	▲	
Confusion/disorientation		●		■		▮
Rash		●		■	▲	▮

PROLONGED USE

Regular use of this drug over several weeks can lead to a reduction in its effect as the body adapts. It may also be habit-forming when taken for extended periods, especially if large doses are taken.

INTERACTIONS

Sedative All drugs, including alcohol, that have a sedative effect on the central nervous system are likely to increase the sedative properties of lorazepam. Such drugs include other anti-anxiety and sleeping drugs, antihistamines, antidepressants, opioid analgesics, scopolamine, and antipsychotics.

LOSARTAN

Product name Cozaar
Used in the following combined preparations Hyzaar, Hyzaar DS

GENERAL INFORMATION

Losartan is a member of the group of vasodilator drugs called angiotensin-II blockers. Used to treat hypertension, the drug works by blocking the action of angiotensin-II (a naturally occurring substance that constricts blood vessels). This action causes the blood vessel walls to relax, thereby easing blood pressure.

Unlike ACE inhibitors, losartan does not cause a persistent dry cough, and its use is now being evaluated in conditions such as heart failure, for which ACE inhibitors are currently being used.

Losartan is prescribed with caution to people with stenosis (narrowing) of the arteries to the kidneys because the initial dose causes a sudden drop in blood pressure. *Adverse effects*, which include diarrhea, dizziness, and fatigue, are rare.

INFORMATION FOR USERS

Your drug prescription is tailored for you. Do not alter dosage without checking with your physician.

How taken

Tablets.

Frequency and timing of doses
Once daily.

Usual adult dosage range
25–100mg. People over 75 years, and other groups that are especially sensitive to the drug's effects, and those with liver dysfunction, may start on 25mg.

Onset of effect
Blood pressure 1–2 weeks, with maximum effect in 3–6 weeks from start of treatment. *Other conditions* Within 1 hour.

Duration of action
12–24 hours.

Diet advice
None.

Storage
Keep in a closed container in a cool, dry place out of the reach of children.

Missed dose
Take as soon as you remember. If your next dose is due within 8 hours, take a single dose now and skip the next.

Stopping the drug
Do not stop the drug without consulting your physician. Stopping the drug may lead to worsening of the underlying condition.

Exceeding the dose
An occasional unintentional extra dose is unlikely to cause problems. Large overdoses may cause dizziness and fainting. Notify your physician.

POSSIBLE ADVERSE EFFECTS

Side effects, of which dizziness and fatigue are the most common, are usually mild.

Symptom/effect	Frequency		Discuss with physician		Stop taking drug now	Call physician now
	Common	Rare	Only if severe	In all cases		
Dizziness/fatigue	●		■			
Migraine		●	■			
Diarrhea		●	■			
Taste disturbance		●	■			
Rash/itching		●		■		
Jaundice		●		■		
Wheezing/facial swelling		●		■	▲	∎

INTERACTIONS

Diuretics There is a risk of a sudden fall in blood pressure when these drugs are taken with losartan.

Potassium supplements, potassium-sparing diuretics, and cyclosporine Losartan increases the effect of these drugs, leading to raised levels of potassium in the blood.

Lithium Losartan may increase the levels and *toxicity* of lithium.

Non-steroidal anti-inflammatory drugs (NSAIDs) Certain NSAIDs may reduce the blood-pressure lowering effect of losartan.

SPECIAL PRECAUTIONS

Be sure to tell your physician if:
▼ You have stenosis of the kidney arteries.
▼ You have liver or kidney problems.
▼ You have congestive heart failure.
▼ You have primary aldosteronism.
▼ You have experienced angioedema.
▼ You are taking other medications.

Pregnancy
▼ Not prescribed. May cause abnormalities in the fetus.

Breast-feeding
▼ Not prescribed. Safety not established.

Infants and children
▼ Not prescribed. Safety not established.

Over 60
▼ Reduced dose may be necessary over 75 years.

Driving and hazardous work
▼ Do not undertake such activities until you have learned how losartan affects you because the drug can cause dizziness and fatigue.

Alcohol
▼ Avoid. Alcohol may raise blood pressure, reducing the effectiveness of losartan. Alcohol also causes blood vessels to dilate, increasing the likelihood of an excessive fall in blood pressure.

PROLONGED USE

No special problems.

Monitoring Periodic checks on blood potassium levels may be performed.

LOVASTATIN

Product names Apo-Lovastatin, Gen-Lovastatin, Mevacor, Novo-Lovastatin, Nu-Lovastatin, PMS-Lovastatin
Used in the following combined preparations Advicor

GENERAL INFORMATION

Lovastatin is a lipid-lowering drug belonging to the class of statins. It blocks the action of an enzyme needed for cholesterol to be manufactured in the liver, and as a result the blood levels of cholesterol are lowered. The drug is prescribed for people with high levels of cholesterol in the blood who have not responded to a special diet, and who are at risk of developing or have existing coronary heart disease.

Lovastatin is usally taken once daily. With higher doses, the daily dosage can be split and taken with the morning and evening meals. Side effects are usually mild. Lovastatin may raise the levels of various liver enzymes. This effect does not usually indicate serious liver damage.

QUICK REFERENCE

Drug group Lipid-lowering drug (p.89)

Overdose danger rating Medium

Dependence rating Low

Prescription needed Yes

Available as generic Yes

INFORMATION FOR USERS

Your drug prescription is tailored for you. Do not alter dosage without checking with your physician.

How taken

Tablets.

Frequency and timing of doses
Usually once daily with the evening meal; higher doses may be split to 2 doses.

Usual adult dosage range
20–80mg daily.

Onset of effect
Within 2 weeks; full beneficial effects may not be felt for 4–6 weeks.

Duration of action
Up to 24 hours.

Diet advice
A low-fat diet is usually recommended.

Storage
Keep in a closed container in a cool, dry place out of the reach of children.

Missed dose
If you miss a dose, take it as soon as you remember. If it is near the time of the next dose, skip the missed dose and resume your using dosing schedule. Do not double up to catch up on a missed dose.

Stopping the drug
Do not stop the drug without consulting your physician. Stopping the drug may lead to worsening of the underlying condition.

Exceeding the dose
An occasional unintentional extra dose is unlikely to cause problems. Large overdoses may cause liver problems. Notify your physician.

SPECIAL PRECAUTIONS

Be sure to tell your physician if:
▼ You have liver or kidney problems.
▼ You have eye or vision problems.
▼ You have muscle weakness.
▼ You have a thyroid disorder.
▼ You have had problems with alcohol abuse.
▼ You have porphyria.
▼ You have angina.
▼ You have high blood pressure.
▼ You are taking other medications.

Pregnancy
▼ Not usually prescribed. Safety in pregnancy not established. Discuss with your physician.

Breast-feeding
▼ Safety not established. Discuss with your physician.

Infants and children
▼ Not recommended.

Over 60
▼ No special problems.

Driving and hazardous work
▼ No special problems.

Alcohol
▼ Avoid excessive amounts. Alcohol may increase the risk of developing liver problems with this drug.

POSSIBLE ADVERSE EFFECTS

Adverse effects are usually mild and do not last long. The most common are those affecting the gastrointestinal system.

Lovastatin may very rarely cause muscle problems, and any muscle pain or weakness should be reported to your physician at once.

Symptom/effect	Frequency		Discuss with physician		Stop taking drug now	Call physician now
	Common	Rare	Only if severe	In all cases		
Abdominal pain		●	■			
Nausea/flatulence		●	■			
Constipation/diarrhea		●	■			
Headache		●	■			
Rash		●		■	▲	
Jaundice		●		■		
Muscle pain/weakness		●		■	▲	▮
Change in cognition		●				▮

PROLONGED USE

Prolonged treatment can adversely affect liver function.

Monitoring Regular blood tests to check liver function are recommended. Tests of muscle function may be carried out if problems are suspected.

INTERACTIONS

Anticoagulants Lovastatin may increase the effect of anticoagulants. Close monitoring and dose adjustment may be required.

Itraconazole, ketoconazole, clarithromycin, erythromycin, and protease inhibitors Simultaneous administration of these drugs with lovastatin may increase the risk of muscle toxicity.

Other lipid-lowering drugs The use of these with lovastatin may increase the risk of muscle toxicity.

Grapefruit juice May increase blood levels of lovastatin.

Cyclosporine and other immuno-suppressant drugs, and antiviral drugs Lovastatin and these drugs are not usually prescribed together because of the risk of muscle toxicity.

MAGNESIUM HYDROXIDE

Product name Phillips' Milk of Magnesia
Used in the following combined preparations Diovol, Gelusil, Maalox, Mylanta, and others

GENERAL INFORMATION

Magnesium hydroxide is a fast-acting antacid given to neutralize stomach acid. The drug is available in a number of over-the-counter preparations for the treatment of indigestion and heartburn. Magnesium hydroxide also prevents pain caused by stomach and duodenal ulcers, gastritis, and reflux esophagitis, although other drugs are normally used for these problems nowadays. It also

acts as a laxative by drawing water into the intestine from the surrounding blood vessels to soften the feces.

Magnesium hydroxide is not often used alone as an antacid because of its laxative effect. However, this effect is countered when the drug is used in combination with aluminum hydroxide, which can cause constipation.

INFORMATION FOR USERS

Follow instructions on the label. Call your physician if symptoms worsen.

How taken

Tablets, liquid, powder.

Frequency and timing of doses
1–4 x daily as needed with water, preferably an hour after food and at bedtime.

Usual adult dosage range
Antacid 2–4 tablets as needed (up to 4 x daily); 5–15ml per dose (liquid).
Laxative 5–20ml per dose (liquid).

Onset of effect
Antacid within 15 minutes.
Laxative 2–8 hours.

Duration of action
2–4 hours.

Diet advice
None.

Storage
Keep in a closed container in a cool (but not cold), dry place out of the reach of children.

Missed dose
Take as soon as you remember.

Stopping the drug
When used as an antacid, can be safely stopped as soon as you no longer need it. When given as ulcer treatment, follow your physician's advice.

Exceeding the dose
An occasional unintentional extra dose is unlikely to be a cause for concern. But if you notice any unusual symptoms, or if a large overdose has been taken, notify your physician.

SPECIAL PRECAUTIONS

Be sure to consult your physician or pharmacist before taking this drug if:
▼ You have a long-term kidney problem.
▼ You have a bowel disorder.
▼ You are taking other medications.

Pregnancy
▼ No evidence of risk, but discuss the most appropriate treatment with your physician.

Breast-feeding
▼ No evidence of risk, but discuss the most appropriate treatment with your physician.

Infants and children
▼ Not recommended under 1 year except on the advice of a physician. Reduced dose necessary for older children.

Over 60
▼ No special problems.

Driving and hazardous work
▼ No known problems.

Alcohol
▼ Avoid excessive alcohol as it irritates the stomach and may reduce the benefits of the drug.

POSSIBLE ADVERSE EFFECTS

Diarrhea is the only common adverse effect of this drug. Dizziness and muscle weakness due to absorption of excess magnesium in

the body may occur in people with poor kidney function.

Symptom/effect	Frequency		Discuss with physician		Stop taking drug now	Call physician now
	Common	Rare	Only if severe	In all cases		
Diarrhea	●		■			

INTERACTIONS

General note Magnesium hydroxide interferes with the absorption of a wide range of drugs taken by mouth, including tetracycline antibiotics, iron supplements, diflunisal, phenytoin, and penicillamine.

Enteric-coated tablets As with other antacids, magnesium hydroxide may allow break-up of the *enteric* coating of tablets, sometimes leading to stomach irritation.

PROLONGED USE

Magnesium hydroxide should not be used for prolonged periods without consulting your physician. If you are over 40 years of age and are experience long-term indigestion or heartburn, your physician will probably refer you to a specialist. Prolonged use in people with kidney damage may cause drowsiness, dizziness, and weakness, resulting from accumulation of magnesium in the body.

MEDROXYPROGESTERONE

Product names Depo-Provera, Provera, Provera-Pak
Used in the following combined preparations Premplus

GENERAL INFORMATION

Medroxyprogesterone is a progestin, a synthetic female sex hormone similar to the natural hormone progesterone. It is used for hormonal replacement therapy to oppose effects of estrogen in women with a uterus. It is also used to treat menstrual disorders such as mid-cycle bleeding and amenorrhea (absence of periods).

Medroxyprogesterone is also often used to treat endometriosis, a condition in which there is abnormal growth of the uterine-lining tissue in the pelvic cavity. *Depot* injections of the drug are used as a contraceptive. However, since they may cause serious *side effects,* such as persistent bleeding from the uterus, amenorrhea, and prolonged infertility, their use remains controversial, and they are recommended for use only under special circumstances.

Medroxyprogesterone may be used to treat some types of cancer, such as cancer of the breast, uterus, or prostate.

QUICK REFERENCE

Drug group Female sex hormone (p.133)

Overdose danger rating Low

Dependence rating Low

Prescription needed Yes

Available as generic Yes

INFORMATION FOR USERS

Your drug prescription is tailored for you. Do not alter dosage without checking with your physician.

How taken

Tablets, depot injection.

Frequency and timing of doses
Usually once daily with plenty of water (by mouth); tablets may need to be taken at certain times during your cycle; follow the instructions you have been given; higher doses are given as individual doses. Every 3 months (depot injection).

Usual adult dosage range
Menstrual disorders 2.5–10mg daily.
Endometriosis 30mg daily or 150mg depot every 6–12 weeks.
Cancer 100–400mg daily.
Contraception 150mg.

Onset of effect
1–2 months (cancer); 1–2 weeks (other conditions).

Duration of action
1–2 days (by mouth); up to some months (depot injection).

Diet advice
None.

Storage
Keep in a closed container in a cool, dry place out of the reach of children.

Missed dose
Take as soon as you remember. If your next dose is due within 3 hours, take a single dose now and skip the next.

Stopping the drug
Do not stop the drug without consulting your physician; symptoms may recur.

Exceeding the dose
An occasional unintentional extra dose is unlikely to be a cause for concern. But if you notice any unusual symptoms, or if a large overdose has been taken, notify your physician.

SPECIAL PRECAUTIONS

Be sure to tell your physician if:
▼ You have high blood pressure.
▼ You have diabetes.
▼ You have had blood clots or a stroke.
▼ You have long-term liver or kidney problems.
▼ You are taking other medications.

Pregnancy
▼ Not prescribed. May cause abnormalities in the unborn baby. Discuss with your physician.

Breast-feeding
▼ The drug passes into the breast milk, but at normal doses adverse effects on the baby are unlikely. Discuss with your physician.

Infants and children
▼ Not usually prescribed.

Over 60
▼ No special problems.

Driving and hazardous work
▼ No known problems.

Alcohol
▼ No known problems.

POSSIBLE ADVERSE EFFECTS

Medroxyprogesterone rarely causes serious adverse effects. Fluid retention may lead to weight gain, swollen feet or ankles, and breast tenderness.

Symptom/effect	Frequency		Discuss with physician		Stop taking drug now	Call physician now
	Common	Rare	Only if severe	In all cases		
Weight gain	●		■			
Swollen ankles	●		■			
Breast tenderness		●	■			
Nausea		●	■			
Fatigue/depression		●		■		
Irregular menstruation		●		■		
Rash/itching/acne		●		■	▲	

INTERACTIONS

Cyclosporine The effects of this drug may be increased by medroxyprogesterone.

PROLONGED USE

Long-term use of this drug may slightly increase the risk of blood clots in the leg veins. Irregular menstrual bleeding or spotting between periods may also occur during long-term use.

Monitoring Periodic checks on blood pressure, yearly cervical smear tests, and breast examinations are usually required.

MEFLOQUINE

Product names Apo-Mefloquine, Lariam
Used in the following combined preparations None

GENERAL INFORMATION

Mefloquine is used for the prevention and treatment of malaria. It is recommended for use in areas where malaria is resistant to other drugs.

However, the use of mefloquine is limited by the fact that it can cause, in some patients, serious *side effects* that include depression, anxiety, nightmares, panic, confusion, hallucinations, paranoid delusions, and convulsions.

For most people, the benefits of the use of mefloquine outweigh the risks, although this should be discussed with your physician.

QUICK REFERENCE

Drug group Antimalarial drug (p.123)
Overdose danger rating High
Dependence rating Low
Prescription needed Yes
Available as generic Yes

INFORMATION FOR USERS

Your drug prescription is tailored for you. Do not alter dosage without checking with your physician.

How taken

Tablets.

Frequency and timing of doses
Prevention Once weekly.
Treatment Up to 3 x daily, every 6–8 hours.

Usual adult dosage range
Prevention 1 tablet once weekly starting 1–3 weeks before departure and continuing until 4 weeks after leaving the malarial area.
Treatment 20–25mg/kg body weight up to a maximum dose of 1.5g.

Onset of effect
2–3 days.

Duration of action
Over 1 week. Low levels of the drug may persist for several months.

Diet advice
None.

Storage
Keep in a cool, dry place out of the reach of children.

Missed dose
Take as soon as you remember. If your next dose is due within 48 hours (if taken once weekly for prevention), take a single dose now and skip the next.

Stopping the drug
If you feel it necessary to stop taking the drug, consult your physician about alternative treatment before the next dose is due.

OVERDOSE ACTION

 Seek immediate medical advice in all cases. Take emergency action if dizziness, palpitations, collapse, or loss of consciousness occur.

See Drug poisoning emergency guide (p.526).

SPECIAL PRECAUTIONS

Be sure to tell your physician if:
▼ You have long-term liver or kidney problems.
▼ You have had epileptic fits.
▼ You have had depression, anxiety, or other psychiatric illness.
▼ You have had a previous allergic reaction to mefloquine or quinine.
▼ You have heart problems.
▼ You are taking other medications.

 Pregnancy
▼ Not usually prescribed. If unavoidable, the drug is given only after the first trimester. Pregnancy must be avoided during and for 3 months after mefloquine use.

 Breast-feeding
▼ Not prescribed. The drug passes into the breast milk.

 Infants and children
▼ Not used in infants under 3 months old. Reduced dose necessary in older children.

 Over 60
▼ Careful monitoring is necessary if liver or kidney problems or heart disease are present.

 Driving and hazardous work
▼ Avoid such activities when taking mefloquine for prevention until you know how the drug affects you. Also avoid during treatment and for 3 weeks afterwards as the drug can cause dizziness or disturb balance.

 Alcohol
▼ Keep consumption low.

PROLONGED USE

May be taken for prevention of malaria for up to one year.

POSSIBLE ADVERSE EFFECTS

Mefloquine commonly causes dizziness, vertigo, nausea, vomiting, and headache. In rare cases, serious adverse effects on the nervous system can occur, including anxiety or panic attacks, depression, hallucinations, and paranoid delusions.

Symptom/effect	Frequency		Discuss with physician		Stop taking drug now	Call physician now
	Common	Rare	Only if severe	In all cases		
Dizziness/vertigo	●		■			
Nausea/vomiting	●		■			
Headache	●		■			
Abdominal pain	●			■		
Depression		●		■	▲	
Anxiety/panic attacks		●		■	▲	
Hallucinations/delusions		●		■	▲	
Hearing disorders		●		■	▲	
Palpitations		●		■	▲	

INTERACTIONS

Anticonvulsant drugs Mefloquine may decrease the effect of these drugs.

Other antimalarial drugs Mefloquine may increase the risk of adverse effects when taken with these drugs.

General note Mefloquine may increase the effects on the heart of drugs such as beta blockers, calcium channel blockers, and digoxin.

MEGESTROL

Product name Megace
Used in the following combined preparations None

GENERAL INFORMATION

Megestrol is a progestin, which is a synthetic female sex hormone similar to the natural hormone progesterone. The drug is used in the treatment of certain types of advanced cancer affecting the breast and uterus that are sensitive to hormone treatment. Megestrol is often prescribed when the tumour cannot be removed by surgery, when the disease has recurred after surgery, or when treatment with other anticancer drugs or radiotherapy have failed.

Successful treatment with megestrol reduces the size of the tumour; the drug may also cause secondary growths to disappear. Improvement usually occurs within two months of starting treatment. Because megestrol does not completely eradicate the cancer, the drug may need to be continued indefinitely.

Megestrol may also be used to prevent weight loss in other types of cancer.

QUICK REFERENCE

Drug group Female sex hormone (p.133) and anticancer drug (p.140)

Overdose danger rating Low

Dependence rating Low

Prescription needed Yes

Available as generic Yes

INFORMATION FOR USERS

Your drug prescription is tailored for you. Do not alter dosage without checking with your physician.

How taken

Tablets, liquid.

Frequency and timing of doses
1–4 x daily.

Usual adult dosage range
Breast cancer 160mg daily.
Cancer of the uterus 40–320mg daily.

Onset of effect
Within 2 months.

Duration of action
1–2 days.

Diet advice
None.

Storage
Keep in a closed container in a cool, dry place out of the reach of children.

Missed dose
Take as soon as you remember.

Stopping the drug
Do not stop the drug without consulting your physician. Stopping the drug may lead to worsening of your underlying condition.

Exceeding the dose
An occasional unintentional extra dose is unlikely to be a cause for concern. But if you notice any unusual symptoms, or if a large overdose has been taken, notify your physician.

SPECIAL PRECAUTIONS

Be sure to tell your physician if:
▼ You have long-term liver or kidney problems.
▼ You have had thrombosis or blood clots.
▼ You have high blood pressure.
▼ You have heart problems.
▼ You are taking other medications.

Pregnancy
▼ Not usually prescribed.

Breast-feeding
▼ Breast-feeding is usually discontinued. Discuss with your physician.

Infants and children
▼ Not usually required.

Over 60
▼ No special problems.

Driving and hazardous work
▼ No known problems.

Alcohol
▼ No known problems.

POSSIBLE ADVERSE EFFECTS

Adverse effects are rare with megestrol. It may cause weight gain owing to increased appetite and food intake. Stop taking the drug and consult your physician if a rash occurs.

Symptom/effect	Frequency		Discuss with physician		Stop taking drug now	Call physician now
	Common	Rare	Only if severe	In all cases		
Weight gain	●		■			
Swollen feet/ankles		●	■			
Nausea		●	■			
Headache		●		■		
Itching		●		■		
Hair loss		●		■		
Rash		●		■	▲	

INTERACTIONS

Cyclosporine The effects of this drug may be increased by megestrol.

PROLONGED USE

Long-term use of this drug may increase the risk of blood clots in the leg veins.

Monitoring Periodic checks on blood pressure may be performed.

341

MELOXICAM

Product name Mobicox
Used in the following combined preparations None

GENERAL INFORMATION

Meloxicam is a member of the non-steroidal anti-inflammatory (NSAID) group of drugs. It reduces pain, stiffness, and inflammation and is used to relieve the symptoms of rheumatoid arthritis, ankylosing spondylitis, and acute episodes of osteoarthritis. Meloxicam does not cure the underlying condition, however.

Meloxicam does not affect the stomach as severely as some other NSAIDs and is therefore less likely to cause gastrointestinal bleeding, ulceration, and perforation. Because elderly people are more sensitive to the drug's effects, they are usually prescribed only half the normal adult dose.

INFORMATION FOR USERS

Your drug prescription is tailored for you. Do not alter dosage without checking with your physician.

How taken

Tablets.

Frequency and timing of doses
Once daily.

Usual adult dosage range
7.5–15mg.

Onset of effect
1 hour. Full anti-inflammatory effect may not be felt for up to 2 weeks.

Duration of action
24 hours.

Diet advice
None.

Storage
Keep in a closed container in a cool, dry place out of the reach of children.

Missed dose
Take as soon as you remember. If your next dose is due within 8 hours, take a single dose now and skip the next.

Stopping the drug
The drug can be safely stopped as soon as you no longer need it (short term). Do not stop taking the drug without consulting your physician (long term).

Exceeding the dose
An occasional unintentional extra dose is unlikely to cause problems. Large overdoses can cause stomach and intestinal pain and damage. Notify your physician.

SPECIAL PRECAUTIONS

Be sure to tell your physician if:
▼ You have asthma.
▼ You are allergic to ASA or other NSAIDs.
▼ You have had a peptic ulcer, esophagitis, or acid indigestion.
▼ You have liver or kidney problems.
▼ You have a bleeding disorder, proctitis, or hemorrhoids.
▼ You are taking other medications.

Pregnancy
▼ Safety not established. May affect the developing foetus. Discuss with your physician.

Breast-feeding
▼ Safety not established. Discuss with your physician.

Infants and children
▼ Not recommended.

Over 60
▼ Increased likelihood of adverse effects. Reduced doses necessary.

Driving and hazardous work
▼ Avoid such activities until you have learned how meloxicam affects you because the drug can cause vertigo and drowsiness.

Alcohol
▼ Keep consumption low. Alcohol may increase the risk of stomach irritation with meloxicam.

Surgery and general anesthetics
▼ Meloxicam may prolong bleeding. Discuss the possibility of stopping treatment temporarily with your physician or dentist.

POSSIBLE ADVERSE EFFECTS

Gastrointestinal disturbance, skin rash, and headache are common *adverse effects*. Black or bloodstained feces and wheezing should be reported to your physician without delay.

Symptom/effect	Frequency		Discuss with physician		Stop taking drug now	Call physician now
	Common	Rare	Only if severe	In all cases		
Abdominal pain/indigestion	●			■		
Headache	●		■			
Diarrhea or constipation	●		■			
Skin rash/itching	●		■			
Lightheadedness/drowsiness	●		■			
Palpitations		●		■		
Vertigo/ringing in the ears		●		■		
Persistent sore throat		●		■		
Wheezing/breathing difficulties		●		■	▲	▮
Black/bloodstained feces		●		■	▲	▮

INTERACTIONS

General note Meloxicam interacts with a wide range of drugs to increase the risk of bleeding and/or peptic ulcers. Such drugs include other NSAIDs, ASA, and also oral anticoagulants, and corticosteroids.

Cyclosporine There is an increased risk of kidney damage when meloxicam is taken with cyclosporine.

Lithium, digoxin, and methotrexate Meloxicam may increase the blood levels of these drugs to an undersirable extent.

Antibacterials Meloxicam may increase the risk of convulsions with ciprofloxacin and similar drugs.

PROLONGED USE

No special problems.

Monitoring Periodic tests on kidney function may be performed.

MEMANTINE

Product name Ebixa
Used in the following combined preparations None

GENERAL INFORMATION

Memantine is used to treat symptoms of moderate to severe Alzheimer's disease. It may be used alone or in combination with other drugs used in this condition called cholinesterase inhibitors. It works by blocking certain receptors in the brain, thereby decreasing abnormal excitement. It can help patients in performing daily activities more easily, but does not decrease the progression of Alzheimer's disease. The dose may be gradually increased. Doses greater than 5mg per day should be administered twice daily.

INFORMATION FOR USERS

Your drug prescription is tailored for you. Do not alter dosage without checking with your physician.

How taken

Tablets.

Frequency and timing of doses
Usually once or twice daily.

Usual adult dosage range
5-20mg daily.

Onset of effect
Within 8 hours.

Duration of action
Up to 24 hours.

Diet advice
None

Storage
Keep in a closed container in a cool, dry place out of the reach of children.

Missed dose
If you miss a dose, take it as soon as you remember. If it is near the time of the next dose, skip the missed dose and resume your usual dosing schedule. Do not double up to catch up on a missed dose.

Stopping the drug
Do not stop the drug without consulting your physician. Stopping the drug may lead to worsening of the underlying condition.

Exceeding the dose
An occasional unintentional extra dose is unlikely to cause problems, but if you notice any unusual symptoms, or if a large overdose has been taken, notify your physician.

SPECIAL PRECAUTIONS

Be sure to tell your physician if:
▼ You have asthma.
▼ You have seizures.
▼ You have kidney disease.
▼ You have repeated urinary tract infections.
▼ You smoke cigarettes.
▼ You are taking other medications.

 Pregnancy
▼ Safety in pregnancy not established. Discuss with your physician.

 Breast-feeding
▼ Safety not established. Discuss with your physician.

 Infants and children
▼ Safety and effectiveness not established.

 Over 60
▼ No special problems.

 Driving and hazardous work
▼ May cause drowsiness. Do not drive a car or operate machinery until the effect of the drug wears off and you feel you are mentally alert.

 Alcohol
▼ Avoid alcohol use as it may increase the effect of drowsiness caused by this drug.

PROLONGED USE

May be continued for as long as there is benefit. Stopping the drug can lead to a gradual loss of the improvements.

Monitoring Periodic checks may be performed to test whether the drug is still providing some benefit.

POSSIBLE ADVERSE EFFECTS

Side effects include dizziness, tiredness, feeling sleepy, headache, and sometimes an increase in blood pressure.

Symptom/effect	Frequency		Discuss with physician		Stop taking drug now	Call physician now
	Common	Rare	Only if severe	In all cases		
High blood pressure		●		■		▮
Headache	●		■			
Blurred vision		●		■		
Dizziness	●		■			
Tiredness/sleepiness		●	■			
Edema		●		■		▮
Change in walk and balance		●				
Constipation or diarrhea	●		■			
Anxiety		●		■		
Loss of appetite		●	■			
Change in behaviour		●		■		

INTERACTIONS

Hydrochlorothiazide Memantine can decrease the amount of hydrochlorothiazide in the blood.

Amantadine, Dextromethorphan (DM), ketamine There is a potential for interaction, as these drugs inhibit the same receptors as memantine.

Cimetidine, nicotine, quinidine These drugs are excreted in a similar manner to memantine in the kidneys and they can affect the levels of memantine; memantine can also affect the levels of these drugs.

Sodium bicarbonate, acetazolamide These drugs can lead to an accumulation of memantine in the body.

MERCAPTOPURINE

Product name Purinethol
Used in the following combined preparations None

GENERAL INFORMATION

Mercaptopurine is an anticancer drug that is widely used in the treatment of certain forms of leukemia. It is usually given in combination with other anticancer drugs.

Nausea and vomiting, mouth ulcers, and loss of appetite are the most common side effects of mercaptopurine. Such symptoms tend to be milder than those caused by other cytotoxic drugs, and often disappear as the body adjusts to the drug.

More seriously, mercaptopurine can interfere with blood cell production, resulting in blood clotting disorders and anemia, and can also cause liver damage. The likelihood of infections is also increased.

INFORMATION FOR USERS

Your drug prescription is tailored for you. Do not alter dosage without checking with your physician.

How taken

Tablets.

Frequency and timing of doses
Once daily.

Usual dosage range
Dosage is determined individually according to body weight and response.

Onset of effect
1–2 weeks.

Duration of action
Side effects may persist for several weeks after stopping treatment.

Diet advice
None.

Storage
Keep in a closed container in a cool, dry place out of the reach of children. Protect from light.

Missed dose
If your next dose is due within 6 hours, take a single dose now and skip the next. Tell your physician that you missed a dose.

Stopping the drug
Do not stop taking the drug without consulting your physician; stopping the drug may lead to worsening of your underlying condition.

Exceeding the dose
An occasional unintentional extra dose is unlikely to cause problems. Large overdoses may cause nausea and vomiting. Notify your physician.

SPECIAL PRECAUTIONS

Be sure to tell your physician if:
▼ You have long-term liver or kidney problems.
▼ You suffer from gout.
▼ You have recently had any infection.
▼ You have porphyria.
▼ You are taking other medications.

Pregnancy
▼ Not usually prescribed. Discuss with your physician.

Breast-feeding
▼ Not advised. The drug passes into the breast milk and may affect the baby adversely. Discuss with your physician.

Infants and children
▼ Reduced dose necessary.

Over 60
▼ Reduced dose may be necessary. Increased risk of adverse effects.

Driving and hazardous work
▼ No known problems.

Alcohol
▼ Avoid. Alcohol may increase the adverse effects of this drug.

POSSIBLE ADVERSE EFFECTS

The most common adverse effects are nausea and vomiting, and loss of appetite. *Jaundice* may also occur, but is reversible on stopping the drug. Because mercaptopurine interferes with the production of blood cells, it may cause anemia and blood clotting disorders; and infections are more likely.

Symptom/effect	Frequency		Discuss with physician		Stop taking drug now	Call physician now
	Common	Rare	Only if severe	In all cases		
Nausea/vomiting	●		■			
Loss of appetite	●		■			
Mouth ulcers	●			■		▌
Jaundice		●		■		▌
Black feces		●		■		▌
Bloodstained vomit		●		■		▌

PROLONGED USE

Prolonged use of this drug may reduce bone marrow activity, leading to a reduction of all types of blood cells.

Monitoring Regular blood checks and tests on liver function are required.

INTERACTIONS

Allopurinol This drug increases blood levels of mercaptopurine.

Warfarin The effects of warfarin may be decreased by mercaptopurine.

Co-trimoxazole and trimethoprim These drugs increase the risk of blood problems with mercaptopurine.

MESALAMINE/5-ASA

Product names Asacol, Mesasal, Pentasa, Salofalk
Used in the following combined preparations None

GENERAL INFORMATION

Mesalamine is prescribed for patients with ulcerative colitis and is sometimes used for Crohn's disease, which affects the large intestine. The drug is given to relieve symptoms in an acute attack and is also taken as a preventative measure. When mesalamine is used to treat severe cases, it is often taken with other drugs such as corticosteroids.

When taken in tablet form, the active component of the drug is released in the large intestine, where its local effect relieves the inflamed mucosa. It is important to stick to the same brand of tablet. Enemas and suppositories are also available and are particularly useful when the disease affects the rectum and lower colon.

This drug produces fewer *side effects* than some older treatments, such as sulfasalazine. Patients who are unable to tolerate sulfasalazine may be able to take mesalamine without any problems. However, those who are hypersensitive to salicylates, for example ASA, should not take mesalamine.

QUICK REFERENCE

Drug group Drug for inflammatory bowel disease (p.98)

Overdose danger rating Low

Dependence rating Low

Prescription needed Yes

Available as generic Yes

INFORMATION FOR USERS

Your drug prescription is tailored for you. Do not alter dosage without checking with your physician.

How taken

Tablets, SR-tablets, rectal suppositories, enema (foam or liquid).

Frequency and timing of doses
3 x daily, swallowed whole and not chewed (tablets); 3 x daily (suppositories); once daily at bedtime (enema).

Usual adult dosage range
800mg–2.4g daily (acute attack); 750mg–2.4g daily (maintenance dose).

Onset of effect
Adverse effects may be noticed within a few days, but full beneficial effects may not be felt for a couple of weeks.

Duration of action
Up to 12 hours.

Diet advice
Your physician may advise you, taking account of the condition affecting you.

Storage
Keep in a closed container in a cool, dry place out of the reach of children. Protect from light. Keep aerosol container out of direct sunlight.

Missed dose
Take as soon as you remember. If your next dose is due within 2 hours, take a single dose now and skip the next.

Stopping the drug
Do not stop taking the drug without consulting your physician; symptoms may recur.

Exceeding the dose
An occasional unintentional extra dose is unlikely to be a cause for concern. But if you notice any unusual symptoms, or if a large overdose has been taken, notify your physician.

SPECIAL PRECAUTIONS

Be sure to tell your physician if:
▼ You have long-term liver or kidney problems.
▼ You are allergic to ASA.
▼ You are taking other medications.

 Pregnancy
▼ Negligible amounts of the drug cross the placenta. However, safety in pregnancy is not established. Discuss with your physician.

 Breast-feeding
▼ Negligible amounts of the drug pass into the breast milk. However, safety is not established. Discuss with your physician.

 Infants and children
▼ Not recommended under 15 years.

 Over 60
▼ Dosage reduction not normally necessary unless there is kidney impairment.

 Driving and hazardous work
▼ No special problems.

 Alcohol
▼ No special problems.

POSSIBLE ADVERSE EFFECTS

The common side effects of mesalamine are on the gastrointestinal tract. Other problems rarely occur. However, unexplained bleeding, bruising, sore throat, fever, or malaise should be reported to your physician, who will carry out a blood test to eliminate blood disorders.

Symptom/effect	Frequency		Discuss with physician		Stop taking drug now	Call physician now
	Common	Rare	Only if severe	In all cases		
Nausea	●		■			
Abdominal pain	●		■			
Diarrhea	●		■			
Fever/wheezing		●		■	▲	▮
Colitis worsening		●		■	▲	
Rash		●		■	▲	
Bleeding/bruising		●		■	▲	▮
Sore throat/malaise		●		■	▲	▮

PROLONGED USE

No problems expected.

INTERACTIONS

Lactulose The release of mesalamine at its site of action may be reduced by lactulose.

Warfarin Mesalamine may reduce the effect of warfarin.

METFORMIN

Product name Glucophage
Used in the following combined preparations None

GENERAL INFORMATION

Metformin is an antidiabetic drug used to treat adult (maturity-onset or Type 2) diabetes in which some insulin-secreting cells are still active in the pancreas.

Metformin lowers blood sugar by reducing the absorption of glucose from the digestive tract into the bloodstream, by reducing the glucose production by cells in the liver and kidneys, and by increasing the sensitivity of cells to insulin so that they take up glucose more effectively from the blood.

The drug is given in conjunction with a special diabetic diet that limits sugar and fat intake. It is often given with another antidiabetic drug that stimulates insulin secretion by the pancreas, or with insulin for treatment of maturity-onset diabetes, especially to obese patients.

QUICK REFERENCE

Drug group Antidiabetic drug (p.128)

Overdose danger rating High

Dependence rating Low

Prescription needed Yes

Available as generic Yes

INFORMATION FOR USERS

Your drug prescription is tailored for you. Do not alter dosage without checking with your physician.

How taken

Tablets.

Frequency and timing of doses
2–4 x daily with food.

Usual adult dosage range
1.5–2.5g daily, with a low dose at the start of treatment.

Onset of effect
Within 2 hours. It may take 2 weeks to achieve control of diabetes.

Duration of action
8–12 hours.

Diet advice
An individualized low-fat, low-sugar diet must be maintained in order for the drug to be fully effective. Follow your physician's advice.

Storage
Keep in a closed container in a cool, dry place out of the reach of children.

Missed dose
Take as soon as you remember. If your next dose is due within 2 hours, take a single dose now and skip the next.

Stopping the drug
Do not stop taking the drug without consulting your physician; stopping the drug may lead to worsening of the underlying condition.

OVERDOSE ACTION

 Seek immediate medical advice in all cases. Take emergency action if fits or loss of consciousness occur.

See Drug poisoning emergency guide (p.526).

SPECIAL PRECAUTIONS

Be sure to tell your physician if:
▼ You have long-term liver or kidney problems.
▼ You have heart failure.
▼ You are a heavy drinker.
▼ You are taking other medications.

 Pregnancy
▼ Not usually prescribed. Insulin is usually substituted because it provides better diabetic control during pregnancy. Discuss with your physician.

 Breast-feeding
▼ Safety not established. Discuss with your physician.

 Infants and children
▼ Not recommended.

 Over 60
▼ Increased likelihood of adverse effects. Reduced dose may therefore be necessary.

 Driving and hazardous work
▼ Usually no problems. Avoid such activities if you have warning signs of low blood sugar.

 Alcohol
▼ Avoid. Alcohol increases the risk of low blood sugar, and can cause coma by increasing the acidity of the blood.

Surgery and general anesthetics
▼ Surgery may reduce the response to this drug. Notify your physician that you are diabetic before any surgery; insulin treatment may need to be substituted. Tell your physician if you are to have a contrast X-ray; metformin should be stopped before the procedure.

POSSIBLE ADVERSE EFFECTS

Minor gastrointestinal symptoms such as nausea, vomiting, and loss of appetite are often helped by taking the drug with food.

Diarrhea usually settles after a few days of continued treatment.

Symptom/effect	Frequency		Discuss with physician		Stop taking drug now	Call physician now
	Common	Rare	Only if severe	In all cases		
Loss of appetite/metallic taste	●		■			
Nausea/vomiting	●		■			
Diarrhea		●	■			
Dizziness/confusion		●		■		
Weakness/sweating		●		■		
Rash		●		■		

INTERACTIONS

General note A number of drugs reduce the effects of metformin. These include corticosteroids, estrogens, and diuretics. Other drugs, notably monoamine oxidase inhibitors (MAOIs) and beta blockers, increase its effects.

Warfarin Metformin may increase the effect of this anticoagulant drug. The dosage of warfarin may need to be adjusted accordingly.

PROLONGED USE

Prolonged treatment with metformin can deplete reserves of vitamin B_{12}, and this may rarely cause anemia.

Monitoring Regular checks on kidney function and on levels of sugar in the urine and/or blood are usually required. Vitamin B_{12} levels may also be checked annually.

METHADONE

Product name Metadol
Used in the following combined preparations None

GENERAL INFORMATION

Methadone is a synthetic drug belonging to the *opioid* analgesic group. It is used in the control of severe pain, and usually used to replace morphine or other opioids in the treatment of *dependence*. For this, methadone can be given once daily to prevent *withdrawal symptoms*. In some cases, dosage can be reduced until the drug is no longer needed.

Tolerance to methadone is marked. Although the initial dose for a person not used to opioids is very low, the dose needed by someone who is dependent could be fatal for a non-user.

QUICK REFERENCE

Drug group Opioid analgesic (p.64)
Overdose danger rating High
Dependence rating High
Prescription needed Yes
Available as generic No

INFORMATION FOR USERS

Your drug prescription is tailored for you. Do not alter dosage without checking with your physician.

How taken

Tablets, liquid.

Frequency and timing of doses
Pain 3–4 x daily; 2 x daily (prolonged use).
Opioid addiction Once daily.

Usual adult dosage range
Pain 5–10mg per dose initially, adjusted according to response.
Opioid addiction 15–30mg (starting dose); 40–60mg daily (maintenance dose).

Onset of effect
15–60 minutes.

Duration of action
36–48 hours.

Diet advice
None.

Storage
Keep in a closed container in a cool, dry place out of the reach of children. Protect liquids from light.

Missed dose
Take as soon as you remember and return to your normal dosing schedule as soon as possible. If you missed the dose because it caused you to vomit, or if you cannot swallow, consult your physician.

Stopping the drug
If the reason for taking the drug no longer exists, it can be safely stopped. Discuss with your physician.

OVERDOSE ACTION

 Seek immediate medical advice in all cases. Take emergency action if symptoms such as slow or irregular breathing, severe drowsiness, or loss of consciousness occur.

See Drug poisoning emergency guide (p.526).

POSSIBLE ADVERSE EFFECTS

Drowsiness and nausea are the most common *side effects* of methadone, but these diminish as the body adapts. Constipation is also common and may be longer lasting.

Symptom/effect	Frequency		Discuss with physician		Stop taking drug now	Call physician now
	Common	Rare	Only if severe	In all cases		
Nausea/vomiting	●		■			
Drowsiness	●		■			
Constipation	●		■			
Dizziness/confusion	●			■		
Loss of consciousness		●		■	▲	▮
Slow, difficult breathing		●		■	▲	▮

INTERACTIONS

Phenytoin, carbamazepine, rifampin, and ritonavir These drugs may reduce the effects of methadone.

Monoamine oxidase inhibitors (MAOIs) and selegiline Taken with methadone, these drugs may produce a dangerous rise or fall in blood pressure.

Sedatives The effects of all drugs that have a sedative effect on the central nervous system are likely to be increased by methadone.

SPECIAL PRECAUTIONS

Be sure to tell your physician if:
▼ You have heart or circulatory problems.
▼ You have liver or kidney problems.
▼ You have lung problems such as asthma or bronchitis.
▼ You have thyroid disease.
▼ You have a history of epileptic fits.
▼ You have problems with alcohol abuse.
▼ You are taking other medications.

 Pregnancy
▼ Not prescribed in late pregnancy if possible. May cause breathing difficulties in the newborn baby. Discuss with your physician.

 Breast-feeding
▼ Safety not established. The drug passes into breast milk and may affect the baby adversely. Discuss with your physician.

 Infants and children
▼ Not recommended.

 Over 60
▼ Not recommended.

 Driving and hazardous work
▼ Your underlying condition may make such activities inadvisable. Discuss with your physician.

 Alcohol
▼ Avoid. Alcohol increases the sedative effects of the drug and may depress breathing.

PROLONGED USE

Treatment with methadone is always closely monitored. If the drug is being taken long term, the dose must be carefully reduced before the drug is stopped.

METHOTREXATE

Product name None
Used in the following combined preparations None

GENERAL INFORMATION

Methotrexate is an anticancer drug used, together with other anticancer drugs, in the treatment of leukemia, lymphoma, and solid cancers such as those of the breast, bladder, head, and neck. It is also used to treat severe uncontrolled psoriasis until less potent drugs can be re-introduced. It is also prescribed for people with rheumatoid arthritis. Once the condition being treated is under control, the dose of methotrexate is reduced to a minimum effective level.

As with most anticancer drugs, methotrexate affects both healthy and cancerous cells, so that its usefulness is limited by its *adverse effects* and *toxicity*. When it is given in high doses, methotrexate is usually given with folinic acid to prevent it from destroying bone marrow cells.

QUICK REFERENCE

Drug group Anticancer drug (p.40), antirheumatic drug (p.103), and drug for psoriasis, (p.166)

Overdose danger rating Medium

Dependence rating Low

Prescription needed Yes

Available as generic Yes

INFORMATION FOR USERS

Your drug prescription is tailored for you. Do not alter dosage without checking with your physician.

How taken

Tablets, injection.

Frequency and timing of doses
Cancer Single dose once weekly or every 3 weeks.
Other conditions Usually, single dose once weekly.

Usual adult dosage range
Cancer Dosage is determined individually according to the nature of the condition, body weight, and response.
Rheumatoid arthritis 7.5–20mg weekly.
Psoriasis 10-25mg weekly.

Onset of effect
30–60 minutes.

Duration of action
Short-term effects last 10–15 hours.

Diet advice
None.

Storage
Keep in a closed container in a cool, dry place out of the reach of children. Wash your hands after handling the tablets.

Missed dose
Take as soon as you remember and consult your physician.

Stopping the drug
Do not stop taking the drug without consulting your physician. Stopping the drug may lead to worsening of the underlying condition.

Exceeding the dose
Tell your physician if you accidentally take an extra tablet. Large overdoses damage the bone marrow and cause nausea and abdominal pain. Notify your physician immediately.

SPECIAL PRECAUTIONS

Be sure to tell your physician if:
▼ You have liver or kidney problems.
▼ You have porphyria.
▼ You have a problem with alcohol abuse.
▼ You have a peptic or other digestive-tract ulcer.
▼ You are taking other medications.

Pregnancy
▼ Not prescribed. Methotrexate may cause birth defects in the unborn baby.

Breast-feeding
▼ Not advised. The drug passes into the breast milk and may affect the baby adversely.

Infants and children
▼ For cancer treatment only. Reduced dose necessary.

Over 60
▼ Increased likelihood of adverse effects. Reduced doses necessary.

Driving and hazardous work
▼ No special problems.

Alcohol
▼ Avoid. Alcohol may increase the adverse effects of methotrexate.

POSSIBLE ADVERSE EFFECTS

Nausea and vomiting may occur within a few hours of taking methotrexate. Diarrhea and mouth ulcers are also common side effects occurring a few days after starting treatment.

Symptom/effect	Frequency		Discuss with physician		Stop taking drug now	Call physician now
	Common	Rare	Only if severe	In all cases		
Nausea/vomiting	●			■		
Diarrhea	●			■		
Dry cough/chest pain	●			■		
Mouth/gum ulcers/inflammation	●			■	▲	∎
Jaundice		●		■		∎
Mood changes/confusion		●		■		
Sore throat/fever		●		■	▲	∎
Rash		●		■	▲	∎

PROLONGED USE

Long-term treatment with methotrexate may be needed for rheumatoid arthritis. Once the condition is controlled, the drug is reduced as much as possible to the lowest effective dose.

Monitoring Full blood counts and kidney and liver function tests will be performed before treatment starts and at intervals during treatment. Blood concentrations of methotrexate may also be measured periodically.

INTERACTIONS

General note Many drugs, including NSAIDs, diuretics, cyclosporine, phenytoin, and probenecid, may increase blood levels and toxicity of methotrexate.

Co-trimoxazole, trimethoprim, and certain antimalarial drugs These drugs may enhance the effects of methotrexate.

METHYLCELLULOSE

Product name Entrocel Solution
Used in the following combined preparations None

GENERAL INFORMATION

Methylcellulose is a laxative used for the treatment of constipation, diverticular disease, and irritable bowel syndrome. Taken by mouth, methylcellulose is not absorbed into the bloodstream but remains in the intestine. It absorbs up to 25 times its volume of water, thereby softening feces and increasing their volume. It is also used to reduce the frequency and increase the firmness of feces in chronic watery diarrhea, and to control the consistency of feces after colostomies and ileostomies.

Methylcellulose preparations are also used with appropriate dieting in some cases of obesity. The bulking agent swells to give a feeling of fullness, thereby encouraging adherence to a reducing diet.

QUICK REFERENCE

Drug group Laxative (p.97) and antidiarrheal drug (p.96)

Overdose danger rating Low

Dependence rating Low

Prescription needed No

Available as generic No

INFORMATION FOR USERS

Follow instructions on the label. Call your physician if symptoms worsen.

How taken

Tablets.

Frequency and timing of doses
1–2 x daily. If being used as a laxative and unless otherwise instructed, take with a full glass of water.

Usual adult dosage range
1.5–6g daily.

Onset of effect
Within 24 hours.

Duration of action
Up to 3 days.

Diet advice
If taken as a laxative, drink plenty of fluids, at least 6–8 glasses daily.

Storage
Keep in a closed container in a cool, dry place out of the reach of children.

Missed dose
Take as soon as you remember. Take the next dose as scheduled.

Stopping the drug
Can be safely stopped as soon as you no longer need it.

Exceeding the dose
An occasional unintentional extra dose is unlikely to be a cause for concern. But if you notice any unusual symptoms, or if a large overdose has been taken, notify your physician.

SPECIAL PRECAUTIONS

Be sure to consult your physician or pharmacist before taking this drug if:
▼ You have severe constipation and/or abdominal pain.
▼ You have unexplained rectal bleeding.
▼ You have difficulty in swallowing.
▼ You vomit readily.
▼ You are taking other medications.

 Pregnancy
▼ No evidence of risk to developing baby, but discuss with your physician.

 Breast-feeding
▼ No evidence of risk.

 Infants and children
▼ Reduced dose necessary, but discuss with your physician.

 Over 60
▼ No special problems.

 Driving and hazardous work
▼ No known problems.

 Alcohol
▼ No known problems.

POSSIBLE ADVERSE EFFECTS

When taken by mouth, the drug may cause bloating and excess wind. Insufficient fluid intake may cause blockage of the esophagus (gullet) or intestine. Consult your physician if you experience severe abdominal pain or if you have no bowel movement for 2 days after taking methylcellulose.

Symptom/effect	Frequency		Discuss with physician		Stop taking drug now	Call physician now
	Common	Rare	Only if severe	In all cases		
Abdominal distension		●	■			
Flatulence		●	■			
Abdominal pain		●		■		

INTERACTIONS

None.

PROLONGED USE

No problems expected.

METHYLDOPA

Product name Apo-Methyldopa
Used in the following combined preparation PMS-Dopazide

GENERAL INFORMATION

Introduced in the 1960s, methyldopa was, for many years, one of the most widely prescribed antihypertensive drugs for the treatment of high blood pressure. In recent years, its use has declined as newer drugs with fewer *side effects* have been introduced. However, it is effective in treating people for whom other, newer drugs are ineffective, and for treating those patients who have taken the drug for many years without experiencing any of the side effects.

Unlike some other antihypertensives, methyldopa does not reduce blood flow to the kidneys and is therefore used for patients with kidney disorders.

Methyldopa does not affect the fetus, so it is often prescribed to pregnant women who have high blood pressure.

INFORMATION FOR USERS

Your drug prescription is tailored for you. Do not alter dosage without checking with your physician.

How taken

Tablets.

Frequency and timing of doses
2–3 x daily.

Usual dosage range
Adults 500mg–3g daily.
Children Reduced dose necessary.

Onset of effect
3–6 hours. Full effect begins in 2–3 days.

Duration of action
6–12 hours. Some effect may last for 1–2 days after stopping the drug.

Diet advice
None.

Storage
Keep in a closed container in a cool, dry place out of the reach of children. Protect from light.

Missed dose
Take as soon as you remember. If your next dose is due within 2 hours, take a single dose now and skip the next.

Stopping the drug
Do not stop the drug without consulting your physician, who will gradually reduce your dose. Suddenly stopping methyldopa may lead to an increase in blood pressure.

Exceeding the dose
An occasional unintentional extra dose is unlikely to cause problems. Large overdoses may cause excessive drowsiness and slow heart beat. Notify your physician.

SPECIAL PRECAUTIONS

Be sure to tell your physician if:
▼ You have long-term liver or kidney problems.
▼ You have anemia.
▼ You have porphyria.
▼ You have angina.
▼ You suffer from depression.
▼ You are taking other medications.

Pregnancy
▼ No evidence of risk.

Breast-feeding
▼ The drug passes into the breast milk, but at normal doses adverse effects on the baby are unlikely. Discuss with your physician.

Infants and children
▼ Reduced dose necessary.

Over 60
▼ Reduced dose necessary.

Driving and hazardous work
▼ Avoid such activities until you have learned how methyldopa affects you because the drug can cause drowsiness.

Alcohol
▼ Avoid. Alcohol may increase the hypotensive and sedative effects of this drug.

Surgery and general anesthetics
▼ Discuss the possibility of stopping methyldopa with your physician or dentist before any surgery.

POSSIBLE ADVERSE EFFECTS

Most adverse effects are uncommon and diminish in time. The fluid retention that occurs during treatment with methyldopa is counteracted by taking a diuretic.

Symptom/effect	Frequency		Discuss with physician		Stop taking drug now	Call physician now
	Common	Rare	Only if severe	In all cases		
Drowsiness	●		■			
Depression/headaches	●			■		
Nightmares	●			■		
Impotence/decreased libido	●		■			
Fever		●		■		
Stuffy nose		●		■		
Dizziness/fainting		●		■		
Nausea/vomiting		●		■		
Rash		●		■	▲	
Jaundice		●		■	▲	■

INTERACTIONS

Antidepressants Tricyclic antidepressants may increase the effects of methyldopa. Monoamine oxidase inhibitors (MAOIs) should not be taken at the same time as methyldopa as they may cause a dangerous drop in blood pressure.

Lithium Concurrent use of methyldopa and lithium may increase the risk of lithium *toxicity*.

Levodopa The effects of methyldopa may be enhanced by levodopa.

PROLONGED USE

Liver and blood problems may occur rarely.

Monitoring Periodic checks on blood and urine are usually required.

METHYLPHENIDATE

Product names Ritalin, Ritalin SR
Used in the following combined preparations None

GENERAL INFORMATION

Methylphenidate is a mild central nervous system stimulant used in the treatment of attention-deficit hyperactivity disorder (ADHD). People with this disorder have difficulty concentrating and are easily distracted. Medication is only one part of an ongoing treatment program, along with psychological, social, and educational interventions.

Methylphenidate tablets are usually given 2 or 3 times daily. Once its effect has worn off there are no residual effects. Slow-release (SR) tablets, and extended-release (ER) and controlled-release (CR)

capsules are also available. These must be swallowed whole. SR starts to work slowly and may have a longer action than the regular tablets. ER and CR capsules are taken once daily.

Insomnia and reduced appetite are the main side effects in children; these can improve with time. Growth may be slowed in children while taking this drug, but their eventual height does not seem to be compromised. This drug is generally not recommended in those with an overactive thyroid gland, high blood pressure, heart disease or abnormality.

QUICK REFERENCE

Drug group Nervous system stimulant (p.72)

Overdose danger rating High

Dependence rating Medium

Prescription needed Yes

Available as generic Yes

INFORMATION FOR USERS

Your drug prescription is tailored for you. Do not alter dosage without checking with your physician.

How taken

Tablets, slow release (SR) tablets, extended and controlled release (ER and CR) capsules.

Frequency and timing of doses
2–3 x daily (tablets), once daily (SR/ER/CR).

Usual dosage range
10–30mg daily, adjusted according to weight and response (regular); 18–54 mg daily (ER).

Onset of effect
30–60 minutes (tablets).

Duration of action
3–5 hrs (tablets), 8 hrs (SR), 24 hrs (ER/CR).

Diet advice
None.

Storage
Keep in a closed container in a cool, dry place out of the reach of children.

Missed dose
Take as needed. Allow at least 4 hours between doses of regular tablets.

Stopping the drug
Can safely be stopped. Consult your physician re: overall management of your ADHD.

OVERDOSE ACTION

 Seek immediate medical advice in all cases. Take emergency action if confusion, palpitations, seizures, or loss of consciousness occur.

See Drug poisoning emergency guide (p.526).

SPECIAL PRECAUTIONS

Be sure to tell your physician if:
▼ You have high blood pressure.
▼ You have heart problems.
▼ You have thyroid disease.
▼ You have glaucoma.
▼ You have a history of seizures/epilepsy.
▼ You have a family history of Tourette's syndrome or motor tics.
▼ You are taking other medications.
▼ You are involved in strenuous exercise or activities.
▼ You have a family history of sudden death related to a heart condition.

 Pregnancy
▼ Safety in pregnancy not established. Discuss with your physician.

 Breast-feeding
▼ It is not known if the drug passes into the breast milk. Discuss with your physician.

 Infants and children
▼ Not recommended for children under 6 years.

 Over 60
▼ Increased likelihood of adverse effects. Reduced dose may therefore be necessary.

 Driving and hazardous work
▼ Avoid such activities until you have learned how the drug affects you; it can cause dizziness.

 Alcohol
▼ No known problems.

POSSIBLE ADVERSE EFFECTS

The main adverse effects in children are insomnia and decreased appetite; these may improve with time. Abdominal pain, headache, and irritability may occur at start of treatment.

Symptom/effect	Frequency		Discuss with physician		Stop taking drug now	Call physician now
	Common	Rare	Only if severe	In all cases		
Decreased appetite	●		■			
Insomnia/nervousness	●		■			
Abdominal pain	●			■		
Headache	●			■		
Fatigue	●			■		
Irritability/anxiety		●		■		
Sadness/social withdrawal		●		■		
Palpitations/chest pain	●			■		■

INTERACTIONS

General note Methylphenidate may interact with many drugs to increase their effects. These include anticoagulants, anticonvulsants, and tricyclic antidepressants.

Antihypertensive drugs Methylphenidate

may reverse the effect of these drugs.

Sympathomimetics and MAOIs May cause severe hypertension when used with methylphenidate (and up to 2 weeks after MAOI discontinuation).

PROLONGED USE

Continuous, long-term use may impair growth. "Drug holidays" may be recommended by your physician.

Monitoring Your physician will assess growth and blood pressure at regular intervals. In addition, periodic checks of blood count may be advised.

METHYLPREDNISOLONE

Product names Depo-Medrol, Medrol, Solu-Medrol
Used in the following combined preparations Depo-Medrol with Lidocaine, Medrol Acne Lotion, Neo-Medrol Acne Lotion

GENERAL INFORMATION

Methylprednisolone, introduced in 1957, is a synthetic corticosteroid drug derived from prednisolone. It is prescribed as a topical lotion to relieve skin conditions such as dermatitis, eczema, psoriasis, and to control acne. Methylprednisolone can be injected into joints to relieve rheumatoid arthritis and other types of joint inflammation (see p.104). It is also prescribed by mouth to replace hormones in pituitary or adrenal gland disorders that reduce the body's natural corticosteroid production. Occasionally, methylprednisolone tablets are given for the long-term control of severe asthma.

Side effects are rare when the drug is administered short-term. However, long-term treatment by mouth can cause adverse effects such as fluid retention, indigestion, fragile bones, and muscle weakness. It may also induce diabetes.

INFORMATION FOR USERS

Your drug prescription is tailored for you. Do not alter dosage without checking with your physician.

How taken

Tablets, injection, topical lotion.

Frequency and timing of doses
Varies according to preparation and condition. Follow your physician's instructions.

Usual dosage range
Considerable variation. Follow your physician's instructions.

Onset of effect
2–4 days.

Duration of action
12–36 hours.

Diet advice
A low-sodium, high-potassium diet may be recommended when the oral or injectable form of the drug is prescribed for extended periods. Follow the advice of your physician.

Storage
Keep in a closed container in a cool, dry place out of the reach of children.

Missed dose
Take as soon as you remember. If your next dose is due within 6 hours, take a single dose now and skip the next.

Stopping the drug
Do not stop tablets without consulting your physician, who may supervise a gradual reduction in dosage. Abrupt cessation may cause adrenal collapse.

Exceeding the dose
An occasional unintentional extra dose is unlikely to be a cause for concern. But if you notice unusual symptoms, or if a large overdose has been taken, notify your physician.

SPECIAL PRECAUTIONS

Be sure to tell your physician if:
▼ You have had glaucoma.
▼ You have high blood pressure.
▼ You have diabetes.
▼ You have had a peptic ulcer.
▼ You have a history of depression.
▼ You have a herpes infection.
▼ You are taking other medications.

Pregnancy
▼ No evidence of risk with topical preparations or joint injections. Prescribed in tablet form in low doses, harm to the baby is unlikely. Discuss with your physician.

Breast-feeding
▼ No evidence of risk with topical solutions or joint injections. Taken regularly by mouth, the drug may adversely affect the baby's growth. Discuss with your physician.

Infants and children
▼ Reduced dose necessary.

Over 60
▼ Reduced dose may be necessary.

Driving and hazardous work
▼ No known problems.

Alcohol
▼ Alcohol may increase the risk of peptic ulcers with methylprednisolone tablets. No special problems with other dosage forms.

POSSIBLE ADVERSE EFFECTS

The rare, but more serious, adverse effects occur only when methylprednisolone is taken by mouth in high doses for long periods of time.

Symptom/effect	Frequency		Discuss with physician		Stop taking drug now	Call physician now
	Common	Rare	Only if severe	In all cases		
Indigestion/weight gain	●		■			
Muscle weakness		●		■		
Mood changes		●		■		
Seizures		●		■	▲	▌
Black/bloody feces		●		■	▲	▌

INTERACTIONS

Oral anticoagulants Methylprednisolone may decrease the effect of anticoagulants.

Vaccines Serious reactions can occur when vaccinations are given with methylprednisolone. Discuss with your physician.

Barbiturates, phenytoin, and rifampin These drugs may reduce the effect of methylprednisolone.

Antidiabetic drugs Methylprednisolone reduces the actions of these drugs.

Antihypertensive drugs Methylprednisolone may reduce the effect of these drugs.

Diuretics Methylprednisolone may increase potassium loss.

PROLONGED USE

Prolonged use of methylprednisolone in high doses by mouth can lead to serious adverse effects, such as diabetes, glaucoma, muscle weakness, cataracts, and fragile bones. The drug may retard growth in children.

METOCLOPRAMIDE

Product names Apo-Metoclop, Metoclopramide Omega, and others
Used in the following combined preparations None

GENERAL INFORMATION

Metoclopramide has a direct action on the gastrointestinal tract. It is used for conditions in which there is a need to encourage normal propulsion of food through the stomach and intestine.

The drug has powerful anti-emetic properties and its most common use is in the prevention and treatment of nausea and vomiting. It is particularly effective for the relief of the nausea that sometimes accompanies migraine headaches, and the nausea caused by treatment with anticancer drugs. It is also prescribed to alleviate symptoms of hiatus hernia caused by acid reflux into the esophagus.

One *side effect* of metoclopramide, muscle spasm of the face and neck, is more likely to occur in children and young adults under 20 years. Other side effects are not usually troublesome.

QUICK REFERENCE

Drug group Gastrointestinal motility regulator and anti-emetic drug (p.74)

Overdose danger rating Medium

Dependence rating Low

Prescription needed Yes

Available as generic Yes

INFORMATION FOR USERS

Your drug prescription is tailored for you. Do not alter dosage without checking with your physician.

How taken

Tablets, liquid, injection.

Frequency and timing of doses
Usually 3 x daily.

Usual adult dosage range
Usually 15–30mg daily; may be higher for nausea caused by anticancer drugs.

Onset of effect
Within 1 hour.

Duration of action
6–8 hours.

Diet advice
Fatty and spicy foods and alcohol are best avoided if nausea is a problem.

Storage
Keep in a closed container in a cool, dry place out of the reach of children.

Missed dose
Take as soon as you remember. If your next dose is due within 3 hours, take a single dose now and skip the next.

Stopping the drug
Can be safely stopped as soon as you no longer need it.

Exceeding the dose
An occasional unintentional extra dose is unlikely to be a cause for concern. Large overdoses may cause drowsiness and muscle spasms. Notify your physician.

SPECIAL PRECAUTIONS

Be sure to tell your physician if:
▼ You have long-term liver or kidney problems.
▼ You have epilepsy.
▼ You have Parkinson's disease.
▼ You have acute porphyria.
▼ You have a history of depression.
▼ You are taking other medications.

 Pregnancy
▼ Safety in pregnancy not established. Discuss with your physician.

 Breast-feeding
▼ The drug passes into the breast milk but at normal doses adverse effects on the baby are unlikely. Discuss with your physician.

 Infants and children
▼ Reduced dose necessary. Restricted use in patients younger than 20 years.

 Over 60
▼ Reduced dose may be necessary.

 Driving and hazardous work
▼ Avoid such activities until you have learned how metoclopramide affects you because the drug can cause drowsiness.

 Alcohol
▼ Avoid. Alcohol may oppose the beneficial effects and increase the sedative effects of this drug.

POSSIBLE ADVERSE EFFECTS

The main adverse effects of metoclopramide are drowsiness and, even less commonly, uncontrolled muscle spasm. Other symptoms rarely occur.

Symptom/effect	Frequency		Discuss with physician		Stop taking drug now	Call physician now
	Common	Rare	Only if severe	In all cases		
Drowsiness		●	■			
Restlessness		●		■		
Diarrhea		●		■		
Muscle tremor/rigidity		●		■		▮
Muscle spasm of face		●		■	▲	▮

INTERACTIONS

Sedatives The sedative properties of metoclopramide are increased by all drugs that have a sedative effect on the central nervous system. Such drugs include anti-anxiety and sleeping drugs, antihistamines, antidepressants, *opioid* analgesics, and antipsychotics.

Cyclosporine Metoclopramide may increase the blood levels of this drug.

Phenothiazine antipsychotics The likelihood of adverse effects from these drugs is increased by metoclopramide.

Lithium Metoclopramide increases the risk of central nervous system side effects.

PROLONGED USE

Not normally used long term, except under specialist supervision for certain gastrointestinal disorders.

METOPROLOL

Product names Betaloc, Lopresor
Used in the following combined preparations None

GENERAL INFORMATION

Metoprolol is a member of the beta-blocker group of drugs. It is used to prevent the heart from beating too quickly in conditions such as angina, hypertension (high blood pressure), arrhythmias (abnormal heart rhythms), and hyperthyroidism (overactive thyroid gland). It is also used to prevent migraine attacks and to protect the heart from further damage following a heart attack.

Because the drug is cardioselective (see p.83), it is less likely to provoke breathing difficulties than other, non-cardioselective, beta blockers. However, it should be used with caution by people with respiratory diseases such as asthma or bronchitis.

INFORMATION FOR USERS

Your drug prescription is tailored for you. Do not alter dosage without checking with your physician.

How taken

Tablets, SR-tablets, injection.

Frequency and timing of doses
1–2 x daily (hypertension); 2–3 x daily (angina/arrhythmias); 4 x daily for 2 days, then 2 x daily (heart attack prevention); 2 x daily (migraine prevention); 4 x daily (hyperthyroidism).

Usual adult dosage range
100–300mg daily.

Onset of effect
1–2 hours.

Duration of action
3–7 hours.

Diet advice
None.

Storage
Keep in a closed container in a cool, dry place out of the reach of children.

Missed dose
Take as soon as you remember. If your next dose is due within 2 hours, take a single dose now and skip the next.

Stopping the drug
Do not stop taking the drug without consulting your physician. Stopping suddenly may lead to worsening of the underlying condition.

OVERDOSE ACTION

 Seek immediate medical advice in all cases. Take emergency action if breathing difficulties, collapse, or loss of consciousness occur.

See Drug poisoning emergency guide (p.526).

POSSIBLE ADVERSE EFFECTS

Like all beta blockers, metoprolol is associated with nightmares and cold fingers and toes.

Other common *adverse effects* include breathing difficulties and slow heart beat.

Symptom/effect	Frequency		Discuss with physician		Stop taking drug now	Call physician now
	Common	Rare	Only if severe	In all cases		
Cold hands and feet	●		■			
Nightmares/drowsiness	●		■			
Fatigue/dizziness/headache	●		■			
Nausea/vomiting/abdominal pain		●	■			
Breathing difficulties/wheezing		●			■	▮
Fainting		●			■	▮

INTERACTIONS

Verapamil When first taken with metoprolol, this drug may seriously slow the heart and lower the blood pressure. Discuss with your physician.

Decongestants Taken with metoprolol, these drugs may increase blood pressure and heart rate.

Ergotamine Taken with metoprolol, this drug increases the constriction of blood vessels in the extremities.

Antidiabetic drugs Taken with metoprolol, these drugs may increase the risk or mask the symptoms of low blood sugar.

Non-steroidal anti-inflammatory drugs (NSAIDs) These drugs may oppose the blood-pressure lowering effects of metoprolol.

SPECIAL PRECAUTIONS

Be sure to tell your physician if:
▼ You have liver or kidney problems.
▼ You have asthma, bronchitis, or emphysema.
▼ You have heart failure.
▼ You have diabetes.
▼ You have hyperthyroidism.
▼ You have pheochromocytoma.
▼ You have psoriasis.
▼ You have poor circulation in the legs.
▼ You are taking other medications.

 Pregnancy
▼ Not usually prescribed. May affect the baby. However, the drug may be given under close supervision. Discuss with your physician.

 Breast-feeding
▼ The drug passes into the breast milk, but at normal doses adverse effects on the baby are unlikely. Discuss with your physician.

 Infants and children
▼ Not recommended.

 Over 60
▼ Reduced dose necessary. There may be an increased risk of adverse effects.

 Driving and hazardous work
▼ Avoid such activities until you have learned how metoprolol affects you because the drug can cause fatigue, dizziness, and drowsiness.

 Alcohol
▼ No special problems.

PROLONGED USE

No special problems.

METRONIDAZOLE

Product names Flagyl, Florazole ER, MetroGel, MetroCream, Noritate, NidaGel
Used in the following combined preparation Flagystatin

GENERAL INFORMATION

Metronidazole is prescribed to fight both protozoal infections and a variety of bacterial infections.

It is widely used in the treatment of trichomonas infection of the vagina. Because the organism responsible for this disorder is sexually transmitted and may not cause any symptoms, a simultaneous course of treatment is usually advised for the sexual partner.

Certain infections of the abdomen, pelvis, and gums also respond well to metronidazole. The drug is used to treat septicemia, infected leg ulcers and pressure sores. Metronidazole may be given to prevent or treat infections after surgery. Because the drug in high doses can penetrate the brain, it is prescribed to treat abscesses occurring there.

Metronidazole is also prescribed for amoebic dysentery and giardiasis, a rare protozoal infection.

Metronidazole may be applied *topically* in the form of a gel or cream to treat some forms of acne, rosacea, infected tumours, and gum disease.

INFORMATION FOR USERS

Your drug prescription is tailored for you. Do not alter dosage without checking with your physician.

How taken

Capsules, tablets, liquid, injection, suppositories, gel, cream, vaginal cream and gel.

Frequency and timing of doses
3 x daily for 5–10 days, depending on the condition being treated. Sometimes a single large dose is prescribed. Tablets should be taken after meals and swallowed whole with plenty of water.

Usual adult dosage range
600–1,500mg daily (by mouth); 3g daily (suppositories); 1.5g daily (injection).

Onset of effect
The drug starts to work within an hour or so, but beneficial effects may not be felt for 1–2 days.

Duration of action
6–12 hours.

Diet advice
None.

Storage
Keep in a closed container in a cool, dry place out of the reach of children. Protect from light.

Missed dose
Take as soon as you remember. If your next dose is due within 2 hours, take a single dose now and skip the next.

Stopping the drug
Take the full course. Even if you feel better, the infection may still be present and symptoms may recur if treatment is stopped too soon.

Exceeding the dose
An occasional unintentional extra dose is unlikely to be a cause for concern. But if you notice unusual symptoms, especially numbness or tingling, or if a large overdose has been taken, notify your physician.

POSSIBLE ADVERSE EFFECTS

Various minor gastrointestinal disturbances are common but tend to diminish with time. The drug may cause a darkening of the urine, which is of no concern. More serious *adverse effects* on the nervous system, causing numbness or tingling, are extremely rare.

Symptom/effect	Frequency		Discuss with physician		Stop taking drug now	Call physician now
	Common	Rare	Only if severe	In all cases		
Nausea/loss of appetite	●		■			
Dark urine	●		■			
Dry mouth/metallic taste		●	■			
Headache/dizziness		●	■			
Numbness/tingling		●		■		

INTERACTIONS

Oral anticoagulants, phenytoin, and fluorouracil Metronidazole may increase the effects of these drugs.

Lithium Metronidazole increases the risk of adverse effects on the kidneys.

Cimetidine This drug may increase the levels of metronidazole in the body.

Phenobarbital This drug may reduce the effects of metronidazole.

SPECIAL PRECAUTIONS

Be sure to tell your physician if:
▼ You have long-term liver problems.
▼ You have a blood disorder.
▼ You have a disorder of the central nervous system, such as epilepsy.
▼ You are taking other medications.

Pregnancy
▼ Safety in pregnancy not established. Discuss with your physician.

Breast-feeding
▼ The drug passes into the breast milk, but at normal doses adverse effects on the baby are unlikely. However, metronidazole may give the milk a bitter taste. Discuss with your physician.

Infants and children
▼ Reduced dose necessary.

Over 60
▼ No special problems.

Driving and hazardous work
▼ Avoid such activities until you have learned how metronidazole affects you because the drug can cause dizziness and drowsiness.

Alcohol
▼ Avoid. Taken with metronidazole, alcohol may cause flushing, nausea, vomiting, abdominal pain, and headache. Avoid alcohol during treatment and for 24 hours after the last dose.

PROLONGED USE

Not usually prescribed for longer than 10 days. Prolonged treatment may cause loss of sensation in the hands and feet (usually temporary), and may also reduce production of white blood cells.

MICONAZOLE

Product names Micatin, Monistat, Micozole
Used in the following combined preparation None

GENERAL INFORMATION

Miconazole is an antifungal drug used to treat candida (yeast) infections of the vagina, and a range of other fungal infections affecting the skin.

The drug is available as a treatment for skin infections, and a variety of vaginal preparations is available.

Side effects are rare because miconazole is absorbed in only very small quantities following topical or vaginal application.

The vaginal suppositories, vaginal ovules, and vaginal cream damage latex condoms and diaphragms.

INFORMATION FOR USERS

Follow instructions on the label. Call your physician if symptoms worsen.

How taken

Vaginal suppositories, vaginal cream, vaginal ovules, cream, spray, ointment.

Frequency and timing of doses
1–2 x daily (vaginal/skin preparations).

Usual adult dosage range
Vaginal infections 1 x 5g applicatorful (cream); 1 x 100mg suppository; 1 x 400mg or 1.2g vaginal ovule.
Skin infections As directed.

Onset of effect
2–3 days.

Duration of action
Up to 12 hours.

Diet advice
None.

Storage
Keep in a closed container in a cool, dry place out of the reach of children.

Missed dose
No cause for concern, but apply missed dose or application as soon as you remember.

Stopping the drug
Apply the full course. Even if you feel better, the original infection may still be present and may recur if treatment is stopped too soon.

Exceeding the dose
An occasional unintentional extra dose is unlikely to cause problems. But if you notice any unusual symptoms or if a large amount has been swallowed, notify your physician.

POSSIBLE ADVERSE EFFECTS

Adverse effects are rare with miconazole.

Symptom/effect	Frequency		Discuss with physician		Stop taking drug now	Call physician now
	Common	Rare	Only if severe	In all cases		
Skin irritation		●	■			
Nausea/vomiting		●	■			
Wheezing/blotchy rash		●		■	▲	▮
Vaginal irritation		●		■		

INTERACTIONS

Oral anticoagulants, cyclosporine, phenytoin, antidiabetics, quinidine, and pimozide Miconazole may increase the effects and *toxicity* of these drugs.

SPECIAL PRECAUTIONS

Be sure to consult your physician or pharmacist before taking this drug if:
▼ You have porphyria.
▼ You have liver problems.
▼ You are taking other medications.

Pregnancy
▼ Discuss with your physician.

Breast-feeding
▼ Safety not established. Discuss with your physician.

Infants and children
▼ Discuss with your physician.

Over 60
▼ No special problems.

Driving and hazardous work
▼ No special problems.

Alcohol
▼ No special problems.

PROLONGED USE

No problems expected. Most types of miconazole are not usually prescribed long term.

MINOCYCLINE

Product name Minocin
Used in the following combined preparations None

GENERAL INFORMATION

Minocycline is a member of the tetracycline group of antibiotics but has a substantially longer duration of action than tetracycline itself. The drug is most commonly used to treat acne.

Minocycline may be given to treat pneumonia or to prevent infection in people with chronic bronchitis. It is also used for the treatment of gonorrhea and non-gonococcal urethritis, and is sometimes prescribed to treat other

sexually transmitted diseases. The drug's most frequent *side effects* are nausea, vomiting, and diarrhea. It also interferes with the functioning of the balance mechanism in the inner ear, with resultant nausea, dizziness, and unsteadiness, but these symptoms generally disappear after the drug is stopped. Minocycline is not prescribed for people with poor kidney function.

QUICK REFERENCE

Drug group Tetracycline antibiotic (p.114)

Overdose danger rating Low

Dependence rating Low

Prescription needed Yes

Available as generic Yes

INFORMATION FOR USERS

Your drug prescription is tailored for you. Do not alter dosage without checking with your physician.

How taken

Capsules.

Frequency and timing of doses
1–2 x daily.

Usual dosage range
Adults 100–200mg daily.
Children Reduced dose according to age and weight.

Onset of effect
4–12 hours.

Duration of action
Up to 24 hours.

Diet advice
Milk products may impair absorption; avoid from 1 hour before to 2 hours after dosage.

Storage
Keep in a closed container in a cool, dry, well-secured place out of the reach of children.

Missed dose
Take as soon as you remember. If your next dose is due within 4 hours, take a single dose now and skip the next.

Stopping the drug
Use the full course. Even if you feel better, the original infection may still be present and symptoms may recur if treatment is stopped too soon.

Exceeding the dose
An occasional unintentional extra dose is unlikely to be a cause for concern. But if you notice any unusual symptoms, or if a large overdose has been taken, notify your physician.

SPECIAL PRECAUTIONS

Be sure to tell your physician if:
▼ You have liver or kidney problems.
▼ You have previously suffered an allergic reaction to a tetracycline antibiotic.
▼ You are taking other medications.

Pregnancy
▼ Not prescribed. May damage the teeth and bones of the developing baby, as well as the mother's liver. Discuss with your physician.

Breast-feeding
▼ The drug passes into the breast milk and may lead to discoloration of the baby's teeth. Discuss with your physician.

Infants and children
▼ Not recommended under 13 years. Reduced dose necessary in older children.

Over 60
▼ No special problems.

Driving and hazardous work
▼ Avoid such activities until you have learned how minocycline affects you because the drug can cause dizziness.

Alcohol
▼ No known problems.

How to take your tablets
▼ To prevent it sticking in your throat, a small amount of water should be taken before, and a full glass of water taken after, each dose of minocycline. Take this medication while sitting or standing and do not lie down immediately afterwards.

POSSIBLE ADVERSE EFFECTS

Minocycline may occasionally cause nausea, vomiting, or diarrhea. Other less common adverse effects are rashes, an increased sensitivity of the skin to sunlight, and, in some cases, dizziness and loss of balance (vertigo).

Symptom/effect	Frequency		Discuss with physician		Stop taking drug now	Call physician now
	Common	Rare	Only if severe	In all cases		
Nausea/vomiting/diarrhea	●		■			
Dizziness/vertigo	●			■	▲	
Rash/itching		●		■	▲	
Light-sensitive rash		●		■	▲	
Headache/blurred vision		●		■	▲	

INTERACTIONS

Oral anticoagulants Minocycline may increase the anticoagulant action of these drugs.

Retinoids Taken with minocycline these drugs may increase the risk of benign intracranial hypertension (high pressure in the skull) leading to headaches, nausea, and vomiting.

Oral contraceptives Minocycline can reduce the effectiveness of these drugs.

Penicillin antibiotics Minocycline interferes with the antibacterial action of these drugs.

Iron may interfere with the absorption of minocycline and may reduce its effectiveness.

Antacids and milk interfere with the absorption of minocycline and may reduce its effectiveness. Doses should be separated by 1–2 hours.

PROLONGED USE

Prolonged use of minocycline may occasionally cause skin darkening and discoloration of the teeth. It can also cause photosensitivity reactions, and use of sunscreen is recommended.

Monitoring Regular blood tests should be carried out to assess liver function.

MINOXIDIL

Product names Apo-Gain, Loniten, Rogaine
Used in the following combined preparations None

GENERAL INFORMATION

Minoxidil is a vasodilator drug (see p.98) that works by relaxing the muscles of artery walls and dilating blood vessels. It is effective in controlling dangerously high blood pressure that is rising very rapidly. Because minoxidil is stronger acting than many other antihypertensive drugs, it is usually recommended for people whose blood pressure is not controlled by other treatment.

Because minoxidil can cause fluid retention and increased heart rate, it should be prescribed with a diuretic and a beta blocker to increase effectiveness and to counteract its *side effects*. Unlike many other drugs in the antihypertensive group, minoxidil rarely causes dizziness and fainting. Its major drawback is that, if it is taken for more than two months, it increases hair growth, especially on the face. Although this effect can be controlled by shaving or depilatories, some people find the abnormal growth distressing. This effect is put to use, however, to treat baldness in men and women, and for this purpose minoxidil is applied locally as a solution.

INFORMATION FOR USERS

Your drug prescription is tailored for you. Do not alter dosage without checking with your physician.

How taken

Tablets, topical solution.

Frequency and timing of doses
Once or twice daily.

Usual adult dosage range
5mg daily initially, increasing gradually. Doses up to 40mg daily may be used.

Onset of effect
Blood pressure Within 1 hour (tablets).
Hair growth Up to 1 year (solution).

Duration of action
Up to 24 hours. Some effect may last for 2–5 days after stopping the drug.

Diet advice
None.

Storage
Keep in a closed container in a cool, dry place out of the reach of children.

Missed dose
Take as soon as you remember (tablets). If your next dose is due within 5 hours, take a single dose now and skip the next.

Stopping the drug
Do not stop the drug without consulting your physician; stopping the drug may lead to worsening of the underlying condition.

Exceeding the dose
An occasional unintentional extra dose is unlikely to cause problems. Large overdoses may cause nausea, vomiting, palpitations, or dizziness. Notify your physician.

SPECIAL PRECAUTIONS

Be sure to tell your physician if:
▼ You have a long-term kidney problem.
▼ You have heart problems.
▼ You retain fluid.
▼ You are taking other medications.

Pregnancy
▼ Safety in pregnancy not established. Discuss with your physician.

Breast-feeding
▼ The drug passes into the breast milk, but at normal doses adverse effects on the baby are unlikely. Discuss with your physician.

Infants and children
▼ Reduced dose necessary.

Over 60
▼ Reduced dose may be necessary.

Driving and hazardous work
▼ Avoid such activities until you have learned how minoxidil affects you because the drug can cause dizziness and lightheadedness.

Alcohol
▼ Avoid. Alcohol may further reduce blood pressure.

Surgery and general anesthetics
▼ Minoxidil treatment may need to be stopped before you have a general anesthetic. Discuss this with your physician or dentist before any surgery.

POSSIBLE ADVERSE EFFECTS

Fluid retention is a common adverse effect of minoxidil, which may lead to an increase in weight. Diuretics are often prescribed to control this adverse effect. Allergic and irritant dermatitis may occur with minoxidil lotion.

Symptom/effect	Frequency		Discuss with physician		Stop taking drug now	Call physician now
	Common	Rare	Only if severe	In all cases		
Increased hair growth	●			■		
Fluid retention/ankle swelling	●			■		
Nausea		●		■		
Breast tenderness		●		■		
Dizziness/lightheadedness		●		■		
Rash		●		■		
Palpitations		●		■	▲	■

INTERACTIONS

Antidepressant drugs The hypotensive effects of minoxidil may be enhanced by antidepressant drugs.

Other antihypertensives These drugs may increase the effects of minoxidil.

Estrogens and progestins (including those in some contraceptive pills) may reduce the effects of minoxidil.

PROLONGED USE

Prolonged use of this drug may lead to swelling of the ankles and increased hair growth.

MIRTAZAPINE

Product names Gen-Mirtazapine, Remeron, Remeron RD
Used in the following combined preparations None

GENERAL INFORMATION

Mirtazapine is an antidepressant chemically different than the SSRIs and tricyclic antidepressants. It is used in the treatment of mild to moderate depression. Mirtazapine is as effective as other antidepressants. It can cause drowsiness and weight gain. It may also cause a decrease in blood pressure on quickly sitting or standing up. Caution should be used; stand up slowly, while supporting oneself.

The RD formulation is an Orally Dispersible Tablet and rapidly disintegrates on the tongue; no water is needed to take these tablets. The regular tablets should be swallowed with water. It is best to take mirtazapine in the evening prior to sleep.

QUICK REFERENCE

Drug group Antidepressant drugs (p.68)

Overdose danger rating High

Dependence rating Low

Prescription needed Yes

Available as generic Yes

INFORMATION FOR USERS

Your drug prescription is tailored for you. Do not alter dosage without checking with your physician.

How taken

Tablets, oral disintegrating tablets.

Frequency and timing of doses
Once daily

Usual adult dosage range
15–45mg.

Onset of effect
The onset of therapeutic response usually occurs within 2 weeks of starting treatment, but full antidepressant effect may not be felt for 4–6 weeks.

Duration of action
Up to 24 hours

Diet advice
None.

Storage
Keep in a closed container in a cool, dry place out of the reach of children.

Missed dose
If you miss a dose, take it as soon as you remember. Do not double up on a dose.

Stopping the drug
Do not stop the drug without consulting your physician. Stopping abruptly can cause withdrawal symptoms. If discontinuation is prescribed by the physician, a gradual reduction in the dose over several weeks is recommended.

Exceeding the dose
An occasional unintentional extra dose is unlikely to be a cause for concern. Large doses may cause drowsiness, disorientation, impaired memory. Notify your physician and seek medical assistance right away.

SPECIAL PRECAUTIONS

Be sure to tell your physician if:
▼ You have long-term liver or kidney problems.
▼ You have a heart problem.
▼ You have had a TIA or stroke.
▼ You have a history of seizures or fits.
▼ You are taking other medications.

Pregnancy
▼ Safety not established. Discuss with your physician.

Breast-feeding
▼ Safety not established. Discuss with your physician.

Infants and children
▼ Not recommended.

Over 60
▼ Increased likelihood of adverse effects. Reduced dose may be necessary.

Driving and hazardous work
▼ Avoid such activities until you have learned how mirtazapine affects you because the drug can cause drowsiness.

Alcohol
▼ Avoid. Alcohol may increase the sedative effects of this drug.

POSSIBLE ADVERSE EFFECTS

Generally well tolerated.

Symptom/effect	Frequency		Discuss with physician		Stop taking drug now	Call physician now
	Common	Rare	Only if severe	In all cases		
Drowsiness	●		■			
Dizziness	●		■			
Increased appetite/weight gain	●			■		
Muscle weakness		●		■		
Dry mouth	●		■			
Constipation		●	■			
Tiredness/fatigue		●		■		

INTERACTIONS

Diazepam and other CNS depressants
These agents will have an additive effect to the sedative effects of mirtazapine.

Monoamine oxidase inhibitors (MAOI)
Mirtazapine should not be used with MOAIs or within 14 days of stopping an MAOI.

PROLONGED USE

No problems expected.

MISOPROSTOL

Product names Apo-Misoprostol, Novo-Misoprostol
Used in the following combined preparations Arthrotec

GENERAL INFORMATION

Misoprostol reduces the amount of acid secreted in the stomach and promotes healing of gastric and duodenal ulcers. The drug is related to naturally occurring chemicals called prostaglandins. Gastric and duodenal ulcers may be caused by ASA and non-steroidal anti-inflammatory drugs (p.102) that block certain prostaglandins, and misoprostol can be used to prevent or cure these ulcers. The ulcers usually heal after a few weeks' treatment with misoprostol. In some cases, misoprostol is given during treatment with these drugs as a preventative measure and combined preparations are available that reduce the likelihood of ulcers occurring. The most likely *adverse effects* are diarrhea and indigestion; if they are severe it may be necessary to stop treatment with the drug. Diarrhea can be made worse by antacids containing magnesium; these should therefore be avoided.

INFORMATION FOR USERS

Your drug prescription is tailored for you. Do not alter dosage without checking with your physician.

How taken

Tablets.

Frequency and timing of doses
2–4 x daily, with milk or food.

Usual adult dosage range
400–800mcg daily.

Onset of effect
Within 24 hours.

Duration of action
Up to 24 hours; some effects may be longer lasting.

Diet advice
None.

Storage
Keep in a closed container in a cool, dry place out of the reach of children.

Missed dose
Take as soon as you remember. If your next dose is due within 3 hours, take a single dose now and skip the next.

Stopping the drug
Do not stop the drug without consulting your physician; symptoms may recur.

Exceeding the dose
An occasional unintentional extra dose is unlikely to be a cause for concern. But if you notice any unusual symptoms, or if a large overdose has been taken, notify your physician.

SPECIAL PRECAUTIONS

Be sure to tell your physician if:
▼ You are pregnant, or intending to become pregnant.
▼ You have had a stroke.
▼ You have heart or circulation problems.
▼ You have high blood pressure.
▼ You have bowel problems.
▼ You are taking other medications.

Pregnancy
▼ Misoprostol should not be taken by women of childbearing years. In exceptional cases, it may be prescribed on the condition that effective contraception is used. If taken during pregnancy, the drug can cause the uterus to contract before the baby is due.

Breast-feeding
▼ Safety not established. Discuss with your physician.

Infants and children
▼ Not recommended.

Over 60
▼ No special problems.

Driving and hazardous work
▼ No problems expected.

Alcohol
▼ No problems expected, but excessive amounts may undermine the desired effect of the drug.

POSSIBLE ADVERSE EFFECTS

Adverse effects on the gastrointestinal tract can occur. These effects may be reduced by spreading the doses out during the day. Taking the drug with food may be recommended.

Symptom/effect	Frequency		Discuss with physician		Stop taking drug now	Call physician now
	Common	Rare	Only if severe	In all cases		
Diarrhea	●		■			
Indigestion	●		■			
Nausea/vomiting		●	■			
Vaginal/intermenstrual bleeding		●		■		
Abdominal pain		●		■		
Skin rashes		●		■	▲	

INTERACTIONS

Magnesium-containing antacids These may increase the severity of any diarrhea caused by misoprostol.

PROLONGED USE

No problems expected.

MOCLOBEMIDE

Product names Apo-moclobemide, Manerix, Novo-moclobemide, Nu-moclobemide
Used in the following combined preparations None

GENERAL INFORMATION

Moclobemide is used in the treatment of depression and it belongs to the class of drugs call MAO inhibitors. This drug works by inhibiting an enzyme in the brain called monoamine oxidase type A (MAO-A), thereby increasing levels of certain neurotransmitters in the brain.

Although restrictions in foods containing tyramine is not strictly required as is for other MAO inhibitors, patients are still advised to minimize excessive use of tyramine-rich foods, such as pickled herring, aged cheeses, salami, tap beer, red wine and, soybean products.

This drug should be discontinued at least 2 days prior to receiving an anesthetic and when receiving epinephrine.

QUICK REFERENCE

Drug group Drugs for depression (p.68)

Overdose danger rating High

Dependence rating Low

Prescription needed Yes

Available as generic Yes

INFORMATION FOR USERS

Your drug prescription is tailored for you. Do not alter dosage without checking with your physician.

How taken

Tablets.

Frequency and timing of doses
Usually twice daily, taken immediately after meals.

Usual adult dosage range
200–600mg daily.

Onset of effect
May take up to 4 weeks to see full benefit from medication.

Duration of action
Up to 12 hours.

Diet advice
Minimize excessive use of tyramine-rich foods.

Storage
Keep in a closed container in a cool, dry place out of the reach of children.

Missed dose
If you miss a dose, take it as soon as you remember. If it is near the time of the next dose, skip the missed dose and resume your using dosing schedule. Do not double-up to catch up on a missed dose.

Stopping the drug
Do not stop the drug without consulting your physician. Stopping the drug may lead to worsening of the underlying condition.

Exceeding the dose
An occasional unintentional extra dose is unlikely to cause problems. Large overdoses may cause serious adverse effects. Get help right away and notify your physician.

SPECIAL PRECAUTIONS

Be sure to tell your physician if:
▼ You have kidney problems.
▼ You have liver problems.
▼ You have thyroid disorder.
▼ You are taking other medications.

Pregnancy
▼ Safety in pregnancy not established. Discuss with your physician.

Breast-feeding
▼ Excreted in breast milk. Discuss with your physician.

Infants and children
▼ Not recommended.

Over 60
▼ No special problems.

Driving and hazardous work
▼ May cause drowsiness. Do not drive a car or operate machinery until the effect of the drug wears off and you feel you are mentally alert.

Alcohol
▼ Avoid alcohol use as it may increase the effect of drowsiness caused by this drug.

POSSIBLE ADVERSE EFFECTS

More common adverse effects include dizziness, headache, dry mouth, nausea, and insomnia.

Symptom/effect	Frequency		Discuss with physician		Stop taking drug now	Call physician now
	Common	Rare	Only if severe	In all cases		
Nausea	●		■			
Insomnia	●		■			
Dizziness	●		■			
Mild headache	●		■			
Sweating		●	■			
Loss of appetite		●	■			
Dry mouth	●		■			
Blurred vision		●		■		
Irregular or rapid heartbeat		●		■		▮
Chest pain		●		■		▮
Sudden and severe headache		●		■		▮

PROLONGED USE

No problems expected.

INTERACTIONS

General note Because of the wide range of possible drug interactions with moclobemide, do not take any medication, whether prescription or nonprescription, without first consulting your physician or pharmacist.

Meperidine, morphine, selegiline, sympathomimetics (in cough and cold preparations), SSRIs, TCAs, antipsychotics, St. John's Wort Taking these with moclobemide can lead to a serious increase in blood pressure and should be avoided.

MOMETASONE

Product names Elocom, Nasonex
Used in the following combined preparations None

GENERAL INFORMATION

Mometasone is a corticosteroid drug used in the form of a nasal spray to relieve the symptoms of allergic rhinitis. The drug is also used *topically* for the treatment of severe inflammatory skin disorders and in conditions such as eczema that have not responded to other corticosteroids (see Topical corticosteroids, p.162).

Serious adverse effects are rare if the drug is used for short periods or in small amounts. However, prolonged or excessive topical use may cause local *side effects* such as thin skin with enlarged capillaries, and *systemic* side effects such as weak bones, muscle weakness, and peptic ulcers. Because corticosteroids can affect growth, children using the nasal spray for prolonged periods may need to have their growth (height) monitored.

INFORMATION FOR USERS

Your drug prescription is tailored for you. Do not alter dosage without checking with your physician.

How taken

Cream, ointment, lotion, nasal spray.

Frequency and timing of doses
Once daily.

Usual dosage range
Nasal spray 100mcg (2 puffs) into each nostril.
Topical preparations As directed, applied thinly.

Onset of effect
12 hours. Full beneficial effect after 48 hours.

Duration of action
24 hours.

Diet advice
None.

Storage
Keep in a cool, dry place out of the reach of children.

Missed dose
Take as soon as you remember. If your next dose/application is due within 8 hours, take a single dose or apply the usual amount now and skip the next.

Stopping the drug
Do not stop the drug without consulting your physician; symptoms may recur.

Exceeding the dose
An occasional unintentional extra dose/application may not be a cause for concern, but if you notice unusual symptoms, notify your physician.

POSSIBLE ADVERSE EFFECTS

Irritation of, and sometimes bleeding from, the nose are the most common side effects.

Symptom/effect	Frequency		Discuss with physician		Stop taking drug now	Call physician now
	Common	Rare	Only if severe	In all cases		
Sore throat	●			■		
Thinning skin	●			■		
Increased capillary size in skin	●			■		
Acne/dermatitis around mouth	●			■		
Nasal irritation/bleeding	●		■			
Loss of skin pigment	●		■			
Weight gain		●		■		
Mood changes		●		■		

INTERACTIONS

None.

SPECIAL PRECAUTIONS

Be sure to tell your physician if:
▼ You have a cold sore, measles, or chickenpox.
▼ You have any other nasal or skin infection.
▼ You have rosacea or acne.

Avoid exposure to chickenpox, measles, or shingles while using mometasone.

Pregnancy
▼ Safety not established. Discuss with your physician.

Breast-feeding
▼ No evidence of risk. Discuss with your physician.

Infants and children
▼ Only used for very short courses in children.

Over 60
▼ No special problems.

Driving and hazardous work
▼ No special problems.

Alcohol
▼ No special problems.

PROLONGED USE

Not advisable. Prolonged use of topical preparations of this drug can cause permanent skin changes and should be avoided whenever possible.

MONTELUKAST

Product name Singulair
Used in the following combined preparations None

GENERAL INFORMATION

Montelukast belongs to the leukotriene receptor antagonist (blocker) group of anti-allergy drugs and is used in the prevention of asthma. It is thought that stimulation of leukotriene receptors by naturally occurring leukotrienes from the mast cells plays a part in causing asthma. Montelukast works by blocking these receptors.

The drug is given as an additional medication when combined treatment with corticosteroids and bronchodilators does not give adequate control. It is usually given by mouth as tablets, and a chewable form is available for children.

Montelukast is not a bronchodilator, and cannot be used to treat an acute attack of asthma.

INFORMATION FOR USERS

Your drug prescription is tailored for you. Do not alter dosage without checking with your physician.

How taken

Tablets, chewable tablets.

Frequency and timing of doses
Once daily at bedtime, on an empty stomach.

Usual adult dosage range
10mg.

Onset of effect
2 hours.

Duration of action
24 hours.

Diet advice
None.

Storage
Keep in a closed container in a cool, dry place out of the reach of children. Protect from light.

Missed dose
Take as soon as you remember. If your next dose is due within 8 hours, take a single dose now and skip the next.

Stopping the drug
Do not stop the drug without consulting your physician, symptoms may recur.

Exceeding the dose
An occasional unintentional extra dose is unlikely to be a cause for concern. But if you notice any unusual symptoms, or if a large overdose has been taken, notify your physician.

SPECIAL PRECAUTIONS

Be sure to tell your physician if:
▼ You have phenylketonuria.
▼ You are taking other medications.

Pregnancy
▼ Safety not established. Discuss with your physician.

Breast-feeding
▼ Safety not established. Discuss with your physician.

Infants and children
▼ Reduced dose necessary.

Over 60
▼ No special problems.

Driving and hazardous work
▼ Avoid such activities until you have learned how montelukast affects you because the drug can cause dizziness.

Alcohol
▼ No special problems.

POSSIBLE ADVERSE EFFECTS

Severe *adverse effects* are rare with montelukast. There seems to be an increase in the incidence of chest infections among people taking this drug.

Symptom/effect	Frequency		Discuss with physician		Stop taking drug now	Call physician now
	Common	Rare	Only if severe	In all cases		
Abdominal pain	●		■			
Headache	●		■			
Diarrhea		●	■			
Dizziness		●	■			
Weakness		●	■			
Fever		●		■		
Productive cough		●		■		
Rash		●		■		
Worsening chest symptoms		●		■		
Numbness/tingling		●		■		

INTERACTIONS

Phenobarbital could decrease level of montelukast. Monitor.

PROLONGED USE

No special problems.

MORPHINE

Product names Kadian, M.O.S. Sulfate, MS Contin, MS IR, Statex, and others
Used in the following combined preparations None

GENERAL INFORMATION

In use since the 19th century, morphine belongs to a group of drugs called the *opioid* analgesics (see p.64). These drugs are derived from opium, which is obtained from the unripe seed capsules of the opium poppy.

The drugs are used to relieve severe pain that can be caused by heart attack, injury, surgery, or chronic diseases such as cancer. They are also sometimes given as *premedication* before surgery.

The drugs' painkilling effect wears off quickly, in contrast to some other opioid analgesics, and they may be given in a special slow-release (long-acting) form to relieve continuous severe pain.

These drugs are habit-forming, and dependence and addiction can occur. However, most patients who are prescribed morphine for pain relief do not become addicted and are able to stop taking them without difficulty.

QUICK REFERENCE

Drug group Opioid analgesic (p.64)
Overdose danger rating High
Dependence rating High
Prescription needed Yes
Available as generic Yes

INFORMATION FOR USERS

Your drug prescription is tailored for you. Do not alter your dosage without checking with your physician.

How taken

Tablets, SR-tablets, capsules, SR-capsules, liquid, SR-granules, injection, suppositories, SR-suppositories.

Frequency and timing of doses
Every 4 hours; every 12–24 hours (SR-preparations).

Usual adult dosage range
5–25mg per dose; however, some patients may need 75mg or more per dose. Doses vary considerably for each individual.

Onset of effect
Within 1 hour; within 4 hours (SR-preparations).

Duration of action
4 hours; up to 24 hours (SR-preparations).

Diet advice
None.

Storage
Keep in a closed container in a cool, dry place out of the reach of children.

Missed dose
Take as soon as you remember. Return to your normal dosing schedule as soon as possible.

Stopping the drug
If the reason for taking the drug no longer exists, you may stop the drug in consultation with your physician.

OVERDOSE ACTION

Seek immediate medical advice in all cases. Take emergency action if symptoms such as slow or irregular breathing, severe drowsiness, or loss of consciousness occur.

See Drug poisoning emergency guide (p.526).

POSSIBLE ADVERSE EFFECTS

Nausea, vomiting, and constipation are common, especially with high doses.

Anti-nausea drugs or laxatives may be needed to counteract these symptoms.

Symptom/effect	Frequency		Discuss with physician		Stop taking drug now	Call physician now
	Common	Rare	Only if severe	In all cases		
Drowsiness	●		■			
Nausea/vomiting	●		■			
Constipation	●		■			
Dizziness	●			■		
Confusion		●		■		
Breathing difficulties		●		■	▲	∎

INTERACTIONS

Monoamine oxidase inhibitors (MAOIs)
These drugs may produce a severe rise in blood pressure when taken with morphine.

Esmolol The effects of this beta blocker may be increased by morphine.

Sedatives Morphine increases the sedative effects of other sedating drugs including antidepressants, antipsychotics, sleeping drugs, and antihistamines.

SPECIAL PRECAUTIONS

Be sure to tell your physician if:
▼ You have long-term liver or kidney problems.
▼ You have heart or circulatory problems.
▼ You have a lung disorder such as asthma or bronchitis.
▼ You have thyroid disease.
▼ You have a history of epileptic fits.
▼ You are taking other medications.

Pregnancy
▼ Not usually prescribed. May cause breathing difficulties in the newborn baby. Discuss with your physician.

Breast-feeding
▼ The drug passes into the breast milk, but at low doses adverse effects on the baby are unlikely. Discuss with your physician.

Infants and children
▼ Reduced dose necessary.

Over 60
▼ Increased likelihood of adverse effects. Reduced dose may therefore be necessary.

Driving and hazardous work
▼ People on morphine treatment are unlikely to be well enough to undertake such activities.

Alcohol
▼ Avoid. Alcohol may increase the sedative effects of this drug.

PROLONGED USE

The effects of this drug usually become weaker during prolonged use as the body adapts. Dependence may occur if it is taken for extended periods although this is unusual in patients taking the correct dose for pain relief.

MOXIFLOXACIN

Product names Avelox, Vigamox
Used in the following combined preparations None

GENERAL INFORMATION

Moxifloxacin is a quinolone antibacterial drug used in the treatment of respiratory infections including sinusitis, bronchitis, and pneumonia. The drug is usually prescribed as oral tablets or given as an intravenous injection. It is also available as a solution for eye infections. The tablets are usually taken once a day for 5 or 10 days. It may be taken with or without food. The tablets should be swallowed whole and should not be split or crushed.

Moxifloxacin may make you more sensitive to sunlight. Protect yourself with sunscreen and appropriate clothing.

INFORMATION FOR USERS

Your drug prescription is tailored for you. Do not alter dosage without checking with your physician.

How taken

Tablets, parenteral (intravenous), ophthalmic solution.

Frequency and timing of doses
Usually once daily.

Usual adult dosage range
Oral: 400mg daily.

Onset of effect
Within one day.

Duration of action
Up to 24 hours.

Diet advice
None.

Storage
Keep in a closed container in a cool, dry place out of the reach of children.

Missed dose
If you miss a dose, take it as soon as you remember. If it is near the time of the next dose, skip the missed dose and resume your using dosing schedule. Do not double-up to catch up on a missed dose.

Stopping the drug
Do not stop the drug without consulting your physician. Stopping the drug may lead to worsening of the underlying condition.

OVERDOSE ACTION

 Seek immediate medical advice. May experience significant gastrointestinal and CNS effects. Get help right away and notify your physician.

SPECIAL PRECAUTIONS

Be sure to tell your physician if:
▼ You have seizure disorders or fits.
▼ You have liver problems.
▼ You are diabetic.
▼ You are allergic to any antibiotics.
▼ You or your family has a history of heart disease, such as irregular rhythms or heart attack.
▼ You are taking other medications.

 Pregnancy
▼ Not usually prescribed. Safety in pregnancy not established. Discuss with your physician.

 Breast-feeding
▼ Safety not established. Discuss with your physician.

 Infants and children
▼ Not recommended.

 Over 60
▼ No special problems.

 Driving and hazardous work
▼ Avoid such activities until you have learned how moxifloxacin affects you because the drug can cause drowsiness and visual disturbances.

 Alcohol
▼ Avoid. Alcohol may increase the sedative effects of moxifloxacin.

POSSIBLE ADVERSE EFFECTS

The most common side effects are nausea and abdominal discomfort.

Symptom/effect	Frequency		Discuss with physician		Stop taking drug now	Call physician now
	Common	Rare	Only if severe	In all cases		
Drowsiness/dizziness	●		■			
Headache	●		■			
Nausea/abdominal pain	●		■			
Diarrhea	●		■			
Skin rash, itching		●				▮
Difficulty breathing/swallowing		●				▮
Yellowing of skin/eyes		●		■		▮
Mood changes		●		■		▮
Fast/irregular heartbeat		●				▮
Seizures		●				▮
Visual changes		●				▮

PROLONGED USE

Usually given for a short course of treatment.

INTERACTIONS

Antacids, multivitamins containing iron or zinc Do not take less than 4 hours before or 8 hours after moxifloxacin.

NSAIDs Increased risk of seizures when these drugs are taken with moxifloxacin.

Antidiabetic drugs. Moxifloxacin can affect blood glucose levels and affect the action of antidiabetic drugs.

Warfarin Close monitoring of INR may be required in individuals on both drugs.

NAPROXEN

Product names Anaprox, Apo-Naproxen, Naprosyn, Novo-Naprox
Used in the following combined preparation None

GENERAL INFORMATION

Naproxen, one of the non-steroidal anti-inflammatory drugs (NSAIDs), is used to reduce pain, stiffness, and inflammation.

The drug relieves the symptoms of adult and juvenile rheumatoid arthritis, ankylosing spondylitis, and osteo-arthritis, although it does not cure the underlying disease.

Naproxen is also used to treat acute attacks of gout, and may sometimes be prescribed for the relief of migraine and pain following orthopedic surgery, dental treatment, strains, and sprains. It is also effective for treating painful menstrual cramps.

Gastrointestinal *side effects* are fairly common, and there is an increased risk of bleeding. However, it may be safer than ASA, and in long-term use it needs to be taken only twice daily.

INFORMATION FOR USERS

Your drug prescription is tailored for you. Do not alter dosage without checking with your physician.

How taken

Tablets, SR-tablets, liquid, suppositories.

Frequency and timing of doses
Every 6–8 hours as required (general pain relief); 1–2 x daily (muscular pain and arthritis); every 8 hours (gout).
All doses should be taken with food.

Usual adult dosage range
Mild to moderate pain, menstrual cramps 500mg (starting dose), then 250mg every 6–8 hours as required. *Muscular pain and arthritis* 500–1,250mg daily. *Gout* 750mg (starting dose), then 250mg every 8 hours until attack has subsided.

Onset of effect
Pain relief begins within 1 hour. Full anti-inflammatory effect may take 2 weeks.

Duration of action
Up to 12 hours.

Diet advice
None.

Storage
Keep in a closed container in a cool, dry place out of the reach of children. Protect from light.

Missed dose
Take as soon as you remember. If your next dose is due within 4 hours, take a single dose now and skip the next.

Stopping the drug
When taken for short-term pain relief, naproxen can be safely stopped as soon as you no longer need it. If prescribed for long-term treatment, however, you should seek medical advice before stopping the drug.

Exceeding the dose
An occasional unintentional extra dose is unlikely to be a cause for concern. But if you notice any unusual symptoms, or if a large overdose has been taken, notify your physician.

SPECIAL PRECAUTIONS

Be sure to tell your physician if:
▼ You have long-term liver or kidney problems.
▼ You have heart problems.
▼ You have a bleeding disorder.
▼ You have high blood pressure.
▼ You have had a peptic ulcer, esophagitis, or acid indigestion.
▼ You are allergic to ASA.
▼ You suffer from asthma.
▼ You are taking other medications.

Pregnancy
▼ Not usually prescribed. When taken in the last three months of pregnancy, may increase the risk of adverse effects on the baby's heart and may prolong labour. Discuss with your physician.

Breast-feeding
▼ The drug passes into the breast milk, but at normal doses adverse effects on the baby are unlikely. Discuss with your physician.

Infants and children
▼ Prescribed only to treat juvenile arthritis. Reduced dose necessary.

Over 60
▼ Increased likelihood of adverse effects. Reduced dose may therefore be necessary.

Driving and hazardous work
▼ Avoid such activities until you have learned how naproxen affects you because the drug may reduce your ability to concentrate.

Alcohol
▼ Keep consumption low. Alcohol may increase the risk of stomach irritation with naproxen.

Surgery and general anesthetics
▼ Naproxen may prolong bleeding. Discuss with your physician or dentist before surgery.

POSSIBLE ADVERSE EFFECTS

Most adverse effects are not serious and may diminish with time. Black or bloodstained bowel movements should be reported to your physician without delay.

Symptom/effect	Frequency		Discuss with physician		Stop taking drug now	Call physician now
	Common	Rare	Only if severe	In all cases		
Gastrointestinal disorders	●		■			
Headache		●	■			
Inability to concentrate		●	■			
Ringing in the ears		●		■		
Swollen feet/ankles		●		■		
Rash/itching		●		■	▲	
Wheezing/breathlessness		●		■	▲	■
Black/bloodstained feces		●		■	▲	■

INTERACTIONS

General note Naproxen interacts with a wide range of drugs to increase the risk of bleeding and/or peptic ulcers. It may also increase the blood levels of lithium, methotrexate, and digoxin to an undesirable extent.

Antihypertensive drugs and diuretics The beneficial effects of these drugs may be reduced by naproxen.

PROLONGED USE

There is an increased risk of bleeding from peptic ulcers and in the bowel when naproxen is used long term.

NICOTINE

Product names Nicoderm, Nicorette
Used in the following combined preparations None

GENERAL INFORMATION

Smoking is a difficult habit to stop due to the addiction to nicotine and the psychological attachment to cigarettes or a pipe. Taking nicotine in a different form can help the smoker deal with the two aspects of the habit separately.

Nicotine comes in the form of chewing gum, skin patches, or an inhaler, and is used for the relief of withdrawal symptoms. The patches should be applied every 24 hours to unbroken, dry, and non-hairy skin on the trunk or the upper arm.

Replacement patches should be placed on a different area, and the same area of application avoided for several days. The strength of the patch is gradually reduced, and abstinence is generally achieved within three months. The chewing gum is used whenever the urge to smoke occurs. Gum is chewed slowly for up to 30 minutes, by which time all available nicotine has been released. Inhaler dose is individualized; the initial dose is usually 6–12 cartridges per day.

QUICK REFERENCE

Drug group Nicotine replacement used in smoking withdrawal.

Overdose danger rating Medium

Dependence rating Low

Prescription needed No

Available as generic Yes

INFORMATION FOR USERS

Follow instructions on the label. Call your physician if symptoms worsen.

How taken

Skin patch, chewing gum, inhaler

Frequency and timing of doses
Every 24 hours, removing the patch after 16 hours (patches); when the urge to smoke is felt (gum); 6–12 cartridges per day (inhaler).

Usual adult dosage range
Will depend on your previous smoking habits. 7–22mg per day (patches); 1 x 2mg piece to 15 x 4mg pieces per day (gum); dose individualized (inhaler).

Onset of effect
A few hours (patches); within minutes (gum).

Duration of action
Up to 24 hours (patches); 30 minutes (gum).

Diet advice
None.

Storage
Keep in a cool, dry place out of the reach of children.

Missed dose
Change your patch as soon as you remember, and keep the new patch on for the required amount of time before removing it.

Stopping the drug
The dose of nicotine is normally reduced gradually.

Exceeding the dose
Application of several nicotine patches at the same time could result in serious overdosage. Remove the patches and seek immediate medical help. Overdosage with the gum can occur only if many pieces of gum are chewed simultaneously. Seek immediate medical help.

SPECIAL PRECAUTIONS

Be sure to consult your physician or pharmacist before taking this drug if:
▼ You have long-term liver or kidney problems.
▼ You have diabetes mellitus.
▼ You have thyroid disease.
▼ You have circulation problems.
▼ You have heart problems.
▼ You have a peptic ulcer.
▼ You have pheochromocytoma.
▼ You have any skin disorders.
▼ You are taking other medications.

Pregnancy
▼ Nicotine should not be used (in any form) during pregnancy.

Breast-feeding
▼ Nicotine should not be used (in any form) while breast-feeding.

Infants and children
▼ Nicotine products should not be administered to children.

Over 60
▼ No special problems.

Driving and hazardous work
▼ Usually no problems.

Alcohol
▼ No special problems.

POSSIBLE ADVERSE EFFECTS

Any skin reaction to patches will usually disappear in a couple of days. The chewing gum may cause local irritation of the throat or nose and increased salivation.

Symptom/effect	Frequency		Discuss with physician		Stop taking drug now	Call physician now
	Common	Rare	Only if severe	In all cases		
Local irritation	●		■			
Headache	●		■			
Dizziness		●	■			
Nausea		●	■			
Cold/flu-like symptoms		●	■			
Insomnia		●	■			
Indigestion		●	■			

INTERACTIONS

General note Nicotine patches and chewing gum should not be used with other nicotine-containing products, including cigarettes.

Stopping smoking may increase the blood levels of some drugs (such as warfarin and theophylline/aminophylline). Discuss with your physician or pharmacist.

PROLONGED USE

Nicotine replacement therapy should not normally be used for more than three months.

NIFEDIPINE

Product names Adalat, Adalat XL
Used in the following combined preparations None

GENERAL INFORMATION

Nifedipine belongs to a group of drugs known as calcium channel blockers (p.87), which interfere with conduction of signals in the muscles of the heart and blood vessels.

Nifedipine is given as a regular medication to help prevent angina attacks. The drug can be used safely by asthmatics, unlike some other anti-angina drugs (such as beta blockers).

Nifedipine is also widely used to reduce high blood pressure and is often helpful in improving circulation to the limbs in disorders such as Raynaud's disease.

Like other drugs of its class, it may cause blood pressure to fall too low, and occasionally causes disturbances of heart rhythm. In rare cases, angina worsens as a result of taking nifedipine, and another drug must be substituted.

INFORMATION FOR USERS

Your drug prescription is tailored for you. Do not alter dosage without checking with your physician.

How taken

Capsules, XL-tablets.

Frequency and timing of doses
3 x daily; 1–2 x daily (XL-preparations).

Usual adult dosage range
15–90mg daily.

Onset of effect
30–60 minutes.

Duration of action
6–24 hours.

Diet advice
Nifedipine should not be taken with grapefruit juice.

Storage
Keep in a closed container in a cool, dry place out of the reach of children. Protect from light.

Missed dose
Take as soon as you remember, or when needed. If your next dose is due within 3 hours, take a single dose now and skip the next.

Stopping the drug
Do not stop the drug without consulting your physician; sudden withdrawal may make angina worse.

Exceeding the dose
An occasional unintentional extra dose is unlikely to cause problems. Large overdoses may cause dizziness. Notify your physician.

SPECIAL PRECAUTIONS

Be sure to tell your physician if:
▼ You have liver or kidney problems.
▼ You have heart failure.
▼ You have had a recent heart attack.
▼ You have aortic stenosis.
▼ You have diabetes.
▼ You are taking other medications.

 Pregnancy
▼ Not usually prescribed. The drug may cause abnormalities in the developing fetus and delay labour. Discuss with your physician.

 Breast-feeding
▼ The drug passes into the breast milk and may affect the baby. Discuss with your physician.

 Infants and children
▼ Not recommended.

 Over 60
▼ Increased likelihood of adverse effects. Reduced dose may therefore be necessary.

 Driving and hazardous work
▼ Avoid such activities until you have learned how nifedipine affects you because the drug can cause dizziness as a result of lowered blood pressure.

 Alcohol
▼ Avoid. Alcohol may further reduce blood pressure, causing dizziness or other symptoms.

Surgery and general anesthetics
▼ Nifedipine may interact with some general anesthetics causing a fall in blood pressure. Discuss this with your physician or dentist before any surgery.

POSSIBLE ADVERSE EFFECTS

Nifedipine can cause a variety of minor *adverse effects*. Dizziness, especially on rising, may be caused by reduced blood pressure. Patients with angina may notice increased severity or frequency of attacks after starting nifedipine. This should always be reported to your physician. An adjustment in dosage or a change of drug may be necessary.

Symptom/effect	Frequency		Discuss with physician		Stop taking drug now	Call physician now
	Common	Rare	Only if severe	In all cases		
Headache	●		■			
Dizziness/fatigue	●			■		
Flushing	●		■			
Ankle swelling	●		■			
Frequency in passing urine		●	■			
Rash		●		■		
Palpitations		●		■		
Increased angina		●		■	▲	▮

INTERACTIONS

Antihypertensive drugs Nifedipine may increase the effects of these drugs.

Phenytoin Nifedipine may increase the effects of phenytoin.

Digoxin Nifedipine may increase the effects and *toxicity* of digoxin.

Rifampin This drug may decrease the effects of nifedipine.

Grapefruit juice This may block the breakdown of nifedipine, increasing its effects.

PROLONGED USE

No problems expected.

NITRAZEPAM

Product names Mogadon, Nitrazadon
Used in the following combined preparations None

GENERAL INFORMATION

Nitrazepam is a long-acting benzo-diazepine, which is used as a sleeping drug and can be used to control seizures. Benzodiazepines relieve tension and nervousness, relax muscles, and encourage sleep. When nitrazepam is taken at night, there are still effects the next day. Taken every night, its effects accumulate. Therefore, short courses of one or two weeks are usually prescribed. Long-term use leads to daytime sedation, tolerance, and dependence.

Stopping nitrazepam after prolonged use gives rebound insomnia, anxiety, and a withdrawal syndrome that may include confusion, toxic psychosis, and convulsions. Nitrazepam should be withdrawn gradually, with a tapering off period. The actual time that is needed for withdrawal can vary from weeks to many months. It is recommended that benzodiazepines should be used to treat insomnia only when the problem is severe, disabling, or very distressing.

QUICK REFERENCE

Drug group Benzodiazepine sleeping drug (p.66)

Overdose danger rating Medium

Dependence rating High

Prescription needed Yes

Available as generic Yes

INFORMATION FOR USERS

Your drug prescription is tailored for you. Do not alter dosage without checking with your physician.

How taken

Tablets.

Frequency and timing of doses
Once daily, at bedtime.

Usual adult dosage range
5–10mg daily.

Onset of effect
30-60 minutes.

Duration of action
24 hours or more.

Diet advice
None.

Storage
Keep in a closed container in a cool, dry place out of the reach of children.

Missed dose
If you fall asleep without having taken a dose and wake some hours later, do not take the missed dose. If necessary, return to your normal dose schedule the following night.

Stopping the drug
If you have taken the drug for 2 weeks or less, it can be safely stopped. If you have been taking the drug for longer, consult your physician, who may supervise a gradual reduction in dosage. Stopping abruptly may lead to withdrawal symptoms.

Exceeding the dose
An occasional unintentional extra dose is unlikely to be a cause for concern. Large overdoses may cause unusual drowsiness. Notify your physician.

SPECIAL PRECAUTIONS

Be sure to tell your physician if:
▼ You have severe respiratory disease.
▼ You have porphyria.
▼ You have kidney or liver problems.
▼ You suffer from depression.
▼ You have myasthenia gravis.
▼ You suffer from sleep apnoea.
▼ You have had problems with alcohol or drug abuse.
▼ You are taking other medications.

Pregnancy
▼ Safety not established. Known to affect the baby in the womb. The baby may be born with dependence and have withdrawal symptoms. Discuss with your physician.

Breast-feeding
▼ Avoid. Nitrazepam passes into the breast milk.

Infants and children
▼ Not recommended.

Over 60
▼ The elderly are more likely to suffer adverse effects. Reduced dose necessary.

Driving and hazardous work
▼ Do not drive. Nitrazepam's effects are still present during the day after taking a dose. It reduces alertness, slows reactions, impairs concentration, and causes drowsiness.

Alcohol
▼ Avoid. Alcohol will add to the sedative effects.

POSSIBLE ADVERSE EFFECTS

The main adverse effects are related primarily to the sedative and tranquillizing properties of nitrazepam.

Symptom/effect	Frequency		Discuss with physician		Stop taking drug now	Call physician now
	Common	Rare	Only if severe	In all cases		
Drowsiness next day	●		■			
Confusion/forgetfulness	●		■			
Uncoordinated walking	●			■		
Dizziness/double vision	●			■		
Headache/vertigo		●	■			
Rash		●		■		
Mood changes/restlessness		●		■		

INTERACTIONS

Sedatives All drugs that have a sedative effect on the central nervous system are likely to increase the sedative properties of nitrazepam. Such drugs include other sleeping drugs, anti-anxiety drugs, antihistamines, opioid analgesics, antidepressants, and antipsychotics.

Rifampin reduces the effect of nitrazepam.

Antiepileptic drugs The side effects and toxicity of these drugs may be increased by nitrazepam.

Macrolide antibacterials and imidazole and triazole antifungals increase levels and toxicity of nitrazepam.

PROLONGED USE

Not recommended. Produces tolerance and dependence.

NITROGLYCERIN

Product names Nitro-Dur, Nitrol, Nitrolingual, Transiderm-Nitro, and others
Used in the following combined preparations None

GENERAL INFORMATION

Introduced in the late 1800s, nitroglycerin is one of the oldest drugs that is still in continual use. It belongs to a group of vasodilator drugs called nitrates that are used to relieve the pain of angina attacks. It is available in short-acting forms (sublingual tablets and spray) and in long-acting forms (slow-release tablets and skin patches). The short-acting forms act very quickly to relieve angina. Nitroglycerin is also given by injection in hospital for severe angina and for controlling blood pressure.

Nitroglycerin may cause a variety of minor symptoms, such as flushing and headache, most of which can be controlled by adjusting the dosage. The drug is best taken for the first time while sitting, as fainting may follow the drop in blood pressure caused by the drug.

An ointment preparation may be used for the specialist treatment of anal fissures.

QUICK REFERENCE

Drug group Anti-angina drug (p.87)

Overdose danger rating Medium

Dependence rating Low

Prescription needed No (most preparations); yes (injection)

Available as generic Yes

INFORMATION FOR USERS

Your drug prescription is tailored for you. Do not alter dosage without checking with your physician.

How taken

SR-tablets, sublingual tablets, injection, ointment, skin patches, spray.

Frequency and timing of doses
Prevention 3 x daily (SR-tablets); once daily (patches); every 3–4 hours (ointment).
Relief Use sublingual tablets or spray at the onset of an attack. Dose may be repeated twice in 5 minutes intervals if further relief is required. If symptoms persist after 3 doses used over 15 minutes, seek immediate medical help. The relief medication (tablets or spray) can be used immediately prior to exercise.

Usual adult dosage range
Prevention 2.6–15mg daily (SR-tablets); 5–15mg daily (patches); as directed (ointment).
Relief 0.3–1mg per dose (sublingual tablets); 1–2 sprays per dose (spray).

Onset of effect
Within minutes (sublingual tablets and spray); 1–3 hours (SR-tablets, patches, and ointment).

Duration of action
20–30 minutes (sublingual tablets and spray); 3–5 hours (ointment); 8–12 hours (SR-tablets); up to 24 hours (patches).

Diet advice
None.

Storage
Keep sublingual tablets in a tightly closed glass container fitted with a foil-lined, screw-on cap in a cool, dry place out of the reach of children. Protect from light. Do not expose to heat. Discard tablets within 3 months of opening. Check label of other preparations for storage conditions.

Missed dose
Take as soon as you remember, or when needed. If your next dose is due within 2 hours, take a single dose now and skip the next.

Stopping the drug
Do not stop taking the drug without consulting your physician.

Exceeding the dose
An occasional unintentional extra dose is unlikely to cause problems. Large overdoses may cause dizziness, vomiting, severe headache, fits, or loss of consciousness. Notify your physician.

SPECIAL PRECAUTIONS

Be sure to tell your physician if:
▼ You have any other heart condition.
▼ You have a lung condition.
▼ You have long-term liver or kidney problems.
▼ You have any blood disorders.
▼ You have glaucoma.
▼ You have thyroid disease.
▼ You are taking other medications.

Pregnancy
▼ Safety in pregnancy not established. Discuss with your physician.

Breast-feeding
▼ It is not known whether the drug passes into the breast milk. Discuss with your physician.

Infants and children
▼ Not usually prescribed.

Over 60
▼ No special problems.

Driving and hazardous work
▼ Avoid such activities until you have learned how nitroglycerin affects you because the drug can cause dizziness.

Alcohol
▼ Avoid excessive intake. Alcohol may increase dizziness due to lowered blood pressure.

POSSIBLE ADVERSE EFFECTS

The most serious *adverse effect* is lowered blood pressure, and this may need to be monitored periodically. Other adverse effects usually decrease in severity after regular use and they can also be controlled by an adjustment in dosage.

Symptom/effect	Frequency		Discuss with physician		Stop taking drug now	Call physician now
	Common	Rare	Only if severe	In all cases		
Headache	●		■			
Flushing	●		■			
Dizziness	●			■		

INTERACTIONS

Antihypertensive drugs These drugs increase the possibility of lowered blood pressure or fainting when taken with nitroglycerin.

Sildenafil The hypotensive effect of nitroglycerin is increased significantly by sildenafil. The two drugs should not be used together.

PROLONGED USE

The effects of the drug usually become slightly weaker during prolonged use as the body adapts. Timing of the doses may be changed to prevent this effect. To ensure continued effectiveness, the 3 daily doses are recommended to be taken 6 hours apart.

Monitoring Periodic checks on blood pressure are usually required.

NORETHINDRONE

Product name None
Used in the following combined preparations Estalis, Estracomb, FemHRT, Loestrin, Minestrin, Brevicon, and others

GENERAL INFORMATION

Norethindrone is a progestin, a synthetic hormone similar to the natural female sex hormone, progesterone. It has a wide variety of uses including the postponement of menstruation and the treatment of menstrual disorders such as endometriosis (p.148). When used for these disorders, it is taken only on certain days during the menstrual cycle. It is also prescribed as hormone replacement therapy (HRT). One of the major uses for norethindrone is as an oral contraceptive. It may be used either on its own or in conjunction with an estrogen. The drug is also available in an injectable contraceptive preparation, which is used in special circumstances.

Adverse effects from norethindrone are rare, but contraceptive preparations containing it may cause "breakthrough" bleeding (see p.151).

endometriosis (p.148)

QUICK REFERENCE

Drug group Female sex hormone (p.133)

Overdose danger rating Low

Dependence rating Low

Prescription needed Yes

Available as generic Yes

INFORMATION FOR USERS

Your drug prescription is tailored for you. Do not alter dosage without checking with your physician.

How taken

Tablets, skin patch.

Frequency and timing of doses
Once daily (tablets); 2 x weekly (skin patch).

Usual adult dosage range
350mcg daily (progestin-only contraceptives); 350–700mcg daily (HRT).

Onset of effect
The drug starts to act within a few hours.

Duration of action
24 hours.

Diet advice
None.

Storage
Keep in a closed container in a cool, dry place out of the reach of children. Protect from light.

Missed dose
Take as soon as you remember. If you are taking the drug for contraception, see What to do if you miss a pill (p.147).

Stopping the drug
The drug can be safely stopped as soon as contraceptive protection is no longer required. If prescribed for an underlying disorder, do not stop taking the drug without consulting your physician.

Exceeding the dose
An occasional unintentional extra dose is unlikely to be a cause for concern. But if you notice any unusual symptoms, or if a large overdose has been taken, notify your physician.

SPECIAL PRECAUTIONS

Be sure to tell your physician if:
▼ You have liver or kidney problems.
▼ You have diabetes.
▼ You have had epileptic fits.
▼ You suffer from migraine.
▼ You have acute porphyria.
▼ You have heart or circulatory problems.
▼ You are taking other medications.

 Pregnancy
▼ Not usually prescribed. May cause defects in the baby. Discuss with your physician.

 Breast-feeding
▼ The drug passes into the breast milk, but at normal doses adverse effects on the baby are unlikely. Discuss with your physician.

 Infants and children
▼ Not prescribed.

 Over 60
▼ Not usually prescribed.

 Driving and hazardous work
▼ No special problems.

 Alcohol
▼ No special problems.

POSSIBLE ADVERSE EFFECTS

Adverse effects of norethindrone are rarely troublesome and are generally typical of drugs of this type. Prolonged treatment may cause *jaundice* due to liver damage.

Symptom/effect	Frequency		Discuss with physician		Stop taking drug now	Call physician now
	Common	Rare	Only if severe	In all cases		
Breakthrough bleeding	●			■		
Swollen feet/ankles		●	■			
Weight gain		●	■			
Depression/headache		●		■		
Jaundice		●		■	▲	

INTERACTIONS

General note Norethindrone may interfere with the beneficial effects of many drugs, including oral anticoagulants, anticonvulsants, antihypertensives, and antidiabetic drugs. Many other drugs may reduce the contraceptive effect of norethindrone-containing pills. These include anticonvulsants, antituberculous drugs, and antibiotics. Be sure to inform your physician that you are taking norethindrone before taking additional prescribed medication.

Cyclosporine Levels of cyclosporine may be raised by norethindrone.

PROLONGED USE

Prolonged use may in rare cases cause liver damage.

Monitoring Blood tests to check liver function may be carried out.

NORFLOXACIN

Product names Apo-Norflox, Co-Norfloxacin, Novo-Floxacin and others
Used in the following combined preparations None

GENERAL INFORMATION

Norfloxacin, a quinolone antibiotic, is effective against several types of bacteria that tend to be resistant to older, more commonly used antibiotics. It is particularly effective against bacteria responsible for urinary tract infections, and it is for this purpose that norfloxacin is usually prescribed. It is also used to treat uncomplicated gonorrhea.

Norfloxacin is generally well tolerated, but occasional side effects occur, the most common of which involves gastrointestinal upset. Allergic reactions may also occur, and those with a history of allergies to quinolone antibiotics are not usually given this drug. Headache, dizziness, and drowsiness sometimes occur. Seizures are a rare possibility.

INFORMATION FOR USERS

Your drug prescription is tailored for you. Do not alter dosage without checking with your physician.

How taken

Tablets.

Frequency and timing of doses
2 x daily at least 1 hour before or 2 hours after meals.

Usual adult dosage range
800mg daily for 7–10 days (acute infections); doses of 400mg daily are used for longer courses of treatment if kidney function is impaired; 800mg as a single dose (gonorrhea).

Onset of effect
1–2 days.

Duration of action
12–24 hours.

Diet advice
Do not get dehydrated. Ensure that you drink fluids regularly.

Storage
Keep in a closed container in a cool, dry place out of the reach of children.

Missed dose
Take as soon as you remember. If your next dose is due within 4 hours, take a single dose now and skip the next.

Stopping the drug
Take the full course. Even if you feel better, the infection may still be present and symptoms may recur if treatment is stopped too soon.

Exceeding the dose
An occasional unintentional extra dose is unlikely to cause problems. But if you notice any unusual symptoms, or if a large overdose has been taken, notify your physician.

SPECIAL PRECAUTIONS

Be sure to tell your physician if:
▼ You have impaired kidney function.
▼ You have had epileptic seizures/fits.
▼ You are allergic to quinolone antibiotics.
▼ You are taking other medications.

Pregnancy
▼ Safety in pregnancy not established. Discuss with your physician.

Breast-feeding
▼ The drug passes into the breast milk and may affect the baby. Discuss with your physician.

Infants and children
▼ Not recommended.

Over 60
▼ Reduced dose may be necessary.

Driving and hazardous work
▼ Avoid such activities until you have learned how the drug affects you; it can cause dizziness, drowsiness, and blurred vision.

Alcohol
▼ Avoid. Alcohol may increase the sedative effects of this drug.

POSSIBLE ADVERSE EFFECTS

The most common side effects with norfloxacin are nausea, headache, dizziness, and lightheadedness. It can also cause fatigue, rash, and drowsiness.

Symptom/effect	Frequency		Discuss with physician		Stop taking drug now	Call physician now
	Common	Rare	Only if severe	In all cases		
Nausea/vomiting	●		■			
Dizziness/lightheadedness	●		■			
Headache		●	■			
Drowsiness/fatigue		●	■			
Rash/itching		●		■		
Light-sensitive rash		●		■		

INTERACTIONS

Oral anticoagulants Norfloxacin may increase the anticoagulant action of these drugs.

Theophylline Norfloxacin may increase the adverse effects with theophylline.

Cyclosporine Norfloxacin may increase the blood levels of cyclosporine.

Caffeine Norfloxacin may increase the effects of caffeine: avoid excessive intake.

Antacids, iron, sucralfate These drugs decrease the absorption of norfloxacin. Avoid taking these within 2 hours of each other.

Probenecid This drug may increase levels of norfloxacin.

PROLONGED USE

No problems expected.

NYSTATIN

Product names Mycostatin, Nyaderm
Used in the following combined preparations Flagystatin, Viaderm-K.C.

GENERAL INFORMATION

Nystatin is an antifungal drug named after the New York State Institute of Health, where it was developed in the early 1950s.

The drug has been used effectively against candidiasis (thrush), an infection caused by the *Candida* yeast. Available in a variety of dosage forms, it is used to treat infections of the skin, mouth, throat, intestinal tract, esophagus, and vagina. As the drug is poorly absorbed into the bloodstream from the digestive tract, it is of little use against *systemic* infections. It is not given by injection.

Nystatin rarely causes *adverse effects* and can be used during pregnancy to treat vaginal candidiasis.

QUICK REFERENCE

Drug group Antifungal drug (p.124)
Overdose danger rating Low
Dependence rating Low
Prescription needed No
Available as generic Yes

INFORMATION FOR USERS

Follow instructions on the label. Call your physician if symptoms worsen.

How taken

Tablets, pastilles, liquid, vaginal suppositories, cream, ointment.

Frequency and timing of doses
Mouth or throat infections 4 x daily. Liquid should be held in the mouth for several minutes before swallowing.
Intestinal infections 4 x daily.
Skin infections 2–4 x daily.
Vaginal infections Once daily for 2 weeks.

Usual adult dosage range
2–4 million units daily (by mouth); 100,000–200,000 units at night (vaginal suppositories); 1–2 applicatorfuls (vaginal cream); as directed (skin preparations).

Onset of effect
Full beneficial effect may not be felt for 7–14 days.

Duration of action
Up to 6 hours.

Diet advice
None.

Storage
Keep in a closed container in a cool, dry place out of the reach of children. Protect from light.

Missed dose
Take as soon as you remember. Take your next dose as usual.

Stopping the drug
Take the full course. Even if the affected area seems to be cured, the original infection may still be present, and symptoms may recur if treatment is stopped too soon.

Exceeding the dose
An occasional unintentional extra dose is unlikely to be a cause for concern. But if you notice any unusual symptoms, or if a large overdose has been taken, notify your physician.

SPECIAL PRECAUTIONS

Be sure to consult your physician or pharmacist before taking this drug if:
▼ You are taking other medications.

Pregnancy
▼ No evidence of risk to developing fetus.

Breast-feeding
▼ No evidence of risk.

Infants and children
▼ Reduced dose necessary.

Over 60
▼ No special problems.

Driving and hazardous work
▼ No known problems.

Alcohol
▼ No known problems.

POSSIBLE ADVERSE EFFECTS

Adverse effects are uncommon, and are usually mild and transient. Nausea and vomiting may occur when high doses of the drug are taken by mouth.

Symptom/effect	Frequency		Discuss with physician		Stop taking drug now	Call physician now
	Common	Rare	Only if severe	In all cases		
Diarrhea		●	■			
Nausea/vomiting		●	■			
Rash		●		■		

INTERACTIONS

None.

PROLONGED USE

No problems expected. Usually given as a course of treatment until the infection is cured.

OLANZAPINE

Product names Zyprexa, Zyprexa Intramuscular, Zyprexa Zydis
Used in the following combined preparations None

GENERAL INFORMATION

Olanzapine is an atypical antipsychotic drug prescribed for the treatment of schizophrenia and mania. It works by blocking several different receptors, including dopamine, histamine, and serotonin receptors.

In schizophrenia, the drug can be used to treat both "positive" symptoms (delusions, hallucinations, and thought disorders) and "negative" symptoms (blunted affect, emotional and social withdrawal). In mania, olanzapine can be used alone or in combination with other drugs.

The drug stays in the body longer in women, non-smokers, and the elderly. Lower starting and maintenance doses may be used in these groups.

INFORMATION FOR USERS

Your drug prescription is tailored for you. Do not alter dosage without checking with your physician.

How taken

Tablets, oral disintegrating tablets, injection.

Frequency and timing of doses
Once daily.

Usual adult dosage range
Schizophrenia 10mg (starting dose).
Mania 15mg if used alone or 10mg if used in combination with other drugs (starting dose). For both conditions, the dose can be adjusted between 5mg and 20mg daily.

Onset of effect
4–8 hours.

Duration of action
30–38 hours, but longer in women than in men, and longer in the elderly.

Diet advice
None.

Storage
Keep in a closed container in a cool, dry place out of the reach of children. Protect from light.

Missed dose
Take as soon as you remember. If your next dose is due within 8 hours take a single dose now and skip the next.

Stopping the drug
Do not stop the drug without consulting your physician; symptoms may recur.

Exceeding the dose
An occasional unintentional extra dose is unlikely to cause problems. Large overdoses may cause unusual drowsiness, depressed breathing, and low blood pressure. Notify your physician.

POSSIBLE ADVERSE EFFECTS

Unusual drowsiness and weight gain are the most common *adverse effects* of olanzapine.

Symptom/effect	Frequency		Discuss with physician		Stop taking drug now	Call physician now
	Common	Rare	Only if severe	In all cases		
Unusual drowsiness	●		■			
Weight gain	●		■			
Dizziness/fainting	●			■		
Parkinsonism		●		■		
Persistent sore throat		●		■		
Sudden weakness/numbness		●				▮
Speech or vision problems		●				▮

INTERACTIONS

Sedatives All drugs that have a *sedative* effect on the central nervous system may increase the sedative effects of olanzapine.

Anticonvulsant drugs Olanzapine opposes the effect of these drugs.

Carbamazepine, phenytoin, and rifampin These drugs decrease the effect of olanzapine.

Anti-arrhythmics There is an increased risk of arrhythmias when certain of these drugs are used with olanzapine.

Diltiazem, fluvoxamine, paroxetine These drugs may increase the effect of olanzapine.

SPECIAL PRECAUTIONS

Be sure to tell your physician if:
▼ You have an enlarged prostate.
▼ You have kidney or liver problems.
▼ You have diabetes.
▼ You have glaucoma.
▼ You have epilepsy.
▼ You are taking other medications.

Pregnancy
▼ Safety not established. Discuss with your physician.

Breast-feeding
▼ Safety not established. Discuss with your physician.

Infants and children
▼ Not recommended.

Over 60
▼ Reduced dose necessary. Higher risk of serious effects including death, reported in those with dementia.

Driving and hazardous work
▼ Avoid. Olanzapine can cause unusual drowsiness.

Alcohol
▼ Avoid. Alcohol increases the sedative effects of this drug.

PROLONGED USE

Prolonged use of olanzapine may, rarely, cause *tardive dyskinesia*, in which there are involuntary movements of the tongue and face.

OMEPRAZOLE

Product name Losec
Used in the following combined preparations Losec 1-2-3 A, Losec 1-2-3 M

GENERAL INFORMATION

Omeprazole is an anti-ulcer drug used to treat stomach and duodenal ulcers as well as reflux esophagitis, a condition in which acid from the stomach rises into the esophagus. It reduces (by about 70 per cent) the amount of acid produced by the stomach and works in a different way from other anti-ulcer drugs that reduce acid secretion. It may also be used to prevent gastroduodenal ulceration sometimes caused by non-steroidal anti-inflammatory drugs (NSAIDS) (p.64).

Treatment is usually given for four to eight weeks, depending on where the ulcer is situated. Omeprazole may also be given with antibiotics to eradicate the *Helicobacter pylori* bacteria that cause many gastric ulcers. Reflux esophagitis may be treated for four to twelve weeks.

Omeprazole causes few serious *side effects*. However, because the drug may affect the actions of enzymes in the liver, where many drugs are broken down, it may increase the effects of cyclosporine, warfarin, and phenytoin, and these drugs require more careful monitoring when used with omeprazole. As with other anti-ulcer drugs, it may mask signs of stomach cancer, so it is used only when the possibility of this disease has been ruled out.

INFORMATION FOR USERS

Your drug prescription is tailored for you. Do not alter dosage without checking with your physician.

How taken

Tablets, capsules, injection, intravenous infusion.

Frequency and timing of doses
Usually once daily.

Usual adult dosage range
10–40mg daily.

Onset of effect
2–5 hours.

Duration of action
24 hours.

Diet advice
None, although spicy foods and alcohol may exacerbate the underlying condition.

Storage
Keep in a closed container in a cool, dry place out of the reach of children. Omeprazole is very sensitive to moisture. It must not be transferred to another container and must be used within 3 months of opening.

Missed dose
Take as soon as you remember. If your next dose is due within 8 hours, take a single dose now and skip the next.

Stopping the drug
Do not stop the drug without consulting your physician; symptoms may recur.

Exceeding the dose
An occasional unintentional extra dose is unlikely to be a cause for concern. But if you notice any unusual symptoms, or if a large overdose has been taken, notify your physician.

POSSIBLE ADVERSE EFFECTS

Adverse effects such as headache and diarrhea are usually mild, and often diminish with continued use of the drug. If you develop a rash, however, you should notify your physician.

Symptom/effect	Frequency		Discuss with physician		Stop taking drug now	Call physician now
	Common	Rare	Only if severe	In all cases		
Nausea		●	■			
Headache	●		■			
Diarrhea	●		■			
Constipation		●	■			
Rash		●		■	▲	

INTERACTIONS

Warfarin The effects of warfarin may be increased by omeprazole.

Phenytoin The effects of phenytoin may be increased by omeprazole.

Cyclosporine Blood levels of cyclosporine are raised by omeprazole.

Ketoconazole Omeprazole may decrease the absorption of ketoconazole.

SPECIAL PRECAUTIONS

Be sure to tell your physician if:
▼ You have liver problems.
▼ You have had an allergic reaction to omeprazole.
▼ You are taking other medications.

Pregnancy
▼ Safety in pregnancy not established. Discuss with your physician.

Breast-feeding
▼ The drug may pass into the breast milk. Safety in breast-feeding not established. Discuss with your physician.

Infants and children
▼ Not recommended.

Over 60
▼ No special problems.

Driving and hazardous work
▼ No special problems.

Alcohol
▼ Avoid. Alcohol may aggravate your underlying condition and reduce the beneficial effects of this drug.

PROLONGED USE

No problems expected.

ONDANSETRON

Product names Zofran, Zofran ODT
Used in the following combined preparations None

GENERAL INFORMATION

Ondansetron, an anti-emetic, is used especially for treating the nausea and vomiting associated with radiotherapy and anticancer drugs such as cisplatin. It may also be prescribed for the nausea and vomiting that occur after surgery.

The dose given and the frequency will depend on which anti-cancer drug you are having and the dose of that drug. In most instances, you will receive a dose of ondansetron, either by mouth or injection, before infusion of the anti-cancer agent, then tablets for up to five days after the treatment has finished. Ondansetron is less effective against the delayed nausea and vomiting that occur several days after chemotherapy than against symptoms that occur soon after anticancer treatment.

To enhance the effectiveness of ondansetron, it is usually taken with other drugs, such as dexamethasone. Serious *adverse effects* are unlikely to occur.

INFORMATION FOR USERS

Your drug prescription is tailored for you. Do not alter dosage without checking with your physician.

How taken

Tablets, oral disintegrating tablets, liquid, injection.

Frequency and timing of doses
Normally 2–3 x daily but the frequency will depend on the reason for which it is being used.

Usual adult dosage range
4–32mg daily depending on the reason for which it is being used.

Onset of effect
Within 1 hour.

Duration of action
Approximately 12 hours.

Diet advice
None.

Storage
Keep in a closed container in a cool, dry place out of the reach of children. Protect from light.

Missed dose
Take as soon as you remember. If your next dose is due within 2 hours, take a single dose now and skip the next.

Stopping the drug
Can be safely stopped as soon as you no longer need it.

Exceeding the dose
An occasional unintentional extra dose is unlikely to be a cause for concern. But if you notice any unusual symptoms, or if a large overdose has been taken, notify your physician.

SPECIAL PRECAUTIONS

Be sure to tell your physician if:
▼ You have a long-term liver problem.
▼ You have phenylketonuria.
▼ You are taking other medications.

 Pregnancy
▼ Safety in pregnancy not established. Discuss with your doctor.

 Breast-feeding
▼ The drug passes into the breast milk. Discuss with your doctor.

 Infants and children
▼ Reduced dose necessary.

 Over 60
▼ No special problems.

 Driving and hazardous work
▼ No problems expected.

 Alcohol
▼ No known problems.

PROLONGED USE

Not generally prescribed for long-term treatment.

POSSIBLE ADVERSE EFFECTS

Ondansetron is considered to be safe and is generally well tolerated. It does not cause sedation and movement disorders – adverse effects of some of the other anti-emetics.

Symptom/effect	Frequency		Discuss with physician		Stop taking drug now	Call physician now
	Common	Rare	Only if severe	In all cases		
Constipation	●		■			
Headache	●		■			
Warm feeling in head/stomach		●	■			
Palpitations		●		■	▲	▮
Dizziness		●		■		
Fits		●		■	▲	▮

INTERACTIONS

None.

ORLISTAT

Product name Xenical
Used in the following combined preparations None

GENERAL INFORMATION

Orlistat blocks the action of stomach and pancreatic enzymes (lipases) that digest fats. This means that the fats are not absorbed into the body but pass through and are excreted in the feces. As a result, the body must burn stored fat from the tissues to provide energy, which should gradually reduce the fat stores and produce weight loss. The effectiveness of orlistat varies from person to person.

Because of the way orlistat works, the feces become oily and this can cause flatulence. Part of the drug's effect may be due to people reducing their fat intake in order to avoid the unpleasantness of these *side effects*.

As fat absorption is greatly reduced, there is a danger that fat soluble vitamins might be lost to the body. Vitamin supplements may be prescribed to compensate for this. The vitamins should be taken at a different time from the orlistat; bedtime might be best, or at least 2 hours apart from any orlistat dose.

QUICK REFERENCE

Overdose danger rating Low
Dependence rating Low
Prescription needed Yes
Available as generic No

INFORMATION FOR USERS

Your drug prescription is tailored for you. Do not alter dosage without checking with your physician.

How taken

Capsules.

Frequency and timing of doses
Just before, during, or up to 1 hour after each main meal (up to 3 x daily). If a meal is omitted or contains no fat, do not take the dose of orlistat.

Usual adult dosage range
120–360mg daily.

Onset of effect
30 minutes; excretion of excess fecal fat begins about 24–48 hours after the first dose.

Duration of action
Orlistat is not absorbed from the gut, and potentially continues to work as it passes through the intestines. If you stop taking the drug, fecal fat returns to normal in 48–72 hours.

Diet advice
Eat a nutritionally balanced diet that does not contain quite enough calories, and that provides about 30 percent of the calories as fat. Eat lots of fruit and vegetables. The intake of fat, carbohydrate, and protein should be distributed over the three main meals.

Storage
Keep in a closed container in a cool dry place. Keep out of the reach of children.

Missed dose
No cause for concern. Take the next dose with the next meal.

Stopping the drug
The drug can be safely stopped as soon as it is no longer needed, but notify your physician.

SPECIAL PRECAUTIONS

Be sure to tell your physician if:
▼ You have diabetes.
▼ You have chronic malabsorption syndrome.
▼ You have gallbladder or liver problems.
▼ You are taking lipid-lowering drugs.
▼ You are taking other medications.

Pregnancy
▼ Safety not established. Discuss with your physician.

Breast-feeding
▼ Safety not established. Discuss with your physician.

Infants and children
▼ Not prescribed.

Over 60
▼ No known problems.

Driving and hazardous work
▼ No special problems.

Alcohol
▼ No special problems.

POSSIBLE ADVERSE EFFECTS

Most of the *side effects* depend on how much fat is eaten, as well as the dose of orlistat.

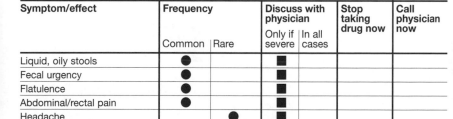

Symptom/effect	Frequency		Discuss with physician		Stop taking drug now	Call physician now
	Common	Rare	Only if severe	In all cases		
Liquid, oily stools	●			■		
Fecal urgency	●			■		
Flatulence	●			■		
Abdominal/rectal pain	●			■		
Headache		●		■		
Menstrual irregularities		●		■		
Anxiety/fatigue/nausea		●		■		

PROLONGED USE

Orlistat treatment should be stopped after 12 weeks if you have not lost 5 percent of your body weight since the start of treatment. If you have, then the drug may be continued, for up to a maximum of 2 years, until your target weight is approached.

When orlistat treatment is stopped, there may be gradual weight gain.

INTERACTIONS

Lipid-lowering drugs Orlistat increases blood levels and *toxicity* of pravastatin.

ORPHENADRINE

Product name Norflex
Used in the following combined preparations None

GENERAL INFORMATION

Orphenadrine possesses significant muscle-relaxant properties. It produces this effect by blocking nerve pathways that are responsible for muscle rigidity and spasm. It has been used for lower back pain and other muscle pain. It may be used along with a medication for pain.

Orphenadrine also has some anticholinergic activity and should be used with caution along with other anticholinergic drugs.

INFORMATION FOR USERS

Your drug prescription is tailored for you. Do not alter dosage without checking with your physician.

How taken

Tablets, injection.

Frequency and timing of doses
2 x daily.

Usual adult dosage range
100–200mg daily (oral); 60mg (injection).

Onset of effect
Within 60 minutes.

Duration of action
8–12 hours.

Diet advice
None.

Storage
Keep in a closed container in a cool, dry place out of the reach of children. Protect from light.

Missed dose
Take as soon as you remember. If your next dose is due within 2 hours, take a single dose now and skip the next.

Stopping the drug
Do not stop the drug without consulting your physician; symptoms may recur.

OVERDOSE ACTION

 Seek immediate medical advice in all cases. Take emergency action if palpitations, fits, or loss of consciousness occur.

See Drug poisoning emergency guide (p.526).

POSSIBLE ADVERSE EFFECTS

The adverse effects of orphenadrine are similar to those of other anticholinergic drugs. The more common symptoms, such as dryness of the mouth and blurred vision, can often be overcome by an adjustment in dosage.

Symptom/effect	Frequency		Discuss with physician		Stop taking drug now	Call physician now
	Common	Rare	Only if severe	In all cases		
Dry mouth/skin	●		■			
Difficulty in passing urine	●		■			
Constipation	●		■			
Dizziness	●			■		
Blurred vision	●			■		
Confusion/agitation		●		■		
Rash/itching		●		■	▲	
Palpitations		●		■	▲	■

INTERACTIONS

Anticholinergic drugs The anticholinergic effects of orphenadrine are likely to be increased by these drugs.

Dextropropoxyphene Confusion, anxiety, and tremors may occur if this drug is taken with orphenadrine.

Metoclopramide and domperidone Orphenadrine opposes the effect of these drugs on the gut.

SPECIAL PRECAUTIONS

Be sure to tell your physician if:
▼ You have long-term liver or kidney problems.
▼ You have heart problems.
▼ You have had glaucoma.
▼ You have difficulty in passing urine and have an enlarged prostate.
▼ You have myasthenia gravis.
▼ You have had peptic ulcers.
▼ You are taking other medications.

 Pregnancy
▼ Safety in pregnancy not established. Discuss with your physician.

 Breast-feeding
▼ The drug passes into the breast milk, but at normal doses adverse effects on the baby are unlikely. Discuss with your physician.

 Infants and children
▼ Not usually prescribed.

 Over 60
▼ Increased likelihood of adverse effects. Reduced dose may therefore be necessary.

 Driving and hazardous work
▼ Avoid such activities until you have learned how orphenadrine affects you because the drug can cause dizziness, lightheadedness, and blurred vision.

 Alcohol
▼ Avoid.

PROLONGED USE

No problems expected.

OSELTAMIVIR

Product name Tamiflu
Used in the following combined preparations None

GENERAL INFORMATION

Oseltamivir is an antiviral drug used to treat influenza (flu), a virus that infects and multiplies in the lungs. The drug works by attacking the virus and preventing it from multiplying and spreading in the lungs. Oseltamivir is not a substitute for flu vaccination, but is used to treat at-risk individuals, for example the elderly and those with long-term illnesses such as chronic heart and lung disease.

Flu causes fever, chills, headache, aches, and pains. Other symptoms include sore throat, cough, and nasal symptoms. Oseltamivir helps to clear these symptoms and may shorten the duration of the illness. Treatment should begin as soon as possible, and certainly within 48 hours of the onset of symptoms.

Symptoms usually subside in two to seven days, unless complications such as a chest infection occur.

In some cases, Oseltamivir may also be used to prevent influenza in those who have had close contact with an infected individual.

Oseltamivir may be taken as a capsule or as an oral suspension.

INFORMATION FOR USERS

Your drug prescription is tailored for you. Do not alter dosage without checking with your physician.

How taken

Capsules, suspension.

Frequency and timing of doses
Once or twice daily.

Usual dosage range
Treatment of influenza 13 years of age or older, 75mg twice daily for 5 days.
Prevention 75mg once daily for up to 14 days.
For children 1–12 years of age, dose is based on the weight of the child.

Onset of effect
Within 7 days.

Duration of action
Up to 12 hours.

Diet advice
May be taken with or without food. Taking it with food may make it easier to tolerate the medication.

Storage
Capsules Keep in a closed container in a cool, dry place out of the reach of children.
Suspension Store in refrigerator at 2–8°C. Suspension should be shaken well before use.

Missed dose
If you miss a dose, take it as soon as you remember. If it is near the time of the next dose, skip the missed dose and resume your using dosing schedule. Do not double-up to catch up on a missed dose.

Stopping the drug
Do not stop the drug without consulting your physician; symptoms may recur.

Exceeding the dose
An occasional unintentional extra dose is unlikely to cause problems. However, if you notice any unusual symptoms, or if a large overdose has been taken, notify your physician.

SPECIAL PRECAUTIONS

Be sure to tell your physician if:
▼ You have ever had an allergic reaction to oseltamivir.
▼ You have a long-term illness.
▼ You have poor immunity to infections.
▼ You have kidney problems or kidney disease.
▼ You are on any other medications.

Pregnancy
▼ Safety in pregnancy not established. Discuss with your physician.

Breast-feeding
▼ Not to be used by women who are breast-feeding children less than one year of age. Discuss use with your physician.

Infants and children
▼ Not recommended in children less than one year of age. For all children, discuss follow-up with your physician.

Over 60
▼ No special problems.

Driving and hazardous work
▼ No known problems.

Alcohol
▼ No known problems.

POSSIBLE ADVERSE EFFECTS

Adverse effects are uncommon. Such effects that occur are similar to signs and symptoms of flu and may therefore sometimes be caused by the influenza virus rather than Oseltamivir.

Symptom/effect	Frequency		Discuss with physician		Stop taking drug now	Call physician now
	Common	Rare	Only if severe	In all cases		
Nausea/vomiting	●		■			
Dizziness	●		■			
Abdominal pain		●	■			
Headache		●	■			
Rash		●		■		▮
Mood changes/abnormal behaviour		●				▮

PROLONGED USE

This drug should only be used for 5 days for treatment or for the appropriate recommended duration for prophylaxis. Not prescribed for long-term use.

INTERACTIONS

Warfarin When Oseltamivir is used in a patient on warfarin, more close monitoring of the effect of warfarin, as measured by INR, is recommended.

OXAZEPAM

Product name Apo-Oxazepam
Used in the following combined preparations None

GENERAL INFORMATION

Oxazepam belongs to a group of drugs known as the benzodiazepines, which help to relieve anxiety and encourage sleep. The actions and adverse effects of this group of drugs are described more fully on page 67.

Oxazepam is used for the short-term treatment of excessive anxiety and may be taken two to four times a day for this condition. When taken 30 minutes to 1 hour before bedtime, it can also help with insomnia. Oxazepam is less likely than some of the other benzodiazepines to accumulate in the body.

Oxazepam, in common with other benzodiazopines, can be habit-forming if taken regularly over a long period of time. Its effects may also diminish with time. For those reasons, treatment should be reviewed regularly.

QUICK REFERENCE

Drug group Benzodiazepine anti-anxiety drug (p.67)

Overdose danger rating Medium

Dependence rating High

Prescription needed Yes

Available as generic Yes

INFORMATION FOR USERS

Your drug prescription is tailored for you. Do not alter dosage without checking with your physician.

How taken

Tablets.

Frequency and timing of doses
1–4 times daily.

Usual adult dosage range
15–120mg daily.

Onset of effect
Within 30–45 minutes.

Duration of action
Several hours.

Diet advice
None.

Storage
Keep in a closed container in a cool, dry place out of the reach of children.

Missed dose
On a daytime schedule, take the missed dose when you remember. If your next dose is due within 2–3 hours, take a single dose now and skip the next. If taken at bedtime only, a missed dose is no cause for concern.

Stopping the drug
If you have been taking the drug continuously for less than 2 weeks, it can be safely stopped as soon as you feel you no longer need it. If you have been taking the drug for longer, consult your physician, who will supervise a gradual reduction in dosage. Stopping abruptly may lead to withdrawal symptoms (see p.66).

Exceeding the dose
An occasional unintentional extra dose is unlikely to cause problems. Large overdoses may cause unusual drowsiness. Notify your physician immediately and seek medical assistance.

SPECIAL PRECAUTIONS

Be sure to tell your physician if:
▼ You have severe respiratory disease or sleep apnea.
▼ You have or have had any problems with alcohol or drug misuse/abuse.
▼ You have myasthenia gravis.
▼ You have glaucoma.
▼ You have had epileptic fits.
▼ You have impaired liver or kidney function.
▼ You are taking other medications.

Pregnancy
▼ Not recommended.

Breast-feeding
▼ Not recommended.

Infants and children
▼ Not recommended.

Over 60
▼ Increased likelihood of adverse effects. Reduced dose may therefore be necessary.

Driving and hazardous work
▼ Avoid such activities until you have learned how oxazepam affects you because the drug can cause drowsiness, reduced alertness, and slowed reactions.

Alcohol
▼ Avoid. Alcohol increases the sedative effects of the drug.

POSSIBLE ADVERSE EFFECTS

The principal adverse effects of this drug are related to its sedative and tranquillizing properties and normally diminish after the first few days of treatment.

Symptom/effect	Frequency		Discuss with physician		Stop taking drug now	Call physician now
	Common	Rare	Only if severe	In all cases		
Daytime drowsiness	●		■			
Dizziness/unsteadiness		●		■		
Headache		●		■		
Nausea/vomiting		●		■		
Amnesia		●		■	▲	
Confusion/disorientation		●		■		▮
Rash		●		■	▲	▮

INTERACTIONS

Sedatives All drugs, including alcohol, that have a sedative effect on the central nervous system are likely to increase the sedative effects of oxazepam. Such drugs include other sleeping and anti-anxiety drugs, antihistamines, antidepressants, opioid analgesics, and antipsychotics.

Antacid May decrease the rate of oxazepam absorption; separate administration times.

Cimetidine May decrease breakdown of oxazepam and increase its effect.

PROLONGED USE

Regular use of this drug over several weeks can lead to a reduction in its effect as the body adapts. It may also be habit-forming when taken for extended periods, especially if large doses are taken.

OXYBUTYNIN

Product names Ditropan, Ditropan XL, Oxytrol, Uromax
Used in the following combined preparations None

GENERAL INFORMATION

Oxybutynin is an *anticholinergic* and *antispasmodic* drug used to treat urinary incontinence and frequency in adults and bedwetting in children. It works by reducing bladder contraction, allowing the bladder to hold more urine. The drug stops bladder spasms and delays the desire to empty the bladder. It also has some local *anesthetic* effect.

It is available as tablets and as a patch that can be applied to the skin. The patch is usually applied twice weekly.

The drug's usefulness is limited to some extent by its *side effects*, especially in children and the elderly. It can aggravate conditions such as an enlarged prostate or coronary heart disease in the elderly. Children are more susceptible to effects on the central nervous system (CNS), such as restlessness, disorientation, hallucinations, and convulsions.

QUICK REFERENCE

Drug group Drug for urinary disorders (p.154)

Overdose danger rating Medium

Dependence rating Low

Prescription needed Yes

Available as generic Yes

INFORMATION FOR USERS

Your drug prescription is tailored for you. Do not alter dosage without checking with your physician.

How taken

Tablets, liquid, patch.

Frequency and timing of doses
2–3 x daily, once daily (XL), twice weekly (patch).

Usual adult dosage range
10–20mg daily.

Onset of effect
1 hour.

Duration of action
Up to 10 hours.

Diet advice
None.

Storage
Keep in a closed container in a cool, dry place out of the reach of children. Protect liquid from light.

Missed dose
Take as soon as you remember. If your next dose is due within 2 hours, take a single dose now and skip the next.

Stopping the drug
Do not stop taking the drug without consulting your physician; symptoms may recur.

Exceeding the dose
An occasional unintentional extra dose is unlikely to cause problems. Larger overdoses may cause restlessness or psychotic behaviour, fall in blood pressure, breathing difficulties, paralysis, or coma. Notify your physician immediately.

SPECIAL PRECAUTIONS

Be sure to tell your physician if:
▼ You have liver or kidney problems.
▼ You have hyperthyroidism.
▼ You have heart problems.
▼ You have an enlarged prostate.
▼ You have hiatus hernia.
▼ You have ulcerative colitis.
▼ You have glaucoma.
▼ You have myasthenia gravis.
▼ You are taking other medications.

Pregnancy
▼ Safety not established. May harm the unborn baby. Discuss with your physician.

Breast-feeding
▼ Safety not established. Discuss with your physician.

Infants and children
▼ Not recommended under 5 years. Reduced dose necessary in older children.

Over 60
▼ Reduced dose necessary.

Driving and hazardous work
▼ Avoid such activities until you have learned how oxybutynin affects you because the drug can cause drowsiness, disorientation, and blurred vision.

Alcohol
▼ Avoid. Alcohol increases the sedative effects of oxybutynin.

POSSIBLE ADVERSE EFFECTS

An adjustment in dosage is necessary in children and the elderly to minimize oxybutynin's adverse effects. The drug can also precipitate glaucoma.

Symptom/effect	Frequency		Discuss with physician		Stop taking drug now	Call physician now
	Common	Rare	Only if severe	In all cases		
Dry mouth	●		■			
Blurred vision/eye pain		●	■			
Constipation	●		■			
Nausea	●		■			
Facial flushing	●		■			
Difficulty in passing urine	●			■		
Headache/confusion		●		■		
Dry skin/rash		●		■		

INTERACTIONS

General note If oxybutynin is taken with other drugs that have anticholinergic effects, the risk of accumulated side effects is increased.

PROLONGED USE

No special problems. The need for continued treatment may be reviewed after six months.

PANTOPRAZOLE

Product names Pantoloc, PANTO IV
Used in the following combined preparations None

GENERAL INFORMATION

Pantoprazole is an anti-ulcer drug used to treat stomach and duodenal ulcers as well as reflux esophagitis, a condition in which acid from the stomach rises into the esophagus. It reduces the amount of acid produced by the stomach and works in a different way from other anti-ulcer drugs that reduce acid secretion. It may also be used to prevent gastroduodenal ulceration sometimes caused by non-steroidal anti-inflammatory drugs (p.64).

Treatment is usually given for four to eight weeks, depending on where the ulcer is situated. Pantoprazole may also be given with antibiotics to eradicate the

Helicobacter pylori bacteria that cause many gastric ulcers. Reflux esophagitis may be treated for four to twelve weeks.

Pantoprazole causes few serious side effects. However, because the drug may affect the actions of enzymes in the liver, where many drugs are broken down, it may increase the effects of cyclosporine, warfarin, and phenytoin, and these drugs require more careful monitoring when used with pantoprazole. As with other anti-ulcer drugs, it may mask signs of stomach cancer, so it is used only when the possibility of this disease has been ruled out.

QUICK REFERENCE

Drug group Anti-ulcer drug (p.95)
Overdose danger rating Low
Dependence rating Low
Prescription needed Yes
Available as generic Yes
(for injection)

INFORMATION FOR USERS

Your drug prescription is tailored for you. Do not alter dosage without checking with your physician.

How taken

Tablets, injection. Tablets should be swallowed whole and should not be chewed or crushed.

Frequency and timing of doses
Once daily in the morning.

Usual adult dosage range
20–40mg daily.

Onset of effect
1–3 hours

Duration of action
24 hours.

Diet advice
None, although spicy foods and alcohol may exacerbate the underlying condition.

Storage
Keep in a closed container in a cool, dry place out of the reach of children.

Missed dose
If you miss a dose, take it as soon as you remember. If your next dose is within 8 hours, take a single dose now and skip the next.

Stopping the drug
Do not stop the drug without consulting your physician; symptoms may recur.

Exceeding the dose
An occasional unintentional extra dose is unlikely to be a cause for concern. But if you notice any unusual symptoms, or if a large overdose has been taken, notify your physician.

SPECIAL PRECAUTIONS

Be sure to tell your physician if:
▼ You have liver problems.
▼ You have had an allergic reaction to pantoprazole.
▼ You are taking other medications.

Pregnancy
▼ Safety has not been established. Discuss with your physician.

Breast-feeding
▼ Safety in breast-feeding not established. Discuss with your physician.

Infants and children
▼ Not recommended.

Over 60
▼ No special problems.

Driving and hazardous work
▼ No special problems.

Alcohol
▼ Avoid. Alcohol may aggravate your underlying condition and reduce the beneficial effects of this drug.

POSSIBLE ADVERSE EFFECTS

Adverse effects such as diarrhea is usually mild, and often diminish with continued use of the drug. If you develop a rash, however, you should notify your physician.

Symptom/effect	Frequency		Discuss with physician		Stop taking drug now	Call physician now
	Common	Rare	Only if severe	In all cases		
Diarrhea	●		■			
Nausea		●	■			
Vomiting		●	■			
Constipation		●	■			
Headaches	●		■			
Dizziness		●	■			
Rash		●		■	▲	▮

PROLONGED USE

No problems expected.

INTERACTIONS

Ketoconazole By decreasing stomach acidity, pantoprazole may decrease the absorption of ketoconazole.

Cyclosporine, warfarin, phenytoin Pantoprazole may increase the effects of these drugs and they may require more careful monitoring.

PAROXETINE

Product name Paxil
Used in the following combined preparations None

GENERAL INFORMATION

Paroxetine is one of the group known as selective serotonin re-uptake inhibitors (SSRIs). It is used in the treatment of mild to moderate depression. It helps control the anxiety often accompanying depression. It is also used to treat generalized anxiety disorder, social phobia, panic disorder, and obsessive-compulsive disorders.

Compared with the older tricyclic antidepressants, paroxetine and other SSRIs are less likely to cause *anti-cholinergic side effects* such as dry mouth, blurred vision, and difficulty in passing urine. They are also much less dangerous if taken in overdose.

The most common *adverse effects* include nausea, diarrhea, drowsiness, sweating, tremor, weakness, insomnia, and sexual problems, such as orgasmic and ejaculation difficulties.

INFORMATION FOR USERS

Your drug prescription is tailored for you. Do not alter dosage without checking with your physician.

How taken

Tablets.

Frequency and timing of doses
Once daily, in the morning.

Usual adult dosage range
10–60mg daily.

Onset of effect
The onset of therapeutic response usually occurs within 7–14 days of starting treatment, but full antidepressant effect may not be felt for 4 weeks.

Duration of action
Up to 24 hours.

Diet advice
None.

Storage
Keep in a closed container in a cool, dry place out of the reach of children.

Missed dose
Take as soon as you remember.

Stopping the drug
Do not stop the drug without consulting your physician. Stopping abruptly can cause withdrawal symptoms.

Exceeding the dose
An occasional unintentional extra dose is unlikely to be a cause for concern. Large doses may cause unusual drowsiness. Notify your physician immediately.

POSSIBLE ADVERSE EFFECTS

Common adverse effects include nausea, diarrhea, drowsiness, sweating, tremor, weakness, insomnia, and sexual dysfunction (lack of orgasm, male ejaculation problems).

Symptom/effect	Frequency		Discuss with physician		Stop taking drug now	Call physician now
	Common	Rare	Only if severe	In all cases		
Nausea	●			■		
Sweating	●			■		
Drowsiness/dizziness	●			■		
Sexual dysfunction (both sexes)	●			■		
Diarrhea	●			■		
Nervousness/anxiety/agitation		●		■		
Rash/itching/hives/joint pain		●		■	▲	∎
Poor appetite/weight loss		●		■		
Convulsions		●		■	▲	∎

INTERACTIONS

General note Any drug that affects the breakdown of others in the liver may alter blood levels of paroxetine or vice versa.

Anticoagulants Paroxetine may increase the effects of these drugs.

Sedatives All sedatives are likely to increase the sedative effects of paroxetine.

Tricyclic antidepressants Paroxetine may increase the *toxicity* of these drugs.

Monoamine oxidase inhibitors (MAOIs) Paroxetine should not be taken during or within 14 days of MAOI treatment because serious reactions may occur.

SPECIAL PRECAUTIONS

Be sure to tell your physician if:
▼ You have long-term liver or kidney problems.
▼ You have a heart problem.
▼ You have a history or a family history of fits.
▼ You are taking other medications.

Pregnancy
▼ Safety in pregnancy not established. Discuss with your physician.

Breast-feeding
▼ The drug passes into the breast milk. Discuss with your physician.

Infants and children
▼ Not recommended under 18 years.

Over 60
▼ Increased likelihood of adverse effects. Reduced dose may be necessary.

Driving and hazardous work
▼ Avoid such activities until you have learned how paroxetine affects you because the drug can cause drowsiness.

Alcohol
▼ Avoid. Alcohol may increase the sedative effects of this drug.

PROLONGED USE

Withdrawal symptoms may occur if the drug is not stopped gradually. Such symptoms include dizziness, electric shock sensations, anxiety, nausea, and insomnia. These rarely last for more than 1–2 weeks.

PENICILLIN V

Product names Apo-Pen VK
Used in the following combined preparations None

GENERAL INFORMATION

Penicillin V, also known as phenoxymethylpenicillin, is a synthetic penicillin-type antibiotic that is prescribed for a wide range of infections.

Various commonly occurring respiratory tract infections, such as some types of tonsillitis and pharyngitis, as well as ear infections, often respond well to this drug. It is also effective for the treatment of the gum disease, Vincent's gingivitis.

Penicillin V is also used to treat less common infections caused by the *Streptococcus* bacterium, such

as scarlet fever. It is also prescribed long term to prevent the recurrence of rheumatic fever, a rare, although potentially serious condition. It is also used long term to prevent infections following removal of the spleen or in sickle cell disease.

As with other penicillin antibiotics, the most serious *adverse effect* that may rarely occur is an allergic reaction that may cause collapse, wheezing, and a rash in susceptible people.

QUICK REFERENCE

Drug group Penicillin antibiotic (p.114)
Overdose danger rating Low
Dependence rating Low
Prescription needed Yes
Available as generic Yes

INFORMATION FOR USERS

Your drug prescription is tailored for you. Do not alter dosage without checking with your physician.

How taken

Tablets, liquid.

Frequency and timing of doses
4 x daily, at least 30 minutes before food.

Usual dosage range
Adults 1.5–2.0 million iu (500,000 iu = 300 mg).
Children Reduced dose according to age

Onset of effect
1–2 days.

Duration of action
Up to 12 hours.

Diet advice
None.

Storage
Keep in a closed container in a cool, dry place out of the reach of children.

Missed dose
Take as soon as you remember. If your next dose is due within 2 hours, take a single dose now and skip the next.

Stopping the drug
Take the full course. Even if you feel better, the original infection may still be present and may recur if the treatment is stopped too soon.

Exceeding the dose
An occasional unintentional extra dose is unlikely to be a cause for concern. But if you notice any unusual symptoms, or if a large overdose has been taken, notify your physician.

SPECIAL PRECAUTIONS

Be sure to tell your physician if:
▼ You have a long-term kidney problem.
▼ You have had a previous allergic reaction to a penicillin or cephalosporin antibiotic.
▼ You have an allergic disorder such as asthma or urticaria.
▼ You are taking other medications.

Pregnancy
▼ No evidence of risk.

Breast-feeding
▼ The drug passes into the breast milk, but at normal doses adverse effects on the baby are unlikely. Discuss with your physician.

Infants and children
▼ Reduced dose necessary.

Over 60
▼ No special problems.

Driving and hazardous work
▼ No known problems.

Alcohol
▼ No known problems.

POSSIBLE ADVERSE EFFECTS

Most people do not experience any serious adverse effects when taking penicillin V.

However, this drug may provoke an allergic reaction in susceptible people.

Symptom/effect	Frequency		Discuss with physician		Stop taking drug now	Call physician now
	Common	Rare	Only if severe	In all cases		
Nausea/vomiting	●		■			
Diarrhea		●	■			
Rash/itching		●		■	▲	▮
Breathing difficulties		●		■	▲	▮

INTERACTIONS

Oral contraceptives Penicillin V may reduce the contraceptive effect of these drugs. Discuss with your physician.

Probenecid increases the level of penicillin V in the blood.

Methotrexate Excretion of this drug may be greatly reduced by penicillin V, leading to toxicity.

PROLONGED USE

Prolonged use may increase the risk of *Candida* infections and diarrhea.

PERINDOPRIL

Product name Coversyl
Used in the following combined preparations Coversyl Plus LD

GENERAL INFORMATION

Perindopril is an ACE inhibitor, a group of drugs used to treat high blood pressure and heart failure. The drug relaxes the muscles around the blood vessels, allowing them to dilate and thereby easing blood flow. Perindopril lowers blood pressure promptly but may need to be taken for several weeks to achieve maximum effect. When treating heart failure, perindopril is usually combined with a diuretic. This can give dramatic improvement, relaxing the muscle in blood vessel walls and reducing the workload on the heart.

At the start of treatment ACE inhibitors can cause a very rapid fall in blood pressure. Therefore, the first dose is usually low and taken at bedtime so that the patient can stay lying down.

The most characteristic adverse effect of perindopril is a persistent dry cough. This may occur in up to 20 per cent of patients. The throat may become irritated, and the voice husky or hoarse.

QUICK REFERENCE

Drug group ACE inhibitor (p.84)
Overdose danger rating Medium
Dependence rating Low
Prescription needed Yes
Available as generic Yes

INFORMATION FOR USERS

Your drug prescription is tailored for you. Do not alter dosage without checking with your physician.

How taken

Tablets.

Frequency and timing of doses
Once daily, 30 minutes before food. Taken in the morning for the treatment of heart failure.

Usual adult dosage range
2mg initially, then 4–8mg daily.

Onset of effect
30–60 minutes.

Duration of action
24 hours.

Diet advice
None.

Storage
Keep in a closed container in a cool, dry place out of the reach of children.

Missed dose
Take as soon as you remember. If your next dose is due within the next 8 hours, take a single dose now, and skip the next.

Stopping the drug
Do not stop the drug without consulting your physician; stopping the drug may lead to worsening of the underlying condition.

Exceeding the dose
An occasional unintentional extra dose is unlikely to cause problems. Large overdoses may cause dizziness or fainting. Notify your physician.

SPECIAL PRECAUTIONS

Be sure to tell your physician if:
▼ You have long-term liver or kidney problems.
▼ You have a history of allergy to any ACE inhibitor.
▼ You are on a low sodium diet.
▼ You are taking other medications.

Pregnancy
▼ Safety in pregnancy not established. Discuss with your physician.

Breast-feeding
▼ Safety in breast-feeding not established. Discuss with your physician.

Infants and children
▼ Not recommended.

Over 60
▼ Elderly people may be more sensitive to the drug. Reduced dose necessary.

Driving and hazardous work
▼ Avoid such activities until you have learned how perindopril affects you. The drug can cause dizziness and fainting.

Alcohol
▼ Avoid. Alcohol may increase the blood pressure-lowering and adverse effects of the drug.

Surgery and general anesthetics
▼ Perindopril may need to be stopped before you have a general anesthetic. Discuss with your physician or dentist before any operation.

POSSIBLE ADVERSE EFFECTS

Perindopril may cause kidney impairment and large falls in blood pressure. Loss of taste and dry cough are two common effects.

Symptom/effect	Frequency		Discuss with physician		Stop taking drug now	Call physician now
	Common	Rare	Only if severe	In all cases		
Loss of taste	●		■			
Nausea/abdominal pain	●		■			
Rash/itching	●		■			
Persistent dry cough	●			■		
Fatigue		●	■			
Sore throat/fever		●		■		
Dizziness/fainting		●		■		

INTERACTIONS

Lithium Blood levels and toxicity of this drug may be raised by perindopril.

Diuretics cause a very rapid fall in blood pressure if taken with perindopril.

Cyclosporine, potassium salts, and potassium-sparing diuretics These drugs increase the risk of high potassium blood levels when taken with perindopril.

Non-steroidal anti-inflammatory drugs (NSAIDs) These drugs may reduce the effects of perindopril. There is also a risk of kidney damage when they are taken together.

Vasodilators (e.g. nitrates) may reduce blood pressure even further if taken with perindopril.

PROLONGED USE

Rarely, long-term use can lead to changes in the blood count or kidney function.

Monitoring Periodic checks on potassium levels, white blood cell count, kidney function, and urine are usually performed.

PERMETHRIN

Product names Kwellada-P, NixCreme Rinse, Nix Dermal Cream
Used in the following combined preparations None

GENERAL INFORMATION

Permethrin is an insecticide used to treat head and pubic lice, and scabies infestations. It works by interfering with the nervous system function of the parasites, causing paralysis and death. Permethrin has the advantage of being less *toxic* than some of the other types of insecticide.

Permethrin is applied *topically* as a liquid to treat head lice and a cream for scabies infestations. In children and elderly people, the entire body surface, including the face, scalp, neck, and ears, may have to be covered; adults are treated from the neck downwards. For pubic lice, the affected area should be treated and the permethrin left on overnight. A second treatment seven days later is needed.

For head lice and scabies, all family members should be treated at the same time, to prevent recontamination, and the process repeated after a week.

There are signs that the parasites are developing resistance to permethrin. If the drug does not work for you, your pharmacist should be able to suggest an alternative treatment.

QUICK REFERENCE

Drug group Drug to treat skin parasites (p.164)

Overdose danger rating Low

Dependence rating Low

Prescription needed No

Available as generic No

INFORMATION FOR USERS

Follow instructions on the label. Call your physician if symptoms worsen.

How taken

Cream, topical liquid (lotion, shampoo, spray).

Frequency and timing of doses
Once only, repeating after 7 days. Avoid contact with eyes and broken or infected skin.

Usual adult dosage range
As directed.

Onset of effect
Liquid should be rinsed off after 10 minutes (head lice) or cream after 8–12 hours (public lice); cream should be washed off after 8–12 hours (scabies).

Duration of action
Until washed off.

Diet advice
None.

Storage
Keep in a closed container in a cool, dry place out of the reach of children. Protect from light.

Missed dose
Timing of the second application is not rigid; use as soon as you remember.

Stopping the drug
Not applicable

Exceeding the dose
An occasional extra application is unlikely to cause problems. If the drug is accidentally swallowed, take emergency action.

SPECIAL PRECAUTIONS

Be sure to consult your physician or pharmacist before taking this drug if:
▼ You are taking other medications.

Pregnancy
▼ Safety not established. Discuss with your physician.

Breast-feeding
▼ Safety not established. Discuss with your physician.

Infants and children
▼ No special problems.

Over 60
▼ No special problems.

Driving and hazardous work
▼ No special problems.

Alcohol
▼ No special problems.

POSSIBLE ADVERSE EFFECTS

In general, permethrin is well tolerated on the skin, although mild skin irritation is common.

Symptom/effect	Frequency		Discuss with physician		Stop taking drug now	Call physician now
	Common	Rare	Only if severe	In all cases		
Itching	●		■			
Reddened skin/stinging	●		■			
Rash		●	■			

INTERACTIONS

None.

PROLONGED USE

Permethrin should not be used for prolonged periods; it is intended for intermittent use only.

PHENOBARBITAL

Product name None
Used in the following combined preparations Bellergal Spacetabs

GENERAL INFORMATION

Phenobarbital belongs to the group of drugs known as barbiturates. It is used mainly in the treatment of epilepsy, but it was also used as a sleeping drug and sedative before the development of safer drugs.

In the treatment of epilepsy, the drug is usually given together with another anticonvulsant drug such as phenytoin. When combined with other drugs, it has been used in anxiety associated with menopausal symptoms. However, there are more effective and safer drugs for this now.

The main disadvantage of the drug is that it often causes unwanted sedation. However, tolerance develops within a week or two. In children and the elderly, it may occasionally cause excessive excitement. Because of their sedative effects, phenobarbital and other barbiturates are sometimes abused.

QUICK REFERENCE

Drug group Barbiturate anticonvulsant drug (p.70)
Overdose danger rating High
Dependence rating High
Prescription needed Yes
Available as generic Yes

INFORMATION FOR USERS

Your drug prescription is tailored for you. Do not alter dosage without checking with your physician.

How taken

Tablets, liquid, injection.

Frequency and timing of doses
Once daily, usually at night.

Usual dosage range
Adults 60–250mg daily (anticonvulsant).

Onset of effect
30–60 minutes (by mouth).

Duration of action
24–48 hours (some effect may persist for up to 6 days).

Diet advice
None.

Storage
Keep in a closed container in a cool, dry place out of the reach of children.

Missed dose
Take as soon as you remember. If the next dose is due within 10 hours, take a single dose now and skip the next.

Stopping the drug
Do not stop taking the drug without consulting your physician, who may supervise a gradual reduction in dosage. Abrupt cessation may cause fits or lead to restlessness, trembling, and insomnia.

OVERDOSE ACTION

 Seek immediate medical advice in all cases. Take emergency action if unsteadiness, severe weakness, confusion, or loss of consciousness occur.

See Drug poisoning emergency guide (p.526).

POSSIBLE ADVERSE EFFECTS

Most of the adverse effects of phenobarbital are the result of its sedative effect. They can sometimes be minimized by a medically supervised reduction of dosage.

Symptom/effect	Frequency		Discuss with physician		Stop taking drug now	Call physician now
	Common	Rare	Only if severe	In all cases		
Drowsiness	●		■			
Clumsiness/unsteadiness	●		■			
Dizziness/faintness	●			■		
Confusion		●		■		
Rash/localized swellings		●		■	▲	▮

INTERACTIONS

Antipsychotics, antidepressants, St John's wort, mefloquine, and chloroquine may reduce the anticonvulsant effect of phenobarbital.

Anticoagulants, corticosteroids, oral contraceptives, and protease inhibitors Phenobarbital may decrease the effect of these drugs.

Sedatives All drugs that have a sedative effect on the central nervous system are likely to increase the sedative properties of phenobarbital. Such drugs include sleeping drugs, antihistamines, opioid analgesics, antidepressants, and antipsychotics.

SPECIAL PRECAUTIONS

Be sure to tell your physician if:
▼ You have long-term liver or kidney problems.
▼ You have heart problems.
▼ You have poor circulation.
▼ You have porphyria.
▼ You have breathing problems.
▼ You are taking other medications.

 Pregnancy
▼ The drug may affect the fetus and increase the tendency of bleeding in the newborn. Discuss with your physician.

 Breast-feeding
▼ The drug passes into the breast milk and could cause drowsiness in the baby. Discuss with your physician.

 Infants and children
▼ Reduced dose necessary.

 Over 60
▼ Increased likelihood of confusion. Reduced dose may therefore be necessary.

 Driving and hazardous work
▼ Your underlying condition, in addition to the possibility of reduced alertness while taking phenobarbital, may make such activities inadvisable. Discuss with your physician.

 Alcohol
▼ Never drink while under treatment with phenobarbital. Alcohol may interact dangerously with this drug.

PROLONGED USE

The sedative effect of phenobarbital can build up, causing excessive drowsiness and lethargy. However, *tolerance* may develop, so reducing these effects. *Dependence* may also result. Withdrawal symptoms may occur if the drug is stopped suddenly.

Monitoring Blood samples may be taken periodically to test blood levels of the drug.

PHENYTOIN/FOSPHENYTOIN

Product names Dilantin, Cerebyx (fosphenytoin)
Used in the following combined preparations None

GENERAL INFORMATION

Phenytoin decreases the likelihood of convulsions by reducing abnormal electrical discharges within the brain. Introduced in the 1930s, it is prescribed for the treatment of epilepsy, including tonic/clonic and temporal lobe epilepsy. Fosphenytoin (Cerebryx) is a new type of phenytoin given by injection for severe fits or for control of seizures, if oral therapy is not temporarily possible.

Some *adverse effects* of phenytoin are more pronounced in children, so it is prescribed for children only when other drugs are unsuitable.

It is recommended that patients remain on the same brand of phenytoin.

INFORMATION FOR USERS

Your drug prescription is tailored for you. Do not alter dosage without checking with your physician.

How taken

Tablets, chewable tablets, capsules, liquid, injection.

Frequency and timing of doses
1–3 x daily with food or plenty of water. Once daily (extended release capsules)

Usual dosage range
Adults 100–500mg daily.
Children According to age and weight.

Onset of effect
Full anticonvulsant effect may not be felt for 7–10 days.

Duration of action
24 hours.

Diet advice
Folic acid and vitamin D deficiency may occasionally occur while taking this drug. Make sure you eat a balanced diet containing fresh, green vegetables.

Storage
Keep in a tightly closed container in a cool, dry place out of the reach of children.

Missed dose
Take as soon as you remember.

Stopping the drug
Do not stop the drug without consulting your physician; symptoms may recur.

Exceeding the dose
An occasional, unintentional extra dose is unlikely to cause problems. However, if you notice excessive drowsiness, slurred speech, or confusion, notify your physician.

SPECIAL PRECAUTIONS

Be sure to tell your physician if:
▼ You have long-term liver or kidney problems.
▼ You have diabetes.
▼ You have porphyria.
▼ You are taking other medications.

Pregnancy
▼ The drug may be associated with malformation and a tendency to bleeding in the newborn baby. Folic acid supplements should be taken by the mother. Discuss with your physician and pharmacist.

Breast-feeding
▼ The drug passes into the breast milk, but at normal doses adverse effects on the baby are unlikely. Discuss with your physician.

Infants and children
▼ Reduced dose necessary. Increased likelihood of overgrowth of the gums and excessive growth of body hair.

Over 60
▼ Reduced dose may be necessary.

Driving and hazardous work
▼ Your underlying condition, as well as the effects of phenytoin, may make such activities inadvisable. Discuss with your physician.

Alcohol
▼ Avoid. Alcohol increases the sedative effects of this drug.

POSSIBLE ADVERSE EFFECTS

Phenytoin has a number of adverse effects, many of which appear only after prolonged use. If they become severe, your physician may prescribe a different anticonvulsant.

Symptom/effect	Frequency		Discuss with physician		Stop taking drug now	Call physician now
	Common	Rare	Only if severe	In all cases		
Dizziness/headache	●			■		
Confusion	●		■			
Nausea/vomiting	●		■			
Insomnia	●		■			
Increased body hair		●	■			
Overgrowth of gums		●		■		
Rash		●		■		▮
Fever/sore throat/mouth ulcers		●		■		▮

INTERACTIONS

General note Many drugs may interact with phenytoin, causing either an increase or a reduction in the phenytoin blood level. The dosage of phenytoin may need to be adjusted. Consult your doctor.

Cyclosporine Blood levels of cyclosporine may be reduced with phenytoin.

Oral contraceptives Phenytoin may reduce their effectiveness.

Antidepressants, antipsychotics, mefloquine, chloroquine, and St John's wort These preparations may reduce the effect of phenytoin.

Warfarin The anticoagulant effect of this drug may be altered. An adjustment in its dosage may be necessary.

PROLONGED USE

There is a slight risk that blood abnormalities may occur. Prolonged use may also lead to adverse effects on skin, gums, and bones. It may also disrupt control of diabetes.

Monitoring Periodic blood tests may be performed to monitor levels of the drug in the body and composition of the blood cells and blood chemistry.

PILOCARPINE

Product names Isopto Carpine, Pilopine HS, Salagen
Used in the following combined preparation None

GENERAL INFORMATION

Pilocarpine is a *miotic* drug used to treat chronic glaucoma and severe glaucoma prior to surgery.

The eye drops are quick-acting but have to be re-applied every four to eight hours. Eye gel is longer acting and needs to be applied only once a day.

Pilocarpine frequently causes blurred vision; and spasm of the eye muscles may cause headaches, particularly at the start of treatment. However, serious *adverse effects* are rare.

Tablets are used to treat dry mouth after radiotherapy to the head and neck.

INFORMATION FOR USERS

Your drug prescription is tailored for you. Do not alter dosage without checking with your physician.

How taken

Tablets, eye drops, eye gel.

Frequency and timing of doses
Eye drops 4 x daily (chronic glaucoma). In acute glaucoma, pilocarpine is given at 5-minute intervals until the condition is controlled.
Eye gel Once daily.
Tablets 3 x daily after food with plenty of water.

Usual dosage range
According to formulation and condition. In general, 1–2 eye drops are used per application.
Tablets 15–20mg daily.

Onset of effect
15–30 minutes.

Duration of action
4–8 weeks for maximum effect (tablets); 3–8 hours (eye drops); up to 24 hours (eye gel).

Diet advice
None.

Storage
Keep in a closed container in a cool, dry place out of the reach of children (tablets/eye drops). Discard eye drops 1 month after opening.

Missed dose
Use as soon as you remember. If not remembered until 2 hours before your next dose, skip the missed dose and take the next dose now.

Stopping the drug
Do not stop the drug without consulting your physician; symptoms may recur.

Exceeding the dose
An occasional unintentional extra application is unlikely to cause problems. Excessive use may cause facial flushing, an increase in the flow of saliva, and sweating. If accidentally swallowed, seek medical attention immediately.

POSSIBLE ADVERSE EFFECTS

Alteration in vision is common. Brow ache and eye pain are common at the start of treatment, but usually wear off after a few days.

Symptom/effect	Frequency		Discuss with physician		Stop taking drug now	Call physician now
	Common	Rare	Only if severe	In all cases		
Eye drops/gel						
Blurred vision/poor night vision	●		■			
Headache/brow ache	●		■			
Sweating/chills	●		■			
Eye pain/irritation	●			■		▮
Red, watery eyes		●	■			
Twitching eyelids		●		■		
Tablets						
Nausea	●		■			
Diarrhea	●		■			
Dizziness	●			■		
Urinary frequency	●		■			

INTERACTIONS

General note A wide range of drugs (including aminoglycoside antibiotics, clindamycin, chloroquine, quinine, quinidine, lithium, and procainamide) may antagonize pilocarpine.

Beta blockers These drugs may reduce the effects of pilocarpine.

Calcium channel blockers These drugs may increase pilocarpine's *systemic* effects.

SPECIAL PRECAUTIONS

Be sure to tell your physician if:
▼ You have asthma.
▼ You have inflamed eyes.
▼ You wear contact lenses.
▼ You have heart, liver, or gastrointestinal problems.
▼ You are taking other medications.

Pregnancy
▼ No evidence of risk at the doses used for chronic glaucoma.

Breast-feeding
▼ The drug passes into the breast milk, but at normal doses adverse effects on the baby are unlikely. Discuss with your physician.

Infants and children
▼ Not usually prescribed.

Over 60
▼ Reduced night vision is particularly noticeable.

Driving and hazardous work
▼ Avoid such activities, especially in poor light, until you have learned how pilocarpine affects you because it may cause short sight and poor night vision.

Alcohol
▼ No known problems.

PROLONGED USE

The effect of the drug may occasionally wear off with prolonged use as the body adapts, but may be restored by changing temporarily to another antiglaucoma drug.

PIOGLITAZONE

Product names Actos, Apo-pioglitazone, Co-pioglitazone, Gen-pioglitazone, Sandoz Pioglitazone
Used in the following combined preparations None

GENERAL INFORMATION

Pioglitazone is used to treat type 2 diabetes mellitus and works by reducing insulin resistance in fatty tissue, skeletal muscle, and in the liver, leading to a decrease in blood glucose levels. It takes 6–12 weeks to reach its full effect. This drug can be used alone or with other antidiabetic drugs such as metformin, but it is not approved for use with insulin. When combined with other antidiabetic drugs, there is a risk of low blood sugar, whose symptoms include shakiness, lightheadedness, sweating, nervousness, sudden change in behaviour, headache, and numbness or tingling around the mouth.

QUICK REFERENCE

Drug group Oral antidiabetic (p.128)
Overdose danger rating High
Dependence rating Low
Prescription needed Yes
Available as generic Yes

INFORMATION FOR USERS

Your drug prescription is tailored for you. Do not alter dosage without checking with your physician.

How taken

Tablets.

Frequency and timing of doses
Usually once daily; may be taken with or without food.

Adult dosage range
Initial dose: 15–30mg once daily; may gradually increase up to a maximum of 45mg daily.

Onset of effect
In 2–4 weeks; full beneficial effects may not be seen until 6–12 weeks.

Duration of action
Up to 24 hours.

Diet advice
An individualized low fat, low carbohydrate diet must be maintained in order for the drug to be fully effective. Follow your physician and dietician's advice.

Storage
Keep in a closed container in a cool, dry place out of the reach of children.

Missed dose
If you remember the same day, take as soon as you remember. If you remember the next day, do not take the missed dose and continue with your regular dosing schedule. Do not double up on your dose.

Stopping the drug
Do not stop the drug without consulting your physician. Stopping the drug may lead to worsening of the underlying condition.

OVERDOSE ACTION

Seek immediate medical advice in all cases. Take emergency action if loss of consciousness occurs.

See Drug poisoning emergency guide (p.526).

SPECIAL PRECAUTIONS

Be sure to tell your physician if:
▼ You have liver problems.
▼ You have heart problems, especially congestive heart failure (CHF).
▼ You have swelling of the ankles.
▼ You have shortness of breath or are easily fatigued.
▼ You have polycystic ovary syndrome.
▼ You are not using birth control, as this drug may increase the chance of conception.
▼ You have osteoporosis or decrease in bone mineral density.
▼ You are taking other medications.

 Pregnancy
▼ Safety in pregnancy not established. Discuss with your physician.

 Breast-feeding
▼ Safety not established. Discuss with your physician.

 Infants and children
▼ Not recommended.

 Over 60
▼ No special problems.

 Driving and hazardous work
▼ No special problems.

 Alcohol
▼ No known problems.

POSSIBLE ADVERSE EFFECTS

If weight gain occurs, especially when used with diabetic drugs, discuss this with your physician.

Symptom/effect	Frequency		Discuss with physician		Stop taking drug now	Call physician now
	Common	Rare	Only if severe	In all cases		
Runny nose	●		■			
Headache	●		■			
Muscle pain	●		■			
Tooth or mouth pain	●		■			
Sore throat	●		■			
Nausea or vomiting		●		■		▮
Loss of appetite		●		■		▮
Dark urine		●		■		
Blurred vision		●		■		▮
Jaundice		●		■		
Edema (swelling)		●		■		▮

INTERACTIONS

Oral contraceptives Pioglitazone may reduce the effectiveness of oral contraceptives by reducing the hormone levels in these products.

Ketoconazole This drug may increase the effects of pioglitazone.

PROLONGED USE

Pioglitazone, like other antidiabetic drugs, is used indefinitely.

Monitoring Blood glucose will be measured regularly when on this medication. A liver function test may be done before starting therapy and periodically. Heart performance will be monitored regularly. Weight will be measured periodically.

PIROXICAM

Product names Apo-Piroxicam, Novo-Pirocam, and others
Used in the following combined preparations None

GENERAL INFORMATION

Piroxicam, introduced in 1980, is a non-steroidal anti-inflammatory drug (NSAID) that, like others in this group, reduces pain, stiffness, and inflammation. Blood levels of the drug remain high for many hours after a dose, so it needs to be taken only once daily.

Piroxicam is used for osteoarthritis, rheumatoid arthritis, acute attacks of gout, and ankylosing spondylitis. It gives relief of the symptoms of arthritis,

although it does not cure the disease. It is sometimes prescribed in conjunction with slow-acting drugs in rheumatoid arthritis to relieve pain and inflammation while these drugs take effect. The drug may also be given for pain relief after sports injuries, for conditions such as tendinitis and bursitis, and following minor surgery.

This drug may be less likely than ASA to cause stomach ulcers.

QUICK REFERENCE

Drug group Non-steroidal anti-inflammatory drug (p.102) and drug for gout (p.105)

Overdose danger rating Medium

Dependence rating Low

Prescription needed Yes

Available as generic Yes

INFORMATION FOR USERS

Your drug prescription is tailored for you. Do not alter dosage without checking with your physician.

How taken

Capsules, suppositories.

Frequency and timing of doses
1–2 x daily with food or plenty of water.

Usual adult dosage range
10–40mg daily.

Onset of effect
Pain relief begins in 3–4 hours. Used for arthritis, the full anti-inflammatory effect develops over 2–4 weeks. Used for gout, this effect develops over 4–5 days.

Duration of action
Up to 2 days. Some effect may last for 7–10 days after treatment has been stopped.

Diet advice
None.

Storage
Keep in a closed container in a cool, dry place out of the reach of children. Protect from light.

Missed dose
Take as soon as you remember. If your next dose is due within 4 hours, take a single dose now and skip the next.

Stopping the drug
When taken for short-term pain relief, the drug can be safely stopped as soon as you no longer need it. If prescribed for the long-term treatment of arthritis, however, you should seek medical advice before stopping the drug.

Exceeding the dose
An occasional unintentional extra dose is unlikely to be a cause for concern. Large overdoses may cause nausea and vomiting. Notify your physician.

SPECIAL PRECAUTIONS

Be sure to tell your physician if:
▼ You have liver or kidney problems.
▼ You have heart problems or high blood pressure.
▼ You have had a peptic ulcer, oesophagitis, or acid indigestion.
▼ You have porphyria.
▼ You have asthma.
▼ You are allergic to ASA.
▼ You are taking other medications.

Pregnancy
▼ Not usually prescribed. When taken in the last three months of pregnancy, the drug increase the risk of adverse effects on the baby's heart and may prolong labour. Discuss with your physician.

Breast-feeding
▼ The drug passes into the breast milk but at normal doses adverse effects are unlikely. Discuss with your physician.

Infants and children
▼ Not recommended under 6 years. Reduced dose necessary.

Over 60
▼ Increased likelihood of adverse effects. Reduced dose may therefore be necessary.

Driving and hazardous work
▼ Avoid such activities until you have learned how piroxicam affects you because the drug can cause dizziness.

Alcohol
▼ Avoid. Alcohol may increase the risk of stomach disorders with piroxicam.

Surgery and general anesthetics
▼ Piroxicam may prolong bleeding. Discuss with your physician or dentist before surgery.

POSSIBLE ADVERSE EFFECTS

Gastrointestinal *side effects*, dizziness, and headache are not generally serious. Black or bloodstained bowel movements should be reported to your physician immediately.

Symptom/effect	Frequency		Discuss with physician		Stop taking drug now	Call physician now
	Common	Rare	Only if severe	In all cases		
Nausea/indigestion	●		■			
Abdominal pain	●			■		
Dizziness/headache		●	■			
Swollen feet/ankles		●		■		
Rash/itching		●		■	▲	
Wheezing/breathlessness		●		■	▲	▮
Black or bloodstained feces		●		■	▲	▮
Bruising or bleeding		●		■	▲	▮

INTERACTIONS

General note Piroxicam interacts with many drugs, including other NSAIDs, corticosteroids, and oral anticoagulant drugs, to increase the risk of bleeding and/or peptic ulcers.

Lithium, digoxin, and methotrexate Piroxicam may raise blood levels of these drugs to an undesirable extent.

Antihypertensive drugs and diuretics The beneficial effects of these drugs may be reduced by piroxicam.

Ciprofloxacin, norfloxacin, and ofloxacin Piroxicam may increase the risk of convulsions when taken with these drugs.

PROLONGED USE

There is an increased risk of bleeding from peptic ulcers and in the bowel.

Monitoring Periodic blood counts and liver function tests may be performed.

PIZOTIFEN

Product names Sandomigran, Sandomigran DS
Used in the following combined preparations None

GENERAL INFORMATION

Pizotifen has a chemical structure similar to that of the tricyclic antidepressants (p.84); it also has similar *anticholinergic* effects. This drug is prescribed for the prevention of migraine headaches in people who suffer frequent, disabling attacks. The drug is thought to work by blocking the chemicals (histamine and serotonin) that act on blood vessels in the brain.

The main disadvantage of prolonged use of pizotifen is that it stimulates the appetite and, as a result, often causes weight gain. It is usually prescribed only for people in whom other measures for migraine prevention, such as avoidance of trigger factors, have failed.

QUICK REFERENCE

Drug group Drug for migraine (p.73)

Overdose danger rating Medium

Dependence rating Low

Prescription needed Yes

Available as generic No

INFORMATION FOR USERS

Your drug prescription is tailored for you. Do not alter dosage without checking with your physician.

How taken

Tablets.

Frequency and timing of doses
Start once a day (at night); gradually increase to 3 x daily.

Adult dosage range
1.5–4.5mg daily. Maximum single dose 3mg.

Onset of effect
Full beneficial effects may not be felt for several days.

Duration of action
Effects of this drug may last for several weeks.

Diet advice
Migraine sufferers may be advised to avoid foods that trigger headaches in their case.

Storage
Keep in a closed container in a cool, dry place out of the reach of children. Protect from light.

Missed dose
Take as soon as you remember. If your next dose is due within 4 hours, take a single dose now and skip the next.

Stopping the drug
Do not stop the drug without consulting your physician; symptoms may recur.

Exceeding the dose
An occasional unintentional extra dose is unlikely to cause problems. Large overdoses may cause drowsiness, nausea, palpitations, and fits. Notify your physician.

SPECIAL PRECAUTIONS

Be sure to tell your physician if:
▼ You have a long-term kidney problem.
▼ You have glaucoma.
▼ You have urinary retention.
▼ You have prostate trouble.
▼ You are taking other medications.

Pregnancy
▼ Safety in pregnancy not established. Discuss with your physician.

Breast-feeding
▼ The drug passes into the breast milk, but at normal doses adverse effects on the baby are unlikely. Discuss with your physician.

Infants and children
▼ Reduced dose usually necessary.

Over 60
▼ No special problems.

Driving and hazardous work
▼ Avoid such activities until you have learned how pizotifen affects you because the drug can cause drowsiness and blurred vision.

Alcohol
▼ Avoid. Alcohol may increase the sedative effects of this drug.

POSSIBLE ADVERSE EFFECTS

Drowsiness is a common *adverse effect* that can often be minimized by starting treatment with a low dose that is gradually increased.

Symptom/effect	Frequency		Discuss with physician		Stop taking drug now	Call physician now
	Common	Rare	Only if severe	In all cases		
Weight gain/increased appetite	●		■			
Drowsiness	●		■			
Nausea/dizziness		●	■			
Muscle pains		●	■			
Dry mouth		●	■			
Blurred vision		●	■			
Depression		●			■	

INTERACTIONS

Anticholinergic drugs The weak anticholinergic effects of pizotifen may be increased by other anticholinergic drugs, including tricyclic antidepressants.

Sedatives All drugs that have a sedative effect on the central nervous system are likely to increase the sedative properties of pizotifen. These include sleeping drugs, anti-anxiety drugs, *opioid* analgesics, and antihistamines.

PROLONGED USE

Pizotifen often causes weight gain during long-term use. Treatment is usually reviewed every 6 months.

PRAMIPEXOLE

Product name Mirapex
Used in the following combined preparations None

GENERAL INFORMATION

Pramipexole helps relieve signs and symptoms of Parkinson's disease by stimulating dopamine receptors in the brain. It is often used with levodopa in the managment of Parkinson's disease, and can help minimize the dose of levodopa that has to be taken.

Pramipexole is quickly absorbed when taken by mouth. Common side effects include dizziness, insomnia, and lightheadedness. Rarely, it can cause hallucinations or fidgety movements (dyskinesia).

QUICK REFERENCE

Drug group Antiparkinsonism drug (p.71)

Overdose danger rating Medium

Dependence rating Low

Prescription needed Yes

Available as generic Yes

INFORMATION FOR USERS

Your drug prescription is tailored for you. Do not alter dosage without checking with your physician.

How taken

Tablets.

Frequency and timing of doses
Up to 3 x daily.

Usual adult dosage range
0.375mg initial dose (0.125mg given 3 x daily); gradually increased. Usual dose: 1.5–3mg. Maximum daily dose: 4.5mg.

Onset of effect
Peak effect: 1–3 hours.

Duration of action
8–12 hours.

Diet advice
None.

Storage
Keep in a closed container in a cool, dry place out of the reach of children. Protect from light.

Missed dose
Take as soon as you remember. Do not double a dose.

Stopping the drug
Do not stop taking the drug without consulting your physician; symptoms may recur. Also, suddenly stopping the drug can cause muscular rigidity and altered consciousness. If these occur, you should seek medical help straight away.

Exceeding the dose
An occasional unintentional extra dose is unlikely to cause problems. But if you notice any unusual symptoms, or if a large overdose has been taken, notify your physician right away.

SPECIAL PRECAUTIONS

Be sure to tell your physician if:
▼ You have kidney problems.
▼ You have unusual conditions relating to your eye.
▼ You have experienced an allergic reaction to pramipexole.
▼ You are taking other medications.

Pregnancy
▼ Safety not established. Discuss with your physician.

Breast-feeding
▼ Safety not established. Discuss with your physician.

Infants and children
▼ Not recommended.

Over 60
▼ Increased likelihood of adverse effects. Reduced dose necessary.

Driving and hazardous work
▼ Avoid such activities until you have learned how pramipexole affects you because the drug can cause dizziness and sudden sleep attacks. Also, your condition may make it difficult to drive. Check with your physician.

Alcohol
▼ Avoid. Alcohol may increase the sedative effects of this drug.

POSSIBLE ADVERSE EFFECTS

Pramipexole can cause lightheadedness on getting up quickly due to a drop in blood pressure. Getting up slowly can prevent this. If nausea occurs, taking the drug with food can minimize this.

Symptom/effect	Frequency		Discuss with physician		Stop taking drug now	Call physician now
	Common	Rare	Only if severe	In all cases		
Dizziness/lightheadedness	●		■			
Nausea/vomiting	●		■			
Drowsiness	●		■			
Movement disorder (dyskinesia)	●			■		
Constipation	●		■			
Difficulty urinating		●		■	▲	▮
Sudden sleep attacks		●		■		

INTERACTIONS

Metoclorpramide, phenothiazines, theophylline These may decrease the effect of pramipexole. Monitor closely.

Cimetidine, diltiazem, quinidine, verapamil, triamterene These may increase the effect of pramipexole. Dose adjustment may be necessary.

Levodopa When pramipexole is initiated, you may have to lower levodopa dose.

Antihypertensives, tricyclic antidepressants, diuretics These drugs can potentiate the lightheadedness caused by pramipexole.

PROLONGED USE

No specific problems expected. However, your condition may change with time and the dose of the drug should be regularly re-evaluated.

Monitoring Regular monitoring of your Parkinsonian symptoms are required. You should report any changes to your physician.

PRAVASTATIN

Product names Apo-Pravastatin, Pravachol, and others
Used in the following combined preparations Pravasa

GENERAL INFORMATION

Pravastatin belongs to the statin group of lipid-lowering drugs. It is prescribed for people with hypercholesterolemia (high levels of cholesterol in the blood) who have not responded to other treatments, such as a special diet, and who are at risk of developing heart disease. The drug works by blocking the action of an enzyme that is needed for the manufacture of cholesterol, mainly in the liver. As a result, blood levels of cholesterol are lowered, which can help to prevent heart disease.

Like most other statins, pravastatin is taken at night because that is when most cholesterol is produced.

Rarely, statins can cause muscle pain, inflammation, and damage. This seems to be more likely if another kind of lipid-lowering drug called a fibrate is given with the statin.

QUICK REFERENCE

Drug group Lipid-lowering drug (p.89)

Overdose danger rating Medium

Dependence rating Low

Prescription needed Yes

Available as generic Yes

INFORMATION FOR USERS

Your drug prescription is tailored for you. Do not alter dosage without checking with your physician.

How taken

Tablets.

Frequency and timing of doses
Once daily at night.

Usual adult dosage range
10–40mg daily, changed after intervals of at least 4 weeks.

Onset of effect
Within 2 weeks. Full beneficial effect may be felt within 4 weeks.

Duration of action
24 hours.

Diet advice
A low fat diet is usually recommended.

Storage
Keep in a closed container in a cool, dry place out of the reach of children. Protect from light.

Missed dose
Take as soon as you remember. If your next dose is due within 8 hours, do not take the missed dose, but take the next dose as usual.

Stopping the drug
Do not stop taking the drug without consulting your physician; stopping the drug may lead to worsening of the underlying condition.

Exceeding the dose
An occasional unintentional extra dose is unlikely to cause problems. Large overdoses may cause liver problems. Notify your physician.

SPECIAL PRECAUTIONS

Be sure to tell your physician if:
▼ You have had liver or kidney problems.
▼ You are taking other medications.
▼ You have thyroid problems.
▼ You are a heavy drinker.
▼ You have a family history of muscular disorders.
▼ You are diabetic.

Pregnancy
▼ Not usually prescribed. Safety not established. Discuss with your physician.

Breast-feeding
▼ Safety not established. Discuss with your physician.

Infants and children
▼ Not recommended.

Over 60
▼ No special problems.

Driving and hazardous work
▼ No special problems.

Alcohol
▼ Avoid excessive amounts. Alcohol may increase the risk of developing liver problems with this drug.

POSSIBLE ADVERSE EFFECTS

Most *adverse effects* are mild and usually disappear with time.

You should report any muscle pains to your physician straight away.

Symptom/effect	Frequency		Discuss with physician		Stop taking drug now	Call physician now
	Common	Rare	Only if severe	In all cases		
Headache	●		■			
Nausea	●		■			
Fatigue		●	■			
Chest pain		●		■		
Jaundice/abdominal pain		●		■		
Rash		●		■	▲	
Muscle pain/weakness		●		■	▲	∎
Change in cognition		●				∎

PROLONGED USE

Long-term use of pravastatin can affect liver function.

Monitoring Regular blood tests to check liver and muscle function are usually required.

INTERACTIONS

Anticoagulants Statins can increase the effect of these drugs, although this is less likely with pravastatin.

Antifungal drugs Taken with statins, itraconazole, ketoconazole, and possibly other antifungal drugs may increase the risk of muscle damage.

Orlistat This drug increases blood levels and *toxicity* of pravastatin.

Other lipid-lowering drugs (fibrates) Taken with pravastatin, these drugs may increase the risk of muscle damage.

Cyclosporine and other immuno-suppressant drugs There is an increased risk of muscle damage if pravastatin is taken with these drugs. They are not usually prescribed together.

PREDNISONE/PREDNISOLONE

Product names Pediapred, Winpred
Used in the following combined preparations [all with prednisolone] Blephamide, Pred Forte, Pred Mild

GENERAL INFORMATION

Prednisolone, the active form of prednisone, is a powerful corticosteroid, and is used for a wide range of conditions, including some skin diseases, rheumatic disorders, allergic states, and certain blood disorders. It is used in the form of eye drops to reduce inflammation in conjunctivitis or iritis. The drug can also be injected into joints to relieve rheumatoid and other forms of arthritis. Prednisolone is also prescribed with fludrocortisone for pituitary or adrenal gland disorders.

Low doses taken short term (by mouth or *topically*) rarely cause serious *side effects*. However, long-term treatment with large doses can cause fluid retention, indigestion, diabetes, hypertension, and acne. *Enteric*-coated tablets reduce the local effects of the drug on the stomach but not the *systemic* effects.

INFORMATION FOR USERS

Your drug prescription is tailored for you. Do not alter dosage without checking with your physician.

How taken

Tablets, liquid, injection, eye drops.

Frequency and timing of doses
1–2 x daily or on alternate days with food (tablets/injection); 2–4 x daily (eye drops).

Usual adult dosage range
Considerable variation. Follow your physician's instructions.

Onset of effect
2–4 days.

Duration of action
12–72 hours.

Diet advice
A low-sodium and high-potassium diet is recommended when the oral or injected form of the drug is prescribed for extended periods. Follow the advice of your physician.

Storage
Keep in a closed container in a cool, dry place out of the reach of children. Protect from light.

Missed dose
Take as soon as you remember. If your next dose is due within 6 hours, take a single dose now and skip the next.

Stopping the drug
Do not stop the drug without consulting your physician. Abrupt cessation of long-term treatment by mouth or injection may be dangerous.

Exceeding the dose
An occasional unintentional extra dose is unlikely to be a cause for concern. But if you notice any unusual symptoms, or if a large overdose has been taken, notify your physician.

POSSIBLE ADVERSE EFFECTS

The rare but more serious adverse effects occur only when high doses are taken by mouth or injection or for long periods. If taking oral forms, you should avoid close personal contact with chickenpox or herpes zoster, and seek urgent medical attention if exposed.

Symptom/effect	Frequency		Discuss with physician		Stop taking drug now	Call physician now
	Common	Rare	Only if severe	In all cases		
Indigestion	●			■		
Acne	●			■		
Weight gain		●	■			
Muscle weakness		●		■		
Mood changes/depression		●		■		
Black/bloodstained feces		●		■	▲	■

INTERACTIONS

Anticonvulsant drugs Carbamazepine, phenytoin, and phenobarbital can reduce the effects of prednisolone/prednisone.

Vaccines Serious reactions can occur when vaccinations are given with this drug. Discuss with your physician.

Anticoagulant drugs Prednisolone may affect the response to these drugs.

Diuretics Prednisolone may increase the adverse effects of these drugs.

Antihypertensive and antidiabetic drugs and insulin Prednisolone may reduce the effects of these drugs.

Cyclosporine increases the effects of prednisolone.

SPECIAL PRECAUTIONS

Be sure to tell your physician if:
▼ You have had a peptic ulcer.
▼ You have glaucoma.
▼ You have had tuberculosis.
▼ You suffer from depression.
▼ You have any infection.
▼ You have diabetes.
▼ You have osteoporosis.
▼ You are taking other medications.

Pregnancy
▼ No evidence of risk with eye drops. Taken as tablets in low doses, harm to the fetus is unlikely. Discuss with your physician.

Breast-feeding
▼ No evidence of risk with drops. Taken by mouth, it passes into the breast milk, but at low doses adverse effects on the baby are unlikely. Discuss with your physician.

Infants and children
▼ Only given when essential. Reduced dose may be necessary.

Over 60
▼ Increased likelihood of adverse effects. Reduced dose may therefore be necessary.

Driving and hazardous work
▼ No known problems.

Alcohol
▼ Keep consumption low. Alcohol may increase the risk of peptic ulcers with prednisolone taken by mouth or injection.

Infection
▼ Avoid exposure to chickenpox, shingles, or measles if you are on systemic treatment.

PROLONGED USE

Prolonged systemic use can lead to such adverse effects as diabetes, glaucoma, cataracts, and fragile bones, and may retard growth in children. Dosages are usually tailored to minimize these effects.

PREGABALIN

Product name Lyrica
Used in the following combined preparations None

GENERAL INFORMATION

Pregabalin is an anti-epileptic drug (see Anticonvulsant drugs, p.70) used to treat pain related to damaged nerves (neuropathic pain) in the hands, fingers, arms, feet, and legs, and other areas as a result of diabetes (diabetic peripheral neuropathy). It is also approved for nerve pain related to rash from shingles (postherpetic neuralgia). Individuals should inform their physician and dentist that they are on this medication.

(see Anticonvulsant drugs, p.70)

QUICK REFERENCE

Drug group An anticonvulsant (p.70)

Overdose danger rating Medium

Dependence rating Low

Prescription needed Yes

Available as generic No

INFORMATION FOR USERS

Your drug prescription is tailored for you. Do not alter dosage without checking with your physician.

How taken

Capsules.

Frequency and timing of doses
Two or three times daily, with or without food.

Adult dosage range
Initial dose: 150mg daily; maximum of 600mg daily.

Onset of effect
Several weeks for pain relief.

Duration of action
8–12 hours.

Diet advice
None.

Storage
Keep in a closed container in a cool, dry place out of the reach of children.

Missed dose
If you miss a dose, take it as soon as you remember. If it is near the time of the next dose, skip the missed dose and resume your usual dosing schedule. Do not double up to catch up on a missed dose.

Stopping the drug
Do not stop the drug without consulting your physician. Stopping the drug may lead to withdrawal symptoms. If the drug is to be discontinued, gradual decrease in dose over a period of weeks is recommended.

Exceeding the dose
An occasional unintentional extra dose is unlikely to cause problems. Large overdoses may cause serious adverse effects. Notify your physician.

SPECIAL PRECAUTIONS

Be sure to tell your physician if:
▼ You have had problems with alcohol or drug abuse.
▼ You have a low number of platelets.
▼ You or your partner plan on becoming pregnant.
▼ You have heart or kidney disease.
▼ You are on rosiglitazone or thioglitazone for diabetes.
▼ You have congestive heart failure.
▼ You are taking other medications.

Pregnancy
▼ Safety in pregnancy not established. Discuss with your physician.

Breast-feeding
▼ Safety not established. Discuss with your physician.

Infants and children
▼ Not recommended.

Over 60
▼ Dose may be adjusted for changes in kidney function.

Driving and hazardous work
▼ May cause drowsiness. Do not drive a car or operate machinery until the effect of the drug wears off and you feel you are mentally alert.

Alcohol
▼ Avoid alcohol use as it may increase the effect of drowsiness caused by this drug.

POSSIBLE ADVERSE EFFECTS

In general, pregabalin is well tolerated. Common side effects include dizziness, tiredness, blurred vision, weight gain, edema (swelling of arms, feet, etc), dry mouth.

Symptom/effect	Frequency		Discuss with physician		Stop taking drug now	Call physician now
	Common	Rare	Only if severe	In all cases		
Dizziness	●			■		
Tiredness	●			■		
Weight gain	●			■		
Dry mouth	●			■		
Constipation	●			■		
Difficulty concentrating		●		■		
Blurred vision or changes in eyesight		●		■		
Swelling of the eyes, face, or throat		●		■		■

INTERACTIONS

CNS depressants Use of pregabalin with central nervous system depressants (such as benzodiazepines, opioids) may result in additional drowsiness and tiredness.

Alcohol May increase drowsiness caused by pregabalin.

PROLONGED USE

No problems expected.

PROBENECID

Product name Benuryl
Used in the following combined preparations None

GENERAL INFORMATION

Probenecid is used in the treatment of high uric acid levels in the blood, associated with gout. As probencid increases the excretion of uric acid through the kidneys, it should not be used in situations where there is an increase in uric acid production, such as in patients receiving chemotherapy. It should also not be used in those with kidney stones or in those with compromised kidney function. Historically, probenecid has also been used in combination with specific beta-lactam antibiotics, such as cefazolin, where it decreases the antibiotic's excretion, thus enhancing its antibacterial effect.

INFORMATION FOR USERS

Your drug prescription is tailored for you. Do not alter dosage without checking with your physician.

How taken

Tablets

Frequency and timing of doses
Gout: twice daily. With antibiotics, may be taken up to 4x daily.

Adult dosage range
Gout: 0.5 to 1gm daily. Start with 250mg twice daily for a week, then increase to 500mg twice daily. Maximum daily dose: 2 G

Onset of effect
Within 4 hours

Duration of action
8–12 hours.

Diet advice
Take with food to minimize stomach upset. Ensure adequate fluid intake.

Storage
Keep in a closed container in a cool, dry place out of the reach of children.

Missed dose
If you miss a dose, take it as soon as you remember. If it is near the time of the next dose, skip the missed dose and resume your usual dosing schedule. Do not double-up to catch up on a missed dose.

Stopping the drug
Do not stop the drug without consulting your physician. Stopping the drug may lead to worsening of the underlying condition.

Exceeding the dose
If you notice any unusual symptoms, or if a large overdose has been taken, call your physician and seek medical assistance.

SPECIAL PRECAUTIONS

Be sure to tell your physician if:
▼ You are taking ASA or Aspirin.
▼ You have kidney problems.
▼ You have a history of kidney stones.
▼ You have a hypersensitivity to probenecid.
▼ You have or will be receiving chemotherapy.
▼ You are taking other medications.

Pregnancy
▼ Safety in pregnancy not established. Discuss with your physician.

Breast-feeding
▼ Limited safety information. Discuss with your physician.

Infants and children
▼ Not recommended in children < 2 years of age. For use in children 2 years and older, consult their physician.

Over 60
▼ Not recommended with reduced kidney function.

Driving and hazardous work
▼ No special problems.

Alcohol
▼ No special problems.

POSSIBLE ADVERSE EFFECTS

Most common side effects include headache, nausea, vomiting, and anorexia. Taking it with food can minimize nausea and vomiting. It can rarely cause a serious blood disorder.

Symptom/effect	Frequency		Discuss with physician		Stop taking drug now	Call physician now
	Common	Rare	Only if severe	In all cases		
Headache	●		■			
Nausea/vomiting	●		■			
Dizziness	●		■			
Decrease in blood pressure/flushing	●			■		
Hypersensitivity reaction/breathing problems		●		■	▲	▮
Kidney stones		●		■	▲	▮
Tiredness/fatigue		●		■		▮
Rash/dermatitis		●		■	▲	▮

INTERACTIONS

Due to its effect on the kidneys, probenecid can alter excretion of many drugs. Please check with your physician or pharmacist before starting any new drug, in particular:

ACE inhibitors, acetaminophen, acyclovir, allopurinol, aminosalicylates, benzodiazepines, cephalosporin antibiotics, dapsone, fexofenedine, furosemide, ganciclovir, ketorolac, morphine, oseltamivir, pramipexole, quinolone antibiotics, sulfinpyrazone, and zidovudine.

PROLONGED USE

Serious problems are unlikely, but prolonged use should be followed closely by a physician. Due to many drug interactions, close monitoring required with changes to drug therapy.

Monitoring Kidney function, uric acid level in the blood and urine.

PROCHLORPERAZINE

Product name Stemetil
Used in the following combined preparations None

GENERAL INFORMATION

Prochlorperazine was introduced in the late 1950s and belongs to a group of drugs called the phenothiazines, which act on the central nervous system.

In small doses, the drug controls nausea and vomiting, especially when they occur as the *side effects* of medical treatment by drugs or radiation, or of anesthesia. Prochlorperazine may also help the nausea that occurs with inner-ear disorders, for example, vertigo. In large doses, it is used as an antipsychotic to tranquillize, reduce aggressiveness, and suppress abnormal behaviour (see p.69). It thus minimizes and controls the abnormal behaviour of schizophrenia, mania, and other mental disorders. Prochlorperazine does not cure any of these diseases, but it helps to relieve symptoms.

QUICK REFERENCE

Drug group Phenothiazine antipsychotic drug (p.69) and anti-emetic (p.74)

Overdose danger rating Medium

Dependence rating Low

Prescription needed Yes

Available as generic Yes

INFORMATION FOR USERS

Your drug prescription is tailored for you. Do not alter the dosage without checking with your physician.

How taken

Tablets, liquid, injection, suppositories.

Frequency and timing of doses
3–4 x daily (tablets); 3–4 x daily (suppositories); 2–3 x daily (injection).

Usual adult dosage range
Nausea and vomiting 20mg initially, then 5–10mg per dose (tablets); 5–25mg per dose (suppositories).
Mental illness 15–40mg daily. Larger doses may be given.

Onset of effect
Within 60 minutes (by mouth or suppository); 10–20 minutes (by injection).

Duration of action
3–6 hours.

Diet advice
None.

Storage
Keep in a closed container in a cool, dry place out of the reach of children. Protect from light.

Missed dose
Take as soon as you remember. If your next dose is due within 2 hours, take a single dose now and skip the next.

Stopping the drug
Do not stop the drug without consulting your physician; symptoms may recur.

Exceeding the dose
An occasional unintentional extra dose is unlikely to be a cause for concern. Large overdoses may cause unusual drowsiness and may affect the heart. Notify your physician.

SPECIAL PRECAUTIONS

Be sure to tell your physician if:
▼ You have heart problems.
▼ You have liver or kidney problems.
▼ You have had epileptic fits.
▼ You have Parkinson's disease.
▼ You have an underactive thyroid gland.
▼ You have prostate problems.
▼ You have glaucoma.
▼ You are taking other medications.

Pregnancy
▼ Safety in pregnancy not established. Discuss with your physician.

Breast-feeding
▼ The drug passes into the breast milk and may affect the baby. Discuss with your physician.

Infants and children
▼ Not recommended in infants weighing less than 10kg and young children. Reduced dose necessary in older children due to increased risk of adverse effects.

Over 60
▼ Increased likelihood of adverse effects. Reduced dose may therefore be necessary.

Driving and hazardous work
▼ Avoid such activities until you have learned how prochlorperazine affects you because it can cause drowsiness and reduced alertness.

Alcohol
▼ Avoid. Alcohol may increase and prolong the sedative effects of this drug.

POSSIBLE ADVERSE EFFECTS

Prochlorperazine has a strong *anticholinergic* effect, which can cause a variety of minor symptoms that often become less marked with time. The most significant adverse effect with high doses is abnormal movements of the face and limbs (*parkinsonism*) caused by changes in the balance of brain chemicals.

Symptom/effect	Frequency		Discuss with physician		Stop taking drug now	Call physician now
	Common	Rare	Only if severe	In all cases		
Drowsiness/lethargy	●		■			
Dry mouth	●		■			
Dizziness/fainting	●			■		
Parkinsonism	●			■		
Rash		●		■	▲	
Jaundice/fever		●		■		■
Tensing of muscles		●		■		

INTERACTIONS

Sedatives All drugs with a sedative effect are likely to increase the sedative effects of prochlorperazine.

Drugs for parkinsonism Prochlorperazine may block the beneficial effect of these.

Anticholinergic drugs Prochlorperazine may increase the side effects of these drugs.

PROLONGED USE

Use of this drug for more than a few months may lead to the development of involuntary, potentially irreversible, eye mouth, and tongue, movements (*tardive dyskinesia*). Occasionally, *jaundice* may occur.

Monitoring Periodic blood tests may be performed.

PROCYCLIDINE

Product name PHL-Procyclidine
Used in the following combined preparations None

GENERAL INFORMATION

Introduced in the 1950s, procyclidine is an *anticholinergic* drug that is used to treat Parkinson's disease. It is especially helpful in the early stages of the disorder for treating muscle rigidity. It also helps to reduce excess salivation. However, the drug has little effect on the shuffling gait and slow muscular movements that characterize Parkinson's disease.

Procyclidine is also often used to treat *parkinsonism* resulting from treatment with antipsychotic drugs.

The drug may cause various minor *adverse effects* (see below), but these are rarely serious enough to warrant stopping treatment.

QUICK REFERENCE

Drug group Anticholinergic drug for parkinsonism (p.71)

Overdose danger rating High

Dependence rating Low

Prescription needed Yes

Available as generic Yes

INFORMATION FOR USERS

Your drug prescription is tailored for you. Do not alter dosage without checking with your physician.

How taken

Tablets, liquid medication.

Frequency and timing of doses
2–3 x daily.

Usual adult dosage range
5–30mg daily. Dosage is determined individually in order to find the best balance between effective relief of symptoms and the occurrence of adverse effects.

Onset of effect
Within 30 minutes.

Duration of action
8–12 hours.

Diet advice
None.

Storage
Keep in a closed container in a cool, dry place out of the reach of children.

Missed dose
Take as soon as you remember. If your next dose is due within 2 hours, take a single dose now and skip the next.

Stopping the drug
Do not stop the drug without consulting your physician; symptoms may recur.

OVERDOSE ACTION

 Seek immediate medical advice in all cases. Take emergency action if palpitations, fits, or unconsciousness occur.

See Drug poisoning emergency guide (p.526).

POSSIBLE ADVERSE EFFECTS

The possible adverse effects of procyclidine are mainly the result of its anticholinergic action. Some of the more common symptoms, such as dry mouth, constipation, and blurred vision, may be overcome by adjustment in dosage. Nausea and vomiting, nervousness, and rash have occasionally been reported.

Symptom/effect	Frequency		Discuss with physician		Stop taking drug now	Call physician now
	Common	Rare	Only if severe	In all cases		
Dry mouth	●		■			
Constipation	●		■			
Nervousness	●		■			
Drowsiness/dizziness	●			■		
Blurred vision	●			■		
Confusion		●		■		
Difficulty in passing urine		●		■		▮
Palpitations		●		■	▲	▮

INTERACTIONS

Anticholinergic and antihistamine drugs These drugs may increase the adverse effects of procyclidine.

Antidepressant drugs may increase the *side effects* of procyclidine.

Nitroglycerin tablets may be less effective in relief of heart pain, since dry mouth may prevent its dissolution under the tongue.

SPECIAL PRECAUTIONS

Be sure to tell your physician if:
▼ You have long-term liver or kidney problems.
▼ You suffer from or have a family history of glaucoma.
▼ You have high blood pressure.
▼ You suffer from constipation.
▼ You have prostate trouble.
▼ You are taking other medications.

 Pregnancy
▼ Safety in pregnancy not established. Discuss with your physician.

 Breast-feeding
▼ The drug passes into the breast milk and may affect the baby. Discuss with your physician.

 Infants and children
▼ Not recommended.

 Over 60
▼ Reduced dose may be necessary.

 Driving and hazardous work
▼ Avoid such activities until you have learned how procyclidine affects you because the drug can cause drowsiness, blurred vision, and mild confusion.

 Alcohol
▼ Avoid. Alcohol may increase the sedative effect of this drug.

PROLONGED USE

Prolonged use of this drug may provoke the onset of glaucoma.

Monitoring Periodic eye examinations are usually advised.

PROGUANIL WITH ATOVAQUONE

Product name Malarone
Used in the following combined preparations None

GENERAL INFORMATION

Proguanil is an antimalarial drug given to prevent the development of malaria. Microbial resistance to its effects can occur and this has led to it being used in combination with other drugs.

Atovaquone is an antiprotozoal drug that is also active against the fungus *Pneumocystis carinii* (a cause of pneumonia in people with poor immunity). Atovaquone is less useful on its own for malaria, but when it is combined with proguanil it rapidly treats the infection. The combination is also used for prevention of malaria,

especially in areas where resistance to other drugs is present.

Used for prevention, you should start taking proguanil with atovaquone a day or two before travelling. Continue taking the tablets during your stay, and for 7 days after your return. It is important to take other precautions, such as using an insect repellent at all times and a mosquito net at night. If you develop an illness after your return from a malarial zone, and especially in the first 3 months, go to your physician immediately and tell him or her where you have been.

INFORMATION FOR USERS

Your drug prescription is tailored for you. Do not alter dosage without checking with your physician.

How taken

Tablets.

Frequency and timing of doses
Prevention Once daily with food or a milky drink, at the same time each day. Start 1–2 days before travel, and continue for 7 days after return.
Treatment Once daily for 3 days, with food or a milky drink.

Usual adult dosage range
Prevention 1 tablet.
Treatment 4 tablets.

Onset of effect
After 24 hours.

Duration of action
24–48 hours.

Diet advice
None.

Storage
Keep in a closed container in a cool, dry place out of the reach of children.

Missed dose
Take as soon as you remember. If your next dose is due at this time, take both doses together.

Stopping the drug
Do not stop taking the drug for 4 weeks after leaving a malaria-infected area, otherwise there is a risk that you may develop the disease.

Exceeding the dose
An occasional unintentional extra dose is unlikely to cause problems. Large overdoses may cause abdominal pain and vomiting. Notify your physician.

SPECIAL PRECAUTIONS

Be sure to tell your physician if:
▼ You have a long-term kidney problem.
▼ You have a liver problem.
▼ You are suffering from diarrhea and vomiting.
▼ You are taking other medications.

 Pregnancy
▼ Safety in pregnancy not established, although benefits are generally considered to outweigh risks. Folic acid supplements must be taken. Discuss with your physician.

 Breast-feeding
▼ The drug passes into breast milk, but at normal doses adverse effects on the baby are unlikely. Breast-feeding while you are on the drug will not protect your baby from malaria. Discuss with your physician.

 Infants and children
▼ Reduced dose necessary.

 Over 60
▼ No known problems.

 Driving and hazardous work
▼ Avoid until you know how the drug affects you because it may cause dizziness.

 Alcohol
▼ No special problems.

POSSIBLE ADVERSE EFFECTS

Adverse effects are generally fairly mild. The most frequent effects are headache, nausea, vomiting, and abdominal pain.

Symptom/effect	Frequency		Discuss with physician		Stop taking drug now	Call physician now
	Common	Rare	Only if severe	In all cases		
Diarrhoea	●		■			
Nausea/vomiting		●	■			
Abdominal pain/indigestion		●	■			
Mouth ulcers		●	■			
Hair loss		●		■		
Jaundice		●		■		
Rash		●		■		
Sore throat/fever		●		■		■

PROLONGED USE

No known problems.

INTERACTIONS

Warfarin The effects of warfarin may be enhanced by proguanil with atovaquone.

Antacids The absorption of proguanil with atovaquone may be reduced by antacids.

Rifampin, metoclopramide, and tetracycline antibiotics These drugs reduce the effect of proguanil with atovaquone.

PROMETHAZINE

Product name Histanil
Used in the following combined preparations None

GENERAL INFORMATION

Promethazine is one of a class of drugs known as the phenothiazines, which were developed in the 1950s for their beneficial effect on abnormal behaviour arising from mental illnesses (see Antipsychotics, p.79). Promethazine was found, however, to have effects more like the antihistamines that are used to treat allergies (see p.110) and some types of nausea and vomiting (see Antiemetics, p.74). The drug is widely used to reduce itching in a variety of skin conditions including urticaria (hives), chickenpox, and eczema. It can also relieve the nausea and vomiting caused by inner ear disturbances such as Ménière's disease and motion sickness. Because of its sedative effect, promethazine is sometimes used for short periods as a sleeping medicine, and is also given as *premedication* before surgery.

Promethazine is used in combined preparations together with *opioid* cough suppressants for the relief of coughs and nasal congestion, and it is given at night for its sedative effect.

QUICK REFERENCE

Drug group Antihistamine (p.110) and anti-emetic (p.74)

Overdose danger rating Medium

Dependence rating Low

Prescription needed No

Available as generic Yes

INFORMATION FOR USERS

Follow instructions on the label. Call your physician if symptoms worsen.

How taken

Tablets, liquid, injection.

Frequency and timing of doses
Allergic symptoms 1–3 x daily or as a single dose at night.
Motion sickness Bedtime on night before travelling, repeating following morning if necessary, then every 6–8 hours as necessary.
Nausea/vomiting Every 4–6 hours as needed.

Usual dosage range (promethazine hydrochloride)
Adults 20–75mg per dose (oral).
Children Reduced dose according to age.

Onset of effect
Within 1 hour. If dose is taken after nausea has started, the onset of effect is delayed.

Duration of action
8–16 hours.

Diet advice
None.

Storage
Keep in a closed container in a cool, dry place out of the reach of children. Protect from light.

Missed dose
No cause for concern, but take as soon as you remember. Adjust the timing of your next dose accordingly.

Stopping the drug
Can be safely stopped as soon as symptoms disappear.

Exceeding the dose
An occasional unintentional extra dose is unlikely to cause problems. Large overdoses may cause drowsiness or agitation, fits, unsteadiness, and coma. Notify your physician.

SPECIAL PRECAUTIONS

Be sure to consult your physician or pharmacist before taking this drug if:
▼ You have liver or kidney problems.
▼ You have had epileptic fits.
▼ You have heart disease.
▼ You have glaucoma.
▼ You suffer from asthma or bronchitis.
▼ You have Parkinson's disease.
▼ You have urinary retention or prostate problems.
▼ You are taking other medications.

 Pregnancy
▼ Safety in pregnancy not established. Discuss with your physician.

 Breast-feeding
▼ The drug passes into the breast milk, but at normal doses adverse effects on the baby are unlikely. Discuss with your physician.

 Infants and children
▼ Not recommended for infants under two years. Reduced dose necessary for older children.

 Over 60
▼ Adverse effects may be more likely.

 Driving and hazardous work
▼ Avoid such activities until you have learned how promethazine affects you because the drug can cause drowsiness.

 Alcohol
▼ Avoid. Alcohol may increase the sedative effects of this drug.

Sunlight
▼ Avoid exposure to strong sunlight.

POSSIBLE ADVERSE EFFECTS

Promethazine usually causes only minor *anticholinergic* effects. More serious *adverse* effects generally occur only during long-term use or with abnormally high doses.

Symptom/effect	Frequency		Discuss with physician		Stop taking drug now	Call physician now
	Common	Rare	Only if severe	In all cases		
Drowsiness/lethargy	●		■			
Dry mouth	●		■			
Blurred vision	●		■			
Urinary retention	●			■		
Palpitations		●		■		
Light-sensitive rash		●		■	▲	

INTERACTIONS

Monamine oxidase inhibitors (MAOIs) These drugs may cause a severe reaction if taken with promethazine. Avoid taking promethazine if MAOIs have been taken in the last 14 days.

Sedatives All drugs that have a sedative effect are likely to increase the sedative properties of promethazine. Such drugs include other antihistamines, sleeping drugs, and antipsychotics.

PROLONGED USE

Use of this drug for long periods is rarely necessary, but may sometimes cause abnormal movements of the face and limbs (*parkinsonism*). The problem normally disappears when the drug is stopped.

PROPRANOLOL

Product names Apo-Propranolol, Inderal-LA, Nu-Propranolol
Used in the following combined preparations None

GENERAL INFORMATION

Propranolol, introduced in 1965, was the first widely available beta blocker. It is most often used to treat hypertension, angina, and abnormal heart rhythms but is also helpful in controlling the fast heart rate and other symptoms of an overactive thyroid gland. Propranolol also helps to reduce the palpitations, sweating, and tremor of severe anxiety and is also used to prevent migraine headaches.

Propranolol is not prescribed to people with asthma, chronic bronchitis, or emphysema because it can cause breathing difficulties. The drug should be used with caution by diabetics, because, like all beta blockers, it affects the body's response to low blood sugar.

INFORMATION FOR USERS

Your drug prescription is tailored for you. Do not alter dosage without checking with your physician.

How taken

Tablets, SR-capsules.

Frequency and timing of doses
2–4 x daily. Once daily (SR-capsules).

Usual adult dosage range
Abnormal heart rhythms 30–160mg daily.
Angina 60–320mg daily.
Hypertension 60–320mg daily.
Migraine prevention and anxiety 40–160mg daily.

Onset of effect
1–2 hours (tablets); after 4 hours (SR-capsules). In hypertension and migraine, it may be several weeks before full benefits of this drug are felt.

Duration of action
6–12 hours (tablets); 24–30 hours (SR-capsules).

Diet advice
None.

Storage
Keep in a closed container in a cool, dry place out of the reach of children. Protect from light.

Missed dose
Take as soon as you remember. If your next dose is due within 2 hours (tablets) or 12 hours (SR-capsules), take a single dose now and skip the next.

Stopping the drug
Do not stop the drug without consulting your physician. Abrupt cessation may lead to worsening of the underlying condition.

OVERDOSE ACTION

 Seek immediate medical advice in all cases. Take emergency action if breathing difficulties, collapse, or loss of consciousness occur.

See Drug poisoning emergency guide (p.526).

SPECIAL PRECAUTIONS

Be sure to tell your physician if:
▼ You have long-term liver or kidney problems.
▼ You have a breathing disorder such as asthma, bronchitis, or emphysema.
▼ You have heart failure.
▼ You have diabetes.
▼ You have poor circulation in the legs.
▼ You are taking other medications.

 Pregnancy
▼ May affect the baby. Discuss with your physician.

 Breast-feeding
▼ The drug passes into the breast milk, but at normal doses adverse effects on the baby are unlikely. Discuss with your physician.

 Infants and children
▼ Reduced dose necessary.

 Over 60
▼ Increased risk of adverse effects.

 Driving and hazardous work
▼ No special problems.

 Alcohol
▼ No special problems.

Surgery and general anesthetics
▼ Propranolol may need to be stopped before you have a general anesthetic. Discuss this with your physician or dentist before any surgery.

PROLONGED USE

No problems expected.

POSSIBLE ADVERSE EFFECTS

Propranolol has *adverse effects* that are common to most beta blockers. Symptoms such as fatigue and nausea are usually temporary and diminish with long-term use. Fainting may be a sign that the drug has slowed the heart beat excessively.

Symptom/effect	Frequency		Discuss with physician		Stop taking drug now	Call physician now
	Common	Rare	Only if severe	In all cases		
Lethargy/fatigue	●		■			
Cold hands and feet	●		■			
Nausea		●	■			
Nightmares/vivid dreams		●		■		
Dry eyes		●		■		
Fainting/breathlessness		●		■		■
Visual disturbances		●		■		

INTERACTIONS

Antihypertensive drugs Propranolol may enhance the blood pressure lowering effect.

Diltiazem and verapamil Combining either of these drugs with propranolol may have adverse effects on heart function.

Cimetidine and hydralazine These drugs may increase the effects of propranolol.

Non-steroidal anti-inflammatory drugs (NSAIDs) e.g., indomethacin may reduce the antihypertensive effect of propranolol.

PROPYLTHIOURACIL

Product name Propyl-Thyracil
Used in the following combined preparations None

GENERAL INFORMATION

Propylthiouracil is an antithyroid drug used to manage an overactive thyroid gland (hyperthyroidism). In some people, particularly those with Graves' disease (the most common form of the disorder), drug treatment alone may bring on a remission. Propylthiouracil may also be prescribed for long-term treatment of the disease in people who may be at special risk from surgery, such as children and pregnant women.

The drug is also used to restore the normal functioning of the thyroid gland before its partial removal by surgery.

Propylthiouracil is preferred to other antithyroid drugs when treatment is essential during pregnancy.

The most important *adverse effect* that sometimes occurs is a reduction in white blood cells, leading to the risk of infection. If you develop a sore throat or mouth ulceration, see your physician immediately; this might be a sign that your blood is being affected.

QUICK REFERENCE

Drug group Drug for thyroid disorders (p.130)

Overdose danger rating Medium

Dependence rating Low

Prescription needed Yes

Available as generic No

INFORMATION FOR USERS

Your drug prescription is tailored for you. Do not alter dosage without consulting your physician.

How taken

Tablets.

Frequency and timing of doses
1–3 x daily.

Usual dosage range
Initially 150–300mg daily. Usually the dose can be reduced to 50–150mg daily.

Onset of effect
10–20 days. Full beneficial effects may not be felt for 6–10 weeks.

Duration of action
24–36 hours.

Diet advice
Your physician may advise you to avoid foods that are high in iodine (see p.473).

Storage
Keep in a closed container in a cool, dry place out of the reach of children. Protect from light.

Missed dose
Take as soon as you remember. If your next dose is due within 3 hours, take a single dose now and skip the next.

Stopping the drug
Do not stop the drug without consulting your physician; stopping the drug may lead to a recurrence of hyperthyroidism.

Exceeding the dose
An occasional unintentional extra dose is unlikely to cause problems. Large overdoses may cause nausea, vomiting, and headache. Notify your physician.

POSSIBLE ADVERSE EFFECTS

Serious side effects are rare with this drug. Skin rashes and itching are fairly common. A sore throat or fever may indicate adverse effects on the blood. If these occur, inform your physician immediately.

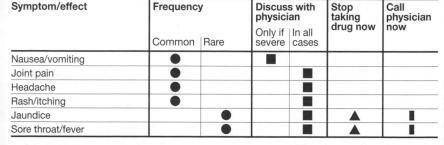

Symptom/effect	Frequency		Discuss with physician		Stop taking drug now	Call physician now
	Common	Rare	Only if severe	In all cases		
Nausea/vomiting	●		■			
Joint pain	●			■		
Headache	●			■		
Rash/itching	●			■		
Jaundice		●		■	▲	▮
Sore throat/fever		●		■	▲	▮

INTERACTIONS

None

SPECIAL PRECAUTIONS

Be sure to tell your physician if:
▼ You have long-term liver or kidney problems.
▼ You are pregnant.
▼ You are taking other medications.

Pregnancy
▼ Prescribed with caution. Risk of goitre and thyroid hormone deficiency (hypothyroidism) in the newborn infant if too high a dose is used. Discuss with your physician.

Breast-feeding
▼ The drug passes into the breast milk and may affect the baby. Discuss with your physician.

Infants and children
▼ Reduced dose necessary.

Over 60
▼ No special problems.

Driving and hazardous work
▼ No problems expected.

Alcohol
▼ No known problems.

PROLONGED USE

High doses of propylthiouracil over a prolonged period may reduce the number of white blood cells.

Monitoring Periodic tests of thyroid function are usually required, and blood cell counts may also be carried out.

PSEUDOEPHEDRINE

Product names Contac Cold 12 Hour Relief Non Drowsy, Eltor 120, Pseudofrin, Sudafed Decongestant 12 Hour, and others
Used in the following combined preparations Dimetapp Daytime Cold, Dristan N.D., Sinutab Sinus Non Drowsy, and others

GENERAL INFORMATION

Pseudoephedrine, a component of many non-prescription remedies, is a sympathomimetic nasal decongestant. It reduces congestion of the nasal passages and sinuses by narrowing blood vessels in the nose.

Apart from its use in nasal congestion, it is also useful for reducing congestion of the eustachian tube (the tube connecting the middle ear with the cavity at the back of the nose). This often occurs with inflammation and infection of the middle ear.

Pseudoephedrine is less likely than other decongestants to cause anxiety, tremor, and restlessness by stimulating the nervous system. But, in common with other drugs in this group, it can cause rebound congestion (worsening of congestion after prolonged use).

INFORMATION FOR USERS

Follow instructions on the label. Call your physician if symptoms worsen.

How taken

Tablets, tablets SR, capsules, oral liquid, powder for solution.

Frequency and timing of doses
Every 3–4 hours (tablets, liquid); every 12 hours (SR tablets).

Usual dosage range
Adults and children 12 years and over Up to 240mg daily.
Children 2–11 years Consult your pharmacist or physician
120mg slow-release preparations are not recommended under 12 years.

Onset of effect
15–30 minutes (tablets and liquid).

Duration of action
4–6 hours (tablets and liquid); 8–12 hours (slow-release preparations).

Diet advice
None.

Storage
Keep in a closed container in a cool, dry place out of the reach of children. Protect from light.

Missed dose
Take as soon as you remember. If your next dose is due within 2 hours, take a single dose now and skip the next.

Stopping the drug
Can be safely stopped as soon as you no longer need it.

OVERDOSE ACTION

 Seek immediate medical advice in all cases. Take emergency action if delirium, seizures, or loss of consciousness occur.

See Drug poisoning emergency guide (p.526).

SPECIAL PRECAUTIONS

Be sure to consult your physician or pharmacist before taking this drug if:
▼ You have heart problems.
▼ You have high blood pressure.
▼ You have had glaucoma.
▼ You have diabetes.
▼ You have an overactive thyroid.
▼ You have urinary difficulties.
▼ You have an enlarged prostate.
▼ You are taking other medications.

 Pregnancy
▼ Safety in pregnancy not established. Discuss with your physician.

 Breast-feeding
▼ The drug passes into the breast milk and may affect the baby. Discuss with your physician.

 Infants and children
▼ Not recommended for children under 2 years. Reduced dose necessary in older children. Consult with your physician or pharmacist.

 Over 60
▼ Reduced dose may need to be given. Increased likelihood of adverse effects.

 Driving and hazardous work
▼ Avoid such activities until you have learned how the drug affects you; it can cause dizziness.

 Alcohol
▼ No known problems.

PROLONGED USE

Pseudoephedrine is not normally taken for prolonged periods. It should not be taken for longer than 7 days except on the advice of your physician.

POSSIBLE ADVERSE EFFECTS

High doses may cause anxiety, nausea, dizziness, and, rarely, a marked rise in blood pressure, causing palpitations, headache, and breathlessness.

Symptom/effect	Frequency		Discuss with physician		Stop taking drug now	Call physician now
	Common	Rare	Only if severe	In all cases		
Nausea/vomiting		●	■			
Dizziness/lightheadedness		●	■			
Nervousness/insomnia		●	■			
Hallucinations		●		■		
Rash		●		■	▲	
Palpitations/breathlessness		●		■		▌
Headache		●		■		▌

INTERACTIONS

Antihypertensive drugs Pseudoephedrine counteracts the lowered blood pressure from antihypertensive drugs.

Other sympathomimetic drugs increase the risk of adverse effects with this drug.

Monoamine oxidase inhibitors (MAOIs) There is a risk of a dangerous rise in blood pressure if pseudoephedrine is taken with these drugs.

PSYLLIUM

Product names Metamucil, Novo-Mucilax, Prodiem Plain
Used in the following combined preparations Prodiem Plus

GENERAL INFORMATION

This bulk-forming laxative has been extracted from the seeds of Plantago plants since 1934. It is used in the treatment of constipation. Taken by mouth, as powder or granules dissolved in water, psyllium passes through the stomach to the intestines, where it absorbs up to 25 times its volume in water, softening and increasing the volume of bowel movements. It may take several days for improved bowel habits to be established.

Psyllium is also used to reduce the frequency and improve the firmness of bowel movements of people with persistent watery diarrhea or those who have had intestinal surgery such as colostomies and ileostomies. Psyllium may dry up and plug the bowel if the intake of fluids is insufficient.

Side effects are rare, but the drug may sometimes cause bloating and excess gas, especially at the start of treatment. It should not be taken without medical advice for constipation that is accompanied by severe abdominal pain because of the risk of obstructing the bowel. People sensitive to inhaled psyllium may experience allergic reactions while mixing it.

QUICK REFERENCE

Drug group Bulk-forming laxative (p.97)

Overdose danger rating Low

Dependence rating Low

Prescription needed No

Available as generic Yes

INFORMATION FOR USERS

Follow instructions on label. Call your physician if symptoms worsen.

How taken

Powder for solution, wafers, granules. (Approximately 3g per tsp; check package.)

Frequency and timing of doses
1–3 x daily with at least 240ml of water or fruit juice. Drink liquid immediately after mixing.

Usual adult dosage range
Adults 2.5g–30g daily.
Children over 6 years on medical advice only.

Onset of effect
12–24 hours.

Duration of action
Up to 24 hours.

Diet advice
Drink plenty of fluids, at least 240ml, with each dose plus additional liquid during the day.

Storage
Keep in a closed container in a cool, dry place out of the reach of children.

Missed dose
Take as soon as you remember. Resume normal dose thereafter.

Stopping the drug
Can be safely stopped as soon as you no longer need it.

Exceeding the dose
An occasional unintentional extra dose is unlikely to be a cause for concern. But if you notice unusual symptoms, or if a large overdose has been taken, notify your physician.

SPECIAL PRECAUTIONS

Be sure to consult your physician or pharmacist before taking this drug if:
▼ You have severe constipation and/or nausea, vomiting, or abdominal pain.
▼ You have unexplained rectal bleeding.
▼ You have difficulty swallowing.
▼ You are allergic to psyllium products.
▼ You have a known narrowing of the bowel.
▼ You are taking other medications.

 Pregnancy
▼ No evidence of risk to the developing baby.

 Breast-feeding
▼ No evidence of risk.

 Infants and children
▼ Given to children over 6 years only on medical advice.

 Over 60
▼ No special problems.

 Driving and hazardous work
▼ No known problems.

 Alcohol
▼ No known problems.

POSSIBLE ADVERSE EFFECTS

Serious adverse effects are rare, but persistent or severe abdominal pain following the use of this (or any) laxative should always receive medical attention.

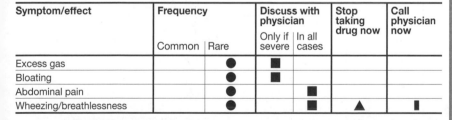

Symptom/effect	Frequency		Discuss with physician		Stop taking drug now	Call physician now
	Common	Rare	Only if severe	In all cases		
Excess gas	●		■			
Bloating	●		■			
Abdominal pain	●			■		
Wheezing/breathlessness	●			■	▲	▮

INTERACTIONS

General note Psyllium may reduce the absorption of oral anticoagulant drugs, digoxin, salicylates, and other drugs. Spacing of doses may be recommended. Ask your pharmacist.

PROLONGED USE

No problems expected.

PYRIDOSTIGMINE

Product names Mestinon, Mestinon-SR
Used in the following combined preparations None

GENERAL INFORMATION

Pyridostigmine is used to treat a rare autoimmune condition involving the faulty transmission of nerve impulses to the muscles, known as myasthenia gravis (p.107). Pyridostigmine improves muscle strength by prolonging nerve signals, although it does not cure the disease. In severe cases, the drug may be prescribed with corticosteroids or other drugs. Pyridostigmine may also be given to reverse temporary paralysis of the bowel and urinary retention following operations.

Side effects, including abdominal cramps, nausea, and diarrhea, usually disappear as a result of reducing the dosage of pyridostigmine.

QUICK REFERENCE

Drug group Drug for myasthenia gravis (p.107)

Overdose danger rating High

Dependence rating Low

Prescription needed Yes

Available as generic No

INFORMATION FOR USERS

Your drug prescription is tailored for you. Do not alter dosage without checking with your physician.

How taken

Tablets, SR-tablets.

Frequency and timing of doses
Every 3–4 hours initially. Thereafter, according to the needs of the individual. SR-tablets 1–2 x daily.

Usual dosage range
Adults 150mg–1g daily (by mouth) according to response and side effects.
Children Reduced dose necessary according to age and weight.

Onset of effect
30–60 minutes.

Duration of action
3–6 hours.

Diet advice
None.

Storage
Keep in a closed container in a cool, dry place out of the reach of children. Protect from light.

Missed dose
Take as soon as you remember. If your next dose is due within 2 hours, take a single dose now and skip the next.

Stopping the drug
Do not stop the drug without consulting your physician; symptoms may recur.

OVERDOSE ACTION

 Seek immediate medical advice in all cases. You may experience severe abdominal cramps, vomiting, weakness, and tremor. Take emergency action if troubled breathing, unusually slow heart beat, fits, or loss of consciousness occur.

See Drug poisoning emergency guide (p.526).

POSSIBLE ADVERSE EFFECTS

Adverse effects of pyridostigmine are usually dose-related and can be avoided by adjusting the dose. In rare cases, hypersensitivity may occur leading to an allergic skin rash.

Symptom/effect	Frequency		Discuss with physician		Stop taking drug now	Call physician now
	Common	Rare	Only if severe	In all cases		
Nausea/vomiting	●		■			
Increased salivation	●		■			
Sweating	●		■			
Abdominal cramps/diarrhea	●			■		
Watering eyes/small pupils		●		■		
Headache		●		■		
Rash		●		■		

INTERACTIONS

General note Drugs that suppress the transmission of nerve signals may oppose the effect of pyridostigmine. Such drugs include aminoglycoside antibiotics, digoxin, procainamide, quinidine, lithium, and chloroquine.

Propranolol antagonizes the effect of pyridostigmine.

SPECIAL PRECAUTIONS

Be sure to tell your physician if:
▼ You have a long-term kidney problem.
▼ You have heart problems.
▼ You have had epileptic fits.
▼ You have asthma.
▼ You have difficulty in passing urine.
▼ You have a peptic ulcer.
▼ You have Parkinson's disease.
▼ You are taking other medications.

 Pregnancy
▼ No evidence of risk to the developing fetus in the first 6 months. Large doses near the time of delivery may cause premature labour and temporary muscle weakness in the baby. Discuss with your physician.

 Breast-feeding
▼ No evidence of risk, but the baby should be monitored for signs of muscle weakness.

 Infants and children
▼ Reduced dose necessary, calculated according to age and weight.

 Over 60
▼ Reduced dose may need to be given. Increased likelihood of adverse effects.

 Driving and hazardous work
▼ Your underlying condition may make such activities inadvisable. Discuss with your physician.

 Alcohol
▼ No special problems.

Surgery and general anesthetics
▼ Pyridostigmine interacts with some anesthetic agents. Make sure your treatment is known to your physician, dentist, and anesthetist before any surgery.

PROLONGED USE

No problems expected.

PYRIMETHAMINE

Product name Daraprim
Used in the following combined preparation None

GENERAL INFORMATION

Pyrimethamine is an antimalarial drug. Because malaria parasites can readily develop resistance to pyrimethamine, the drug is now always given combined with the antibacterial drug sulfadoxine for the treatment of malaria. The activity of the combination greatly exceeds that of either drug alone. Pyrtimethamine and sulfadoxine are used with quinine in the treatment of malaria. Pyrimethamine is not used for the prevention of malaria.

Pyrimethamine is sometimes given with another drug, sulfadiazine, to treat toxoplasmosis in people with lowered immunity. Such treatment must be supervised by an expert.

Blood disorders can sometimes arise during prolonged treatment with pyrimethamine, and, because of this, blood counts are monitored regularly and vitamin supplements are given.

QUICK REFERENCE

Drug group Antimalarial drug (p.123)

Overdose danger rating Medium

Dependence rating Low

Prescription needed Yes

Available as generic No

INFORMATION FOR USERS

Your drug prescription is tailored for you. Do not alter dosage without checking with your physician.

How taken

Tablets.

Frequency and timing of doses
Taken once only.

Usual dosage range
Adults 2–3 tablets.
Children Reduced dose necessary according to age.

Onset of effect
24 hours.

Duration of action
Up to 1 week.

Diet advice
None.

Storage
Keep in a closed container in a cool, dry place out of the reach of children. Protect from light.

Missed dose
If you are being treated for toxoplasmosis, take as soon as you remember. If your next dose is due within 24 hours, take a single dose now and alter the dosing day so that your next dose is one week later.

Stopping the drug
Do not stop taking the drug without discussing it with your physician.

Exceeding the dose
An occasional unintentional extra dose is unlikely to cause problems. Large overdoses may cause trembling, breathing difficulty, fits, and blood disorders. Notify your physician.

SPECIAL PRECAUTIONS

Be sure to tell your physician if:
▼ You have long-term liver or kidney problems.
▼ You have had epileptic fits.
▼ You have anemia.
▼ You are allergic to sulfonamides.
▼ You have glucose-6-phosphate dehydrogenase (G6PD) deficiency.
▼ You are taking other medications.

Pregnancy
▼ Pyrimethamine can cause folic acid deficiency in the unborn baby. Discuss with your physician.

Breast-feeding
▼ The drug passes into the breast milk, but at normal doses adverse effects on the baby are unlikely. Discuss with your physician.

Infants and children
▼ Reduced dose necessary.

Over 60
▼ No special problems.

Driving and hazardous work
▼ No special problems.

Alcohol
▼ No known problems.

POSSIBLE ADVERSE EFFECTS

Unusual tiredness, weakness, bleeding, bruising, and sore throat may be signs of a blood disorder. Notify your physician promptly if they occur. Breathing difficulties or signs of chest infection should be reported to your physician immediately.

Symptom/effect	Frequency		Discuss with physician		Stop taking drug now	Call physician now
	Common	Rare	Only if severe	In all cases		
Loss of appetite	●		■			
Insomnia	●		■			
Gastric irritation	●			■		
Rash	●			■		▮
Unusual bleeding/bruising	●			■		▮
Sore throat/fever	●			■		▮
Breathing problems	●			■		▮

INTERACTIONS

General note Drugs that suppress the bone marrow or cause folic acid deficiency may increase the risk of serious blood disorders when taken with pyrimethamine.

Such drugs include anticancer and antirheumatic drugs, sulfasalazine, co-trimoxazole, trimethoprim, phenytoin, and phenylbutazone.

PROLONGED USE

Prolonged use of this drug may cause folic acid deficiency, leading to serious blood disorders. Supplements of folic acid may be recommended (in the form of folinic acid).

Monitoring Regular blood cell counts are required during high-dose or long-term treatment.

QUETIAPINE

Product name Seroquel
Used in the following combined preparations None

GENERAL INFORMATION

Quetiapine is an atypical antipsychotic drug that is prescribed for the treatment of schizophrenia. It can be used to treat "positive" symptoms (thought disorders, delusions, and hallucinations) and "negative" symptoms (blunted affect and emotional and social withdrawal).

The drug may be more effective when used for positive symptoms, however.

Elderly people excrete the drug up to 50 per cent more slowly than the usual adult rate. They, therefore, need to be prescribed much lower doses in order to avoid *adverse effects*.

QUICK REFERENCE

Drug group Antipsychotic drug (p.69)
Overdose danger rating Medium
Dependence rating Low
Prescription needed Yes
Available as generic No

INFORMATION FOR USERS

Your drug prescription is tailored for you. Do not alter dosage without checking with your physician.

How taken

Tablets.

Frequency and timing of doses
2 x daily.

Usual adult dosage range
50mg daily (day 1), 100mg daily (day 2), 200mg daily (day 3), 300mg daily (day 4), then changing according to response.
Usual dose: 300–600mg daily.

Onset of effect
1 hour.

Duration of action
Up to 12 hours.

Diet advice
None.

Storage
Keep in a closed container in a cool, dry place out of the reach of children.

Missed dose
Take as soon as you remember. If your next dose is due within 4 hours take a single dose now and skip the next.

Stopping the drug
Do not stop the drug without consulting your physician; symptoms may recur.

Exceeding the dose
An occasional unintentional extra dose is unlikely to cause problems. Large overdoses may cause unusual drowsiness, palpitations, and low blood pressure. Notify your physician.

SPECIAL PRECAUTIONS

Be sure to tell your physician if:
▼ You have epilepsy.
▼ You have Parkinson's disease.
▼ You have liver or kidney problems.
▼ You have heart problems.
▼ You have blood problems.
▼ You are taking other medications.

Pregnancy
▼ Safety not established. Discuss with your physician.

Breast-feeding
▼ Safety not established. Discuss with your physician.

Infants and children
▼ Not recommended.

Over 60
▼ Reduced doses necessary. The elderly eliminate quetiapine much more slowly than younger adults.

Driving and hazardous work
▼ Avoid. Quetiapine can cause drowsiness.

Alcohol
▼ Avoid. Alcohol increases the sedative effects of this drug.

POSSIBLE ADVERSE EFFECTS

Unusual drowsiness and weight gain are common adverse effects of quetiapine.

Symptom/effect	Frequency		Discuss with physician		Stop taking drug now	Call physician now
	Common	Rare	Only if severe	In all cases		
Unusual drowsiness	●		■			
Weight gain	●		■			
Digestive upset	●		■			
Parkinsonism	●			■		
Dizziness/fainting		●		■		
Persistent sore throat		●		■		
Palpitations		●		■		■

PROLONGED USE

Prolonged use of quetiapine has been reported to produce *tardive dyskinesia* (in which there are involuntary movements of the tongue and face).

INTERACTIONS

Antiepileptics Quetiapine opposes the effect of these drugs but phenytoin decreases the effect of quetiapine. Other liver enzyme-inducing antiepileptic drugs, such as carbamazepine and barbiturates, may have a similar effect.

Sedatives All drugs that have a sedative effect on the central nervous system are likely to increase the sedative properties of quetiapine.

QUINIDINE

Product name Biquin Durules
Used in the following combined preparations None

GENERAL INFORMATION

Although quinidine is one of the oldest of the anti-arrhythmic drugs, it is still used to treat many different abnormal heart rhythms, particularly in cases where a rapid heartbeat causes important symptoms or is life-threatening.

When taken by mouth, the onset of action is slow. It can be given by injection in emergencies when rapid control of an abnormal heart rhythm is required.

Quinidine has several possible adverse effects. Diarrhea, nausea, and vomiting, which are common, may be due to its irritant effect. Serious allergic reactions have also occurred. The most serious adverse effect is the possibility of further abnormal heart rhythms that may give rise to palpitations.

INFORMATION FOR USERS

Your drug prescription is tailored for you. Do not alter dosage without checking with your physician.

How taken

Tablets, slow-release (S-R) tablets, injection.

Frequency and timing of doses
Every 6 hours (tablets); every 8–12 hours (S-R tablets). In some situations, higher doses may be used initially.

Usual adult dosage range
600mg–2.4g daily.

Onset of effect
Within 3 hours.

Duration of action
6–8 hours (tablets); up to 12 hours (SR-tablets).

Diet advice
None.

Storage
Keep in a closed container in a cool, dry place out of the reach of children. Protect from light.

Missed dose
Take as soon as you remember. If your next dose is due within 2 hours, take a single dose now and skip the next.

Stopping the drug
Do not stop taking the drug without consulting your physician; symptoms may recur.

OVERDOSE ACTION

 Seek immediate medical advice in all cases. Take emergency action if breathing problems, seizures, or collapse occurs.

See Drug poisoning emergency guide (p.526).

SPECIAL PRECAUTIONS

Be sure to tell your physician if:
▼ You have impaired liver or kidney function.
▼ You have heart failure.
▼ You have myasthenia gravis.
▼ You have had a rash following quinidine on a previous occasion.
▼ You are taking digoxin.
▼ You are taking other medications.

 Pregnancy
▼ Safety in pregnancy not established. Discuss with your physician.

 Breast-feeding
▼ The drug passes into the breast milk and may affect the baby. Discuss with your physician.

 Infants and children
▼ Not usually prescribed.

 Over 60
▼ Reduced dose necessary.

 Driving and hazardous work
▼ Avoid such activities until you know how quinidine affects you; it can cause dizziness and blurred vision.

 Alcohol
▼ No known problems.

PROLONGED USE

Sudden onset of abnormal heart rhythms or abnormalities of the blood may occur.

Monitoring Periodic checks on blood levels of the drug may be required.

POSSIBLE ADVERSE EFFECTS

The most common adverse effects are diarrhea, nausea, and vomiting. If they become severe, a change of drug may be necessary. Vertigo or palpitations may indicate the dose is too high; notify your physician promptly.

Symptom/effect	Frequency		Discuss with physician		Stop taking drug now	Call physician now
	Common	Rare	Only if severe	In all cases		
Diarrhea	●		■			
Nausea/vomiting	●		■			
Dizziness	●		■			
Ringing in the ears		●		■		
Headache/vertigo		●		■		
Palpitations		●		■		▮
Lightheadedness		●		■		▮
Rash		●		■		
Blurred vision		●		■		▮

INTERACTIONS

Antihypertensive drugs Quinidine may increase the effects of these drugs.

Anticoagulant drugs Quinidine increases the effects of these drugs.

Phenobarbital and phenytoin reduce the effect of quinidine.

Digoxin Quinidine increases the effects of digoxin; blood levels must be checked.

QUININE

Product name Quinine-Odan
Used in the following combined preparations None

GENERAL INFORMATION

Quinine, obtained from the bark of the cinchona tree, is the earliest antimalarial drug. It often causes *side effects*, but is still given for cases of malaria that are resistant to safer treatments. Owing to the resistance of malaria parasites to chloroquine and some of the more modern antimalarials, quinine remains the mainstay of treatment, but it is not used as a preventative.

At the high doses used to treat malaria, quinine may cause ringing in the ears, headaches, nausea, hearing loss, and blurred vision: a group of symptoms known as cinchonism. In rare cases, it may cause bleeding into the skin due to reduced blood platelets.

Quinine is also often used, in small doses, to prevent painful night-time leg cramps.

QUICK REFERENCE

Drug group Antimalarial drug (p.123)

Overdose danger rating High

Dependence rating Low

Prescription needed Yes

Available as generic Yes

INFORMATION FOR USERS

Your drug prescription is tailored for you. Do not alter dosage without checking with your physician.

How taken

Tablets, capsules.

Frequency and timing of doses
Malaria Every 8 hours after meals.
Muscle cramps Once daily at bedtime.

Usual adult dosage range
1.8g daily for 3–7 days (malaria);
200–300mg daily at bedtime (cramps).

Onset of effect
1–2 days (malaria); up to 4 weeks (cramps).

Duration of action
Up to 24 hours.

Diet advice
None.

Storage
Keep in a closed container in a cool, dry place out of the reach of children. Protect from light.

Missed dose
Take as soon as you remember. If your next dose is due within 4 hours, skip the missed one and return to your normal dosing schedule thereafter.

Stopping the drug
If prescribed for malaria, take the full course. Even if you feel better, the original infection may still be present and may recur if treatment is stopped too soon. If taken for muscle cramps, the drug can safely be stopped as soon as you no longer need it.

OVERDOSE ACTION

Seek immediate medical advice in all cases. Take emergency action if breathing problems, fits, or loss of consciousness occur.

See Drug poisoning emergency guide (p.526).

SPECIAL PRECAUTIONS

Be sure to consult your physician if:
▼ You have a long-term kidney problem.
▼ You have tinnitus (ringing in the ears).
▼ You have optic neuritis.
▼ You have myasthenia gravis.
▼ You have glucose-6-phosphate dehydrogenase (G6PD) deficiency.
▼ You have heart problems.
▼ You are taking other medications.

Pregnancy
▼ Not usually prescribed. May cause defects in the unborn baby. Discuss with your physician.

Breast-feeding
▼ The drug passes into the breast milk, but at normal doses adverse effects on the baby are unlikely. Discuss with your physician.

Infants and children
▼ Reduced dose necessary.

Over 60
▼ No special problems.

Driving and hazardous work
▼ Avoid these activities until you know how quinine affects you because the drug's side effects may distract you.

Alcohol
▼ No known problems.

POSSIBLE ADVERSE EFFECTS

Adverse effects are unlikely with low doses. At antimalarial doses, hearing disturbances, headache, and blurred vision are more common. Nausea and diarrhea may occur.

Symptom/effect	Frequency		Discuss with physician		Stop taking drug now	Call physician now
	Common	Rare	Only if severe	In all cases		
Nausea/vomiting/diarrhea		●		■		
Headache		●		■		
Ringing in ears/giddiness		●		■		
Rash/itching		●		■	▲	❚
Loss of hearing		●		■	▲	❚
Blurred vision		●		■	▲	❚

INTERACTIONS

Cimetidine This drug increases the blood levels of quinine.

Mefloquine may cause increased effect on the heart. Do not use with quinine.

Digoxin Quinine increases the blood levels of digoxin, and so the dose of digoxin should be reduced. Discuss with your physician.

PROLONGED USE

No problems expected with low doses used to control night-time leg cramps. Treatment may be stopped after 3 months to assess the need to continue.

RALOXIFENE

Product name Evista
Used in the following combined preparations None

GENERAL INFORMATION

Raloxifene is a non-steroidal drug that acts on some estrogen receptors (estrogen is a naturally occurring female sex hormone, see p.133). It is a selective estrogen receptor modulator (SERM), which acts like estrogen on bone. It is prescribed to prevent vertebral fractures in postmeno-pausal women who are at increased risk of osteoporosis. There is evidence that the drug may also be useful for preventing hip fractures, but its use in prevention of other bone fractures is uncertain.

Raloxifene has no beneficial effect on other menopausal problems such as hot flushes. It is not prescribed to women who might become pregnant because it may harm the unborn baby, and it is not prescribed to men.

There is an increased risk of a thrombosis (blood clot) developing in a vein in the leg, but the risk is similar to that due to HRT (see p.133). However, because of this risk, raloxifene is usually stopped if the woman taking it becomes immobile or bedbound, when clots are more likely to form. Treatment is restarted when full activity is resumed.

(see p.133)

QUICK REFERENCE

Drug group Drug for bone disorders (p.108)

Overdose danger rating Low

Dependence rating Low

Prescription needed Yes

Available as generic No

INFORMATION FOR USERS

Your drug prescription is tailored for you. Do not alter dosage without checking with your physician.

How taken

Tablets.

Frequency and timing of doses
Once daily.

Usual adult dosage range
60mg daily.

Onset of effect
1–4 hours.

Duration of action
24–48 hours.

Diet advice
Calcium supplements are recommended if dietary calcium is low.

Storage
Keep in a closed container in a cool, dry place out of the reach of children. Protect from light.

Missed dose
Take as soon as you remember. If your next dose is due within 8 hours, take a single dose now and skip the next.

Stopping the drug
Do not stop the drug without consulting your physician except under conditions specified in advance, such as immobility, which increases the risk of blood clots forming.

Exceeding the dose
An occasional unintentional extra dose is unlikely to be a cause for concern. But if you notice any unusual symptoms, or if a large overdose has been taken, notify your physician.

SPECIAL PRECAUTIONS

Be sure to tell your physician if:
▼ You have had a blood clot in a vein.
▼ You have uterine bleeding.
▼ You have liver or kidney problems.
▼ You are taking other medications.
▼ You have a history of stroke.
▼ You have heart rhythm problems.

Pregnancy
▼ Not prescribed to premenopausal women.

Breast-feeding
▼ Not prescribed to premenopausal women.

Infants and children
▼ Not prescribed.

Over 60
▼ No special problems.

Driving and hazardous work
▼ No special problems.

Alcohol
▼ No special problems.

PROLONGED USE

No special problems. Raloxifene is normally used long term.

Monitoring Liver function tests may be performed periodically.

POSSIBLE ADVERSE EFFECTS

Some adverse effects of raloxifene are indications of a thrombosis (blood clot) in a vein in the leg. If a clot occurs somewhere else in the body, there might not be any obvious symptoms.

Symptom/effect	Frequency		Discuss with physician		Stop taking drug now	Call physician now
	Common	Rare	Only if severe	In all cases		
Hot flushes	●		■			
Leg cramps	●		■			
Swollen ankles/feet	●			■		
Headache		●		■		
Rash		●		■		
Leg pain/tenderness		●		■	▲	∎
Leg swelling		●		■	▲	∎
Leg discoloration/ulceration		●		■	▲	∎
Inflammation of capillaries		●		■	▲	∎

INTERACTIONS

Anticoagulants Raloxifene reduces the effect of warfarin.

Cholestyramine This drug reduces the absorption of raloxifene by the body.

RAMIPRIL

Product name Altace
Used in the following combined preparations Altace HCT

GENERAL INFORMATION

Ramipril belongs to a group of drugs known as ACE (angiotensin converting enzyme) inhibitors. It works by dilating the blood vessels, which enables the blood to circulate more easily. The drug is used to treat high blood pressure (p.88) and to reduce the strain on the heart in patients with heart failure after a heart attack. The first dose of an ACE inhibitor can cause the blood pressure to drop very suddenly, so a few hours' bed rest afterwards may be advised. You may need to stay in hospital until you are stabilized on the treatment.

Side effects such as headache, nausea, and dizziness are usually mild. Like all ACE inhibitors, however, ramipril causes the body to retain potassium, an excess of which can cause a number of *adverse effects*.

INFORMATION FOR USERS

Your drug prescription is tailored for you. Do not alter dosage without checking with your physician.

How taken

Capsules.

Frequency and timing of doses
With water, with or without food.
High blood pressure Usually once daily.
Heart failure after a heart attack 2 x daily.

Usual adult dosage range
High blood pressure 1.25–10mg daily.
Heart failure after a heart attack 5–10mg daily.

Onset of effect
Within 2 hours.

Duration of action
Up to 24 hours.

Diet advice
Your physician may advise you to decrease your salt intake to help control your blood pressure.

Storage
Keep in a closed container in a cool, dry place out of the reach of children.

Missed dose
Take as soon as you remember. If your next dose is due within 6 hours, take a single dose now and skip the next. Subsequently, continue with your usual routine.

Stopping the drug
Do not stop taking the drug without consulting your physician. Treatment of hypertension and heart failure is normally lifelong, it may be necessary to substitute alternative therapy.

Exceeding the dose
If you notice any unusual symptoms or if a large overdose has been taken, notify your physician.

SPECIAL PRECAUTIONS

Be sure to tell your physician if:
▼ You have long-term liver or kidney problems.
▼ You have ever suffered from severe allergies.
▼ You have had heart-valve problems.
▼ You have peripheral vascular disease or atherosclerosis.
▼ You suffer from systemic lupus erythematosus or scleroderma.
▼ You are taking other medications.

Pregnancy
▼ Not usually prescribed. May cause defects in the unborn baby. Discuss with your physician.

Breast-feeding
▼ The drug passes into the breast milk and may affect the baby. Discuss with your physician.

Infants and children
▼ Not recommended.

Over 60s
▼ Reduced dose may be necessary.

Driving and hazardous work
▼ Avoid such activities until you have learned how ramipril affects you because the drug may cause dizziness due to low blood pressure.

Alcohol
▼ Avoid. Alcohol may reduce blood pressure further at first dose or dosage adjustment.

Surgery and general anesthetics
▼ Notify your physician or dentist that you are taking ramipril as anesthetics can increase the effects of this drug.

POSSIBLE ADVERSE EFFECTS

Nausea, dizziness, and headache are common but are usually mild and transient. An irritating dry cough may necessitate withdrawal of the drug. High potassium levels may occur. Rarely, ramipril may cause deterioration of kidney function, digestive tract disturbance, severe rash, or severe swelling of the face accompanied by breathing difficulties.

Symptom/effect	Frequency		Discuss with physician		Stop taking drug now	Call physician now
	Common	Rare	Only if severe	In all cases		
Nausea	●		■			
Dizziness/headache	●		■			
Cough	●		■			
Dry mouth/taste disturbance	●		■			
Jaundice		●		■		
Rash/itching		●		■		▌
Swelling of face/mouth		●		■	▲	▌
Difficulty in breathing		●		■	▲	▌
Chest pain/unconsciousness		●		■	▲	▌

INTERACTIONS

Non-steroidal anti-inflammatory drugs (NSAIDs) (e.g., ibuprofen) may reduce the antihypertensive effect of ramipril and increase the risk of kidney damage.

Cyclosporine increases the risk of high potassium levels in the blood.

Potassium supplements and potassium-sparing diuretics may cause excess levels of potassium in the body.

Lithium Like other ACE inhibitors, ramipril may cause raised blood lithium levels and *toxicity*.

PROLONGED USE

No problems expected.

Monitoring If you have other medical conditions, blood counts and kidney function tests may be performed at intervals.

RANITIDINE

Product names Apo-Ranitidine, CO Ranitidine, Gen-Ranitidine, Novo-Ranidine, Zantac
Used in the following combined preparations None

GENERAL INFORMATION

Ranitidine is prescribed in the treatment of stomach and duodenal ulcers. In combination with antibiotics, the drug is used for ulcers caused by *Helicobacter pylori* infection. It is also used to protect against duodenal (but not stomach) ulcers in people taking NSAIDs (p.102), who may be prone to ulcers. This drug reduces the discomfort and ulceration of reflux esophagitis, and may prevent stress ulceration and gastric bleeding in severely ill patients. Ranitidine reduces the amount of stomach acid produced, allowing ulcers to heal. It is usually given in courses lasting four to eight weeks, with further courses if symptoms recur.

Unlike the similar drug cimetidine, ranitidine does not increase blood levels of other drugs such as anticoagulants and anti-convulsants, which might reduce the effectiveness of treatment. It is available in smaller doses over-the-counter for self-management of the discomfort of acid indigestion.

Most people experience no serious effects during ranitidine treatment. As it promotes healing of the stomach lining, there is a risk that ranitidine may mask stomach cancer, delaying diagnosis. It is therefore usually prescribed only when the possibility of stomach cancer has been ruled out.

INFORMATION FOR USERS

Follow instructions on the label. Call your physician if symptoms worsen.

How taken

Tablets, oral liquid, injection.

Frequency and timing of doses
Once daily at bedtime or 2–3 x daily.

Usual adult dosage range
150–600mg daily, depending on the condition being treated. Usual dose is 150mg twice daily.

Onset of effect
Within 1 hour.

Duration of action
12 hours.

Diet advice
None.

Storage
Keep in a closed container in a cool, dry place out of the reach of children. Protect from light.

Missed dose
Take as soon as you remember. If your next dose is due within 3 hours, take a single dose now and skip the next.

Stopping the drug
Do not stop the drug without consulting your physician; symptoms may recur.

Exceeding the dose
An occasional unintentional extra dose is unlikely to be a cause for concern. But if you notice any unusual symptoms, or if a large overdose has been taken, notify your physician.

POSSIBLE ADVERSE EFFECTS

The *adverse effects* of ranitidine, of which headache is the most common, are usually related to dosage level and almost always disappear when treatment finishes.

Symptom/effect	Frequency		Discuss with physician		Stop taking drug now	Call physician now
	Common	Rare	Only if severe	In all cases		
Headache/dizziness	●		■			
Nausea/vomiting		●	■			
Constipation		●	■			
Diarrhea		●	■			
Jaundice		●		■		
Mental problems		●		■		
Sore throat/fever		●		■		■

INTERACTIONS

Ketoconazole Ranitidine may reduce the absorption of ketoconazole. Ranitidine should be taken at least 2 hours after ketoconazole.

Sucralfate High doses (2g) of sucralfate may reduce the absorption of ranitidine. Sucralfate should be taken at least 2 hours after ranitidine.

SPECIAL PRECAUTIONS

Be sure to tell your physician or pharmacist if:
▼ You have long-term liver or kidney problems.
▼ You have porphyria.
▼ You have had an allergic reaction to ranitidine or to another H_2 blocker.
▼ You are taking other medications.

Pregnancy
▼ Safety in pregnancy not established. Discuss with your physician.

Breast-feeding
▼ The drug passes into the breast milk and may affect the baby. Discuss with your physician.

Infants and children
▼ Reduced dose necessary.

Over 60
▼ No special problems.

Driving and hazardous work
▼ No known problems. Dizziness can occur in a very small proportion of patients.

Alcohol
▼ Avoid. Alcohol may aggravate your underlying condition and reduce the beneficial effects of this drug.

PROLONGED USE

No problems expected.

RASAGILINE

Product name Azilect
Used in the following combined preparations None

GENERAL INFORMATION

Rasagiline is used alone or in combination with another medication to treat Parkinson's disease. It works by inhibiting an enzyme called monoamine oxidase type B (MAO-B), which increases dopamine in the brain. It can be used early on in the disease to control symptoms. It can be used with medications such as levodopa as it helps prolong its effect.

While on this medication, it is advised that you get up slowly while supporting yourself, to minimize dizziness or lightheadedness. As rasagiline blocks the MAO-B enzyme, it can prevent the breakdown of tyramine, which is a by-product of some foods. When these foods are taken while on this medication, serious side effects can occur (see below).

QUICK REFERENCE

Drug group Drugs for Parkinsonism (p. 71)

Overdose danger rating High

Dependence rating Low

Prescription needed Yes

Available as generic No

INFORMATION FOR USERS

Your drug prescription is tailored for you. Do not alter dosage without checking with your physician.

How taken

Tablets.

Frequency and timing of doses
Usually once daily.

Adult dosage range
0.5–1mg daily.

Onset of effect
1 hour.

Duration of action
Up to 24 hours.

Diet advice
Avoid foods rich in tyramine while on, and for 14 days after stopping, rasagiline. These include aged cheeses, salami, fava beans, red wine, soybean products. Consult your dietician.

Storage
Keep in a closed container in a cool, dry place out of the reach of children.

Missed dose
If you miss a dose, take it as soon as you remember. If it is near the time of the next dose, skip the missed dose and resume your usual dosing schedule. Do not double up to catch up on a missed dose.

Stopping the drug
Do not stop the drug without consulting your physician. Stopping the drug may lead to worsening of the underlying condition.

OVERDOSE ACTION

 Seek immediate medical advice in all cases. Take emergency action if chest pain or loss of consciousness occurs.

See Drug poisoning emergency guide (p.526).

SPECIAL PRECAUTIONS

Be sure to tell your physician if:
▼ You have pheochromocytoma.
▼ You have kidney or liver disease.
▼ You have had melanoma.
▼ You are taking herbal remedies such as St. John's Wort.
▼ You are taking other medications.

 Pregnancy
▼ Not usually prescribed. Safety in pregnancy not established. Discuss with your physician.

 Breast-feeding
▼ Safety not established. Discuss with your physician.

 Infants and children
▼ Not recommended.

 Over 60
▼ No special problems.

 Driving and hazardous work
▼ May cause drowsiness. Do not drive a car or operate machinery until the effect of the drug wears off and you feel you are mentally alert.

 Alcohol
▼ Avoid alcohol use as it may increase the effect of drowsiness caused by this drug.

PROLONGED USE

No problems expected.

POSSIBLE ADVERSE EFFECTS

Rasigiline may cause some drowsiness and change in bowel pattern.

Symptom/effect	Frequency		Discuss with physician		Stop taking drug now	Call physician now
	Common	Rare	Only if severe	In all cases		
Mild headache		●	■			
Constipation or diarrhea	●		■			
Drowsiness	●		■			
Loss of appetite		●	■			
Unsteadiness,		●	■			
Severe headache/ chest pain/blurred vision		●		■	▲	▌
Hallucinations		●		■	▲	▌
Shortness of breath		●		■		▌
Slow or difficult speech		●		■		▌

INTERACTIONS

General note Because of the wide range of possible drug interactions with rasagiline, do not take any medication, whether prescription or nonprescription, without first consulting your physician or pharmacist.

Antidepressants, St. John's wort, dextromethorphan, pseudoephedrine meperidine The combination of rasagiline with these may cause severe and dangerous reactions. Allow at least 14 days after stopping rasagiline before taking these.

REPAGLINIDE

Product name GlucoNorm
Used in the following combined preparations None

GENERAL INFORMATION

Repaglinide is a drug used to treat non-insulin dependent diabetes that cannot be adequately controlled by diet and exercise alone. It acts in a similar manner to sulfonylurea drugs by stimulating the release of insulin from the pancreas. Therefore, some of the pancreatic cells need to be functioning in order for it to be effective.

Repaglinide is quick acting, but its effects last for only about four hours. The drug is sometimes given with metformin if that drug is not providing adequate diabetic control.

Repaglinide is best taken just before a meal in order for the insulin that is released to cope with the food. If a meal is likely to be missed, the dose of repaglinide should not be taken. If a tablet has been taken and a meal is not forthcoming, some carbohydrate (as specified by your physician or dietician) should be eaten as soon as possible.

QUICK REFERENCE

Drug group Oral antidiabetic drug (p.128)

Overdose danger rating Medium

Dependence rating Low

Prescription needed Yes

Available as generic No

INFORMATION FOR USERS

Your drug prescription is tailored for you. Do not alter dosage without checking with your physician.

How taken

Tablets.

Frequency and timing of doses
1–4 x daily (up to 30 minutes before a meal, and up to 4 meals a day). If you are going to miss a meal, do not take the tablet.

Usual adult dosage range
500mcg (starting dose), increased at intervals of 1–2 weeks according to response; 4–16mg daily (maintenance dose).

Onset of effect
30 minutes.

Duration of action
4 hours.

Diet advice
Follow the diet advised by your physician or dietician.

Storage
Keep in a closed container in a cool, dry place out of the reach of children.

Missed dose
Do not take tablets between meals. Discuss with your physician.

Stopping the drug
Do not stop taking the drug without consulting your physician.

Exceeding the dose
An overdose will cause hypoglycaemia with dizziness, sweating, trembling, confusion, and headache. Notify your physician.

SPECIAL PRECAUTIONS

Be sure to tell your physician if:
▼ You have liver or kidney problems.
▼ You are taking other medications.

Pregnancy
▼ Safety not established. Discuss with your physician.

Breast-feeding
▼ Safety not established. Discuss with your physician.

Infants and children
▼ Not recommended.

Over 60
▼ No special problems, but safety not established over 75 years.

Driving and hazardous work
▼ Avoid if low blood sugar without warning signs is likely.

Alcohol
▼ Avoid. Alcohol may upset diabetic control and may increase and prolong the effects of repaglinide.

POSSIBLE ADVERSE EFFECTS

Intestinal problems are common at the start of treatment with repaglinide. However, such adverse effects tend to become less troublesome as treatment continues.

Symptom/effect	Frequency		Discuss with physician		Stop taking drug now	Call physician now
	Common	Rare	Only if severe	In all cases		
Nausea/vomiting	●		■			
Abdominal pain	●		■			
Diarrhea/constipation	●		■			
Rash/itching		●		■		

INTERACTIONS

Monoamine oxidase inhibitors (MAOIs), beta-blockers, ACE inhibitors, and NSAIDs These drugs may increase the effect of repaglinide.

Ketoconazole and erythromycin may increase the effect of repaglinide.

Oral contraceptives, thiazide diuretics, corticosteroids, danazol, thyroid hormones, and sympathomimetics These drugs may decrease the effect of repaglinide.

Rifampin and carbamazepine may decrease the effect of repaglinide.

PROLONGED USE

Repaglinide is usually prescribed indefinitely. No special problems.

RIFAMPIN

Product name Rofact
Used in the following combined preparation Rifater

GENERAL INFORMATION

Rifampin is an antibacterial drug that is highly effective in the treatment of tuberculosis. Taken by mouth, the drug is well absorbed in the intestine and widely distributed throughout the body, including the brain. As a result, it is particularly useful in the treatment of tuberculous meningitis.

Rifampin has also been used to prevent infection in close contacts of those with meningococcal meningitis.

Rifampin is always prescribed with other antibiotics or antituberculous drugs because of the rapid development of resistance in some bacteria.

A harmless red-orange coloration may be imparted to the urine, saliva, and tears, and soft contact lenses may become permanently stained.

QUICK REFERENCE

Drug group Antituberculous drug (p.118)

Overdose danger rating Medium

Dependence rating Low

Prescription needed Yes

Available as generic Yes

INFORMATION FOR USERS

Your drug prescription is tailored for you. Do not alter dosage without checking with your physician.

How taken

Tablets, capsules, injection (available through Special Access Programme).

Frequency and timing of doses
1 x daily, 30 minutes before breakfast (tuberculosis); 2 x daily (prevention of meningococcal meningitis); 2–4 x daily, 30 minutes before or 2 hours after meals (other serious infections).

Usual adult dosage range
According to weight; usually 450–600mg daily (tuberculosis); 600mg–1.2g daily (other serious infections); 1.2g daily for 2 days (meningococcal meningitis).

Onset of effect
Over several days.

Duration of action
Up to 24 hours.

Diet advice
None.

Storage
Keep in a closed container in a cool, dry place out of the reach of children. Protect from light.

Missed dose
Take as soon as you remember. If your next dose is due within 6 hours, take a single dose now, then return to normal dosing schedule.

Stopping the drug
Take the full course. Even if you feel better, the original infection may still be present and symptoms may recur if treatment is stopped too soon. In rare cases stopping the drug suddenly after high-dose treatment can lead to a severe flu-like illness.

Exceeding the dose
An occasional unintentional extra dose is unlikely to cause problems. Large overdoses may cause liver damage, nausea, vomiting, and lethargy. Notify your physician immediately.

SPECIAL PRECAUTIONS

Be sure to tell your physician if:
▼ You have a long-term liver or kidney problem.
▼ You have porphyria.
▼ You wear contact lenses.
▼ You are taking other medications.

 Pregnancy
▼ Safety in pregnancy not established. Discuss with your physician.

 Breast-feeding
▼ The drug passes into the breast milk, but at normal doses adverse effects on the baby are unlikely. Discuss with your physician.

 Infants and children
▼ Reduced dose necessary.

 Over 60
▼ Increased risk of adverse effects. Reduced dose may therefore be necessary.

 Driving and hazardous work
▼ No problems expected.

 Alcohol
▼ Avoid excessive amounts. Heavy alcohol consumption may increase the risk of liver damage.

POSSIBLE ADVERSE EFFECTS

A harmless red-orange discoloration of body fluids normally occurs. Serious adverse effects are rare. *Jaundice* usually improves during treatment but should be reported to your physician. Headache and breathing difficulties may occur after stopping high-dose treatment.

Symptom/effect	Frequency		Discuss with physician		Stop taking drug now	Call physician now
	Common	Rare	Only if severe	In all cases		
Muscle cramps/aches		●		■		
Nausea/vomiting/diarrhea		●	■			
Jaundice		●		■		❚
Flu-like illness		●		■	▲	❚
Rash/itching		●		■		

INTERACTIONS

General note Rifampin may reduce the effectiveness of a wide variety of drugs, such as oral contraceptives (in which case alternative contraceptive methods may be necessary), phenytoin, corticosteroids, oral antidiabetics, disopyramide, and oral anticoagulants. Dosage adjustment of these drugs may be necessary at the start or end of treatment with rifampin. Consult your physician or pharmacist for advice.

PROLONGED USE

Prolonged use of rifampin may cause liver damage.

Monitoring Periodic blood tests may be performed to monitor liver function.

RISEDRONATE

Product name Actonel
Used in the following combined preparations Actonel Plus

GENERAL INFORMATION

Risedronate is given for the prevention and treatment of osteoporosis in post-menopausal women and osteoporosis due to long-term use of corticosteroid drugs in men and women. Risedronate is also beneficial in individuals with Paget's disease.

A calcium supplement and vitamin D may be prescribed with the drug if dietary amounts are not adequate. However, calcium should not be taken at the same time as risedronate because calcium is one of the many substances that reduces its absorption.

Generally, the drug's side effects are mild. The most common are diarrhea, nausea and abdominal pain.

QUICK REFERENCE

Drug group Drug for bone disorders (p.108)
Overdose danger rating Medium
Dependence rating Low
Prescription needed Yes
Available as generic No

INFORMATION FOR USERS

Your drug prescription is tailored for you. Do not alter dosage without checking with your physician.

How taken

Tablets.

Frequency and timing of doses
Once daily or once weekly; take with a full glass of water (not with juice or other drinks) 30 minutes before breakfast or at least 2 hours before or after food. Remain upright for 30 minutes after taking the drug.

Usual adult dosage range
Osteoporosis 5mg daily or 30mg once weekly.
Paget's disease 30mg daily for 2 months.

Onset of effect
It may take months to notice an improvement.

Duration of action
Some effects may persist for months or years.

Diet advice
Absorption of risedronate is reduced by foods and drinks, including dairy products such as milk. The drug should be taken on an empty stomach. The diet must contain adequate calcium and vitamin D; supplements may be given.

Storage
Keep in a closed container in a cool, dry place out of the reach of children.

Missed dose
Daily dose If you missed the dose by a few hours and you can take it on an empty stomach and remain upright for 30 minutes, take the missed dose now. If not, take the next dose at the usual time next morning.
Weekly dose Take the missed dose at the usual time on the next day. Do not take the weekly dose more than once a week.

Stopping the drug
Do not stop taking the drug without consulting your physician; the underlying condition may worsen.

Exceeding the dose
An occasional unintentional extra dose is unlikely to cause problems. Large overdoses may cause stomach problems including heartburn, irritation, and ulcers. Notify your physician at once, and try to remain upright.

SPECIAL PRECAUTIONS

Be sure to tell your physician if:
▼ You have an abnormality of the esophagus.
▼ You have stomach problems or a history of ulcers.
▼ You have unusual bone pain.
▼ You have impaired kidney function.
▼ You have had a previous allergic reaction to risedronate or other bisphosphonates.
▼ You have problems swallowing.
▼ You are unable to stay upright for 30 minutes.
▼ You have hypocalcemia.
▼ You are taking other medications.

Pregnancy
▼ Not recommended.

Breast-feeding
▼ Not recommended.

Infants and children
▼ Not recommended.

Over 60
▼ No special problems.

Driving and hazardous work
▼ No special problems.

Alcohol
▼ May cause stomach irritation.

POSSIBLE ADVERSE EFFECTS

The most common side effect caused by risedronate is diarrhea, which is more likely with higher doses.

Symptom/effect	Frequency		Discuss with physician		Stop taking drug now	Call physician now
	Common	Rare	Only if severe	In all cases		
Diarrhea	●		■			
Abdominal pain	●		■			
Nausea		●	■			
Rash/itching		●		■		
Bone pain	●		■			
Eye pain/redness/blurred vision		●		■		

INTERACTIONS

Antacids, calcium, and dairy products can decrease the absorption of risedronate. Take risedronate at least 30 minutes before any calcium tablets, calcium-rich foods or calcium-containing antacids.

Warfarin Risedronate could increase warfarin's effect. Careful monitoring is required.

PROLONGED USE

Treatment for osteoporosis may be given for several years. Initial response to therapy should be assessed by measuring bone mineral density after 1–2 years of use.

Monitoring Blood and urine tests may be carried out at intervals.

RISPERIDONE

Product name Risperdal
Used in the following combined preparations None

GENERAL INFORMATION

Risperidone is used to treat patients with acute psychiatric disorders, and long-term psychotic illness such as schizophrenia, and, in small doses, is used to manage behavioural disturbances in geriatric patients with dementia. Although not a cure, it helps to alleviate distressing symptoms. It is effective for relieving "positive" symptoms (such as hostility, and hallucinations) and "negative" symptoms (such as emotional and social withdrawal). It may also help with other symptoms often associated with schizophrenia, such as depression and anxiety. Risperidone has less of a sedative effect and is less likely to cause movement disorders as a *side effect* than some other antipsychotics.

QUICK REFERENCE

Drug group Antipsychotic drug (p.69)
Overdose danger rating Medium
Dependence rating Low
Prescription needed Yes
Available as generic Yes

INFORMATION FOR USERS

Your drug prescription is tailored for you. Do not alter dosage without checking with your physician.

How taken

Tablets, liquid.

Frequency and timing of doses
1–2 x daily.

Usual adult dosage range
Schizophrenia and related disorders 2mg daily (starting dose) increasing gradually to 4–6mg daily (usual maintenance dose); maximum 10mg daily.
Behavioural disturbances 0.25–0.5mg daily (starting dose) to a maximum of 2mg daily.

Onset of effect
Tablets Within 2–3 days, but may take up to 4 weeks before maximum effect is seen.

Duration of action
Approximately 2 days.

Diet advice
None.

Storage
Keep in a closed container in a cool, dry place out of the reach of children. Protect from light.

Missed dose
Take as soon as you remember. If your next dose is due within 3 hours, take a single dose now and skip the next.

Stopping the drug
Do not stop taking the drug without consulting your physician; symptoms may recur.

Exceeding the dose
An occasional unintentional extra dose is unlikely to cause problems. If larger doses have been taken, notify your physician.

SPECIAL PRECAUTIONS

Be sure to tell your physician if:
▼ You have liver or kidney problems.
▼ You have heart or circulation problems.
▼ You have had epileptic fits.
▼ You have Parkinson's disease.
▼ You are taking other medications.

Pregnancy
▼ Safety in pregnancy not established. Discuss with your physician.

Breast-feeding
▼ The drug probably passes into breast milk. Discuss with your physician.

Infants and children
▼ Not recommended under 15 years.

Over 60
▼ Reduced dose necessary.

Driving and hazardous work
▼ Avoid such activities until you have learned how risperidone affects you because the drug may cause difficulty in concentration and slowed reactions.

Alcohol
▼ Avoid. Alcohol may increase the sedative effects of this drug.

Surgery and general anesthetics
▼ Risperidone treatment may need to be stopped before you have a general anesthetic. Discuss this with your physician or dentist before any operation.

POSSIBLE ADVERSE EFFECTS

Risperidone is generally well tolerated with a low incidence of movement disorders. This drug is less sedating than some of the other antipsychotics.

Symptom/effect	Frequency		Discuss with physician		Stop taking drug now	Call physician now
	Common	Rare	Only if severe	In all cases		
Insomnia/anxiety/agitation	●		■			
Headache	●		■			
Difficulty in concentration	●		■			
Weight gain	●		■			
Shakiness/tremor	●			■		
Dizziness/drowsiness		●		■		
Rash		●		■		
Unusual thirst		●		■		
High fever/rigid muscles		●		■	▲	∎

INTERACTIONS

Sedatives All drugs that have a sedative effect on the central nervous system are likely to increase any sedative effect of risperidone.

Fluoxetine This drug increases the blood levels of risperidone and the risk of side effects.

Carbamazepine This drug reduces the effects of risperidone. Other liver-enzyme inducing drugs, e.g., phenytoin, may have the same effect.

Drugs for parkinsonism Risperidone may reduce the effect of these drugs.

PROLONGED USE

If used long term, permanent movement disorders (*tardive dyskinesia*) may occur, although they are less likely than with many other antipsychotic drugs.

RITUXIMAB

Product name Rituxan
Used in the following combined preparations None

GENERAL INFORMATION

Rituximab is in a class of medications called biologic agents. It is used to treat non-Hodgkin's lymphoma (NHL), a type of cancer which develops in white blood cells. In combination with another drug, methotrexate, it is also used in the treatment of rheumatoid arthritis (RA). This medication is given by injection as an intravenous infusion and is administered by a physician or a nurse. Infusion reactions, which include fever, shaking, chills, and a headache, may occur when the drug is administered. Medications such as acetaminophen and diphenhydramine are usually given prior to the infusion to minimize any infusion reaction.

INFORMATION FOR USERS

Your drug prescription is tailored for you. Do not alter dosage without checking with your physician.

How taken

Intravenous.

Frequency and timing of doses
For Non-Hodgkin's lymphoma: once weekly, initially for four doses; maintenance dose: every 3 months up to 2 years; dose may vary for other types of non-Hodgkin's disease medications. RA: 2 doses, 2 weeks apart.

Adult dosage range
Dose based on body surface area and calculated individually.

Onset of effect
Several days.

Duration of action
Several days.

Diet advice
None.

Storage
Usually stored at 2–8°C. Protect from light.

Missed dose
As this medication is administered by your physician or nurse, it is unlikely to be missed.

Stopping the drug
Do not stop the drug without consulting your physician. Stopping the drug may lead to worsening of the underlying condition.

OVERDOSE ACTION

 Seek immediate medical advice. Get help right away and notify your physician.

POSSIBLE ADVERSE EFFECTS

Infusion reactions such as fever, chills, and headache are common in the first few hours.

Symptom/effect	Frequency		Discuss with physician		Stop taking drug now	Call physician now
	Common	Rare	Only if severe	In all cases		
Rash, swollen lips/tongue		●				▮
Difficulty breathing/swallowing		●				▮
Blurred vision, headache		●				▮
Irregular heartbeat		●				▮
Fast breathing/anxiety		●				▮
Chest pain/weakness		●				▮
Skin blisters, sores		●				▮
Nausea/vomiting/heartburn	●		▮			
Sore throat, fever, chills		●		▮		▮
Muscle or back pain	●		▮			
Night sweats	●		▮			
Burning/tingling of hands /feet	●		▮			
Diarrhea	●		▮			
Abdominal pain		●				▮

INTERACTIONS

Biologic agents and disease modifying drugs (except methotrexate) If used together, monitor for signs of infection.

Cisplatin Caution in using this drug with rituximab as it may affect kidney function.

SPECIAL PRECAUTIONS

Be sure to tell your physician if:
▼ You have had a cancer of the white blood cells or of the immune system.
▼ You have an irregular heartbeat.
▼ You have any type of infection now or previously that took a long time to be treated.
▼ You have hepatitis B or an infection with other viruses such as chicken pox or West Nile virus.
▼ You have heart or lung disease.
▼ You are taking other medications.
▼ You have an autoimmune disease.

 Pregnancy
▼ Not usually prescribed. Safety in pregnancy not established. Discuss with your physician.

 Breast-feeding
▼ Safety not established. Discuss with your physician.

 Infants and children
▼ Not recommended.

 Over 60
▼ No special problems.

 Driving and hazardous work
▼ No special problems.

 Alcohol
▼ Avoid excessive amounts. Alcohol may increase the risk of developing liver problems with this drug.

PROLONGED USE

Usually only used for a defined period. Due to many potential side effects, close monitoring required.

Monitoring Regular monitoring of blood cells and for signs of infection.

RIVASTIGMINE

Product name Exelon
Used in the following combined preparations None

GENERAL INFORMATION

Rivastigmine is an inhibitor of the enzyme anticholinesterase. This enzyme breaks down the naturally occurring *neurotransmitter* acetylcholine to limit its effects. Blocking the enzyme raises the levels of acetylcholine which, in the brain, increases alertness. It has been found that rivastigmine can improve the symptoms of mild to moderate dementia in Alzheimer's disease, and is used to slow the rate of deterioration in that disease. The drug is not currently recommended for dementia due to other causes. It is usual to assess anyone being treated with rivastigmine after about three months to decide whether the drug is helping and whether it is worth continuing the treatment. As the disease progresses, the benefit obtained may diminish.

Side effects may include agitation, confusion and depression, which could be thought due to Alzheimer's disease. Weight loss should be monitored.

INFORMATION FOR USERS

Your drug prescription is tailored for you. Do not alter dosage without checking with your physician.

How taken

Capsules, liquid, skin patch.

Frequency and timing of doses
2 x daily.

Usual adult dosage range
3mg daily (starting dose); 6–12mg daily (maintenance dose).

Onset of effect
30–60 minutes.

Duration of action
8–12 hours.

Diet advice
None.

Storage
Keep in a closed container in a cool, dry place out of the reach of children.

Missed dose
Take as soon as you remember. If your next dose is due within 4 hours, take a single dose now and skip the next. A carer should be overseeing the taking of tablets.

Stopping the drug
Do not stop the drug without consulting your physician; symptoms may recur.

Exceeding the dose
An occasional unintentional extra dose is unlikely to be a problem. Large overdoses may cause nausea, vomiting, and diarrhea. Notify your physician.

POSSIBLE ADVERSE EFFECTS

Adverse effects include mental changes and intestinal problems. Although common, these effects are usually quite mild. However, women may be more susceptible to nausea, vomiting, and weight loss.

Symptom/effect	Frequency		Discuss with physician		Stop taking drug now	Call physician now
	Common	Rare	Only if severe	In all cases		
Reduced appetite/weight loss	●			■		
Nausea/abdominal pain	●			■		
Agitation/confusion/depression	●			■		
Drowsiness/dizziness	●			■		
Weakness/trembling	●			■		
Headache/insomnia	●		■			
Sweating/malaise	●		■			
Convulsions		●		■		

INTERACTIONS

General note Rivastigmine is a relatively new drug and known interactions with other drugs are not fully established. If you notice changes in the effect of the drug after taking or stopping other medications, discuss this with your physician.

Muscle relaxants used in surgery Rivastigmine may increase the effects of some muscle relaxants, but it may also block the effects of some others.

SPECIAL PRECAUTIONS

Be sure to tell your physician if:
▼ You have a heart problem.
▼ You have liver or kidney problems.
▼ You have asthma or respiratory problems.
▼ You have had a gastric or duodenal ulcer.
▼ You are taking other medications.

Pregnancy
▼ Safety in pregnancy not established.

Breast-feeding
▼ Not recommended.

Infants and children
▼ Not recommended.

Over 60
▼ No special problems.

Driving and hazardous work
▼ Your underlying condition may make such activities inadvisable. Discuss with your physician.

Alcohol
▼ Avoid. Alcohol increases the sedative effects of rivastigmine.

Surgery and general anesthetics
▼ Treatment with rivastigmine may need to be stopped before you have a general anesthetic. Discuss this with your physician or dentist before any operation.

PROLONGED USE

May be continued for as long as there is benefit. Stopping the drug leads to a gradual loss of the improvements.

Monitoring Periodic checks may be performed to test whether the drug is still providing some benefit.

RIZATRIPTAN

Product names Maxalt, Maxalt RPD
Used in the following combined preparations None

GENERAL INFORMATION

Rizatriptan is a highly effective drug for migraine, usually given when people fail to respond to analgesics (such as ASA and acetaminophen). The drug is very beneficial in the treatment of acute migraine attacks, whether or not they are preceded by an aura, but is not meant to be taken regularly to prevent attacks. Rizatriptan is also used for the acute treatment of cluster headache

(a form of migraine headache). It should be taken as soon as possible after the onset of the attack. Rizatriptan relieves the symptoms of migraine by preventing the dilation of blood vessels in the brain that causes the attack.

The recommended daily maximum is 20mg per day. If you need to use rizatriptan for more than 10 days per month, discuss this with your physician.

INFORMATION FOR USERS

Your drug prescription is tailored for you. Do not alter dosage without checking with your physician.

How taken

Tablets, rapidly disintegrating tablet-wafer (RPD).

Frequency and timing of doses
Should be taken as soon as possible after the onset of an attack. However, it is equally effective at whatever stage it is taken. The dose may be repeated once no sooner than TWO HOURS AFTER; no more than 20mg should be taken in any 24 hour period. RPD to be placed on the tongue (will dissolve).

Usual adult dosage range
Tablets or wafers usual dose: 5mg; some may require 10mg (maximum 24 hour dose: 20mg).

Onset of effect
1–2.5 hours.

Duration of action
3–6 hours.

Diet advice
None unless otherwise advised.

Storage
Keep in a closed container in a cool, dry place out of the reach of children. Protect from light.

Missed dose
Not applicable (taken only to treat a migraine attack).

Stopping the drug
Taken only to treat a migraine attack.

Exceeding the dose
An occasional unintentional extra dose is unlikely to cause concerns. But if you notice any unusual symptoms or if a large overdose has been taken, notify your physician.

POSSIBLE ADVERSE EFFECTS

Many of the adverse effects will disappear after about 1 hour as your body becomes adjusted to the medicine. If the symptoms persist or are severe, contact your physician.

Symptom/effect	Frequency		Discuss with physician		Stop taking drug now	Call physician now
	Common	Rare	Only if severe	In all cases		
Nausea	●		■			
Drowsiness/dizziness	●		■			
Tiredness	●		■			
Headache	●		■			
Dry mouth	●		■			
Chest pain		●		■		▮
Mental/mood changes		●		■		▮
Vision changes		●		■		▮
Cold/tingling/numb hand		●		■		▮

INTERACTIONS

Propranolol, SSRI type of antidepressants These drugs may increase the effect of rizatriptan. A lower dose of rizatriptan is recommended for those on these medications. Discuss with your physician or pharmacist.

Almotriptan, dihydroergotamine, eletriptan, ergotamine, methysergide,
naratriptan, sumatriptan, zolmitriptan Rizatriptan should not be taken within 24 hours of having used one of these drugs.

Moclobemide, phenelzine, tranylcypromine Rizatriptan should not be used within 2 weeks of having used these drugs.

SPECIAL PRECAUTIONS

Be sure to tell your physician if:
▼ You have liver or kidney problems.
▼ You have heart problems.
▼ You have high blood pressure.
▼ You have high cholesterol.
▼ You have had a heart attack.
▼ You have angina.
▼ You have phenylketonuria.
▼ You are allergic to some medicines or other triptans.
▼ You are taking other medications.

Pregnancy
▼ Safety in pregnancy not established. Discuss with your physician.

Breast-feeding
▼ Safety in breast-feeding not established. Discuss with your physician.

Infants and children
▼ Not recommended.

Over 60
▼ Not recommended for patients over 65 years of age.

Driving and hazardous work
▼ Avoid such activities until you have learned how rizatriptan affects you because the drug can cause drowsiness.

Alcohol
▼ No special problems, but some drinks may provoke migraine in some people (p.69).

Surgery and general anesthetics
▼ Notify your physician or dentist if you have used rizatriptan within 48 hours prior to surgery.

PROLONGED USE

Rizatriptan should not be used continuously to prevent migraine but only to treat migraine attacks.

ROSIGLITAZONE

Product name Avandia
Used in the following combined preparation Avandamet, Avandaryl

GENERAL INFORMATION

Rosiglitazone is used to treat non-insulin-dependent diabetes mellitus (NIDDM, Type 2 diabetes). It works by reducing insulin resistance in fatty tissue, skeletal muscle, and in the liver, which leads to a reduction of blood glucose levels. The effects appear gradually and reach their full extent in about 8 weeks.

The drug is usually prescribed with metformin or a sulfonylurea (p.128)

if metformin is contraindicated. The combined treatment can produce a significant improvement in diabetic control. Rosiglitazone works better in obese diabetics, although it often causes weight gain. Anemia is another adverse effect.

Rosiglitazone is not approved for use with insulin. This drug is not used in individuals with heart failure.

INFORMATION FOR USERS

Your drug prescription is tailored for you. Do not alter dosage without checking with your physician.

How taken

Tablets.

Frequency and timing of doses
1–2 x daily.

Usual adult dosage range
4–8mg daily.

Onset of effect
60 minutes; it can take 8 weeks for full effects to appear.

Duration of action
12–24 hours.

Diet advice
An individualized low fat, low sugar diet must be maintained in order for the drug to be fully

effective. Follow your physician's advice.

Storage
Keep in a closed container in a cool dry place out of the reach of children.

Missed dose
Take as soon as you remember. If your next dose is due within 2 hours, take a single dose now and skip the next.

Stopping the drug
Do not stop taking the drug without consulting your physician; stopping the drug may lead to worsening of the underlying condition.

OVERDOSE ACTION

 Seek immediate medical advice in all cases. Take emergency action if loss of consciousness occurs.

See Drug poisoning emergency guide (p.526).

SPECIAL PRECAUTIONS

Be sure to tell your physician if:
▼ You have liver problems.
▼ You are anemic.
▼ You have heart failure.
▼ You have severe kidney failure.
▼ You are taking other medications.
▼ You are not using birth control.
▼ You have shortness of breath or are easily fatigued.
▼ You have osteoporosis or a decrease in bone mineral density.

 Pregnancy
▼ Safety not established. Discuss with your physician.

 Breast-feeding
▼ Safety not established. Discuss with your physician.

 Infants and children
▼ Not recommended.

 Over 60
▼ No special problems.

 Driving and hazardous work
▼ No known problems.

 Alcohol
▼ No known problems.

POSSIBLE ADVERSE EFFECTS

Fatigue and weakness (as a result of anemia) and weight gain (even on a strict diabetic diet) are two of the more common side effects of rosiglitazone.

Symptom/effect	Frequency		Discuss with physician		Stop taking drug now	Call physician now
	Common	Rare	Only if severe	In all cases		
Nausea/abdominal pain		●	■			■
Indigestion/flatulence	●		■			
Fatigue/weakness	●			■		
Headache	●			■		
Weight gain	●			■		
Dark urine		●		■		
Dizziness/pins and needles		●		■		
Sleepiness		●		■		
Edema (swelling)		●		■		■
Painful breathing/night cough		●		■		
Blurred vision		●		■		

PROLONGED USE

Rosiglitazone, like other antidiabetic drugs, is used indefinitely.

Monitoring Periodic blood tests of liver function and hemoglobin levels will be performed. Heart performance will be monitored regularly. Weight will be measured at intervals

INTERACTIONS

Paclitaxel may reduce the metabolism and increase the effects of rosiglitazone.

ACE inhibitors may increase the effects of rosiglitazone.

Diazoxide reduces the effects of rosiglitazone.

ROSUVASTATIN

Product name Crestor
Used in the following combined preparations None

GENERAL INFORMATION

Rosuvastatin is a lipid-lowering drug belonging to the class of drugs called statins. It blocks the action of an enzyme needed for the formation of cholesterol in the liver, and as a result the blood levels of cholesterol are lowered. The drug is prescribed for people who will benefit from the lowering of their blood cholesterol level and have not responded to a special diet, and are at risk of developing or have existing coronary heart disease.

Rosuvastatin is usually taken once a day, with or without food, and should be taken at the same time daily. The drug should be continued even when cholesterol levels are normal as the benefits seen with this class of drugs are long-term. Side effects are usually mild. Rosuvastatin may raise the levels of various liver enzymes. These enzymes are monitored periodically and do not usually indicate serious liver damage.

INFORMATION FOR USERS

Your drug prescription is tailored for you. Do not alter dosage without checking with your physician.

How taken

Tablets.

Frequency and timing of doses
Usually once daily.

Adult dosage range
5–40mg daily.

Onset of effect
2–4 weeks to see a change in cholesterol levels.

Duration of action
Up to 24 hours.

Diet advice
A diet low in saturated fat and cholesterol.

Storage
Keep in a closed container in a cool, dry place out of the reach of children.

Missed dose
If you miss a dose, take it as soon as you remember. If it is near the time of the next dose, skip the missed dose and resume your usual dosing schedule.

Stopping the drug
Do not stop the drug without consulting your physician. Stopping the drug may lead to worsening of the underlying condition.

Exeeding the dose
An occasional unintentional extra dose is unlikely to cause problems. Large overdoses may cause liver problems. Notify your physician.

SPECIAL PRECAUTIONS

Be sure to tell your physician if:
▼ You have liver or kidney problems.
▼ You have eye or vision problems.
▼ You have muscle weakness.
▼ You have a thyroid disorder.
▼ You have had problems with alcohol abuse.
▼ You have porphyria.
▼ You have angina.
▼ You have high blood pressure.
▼ You are taking other medications.

Pregnancy
▼ Contraindicated in pregnancy.

Breast-feeding
▼ Safety not established. Discuss with your physician.

Infants and children
▼ Not recommended.

Over 60
▼ No special problems.

Driving and hazardous work
▼ No special problems.

Alcohol
▼ Avoid excessive amounts. Alcohol may increase the risk of developing liver problems with this drug.

POSSIBLE ADVERSE EFFECTS

Common side effects of Rosuvastatin include nausea and constipation. If muscle pain or weakness occurs, talk to your doctor.

Symptom/effect	Frequency		Discuss with physician		Stop taking drug now	Call physician now
	Common	Rare	Only if severe	In all cases		
Abdominal pain	●		■			
Nausea	●		■			
Constipation	●		■			
Headache	●		■			
Rash		●		■	▲	
Jaundice		●		■		
Muscle pain/weakness		●		■		■

INTERACTIONS

Antacids These may decrease the amount of rosuvastatin that is absorbed. Take antacid at least 2 hours after taking rosuvastatin.

Cyclosporine and Gemfibrozil Both can increase the level of rosuvastatin in the blood and increase the risk for adverse effects; dosage adjustment is recommended.

Warfarin Rosuvastatin may increase the effect of warfarin. INR should be monitored before starting rosuvastatin and periodically after.

Lopinavir/ritonavir These drugs can increase the level of rosuvastatin and increase its adverse effects.

PROLONGED USE

Prolonged treatment can adversely affect liver function.

Monitoring Regular blood tests to check liver enzymes are recommended. Tests of muscle enzymes may be carried out if problems are suspected.

SALBUTAMOL

Product names Airomir, Ventodisks, Ventolin, and others
Used in the following combined preparations Combivent

GENERAL INFORMATION

Salbutamol is a *sympathomimetic bronchodilator* that relaxes the muscle surrounding the bronchioles (airways in the lungs).

This drug is used to relieve symptoms of asthma, chronic bronchitis, and emphysema. Although it can be taken by mouth, inhalation is considered more effective because the drug is delivered directly to the bronchioles, thus giving rapid relief, allowing smaller doses, and causing fewer *side effects*.

Compared with some similar drugs, it has little stimulant effect on the heart rate and blood pressure, making it safer for people with heart problems or high blood pressure. Because salbutamol relaxes the muscles of the uterus, it may also be used to prevent premature labour.

The most common side effect of salbutamol is fine tremor of the hands, which may interfere with precise manual work. Anxiety, tension, and restlessness may also occur.

INFORMATION FOR USERS

Your drug prescription is tailored for you. Do not alter dosage without checking with your physician.

How taken

Liquid, injection, inhaler, powder for inhalation, inhalation solution.

Frequency and timing of doses
1–2 inhalations 3–4 x daily (inhaler); 3–4 x daily (liquid).

Usual adult dosage range
400–800mcg daily (inhaler); 6–16mg daily (by mouth).

Onset of effect
Within 5–15 minutes (inhaler); within 30–60 minutes (by mouth).

Duration of action
Up to 6 hours (inhaler); up to 8 hours (by mouth).

Diet advice
None.

Storage
Keep in a closed container in a cool, dry place out of the reach of children. Protect from light. Do not puncture or burn inhalers.

Missed dose
Take as soon as you remember if you need it. If your next dose is due within 2 hours, take a single dose now and skip the next.

Stopping the drug
Do not stop the drug without consulting your physician; symptoms may recur.

Exceeding the dose
An occasional unintentional extra dose is unlikely to be a cause for concern. But if you notice any unusual symptoms, or if a large overdose has been taken, notify your physician.

SPECIAL PRECAUTIONS

Be sure to tell your physician if:
▼ You have heart problems.
▼ You have high blood pressure.
▼ You have an overactive thyroid gland.
▼ You have diabetes.
▼ You are taking other medications.

Pregnancy
▼ No evidence of risk when used to treat asthma, or to treat or prevent premature labour. Discuss with your physician.

Breast-feeding
▼ The drug passes into the breast milk, but at normal doses adverse effects on the baby are unlikely. Discuss with your physician.

Infants and children
▼ Reduced dose necessary.

Over 60
▼ Increased likelihood of adverse effects. Reduced dose may therefore be necessary.

Driving and hazardous work
▼ Avoid such activities until you have learned how salbutamol affects you because the drug can cause tremors.

Alcohol
▼ No known problems.

POSSIBLE ADVERSE EFFECTS

Muscle tremor, which particularly affects the hands, anxiety, and restlessness are the most common adverse effects. Palpitations and headache are rare.

Symptom/effect	Frequency		Discuss with physician		Stop taking drug now	Call physician now
	Common	Rare	Only if severe	In all cases		
Anxiety/nervous tension	●		■			
Tremor	●		■			
Restlessness	●		■			
Headache		●		■		
Palpitations		●		■	▲	
Muscle cramps		●		■		

INTERACTIONS

Theophylline There is a risk of low potassium levels in the blood occurring if this drug is taken with salbutamol.

Monoamine oxidase inhibitors (MAOIs) can interact with salbutamol to produce a dangerous rise in blood pressure.

Other sympathomimetic drugs may increase the effects of salbutamol, thereby also increasing the risk of adverse effects.

Beta blockers Drugs in this group may reduce the action of salbutamol.

PROLONGED USE

No problems expected. However, you should contact your physician if you find you are needing to use your salbutamol inhaler more than usual or are increasing frequency of use to more than 8 puffs in 24 hours. Failure to respond to the drug may be a result of worsening asthma that requires urgent medical attention.

Monitoring Periodic blood tests for potassium may be needed in people on high-dose treatment with salbutamol combined with other asthma drugs.

SALMETEROL

Product name Serevent
Used in the following combined preparation Advair

GENERAL INFORMATION

Salmeterol is a *sympathomimetic* bronchodilator used to treat conditions, such as asthma and bronchospasm, in which the airways become constricted. Its advantage over salbutamol (p.424) is that it is longer acting.

Salmeterol relaxes the muscle surrounding the airways in the lungs but, because of its slow onset of effect,

it is not used for immediate relief of symptoms of asthma. It is prescribed to prevent attacks, however, and can be helpful in preventing night-time asthma.

Taken by inhalation, salmeterol is delivered directly to the airways. This allows smaller doses to be taken and reduces the risk of *adverse effects*.

QUICK REFERENCE

Drug group Bronchodilator (p.76), and drug to treat asthma (p.77)

Overdose danger rating Low

Dependence rating Low

Prescription needed Yes

Available as generic No

INFORMATION FOR USERS

Your drug prescription is tailored for you. Do not alter dosage without checking with your physician.

How taken

Inhaler, powder for inhalation.

Frequency and timing of doses
2 x daily.

Usual adult dosage range
100mcg daily (2 inhalations twice daily).

Onset of effect
10–20 minutes.

Duration of action
12 hours.

Diet advice
None.

Storage
Keep in a cool, dry place out of the reach of children.

Missed dose
Take as soon as you remember. If your next dose is due within 4 hours, take a single dose now and skip the next.

Stopping the drug
Do not stop the drug without consulting your physician; symptoms may recur.

Exceeding the dose
An occasional unintentional extra dose is unlikely to be a cause for concern. But if you notice any unusual symptoms, or if a large overdose has been taken, notify your physician.

SPECIAL PRECAUTIONS

Be sure to tell your physician if:
▼ You have heart problems.
▼ You have high blood pressure.
▼ You have an overactive thyroid.
▼ You have diabetes.
▼ You are taking other medications.

Pregnancy
▼ No evidence of risk when used to treat asthma. Discuss with your physician.

Breast-feeding
▼ The drug passes into the breast milk, but at normal doses adverse effects on the baby are unlikely. Discuss with your physician.

Infants and children
▼ Reduced dose necessary. Not recommended for children under 4 years.

Over 60
▼ No special problems.

Driving and hazardous work
▼ No special problems.

Alcohol
▼ No known problems.

POSSIBLE ADVERSE EFFECTS

Side effects are usually mild. If wheezing and breathlessness (paradoxical bronchospasm) occur, stop taking the drug and notify your physician immediately.

Symptom/effect	Frequency		Discuss with physician		Stop taking drug now	Call physician now
	Common	Rare	Only if severe	In all cases		
Tremor	●		■			
Palpitations		●		■		
Headache		●		■		
Sudden breathlessness		●		■	▲	■

INTERACTIONS

Corticosteroids, theophylline, and diuretics There is an increased risk of low blood potassium levels when high doses of salmeterol are taken with these drugs.

PROLONGED USE

Salmeterol is intended to be used long term. The main problem comes from using combinations of anti-asthma drugs, leading to low blood potassium levels.

Monitoring Periodic blood tests are usually carried out to monitor potassium levels.

SELEGILINE

Product name Novo-Selegiline
Used in the following combined preparation None

GENERAL INFORMATION

Selegiline, also known as deprenyl, is an inhibitor of an enzyme in the brain called monoamine oxidase type B (MAO-B). It is used alone or together with levodopa or levodopa-carbidopa combination to treat Parkinson's disease. In patients newly diagnosed with Parkinson's disease, selegiline may delay the need to start levodopa treatment and may help to slow the progress of the disease itself. In combination with levodopa, it works to increase and extend the effects of levodopa.

At usual doses of up to 10mg, there are no dietary restrictions. However, if the maximum recommended daily dose of 10mg is exceeded, the risk of dangerous reactions, such as sudden elevation of blood pressure, is increased if selegiline is taken with foods that are high in tyramine content. These foods include mature cheeses, pickled herring, red wine, and other foods that are aged or fermented, including beer.

QUICK REFERENCE

Drug group Antiparkinsonism drug (p.71)
Overdose danger rating High
Dependence rating Low
Prescription needed Yes
Available as generic Yes

INFORMATION FOR USERS

Your drug prescription is tailored for you. Do not alter dosage without checking with your physician.

How taken

Tablets.

Frequency and timing of doses
2 x daily (breakfast and lunch).

Usual adult dosage range
2.5–10mg daily.

Onset of effect
30 minutes to 2 hours.

Duration of action
Variable.

Diet advice
No restrictions on food or beverages when taken in doses of 10mg/day or less.

Storage
Keep in a cool, dry place out of the reach of children. Protect from light.

Missed dose
Take as soon as you remember. If your next dose is due within 2 hours, take a single dose now and skip the next.

Stopping the drug
Do not stop the drug without consulting your physician; symptoms may recur.

OVERDOSE ACTION

 Seek immediate medical advice in all cases. Take emergency action if chest pain or loss of consciousness occurs.

See Drug poisoning emergency guide (p.526).

POSSIBLE ADVERSE EFFECTS

The adverse effects associated with selegiline, when taken in combination with levodopa, are usually related to excess levodopa and may require a dosage adjustment. Some of the most serious adverse reactions occurring with the combination are hallucinations and confusion, particularly visual hallucinations.

Severe headache, nausea, and/or vomiting or unexplained sweating require immediate medical attention.

Symptom/effect	Frequency		Discuss with physician		Stop taking drug now	Call physician now
	Common	Rare	Only if severe	In all cases		
Nausea	●			■		
Dizziness/faintness	●			■		
Hallucinations		●		■		▌
Dry mouth		●	■			
Severe headache/chest pains		●		■	▲	▌
Diarrhea		●		■		

INTERACTIONS

General note Because of the wide range of possible drug interactions with selegiline, do not take any medication, whether prescription or nonprescription, without first consulting your physician or pharmacist.

Meperidine, SSRIs, e.g. fluoxetine, and tricyclic antidepressants The combination of selegiline with any of these drugs may cause severe and dangerous reactions. Allow at least 14 days after stopping selegiline before taking fluoxetine.

SPECIAL PRECAUTIONS

Be sure to tell your physician if:
▼ You have impaired liver function.
▼ You have a peptic ulcer.
▼ You are taking other medications.

 Pregnancy
▼ Safety in pregnancy not established. Discuss with your physician.

 Breast-feeding
▼ It is not known if the drug passes into the breast milk. Discuss with your physician.

 Infants and children
▼ Not recommended.

 Over 60
▼ Increased likelihood of adverse effects. Reduced dose may therefore be necessary.

 Driving and hazardous work
▼ Avoid such activities until you have learned how the drug affects you; it can cause dizziness.

 Alcohol
▼ Avoid. Alcohol may increase the risk of adverse effects.

Surgery and general anesthetics
▼ Selegiline treatment should be withdrawn at least 2 weeks before you have a general anesthetic and some dental treatments. Discuss this with your physician or dentist before any surgery.

PROLONGED USE

No problems expected.

SERTRALINE

Product name Zoloft
Used in the following combined preparations None

GENERAL INFORMATION

Sertraline is a member of the group of antidepressants called selective serotonin re-uptake inhibitors (SSRIs). These drugs tend to cause less sedation and have different side effects from older types of antidepressants. Sertraline elevates mood, increases physical activity, and restores interest in everyday activities. It is used to treat depression, including accompanying anxiety, and obsessive-compulsive disorder. Sertraline is also prescribed for post-traumatic stress disorder in women; it has not been shown to work in men with this condition.

The drug is usually stopped gradually, because symptoms such as headache, nausea, and dizziness may occur if sertraline is withdrawn suddenly.

QUICK REFERENCE

Drug group Antidepressant (p.68)
Overdose danger rating Medium
Dependence rating Low
Prescription needed Yes
Available as generic Yes

INFORMATION FOR USERS

Your drug prescription is tailored for you. Do not alter dosage without checking with your physician.

How taken

Capsules.

Frequency and timing of doses
Once daily, with meal.

Usual adult dosage range
50–200mg daily.

Onset of effect
Some benefits may appear within 14 days, but full effects may take up to 4 weeks.

Duration of action
24 hours.

Diet advice
None.

Storage
Keep in a closed container in a cool, dry place out of the reach of children.

Missed dose
Take as soon as you remember. If your next dose is due within 8 hours, take a single dose now and skip the next.

Stopping the drug
Do not stop the drug without consulting your physician, who may supervise a gradual reduction in dosage.

Exceeding the dose
An occasional unintentional extra dose is unlikely to cause problems. Large overdoses may cause adverse effects. Notify your physician.

POSSIBLE ADVERSE EFFECTS

The most common side effects caused by sertraline are restlessness, insomnia, and gastrointestinal problems.

Symptom/effect	Frequency		Discuss with physician		Stop taking drug now	Call physician now
	Common	Rare	Only if severe	In all cases		
Nausea	●		■			
Diarrhea/loose stools	●		■			
Loss of appetite/indigestion	●		■			
Insomnia/sleepiness/anxiety	●		■			
Dizziness/tremor/confusion		●		■		
Palpitations/fainting		●		■		
Sexual dysfunction		●		■		
Rash/itching/skin eruptions		●	■		▲	▮

INTERACTIONS

General note Any drug that affects the breakdown of others in the liver may alter blood levels of sertraline, and vice versa.

St John's wort There is a danger of greatly increasing the effects of both substances.

Monoamine oxidase inhibitors (MAOIs) Sertraline's effects and toxicity are greatly increased by MAOIs.

Antiepileptics Sertraline opposes the effects of these drugs and increases the risk of seizures.

Clozapine and haloperidol The levels and effects of these drugs are increased by sertraline.

SPECIAL PRECAUTIONS

Be sure to tell your physician if:
▼ You have long-term liver or kidney problems.
▼ You have had epileptic fits.
▼ You have heart problems.
▼ You have a history of bleeding disorders.
▼ You have diabetes.
▼ You have glaucoma.
▼ You have had an allergic reaction to any SSRI.
▼ You have a history of mania.
▼ You are taking other medications.

Pregnancy
▼ Safety not established. Discuss with your physician.

Breast-feeding
▼ Safety not established. Discuss with your physician.

Infants and children
▼ Not recommended for children under 6 years. For children over 6 years with obsessive-compulsive disorder, reduced dose necessary.

Over 60
▼ No special problems.

Driving and hazardous work
▼ Avoid such activities until you know how sertraline affects you because the drug can cause drowsiness, dizziness, visual disturbances, and hallucinations.

Alcohol
▼ Avoid. SSRIs may increase the sedative effects of alcohol.

PROLONGED USE

No known problems.

SIBUTRAMINE

Product name Meridia
Used in the following combined preparations None

GENERAL INFORMATION

Sibutramine acts on brain *neuro-transmitters*. The drug is used to suppress appetite in people who are obese (*Body Mass Index (BMI)* of 30 or higher) or overweight (BMI greater than 27) and who have a condition such as Type 2 diabetes (p.128) or high blood lipid levels (p.89). Losing weight reduces the risk of stroke, improves the control of diabetes and gallstones, and reduces the load on joints in conditions such as osteoarthritis.

The drug treatment must be accompanied by a suitable diet. The drug is prescribed when diet alone has failed. Lifestyle changes also need to be made to avoid weight being regained when the drug is withdrawn. Psychological help from a support group is beneficial for some people.

INFORMATION FOR USERS

Your drug prescription is tailored for you. Do not alter dosage without checking with your physician.

How taken

Capsules.

Frequency and timing of doses
Once daily, in the morning.

Usual adult dosage range
10–15mg daily.

Onset of effect
30–60 minutes.

Duration of action
24 hours.

Diet advice
Low fat, low calorie diet.

Storage
Keep in a closed container (the original pack) in a cool, dry place out of the reach of children.

Missed dose
Take as soon as you remember. If your next dose is due within 12 hours, wait until you are due to take the next dose.

Stopping the drug
Do not stop taking the drug without consulting your physician. Stopping the drug may result in your gaining weight again.

Exceeding the dose
An occasional unintentional extra dose is unlikely to cause problems. Large overdoses may cause adverse effects. Notify your physician.

SPECIAL PRECAUTIONS

Be sure to tell your physician if:
▼ You have high blood pressure.
▼ You have a psychiatric illness.
▼ You have heart problems.
▼ You have an overactive thyroid.
▼ You have prostate problems.
▼ You have pheochromocytoma.
▼ You have glaucoma.
▼ You have a history of drug abuse.
▼ You are taking other medications.
▼ You have had a stroke.
▼ You have a history of an eating disorder such as anorexia or bulimia.

 Pregnancy
▼ Safety not established. Weight reducing drugs should not be used in pregnancy.

 Breast-feeding
▼ It is not known whether sibutramine is secreted in breast milk. Do not use the drug during the period when you are breast-feeding.

 Infants and children
▼ Not recommended under 18 years.

 Over 60
▼ Not recommended for people over 65 years.

 Driving and hazardous work
▼ Avoid until you have learned how sibutramine affects you because the drug may cause light-headedness, blurred vision, seizures, and impaired thinking.

 Alcohol
▼ Alcohol contains calories and should not be part of a diet supported by sibutramine.

POSSIBLE ADVERSE EFFECTS

The most common side effects are on the cardiovascular system.

Symptom/effect	Frequency		Discuss with physician		Stop taking drug now	Call physician now
	Common	Rare	Only if severe	In all cases		
Constipation/hemorrhoids	●		■			
Dry mouth	●		■			
Nausea	●		■			
Insomnia/anxiety	●		■			
Palpitations/rapid heart beat	●			■		
Lightheadedness	●		■			
Headache	●		■			
Hot flushes/sweating	●		■			

INTERACTIONS

Erythromycin, clarithromycin, cyclosporine, ketoconazole, and itraconazole These drugs increase blood levels and the effects of sibutramine.

Cough and cold remedies may possibly add to sibutramine's blood pressure-raising effect.

Dihydroergotamine, sumatriptan, SSRIs, St John's wort, and some opioid analgesics Not recommended to be used with sibutramine. All these drugs inhibit serotonin re-uptake and can increase the effects of sibutramine.

PROLONGED USE

Sibutramine is used for up to 1 year only.

Monitoring Pulse rate and blood pressure will be checked regularly. Body weight will be checked at intervals. If weight loss is insufficient (less than 5 per cent of body weight), the drug will be stopped.

SILDENAFIL

Product names Revatio, Viagra
Used in the following combined preparations None

GENERAL INFORMATION

Sildenafil is a drug that is used to treat impotence. It does not cause an erection directly, but it produces a chemical change that prevents the muscle walls of the blood-filled chambers in the penis from relaxing. This drug is also used in the treatment of pulmonary arterial hypertension (PAH).

When used for impotence, sildenafil only needs to be taken before sexual activity to produce an erection.

Because it is a vasodilator, sildenafil can cause a small fall in blood pressure while it is active, and it may increase the effect of antihypertensive drugs. The drug is not usually prescribed with nitrates (see p.84) because it greatly increases their effects.

(see p.84)

QUICK REFERENCE

Drug group Drug for impotence (p.152)

Overdose danger rating Medium

Dependence rating Low

Prescription needed Yes

Available as generic No

INFORMATION FOR USERS

Your drug prescription is tailored for you. Do not alter dosage without checking with your physician.

How taken

Tablets.

Frequency and timing of doses
Erectile dysfunction (ED): maximum once daily, usually 1 hour before sexual activity; pulmonary hypertension (PH): 3 x daily.

Usual adult dosage range
ED: 25–100mg; PH: 60mg.

Onset of effect
30 minutes.

Duration of action
4 hours.

Diet advice
None, although sildenafil will take longer to work after a meal, especially a high fat meal. It is absorbed faster on an empty stomach.

Storage
Keep in a closed container in a cool, dry place out of the reach of children.

Missed dose
Take the next dose when you need to. Do not use more than one dose in a 24-hour period.

Stopping the drug
Can be safely stopped as soon as you no longer need it.

Exceeding the dose
An occasional unintentional extra dose is unlikely to cause problems. Large overdoses may cause headache, dizziness, flushing, altered vision, and nasal congestion. Notify your physician.

SPECIAL PRECAUTIONS

Be sure to tell your physician if:
▼ You have heart problems.
▼ You have had a stroke or heart attack.
▼ You have sickle cell anemia.
▼ You have multiple myeloma.
▼ You have leukemia.
▼ You have liver or kidney problems.
▼ You have an inherited eye problem.
▼ You have an abnormality of the penis.
▼ You are taking a nitrate drug.
▼ You are taking other medications.

Pregnancy
▼ Not prescribed.

Breast-feeding
▼ Not prescribed.

Infants and children
▼ Not prescribed under 18 years.

Over 60
▼ Reduced dose may be necessary.

Driving and hazardous work
▼ Avoid such activities until you have learned how sildenafil affects you because the drug can cause dizziness and altered vision.

Alcohol
▼ No special problems.

PROLONGED USE

No problems expected.

POSSIBLE ADVERSE EFFECTS

Most *adverse effects* of sildenafil are common. However, if priapism (a persistent, painful erection) occurs, you should discontinue the drug and consult your physician.

Symptom/effect	Frequency		Discuss with physician		Stop taking drug now	Call physician now
	Common	Rare	Only if severe	In all cases		
Headache	●		■			
Flushing	●		■			
Dizziness	●		■			
Indigestion	●		■			
Nasal congestion	●		■			
Blurred vision	●		■			
Altered colour vision	●		■			
Sudden decrease or loss of vision		●		■		▌
Persistent erection		●		■	▲	▌
Chest pain		●		■	▲	▌

INTERACTIONS

Nitrates The effects of these drugs are greatly increased by sildenafil, and they are therefore not prescribed with it.

Antihypertensive drugs Sildenafil may enhance the blood pressure-lowering effect of these drugs.

Cimetidine, erythromycin, nicorandil, ketoconazole (oral), and antivirals (ritonavir) These drugs increase the blood levels and *toxicity* of sildenafil.

Other drugs for impotence Safety not established. Not recommended.

SIMVASTATIN

Product name Zocor
Used in the following combined preparations None

GENERAL INFORMATION

Simvastatin is a lipid-lowering drug belonging to the class of statins. It blocks the action of an *enzyme* needed for cholesterol to be manufactured in the liver, and as a result the blood levels of cholesterol are lowered. The drug is prescribed for people with hypercholesterolemia (high levels of cholesterol in the blood) who have not responded to other forms of therapy, such as a special diet, and who are at risk of developing or have existing coronary heart disease. At present it is used only for patients with a high cholesterol level that is not caused by another disease; these high levels are often hereditary.

Side effects are usually mild and often wear off with time. In the body, simvastatin is found mainly in the liver, and it may raise the levels of various liver enzymes. This effect does not usually indicate serious liver damage.

INFORMATION FOR USERS

Your drug prescription is tailored for you. Do not alter dosage without checking with your physician.

How taken

Tablets.

Frequency and timing of doses
Once daily in the evening.

Usual adult dosage range
10–80mg daily.

Onset of effect
Within 2 weeks; full beneficial effects may not be felt for 4–6 weeks.

Duration of action
Up to 24 hours.

Diet advice
A low-fat diet is usually recommended.

Storage
Keep in a closed container in a cool, dry place out of the reach of children. Protect from light.

Missed dose
Take as soon as you remember. If your next dose is due within 8 hours, do not take the missed dose, but take the next dose on schedule.

Stopping the drug
Do not stop taking the drug without consulting your physician. Stopping the drug may lead to worsening of the underlying condition.

Exceeding the dose
An occasional unintentional extra dose is unlikely to cause problems. Large overdoses may cause liver problems. Notify your physician.

SPECIAL PRECAUTIONS

Be sure to tell your physician if:
▼ You have liver or kidney problems.
▼ You have eye or vision problems.
▼ You have muscle weakness.
▼ You have a family history of muscular disorders.
▼ You have a thyroid disorder.
▼ You have had problems with alcohol abuse.
▼ You have porphyria.
▼ You have angina.
▼ You have high blood pressure.
▼ You are taking other medications.

Pregnancy
▼ Not usually prescribed. Safety in pregnancy not established. Discuss with your physician.

Breast-feeding
▼ Safety not established. Discuss with your physician.

Infants and children
▼ Not recommended.

Over 60
▼ No special problems.

Driving and hazardous work
▼ No special problems.

Alcohol
▼ Avoid excessive amounts. Alcohol may increase the risk of developing liver problems with this drug.

POSSIBLE ADVERSE EFFECTS

Adverse effects are usually mild and do not last long. The most common are those affecting the gastrointestinal system.

Simvastatin may very rarely cause muscle problems, and any muscle pain or weakness should be reported to your physician at once.

Symptom/effect	Frequency		Discuss with physician		Stop taking drug now	Call physician now
	Common	Rare	Only if severe	In all cases		
Abdominal pain		●	■			
Constipation/diarrhea		●	■			
Nausea/flatulence		●	■			
Headache		●	■			
Rash		●		■	▲	
Jaundice		●		■		
Muscle pain/weakness		●		■	▲	∎
Change in cognition	●					∎

INTERACTIONS

Anticoagulants Simvastatin may increase the effect of these. Close monitoring dose adjustment may be required

Other lipid-lowering drugs The use of other lipid-lowering drugs with simvastatin may increase the risk of muscle toxicity.

Grapefruit juice may increase blood levels of simvastatin.

Cyclosporine, immunosuppressants, antivirals These, given with simvastatin, can increase the risk of muscle toxicity; not usually prescribed together.

Itraconazole, ketoconazole erythromycin, protease inhibitors These, given with a statin, may increase the risk of muscle damage.

PROLONGED USE

Prolonged treatment can adversely affect liver function.

Monitoring Regular blood tests to check liver function are recommended. Tests of muscle function may be carried out if problems are suspected.

SODIUM CROMOGLYCATE

Product names Intal, Nalcrom, Opticrom
Used in the following combined preparations None

GENERAL INFORMATION

Sodium cromoglycate, introduced in the 1970s, is used primarily to prevent asthma and allergic conditions.

When taken by inhaler as a powder (Spinhaler) or spray, it is commonly used to reduce the frequency and severity of asthma attacks, and is also effective in helping to prevent attacks induced by exercise or cold air. The drug has a slow onset of action, and it may take up to six weeks to produce its full anti-asthmatic effect. It is not effective for the relief of an asthma attack, and aside from its use in asthma prevention, it is also given as eye drops to prevent allergic conjunctivitis. It is also given, in the form of capsules, for food allergy.

Side effects are mild. Coughing and wheezing occurring on inhalation of the drug may be prevented by using a *sympathomimetic bronchodilator* (p.76) first. Hoarseness and throat irritation can be avoided by rinsing the mouth with water after inhalation.

QUICK REFERENCE

Drug group Anti-allergy drug (p.109)

Overdose danger rating Low

Dependence rating Low

Prescription needed No (some preparations)

Available as generic Yes

INFORMATION FOR USERS

Follow instructions on the label. Call your physician if symptoms worsen.

How taken

Capsules, inhaler (various types), eye drops.

Frequency and timing of doses
Capsules 4 x daily before meals, swallowed whole or dissolved in water.
Inhaler 4–6 x daily.
Eye preparations 4 x daily (drops).

Usual dosage range
800mg daily (capsules); as directed (inhaler); 1–2 drops in each eye per dose (eye drops).

Onset of effect
Varies with dosage, form, and condition treated. Eye conditions and allergic rhinitis may respond after a few days' treatment with drops, while asthma and chronic allergic rhinitis may take take 2–6 weeks to show improvement.

Duration of action
4–6 hours. Some effect persists for several days after treatment is stopped.

Diet advice
Capsules: you may be advised to avoid certain foods. Follow your physician's advice.

Storage
Keep in a closed container in a cool, dry place out of the reach of children. Protect from light.

Missed dose
Take as soon as you remember. If your next dose is due within 2 hours, take a single dose now and skip the next.

Stopping the drug
Do not stop the drug without consulting your physician; symptoms may recur.

Exceeding the dose
An occasional unintentional extra dose is unlikely to be a cause for concern. But if you notice any unusual symptoms, or if a large overdose has been taken, notify your physician.

POSSIBLE ADVERSE EFFECTS

Coughing and hoarseness are common with inhalation of sodium cromoglycate. These symptoms usually diminish with continued use.

Symptom/effect	Frequency		Discuss with physician		Stop taking drug now	Call physician now
	Common	Rare	Only if severe	In all cases		
Coughing/hoarseness	●		■			
Local irritation	●		■			
Nausea/vomiting (capsules)		●		■		
Joint pain (capsules)		●		■		
Wheezing/breathlessness		●		■		
Rash (capsules)		●		■	▲	

INTERACTIONS

None.

SPECIAL PRECAUTIONS

Be sure to consult your physician or pharmacist before taking this drug if:
▼ You are taking other medications.

 Pregnancy
▼ No evidence of risk.

 Breast-feeding
▼ No evidence of risk.

 Infants and children
▼ Reduced dose necessary.

 Over 60
▼ No special problems.

 Driving and hazardous work
▼ No known problems.

 Alcohol
▼ No known problems.

PROLONGED USE

No problems expected.

SOTALOL

Product name Novo-Sotalol
Used in the following combined preparations None

GENERAL INFORMATION

Sotalol is a non-cardioselective beta blocker used in the prevention and treatment of ventricular and supra-ventricular arrhythmias (see p.86). It has an additional anti-arrhythmic action to other beta blockers.

Sotalol is no longer prescribed for the other conditions that beta blockers are prescribed for. This is due to a serious *side effect* called 'torsades de pointes', a kind of ventricular arrhythmia that is serious enough to produce symptoms and, rarely, death. For this reason, anyone taking sotalol will be carefully monitored.

(see p.86)

QUICK REFERENCE

Drug group Beta blocker (p.83)
Overdose danger rating Medium
Dependence rating Low
Prescription needed Yes
Available as generic Yes

Beta blocker (p.83)

INFORMATION FOR USERS

Your drug prescription is tailored for you. Do not alter dosage without checking with your physician.

How taken

Tablets.

Frequency and timing of doses
2 x daily.

Usual adult dosage range
80mg daily initially, increased at 2–3-day intervals to 160–320mg daily. Higher doses under specialist supervision.

Onset of effect
30–60 minutes.

Duration of action
12 hours.

Diet advice
None.

Storage
Keep in a closed container in a cool, dry place out of the reach of children. Protect from light.

Missed dose
Take as soon as you remember. If your next dose is due within 3 hours, take a single dose now and skip the next.

Stopping the drug
Do not stop the drug without consulting your physician, who will supervise a gradual reduction in dosage. Sudden withdrawal may lead to worsening of your condition.

Exceeding the dose
An occasional unintentional extra dose is unlikely to be a cause for concern. Large overdoses may cause low blood pressure, slow heart rate, heart block, bronchospasm, and heart arrhythmias. Notify your physician immediately.

SPECIAL PRECAUTIONS

Be sure to tell your physician if:
▼ You have liver or kidney problems.
▼ You have a breathing disorder such as asthma, bronchitis, or emphysema.
▼ You have heart failure.
▼ You have diabetes.
▼ You have poor circulation in the legs.
▼ You are taking other medications.

Pregnancy
▼ Not usually prescribed. May affect the unborn baby. Discuss with your physician.

Breast-feeding
▼ The drug passes into the breast milk and may affect the baby. Discuss with your physician.

Infants and children
▼ Not prescribed.

Over 60
▼ Reduced dose may be necessary.

Driving and hazardous work
▼ Do not undertake such activities until you have learned how sotalol affects you because the drug can cause dizziness and fatigue.

Alcohol
▼ No special problems.

POSSIBLE ADVERSE EFFECTS

A very fast heart rate with palpitations could be a symptom of torsades de pointes; if you experience this you should notify your physician immediately.

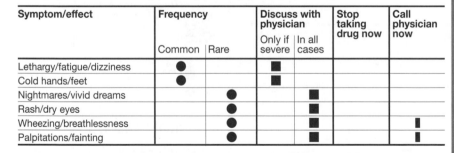

Symptom/effect	Frequency		Discuss with physician		Stop taking drug now	Call physician now
	Common	Rare	Only if severe	In all cases		
Lethargy/fatigue/dizziness	●		■			
Cold hands/feet	●		■			
Nightmares/vivid dreams		●		■		
Rash/dry eyes		●		■		
Wheezing/breathlessness		●		■		▮
Palpitations/fainting		●		■		▮

INTERACTIONS

Phenothiazines, antidepressants, and erythromycin (IV) These drugs increase the risk of torsades de pointes with sotalol.

Verapamil and diltiazem Combining these drugs with sotalol will have very adverse effects on heart function.

Anti-arrhythmics such as amiodarone, disopyramide, quinidine, lidocaine, and procainamide Taking any of these drugs with sotalol may slow the heart rate and affect heart function.

Calcium channel blockers These may cause low blood pressure, slow heartbeats and heart failure if taken with sotalol.

Diuretics, amphotericin, corticosteroids, and some laxatives These drugs may lower blood potassium levels, increasing the risk of torsades de pointes.

Sympathomimetics such as epinephrine (adrenaline), norepinephrine (noradren-aline), and dobutamine There is a risk of severe high blood pressure if these drugs are taken with sotalol.

PROLONGED USE

Sotalol may be taken indefinitely for prevention of ventricular arrhythmias.

Monitoring Periodic blood tests are usually performed to monitor levels of potassium and magnesium. The heartbeat is usually monitored for signs of development of torsades de pointes.

SPIRONOLACTONE

Product names Aldactone, Novo-Spiroton
Used in the following combined preparations Aldactazide, Novo-Spirozine

GENERAL INFORMATION

Spironolactone is a diuretic. It acts by inhibiting a hormone called aldosterone, which then results in an increase in the amount of urine that is passed through the kidneys. It is used in the treatment of edema (fluid retention), which can result from heart failure or liver disease (liver cirrhosis) and for hypertension (high blood pressure). It can also be used to counteract overproduction of the hormone aldosterone, which can occur with certain adrenal gland tumors.

Spironolactone causes the kidneys to conserve potassium (potassium-sparing diuretic) and should not be used when there is a high blood level of potassium. The drug is prescribed cautiously in people taking potassium supplements or those with kidney disease. When used for hypertension, it is usually combined with other diuretics.

QUICK REFERENCE

Drug group Potassium-sparing diuretic (p.85)

Overdose danger rating Low

Dependence rating Low

Prescription needed Yes

Available as generic Yes

INFORMATION FOR USERS

Your drug prescription is tailored for you. Do not alter dosage without checking with your physician.

How taken

● Tablets.

Frequency and timing of doses
Once daily (with higher doses, the daily dose may be divided into two doses).

Usual adult dosage range
50–100mg (starting dose); may increase up to 200mg.

Onset of effect
Within 2–4 hours.

Duration of action
12–24 hours.

Diet advice
Avoid foods that are high in potassium; for example, dried fruit, bananas, tomatoes, and salt substitutes.

Storage
Keep in a closed container in a cool, dry place out of the reach of children.

Missed dose
If you miss a dose, take it as soon as you remember. However, if it is late in the day, do not take the missed dose. Take the next scheduled dose as usual.

Stopping the drug
Do not stop the drug without consulting your physician; symptoms may recur.

Exceeding the dose
An occasional unintentional extra dose is unlikely to be a cause for concern. But if you notice any unusual symptoms, or if a large overdose has been taken, notify your physician.

POSSIBLE ADVERSE EFFECTS

Generally well tolerated. The main problem is that potassium may be retained by the body, causing muscle weakness and numbness. Rarely, breast enlargement can occur; this is related to the length of therapy and the dose. This is usually resolved by discontinuation of spironolactone.

Symptom/effect	Frequency		Discuss with physician		Stop taking drug now	Call physician now
	Common	Rare	Only if severe	In all cases		
Muscle weakness/cramps		●		■		
Breast enlargement		●		■		
Drowsiness/tiredness		●	■			
Nausea, vomiting		●		■		

INTERACTIONS

Diuretic Spironolactone is commonly used with other diuretics; however, the effect is additive and the dose of other diuretics may need to be decreased.

Lisinopril, ramipril, etc. ACE-inhibitors such as lisinopril, ramipril, etc. can increase blood potassium and this effect will be additive to the effect of spironolactone.

Non-steroidal anti-inflammatory drugs These drugs can counteract the antihypertensive effect of spironolactone, as well as increasing the risk of potassium retention.

SPECIAL PRECAUTIONS

Be sure to tell your physician if:
▼ You have long-term liver or kidney problems.
▼ You are taking potassium supplements.
▼ You have diabetes.
▼ You are taking other medications.

 Pregnancy
▼ Safety in pregnancy is not established. Also, diuretics in general may cause a reduction in the blood supply to the developing baby. Discuss with your physician.

 Breast-feeding
▼ Not recommended during breast-feeding. Discuss with your physician.

 Infants and children
▼ Not recommended.

 Over 60
▼ Increased likelihood of adverse effects. Reduced dose necessary.

 Driving and hazardous work
▼ No known problems.

 Alcohol
▼ No special problems.

PROLONGED USE

Monitoring Blood tests may be carried out to monitor levels of electrolytes in the blood.

STREPTOKINASE

Product name Streptase
Used in the following combined preparations None

GENERAL INFORMATION

Streptokinase, an *enzyme* produced by the streptococcus bacteria, is used in hospitals to dissolve the fibrin (see p.91) of blood clots, especially those in the arteries of the heart and lungs. It is also used on the clots formed in shunts during kidney dialysis.

A fast-acting drug, streptokinase is most effective in dissolving any newly formed clots, and it is often released at the site of the clot via a catheter inserted into an artery. Administered in the early stages of a heart attack to dissolve a clot (thrombosis) in the coronary arteries, it can reduce the amount of damage to heart muscle. Because excessive bleeding is a common *side effect*, treatment is closely supervised.

Streptokinase is also used to treat wounds and ulcers in combination with another enzyme called streptodornase.

Streptokinase is a protein, and can cause allergic reactions. To reduce this risk, antihistamines may be given at the start of treatment.

QUICK REFERENCE

Drug group Thrombolytic drug (p.91).

Overdose danger rating Medium

Dependence rating Low

Prescription needed Yes

Available as generic Yes

INFORMATION FOR USERS

The drug is only given under medical supervision and is not for self-administration.

How taken

Injection.

Frequency and timing of doses
By a single injection or continuously over a period of 24–72 hours.

Usual dosage range
Dosage is determined individually by the patient's condition and response.

Onset of effect
As soon as streptokinase reaches the blood clot, it begins to dissolve within minutes. Most of the blood clot will be dissolved within a few hours.

Duration of action
Effect disappears within a few minutes of stopping the drug.

Diet advice
None.

Storage
Not applicable. This drug is not normally kept in the home.

Missed dose
Not applicable. This drug is given only in hospital under close medical supervision.

Stopping the drug
The drug is usually given for up to 3 days.

Exceeding the dose
Overdosage is unlikely since treatment is carefully monitored.

SPECIAL PRECAUTIONS

Streptokinase is only prescribed under close medical supervision, usually only in life-threatening circumstances.

Pregnancy
▼ Not usually prescribed. If used during the first 18 weeks of pregnancy there is a risk that the placenta may separate from the wall of the uterus.

Breast-feeding
▼ No evidence of risk.

Infants and children
▼ Reduced dose necessary.

Over 60
▼ Increased likelihood of bleeding into the brain.

Driving and hazardous work
▼ Not applicable.

Alcohol
▼ Not applicable.

POSSIBLE ADVERSE EFFECTS

Streptokinase is given under strict supervision and all adverse effects are closely monitored so that any of the symptoms below can be quickly dealt with.

Symptom/effect	Frequency		Discuss with physician		Stop taking drug now	Call physician now
	Common	Rare	Only if severe	In all cases		
Excessive bleeding	●			■		
Nausea/vomiting	●			■		
Fever		●		■		
Wheezing		●		■		
Abnormal heart rhythms		●		■		
Collapse		●		■		
Rash/itching		●		■	▲	▮

PROLONGED USE

Streptokinase is never used long term.

Further instructions Once you have had a dose, you will be given a card which you must keep with you at all times, and present to any doctor in case further treatment is required. A second course of treatment with streptokinase would not normally be given within 6 months of the first course of treatment.

INTERACTIONS

Anticoagulant drugs There is an increased risk of bleeding when these are taken at the same time as streptokinase.

Antiplatelet drugs There is an increased risk of bleeding if these drugs are given with streptokinase.

SUCRALFATE

Product name Sulcrate
Used in the following combined preparations None

GENERAL INFORMATION

Sucralfate, a drug partly derived from aluminium, is prescribed to treat gastric and duodenal ulcers. The drug does not neutralize stomach acid, but it forms a protective barrier over the ulcer that protects it from attack by digestive juices, giving it time to heal.

If it is necessary during treatment to take antacids to relieve pain, they should be taken at least half an hour before or after taking sucralfate.

There are a few reports of seriously ill patients developing bezoars (balls of indigestible material) in their stomachs while on sucralfate. The safety of the drug for long-term use has not yet been confirmed. Therefore, courses of more than 12 weeks are not recommended.

QUICK REFERENCE

Drug group Ulcer-healing drug (p.95).

Overdose danger rating Low

Dependence rating Low

Prescription needed Yes

Available as generic Yes

INFORMATION FOR USERS

Your drug prescription is tailored for you. Do not alter dosage without checking with your physician.

How taken

Tablets, liquid.

Frequency and timing of doses
2–4 x daily, 1 hour before each meal and at bedtime, at least 2 hours after food.

Usual dosage range
4–8g daily.

Onset of effect
Some improvement may be noted after one or two doses, but it takes a few weeks for an ulcer to heal.

Duration of action
Up to 5 hours.

Diet advice
Your physician will advise if supplements are needed.

Storage
Keep in a closed container in a cool, dry place out of the reach of children.

Missed dose
Do not make up the dose you missed. Take your next dose on your original schedule.

Stopping the drug
Do not stop the drug without consulting your physician; symptoms may recur.

Exceeding the dose
An occasional unintentional extra dose is unlikely to be a cause for concern. But if you notice any unusual symptoms, or if a large overdose has been taken, notify your physician.

SPECIAL PRECAUTIONS

Be sure to tell your physician if:
▼ You have a long-term kidney problem.
▼ You are taking other medications.

Pregnancy
▼ Safety in pregnancy not established. Discuss with your physician.

Breast-feeding
▼ No evidence of risk.

Infants and children
▼ Not usually prescribed.

Over 60
▼ No special problems.

Driving and hazardous work
▼ Usually no problems, but sucralfate may cause dizziness in some people.

Alcohol
▼ Avoid. Alcohol may counteract the beneficial effect of this drug.

POSSIBLE ADVERSE EFFECTS

Most people do not experience any adverse effects while they are taking sucralfate. The most common is constipation, which will diminish as your body adjusts to the drug.

Symptom/effect	Frequency		Discuss with physician		Stop taking drug now	Call physician now
	Common	Rare	Only if severe	In all cases		
Indigestion	●		■			
Constipation	●		■			
Diarrhea		●	■			
Dry mouth		●	■			
Nausea		●		■		
Rash/itching		●		■		
Dizziness/vertigo		●		■		
Insomnia		●		■		

PROLONGED USE

Not usually prescribed for periods longer than 12 weeks at a time. Prolonged use may lead to deficiencies of vitamins A, D, E, and K.

INTERACTIONS

General note Sucralfate may reduce the absorption and effect of a range of drugs, including ranitidine, digoxin, phenytoin, warfarin, levothyroxine, and antibacterials. Take these and other medications at least 30 minutes before or after sucralfate.

Antacids and other indigestion remedies These reduce the effectiveness of sucralfate and should be taken more than 30 minutes before or after sucralfate.

SULFASALAZINE

Product names Salazopyrin, Salazopyrin En-Tabs
Used in the following combined preparations None

GENERAL INFORMATION

Sulfasalazine, a chemical combination of a sulfonamide and a salicylate, is used to treat two inflammatory disorders affecting the bowel. One is ulcerative colitis (which mainly affects the large intestine); the other is Crohn's disease (which usually affects the small intestine). Sulfasalazine is also effective in the treatment of rheumatoid arthritis.

Adverse effects such as nausea, loss of appetite, and general discomfort are more likely when higher doses are taken. *Side effects* caused by stomach irritation may be avoided by changing to a specially coated tablet form of the drug. Allergic reactions such as fever and skin rash may be avoided or minimized by low initial doses of the drug, followed by gradual increases. Maintenance of adequate fluid intake is important while taking this drug. In rare cases among men, temporary sterility may occur.

INFORMATION FOR USERS

Your drug prescription is tailored for you. Do not alter dosage without checking with your physician.

How taken

Tablets.

Frequency and timing of doses
4 x daily after meals with a glass of water.

Usual adult dosage range
4–8g daily (Crohn's disease/ulcerative colitis); 500mg–2g daily (rheumatoid arthritis).

Onset of effect
Adverse effects may occur within a few days, but full beneficial effects may take 1–3 weeks, depending on the severity of the condition.

Duration of action
Up to 24 hours.

Diet advice
It is important to drink plenty of liquids (at least 1.5 litres a day) during treatment unless otherwise directed by your physician. Sulfasalazine may reduce the absorption of folic acid from the intestine, leading to a deficiency of this vitamin. Eat plenty of green vegetables.

Storage
Keep in a closed container in a cool, dry place out of the reach of children.

Missed dose
Take as soon as you remember. If your next dose is due within 2 hours, take a single dose now and skip the next.

Stopping the drug
Do not stop the drug without consulting your physician; symptoms may recur.

Exceeding the dose
An occasional unintentional extra dose is unlikely to be a cause for concern. But if you notice any unusual symptoms, or if a large overdose has been taken, notify your physician.

SPECIAL PRECAUTIONS

Be sure to tell your physician if:
▼ You have long-term liver or kidney problems.
▼ You have glucose-6-phosphate dehydrogenase (G6PD) deficiency.
▼ You have a blood disorder.
▼ You suffer from porphyria.
▼ You are allergic to sulfonamides or salicylates.
▼ You wear soft contact lenses.
▼ You are taking other medications.

Pregnancy
▼ No evidence of risk to developing fetus. Folic acid supplements may be required. Discuss with your physician.

Breast-feeding
▼ The drug passes into the breast milk and may affect the baby. Discuss with your physician.

Infants and children
▼ Not recommended under 2 years. Reduced dose necessary for older children, according to body weight.

Over 60
▼ No special problems.

Driving and hazardous work
▼ No special problems.

Alcohol
▼ No known problems.

POSSIBLE ADVERSE EFFECTS

Adverse effects are common with high doses, but may disappear with a reduction in the dose. Symptoms such as nausea and vomiting may be helped by taking the drug with food. Orange or yellow discoloration of the urine is no cause for alarm.

Symptom/effect	Frequency		Discuss with physician		Stop taking drug now	Call physician now
	Common	Rare	Only if severe	In all cases		
Nausea/vomiting	●		■			
Malaise/loss of appetite	●		■			
Headache	●			■		
Joint pain	●			■		
Ringing in the ears		●	■			
Fever/rash		●		■		▮
Bleeding/bruising		●		■		▮

INTERACTIONS

General note 1 Sulfasalazine may increase the effects of a variety of drugs, including oral anticoagulants, oral antidiabetics, anticonvulsants, and methotrexate.

General note 2 Sulfasalazine reduces the absorption and effect of some drugs, including digoxin, folic acid, and iron.

PROLONGED USE

Blood disorders may occur with prolonged use of this drug. Maintenance dosage is usually continued indefinitely.

Monitoring Periodic tests of blood composition and liver function are usually required.

SUMATRIPTAN

Product name Imitrex
Used in the following combined preparations None

GENERAL INFORMATION

Sumatriptan is a highly effective drug for migraine, usually given when people fail to respond to analgesics (such as ASA and acetaminophen). The drug is of considerable value in the treatment of acute migraine attacks, whether or not they are preceded by an aura, but is not meant to be taken regularly to prevent attacks. Sumatriptan is also used for the acute treatment of cluster headache (a form of migraine headache). It should be taken as soon as possible after the onset of the attack, although it will still be of benefit at whatever stage of the attack it is taken.

Sumatriptan relieves the symptoms of migraine by preventing the dilation of blood vessels in the brain, which causes the attack.

QUICK REFERENCE

Drug group Drug for migraine (p.73)

Overdose danger rating Medium

Dependence rating Low

Prescription needed Yes

Available as generic Yes

INFORMATION FOR USERS

Your drug prescription is tailored for you. Do not alter dosage without checking with your physician.

How taken

Tablets, injection, nasal spray.

Frequency and timing of doses
Should be taken as soon as possible after the onset of an attack. However, it is equally effective at whatever stage it is taken. If partial response only, the dose may be repeated once after 2 hours. The tablets should be swallowed whole with water.

Usual adult dosage range
Tablets 25–100mg per attack, up to maximum of 200mg in 24 hours if another attack occurs. *Injection* 6mg per attack, up to maximum of 12mg (two injections) in 24 hours if another attack occurs. *Nasal spray* 5–20mg per attack, up to maximum of 40mg (2 puffs) in 24 hours if another attack occurs.

Onset of effect
30 minutes (tablets);10–15 minutes (injection).

Duration of action
Tablets The maximum effect occurs after 2–4 hours.
Injection The maximum effect occurs after 1½–2 hours.

Diet advice
None unless otherwise advised.

Storage
Keep in a closed container in a cool, dry place out of the reach of children. Protect from light.

Missed dose
Not applicable, as it is taken only to treat a migraine attack.

Stopping the drug
Taken only to treat a migraine attack.

Exceeding the dose
An occasional unintentional extra tablet or injection is unlikely to cause problems. But if you notice any unusual symptoms, or if a large overdose has been taken, notify your physician.

SPECIAL PRECAUTIONS

Be sure to tell your physician if:
▼ You have liver or kidney problems.
▼ You have heart problems.
▼ You have high blood pressure.
▼ You have had a heart attack.
▼ You have angina.
▼ You are allergic to some medicines.
▼ You are taking other medications.

 Pregnancy
▼ Safety in pregnancy not established. Discuss with your physician.

 Breast-feeding
▼ Safety not established. Discuss with your physician.

 Infants and children
▼ Not recommended.

 Over 60
▼ Not recommended for patients over 65 years.

 Driving and hazardous work
▼ Avoid such activities until you have learned how sumatriptan affects you because the drug can cause drowsiness.

 Alcohol
▼ No special problems, but some drinks may provoke migraine in some people (see p.69).

Surgery and general anesthetics
▼ Notify your physician or dentist if you have used sumatriptan within 48 hours prior to surgery.

POSSIBLE ADVERSE EFFECTS

Many of the adverse effects will disappear after about 1 hour as your body becomes adjusted to the medicine. If the symptoms persist or are severe, contact your physician.

Symptom/effect	Frequency		Discuss with physician		Stop taking drug now	Call physician now
	Common	Rare	Only if severe	In all cases		
Pain at injection site	●		■			
Feeling of tingling/heat	●		■			
Flushing	●		■			
Feeling of heaviness/weakness	●		■			
Dizziness		●	■			
Fatigue/drowsiness		●	■			
Palpitations/chest pain		●		■	▲	▌

PROLONGED USE

Sumatriptan should not be used continuously to prevent migraine but only to treat migraine attacks.

INTERACTIONS

Antidepressants Monoamine oxidase inhibitors (MAOIs) and some other antidepressants, such as fluvoxamine, fluoxetine, paroxetine, and sertraline, increase the risk of adverse effects with sumatriptan.

Lithium Patients taking lithium should not take sumatriptan due to the high risk of adverse effects.

Ergotamine must be taken at least 6 hours after sumatriptan, and sumatriptan must be taken at least 24 hours after ergotamine.

TAMOXIFEN

Product names Nolvadex, Tamofen
Used in the following combined preparations None

GENERAL INFORMATION

Tamoxifen is an anti-estrogen drug (estrogen is a naturally occurring female sex hormone, see p.133). It is used as an anticancer drug for breast cancer because it works against estrogens. By latching on to cells that recognize these hormones, it can slow the growth of the tumour and even shrink it. It can also be used to prevent the recurrence of breast cancer that has been surgically removed.

As its effect is specific, tamoxifen has fewer *adverse effects* than most other drugs used for breast cancer. However, it may cause eye damage if high doses are taken for long periods.

QUICK REFERENCE

Drug group Anticancer drug (p.140)
Overdose danger rating Low
Dependence rating Low
Prescription needed Yes
Available as generic Yes

INFORMATION FOR USERS

Your drug prescription is tailored for you. Do not alter dosage without checking with your physician.

How taken

Tablets.

Frequency and timing of doses
1–2 x daily.

Usual adult dosage range
20–40mg daily.

Onset of effect
Side effects may be felt within days, but beneficial effects may take 4–10 weeks.

Duration of action
Effects may be felt for several weeks after stopping the drug.

Diet advice
None.

Storage
Keep in a closed container in a cool, dry place out of the reach of children. Protect from light.

Missed dose
Take as soon as you remember. If your next dose is due within 2 hours, take a single dose now and skip the next.

Stopping the drug
Do not stop the drug without consulting your physician; stopping the drug may lead to worsening of your underlying condition.

Exceeding the dose
An occasional unintentional extra dose is unlikely to be a cause for concern. But if you notice any unusual symptoms, or if a large overdose has been taken, notify your physician.

SPECIAL PRECAUTIONS

Be sure to tell your physician if:
▼ You have cataracts or poor eyesight.
▼ You suffer from porphyria.
▼ You are taking other medications.

Pregnancy
▼ Not usually prescribed. May have effects on the developing baby. Discuss with your physician.

Breast-feeding
▼ Not usually prescribed. Discuss with your physician.

Infants and children
▼ Not prescribed.

Over 60
▼ No special problems.

Driving and hazardous work
▼ Do not drive until you have learned how tamoxifen affects you because the drug can cause dizziness and blurred vision.

Alcohol
▼ No known problems.

POSSIBLE ADVERSE EFFECTS

These are rarely serious and do not usually require treatment to be stopped. Nausea, vomiting, and hot flushes are the most common reactions. There is a small risk of endometrial cancer (cancer of the uterine lining) developing, so you should notify your physician of any symptoms such as irregular vaginal bleeding as soon as possible.

Symptom/effect	Frequency		Discuss with physician		Stop taking drug now	Call physician now
	Common	Rare	Only if severe	In all cases		
Nausea/vomiting	●		■			
Hot flushes	●		■			
Irregular vaginal bleeding	●			■		▮
Irregular vaginal discharge	●			■		▮
Swollen feet/ankles		●	■			
Bone and tumour pain		●		■		
Rash/itching		●		■		
Blurred vision/headache		●		■		

INTERACTIONS

Anticoagulants People treated with anticoagulants such as warfarin usually need a lower dose of the anticoagulant.

PROLONGED USE

There is a risk of damage to the eye with long-term, high-dose treatment.

There is a small increased risk of endometrial cancer with long-term treatment but this is far outweighed by the benefits of treatment.

Monitoring Eyesight may be tested periodically.

TAMSULOSIN

Product names Flomax, Flomax CR, Novo-Tamsulosin, Sandoz Tamsulosin, and others
Used in the following combined preparations None

GENERAL INFORMATION

Tamsulosin is a selective alpha-blocker drug used to treat urinary retention due to benign prostatic hypertrophy, or BPH (enlarged prostate gland). The drug, as it passes through the prostate, relaxes the muscle in the wall of the urethra, thereby increasing urine flow.

To exclude other conditions with similar symptoms, your physician will arrange for you to have a physical examination and a special blood test, which may be repeated at intervals during treatment.

Like other alpha-blockers, tamsulosin may lower blood pressure rapidly after the first dose. For this reason, the first dose should be taken at home so that, if dizziness or weakness occur, you can lie down until they have disappeared.

INFORMATION FOR USERS

Your drug prescription is tailored for you. Do not alter dosage without checking with your physician.

How taken

SR capsules, extended release (ER) tablets.

Frequency and timing of doses
Once daily after breakfast.

Usual adult dosage range
400–800mcg.

Onset of effect
1–2 hours.

Duration of action
24 hours.

Diet advice
None.

Storage
Keep in a closed container in a cool, dry place out of the reach of children.

Missed dose
Taken as soon as you remember. If your next dose is due within 4 hours, take a single dose now and skip the next.

Stopping the drug
Do not stop taking the drug without consulting your physician; stopping suddenly may lead to a rise in blood pressure.

Exceeding the dose
An occasional unintentional extra dose is unlikely to cause problems. Large overdoses may produce sedation, dizziness, low blood pressure, and rapid pulse. Notify your physician immediately.

SPECIAL PRECAUTIONS

Be sure to tell your physician if:
- ▼ You have had low blood pressure.
- ▼ You have liver or kidney problems.
- ▼ You have heart failure.
- ▼ You have a history of depression.
- ▼ You are taking an MAOI drug.
- ▼ You are taking drugs for high blood pressure.
- ▼ You are taking other medications.

Pregnancy
▼ Not prescribed.

Breast-feeding
▼ Not prescribed.

Infants and children
▼ Not prescribed.

Over 60
▼ No special problems.

Driving and hazardous work
▼ Avoid such activities until you have learned how tamsulosin affects you because the drug can cause drowsiness and dizziness.

Alcohol
▼ Avoid until you know how tamsulosin affects you because alcohol can further lower blood pressure.

Surgery and general anesthetics
▼ Tamsulosin may need to be stopped. Discuss with your physician or dentist before you have any surgery.

POSSIBLE ADVERSE EFFECTS

Dizziness seems to be the most common adverse effect, but this usually improves after the first few doses.

Symptom/effect	Frequency		Discuss with physician		Stop taking drug now	Call physician now
	Common	Rare	Only if severe	In all cases		
Dizziness/weakness/fainting	●			■		
Ejaculatory problems	●		■			
Headache	●		■			
Drowsiness	●		■			
Palpitations	●			■		
Nausea/vomiting		●	■			
Diarrhea/constipation		●	■			
Rash/itching		●		■		

INTERACTIONS

Antidepressants, beta blockers, calcium channel blockers, and diuretics These drugs are likely to increase the blood pressure-lowering effect of tamsulosin.

PROLONGED USE

No special problems.

TEMAZEPAM

Product names Apo-Temazepam, Novo-Temazepam, Restoril, and others
Used in the following combined preparations None

GENERAL INFORMATION

Temazepam belongs to a group of drugs known as the benzodiazepines. The actions and *adverse effects* of this group of drugs are described more fully under Anti-anxiety drugs (p.67).

Temazepam is used in the short-term treatment of insomnia. Because it is a short-acting drug compared with some other benzodiazepines, it is less likely to cause drowsiness and/or lightheadedness the following day.

For this reason, the drug is not usually effective in preventing early wakening, but hangover is less common than with other benzodiazepines.

Like other benzodiazepine drugs, temazepam can be habit-forming if taken regularly over a long period. Its effects also grow weaker with time. For these reasons, treatment with temazepam is usually only continued for a few days at a time.

QUICK REFERENCE

Drug group Benzodiazepine sleeping drug (p.66)

Overdose danger rating Medium

Dependence rating High

Prescription needed Yes

Available as generic Yes

INFORMATION FOR USERS

Your drug prescription is tailored for you. Do not alter dosage without checking with your physician.

How taken

Capsules.

Frequency and timing of doses
Once daily, 30 minutes before bedtime.

Usual adult dosage range
10–40mg.

Onset of effect
15–40 minutes, or longer.

Duration of action
6–8 hours.

Diet advice
None.

Storage
Keep in a closed container in a cool, dry place out of the reach of children. Protect from light.

Missed dose
If you fall asleep without having taken a dose and wake some hours later, do not take the missed dose. If necessary, return to your normal dose schedule the following night.

Stopping the drug
If you have been taking the drug continuously for less than 2 weeks, it can be safely stopped as soon as you no longer need it. If you have been taking the drug for longer, consult your physician, who may supervise a gradual reduction in dosage. Stopping abruptly may lead to *withdrawal symptoms* (see p.66).

Exceeding the dose
An occasional unintentional extra dose is unlikely to be a cause for concern. Large overdoses may cause unusual drowsiness. Notify your physician.

POSSIBLE ADVERSE EFFECTS

The principal adverse effects of this drug are related to its sedative and tranquillizing properties. These effects normally diminish after the first few days of treatment.

Symptom/effect	Frequency		Discuss with physician		Stop taking drug now	Call physician now
	Common	Rare	Only if severe	In all cases		
Daytime drowsiness	●		■			
Dizziness/unsteadiness		●		■		
Headache		●		■		
Vivid dreams/nightmares		●		■		
Forgetfulness/confusion		●		■		■

INTERACTIONS

Sedatives All drugs that have a sedative effect on the central nervous system are likely to increase the sedative properties of temazepam. Such drugs include other anti-anxiety and sleeping drugs, *opioid* analgesics, antidepressants, antihistamines, and antipsychotics.

SPECIAL PRECAUTIONS

Be sure to tell your physician if:
▼ You have severe respiratory disease.
▼ You suffer from porphyria.
▼ You suffer from depression.
▼ You have liver or kidney problems.
▼ You have myasthenia gravis.
▼ You have had problems with alcohol or drug abuse.
▼ You are taking other medications.

Pregnancy
▼ Safety in pregnancy not established. Discuss with your physician.

Breast-feeding
▼ The drug passes into the breast milk, but at normal doses adverse effects on the baby are unlikely. Discuss with your physician.

Infants and children
▼ Not recommended.

Over 60
▼ Reduced dose may be necessary. Increased likelihood of adverse effects.

Driving and hazardous work
▼ Avoid such activities until you have learned how temazepam affects you because the drug can cause reduced alertness and slowed reactions.

Alcohol
▼ Avoid. Alcohol may increase the sedative effect of this drug.

PROLONGED USE

Regular use of this drug over several weeks can lead to a reduction in its effect as the body adapts. It may also be habit-forming when taken for extended periods. Temazepam should not normally be used for longer than 1–2 weeks.

TENECTEPLASE

Product name TNKase
Used in the following combined preparations None

GENERAL INFORMATION

Tenecteplase is a fibrinolytic (or thrombolytic, see p.91) drug. It dissolves blood clots (thrombi) by boosting the action of the blood enzyme plasmin in breaking up the strands of fibrin that hold the clot together. It is given by intravenous injection. The sooner this is done after formation of the clot, the greater the success rate in clearing the clot from the coronary arteries in the heart, and reducing the damage to heart muscle. Tenecteplase is licensed only for treatment of heart attacks. Fibrinolytics are usually given in

hospitals, where all the resources needed for this kind of urgent action are held in readiness.

After the tenecteplase has been given, ASA and heparin are used to maintain the anticoagulant effect and stop further clotting. Low-dose ASA will usually be prescribed long term, and heparin will be given for a few days until the situation is stable.

Because tenecteplase activates the destruction of the body's fibrin (which causes clotting), the main side effect is bleeding, most often at the injection site.

INFORMATION FOR USERS

The drug is only given under medical supervision and is not for self-administration.

How taken

Injection.

Frequency and timing of doses
A single intravenous injection over 5 seconds.

Usual adult dosage range
30–50mg (6000–10000 units) depending on body weight.

Onset of effect
The drug reaches begins to dissolve the blood clot within minutes. Most of the clot will be gone within a few hours.

Duration of action
25–30 minutes.

Diet advice
None.

Storage
Not applicable. The drug is not normally kept in the home.

Missed dose
Not applicable. The drug is given once, in urgent circumstances, in hospital.

Stopping the drug
Not applicable.

Exceeding the dose
Overdose is unlikely because dosage is carefully monitored.

SPECIAL PRECAUTIONS

Tenecteplase is prescribed only under close medical supervision, usually only under life-threatening circumstances.

Pregnancy
▼ Safety not established. The benefit of treatment must be weighed against the likelihood of bleeding and fetal loss.

Breast-feeding
▼ Breast milk should be discarded for the first 24 hours after tenecteplase treatment, because it is not known whether the drug enters breast milk, or is harmful.

Infants and children
▼ Reduced dose necessary.

Over 60
▼ No known problems.

Driving and hazardous work
▼ Not applicable.

Alcohol
▼ Not applicable.

POSSIBLE ADVERSE EFFECTS

Tenecteplase is given under close medical supervision, so any of the symptoms listed below can be quickly dealt with. Tenecteplase is a protein, and can, therefore, produce allergic reactions.

Symptom/effect	Frequency		Discuss with physician		Stop taking drug now	Call physician now
	Common	Rare	Only if severe	In all cases		
Nausea/vomiting	●			■		
Bleeding	●			■		
Palpitations	●			■		
Chest pain	●			■		
Fainting/dizziness	●			■		
Wheezing		●		■		
Rash/itching		●		■		

INTERACTIONS

Anticoagulants and drugs affecting platelet function may increase bleeding tendency.

PROLONGED USE

Not applicable.

TERAZOSIN

Product name Hytrin
Used in the following combined preparations None

GENERAL INFORMATION

Terazosin belongs to the group of antihypertensive drugs known as alpha blockers and is used to treat high blood pressure (hypertension). The drug works by relaxing the muscles in the blood vessel walls. Terazosin is also used to relieve the obstruction caused by an enlarged prostate (benign prostatic hypertrophy, or BPH), thereby improving the flow of urine.

Dizziness and fainting, especially on standing up, are common at the start of treatment with terazosin because the first dose may cause a marked drop in blood pressure. For this reason, the initial dose that is prescribed is usually low. To avoid experiencing these effects, it is advisable to take the drug just before going to bed.

QUICK REFERENCE

Drug group Antihypertensive drug (p.88) and drug for urinary disorders (p.154)

Overdose danger rating Medium

Dependence rating Low

Prescription needed Yes

Available as generic Yes

INFORMATION FOR USERS

Your drug prescription is tailored for you. Do not alter dosage without checking with your physician.

How taken

Tablets.

Frequency and timing of doses
Once daily.

Usual adult dosage range
Hypertension 1mg at bedtime (starting dose) doubled after 7 days if necessary. Usual dosage range 1–5mg.
Benign prostatic hypertrophy 1mg at bedtime (starting dose) doubled after 1–2 weeks if necessary. Usual dosage range 5–10mg.

Onset of effect
Hypertension Within 3 hours.
Benign prostatic hypertrophy Improvements in symptoms can occur as early as 2 weeks after starting treatment. Full beneficial effects may not be felt for 4–6 weeks.

Duration of action
24 hours.

Diet advice
None.

Storage
Keep in a closed container in a cool dry place out of the reach of children.

Missed dose
Do not double up on a dose. Take the next dose at the usual time.

Stopping the drug
Do not stop the drug without consulting your physician. Stopping the drug may lead to an increase in blood pressure.

Exceeding the dose
An occasional unintentional extra dose is unlikely to be a cause for concern. Large overdoses may drop blood pressure and cause dizziness or fainting. Notify your physician.

SPECIAL PRECAUTIONS

Be sure to tell your physician if:
▼ You are taking other medications.

 Pregnancy
▼ Safety in pregnancy not established. Discuss with your physician.

 Breast feeding
▼ Safety in breast feeding not established. Discuss with your physician.

 Infants and children
▼ Not recommended.

 Over 60
▼ No special problems.

 Driving and hazardous work
▼ Avoid such activities until you have learned how terazosin affects you because the drug can cause dizziness, lightheadedness, or drowsiness.

 Alcohol
▼ Avoid. Alcohol may increase some of the *adverse effects* of terazosin, such as drowsiness.

Surgery and general anesthetics
▼ Terazosin may need to be stopped. Discuss with your physician or dentist before you have any surgery.

PROLONGED USE

No problems expected.

POSSIBLE ADVERSE EFFECTS

Rarely, headaches occur with terazosin treatment. A common problem with the drug, however, is that it may cause dizziness or fainting when you stand up.

Symptom/effect	Frequency		Discuss with physician		Stop taking drug now	Call physician now
	Common	Rare	Only if severe	In all cases		
Dizziness/faintness	●			■		
Weakness	●		■			
Palpitations	●			■		
Nausea	●		■			
Drowsiness	●		■			
Stuffy nose	●		■			
Ankle swelling	●			■		
Blurred vision	●			■		
Headache		●	■			

INTERACTIONS

Anesthetics, antidepressants, and hypotensive drugs These drugs may enhance the blood pressure-lowering effect of terazosin.

TERBINAFINE

Product name Lamisil
Used in the following combined preparations None

GENERAL INFORMATION

Terbinafine is an antifungal drug used to treat fungal infections of the skin and nails, particularly tinea (ringworm). It is also used as a cream for candida (yeast) infections.

Terbinafine has largely replaced older drugs such as griseofulvin because it is more easily absorbed and is therefore more effective.

Tinea infections are treated in two to six weeks, but treatment of nail infections may take up to 6 months.

Rare *adverse effects* of terbinafine include *jaundice* and a severe skin rash, both of which should be reported to your physician without delay.

INFORMATION FOR USERS

Your drug prescription is tailored for you. Do not alter dosage without checking with your physician.

How taken

Tablets, cream, skin spray.

Frequency and timing of doses
Once daily (tablets); 1–2 x daily (cream).

Usual adult dosage range
Tinea infections 250mg (tablets).
Candida infections As directed (cream).

Onset of effect
1 hour.

Duration of action
24 hours.

Diet advice
None.

Storage
Keep in a closed container in a cool, dry place out of the reach of children. Protect from light.

Missed dose
Take as soon as you remember. If your next dose is due within 4 hours, take a single dose now and skip the next.

Stopping the drug
Take the full course. Even if you feel better, the original infection may still be present and may recur if treatment is stopped too soon.

Exceeding the dose
An occasional unintentional extra dose is unlikely to be a cause for concern. But if you notice any unusual symptoms, or if a large overdose has been taken, notify your physician.

POSSIBLE ADVERSE EFFECTS

Side effects of terbinafine are generally mild and transient.

Symptom/effect	Frequency		Discuss with physician		Stop taking drug now	Call physician now
	Common	Rare	Only if severe	In all cases		
Nausea/indigestion/bloating	●		■			
Mild abdominal pain/diarrhea	●		■			
Headache	●		■			
Taste disturbance/loss		●	■			
Dizziness		●	■			
"Pins and needles"		●	■			
Muscle or joint pain		●		■		
Severe skin rash		●		■	▲	▮
Sore mouth/throat		●		■	▲	▮
Bruising/bleeding in mouth		●		■	▲	▮
Jaundice		●		■	▲	▮

INTERACTIONS

Oral contraceptives "Breakthrough" bleeding may occur when these are taken with terbinafine.

Rifampin This drug may reduce the blood level and effect of terbinafine.

Cimetidine This drug may increase the blood level of terbinafine.

SPECIAL PRECAUTIONS

Be sure to tell your physician if:
▼ You have liver or kidney problems.
▼ You have psoriasis.
▼ You are taking other medications.

Pregnancy
▼ Safety in pregnancy not established. Discuss with your physician.

Breast-feeding
▼ The drug passes into the breast milk and may affect the baby. Discuss with your physician.

Infants and children
▼ Safety not established. Discuss with your physician.

Over 60
▼ No special problems.

Driving and hazardous work
▼ No known problems.

Alcohol
▼ No known problems.

PROLONGED USE

No special problems.

TERBUTALINE

Product name Bricanyl
Used in the following combined preparations None

GENERAL INFORMATION

Terbutaline is a *sympathomimetic bronchodilator* that dilates the small airways in the lungs. The drug is used in the treatment and prevention of the bronchospasm occurring with asthma, chronic bronchitis, and emphysema.

Muscle tremor, especially of the hands, is common with terbutaline and usually disappears on reduction of the dose or with continued use as the body adapts to the drug. In common with the other sympathomimetic drugs, it may produce nervousness and restlessness.

INFORMATION FOR USERS

Your drug prescription is tailored for you. Do not alter dosage without checking with your physician.

How taken

Inhaler.

Frequency and timing of doses
As necessary.

Usual dosage range
Adults 0.5–3mg daily.
Children Reduced dose according to age and weight.

Onset of effect
Within a few minutes.

Duration of action
4–8 hours.

Diet advice
None.

Storage
Keep in a closed container in a cool, dry place out of the reach of children. Protect from light. Do not puncture or burn aerosol containers.

Missed dose
Do not take the missed dose. Take your next dose as usual.

Stopping the drug
Do not stop the drug without consulting your physician; symptoms may recur.

Exceeding the dose
An occasional unintentional extra dose is unlikely to be a cause for concern. But if you notice any unusual symptoms, or if a large overdose has been taken, notify your physician.

SPECIAL PRECAUTIONS

Be sure to tell your physician if:
▼ You have heart problems.
▼ You have high blood pressure.
▼ You have diabetes.
▼ You have an overactive thyroid.
▼ You are taking other medications.

Pregnancy
▼ Safety in early pregnancy not established, although it is used in late pregnancy to prevent premature labour. Discuss with your physician.

Breast-feeding
▼ The drug passes into the breast milk and may affect the baby. Discuss with your physician.

Infants and children
▼ Reduced dose necessary.

Over 60
▼ Increased likelihood of adverse effects. Reduced dose may therefore be necessary.

Driving and hazardous work
▼ Avoid such activities until you have learned how terbutaline affects you because the drug can cause tremor of the hands.

Alcohol
▼ No special problems.

POSSIBLE ADVERSE EFFECTS

Possible *adverse effects* include tremor, nervousness, restlessness, and nausea. These may be reduced by adjustment of dosage.

Palpitations and headache, resulting from stimulation of the heart and narrowing of the blood vessels, are rare.

Symptom/effect	Frequency		Discuss with physician		Stop taking drug now	Call physician now
	Common	Rare	Only if severe	In all cases		
Nausea/vomiting	●		■			
Tremor	●		■			
Restlessness/anxiety	●		■			
Headache		●	■			
Palpitations		●		■		
Muscle cramps		●		■		

INTERACTIONS

Other sympathomimetics may add to the effects of terbutaline and vice versa, so increasing the risk of adverse effects.

Monoamine oxidase inhibitors (MAOIs) Terbutaline may interact with these drugs to cause a dangerous rise in blood pressure.

Beta blockers may reduce the beneficial effects of terbutaline.

PROLONGED USE

Prolonged use may result in tolerance to the effects of terbutaline. However, failure to respond to the drug may be a result of worsening asthma, requiring prompt medical attention.

TERIPARATIDE

Product name Forteo
Used in the following combined preparations None

GENERAL INFORMATION

Teriparatide, a recombinant human analogue of parathyroid hormone, is used in severe osteoporosis in men and in post-menopausal women. It increases the amount of bone formed and increases bone strength and thickness. In studies in severe osteoporosis, when used for 18 months, it increased bone density and decreased the incidence of new fractures. This drug is not advised for individuals with calcium disorders, Paget's disease, and bone tumors.

Teriparatide is given as an injection into the subcutaneous tissue of the thigh or abdominal wall. It comes as a prefilled delivery device containing 28 doses. The individual should be seated or lying down when receiving this drug as it can cause lightheadedness. It can be self-administered. Daily calcium intake in those using teriparatide should be limited to 500mg to prevent high calcium levels. Discuss your calcium and vitamin D intake with your physician.

QUICK REFERENCE

Drug group A drug for bone disorders (p.108)

Overdose danger rating Medium

Dependence rating Low

Prescription needed Yes

Available as generic No

INFORMATION FOR USERS

Your drug prescription is tailored for you. Do not alter dosage without checking with your physician.

How taken

Injection (subcutaneous).

Frequency and timing of doses
Once daily.

Adult dosage range
20mcg subcutaneously daily for 18 months.

Onset of effect
Several weeks to see effect on bone density.

Duration of action
Up to 24 hours.

Diet advice
A diet with calcium (no more than 500mg daily) and vitamin D (800 IU daily)

is recommended. Supplements may be used.

Storage
Store this medication in the refrigerator at all times. Do not freeze it. Protect it from light. Keep out of the reach of children.

Missed dose
If you miss a dose and remember it on that day, take it as soon as you remember. If it is the next day, skip the missed dose and resume your usual dosing schedule. Do not double up to catch up on a missed dose.

Stopping the drug
Do not stop the drug without consulting your physician.

Exeeding the dose
An occasional unintentional extra dose is unlikely to cause problems. Large overdoses may cause changes to calcium levels in the blood and toxicity related to this.

SPECIAL PRECAUTIONS

Be sure to tell your physician if:
▼ You have Paget's disease.
▼ You have other bone disorders including bone tumors.
▼ You have had radiation treatment.
▼ You have had high calcium levels or parathyroid disorder.
▼ You have kidney or liver disorder or heart disease.
▼ You are allergic to mannitol or other medications.
▼ You are taking other medications.

Pregnancy
▼ Safety not established. Discuss with your physician.

Breast-feeding
▼ Safety not established. Not to be used in pre-menopausal women.

Infants and children
▼ Not recommended in children and adolescents.

Over 60
▼ No special problems.

Driving and hazardous work
▼ No special problems.

Alcohol
▼ No special problems. Individuals with osteoporosis should ensure that strategies are in place to prevent falling, which can result in fractures.

POSSIBLE ADVERSE EFFECTS

This drug is generally well tolerated. Its side effects include muscle cramps and, rarely, high calcium levels, nausea, and dizziness.

Symptom/effect	Frequency		Discuss with physician		Stop taking drug now	Call physician now
	Common	Rare	Only if severe	In all cases		
Pain at injection site	●		■			
Weakness	●		■			
Nausea	●		■			
Dizziness	●		■			
Heart burn	●		■			
Fainting		●		■		
Tooth disorder		●		■		
Leg cramps		●		■		
Chest pain		●		■	▲	▮
Difficulty breathing		●		■	▲	▮
Fever, chills		●		■		▮

PROLONGED USE

This medication is usually recommended up to 18 months only.

Monitoring Calcium levels will be measured prior to starting therapy and periodically while on the medication. Bone density may be measured yearly.

INTERACTIONS

Digoxin Teriparatide should be used cautiously in those on digoxin; increase in calcium levels can result in adverse effects from digoxin.

TESTOSTERONE

Product names Andriol, Androderm, AndroGel, Delatestryl
Used in the following combined preparation None

GENERAL INFORMATION

Testosterone is a male sex hormone produced by the testes and, in small quantities, by the ovaries in women. The hormone encourages bone and muscle growth in both men and women and stimulates sexual development in men.

The drug is used to initiate puberty in male adolescents if it has been delayed because of a deficiency of the natural hormone. It may help to increase fertility in men suffering from either pituitary or testicular disorders. Rarely, testosterone is used to treat breast cancer.

Testosterone can interfere with growth or cause over-rapid sexual development in adolescents. High doses may cause deepening of the voice, excessive hair growth, or hair loss in women.

INFORMATION FOR USERS

Your drug prescription is tailored for you. Do not alter dosage without checking with your physician.

How taken

Capsules, injection, patch, topical gel.

Frequency and timing of doses
2 x daily (capsules); once every 2 weeks to 2 x weekly (injection) depending on condition being treated; once daily (patch); once daily (gel).

Usual dosage range
Varies with method of administration and the condition being treated.

Onset of effect
2–3 days.

Duration of action
1–2 days (capsules and patch); 1–3 weeks (injection); approximately 6 months (implant).

Diet advice
None.

Storage
Keep in a closed container in a cool, dry place out of the reach of children. Protect from light.

Missed dose
No cause for concern, but take as soon as you remember. If your next dose (by mouth) is due within 3 hours, take a single dose now and skip the next.

Stopping the drug
Do not stop taking the drug without consulting your physician.

Exceeding the dose
An occasional unintentional extra dose is unlikely to be a cause for concern. But if you notice unusual symptoms, or if a large overdose was taken, notify your physician.

SPECIAL PRECAUTIONS

Be sure to tell your physician if:
▼ You have long-term liver or kidney problems.
▼ You have heart problems.
▼ You have prostate trouble.
▼ You have high blood pressure.
▼ You have epilepsy or migraine headaches.
▼ You have diabetes.
▼ You are taking other medications.

Pregnancy
▼ Not prescribed.

Breast-feeding
▼ Not prescribed.

Infants and children
▼ Not prescribed for infants and young children. Reduced dose necessary in adolescents.

Over 60
▼ Rarely required. Increased risk of prostate problems in elderly men. Reduced dose may therefore be necessary.

Driving and hazardous work
▼ No special problems.

Alcohol
▼ No special problems.

POSSIBLE ADVERSE EFFECTS

Most of the more serious *adverse effects* are likely to occur only with long-term treatment with testosterone, and may be helped by a reduction in dosage.

Symptom/effect	Frequency		Discuss with physician		Stop taking drug now	Call physician now
	Common	Rare	Only if severe	In all cases		
Jaundice		●		■	▲	
Water retention		●	■			
Men only						
Difficulty in passing urine		●		■		
Abnormal erection	●			■		
Women only						
Unusual hair growth/loss		●	■			
Voice changes		●		■		
Enlarged clitoris		●		■		

INTERACTIONS

Anticoagulant drugs Testosterone may increase the effect of these drugs. Dosage of anticoagulant drugs may need to be adjusted accordingly.

Antidiabetic agents As testosterone may lower the blood sugar, dosage of antidiabetic drugs and insulin may need to be reduced.

PROLONGED USE

Prolonged use of this drug may lead to reduced growth in adolescents.

Monitoring Regular blood tests for the effects of testosterone treatment are required.

TETRACYCLINE

Product names Apo-Tetra, Novo-Tetra, and others
Used in the following combined preparations None

GENERAL INFORMATION

Tetracycline is a very widely used antibiotic. However, the development of drug-resistant bacteria has reduced its effectiveness in many types of infection. Tetracycline is still used for chest infections caused by chlamydia (for example, psittacosis) and mycoplasma microorganisms. Tetracycline is also used in non-specific urethritis and a number of rarer conditions, such as Q fever, Rocky Mountain spotted fever, cholera, and brucellosis. Acne improves with long-term treatment with tetracycline either taken by mouth or applied to the skin.

Common *side effects* of this drug are nausea, vomiting, and diarrhea. Rashes may also occur. Tetracycline may discolour developing teeth if it is taken by children or by the mother during pregnancy. People with poor kidney function are not prescribed tetracycline because it can cause further deterioration.

QUICK REFERENCE

Drug group Tetracycline antibiotic (p.114)

Overdose danger rating Low

Dependence rating Low

Prescription needed Yes

Available as generic Yes

INFORMATION FOR USERS

Your drug prescription is tailored for you. Do not alter your dosage without checking with your physician.

How taken

Tablets, capsules, ointment.

Frequency and timing of doses
By mouth 4 x daily, at least 1 hour before or 2 hours after meals.
Long-term treatment of acne may require only a single dose daily.
Skin preparations 1–3 times daily as directed.

Usual adult dosage range
Infections 1–2g daily.
Acne 250mg–1g daily.

Onset of effect
4–12 hours. Improvement in acne may not be noticed for up to 4 weeks.

Duration of action
Up to 6 hours.

Diet advice
Milk products should be avoided for 1 hour before and 2 hours after taking the drug, since they may impair its absorption.

Storage
Keep in a closed container in a cool, dry place out of the reach of children.

Missed dose
Take as soon as you remember. If your next dose is due within 2 hours, take a single dose now and skip the next.

Stopping the drug
Take the full course. Even if you feel better, the original infection may still be present and may recur if treatment is stopped too soon.

Exceeding the dose
An occasional unintentional extra dose is unlikely to be a cause for concern. But if you notice any unusual symptoms, or if a large overdose has been taken, notify your physician.

SPECIAL PRECAUTIONS

Be sure to tell your physician if:
▼ You have long-term liver or kidney problems.
▼ You have previously suffered an allergic reaction to a tetracycline antibiotic.
▼ You have myasthenia gravis.
▼ You have systemic lupus erythematosus.
▼ You are taking other medications.

Pregnancy
▼ Not usually prescribed. May cause discoloured teeth and damage bones of the developing fetus. Discuss with your physician.

Breast-feeding
▼ The drugs pass into the breast milk and may damage developing bones and discolour the baby's teeth. Discuss with your physician.

Infants and children
▼ Not recommended under 12 years. Reduced dose necessary in older children. May discolour developing teeth.

Over 60
▼ No special problems.

Driving and hazardous work
▼ No known problems.

Alcohol
▼ No known problems.

Taking your tablets
▼ To prevent irritation to the esophagus, each dose of the drug should be taken with a full glass of water while standing.

POSSIBLE ADVERSE EFFECTS

Adverse effects from skin preparations are rare. When tetracyclines are given by mouth, however, they may cause nausea, vomiting, or diarrhea.

Symptom/effect	Frequency		Discuss with physician		Stop taking drug now	Call physician now
	Common	Rare	Only if severe	In all cases		
Nausea/vomiting	●		■			
Diarrhea	●		■			
Light-sensitive rash		●		■	▲	
Rash/itching		●		■	▲	
Jaundice		●		■	▲	
Headache/visual disturbance		●		■	▲	■

INTERACTIONS

Iron may reduce the effectiveness of tetracycline.

Oral anticoagulants Tetracycline may increase the action of these drugs.

Retinoids may increase the adverse effects of tetracycline.

Oral contraceptives Tetracycline may reduce the effectiveness of oral contraceptives.

Antacids and milk These interfere with the absorption of tetracycline and may reduce their effectiveness. Doses should be separated by 1–2 hours.

PROLONGED USE

No problems expected.

THEOPHYLLINE/AMINOPHYLLINE

Product names [theophylline], Phyllocontin, Theolair, Uniphyl
Used in the following combined preparations [theophylline] ratio-Theo-Bronc

GENERAL INFORMATION

Theophylline (and aminophylline, which breaks down to theophylline in the body) is used to treat bronchospasm (constriction of the air passages) in patients suffering from asthma, bronchitis, and emphysema.

It is usually taken continuously as a preventative measure, and is added to standard therapy. It can also be used to treat acute attacks in hospital.

Slow-release formulations of the drugs produce beneficial effects lasting for up to 12 hours. These preparations may be prescribed twice daily, but they are also useful as a single dose taken at night to prevent night-time asthma.

Treatment with theophylline must be monitored because the effective dose is very close to the *toxic* dose. Some *adverse effects*, such as indigestion, nausea, headache, and agitation, can be controlled by regulating the dosage and checking blood levels of the drug.

INFORMATION FOR USERS

Your drug prescription is tailored for you. Do not alter dosage without checking with your physician.

How taken

Tablets, SR-tablets, liquid, injection.

Frequency and timing of doses
3–4 x daily (tablets, liquid); every 12 or 24 hours (SR-tablets). The drug should be taken at the same time each day in relation to meals.

Usual dosage range
Adults 200–600mg daily, depending on which product is used.

Onset of effect
Within 30 minutes (by mouth); within 90 minutes (SR-tablets).

Duration of action
Up to 8 hours (by mouth); 12–24 hours (SR-tablets).

Diet advice
None.

Storage
Keep in a closed container in a cool, dry place out of the reach of children.

Missed dose
Take as soon as you remember. If your next dose is due within 2 hours, take half the dose now (short-acting preparations) or forget about the missed dose and take your next dose now (SR-preparations). Return to your normal dose schedule thereafter.

Stopping the drug
Do not stop taking the drug without consulting your physician; stopping the drug may lead to worsening of the underlying condition.

OVERDOSE ACTION

 Seek immediate medical advice in all cases. Take emergency action if chest pains, confusion, or loss of consciousness occur.

See Drug poisoning emergency guide (p.526).

SPECIAL PRECAUTIONS

Be sure to tell your physician if:
▼ You have a long-term liver problem.
▼ You have angina or irregular heart beat.
▼ You have high blood pressure.
▼ You have epilepsy.
▼ You have hyperthyroidism.
▼ You have porphyria.
▼ You have stomach ulcers.
▼ You smoke.
▼ You are taking other medications.

 Pregnancy
▼ Safety in pregnancy not established. Discuss with your physician.

 Breast-feeding
▼ The drug passes into the breast milk and may affect the baby. Discuss with your physician.

 Infants and children
▼ Reduced dose necessary according to age and weight.

 Over 60
▼ Reduced dose may be necessary.

 Driving and hazardous work
▼ No known problems

 Alcohol
▼ Avoid excess as this may alter levels of the drug and may increase gastrointestinal symptoms.

PROLONGED USE

No problems expected.

Monitoring Periodic checks on blood levels of this drug are usually required.

POSSIBLE ADVERSE EFFECTS

Most adverse effects of this drug are related to dosage. These include effects related to the drug's action on the central nervous system, such as agitation and insomnia.

Symptom/effect	Frequency		Discuss with physician		Stop taking drug now	Call physician now
	Common	Rare	Only if severe	In all cases		
Agitation		●		■		
Headache	●			■		
Nausea/vomiting	●		■			
Diarrhea		●	■			
Insomnia		●	■			
Palpitations		●		■	▲	▮

INTERACTIONS

General note Many drugs increase the effect of theophylline (e.g., erythromycin, cimetidine, acyclovir, oral contraceptives, ciprofloxacin, and clarithromycin); others reduce its effect (e.g., carbamazepine, phenytoin, and rifampin). Discuss with your physician.

TIMOLOL

Product names Timoptic, Timoptic-XE
Used in the following combined preparations Combigan, Cosopt

GENERAL INFORMATION

Timolol is a beta blocker prescribed to treat hypertension (high blood pressure) and angina (pain due to narrowing of the coronary arteries). It may be given after a heart attack to prevent further damage to the heart muscle. When used to treat hypertension, it may also be given with a diuretic. Timolol is commonly administered as eye drops to people with certain types of glaucoma, and is occasionally given to prevent migraine.

Timolol can cause breathing difficulties, especially in people who have asthma, chronic bronchitis, or emphysema. This problem is more likely in people taking the drug in tablet form, although it can also occur in individuals using timolol eye drops. As with other beta blockers, timolol may mask the body's response to low blood sugar and, for that reason, is prescribed with caution to diabetics.

QUICK REFERENCE

Drug group Beta blocker (p.83) and drug for glaucoma (p.156)

Overdose danger rating High

Dependence rating Low

Prescription needed Yes

Available as generic Yes

INFORMATION FOR USERS

Your drug prescription is tailored for you. Do not alter dosage without checking with your physician.

How taken

Tablets, eye drops.

Frequency and timing of doses
1–2 x daily.

Usual adult dosage range
By mouth 10–40mg daily (hypertension); 10–45mg daily (angina); 10–20mg daily (after a heart attack); 10–20mg daily (migraine prevention).

Onset of effect
Within 30 minutes (by mouth).

Duration of action
Up to 24 hours.

Diet advice
None.

Storage
Keep in a closed container in a cool, dry place out of the reach of children.

Missed dose
Take as soon as you remember. If your next dose is due within 3 hours, take a single dose now and skip the next.

Stopping the drug
Do not stop the drug without consulting your physician; stopping the drug may lead to worsening of the underlying condition.

OVERDOSE ACTION

 Seek immediate medical advice in all cases of overdose by mouth. Take emergency action if breathing difficulties, palpitations, or loss of consciousness occur.

See Drug poisoning emergency guide (p.526).

POSSIBLE ADVERSE EFFECTS

Timolol taken by mouth can occasionally provoke or worsen heart problems and asthma. Fainting may be a sign that the drug has slowed the heartbeat excessively. Eye drops cause these problems only rarely; headache or blurred vision is more likely.

Symptom/effect	Frequency		Discuss with physician		Stop taking drug now	Call physician now
	Common	Rare	Only if severe	In all cases		
Lethargy/fatigue/headache	●		■			
Blurred vision (eye drops)	●		■			
Eye irritation (eye drops)		●	■			
Cold hands/feet		●	■			
Dizziness/fainting		●		■		
Nightmares/vivid dreams		●		■		
Wheezing/breathlessness		●		■	▲	■

INTERACTIONS

Sympathomimetics Present in many cough and cold remedies, these drugs can cause a dangerous rise in blood pressure when taken with timolol.

Salbutamol, salmeterol, and other beta agonists The effects of these drugs may be reduced by timolol.

SPECIAL PRECAUTIONS

Be sure to tell your physician if:
▼ You have a lung disorder such as asthma, bronchitis, or emphysema.
▼ You have diabetes.
▼ You have myasthenia gravis.
▼ You have poor circulation.
▼ You have allergies.
▼ You are taking other medications.

 Pregnancy
▼ Safety in pregnancy not established. Discuss with your physician.

 Breast-feeding
▼ The drug passes into the breast milk, but at normal doses *adverse effects* on the baby are unlikely. Discuss with your physician.

 Infants and children
▼ Not usually prescribed.

 Over 60
▼ Reduced dose may be necessary.

 Driving and hazardous work
▼ Avoid such activities until you have learned how timolol affects you because the tablets may cause drowsiness and the eye drops may cause blurred vision.

 Alcohol
▼ May enhance lowering of blood pressure; avoid excessive amounts.

Surgery and general anesthetics
▼ Timolol by mouth may need to be stopped before you have a general anesthetic. Discuss with your physician or dentist before any surgery.

PROLONGED USE

No problems expected.

TIOTROPIUM

Product name Spiriva
Used in the following combined preparations None

GENERAL INFORMATION

Tiotropium is an *anticholinergic* bronchodilator that relaxes the muscles surrounding the bronchioles (airways in the lung). It is used in the maintenance treatment of reversible airway disorders, such as chronic bronchitis. Tiotropium is a long-acting drug, but its effects are felt after only 5 minutes or so. It is not suitable for acute attacks of wheezing or in the emergency treatment of asthma. Tiotropium is taken by inhalation of a powder, and it acts directly and locally on the internal surface of the lungs and not via the blood. The most common side effect is a dry mouth.

QUICK REFERENCE

Drug group Bronchodilator (p.76)
Overdose danger rating Low
Dependence rating Low
Prescription needed Yes
Available as generic No

INFORMATION FOR USERS

Your drug prescription is tailored for you. Do not alter dosage without checking with your physician.

How taken

Powder in capsules for inhaler.

Frequency and timing of doses
Once daily, at the same time each day.

Usual adult dosage range
18mcg daily.

Onset of effect
5 minutes.

Duration of action
24 hours.

Diet advice
None.

Storage
Keep in a closed container in a cool, dry place out of the reach of children.

Missed dose
Take as soon as you remember. If your next dose is due within 8 hours, take a single dose now and skip the next.

Stopping the drug
Do not stop taking the drug without consulting your physician. Symptoms may recur.

Exceeding the dose
An occasional unintentional extra dose is unlikely to be a cause for concern. But if you notice any unusual symptoms, or if a large overdose has been taken, notify your physician.

SPECIAL PRECAUTIONS

Be sure to tell your physician if:
▼ You are allergic to atropine or ipratropium.
▼ You have prostate problems.
▼ You have urinary retention.
▼ You have glaucoma.
▼ You have kidney problems.
▼ You are taking other medications.

Pregnancy
▼ Safety not established.

Breast-feeding
▼ Safety not established.

Infants and children
▼ Not recommended under 18 years of age.

Over 60
▼ No known problems.

Driving and hazardous work
▼ No known problems.

Alcohol
▼ No known problems.

Protecting your eyes
▼ Care must be taken to avoid getting the powder into the eyes as it could trigger glaucoma or make existing glaucoma worse. If you develop eye or vision problems, call your physician immediately.

POSSIBLE ADVERSE EFFECTS

Dry mouth is the most common side effect. If you get the powder in your eyes, it could trigger glaucoma; you should call the physician immediately.

Symptom/effect	Frequency		Discuss with physician		Stop taking drug now	Call physician now
	Common	Rare	Only if severe	In all cases		
Dry mouth/sore throat	●		■			
Constipation	●		■			
Fast heart beat/palpitations		●		■		
Difficulty passing urine		●		■		
Rash		●		■		
Wheezing after inhalation		●		■		
Eye pain/blurred vision		●		■		▮
Visual halos		●		■		▮

INTERACTIONS

Atropine and ipratropium The effects and toxicity of tiotropium are likely to be increased if it is used at the same time as these drugs.

PROLONGED USE

No known problems.

TIZANIDINE

Product names Apo-Tizanidine, Zanaflex
Used in the following combined preparations None

GENERAL INFORMATION

Tizanadine is a medication used to treat muscle spasms. It can be used in many conditions where spasticity or muscle tone needs to be controlled. The dose should be scheduled such that the peak effect coincides with the time when relief of spasticity is most desirable.

Generally, the drug is well tolerated. The most common side effects are constipation, dry mouth, drowsiness, dizziness, and decrease in blood pressure. To minimize side effects, especially the decrease in blood pressure, the dose should be increased gradually.

INFORMATION FOR USERS

Your drug prescription is tailored for you. Do not alter dosage without checking with your physician.

How taken

Tablets.

Frequency and timing of doses
Up to three or four times daily.

Usual adult dosage range
4–8mg (1–2 tablets) two to four times daily; starting dose 4mg once daily.

Onset of effect
Peak effect usually occurs in 1–2 hours.

Duration of action
Effect may last between 3–6 hours.

Diet advice
None.

Storage
Keep in a closed container in a cool, dry place out of the reach of children.

Missed dose
If you miss a dose, take it as soon as you remember. If it is near the time of the next dose, skip the missed dose and resume your using dosing schedule. Do not double-up to catch up on a missed dose.

Stopping the drug
Do not stop the drug without consulting your physician. Stopping the drug may lead to worsening of the underlying condition.

Exceeding the dose
An occasional unintentional extra dose is unlikely to cause problems. Large overdoses may cause severe drowsiness, fainting, or trouble breathing. If overdose is suspected, notify your local poison control centre right away.

SPECIAL PRECAUTIONS

Be sure to tell your physician if:
▼ You are allergic to tizanidine.
▼ You are taking blood pressure medications.
▼ You have fainted before or have low blood pressure.
▼ You have kidney problems.
▼ You are on any other medications.

 Pregnancy
▼ Safety in pregnancy not established. Discuss with your physician.

 Breast-feeding
▼ Safety in breast-feeding not established. Discuss with your physician.

 Infants and children
▼ Not recommended.

 Over 60
▼ Increased likelihood of adverse effects. Reduced dose may therefore be necessary. Dose should be adjusted for any changes in kidney function.

 Driving and hazardous work
▼ Do not undertake such activities until you have learned how the drug affects you; it can cause reduced alertness and slowed reactions.

 Alcohol
▼ Avoid. Can increase side effects of tizanidine. Alcohol increases the sedative effects of this drug.

POSSIBLE ADVERSE EFFECTS

The most common side effects caused by tizanidine are dizziness and dry mouth. Blood pressures can decrease more significantly with higher doses. To minimize dizziness, stand up slowly when arising from a sitting or lying position.

Symptom/effect	Frequency		Discuss with physician		Stop taking drug now	Call physician now
	Common	Rare	Only if severe	In all cases		
Dizziness	●		■			
Drowsiness	●		■			
Nausea	●		■			
Dry mouth	●		■			
Constipation	●		■			
Muscle fatigue/weakness	●		■			
Stomach pain, vomiting		●		■		▮
Yellowing of skin or eyes		●		■		▮
Vision/hearing changes		●		■		▮

INTERACTIONS

All drugs, including alcohol, that cause drowsiness such as anti-anxiety and sleeping drugs, antihistamines, antidepressants, opioid analgesics, and antipsychotics These can increase the sedative properties of tizanidine.

Antihypertensive and diuretic drugs The effect of such drugs may be increased.

Oral contraceptives These may increase the effect of tizanidine; dose of tizanidine may need to be adjusted.

PROLONGED USE

If this medication has been taken for a prolonged time, it should not be stopped suddenly without consulting with your physician.

Monitoring Periodic blood tests may be performed to check for liver function.

TOLTERODINE

Product names Detrol, Detrol LA
Used in the following combined preparations None

GENERAL INFORMATION

Tolterodine is an *anticholinergic* and antispasmodic drug that is similar to oxybutynin. It is used to treat urinary frequency and incontinence in adults. Tolterodine works by reducing contraction of the bladder, allowing it to expand and hold more. It also stops spasms and delays the desire to empty the bladder.

Tolterodine's usefulness is limited to some extent by its *side effects*, and dosage needs to be reduced in the elderly. Children are more susceptible than adults to the drug's anticholinergic effects. Tolterodine can also trigger glaucoma.

QUICK REFERENCE

Drug group Drug for urinary disorders (p.154)

Overdose danger rating Medium

Dependence rating Low

Prescription needed Yes

Available as generic No

INFORMATION FOR USERS

Your drug prescription is tailored for you. Do not alter dosage without checking with your physician.

How taken

Tablets, ER capsules.

Frequency and timing of doses
2 x daily, once daily for extended release.

Usual adult dosage range
4mg daily, reduced to 2mg daily, if necessary, to minimize side effects.

Onset of effect
1 hour.

Duration of action
12 hours.

Diet advice
None.

Storage
Keep in a closed container in a cool, dry place out of the reach of children.

Missed dose
Take as soon as you remember. If your next dose is due within 2 hours, take a single dose now and skip the next.

Stopping the drug
Do not stop taking the drug without consulting your physician; symptoms may recur.

Exceeding the dose
An occasional unintentional extra dose is unlikely to cause problems. Large overdoses may cause visual disturbances, urinary difficulties, hallucinations, convulsions, and breathing difficulties. Notify your physician.

SPECIAL PRECAUTIONS

Be sure to tell your physician if:
▼ You have liver or kidney problems.
▼ You have thyroid problems.
▼ You have heart problems.
▼ You have porphyria.
▼ You have hiatus hernia.
▼ You have prostate problems or urinary retention.
▼ You have ulcerative colitis.
▼ You have glaucoma.
▼ You have myasthenia gravis.
▼ You are taking other medications.

Pregnancy
▼ Safety in pregnancy not established. May harm the unborn baby. Discuss with your physician.

Breast-feeding
▼ Safety not established. Discuss with your physician.

Infants and children
▼ Not recommended. Safety not established.

Over 60
▼ Reduced dose may be necessary.

Driving and hazardous work
▼ Avoid. Tolterodine may cause drowsiness, disorientation, and blurred vision.

Alcohol
▼ Avoid. Alcohol increases the drug's sedative effects.

POSSIBLE ADVERSE EFFECTS

The most common side effects, such as dry mouth, digestive upset, and dry eyes, are the result of the drug's anticholinergic action.

Symptom/effect	Frequency		Discuss with physician		Stop taking drug now	Call physician now
	Common	Rare	Only if severe	In all cases		
Dry mouth/digestive upset	●		■			
Constipation/abdominal pain	●		■			
Headache	●		■			
Dry eyes/blurred vision	●		■			
Drowsiness/nervousness	●		■			
Chest pain		●		■		
Confusion		●		■		
Urinary difficulties		●		■		

INTERACTIONS

General note All drugs that have an anticholinergic effect will have increased side effects when taken with tolterodine.

Domperidone and metoclopramide The effects of these drugs may be decreased by tolterodine.

Erythromycin, clarithromycin, itraconazole, ketoconazole, and miconazole These drugs may increase blood levels of tolterodine.

PROLONGED USE

No special problems. Effectiveness of the drug, and continuing clinical need for it, are usually reviewed after 6 months.

Monitoring Periodic eye tests for glaucoma may be performed.

TOPIRAMATE

Product names Dom-Topiramate, Gen-Topiramate, PMS-Topiramate, Sandoz Topiramate, Topamax
Used in the following combined preparations None

GENERAL INFORMATION

Topiramate is an anticonvulsant drug, usually prescribed in combination with other anticonvulsants, such as valproic acid, carbamazepine, or phenytoin, for the treatment of epilepsy. It may also be used to prevent migraine headaches and can reduce the frequency of migraines. It is not recommended in children less than 2 years of age.

Tablets should be swallowed whole. Sprinkle capsules can be swallowed whole or sprinkled on a teaspoonful of food and swallowed without chewing. Topiramate may cause a number of dose-related side effects. Some individuals may experience weight loss; if this occurs, an increase in food intake or dietary supplements may be helpful.

INFORMATION FOR USERS

Your drug prescription is tailored for you. Do not alter dosage without checking with your physician.

How taken

Tablets, Sprinkle capsules.

Frequency and timing of doses
Usually twice daily; can sprinkle capsule contents on soft food or swallow whole.

Usual adult dosage range
50mg (starting); 200–400mg daily (maintenance).

Onset of effect
Approximately 4–8 days at a constant dose.

Duration of action
Up to 24 hours.

Diet advice
None.

Storage
Keep in a closed container in a cool, dry place out of the reach of children.

Missed dose
If it is almost time for the next dose, take a single dose now and skip the next. Do not double up on a dose.

Stopping the drug
Do not stop taking the drug without consulting your physician. A gradual reduction is necessary to reduce the risk of rebound fits.

Exceeding the dose
An occasional unintentional extra dose is unlikely to be a cause for concern. Large overdoses may cause sedation, loss of muscular coordination, nausea, and vomiting. Contact your physician immediately.

POSSIBLE ADVERSE EFFECTS

Generally well tolerated.

Symptom/effect	Frequency		Discuss with physician		Stop taking drug now	Call physician now
	Common	Rare	Only if severe	In all cases		
Headache	●		■			
Dizziness/drowsiness	●		■			
Nervousness	●			■		
Difficulty coordinating muscle movements/speech problems	●			■		
Difficulty concentrating/with memory	●			■		
Tingling in fingers/toes		●		■		
Confusion/mood changes		●		■		
Vision changes		●		■		
Decreased sweating		●		■		

INTERACTIONS

Phenytoin and carbamazepine These drugs can decrease the effectiveness of topiramate and the dose of topiramate may need to be adjusted.

Acetazolamide When taken with topiramate, can increase the risk of kidney stones.

Oral contraceptives Topiramate may decrease the amount of estrogen in the bodies of women taking oral contraceptives, possibly decreasing their effectiveness.

Metformin When metformin (used in diabetic management) is given with topiramate, blood glucose levels should be closely followed.

CNS depressants Any drugs that affect the CNS can have an additive effect with topiramate.

SPECIAL PRECAUTIONS

Be sure to tell your physician if:
▼ You have long-term liver or kidney problems.
▼ You have a heart condition.
▼ You are taking other medications.

Pregnancy
▼ Safety not established. Discuss with your physician.

Breast-feeding
▼ Safety not established. Discuss with your physician.

Infants and children
▼ Not recommended in children younger than 2 years. Reduced dose recommended in children between 2 and 18 years of age.

Over 60
▼ Increased likelihood of adverse effects. Reduced dose may be necessary.

Driving and hazardous work
▼ Avoid such activities until you have learned how topiramate affects you because the drug can cause drowsiness.

Alcohol
▼ Avoid. Alcohol may increase the adverse effects of this drug.

PROLONGED USE

No problems expected.

TRAMADOL

Product names Ralivia, Tridural, Zytram XL
Used in the following combined preparations Tramacet

GENERAL INFORMATION

Tramadol is a type of opioid analgesic (p.64) used to relieve moderate to severe pain. It is available as regular (RR) and extended release (ER) tablets. The ER tablets should only be used when round-the-clock pain relief is needed in someone who has already been on the regular tablets. There are different forms of ER available. These should be swallowed whole and should not be split, chewed, or crushed.

Tramadol can cause lightheadedness; it is best to get up slowly from a lying or sitting position, while supporting oneself. These drugs are habit-forming. However, most patients prescribed tramadol for pain relief do not become addicted and are able to stop taking them without difficulty.

INFORMATION FOR USERS

Your drug prescription is tailored for you. Do not alter dosage without checking with your physician.

How taken

Tablets, regular (RR) and extended release (ER).

Frequency and timing of doses
RR: every 4–6 hour; ER taken once daily.

Adult dosage range
150–400mg per day.

Onset of effect
Usually within an hour.

Duration of action
RR: 4–6 hours; ER: up to 24 hours, depending on product.

Diet advice
None.

Storage
Keep in a closed container in a cool, dry place out of the reach of children.

Missed dose
If you have been instructed to take the medication regularly, take the missed dose as soon as you remember. However, if it is near the time of the next dose, skip the missed dose and resume your usual dosing schedule. Do not double up to catch up on a missed dose.

Stopping the drug
Do not stop the drug without consulting your physician. Stopping the drug may lead to withdrawal symptoms. Tramadol requires a gradual withdrawal.

OVERDOSE ACTION

Seek immediate medical advice in all cases. Take emergency action if loss of consciousness occurs. Notify your physician.

See Drug poisoning emergency guide (p. 526).

POSSIBLE ADVERSE EFFECTS

The most common side effects are dizziness, nausea, constipation, and headache.

Symptom/effect	Frequency		Discuss with physician		Stop taking drug now	Call physician now
	Common	Rare	Only if severe	In all cases		
Nausea	●		■			
Agitation/anxiety	●			■		
Constipation	●		■			
Dizziness	●		■			
Dry mouth	●		■			
Headache	●		■			
Changes in walking or balance		●		■		
Shortness of breath		●		■		▮
Seizures		●		■		▮
Trouble concentrating/sleeping		●		■		

INTERACTIONS

CNS depressants Can have drowsiness and other additive effects.

SSRIs, TCAs, MAOIs, carbamazepine Can increase the potential for seizures.

MAOIs Tramadol must not to be used with, or for 14 days after stopping, MAOIs.

Quinidine, Cimetidine, Ritonavir These drugs can increase the effect of tramadol.

Warfarin Warfarin's effect may change with tramadol; monitor INR.

SPECIAL PRECAUTIONS

Be sure to tell your physician if:
▼ You have an allergic reaction or sensitivity to the opioid class of drugs.
▼ You have a history of seizures or epileptic fits.
▼ You have liver or kidney problems.
▼ You have a lung disorder such as asthma or bronchitis.
▼ You have sleep apnea.
▼ You have had problems with alcohol or drug abuse.
▼ You are taking herbal products such as St. John's Wort.
▼ You are taking other medications.

Pregnancy
▼ Safety in pregnancy not established. Discuss with your physician.

Breast-feeding
▼ Safety not established. Discuss with your physician.

Infants and children
▼ Safety not established in children at or below 16 years of age. For those 16 and over, see adult dosage and discuss with your physician.

Over 60
▼ A lower starting dose may be recommended.

Driving and hazardous work
▼ May cause drowsiness. Do not drive a car or operate machinery until the effect of the drug wears off and you feel you are mentally alert.

Alcohol
▼ Avoid alcohol use as it may increase the effect of drowsiness caused by this drug.

PROLONGED USE

Dependence may occur if it is taken for extended periods, although this is unusual in patients taking the correct dose for pain relief.

TRIAMTERENE

Product name Only available as combination product
Used in the following combined preparations Apo-Triazide, Novo-Triamzide

GENERAL INFORMATION

Triamterene belongs to the class of drugs known as potassium-sparing diuretics. In combination with thiazide or loop diuretics, this drug is given for the treatment of hypertension and oedema (fluid retention). Triamterene, either on its own or, more commonly, with a thiazide diuretic, may be used to treat edema as a complication of heart failure, nephrotic syndrome, or cirrhosis of the liver.

Triamterene is quick to act; its effect on urine flow is apparent within two hours. For this reason, you should avoid taking the drug after about 4 pm. As with other potassium-sparing diuretics, unusually high levels of potassium may build up in the blood if the kidneys are functioning abnormally. Therefore, triamterene is prescribed with caution to people with kidney failure.

INFORMATION FOR USERS

Your drug prescription is tailored for you. Do not alter dosage without checking with your physician.

How taken

Tablets.

Frequency and timing of doses
1–2 x daily after meals or on alternate days.

Usual adult dosage range
50–250mg daily.

Onset of effect
Within 2 hours.

Duration of action
9–12 hours.

Diet advice
Avoid foods that are high in potassium, such as dried fruit and salt substitutes.

Storage
Keep in a closed container in a cool, dry place out of the reach of children.

Missed dose
Take as soon as you remember. However, if it is late in the day, do not take the missed dose, or you may need to get up at night to pass urine. Take the next scheduled dose as usual.

Stopping the drug
Do not stop the drug without consulting your physician; symptoms may recur.

Exceeding the dose
An occasional unintentional extra dose is unlikely to be a cause for concern. But if you notice any unusual symptoms, or if a large overdose has been taken, notify your physician.

SPECIAL PRECAUTIONS

Be sure to tell your physician if:
▼ You have long-term liver or kidney problems.
▼ You have had kidney stones.
▼ You have gout.
▼ You are taking other medications.

Pregnancy
▼ Not usually prescribed. May cause a reduction in the blood supply to the developing fetus. Discuss with your physician.

Breast-feeding
▼ The drug passes into breast milk and may affect the baby. It could also reduce your milk supply. Discuss with your physician.

Infants and children
▼ Not usually prescribed. Reduced dose necessary.

Over 60
▼ Increased likelihood of adverse effects. Reduced dose may therefore be necessary.

Driving and hazardous work
▼ No special problems.

Alcohol
▼ No known problems.

POSSIBLE ADVERSE EFFECTS

Triamterene has few adverse effects; the main problem is the possibility of potassium being retained by the body, causing muscle weakness and numbness. Triamterene may colour your urine blue but this is not a cause for concern.

Symptom/effect	Frequency		Discuss with physician		Stop taking drug now	Call physician now
	Common	Rare	Only if severe	In all cases		
Digestive disturbance		●	■			
Headache		●	■			
Muscle weakness		●		■		
Rash		●		■		
Dry mouth		●	■			

INTERACTIONS

Lithium Triamterene may increase the blood levels of lithium, leading to an increased risk of lithium *toxicity*.

Non-steroidal anti-inflammatory drugs (NSAIDs) may increase the risk of raised blood levels of potassium.

ACE inhibitors These drugs increase the risk of raised blood levels of potassium with triamterene.

Cyclosporine This drug may increase levels of potassium with triamterene.

PROLONGED USE

Serious problems are unlikely, but levels of salts such as sodium and potassium may occasionally become abnormal during prolonged use.

Monitoring Blood tests may be performed to check on kidney function and levels of body salts.

TRIFLUOPERAZINE

Product name Apo-Trifluoperazine
Used in the following combined preparations None

GENERAL INFORMATION

Trifluoperazine belongs to a group of drugs called the phenothiazines. These drugs act on the brain to modify abnormal behavior (see Antipsychotics p.69). It is effective in suppressing abnormal behavior, reducing aggression, and tranquillizing agitation.

Trifluoperazine is used in the treatment of schizophrenia, mania, dementia, and other disorders where confusion, aggression, hallucinations, or abnormal behavior may occur. It is sometimes used to treat nausea and vomiting caused by drug or radiation therapy.

Trifluoperazine causes less drowsiness and *anticholinergic* side effects than most phenothiazines, but it can produce stiffness and shaking (*parkinsonism*), and abnormal movements of the face, limbs, and body (*tardive dyskinesia*).

QUICK REFERENCE

Drug group Antipsychotic (p.69), anti-emetic drug (p.74)

Overdose danger rating Medium

Dependence rating Low

Prescription needed Yes

Available as generic Yes

INFORMATION FOR USERS

Your drug prescription is tailored for you. Do not alter dosage without checking with your physician.

How taken

Tablets.

Frequency and timing of doses
2–4 x daily.

Usual adult dosage range
Mental illness 2–6mg daily (starting dose), increasing to 20mg daily (maintenance dose). Dose may be increased in cases of extreme agitation. Higher doses may be used under supervision in hospital.

Onset of effect
2–3 hours.

Duration of action
6–24 hours. Some effects may persist for weeks when stopping the drug after regular use.

Diet advice
None.

Storage
Keep in a closed container in a cool, dry place out of the reach of children. Protect from light and from freezing.

Missed dose
Take as soon as you remember. If your next dose is due within 2 hours, take a single dose now and skip the next.

Stopping the drug
Do not stop the drug without consulting your physician; symptoms may recur.

Exceeding the dose
An occasional unintentional extra dose is unlikely to be a cause for concern. Larger overdoses may cause unusual drowsiness, muscle weakness or rigidity, and/or faintness. Notify your physician.

SPECIAL PRECAUTIONS

Be sure to tell your physician if:
▼ You have impaired liver or kidney function.
▼ You have heart or circulation problems.
▼ You have had epileptic seizures.
▼ You have an overactive thyroid gland.
▼ You have Parkinson's disease.
▼ You have had glaucoma.
▼ You have prostate trouble.
▼ You are taking other medications.

Pregnancy
▼ Safety in pregnancy not established. Discuss with your physician.

Breast-feeding
▼ The drug passes into breast milk. Its effects on the baby are not known. Discuss with your physician.

Infants and children
▼ Rarely required. Reduced dose necessary.

Over 60
▼ Reduced dose may be necessary.

Driving and hazardous work
▼ Avoid such activities until you have learned how the drug affects you; it can cause drowsiness and slowed reactions.

Alcohol
▼ Avoid. Alcohol may increase the sedative effect of this drug.

POSSIBLE ADVERSE EFFECTS

Trifluoperazine can cause a variety of minor anticholinergic symptoms that often become less marked with time. The most significant adverse effect is abnormal movements of the face and limbs (parkinsonism). This may be controlled by dosage adjustment.

Symptom/effect	Frequency		Discuss with physician		Stop taking drug now	Call physician now
	Common	Rare	Only if severe	In all cases		
Drowsiness/lethargy	●		■			
Parkinsonism	●			■		
Dizziness/fainting	●			■		
Infrequent periods		●		■		
Rash		●		■	▲	
High fever/confusion		●		■	▲	■

INTERACTIONS

Anticonvulsants and antiparkinsonian drugs Trifluoperazine may reduce the effectiveness of such drugs.

Anticholinergic drugs Their side effects may be increased by trifluoperazine.

Sedatives All drugs, including alcohol, that have a sedative effect on the central nervous system are likely to increase the sedative effects of trifluoperazine.

PROLONGED USE

Use of this drug for more than a few months may lead to tardive dyskinesia, i.e., abnormal, involuntary movements of the eyes, face, and tongue. Occasionally, jaundice may occur.

Monitoring Periodic blood tests may be performed.

TRIMETHOPRIM

Product name Apo-Trimethoprim
Used in the following combined preparations Apo-Sulfatrim, Apo-Sulfatrim DS, Novo-Trimel DS, PMS-Polytrimethoprim

GENERAL INFORMATION

Trimethoprim is an antibacterial drug that became popular in the 1970s for prevention and treatment of infections of the urinary and respiratory tracts. The drug has been used for many years in combination with another antibacterial, sulfamethoxazole, in a preparation known as co-trimoxazole (see p.245). Trimethoprim, however, has fewer *adverse effects* than co-trimoxazole and is equally effective in treating many conditions. The drug can also be given by injection to treat severe infections.

Although *side effects* of trimethoprim are not usually troublesome, tests to monitor blood composition are often advised when the drug is taken for prolonged periods.

QUICK REFERENCE

Drug group Antibacterial drug (p.117)

Overdose danger rating Low

Dependence rating Low

Prescription needed Yes

Available as generic Yes

INFORMATION FOR USERS

Your drug prescription is tailored for you. Do not alter dosage without checking with your physician.

How taken

Tablets, liquid, injection, eye drops.

Frequency and timing of doses
Oral: 1–2 x daily; eye drops: up to 6 x per day

Usual adult dosage range
Oral: 200mg daily.
Eye drops: one drop in affected eye every 3 hours (maximum 6 doses per day)

Onset of effect
1–4 hours.

Duration of action
Up to 24 hours.

Diet advice
None.

Storage
Keep in a closed container in a cool, dry place out of the reach of children. Protect from light.

Missed dose
Take as soon as you remember.

Stopping the drug
Take the full course. Even if you feel better, the original infection may still be present and symptoms may recur if treatment is stopped too soon.

Exceeding the dose
An occasional unintentional extra dose is unlikely to be a cause for concern. But if you notice any unusual symptoms, or if a large overdose has been taken, notify your physician.

POSSIBLE ADVERSE EFFECTS

Trimethoprim taken on its own rarely causes side effects. However, additional adverse effects may occur when trimethoprim is taken in combination with sulfamethoxazole.

Symptom/effect	Frequency		Discuss with physician		Stop taking drug now	Call physician now
	Common	Rare	Only if severe	In all cases		
Nausea/vomiting		●	■			
Rash/itching		●		■	▲	
Sore throat/fever		●		■	▲	
Bruising/bleeding		●		■	▲	

INTERACTIONS

Cytotoxic drugs Trimethoprim increases the risk of blood problems if taken with azathioprine or mercaptopurine. Taken with methotrexate, there is an increased risk of folate deficiency.

Warfarin Trimethoprim may increase the anticoagulant effect of warfarin.

Cyclosporine Trimethoprim increases the risk of this drug causing kidney damage.

Phenytoin Taken with trimethoprim, this drug may increase the risk of folic acid deficiency, resulting in blood abnormalities.

Antimalarials containing pyrimethamine Drugs such as maloprim may increase the risk of folic acid deficiency, resulting in blood abnormalities, if they are taken with trimethoprim.

SPECIAL PRECAUTIONS

Be sure to tell your physician if:
▼ You have long-term liver or kidney problems.
▼ You have a blood disorder.
▼ You have porphyria.
▼ You are taking other medications.

Pregnancy
▼ Safety in pregnancy not established. Discuss with your physician.

Breast-feeding
▼ The drug passes into the breast milk, but at normal doses adverse effects on the baby are unlikely. Discuss with your physician.

Infants and children
▼ Reduced dose necessary.

Over 60
▼ Increased likelihood of adverse effects. Reduced dose may be required.

Driving and hazardous work
▼ No known problems.

Alcohol
▼ No known problems.

PROLONGED USE

Long-term use of this drug may lead to folate deficiency, which, in turn, may lead to blood abnormalities. Folate supplements may be prescribed.

Monitoring Periodic blood tests to monitor blood composition are usually advised.

VALPROIC ACID

Product names Depakene, Epival (divalproex sodium)
Used in the following combined preparations None

GENERAL INFORMATION

Valproic acid is an anticonvulsant drug that is often used for the treatment of different types of epilepsy. Divalproex, also an anticonvulsant, is chemically related to valproic acid. The action of valproic acid is similar to that of other anticonvulsants, reducing electrical discharges in the brain to prevent the excessive build-up of discharges that can lead to epileptic fits.

Beneficial in long-term treatment, this drug does not have a sedative effect. This makes it particularly suitable for children who suffer either from atonic epilepsy (the sudden relaxing of the muscles throughout the body) or from absence seizures (during which the person appears to be daydreaming).

Care should be taken if changing brands.

QUICK REFERENCE

Drug group Anticonvulsant drug (p.70)

Overdose danger rating Medium

Dependency rating Low

Prescription needed Yes

Available as generic Yes

INFORMATION FOR USERS

Your drug prescription is tailored for you. Do not alter dosage without checking with your physician.

How taken

Capsules, tablets (divalproex), liquid, injection.

Frequency and timing of doses
1–2 x daily, after food.

Usual dosage range
15mg/kg/day (starting dose), gradually increasing until seizures controlled. Maximum dose of 60mg/kg/day.

Onset of effect
Within 60 minutes.

Duration of action
12 hours or more.

Diet advice
None.

Storage
Keep in a tightly closed container in a cool, dry place out of the reach of children. Protect from light.

Missed dose
Take as soon as you remember. If your next dose is due within 2 hours, take a single dose now and skip the next.

Stopping the drug
Do not stop the drug without consulting your physician; symptoms may recur.

Exceeding the dose
An occasional unintentional extra dose is unlikely to cause problems. Large overdoses may lead to coma. Notify your physician.

SPECIAL PRECAUTIONS

Be sure to tell your physician if:
▼ You have long-term liver or kidney problems.
▼ You are taking other medications.
▼ You have porphyria.
▼ You have diabetes.

Pregnancy
▼ Not usually prescribed. May cause abnormalities in the unborn baby. If prescribed, extra folic acid supplements should also be taken. Discuss with your physician and pharmacist.

Breast-feeding
▼ The drug passes into the breast milk, but at normal doses adverse effects on the baby are unlikely. Discuss with your physician.

Infants and children
▼ Reduced dose necessary.

Over 60
▼ Reduced dose may be necessary.

Driving and hazardous work
▼ Your underlying condition, as well as the possibility of reduced alertness while taking valproic acid, may make such activities inadvisable. Discuss with your physician.

Alcohol
▼ Avoid. Alcohol may increase the sedative effects of this drug.

POSSIBLE ADVERSE EFFECTS

Most of the *adverse effects* of valproic acid are uncommon and the most serious ones are rare. They include liver failure, and platelet and bleeding abnormalities.

Menstrual periods may become irregular or cease altogether.

Symptom/effect	Frequency		Discuss with physician		Stop taking drug now	Call physician now
	Common	Rare	Only if severe	In all cases		
Temporary loss of hair	●		■			
Weight gain	●		■			
Nausea/indigestion		●		■		
Rash		●		■		▮
Drowsiness		●		■		▮
Jaundice		●		■		▮
Vomiting		●		■		▮

INTERACTIONS

Other anticonvulsant drugs These drugs may reduce blood levels of valproic acid.

ASA This drug may increase the effects of valproic acid.

Antidepressants, antipsychotics, mefloquine, and chloroquine These drugs may reduce the effectiveness of valproic acid.

Cholestyramine This drug may reduce the absorption of oral valproic acid.

Cimetidine and erythromycin These drugs may increase the effects of valproic acid.

Zidovudine When zidovudine and valproic acid are taken together, the blood levels of zidovudine may increase, leading to increased adverse effects.

PROLONGED USE

Use of this drug may cause liver damage, which is more likely in the first 6 months of use.

Monitoring Periodic blood tests of liver function and blood composition may be carried out.

VALSARTAN

Product name Diovan
Used in the following combined preparations Diovan-HCT

GENERAL INFORMATION

Valsartan is a member of the group of vasodilator drugs called angiotensin-II blockers. Used to treat hypertension, the drug works by blocking the action of angiotensin-II (a naturally occurring substance that constricts blood vessels). This action causes the blood vessel walls to relax, thereby easing blood pressure. It can also be used after a heart attack to improve prognosis in those with heart failure, who cannot take ACE inhibitors. Valsartan is prescribed with caution to people with stenosis (narrowing) of the arteries of the kidneys. A small starting dose may be used initially to minimize the risk of a sudden drop in blood pressure seen early in therapy. This drug is taken once daily when taken for high blood pressure; it is usually taken twice daily in those with heart failure.

INFORMATION FOR USERS

Your drug prescription is tailored for you. Do not alter dosage without checking with your physician.

How taken

Tablets and capsules.

Frequency and timing of doses
Once to twice daily.

Adult dosage range
40–320mg daily.

Onset of effect
Within 2 hours; to see changes in blood pressure, it may take 1–2 weeks, with maximum effect in 3–6 weeks.

Duration of action
Up to 24 hours.

Diet advice
None.

Storage
Keep in a closed container in a cool, dry place out of the reach of children.

Missed dose
Take as soon as you remember. If you take the dose daily and your next dose is within 8 hours, take a single dose now and skip the next.

Stopping the drug
Do not stop the drug without consulting your physician. Stopping the drug may lead to worsening of the underlying condition.

Exceeding the dose
An occasional unintentional extra dose is unlikely to cause problems. Large overdoses may cause dizziness and fainting. Notify your physician.

POSSIBLE ADVERSE EFFECTS

A common side effect of this drug is dizziness. When getting out of bed or up from a chair, you should be sure to get up slowly while supporting yourself.

Symptom/effect	Frequency		Discuss with physician		Stop taking drug now	Call physician now
	Common	Rare	Only if severe	In all cases		
Dizziness/fatigue	●		■			
Headache		●	■			
Chills, fever, sore throat		●		■		
Diarrhea	●		■			
Abdominal pain	●		■			
Rash/itching		●		■		
Jaundice		●		■		
Wheezing/facial swelling		●		■	▲	■

INTERACTIONS

Diuretics There is a risk of a sudden fall in blood pressure when these drugs are taken with valsartan.

Potassium supplements, potassium-sparing diuretics, cyclosporine Valsartan increases the effect of these drugs, leading to raised levels of potassium in the blood.

Lithium Valsartan may increase the levels and toxicity of lithium.

Warfarin Valsartan may increase the effect of warfarin. Close monitoring of INR levels are required, with possible dose adjustment.

Non-steroidal anti-inflammatory drugs (NSAIDs) Certain NSAIDs may interfere with the blood-pressure lowering effect of valsartan.

SPECIAL PRECAUTIONS

Be sure to tell your physician if:
▼ You have kidney or liver problems.
▼ You are at risk for dehydration.
▼ You are allergic to valsartan or any other medications.
▼ You are taking other medications.

Pregnancy
▼ Not prescribed. May cause abnormalities in the fetus.

Breast-feeding
▼ Not prescribed. Safety not established.

Infants and children
▼ Not recommended.

Over 60
▼ A reduced dose may be necessary.

Driving and hazardous work
▼ Do not undertake such activities until you have learned how valsartan affects you because the drug can cause dizziness and fatigue.

Alcohol
▼ Avoid. Alcohol may raise blood pressure, reducing the effectiveness of valsartan. Alcohol can cause blood vessels to dilate, increasing the likelihood of an excessive fall in blood pressure.

PROLONGED USE

No special problems.

Monitoring Periodic checks on blood potassium levels may be performed.

VARENICLINE

Product name Champix
Used in the following combined preparations None

GENERAL INFORMATION

Varenicline relieves symptoms of nicotine withdrawal and craving by partially activating nicotinic receptors in the brain by binding to these receptors. This blocks the rewarding and habituating effects of nicotine. Varenicline should be started one week prior to the date when an individual decides to stop smoking. A dose of 0.5mg once daily is initially started; the dose is then gradually increased to twice daily over a week. The medication is continued for 12 weeks. If needed, the medication may be continued for another 12-week cycle. Individuals should continue any other quit-smoking educational strategies or counseling that may be recommended by their physician or pharmacist.

QUICK REFERENCE

Drug group Drug for treatment of tobacco dependence

Overdose danger rating Medium

Dependence rating Low

Prescription needed Yes

Available as generic No

INFORMATION FOR USERS

Your drug prescription is tailored for you. Do not alter dosage without checking with your physician.

How taken

Tablets.

Frequency and timing of doses
Once to twice daily. Take after a meal, with a full glass of water.

Adult dosage range
0.5–2mg daily.

Onset of effect
3–4 hours.

Duration of action
Up to 24 hours.

Diet advice
None.

Storage
Keep in a closed container in a cool, dry place out of the reach of children.

Missed dose
If you miss a dose, take it as soon as you remember. If it is almost time for the next dose, skip the missed dose and continue your usual dosing schedule. Do not double up to catch up on a missed dose.

Stopping the drug
Do not stop the drug without consulting your physician. Stopping the drug may lead to worsening of the underlying condition.

Exceeding the dose
An occasional unintentional extra dose is unlikely to cause problems. With large overdoses, notify your physician immediately.

SPECIAL PRECAUTIONS

Be sure to tell your physician if:
▼ You are taking nicotine replacement therapy.
▼ You have kidney disease.
▼ You are allergic to varenicline.
▼ You have had problems with alcohol abuse.
▼ You are taking other medications.

Pregnancy
▼ Not recommended in pregnancy; safety in pregnancy not established. Discuss with your physician.

Breast-feeding
▼ Safety not established. Discuss with your physician.

Infants and children
▼ Not recommended.

Over 60
▼ If there is compromised kidney function, a smaller dose may be recommended.

Driving and hazardous work
▼ May cause drowsiness or dizziness. Do not drive a car or operate machinery until you feel you are mentally alert.

Alcohol
▼ Alcohol may increase the risk of drowsiness caused by this drug.

POSSIBLE ADVERSE EFFECTS

Nausea is the most commonly reported adverse effect and is related to the dose. With continued use, the incidence of nausea can decrease.

Symptom/effect	Frequency Common	Frequency Rare	Discuss with physician Only if severe	Discuss with physician In all cases	Stop taking drug now	Call physician now
Nausea	●		■			
Vomiting	●		■			
Abnormal dreams	●			■		
Constipation	●		■			
Flatulence	●		■			
Taste changes	●		■			
Sleep disturbance		●		■		
Dizziness/drowsiness		●		■		
Unusual tiredness/weakness		●		■		
Abdominal pain		●		■		
Allergic reaction (puffy, swollen eyelids, lips, throat, or hands, shortness of breath)		●			▲	▮
Changes in your usual thought or behaviour or thinking of harming yourself		●		■		▮

PROLONGED USE

Varenicline is not normally used for prolonged periods.

INTERACTIONS

Nicotine When used with nicotine products, side effects such as nausea, vomiting, headache, and dizziness may be higher. Combined therapy is not recommended.

VENLAFAXINE

Product names Effexor, Effexor XR
Used in the following combined preparations None

GENERAL INFORMATION

Venlafaxine is an antidepressant with a chemical structure unlike any other available antidepressant. It combines the therapeutic properties of both the tricyclic antidepressants and selective serotonin reuptake inhibitors (SSRIs), without *anticholinergic adverse effects*.

As with other antidepressants, this drug acts to elevate mood, increase physical activity, and restore interest in everyday pursuits.

Nausea, dizziness, drowsiness or insomnia, and restlessness are common adverse effects. Weight loss may occur due to decreased appetite. At high doses, the drug can cause an elevation of blood pressure, which should be monitored during treatment.

INFORMATION FOR USERS

Your drug prescription is tailored for you. Do not alter dosage without checking with your physician.

How taken

Tablets, SR-capsules.

Frequency and timing of doses
Twice daily (tablets); once daily (SR-capsules). The drug should be taken with food.

Usual dosage range
75–150mg daily for outpatients; up to 375mg daily in severely depressed patients.

Onset of effect
Full antidepressant effect may not be felt for 2–4 weeks or more.

Duration of action
About 8–12 hours; up to 24 hours for SR-capsules. Following prolonged treatment, antidepressant effects may persist for up to 6 weeks.

Diet advice
None.

Storage
Keep in the original container in a cool, dry place out of the reach of children.

Missed dose
Do not make up for a missed dose. Just take your next regularly scheduled dose.

Stopping the drug
Do not stop the drug without consulting your physician. Stopping abruptly can cause withdrawal symptoms.

OVERDOSE ACTION

 Seek immediate medical advice in all cases. Take emergency action if fits, slow or irregular pulse, or loss of consciousness occur.

See Drug poisoning emergency guide (p.526).

SPECIAL PRECAUTIONS

Be sure to tell your physician if:
▼ You have had an adverse reaction to any other antidepressants.
▼ You have long-term liver or kidney problems.
▼ You have a heart problem or elevated blood pressure.
▼ You have had epileptic fits.
▼ You have had problems with alcohol or drug misuse/abuse.
▼ You are taking other medications.

 Pregnancy
▼ Safety in pregnancy not established. Discuss with your physician.

 Breast-feeding
▼ Not recommended. Discuss with your physician.

 Infants and children
▼ Not recommended under 18 years.

 Over 60
▼ Increased likelihood of adverse effects. Reduced dose may therefore be necessary.

 Driving and hazardous work
▼ Avoid such activities until you have learned how venlafaxine affects you because the drug can cause dizziness, drowsiness, and blurred vision.

 Alcohol
▼ Avoid. Alcohol may increase the sedative effects of this drug.

POSSIBLE ADVERSE EFFECTS

The most common adverse effects are weakness, nausea, restlessness, and drowsiness. Some of these effects may wear off within a few days. Restlessness may include anxiety, nervousness, tremor, abnormal dreams, agitation, and confusion.

Symptom/effect	Frequency		Discuss with physician		Stop taking drug now	Call physician now
	Common	Rare	Only if severe	In all cases		
Nausea	●			■		
Restlessness/insomnia	●			■		
Weakness/blurred vision	●			■		
Drowsiness/dizziness	●			■		
Decreased appetite		●		■		
Sexual dysfunction		●		■	▲	
Rash/itching		●		■	▲	
High blood pressure		●		■		

INTERACTIONS

General note Drugs that affect breakdown of others in the liver may alter blood levels of venlafaxine, and vice versa.

Sedatives All drugs with a sedative effect may increase sedative effects of venlafaxine.

Antihypertensive drugs Venlafaxine may reduce the effectiveness of these drugs.

MAOIs Venlafaxine may interact with these drugs to produce a dangerous rise in blood pressure. MAOIs should be stopped at least 14 days before starting venlafaxine.

PROLONGED USE

Withdrawal symptoms may occur if the drug is not stopped gradually. Symptoms may include dizziness, electric shock sensations, anxiety, nausea, and insomnia. These rarely last for more than 1–2 weeks.

Monitoring Blood pressure should be measured periodically if high doses of venlafaxine are prescribed.

VERAPAMIL

Product name Isoptin
Used in the following combined preparation Tarka

GENERAL INFORMATION

Verapamil belongs to a group of drugs known as calcium channel blockers, which interfere with the conduction of signals in the muscles of the heart and blood vessels. It is used in the treatment of hypertension, abnormal heart rhythms, and angina. It reduces the frequency of angina attacks but does not help relieve pain while an attack is in progress. Verapamil increases the ability to tolerate physical exertion, and unlike

some drugs it does not affect breathing so it can be used safely by asthmatics.

Verapamil is also prescribed for certain types of abnormal heart rhythm. It can be administered by injection as well as in tablet form for such disorders.

Verapamil is not generally prescribed for people with low blood pressure, slow heart beat, or heart failure because it may worsen these conditions. The drug may also cause constipation.

QUICK REFERENCE

Drug group Anti-angina drug (p.87), anti-arrhythmic drug (p.86), and antihypertensive drug (p.88)

Overdose danger rating Medium

Dependence rating Low

Prescription needed Yes

Available as generic Yes

INFORMATION FOR USERS

Your drug prescription is tailored for you. Do not alter dosage without checking with your physician.

How taken

Tablets, SR-tablets, injection.

Frequency and timing of doses
2–3x daily (tablets); 1–2x daily (SR-tablets). Injection: as directed by physician.

Usual adult dosage range
120–480mg daily.

Onset of effect
1–2 hours (tablets); 2–3 minutes (injection).

Duration of action
6–8 hours. During prolonged treatment some beneficial effects may last for up to 12 hours. SR-tablets act for 12–24 hours.

Diet advice
Avoid grapefruit juice which may increase blood levels of verapamil.

Storage
Keep in a closed container in a cool, dry place out of the reach of children.

Missed dose
Take as soon as you remember. If your next dose is due within 3 hours (tablets) or 8 hours (SR-tablets), take a single dose now and skip the next.

Stopping the drug
Do not stop the drug without consulting your physician; symptoms may recur.

Exceeding the dose
An occasional unintentional extra dose is unlikely to be a cause for concern. Large overdoses may cause dizziness. Notify your physician.

SPECIAL PRECAUTIONS

Be sure to tell your physician if:
▼ You have a long-term liver problem.
▼ You have heart failure.
▼ You have porphyria.
▼ You are taking other medications.

Pregnancy
▼ Not usually prescribed. May inhibit labour if taken during later stages of pregnancy. Discuss with your physician.

Breast-feeding
▼ The drug passes into the breast milk, but at normal doses adverse effects on the baby are unlikely. Discuss with your physician.

Infants and children
▼ Usually given on specialist advice only. Reduced dose necessary.

Over 60
▼ No special problems.

Driving and hazardous work
▼ Avoid such activities until you have learned how verapamil affects you because the drug can cause dizziness.

Alcohol
▼ Avoid. Alcohol may further reduce blood pressure, causing dizziness or other symptoms.

Surgery and general anesthetics
▼ Verapamil may need to be stopped before surgery. Consult your physician or dentist.

POSSIBLE ADVERSE EFFECTS

Verapamil may cause gynecomastia (breast enlargement in males) and an increase in gum tissue after long-term use.

Symptom/effect	Frequency		Discuss with physician		Stop taking drug now	Call physician now
	Common	Rare	Only if severe	In all cases		
Constipation	●		■			
Headache	●		■			
Nausea/vomiting	●		■			
Ankle swelling	●			■		
Flushing		●	■			
Dizziness		●		■		
Breast/gum enlargement		●		■		
Rash		●		■		■

PROLONGED USE

No problems expected.

INTERACTIONS

Beta blockers When verapamil is taken with these drugs, there is a slight risk of abnormal heart beat and heart failure.

Carbamazepine The effects of this drug may be enhanced by verapamil.

Cyclosporine The blood levels of this drug may be increased by verapamil and its dose may need to be reduced.

Antihypertensive drugs Blood pressure may be further lowered when these drugs are taken with verapamil.

Digoxin The effects of this drug may be increased if it is taken with verapamil. The dosage of digoxin may need to be reduced.

WARFARIN

Product name Coumadin
Used in the following combined preparations None

GENERAL INFORMATION

Warfarin is an anticoagulant used to prevent blood clots, mainly in areas where blood flow is slowest, particularly in the leg and pelvic veins. Such clots can break off and travel through the bloodstream to the lungs, where they lodge and cause pulmonary embolism. The drug is also used to reduce the risk of clots forming in the heart in people with atrial fibrillation, or after insertion of artificial heart valves. These clots may travel to the brain and cause a stroke.

A widely used oral anticoagulant drug, warfarin requires regular monitoring to ensure proper maintenance dosage. As its full beneficial effects are not felt for two to three days, a faster-acting drug such as heparin is often used to complement the effects of warfarin at the start of treatment.

The most serious *adverse effect*, as with all anticoagulants, is the risk of excessive bleeding, which is usually the result of excessive dosage.

INFORMATION FOR USERS

Your drug prescription is tailored for you. Do not alter dosage without checking with your physician.

How taken

Tablets.

Frequency and timing of doses
Once daily, taken at the same time each day.

Usual dosage range
10 mg for 2 days (starting dose); 2–9 mg daily at the same time, as determined by blood tests (maintenance dose).

Onset of effect
Within 24–48 hours, with full effect after several days.

Duration of action
2–3 days.

Diet advice
None.

Storage
Keep in a closed container in a cool, dry place out of the reach of children. Protect from light.

Missed dose
Take as soon as you remember. Take the following dose on your original schedule.

Stopping the drug
Do not stop taking the drug without consulting your physician; stopping the drug may lead to worsening of the underlying condition.

OVERDOSE ACTION

 Seek immediate medical advice in all cases. Take emergency action if severe bleeding or loss of consciousness occur.

See Drug poisoning emergency guide (p.526).

POSSIBLE ADVERSE EFFECTS

Bleeding is the most common adverse effect with warfarin. Any bruising, dark stools, dark urine, or bleeding should be reported to your physician at once.

Symptom/effect	Frequency		Discuss with physician		Stop taking drug now	Call physician now
	Common	Rare	Only if severe	In all cases		
Bleeding/bruising	●			■	▲	▮
Fever		●		■	▲	▮
Nausea/vomiting		●		■	▲	▮
Abdominal pain/diarrhea		●		■		
Rash		●		■		
Hair loss		●		■		
Jaundice		●		■		▮

INTERACTIONS

General note A wide variety of drugs, such as ASA, barbiturates, oral contraceptives, cimetidine, diuretics, certain laxatives, certain antidepressants, and certain antibiotics interact with warfarin, either by increasing or decreasing the anticlotting effect. Consult your pharmacist before using over-the-counter medicines.

SPECIAL PRECAUTIONS

Be sure to tell your physician if:
▼ You have long-term liver or kidney problems.
▼ You have high blood pressure.
▼ You have peptic ulcers.
▼ You bleed easily.
▼ You are taking other medications.

 Pregnancy
▼ Not usually prescribed. If given in early pregnancy, the drug can cause malformations in the unborn child. Taken near the time of delivery, it may cause the mother to bleed excessively. Discuss with your physician.

 Breast-feeding
▼ The drug passes into the breast milk, but at normal doses adverse effects on the baby are unlikely. Discuss with your physician.

 Infants and children
▼ Reduced dose necessary.

 Over 60
▼ No special problems.

 Driving and hazardous work
▼ Use caution. Even minor bumps can cause bad bruises and excessive bleeding.

 Alcohol
▼ Avoid excessive amounts. Alcohol may increase the effects of this drug.

Surgery and general anesthetics
▼ Warfarin may need to be stopped before surgery. Discuss with your physician or dentist.

PROLONGED USE

No special problems.

Monitoring Regular blood tests are performed during treatment.

XYLOMETAZOLINE

Product names Balminil Nasal Decongestant, Otrivin
Used in the following combined preparation None

GENERAL INFORMATION

Xylometazoline is a sympathomimetic nasal decongestant that can be bought over-the-counter to relieve a stuffy nose caused by colds, hayfever, or sinusitis. It works by constricting the small blood vessels in the nose, thereby reducing inflammation and swelling.

Because the effect of xylometazoline may last for up to 10 hours, it needs to be used only two or three times daily.

Using the drug more often than this will increase the likelihood of adverse effects such as headache, palpitations, and drowsiness. Nor should xylometazoline be used for more than a few days at a time; this may cause "rebound" congestion, making nasal stuffiness worse.

QUICK REFERENCE

Drug group Decongestant (p.79)
Overdose danger rating Medium
Dependence rating Low
Prescription needed No
Available as generic Yes

INFORMATION FOR USERS

Follow instructions on the label. Call your physician if symptoms worsen.

How taken

Nose drops, nasal spray.

Frequency and timing of doses
As needed up to 3 x daily.

Usual dosage range
Adults 2–3 drops or 1–2 sprays in each nostril (0.1 per cent solution).
Children 2-5 years 1 drop or 1 spray in each nostril (0.05 per cent solution).
Children 6 years and over 2–3 drops or 1–2 sprays in each nostril (0.05 per cent solution).

Onset of effect
Within 10 minutes.

Duration of action
Up to 10 hours.

Diet advice
None.

Storage
Keep in a closed container in a cool, dry place out of the reach of children. Protect from light.

Missed dose
No cause for concern. Take only if needed.

Stopping the drug
Can be safely stopped as soon as you no longer need it. Seek medical advice if symptoms persist for more than a few days.

Exceeding the dose
An occasional unintentional extra dose is unlikely to cause problems. Large overdoses or accidental poisoning may cause headaches, insomnia, and drowsiness. Notify your physician.

POSSIBLE ADVERSE EFFECTS

The adverse effects of xylometazoline are mild and infrequent when the medication is taken for short periods of time. When they do occur it is usually a signal that too much of the drug is being absorbed into the body, and this can be helped by reducing the dose.

Symptom/effect	Frequency		Discuss with physician		Stop taking drug now	Call physician now
	Common	Rare	Only if severe	In all cases		
Headache/lightheadedness		●		■		
Nasal discomfort		●	■			
Insomnia		●		■		
Blurred vision		●	■			
Excessive sneezing		●	■			
Drowsiness		●	■			
Palpitations/tremor		●		■	▲	

INTERACTIONS

Sympathomimetic drugs There is an increased risk of adverse effects when drugs such as ephedrine and pseudoephedrine are taken with xylometazoline.

Monoamine oxidase inhibitors (MAOIs) increase the risk of high blood pressure with xylometazoline, with potentially serious effects. Xylometazoline should not be taken during or within 14 days of MAOI treatment.

SPECIAL PRECAUTIONS

Be sure to consult your physician or pharmacist before using this drug if:
▼ You have glaucoma.
▼ You have heart problems.
▼ You have high blood pressure.
▼ You are taking other medications.

Pregnancy
▼ No evidence of risk if used sparingly. However, overuse can cause a rise in blood pressure that could harm the developing baby. Discuss with your physician.

Breast-feeding
▼ The drug passes into the breast milk, but at normal doses adverse effects on the baby are unlikely. Discuss with your physician.

Infants and children
▼ Reduced dose necessary. For children in general, but especially for those under 2 years of age, consult with your health care provider. Reduced dose necessary for all children.

Over 60
▼ Increased likelihood of adverse effects. Reduced dose may therefore be necessary.

Driving and hazardous work
▼ Exercise caution if blurred vision or drowsiness occurs.

Alcohol
▼ No special problems

PROLONGED USE

Long-term use of this drug may lead to worsening of the condition. Also, it may lead to a rise in blood pressure. The drug increases the risk of lightheadedness, sleeplessness, and palpitations. Courses of longer than a few days are not recommended.

ZANAMIVIR

Product name Relenza
Used in the following combined preparations None

GENERAL INFORMATION

Zanamivir is an antiviral drug used to treat influenza (flu), a virus that infects and multiplies in the lungs. The drug works by attacking the virus and preventing it from multiplying and spreading in the lungs. Zanamivir is not a substitute for flu vaccination, but is used to treat at-risk individuals, for example the elderly and people with long-term illnesses such as chronic heart and lung disease.

Flu causes fever, chills, headache, aches and pains. Other symptoms include sore throat, cough, and nasal symptoms. Taken by inhaler, zanamivir helps to clear these symptoms and may shorten the duration of the illness. There is no benefit, however, if you do not have a fever. Therefore, treatment should begin as soon as possible, and certainly within 48 hours of the onset of symptoms.

Symptoms usually subside in two to seven days, unless complications such as a chest infection occur.

Zanamivir should be used with caution by asthmatic patients because it may provoke wheezing requiring urgent use of a *bronchodilator*.

QUICK REFERENCE

Drug group Antiviral drug (p.119)
Overdose danger rating Low
Dependence rating Low
Prescription needed Yes
Available as generic No

INFORMATION FOR USERS

Your drug prescription is tailored for you. Do not alter dosage without checking with your physician.

How taken

Inhaled via Diskhaler.

Frequency and timing of doses
2 x daily. Inhale the contents of the blisters one at a time.

Usual dosage range
Adults 20mg (4 x 5mg blisters) daily for 5 days.
Children ≥ 7 years Same dose as in adults.

Onset of effect
Within 7 days.

Duration of action
Up to 12 hours.

Diet advice
None.

Storage
Keep in a cool, dry place out of the reach of children.

Missed dose
Take as soon as you remember. If your next dose is due within 2 hours, take a single dose now and skip the next.

Stopping the drug
Do not stop taking the drug without consulting your physician; symptoms may recur.

Exceeding the dose
An occasional unintentional dose is unlikely to cause problems. However, if you notice any unusual symptoms, or if a large overdose has been taken, notify your physician.

SPECIAL PRECAUTIONS

Be sure to tell your physician if:
▼ You have ever had an allergic reaction to zanamivir or lactose monohydrate.
▼ You have a long-term illness.
▼ You have a lung disease such as asthma.
▼ You have poor immunity to infections.
▼ You are taking other medications.

 Pregnancy
▼ Safety in pregnancy not established. Discuss with your physician.

 Breast-feeding
▼ Safety in breast-feeding not established. Discuss with your physician.

 Infants and children
▼ Not recommended in children < 7 years of age.

 Over 60
▼ No special problems.

 Driving and hazardous work
▼ No known problems.

 Alcohol
▼ No known problems.

POSSIBLE ADVERSE EFFECTS

Adverse effects are uncommon. Such effects that occur are similar to signs and symptoms of flu and may therefore sometimes be caused by the influenza virus rather than zanamivir.

Symptom/effect	Frequency		Discuss with physician		Stop taking drug now	Call physician now
	Common	Rare	Only if severe	In all cases		
Headache		●	■			
Sore throat		●	■			
Cough		●	■			
Nasal symptoms		●	■			
Wheezing/breathlessness		●		■	▲	

INTERACTIONS

Inhaled drugs (e.g., salbutamol and beclomethasone) These should be inhaled just before zanamivir is administered.

PROLONGED USE

This drug should only be used for 5 days and is not prescribed for long-term use.

ZIDOVUDINE/LAMIVUDINE

Product names Retrovir (zidovudine); Heptovir (lamivudine)
Used in the following combined preparations Combivir, Trizivir

GENERAL INFORMATION

Zidovudine and lamivudine are from the same class of drugs – nucleoside analogues – and are used in the treatment of HIV infection. The two drugs are combined in one tablet, which is usually prescribed with another class of drug to treat HIV, either a non-nucleoside reverse transcriptase inhibitor or a protease inhibitor. This combination of three drugs is more effective at treating HIV than either a single or double regime of drugs.

Although not a cure for HIV, combination retroviral therapy slows down production of the virus and, therefore, reduces the damage done to the immune system. The drugs need to be taken regularly and on a long-term basis to remain effective.

QUICK REFERENCE

Drug group Drug for HIV and immune deficiency (p.144)

Overdose danger rating Medium

Dependence rating Low

Prescription needed Yes

Available as generic No

INFORMATION FOR USERS

Your drug prescription is tailored for you. Do not alter dosage without checking with your physician.

How taken

Tablets.

Frequency and timing of doses
Every 12 hours.

Usual adult dosage range
One tablet.

Onset of effect
1 hour.

Duration of action
12 hours.

Diet advice
None.

Storage
Keep in the original container in a cool, dry place out of the the reach of children.

Missed dose
Take as soon as you remember. If your next dose is due within 2 hours, take a single dose now and skip the next. It is very important not to miss doses on a regular basis as this can lead to the development of drug-resistant HIV.

Stopping the drug
Do not stop taking the drug without consulting your physician.

Exceeding the dose
An occasional unintentional extra dose is unlikely to cause problems. But if you notice any unusual symptoms, or if a large overdose has been taken, notify your physician.

POSSIBLE ADVERSE EFFECTS

The most common adverse effects of zidovudine/lamivudine are nausea, vomiting, and diarrhea. Sometimes, anemia may develop with prolonged use.

Symptom/effect	Frequency		Discuss with physician		Stop taking drug now	Call physician now
	Common	Rare	Only if severe	In all cases		
Nausea/vomiting	●		■			
Diarrhea	●		■			
Fatigue	●		■			
Skin discoloration		●	■			
Anemia		●		■		
Severe abdominal pain		●		■		▮

INTERACTIONS

General note A wide range of drugs may interact with zidovudine and lamivudine causing either an increase in adverse effects or a reduction in the effect of the antiretroviral drugs. Check with your physician or pharmacist before taking any new drugs, including those from the dentist and supermarket, and herbal medicines.

SPECIAL PRECAUTIONS

Be sure to tell your physician if:
▼ You have liver or kidney problems.
▼ You have other infections, such as hepatitis B or C.
▼ You are taking other medications.

Pregnancy
▼ Safety in pregnancy not established. If you are pregnant or planning pregnancy, discuss with your physician.

Breast-feeding
▼ Safety in breast-feeding not established. Breast-feeding is not recommended by HIV-positive mothers as the virus may be passed to the baby.

Infants and children
▼ Reduced dose necessary.

Over 60
▼ Increased likelihood of adverse effects. Reduced dose may therefore be necessary.

Driving and hazardous work
▼ No special problems.

Alcohol
▼ No known problems.

PROLONGED USE

There is an increased risk of serious blood disorders, such as anemia, with long-term use of zidovudine and lamivudine.

Monitoring Regular blood checks will be carried out to monitor the drugs' effects on the virus and to look for signs of anemia.

ZOPICLONE

Product names Apo-Zopiclone, Imovane, Rhovane, and others
Used in the following combined preparations None

GENERAL INFORMATION

Zopiclone is a hypnotic (sleeping drug) used for the short-term treatment of insomnia. Sleep problems can take the form of difficulty in falling asleep, frequent night-time awakenings, and/or early morning awakenings. Hypnotic drugs are given only when non-drug measures – for example, avoidance of caffeine – have proved ineffective.

Unlike benzodiazepines, zopiclone possesses no anti-anxiety properties. Therefore, it may be suited for instances of insomnia that are not accompanied by anxiety – for example, international travel or change in shift work routine.
    Hypnotics are intended for occasional use only. *Dependence* can develop after as little as one week of continuous use.

QUICK REFERENCE

Drug group Sleeping drug (p.66)
Overdose danger rating Medium
Dependence rating Medium
Prescription needed Yes
Available as generic Yes

INFORMATION FOR USERS

Your drug prescription is tailored for you. Do not alter dosage without checking with your physician.

How taken

Tablets.

Frequency and timing of doses
Once daily at bedtime when required.

Usual dosage range
3.75–7.5mg.

Onset of effect
Within 30 minutes.

Duration of action
4–6 hours.

Diet advice
None.

Storage
Keep in a closed container in a cool, dry place out of the reach of children. Protect from light.

Missed dose
If you fall asleep without having taken a dose and wake some hours later, do not take the missed dose.

Stopping the drug
If you have been taking the drug continuously for less than 1 week, it can be safely stopped as soon as you feel you no longer need it. However, if you have been taking the drug for longer, consult your physician.

Exceeding the dose
An occasional, unintentional extra dose is unlikely to cause problems. Large overdoses may cause prolonged sleep, drowsiness, lethargy, and poor muscle coordination and reflexes. Notify your physician immediately.

SPECIAL PRECAUTIONS

Be sure to tell your physician if:
▼ You have or have had any problems with alcohol or drug misuse/abuse.
▼ You have myasthenia gravis.
▼ You have had epileptic fits.
▼ You have liver or kidney problems.
▼ You are taking other medications.

 Pregnancy
▼ Not recommended.

 Breast-feeding
▼ Not recommended.

 Infants and children
▼ Not recommended.

 Over 60
▼ Increased likelihood of adverse effects. Reduced dose may therefore be necessary.

 Driving and hazardous work
▼ Avoid such activities until you have learned how zopiclone affects you because the drug can cause drowsiness, reduced alertness, and slowed reactions.

 Alcohol
▼ Avoid. Alcohol increases the sedative effects of this drug.

POSSIBLE ADVERSE EFFECTS

The most common *adverse effects* of zopiclone are daytime drowsiness, which normally diminishes after the first few days of treatment, and a bitter taste in the mouth. Persistent morning drowsiness or impaired coordination are signs of excessive dose.

Symptom/effect	Frequency		Discuss with physician		Stop taking drug now	Call physician now
	Common	Rare	Only if severe	In all cases		
Bitter taste	●		■			
Dizziness/weakness		●	■			
Nausea/vomiting/diarrhea		●	■			
Daytime drowsiness/headache	●			■		
Amnesia/confusion		●		■	▲	
Rash		●		■	▲	■

INTERACTIONS

Sedatives All drugs, including alcohol, that have a sedative effect on the central nervous system are likely to increase the sedative effects of zopiclone. Such drugs include other sleeping and anti-anxiety drugs, antihistamines, antidepressants, *opioid* analgesics, and antipsychotics.

PROLONGED USE

Intended for occasional use only. Continuous use of zopiclone – or any other sleeping drug – for as little as one week may cause *dependence*.

A–Z OF VITAMINS, MINERALS, AND SUPPLEMENTS

This section gives detailed information on the major vitamins and minerals that are required by the body for good health – essential chemicals that the body cannot make by itself. These include the main vitamins – A, C, D, E, K, H (biotin), and the B vitamins – together with 11 essential minerals. Information on selected supplements is also included. The section on vitamins in Part 3 (p.135) gives in general terms the main sources of the major vitamins and minerals and their roles in the body, while the following profiles discuss each vitamin and mineral in detail.

The following pages may be particularly useful as a guide for those who think their diet lacks sufficient amounts of a certain vitamin or mineral, and for those with disorders of the digestive tract or liver, who may need larger amounts of certain vitamins. The table on p.136 gives the good dietary sources of each one.

The profiles

The vitamin, mineral, and supplement profiles are arranged in alphabetical order and give information under standard headings. These include the different names by which each chemical is known; whether it is available over-the-counter or by prescription only; its role in body maintenance; specific foods in which it can be found; recommended daily amounts; how to detect a deficiency; how and when to supplement your diet; and the risks associated with excessive intake of a particular vitamin, mineral, or supplement.

Normal daily vitamin and mineral requirements are usually based on the Recommended Daily Allowance (RDA). This measurement is the amount of the nutrient thought to be enough for about 97 per cent of people. The dosages for treating a vitamin or mineral deficiency are usually much higher, but the precise doses need to be determined by your physician.

HOW TO UNDERSTAND THE PROFILES

Each vitamin, mineral, and supplement profile contains information arranged under standard headings to enable you to find the information you need.

Availability
Tells you whether the vitamin, mineral, or supplement is available over the counter or only by prescription.

Other names
Lists the chemical and non-chemical names by which the vitamin or mineral is also known.

Dietary and other natural sources
Tells you how the vitamin or mineral is obtained naturally.

When supplements are helpful
Suggests when your physician may recommend that you take supplements.

Dosage range for treating deficiency
Gives a usual recommended dosage of vitamin or mineral supplements.

Actions on the body
Explains the role played by each vitamin or mineral in maintaining healthy body function.

Normal daily requirement
Gives you a guide to the recommended daily allowance (RDA) of each vitamin or mineral.

Symptoms of deficiency
Describes the common signs of deficiency.

Symptoms and risks of excessive intake
Explains the risks that may accompany excessive intake of each vitamin or mineral and warning signs to look out for.

PANTOTHENIC ACID

Other names Calcium pantothenate, vitamin B₅

Availability
Pantothenic acid, calcium pantothenate, and panthenol are available without prescription in a variety of multivitamin and mineral preparations.

Actions on the body
Pantothenic acid plays a vital role in the activities of many enzymes. It is essential for the production of energy from sugars and fats, for the manufacture of fats, corticosteroids, and sex hormones, for the utilization of other vitamins, for the proper function of the nervous system and the adrenal glands, and for normal growth and development.

Dietary and other natural sources
Pantothenic acid is present in almost all vegetables, cereals, and animal foods. Liver, kidney, heart, fish, and egg yolks are good dietary sources. Brewer's yeast, wheat germ, and royal jelly (the substance on which queen bees feed) are also rich in the vitamin.

Normal daily requirement
No recommended daily allowance (RDA) for pantothenic acid has ever been established, but adult requirements are met by a 4–7mg intake daily.

When supplements are helpful
Most diets provide adequate amounts of pantothenic acid. Any deficiency is likely to occur in malnutrition together with other B vitamin deficiency diseases such as pellagra (see niacin), beriberi (see thiamine), or with alcoholism, and will be treated with B complex supplements. There is no firm evidence that large doses help, as some believe, in the prevention of greying hair, nerve disorders in diabetes, or psychiatric illness.

Symptoms of deficiency
Pantothenic acid deficiency is unlikely to occur unless a person is suffering from malnutrition. However, deficiency produced under experimental conditions can cause malaise, abdominal discomfort, and burning feet.

Dosage range for treating deficiency
Usually 5–10mg per day.

Symptoms and risks of excessive intake
In tests, doses of 1,000mg or more of pantothenic acid have not caused toxic effects. The risk of toxicity is considered to be very low, since pantothenic acid is a water-soluble vitamin that does not accumulate in the tissues. Any excess is eliminated rapidly in the urine. However, very high intakes of 10–20g can cause diarrhea.

476

POTASSIUM

Other names Potassium chloride, potassium citrate, potassium gluconate

Availability
Salts of potassium in small doses are available in a number of multivitamin and mineral supplements. They are available at higher doses as supplements and in an injectable form, both to be used under medical supervision. Potassium salts are also widely available in sodium-free salt (used as a salt substitute).

Actions on the body
Potassium works together with sodium in the control of the body's water balance, conduction of nerve impulses, contraction of muscle, and maintenance of a normal heart rhythm. Potassium is essential for maintenance of normal blood sugar.

Dietary and other natural sources
The best dietary sources of potassium are leafy green vegetables, tomatoes, oranges, potatoes, and bananas. Lean meat, pulses, chocolate, coffee, and milk are also rich in the mineral. Many methods of food processing may lower the potassium levels found in fresh food.

Normal daily requirement
The recommended daily allowance (RDA) is 2,000mg in adults. There are no extra requirements in pregnancy or breast-feeding.

When supplements are helpful
Most diets contain adequate amounts of potassium, and supplements are rarely required in normal circumstances. However, people who drink large amounts of alcohol or eat lots of salty foods may become marginally deficient. People with a condition called diabetic ketoacidosis or with certain types of kidney disease may be deficient in potassium, but the most common cause is prolonged treatment with diuretics. Long-term use of corticosteroids may also deplete the body's potassium. Prolonged vomiting and diarrhea also cause potassium deficiency, so people who abuse laxatives may be affected. Supplements are usually advised only when symptoms suggest deficiency, or for people at particular risk.

Symptoms of deficiency
Early symptoms of potassium deficiency may include muscle weakness, fatigue, dizziness, and mental confusion. Impairment of nerve and muscle function may progress to cause disturbances of the heart rhythm and paralysis of the skeletal muscles and those of the bowel, which leads to constipation.

Dosage range for treating deficiency
Depends on the preparation, the individual, and the cause and severity of deficiency. In general, daily doses equivalent to 20–40mmol/day of potassium chloride are given to prevent deficiency (for example, in people treated with diuretics that deplete potassium). Doses equivalent to 40–60mmol of potassium chloride daily are used to treat deficiency. Potassium supplements should be taken with a full glass of water, and may be taken after a meal to avoid gastric irritation.

Symptoms and risks of excessive intake
Blood potassium levels are normally regulated by the kidneys, and any excess is rapidly eliminated in the urine. Massive doses cause serious disturbances of the heart rhythm and muscular paralysis. In people with impaired kidney function, excess potassium may build up and the risk of potassium poisoning is increased. People on hemodialysis treatment need to take a carefully controlled low-potassium diet.

BIOTIN

Other names Coenzyme R, vitamin H

Availability
Biotin is available without a prescription, alone and in a wide variety of multivitamin and mineral preparations.

Actions on the body
Biotin plays a vital role in the activities of several *enzymes*. It is essential for the breakdown of carbohydrates and fatty acids in the diet for conversion into energy, for the manufacture of fats, and for excretion of the products of protein breakdown.

Dietary and other natural sources
Traces of biotin are present in a wide variety of foods. Dietary sources rich in this vitamin include liver, nuts, peas, beans, egg yolks, cauliflower, and mushrooms. A large proportion of the biotin we require is manufactured by bacteria in the intestine.

Normal daily requirement
The recommended daily allowance (RDA) has not been clearly established, but a daily dietary intake of 30mcg is considered appropriate.

When supplements are helpful
Adequate amounts of biotin are provided in most diets and by the bacteria living in the intestine, so supplements are rarely needed. However, deficiency can occur with prolonged, excessive consumption of raw egg whites (as in eggnogs), because these contain a protein – avidin – that prevents absorption of the vitamin in the intestine. The risk of deficiency is also increased during long-term treatment with antibiotics or sulfonamide antibacterial drugs, which may destroy the biotin-producing bacteria in the intestine. However, additional biotin is not usually necessary with a balanced diet.

Symptoms of deficiency
Deficiency symptoms include weakness, tiredness, poor appetite, hair loss, muscle pain, and depression. Severe deficiency may cause eczema of the face and body, and inflammation of the tongue.

Dosage range for treating deficiency
Depends on the individual and on the nature and severity of the disorder. Dietary deficiency can be treated with doses of 150–300mcg of biotin daily. Deficiency of biotin resulting from a genetic defect that limits use of the vitamin by body cells can be treated with very large doses of 5mg given once or twice daily.

Symptoms and risks of excessive intake
None known.

CALCIUM

Other names Calcium acetate, calcium carbonate, calcium chloride, calcium citrate, calcium gluconeptonate, calcium gluconate, calcium lactate, calcium phosphate

Availability
Oral forms are available without a prescription. Injectable forms of calcium are available only under medical supervision.

Actions on the body
The most abundant mineral in the body, calcium makes up more than 90 per cent of the hard matter in bones and teeth. It is essential for the formation and maintenance of strong bones and healthy teeth, as well as blood clotting, transmission of nerve impulses, and muscle contraction.

Dietary and other natural sources
The main dietary sources of calcium are milk and dairy products, sardines, dark green leafy vegetables, beans, peas, and nuts. Calcium may also be obtained by drinking water in hard water areas.

Normal daily requirement
The recommended daily requirements for elemental calcium are: 270mg (birth–1 year); 500mg (1–3 years); 800mg (4–8 years); 1,300mg (9–18 years); 1,000mg (19–50 years); and 1,500mg (over 50 years). The daily requirement of elemental calcium during pregnancy and during breast-feeding is 1,000mg.

When supplements are helpful
Unless a sufficient amount of dairy products is consumed (a glass of milk contains approximately 300mg) the diet may not contain enough calcium, and supplements may be needed. Breast-feeding women are especially vulnerable to calcium deficiency because breast-feeding demands large amounts of calcium, which may be extracted from the skeleton if intake is not adequate. Osteoporosis (fragile bones) has been linked to dietary calcium deficiency in some cases, but may not be helped by supplements in all women. Other treatment may also be necessary (see Drugs for bone disorders, p.108).

Symptoms of deficiency
When dietary intake is inadequate, the body obtains the calcium it needs from the skeleton. Long-term deficiency of calcium may lead to increased fragility of the bones. Osteoporosis results in increased risk of fractures, particularly of the vertebrae, hip, and wrist. Severe deficiency, resulting in low levels of calcium in the blood, causes abnormal stimulation of the nervous system, resulting in cramp-like spasms in the hands, feet, and face. Vitamin D deficiency is the main cause of the bone-softening diseases rickets and osteomalacia.

Dosage range for treating deficiency
Vitamin D helps with calcium absorption and is needed for treatment of rickets and osteomalacia (p.108). Oral supplements of up to 800IU vitamin D daily may be advised for children with rickets, and 800IU to 1,000IU daily may be given for osteoporosis and osteomalacia. Severe calcium deficiency is treated in hospital by intravenous injection of calcium.

Symptoms and risks of excessive intake
Excessive intake of calcium may reduce the amount of iron and zinc absorbed and may also cause constipation and nausea. There is an increased risk of palpitations and, for susceptible people, of calcium deposits in the kidneys leading to kidney stones and kidney damage. These symptoms do not usually develop unless calcium is taken with large amounts of vitamin D.

CHROMIUM

Other name Chromium picolinate

Availability
Chromium supplements are available without prescription.

Actions on the body
Chromium plays a vital role in the activities of several *enzymes*. It is involved in the breakdown of sugar for conversion into energy and in the manufacture of certain fats. The mineral works together with insulin and is thus essential to the body's ability to use sugar. Chromium may also be involved in the manufacture of proteins in the body.

Dietary and other natural sources
Traces of chromium are present in a wide variety of foods. Meat, dairy products, and wholemeal cereals are good sources of this mineral.

Normal daily requirement
Only minute quantities of chromium are required. A recommended daily allowance (RDA) has not been determined, but a safe intake for adults is about 25mcg.

When supplements are helpful
Most people who eat a healthy diet containing plenty of fresh or unprocessed foods receive adequate amounts of chromium. The use of chromium in diabetes is under investigation, but diabetics and those with diabetes-like symptoms may benefit from additional chromium. Supplements may also be helpful if symptoms suggest chromium deficiency.

Symptoms of deficiency
Chromium deficiency is very rare in Canada. A diet of too many processed foods may contribute to chromium deficiency. Inadequate intake of chromium over a prolonged period may impair the body's ability to use sugar, leading to high blood sugar levels. However, in most cases, there are no symptoms. In some people, there may be diabetes-like symptoms such as tiredness, mental confusion, and numbness or tingling of the hands and feet. Deficiency may worsen pre-existing diabetes and may depress growth in children. It has also been suggested that chromium deficiency may contribute to the development of atherosclerosis (narrowing of the arteries).

Dosage range for treating deficiency
Severe chromium deficiency may be treated with daily doses of up to 10mcg.

Symptoms and risks of excessive intake
Chromium is poisonous in excess. Levels that produce symptoms are usually obtained from occupational exposure or industrial waste in drinking water or the atmosphere, not from excessive dietary intake. Symptoms include inflammation of the skin and, if inhaled, damage to the nasal passages. People who are repeatedly exposed to chromium fumes have a higher-than-average risk of developing lung cancer. High levels may reduce kidney function.

CO-ENZYME Q_{10}

Other names Ubiquinone-10, ubidecarenone, CoQ_{10}

Availability
Co-enzyme Q_{10} is considered to be a natural health product in Canada and is regulated by the Natural Health Products Directorate. Supplements may not be standardized in how they are manufactured, and the amount of the active substance may vary between products (and from the product used to conduct research upon which health claims are based). Co-enzyme Q_{10}, also known as CoQ_{10}, is available without a prescription.

Actions on the body
Co-enzyme Q_{10} is a natural substance in the body and is used to produce energy for cell growth. It is also an antioxidant, protecting cells from damage caused by harmful molecules. CoQ_{10} is naturally present in foods.

Dietary and other natural sources
Peanuts, soy oil, fish such as sardines and mackerel, and organ meats (heart, liver) are particularly high in CoQ_{10}.

Normal daily requirement
There is no specific recommended daily allowance for Co-enzyme Q_{10}.

When supplements are helpful
CoQ_{10} has been studied in patients with heart failure and is thought to protect the heart muscle from damage caused by some prescription drugs. However, not all scientists agree that it has beneficial effects. In general, it may have potential benefits for heart health and as an antioxidant. It has also been studied in patients with lymphoma (a type of cancer), although it has not been shown to be beneficial. Excessive exercise is not recommended while on CoQ_{10}, especially by people with heart disease, as it may negatively affect tissue oxygenation.

Symptoms of deficiency
No specific deficiency noted.

Dosage range for treating deficiency
There is no specific deficiency range. When used for heart health, CoQ_{10} has been used in doses ranging from 30–100 mg, taken one to three times daily. Rarely, CoQ_{10} may increase liver enzymes or affect thyroid hormone levels. CoQ_{10} may decrease the effect of some drugs when taken concurrently, such as warfarin. Other drugs, such as those used for high cholesterol (statins) or for diabetes, may decrease the level of CoQ_{10}. Liver function tests and blood glucose levels may need to be periodically monitored. Individuals on co-enzyme Q_{10} should be monitored by their physician and pharmacist. Pregnant women and women who are breast-feeding should consult their physician as safety in these situations has not been established.

Symptoms and risks of excessive intake
No specific adverse effects related to high doses have been reported. May adversely affect liver function.

COPPER

Other names Copper chloride, copper chloride dihydrate, copper gluconate, copper sulfate

Availability
Copper supplements are available in oral forms without a prescription.

Actions on the body
Copper is an essential constituent of several proteins and *enzymes*. It plays an important role in the development of red blood cells, helps to form the dark pigment that colours hair and skin, and helps the body to use vitamin C. It is essential for the formation of collagen and elastin – proteins found in ligaments, blood vessel walls, and the lungs – and for the proper formation and maintenance of strong bones. It is also required for central nervous system activity.

Dietary and other natural sources
Most unprocessed foods contain copper. Liver, shellfish, nuts, mushrooms, wholemeal cereals, and dried pulses are particularly rich sources. Soft water may dissolve copper from pipes.

Normal daily requirement
The recommended daily allowances (RDA) for copper are: 0.2mg (birth–6 months); 0.22mg (7 months–1 year); 0.34mg (1–3 years); 0.44mg (4–8 years); 0.7mg (9–13 years); 0.89mg (14–18 years); and 0.9mg (19 years and over). Daily requirement during pregnancy is 1mg, and rises to 1.3mg when breast-feeding.

When supplements are helpful
A diet that regularly includes a selection of the foods mentioned above provides sufficient copper. Supplements are rarely necessary. However, physicians may advise additional copper for malnourished infants and children.

Symptoms of deficiency
Copper deficiency is very rare. The major change is *anemia* due to failure of production of red blood cells, the main symptoms of which are pallor, fatigue, shortness of breath, and palpitations. In severe cases, abnormal bone changes may occur. An inherited copper deficiency disorder called Menke's syndrome (kinky hair disease) results in brain degeneration, retarded growth, sparse and brittle hair, and weak bones.

Dosage range for treating deficiency
This depends on the individual and on the nature and severity of the disorder.

Symptoms and risks of excessive intake
As little as 250mg of copper sulphate taken by mouth in a single dose can produce toxic effects. Symptoms of poisoning include nausea, vomiting, abdominal pain, diarrhea, and general aches and pains. Large overdoses of copper may cause destruction of red blood cells (hemolytic anemia), and liver and kidney damage. In Wilson's disease, an inherited disorder, the patient cannot excrete copper and suffers from long-term copper poisoning and gradually develops liver and brain damage. The disease is treated with *chelating agents* such as penicillamine. Acute copper poisoning may occur in people who regularly drink homemade alcohol distilled through copper tubing.

FLUORIDE

Other name Sodium fluoride

Availability
Sodium fluoride may be added to drinking water and is available over-the-counter in single- or multiple-ingredient preparations. It is also available in mouth rinses, toothpastes, tablets, gels, and oral drops.

Actions on the body
Fluoride helps to prevent tooth decay and contributes to the strength of bones. It is thought to work on the teeth by strengthening the mineral composition of the tooth enamel, making it more resistant to attack by acid in the mouth. Fluoride is most effective when taken during the formation of teeth in childhood, since it is then incorporated into the tooth itself. It may also strengthen developing bones.

Dietary and other natural sources
Fluoride has been added to drinking water in many areas, and water is therefore a prime source of this mineral (fluoride levels in water vary from area to area, and untreated water also contains a small amount of fluoride). Foods and beverages grown or prepared in areas with fluoride-treated water may also contribute fluoride. Tea and sea fish are also rich in fluoride.

Normal daily requirement
No recommended daily allowance (RDA) has been established.

When supplements are helpful
Fluoride supplements are not usually necessary for adults, particularly those who use a fluoride toothpaste, although a dentist may recommend supplements for people who are especially prone to tooth decay. For children, supplements are not generally advised unless the drinking water contains a very low level of fluoride; infants less than 6 months old should not be given supplements even if the drinking water is low in fluoride. In all cases, supplements should only be used on the advice of a dentist. See below for more information about dosage ranges for supplements.

Symptoms of deficiency
Fluoride deficiency increases the risk of tooth decay, especially in children.

Dosage range for treating deficiency
Dietary supplements are not usually advised unless the drinking water contains less than 0.7 parts per million (ppm) of fluoride. In such cases, the recommended dosage depends on the level of fluoride in the water and the age of the child; supplements are not recommended for infants under 6 months old. When the drinking water contains less than 0.3ppm, the recommended daily dose is: 0.5–0.7mg (6 months–3 years); 1mg (4–8 years); and 2mg (9–13 years). When the drinking water contains 0.3–0.7ppm, supplements are not recommended for children under 3 years old; the recommended daily dose for older children is 0.25mg (3–6 years) and 0.5mg (over 6 years).

Symptoms and risks of excessive intake
Prolonged intake of water containing high concentrations of fluoride may lead to mottled or brown discoloration of the enamel in developing teeth, a condition known as fluorosis. Suggestions of a link between fluoridation of the water supply and cancer are without foundation. A child or adult who has taken a number of fluoride tablets may become seriously unwell and eventually lose consciousness. Give milk if the person is conscious, and seek immediate medical help (see p.526).

FOLIC ACID

Other names Folacin, vitamin B$_9$, folate, pteroylglutamic acid

Availability
Folic acid is available without prescription, alone and in a variety of multivitamin and mineral preparations. Strengths of 1,000mcg (1mg) and over are available only on prescription.

Actions on the body
Folic acid is essential for the activities of several *enzymes*. It is required for the manufacture of nucleic acids – the genetic material of cells – and thus for the processes of growth and reproduction. It is vital for the formation of red blood cells by the bone marrow and the development and function of the central nervous system.

Dietary and other natural sources
The best sources are leafy green vegetables, yeast extract, and liver. Root vegetables, oranges, nuts, dried pulses, and egg yolks are also rich sources.

Normal daily requirement
Recommended daily allowances as folate are: 0.065mg (birth–6 months); 0.08mg (7 months–1 year); 0.15mg (1–3 years); 0.20mg (4–8 years); 0.30mg (9–13 years); 0.40mg (14 years and over). For women considering pregnancy, the following are recommended to decrease incidence of fetal congenital problems; women with no personal health risks, on a healthy folate-rich diet, should take a daily supplement of a multivitamin with folic acid (0.4–1mg) for at least 2-3 months before conception, to be continued throughout pregnancy and after childbirth for 4–6 weeks and while breast-feeding; women with health risks (epilepsy, Type 1 Diabetes mellitus, obesity, family history of neural tube defect) should consume a folate-rich diet and a daily multivitamin with 5mg folic acid to be started 3 months before conception and for the first 10–12 weeks of pregnancy. Folic acid dose of 0.4–1mg to be taken for the remainder of pregnancy and for 4–6 weeks after childbirth while breast-feeding.

When supplements are helpful
A varied diet containing fresh fruit and vegetables usually provides adequate amounts. However, minor deficiency is fairly common, and can be corrected by the addition of one uncooked fruit or vegetable or a glass of fruit juice daily. Supplements are now routinely recommended for women planning a pregnancy and during the first 12 weeks of pregnancy for the prevention of neural tube defects such as spina bifida. Supplements may also be needed in premature or low-birth-weight infants and those fed on goat's milk (breast and cow's milk contain adequate amounts of the vitamin). Physicians may recommend additional folic acid for people on hemodialysis, those who have certain blood disorders, psoriasis, certain conditions in which absorption of nutrients from the intestine is impaired, severe alcoholism, or liver disease. Supplements may be helpful if you are a heavy drinker or if you are taking certain drugs that deplete folic acid. Such drugs include anticonvulsants, antimalarial drugs, estrogen-containing contraceptives, certain analgesics, corticosteroids, and sulfonamide antibacterial drugs.

Symptoms of deficiency
Folic acid deficiency leads to abnormally low numbers of red blood cells (*anemia*). The main symptoms include fatigue, loss of appetite, nausea, diarrhea, and hair loss. Mouth sores are common and the tongue is often sore. Deficiency may also cause poor growth in infants and children.

Dosage range for treating deficiency
Symptoms of anemia are usually treated with 0.25–1mg of folic acid daily (some may need higher doses), together with vitamin B$_{12}$. A lower maintenance dose may be substituted once the anemia has responded.

Symptoms and risks of excessive intake
Excessive folic acid is not toxic. However, it may worsen the symptoms of a coexisting vitamin B$_{12}$ deficiency and should never be taken to treat anemia without a full medical investigation of the cause of the anemia.

GLUCOSAMINE

Other names Glucosamine sulfate, Glucosamine hydrochloride

Availability
Glucosamine is considered a natural health product in Canada and is regulated by the Natural Health Products Directorate. Supplements such as these may not be standardized in how they are manufactured, and the amount of the active substance may vary between products (and from the product used to conduct research). Glucosamine is available without a prescription. It is available mainly as tablets or capsules, and as a sulfate salt (glucosamine sulfate) or hydrochloride or hydroiodide. Most of the studies have been conducted with glucosamine sulfate. It is also available in combination with another natural product, chondroitin.

Actions on the body
Glucosamine is a natural component of cartilage found in human joints and is thought to be able to provide some protection from damage to the cartilage.

Dietary and other natural sources
There are no food sources of glucosamine. Supplements are generally derived from the outer shells of crabs, shrimp, and lobsters.

Normal daily requirement
There are no specific recommended daily allowances for glucosamine.

When supplements are helpful
Glucosamine has been studied in the treatment of osteoarthritis, especially of the knee. It is thought to provide benefit by strengthening the cartilage in the joints. Although some smaller studies with glucosamine have shown improvement in pain and joint movement associated with osteoarthritis, others have not shown a benefit. In the studies where benefit was observed, there was some indication that glucosamine may allow for reduced doses of pain medications such as non-steroidal anti-inflammatory drugs.

Symptoms of deficiency
No specific deficiency noted.

Dosage range for treating deficiency
In studies with glucosamine sulfate in osteoarthritis, doses of 1500mg daily have been used; this is usually recommended to be taken as 500mg three times daily with food. There is some indication that a higher dose, up to 2000mg a day, may be needed with glucosamine hydrochloride. Glucosamine may need to be tried for at least 4 weeks in order to evaluate its beneficial effects. Blood glucose may need to be monitored in those with diabetes or on medications that can affect blood glucose. Glucosamine may increase the effect of anti-inflammatory drugs and doses may need adjustment. Individuals on glucosamine may require ongoing monitoring by their physician and pharmacist. Pregnant women or women who are breast-feeding should consult their physician, as safety in these situations has not been established.

Symptoms and risks of excessive intake
Upset stomach, heart burn, and diarrhea are some of its side effects. It is unclear whether there are any serious effects of excessive intake.

IODINE

Other names Potassium iodide, potassium iodate, sodium iodide

Availability
Iodine supplements are available without prescription as kelp tablets and in several multivitamin and mineral preparations. Iodine skin preparations are also available without a prescription for antiseptic use. A small amount of iodine is routinely added to most table salts in order to prevent iodine deficiency from occurring. Treatments for thyroid suppression are available only on prescription.

Actions on the body
Iodine is essential for the formation of thyroid hormone, which regulates the body's energy production, promotes growth and development, and helps burn excess fat.

Dietary and other natural sources
Seafood is the best source of iodine, but bread and dairy products such as milk are the main sources of this mineral in most diets. Iodized table salt is also a good source. Iodine may also be inhaled from the atmosphere in coastal regions.

Normal daily requirement
The recommended daily allowances (RDA) for iodine in micrograms (mcg) are: 110mcg (birth–6 months); 130mcg (7–12 months); 90mcg (1–3 years); 90mcg (4–8 years); 120mcg (9–13 years); and 150mcg (14 years and over). Requirements increase very slightly during breast-feeding; one vitamin tablet with calcium and iodine daily is recommended for nursing mothers.

When supplements are helpful
Most diets contain adequate amounts of iodine and use of iodized table salt can usually make up for any deficiency. Supplements are rarely necessary except on medical advice. However, excessive intake of raw cabbage or nuts reduces uptake of iodine into the thyroid gland and it may lead to deficiency if iodine intake is otherwise low. Kelp supplements may be helpful.

Adults exposed to radiation from radioactive iodine released into the environment may be given 100mg of iodine as a single dose (as potassium iodate 170mg) to prevent their thyroid gland absorbing the radioactive material; a lower dose is given to children according to age.

Iodine is used to treat people with thyrotoxicosis before surgery on the thyroid gland.

Symptoms of deficiency
Deficiency may result in a goitre (enlargement of the thyroid gland) and hypothyroidism (deficiency of thyroid hormone). Symptoms of hypothyroidism include tiredness, physical and mental slowness, weight gain, facial puffiness, and constipation. Babies born to iodine-deficient mothers are lethargic and difficult to feed. Left untreated, many show poor growth and mental retardation.

Dosage range for treating deficiency
Iodine deficiency may be treated with doses of 150mcg of iodine daily, and then followed up by ensuring that iodized table salt is used.

Symptoms and risks of excessive intake
The amount of iodine that occurs naturally in food is non-toxic, but prolonged use of large amounts (6mg or more daily) may suppress the activity of the thyroid gland. Large overdoses of iodine compounds may cause abdominal pain, vomiting, bloody diarrhea, and swelling of the thyroid and salivary glands.

IRON

Other names Ferrous fumarate, ferrous gluconate, ferrous sulfate, iron dextran, iron-polysaccharide complex, sodium ferric gluconate complex

Availability
Ferrous sulfate, ferrous fumarate, ferrous gluconate, and iron-polysaccharide complex are all available without prescription, alone and in multivitamin and mineral preparations. Iron dextran, an injectable form, is available only on prescription.

Actions on the body
Iron has an important role in the formation of red blood cells (which contain two-thirds of the body's iron) and is a vital component of the oxygen-carrying pigment hemoglobin. It is involved in the formation of myoglobin, a pigment that stores oxygen in muscles for use during exercise. It is also an essential component of several *enzymes*, and is involved in the uptake of oxygen by the cells and the conversion of blood sugar to energy.

Dietary and other natural sources
Liver is the best dietary source of iron. Meat (especially organ offal), eggs, chicken, fish, leafy green vegetables, dried fruit, enriched or wholemeal cereals, breads and pastas, nuts, and dried pulses are also rich sources. Iron is better absorbed from meat, eggs, chicken, and fish than from vegetables. Foods containing vitamin C enhance iron absorption.

Normal daily requirement
The recommended daily allowances (RDA) for elemental iron are: 0.27mg (birth–6 months); 11mg (7–12 months); 7mg (1–3 years); 10mg (4–8 years); 8mg (9–13 years); 11mg (males aged 14–18 years); 15mg (females aged 14–18 years); 8mg (males aged 19 years and over); 18mg (females 19–50 years); and 8mg (females 51 years and over). Requirements may be increased during pregnancy (27mg/day) and for 2 to 3 months after childbirth.

When supplements are helpful
Most diets supply adequate amounts of iron. However, larger amounts are necessary during pregnancy. Supplements may be given throughout pregnancy and for 2 to 3 months after childbirth to maintain and replenish adequate iron stores in the mother. Premature babies may be prescribed supplements from a few weeks after birth to prevent deficiency. Supplements may be helpful in young vegetarians, women with heavy menstrual periods, and people with chronic blood loss due to disease (for example, peptic ulcer). Iron is available as iron salts (e.g., ferrous sulfate or ferrous gluconate). Always clarify whether a dosage refers to elemental iron or a specific salt of iron.

Symptoms of deficiency
Iron deficiency causes *anemia*. Symptoms of anemia include pallor, fatigue, shortness of breath, and palpitations. Apathy, irritability, and lowered resistance to infection may also occur. Iron deficiency may also affect intellectual performance and behaviour.

Dosage range for treating deficiency
Depends on the individual and the nature and severity of the condition. In adults, iron-deficiency anemia is usually treated with 100mg of elemental iron (usually as ferrous sulphate or gluconate) daily. In children, the dose is reduced according to age and weight. Iron supplements of 30–60mg daily may be given during pregnancy.

Symptoms and risks of excessive intake
An overdose of iron tablets is extremely dangerous. Pain in the abdomen, nausea, and vomiting may be followed by abdominal bloating, dehydration, and dangerously lowered blood pressure. Immediate medical attention must be sought (see p.526). Keep out of the reach of children.

Excessive long-term intake, especially when it is taken with large amounts of vitamin C, may in susceptible individuals cause iron to accumulate in organs, causing congestive heart failure, cirrhosis of the liver, and diabetes mellitus. This condition is known as hemochromatosis.

LUTEIN

Other names Luteol, xanthophyll; also as a combined product with zeaxanthin

Availability
Lutein is considered to be a natural health product in Canada and is regulated by the Natural Health Products Directorate. Supplements may not be standardized in how they are manufactured, and the amount of the active substance may vary between products (and from the product used to conduct research on which health claims are based). Lutein is available without a prescription, alone or combined with zeaxanthin. It may also be included as an additive in some food products.

Actions on the body
Lutein is a component of the lens and retina of the eye. Along with fatty acids, which are components of these tissues, lutein is thought to act as an antioxidant and absorb certain types of harmful light.

Dietary and other natural sources
Lutein is naturally found in dark green, leafy vegetables such as spinach, kale, turnip greens, collard greens, broccoli, and also in highly coloured foods such as corn and egg yolks.

Normal dietary requirement
There is no specific recommended daily allowance for lutein.

When supplements are helpful
Some tissues in the eyes are susceptible to damage. Research has been conducted to see if lutein, and zeaxanthin, can prevent macular degeneration and cataract formation. Studies to-date indicate that there may be some benefit. However, better controlled studies are needed to demonstrate conclusively such a benefit.

Symptoms of deficiency
No specific deficiency noted.

Dosage range for treating deficiency
There is no specific deficiency range. Studies that examined the use of lutein in people with age-related macular degeneration used doses ranging from 5mg to 20mg per day. Individuals on lutein may need ongoing monitoring by their physician and pharmacist. Pregnant women and women who are breast-feeding should consult their physician as the safety in these situations has not been established.

Symptoms and risks of excessive intake
No specific adverse effects have been reported.

MAGNESIUM

Other names Magnesium carbonate, magnesium citrate, magnesium hydroxide, magnesium sulfate

Availability
Magnesium is available without prescription in a variety of multivitamin and mineral preparations. Magnesium is also an ingredient of numerous over-the-counter antacid and laxative preparations, but it is not absorbed well from these sources.

Actions on the body
About 60 per cent of the body's magnesium is found in bones and teeth. Magnesium is essential for the formation of healthy bones and teeth, the transmission of nerve impulses, and the contraction of muscles. It activates several *enzymes*, and is important in the conversion of carbohydrates, fats, and proteins into energy.

Dietary and other natural sources
The best dietary sources of magnesium are leafy green vegetables. Nuts, wholemeal cereals, soya beans, cheese, and seafood are also rich in magnesium. Drinking water in hard water areas is also a source of this mineral.

Normal daily requirement
The recommended daily allowances (RDA) for magnesium are: 30mg (birth–6 months); 75mg (7–12 months); 80mg (1–3 years); 130mg (4–8 years); 240mg (9–13 years); 410mg (males aged 14–18 years); 360mg (females aged 14–18 years); 400mg (males aged 19–30); 310mg (females aged 19–30); 420mg (males aged 31 years and over); and 320mg (females aged 31 years and over). Daily requirements do not increase much during pregnancy but rise by 50mg during breast-feeding.

When supplements are helpful
A varied diet provides adequate amounts of magnesium, particularly in hard water areas. Supplements are usually necessary only on medical advice for deficiency of magnesium associated with certain conditions in which absorption from the intestine is impaired, which occurs in repeated vomiting or diarrhea, advanced kidney disease, severe alcoholism, or prolonged treatment with certain diuretic drugs. Magnesium is used to treat eclampsia, cardiac arrhythmias, and myocardial infarction.
Estrogens and estrogen-containing oral contraceptives may reduce blood magnesium levels, but women who are on adequate diets do not need supplements.

Symptoms of deficiency
The symptoms of magnesium deficiency include anxiety, restlessness, tremors, confusion, palpitations, irritability, depression, and disorientation. Severe magnesium deficiency causes marked overstimulation of the nervous system, and results in fits and cramp-like spasms of the hands and feet. Inadequate intake may be a factor in the development of coronary heart disease, and may also lead to calcium deposits in the kidneys, resulting in kidney stones.

Dosage range for treating deficiency
This depends on the individual and on the nature and severity of the disorder. Severe deficiency is usually treated in hospital by injection of magnesium sulfate.

Symptoms and risks of excessive intake
Magnesium toxicity (hypermagnesemia) is rare, but can occur in people with impaired kidney function after prolonged intake of the large amounts that are found in antacid or laxative preparations. Symptoms include nausea, vomiting, dizziness (due to a drop in blood pressure), and muscle weakness. Very large increases in magnesium in the blood may cause fatal respiratory failure or heart arrest.

NIACIN

Other names Niacinamide, nicotinamide, nicotinic acid, vitamin B₃

Availability
Niacin is available without prescription in a wide variety of single-ingredient and multivitamin and mineral preparations. However, high doses of nicotinic acid are available only on prescription.

Actions on the body
Niacin plays a vital role in the activities of many *enzymes* and is important in producing energy from blood sugar, and in the manufacture of fats. Niacin is essential for the proper working of the nervous system, for a healthy skin and digestive system, and for the manufacture of steroid hormones.

Dietary and other natural sources
Liver, lean meat, poultry, fish, wholemeal cereals, nuts, and dried pulses are the best dietary sources of niacin.

Normal daily requirement
The recommended daily allowances (RDA) for niacin are: 2mg (birth–6 months); 4mg (7–12 months); 6mg (1–3 years); 8mg (4–8 years); 12mg (9–13 years); 16mg (males aged 14 years and over); and 14mg (females aged 14 years and over). Daily requirements increase during pregnancy and during breast-feeding.

When supplements are helpful
Most Canadian diets provide adequate amounts of niacin, and dietary deficiency is rare. Supplements are required for niacin deficiency associated with bowel disorders in which absorption from the intestine is impaired, and for people with liver disease or severe alcoholism. They may also be required for elderly people on poor diets. Large doses of niacin (up to 6g daily) are sometimes used in the treatment of hyperlipidemia (high cholesterol). There is no convincing medical evidence that niacin helps psychiatric disorders (except those associated with pellagra).

Symptoms of deficiency
Severe niacin deficiency causes pellagra (literally, rough skin). Symptoms include sore, red, cracked skin in areas exposed to sun, friction, or pressure, inflammation of the mouth and tongue, abdominal pain and distension, nausea, diarrhea, and mental disturbances such as depression, anxiety, and dementia.

Dosage range for treating deficiency
For severe pellagra, adults are usually treated with 300–500mg daily by mouth, and children are usually given 100–300mg daily. For less severe deficiency, doses of 25–50mg are given.

Symptoms and risks of excessive intake
At doses of over 50mg, niacin may cause transient itching, flushing, tingling, or headache. Niacin in the form that occurs naturally in the body (nicotinamide), is free of these effects. Large doses of niacin may cause nausea and may aggravate a peptic ulcer. Side effects may be reduced by taking the drug on a full stomach. At doses of over 2g daily (which have been used to treat hyperlipidemia), there is a risk of gout, liver damage, and high blood sugar levels, leading to extreme thirst.

OMEGA-3 FATTY ACIDS

Other names Omega-3 acid ethyl esters, Omega-3 oils

Availability
Omega-3 fatty acids (OFA) is considered a natural health product in Canada and is regulated by the Natural Health Products Directorate. Supplements such as these may not be standardized in how they are manufactured, and the amount of the active substance may vary between products (and from the product used to conduct research). OFAs are available without a prescription. Preparations include capsules, oil, and liquid.

Actions on the body
There are many types of OFAs; some are found in plants and some in fish. Plant OFAs (such as flaxseed and soy bean oil) are broken down and used differently in the body from the longer-chain OFAs found in fish. Fish oil fatty acids contain a combination of omega-3 ethyl esters called eicosapentaenoic acid (EPA) and docosahexaenoic acid (DHA). Omega-3-acids are polyunsaturated and are considered an essential fatty acid, as these cannot be made by the body. They may have many potential benefits and continue to be researched (see When supplements are helpful, below).

Dietary and other natural sources
Eicosapentaenoic acid (EPA) and docosahexaenoic acid (DHA): are found in salmon, trout, mackerel, sardines, and herring. Plant OFAs are found in flax seeds, walnuts, and canola oil.

Normal daily requirement
There is no specific recommended daily allowance for OFAs.

When supplements are helpful
It appears that omega-3 fatty acids can reduce the risk of some types of heart disease. However, studies indicate that the fish oils may have a more positive benefit in those with heart problems than the plant fatty acids, especially after a heart attack. A small percent of the plant oils is converted to the longer chain fatty acids in the body. Fish oils can decrease the amount of triglycerides (TG) (a type of cholesterol) in the blood. These may be used along with lifestyle changes, an appropriate diet, and exercise to decrease high triglycerides. There are several studies that are currently ongoing in evaluating the specific benefit of these in decreasing the risk of heart disease. Omega-3 oils are also being evaluated in decreasing the risk of eye problems such as macular degeneration and in inflammatory conditions such as arthritis. Although this product is available without a prescription, its use should be considered in conjunction with the individual's other medical conditions and medications in consultation with a physician.

Symptoms of deficiency
No specific deficiency noted.

Dosage range for treating deficiency
As there is no specific deficiency range, there are no recommendations to treat deficiency to-date. One study evaluating the potential benefits of omega-3 oils had participants eat 2 servings of fatty fish per week; in another study, participants took 850mg of omega-3 fatty acids daily. The American Heart Association recommends that eating fish twice weekly or taking 1g of EPA plus DHA in those with heart disease may be beneficial. Higher doses may be needed to decrease high triglycerides and for use in other conditions. Individuals on omega-3 oils may require monitoring by their health care provider. There is also potential for interaction with medicines such as warfarin. Pregnant or breast-feeding women should consult their physician, as safety in these situations has not been established.

Symptoms and risks of excessive intake
High doses may cause excessive bleeding in some. There is concern about contaminants like mercury in some types of fish.

PANTOTHENIC ACID

Other names Calcium pantothenate, vitamin B.

Availability
Pantothenic acid, calcium pantothenate, and panthenol are available without prescription in a variety of multivitamin and mineral preparations.

Actions on the body
Pantothenic acid plays a vital role in the activities of many *enzymes*. It is essential for the production of energy from sugars and fats, for the manufacture of fats, corticosteroids, and sex hormones, for the utilization of other vitamins, for the proper function of the nervous system and the adrenal glands, and for normal growth and development.

Dietary and other natural sources
Pantothenic acid is present in almost all vegetables, cereals, and animal foods. Liver, kidney, heart, fish, and egg yolks are good dietary sources. Brewer's yeast, wheat germ, and royal jelly (the substance on which queen bees feed) are also rich in the vitamin.

Normal daily requirement
No recommended daily allowance (RDA) for pantothenic acid has ever been established, but adult requirements are met by a 4–7mg intake daily.

When supplements are helpful
Most diets provide adequate amounts of pantothenic acid. Any deficiency is likely to occur in malnutrition together with other B vitamin deficiency diseases such as pellagra (see niacin), beriberi (see thiamine), or with alcoholism, and will be treated with B complex supplements. There is no firm evidence that large doses help, as some believe, in the prevention of greying hair, nerve disorders in diabetes, or psychiatric illness.

Symptoms of deficiency
Pantothenic acid deficiency is unlikely to occur unless a person is suffering from malnutrition. However, deficiency produced under experimental conditions can cause malaise, abdominal discomfort, and burning feet.

Dosage range for treating deficiency
Usually 5–10mg per day.

Symptoms and risks of excessive intake
In tests, doses of 1,000mg or more of pantothenic acid have not caused toxic effects. The risk of toxicity is considered to be very low, since pantothenic acid is a water-soluble vitamin that does not accumulate in the tissues. Any excess is eliminated rapidly in the urine. However, very high intakes of 10–20g can cause diarrhea.

POTASSIUM

Other names Potassium chloride, potassium citrate, potassium gluconate

Availability
Salts of potassium in small doses are available in a number of multivitamin and mineral supplements. They are available at higher doses as supplements and in an injectable form, both to be used under medical supervision. Potassium salts are also widely available in sodium-free salt (used as a salt substitute).

Actions on the body
Potassium works together with sodium in the control of the body's water balance, conduction of nerve impulses, contraction of muscle, and maintenance of a normal heart rhythm. Potassium is essential for maintenance of normal blood sugar.

Dietary and other natural sources
The best dietary sources of potassium are leafy green vegetables, tomatoes, oranges, potatoes, and bananas. Lean meat, pulses, chocolate, coffee, and milk are also rich in the mineral. Many methods of food processing may lower the potassium levels found in fresh food.

Normal daily requirement
The recommended daily allowance (RDA) is 2,000mg in adults. There are no extra requirements in pregnancy or breast-feeding.

When supplements are helpful
Most diets contain adequate amounts of potassium, and supplements are rarely required in normal circumstances. However, people who drink large amounts of alcohol or eat lots of salty foods may become marginally deficient. People with a condition called diabetic ketoacidosis or with certain types of kidney disease may be deficient in potassium, but the most common cause is prolonged treatment with diuretics. Long-term use of corticosteroids may also deplete the body's potassium. Prolonged vomiting and diarrhea also cause potassium deficiency, so people who abuse laxatives may be affected. Supplements are usually advised only when symptoms suggest deficiency, or for people at particular risk.

Symptoms of deficiency
Early symptoms of potassium deficiency may include muscle weakness, fatigue, dizziness, and mental confusion. Impairment of nerve and muscle function may progress to cause disturbances of the heart rhythm and paralysis of the skeletal muscles and those of the bowel, which leads to constipation.

Dosage range for treating deficiency
Depends on the preparation, the individual, and the cause and severity of deficiency. In general, daily doses equivalent to 20-40mmol/day of potassium chloride are given to prevent deficiency (for example, in people treated with diuretics that deplete potassium). Doses equivalent to 40–60mmol of potassium chloride daily are used to treat deficiency. Potassium supplements should be taken with a full glass of water, and may be taken after a meal to avoid gastric irritation.

Symptoms and risks of excessive intake
Blood potassium levels are normally regulated by the kidneys, and any excess is rapidly eliminated in the urine. Massive doses cause serious disturbances of the heart rhythm and muscular paralysis. In people with impaired kidney function, excess potassium may build up and the risk of potassium poisoning is increased. People on hemodialysis treatment need to take a carefully controlled low-potassium diet.

PYRIDOXINE

Other names Pyridoxine hydrochloride, vitamin B₆

Availability
Pyridoxine and pyridoxine hydrochloride are available without prescription in a variety of single-ingredient and multivitamin and mineral preparations. Pyroxidine is also available as an injection to be used under medical supervision.

Actions on the body
Pyridoxine plays a vital role in the activities of many enzymes. This B vitamin is essential for the release of carbohydrates stored in the liver and muscles for energy; for the breakdown and use of proteins, carbohydrates, and fats from food; and for the manufacture of niacin (vitamin B₃). It is needed for the production of red blood cells and antibodies, for healthy skin. It is also important for normal function of the central nervous system.

Dietary and other natural sources
Liver, chicken, fish, wholemeal cereals, wheat germ, and eggs are rich in this vitamin. Bananas, avocados, and potatoes are also good sources.

Normal daily requirement
The recommended daily allowances (RDA) for pyridoxine are: 0.1mg (birth–6 months); 0.3mg (7–12 months); 0.5mg (1–3 years); 0.6mg (4–8 years); 1.0mg (9–13 years); 1.3mg (males aged 14–50 years); 1.2mg (females aged 14–18 years); 1.3mg (females aged 19–50 years); 1.7mg (males aged 51 and over); and 1.5mg (females aged 51 and over). There are no extra requirements in pregnancy or breast-feeding.

When supplements are helpful
Most balanced diets contain adequate amounts of pyridoxine, and it is also manufactured in small amounts by bacteria that live in the intestine. However, breast-fed infants and elderly people may require additional pyridoxine. Supplements may be given on medical advice together with other B vitamins to people with certain conditions in which absorption from the intestine is impaired. They may also be used to treat a form of anemia (sideroblastic) and certain rare genetic disorders termed pyridoxine dependency conditions. Supplements may also be recommended to prevent or treat deficiency caused by alcoholism, oral contraceptives, and treatment with drugs such as isoniazid, penicillamine, and hydralazine.

Symptoms of deficiency
Pyridoxine deficiency is rare unless it is due to drug treatment Deficiency may cause weakness, nervousness, irritability, depression, skin disorders, inflammation of the mouth and tongue, and cracked lips. In adults, it may cause *anemia* (abnormally low levels of red blood cells). Convulsions may occur in infants.

Dosage range for treating deficiency
Depends on the individual and the nature and severity of the disorder. In general, deficiency is treated with 2.5–10mg daily in adults. Once signs of deficiency are corrected, a lower dose of 2.5mg daily can be used. Deficiency resulting from genetic defects that prevent use of the vitamin is treated with doses of 10–100mg daily in infants and 10–250mg daily in adults and children. More studies are needed to determine whether pyroxidine has a clear benefit in the treatment of premenstrual syndrome.

Symptoms and risks of excessive intake
Daily doses of over 500mg taken over a prolonged period may severely damage the nervous system, resulting in unsteadiness, numbness, and clumsiness of the hands.

RIBOFLAVIN

Other names Vitamin B₂, vitamin G

Availability
Riboflavin is available without a prescription, alone and in a wide variety of multivitamin and mineral preparations.

Actions on the body
Riboflavin plays a vital role in the activities of several *enzymes*. It is involved in the breakdown and utilization of carbohydrates, fats, and proteins and in the production of energy in cells using oxygen. It is needed for utilization of other B vitamins and for production of steroid hormones (by the adrenal glands).

Dietary and other natural sources
Riboflavin is found in most foods. Good dietary sources are liver, milk, cheese, eggs, leafy green vegetables, wholemeal cereals, and pulses. Brewer's yeast is also a rich source of the vitamin.

Normal daily requirement
The recommended daily allowances (RDA) for riboflavin are: 0.3mg (birth–6 months); 0.4mg (7–12 months); 0.5mg (1–3 years); 0.6mg (4–8 years); 0.9mg (9–13 years); 1.3mg (males aged 14 and over); 1mg (females 14–18 years); and 1.1mg (females aged over 18 years). Daily requirements rise by 0.3mg in pregnancy and by 0.5mg when breast-feeding.

When supplements are helpful
A balanced diet generally provides adequate amounts of riboflavin. Supplements may be beneficial in people on very low-calorie diets and elderly people on poor diets. Riboflavin requirements may also be increased by prolonged use of phenothiazine antipsychotics, tricyclic antidepressants, and estrogen-containing oral contraceptives. Supplements are required for riboflavin deficiency associated with chronic diarrheal illnesses in which absorption of nutrients from the intestine is impaired. Riboflavin deficiency is also common among alcoholics. As with other B vitamins, the need for riboflavin is increased by injury, surgery, severe illness, and psychological stress. In all cases, treatment with supplements works best in a complete B-complex formulation.

Symptoms of deficiency
Prolonged deficiency may lead to chapped lips, cracks, and sores in the corners of the mouth, a red, sore tongue, and skin problems in the genital area. The eyes may itch, burn, and become unusually sensitive to light.

Dosage range for treating deficiency
Usually treated with 1–2mg daily in combination with other B vitamins.

Symptoms and risks of excessive intake
Excessive intake does not appear to have harmful effects.

SELENIUM

Other name Selenium sulfide

Availability
Selenium is available without a prescription alone and in a multivitamin and mineral preparation. Selenium sulfide is the active ingredient of several antidandruff shampoos.

Actions on the body
Selenium is an trace element that is an essential part of an enzyme system that protects cells against damage by oxygen radicals (it is an *antioxidant* like vitamins A, C, and E).

Dietary and other natural sources
Meat, fish, wholemeal cereals, and dairy products are good dietary sources. The amount of selenium found in vegetables depends on the content of the mineral in the soil where they were grown. Selenium is found in foodstuffs combined in amino acids.

Normal daily requirement
The recommended daily allowances (RDA) for selenium are: 15mcg (birth–6 months); 20mcg (7–12 months); 20mcg (1–3 years); 30mcg (4–8 years); 40mcg (9–13 years); and 55mcg (14 years and over). There is a slight extra requirement during pregnancy, and 15mcg extra daily are required when breast-feeding.

When supplements are helpful
Most normal diets provide adequate amounts of selenium, and supplements are, therefore, rarely necessary. At present, there is no conclusive medical evidence to support some claims that selenium may provide protection against cancer or that it prolongs life. A daily intake of more than 150mcg is not recommended, except on the advice of a physician.

Symptoms of deficiency
Long-term lack of selenium may result in loss of stamina and degeneration of tissues, leading to premature ageing. Severe deficiency may cause muscle pain and tenderness, and can eventually lead to a fatal form of heart disease in children in areas where selenium levels in the diet are very low – for example in one remote part of China.

Dosage range for treating deficiency
Depends on the individual and on the nature and severity of the disorder. Severe selenium deficiency may be treated under medical supervision with doses of up to 200mcg daily.

Symptoms and risks of excessive intake
Excessive intake may cause hair and nail loss, tooth decay and loss, fatigue, nausea, vomiting, and garlic breath. Total daily intake should not exceed 400mcg; large overdoses may be fatal.

SODIUM

Other names Sodium bicarbonate (baking soda), sodium chloride (table salt), sodium phosphate

Availability
Sodium is widely available in the form of common table salt (sodium chloride). Sodium bicarbonate is used in many over-the-counter antacids and is available as an injection. Sodium phosphate is a laxative to be used under medical supervision. Sodium chloride is also available as an injection and an inhalation solution.

Actions on the body
Sodium works with potassium in control of the water balance in the body, conduction of nerve impulses, contraction of muscles, and maintenance of a normal heart rhythm.

Dietary and other natural sources
Sodium is present in almost all foods as a natural ingredient, or as an extra ingredient added during processing. The main sources are table salt, processed foods, cheese, breads and cereals, and smoked, pickled, or cured meats and fish. High concentrations are found in pickles and snack foods, including potato crisps and olives. Sodium is also present in water that has been treated with water softeners. Manufactured foods may also contain sodium compounds such as monosodium glutamate.

Normal daily requirement
There is no clearly defined recommended daily allowance (RDA) for sodium. Most diets contain far more sodium than what may be needed: the average consumption of sodium is 3–7g daily. One teaspoon of table salt contains about 2g of sodium.

When supplements are helpful
The need for supplementation is rare in temperate climates, even with "low-salt" diets. In tropical climates, however, sodium supplements may help to prevent cramps and possibly heatstroke occurring as a result of sodium lost through excessive perspiration during heavy work. Sodium supplements may be given on medical advice to replace salt loss due to prolonged diarrhea and vomiting, particularly in infants. They may also be given to prevent or treat deficiency due to certain kidney disorders, cystic fibrosis, adrenal gland insufficiency, use of diuretics, or severe bleeding (as intravenous infusion).

Symptoms of deficiency
Sodium deficiency caused by dietary insufficiency is rare. It is usually a result of conditions that increase loss of sodium from the body, such as diarrhea, vomiting, and excessive perspiration. Early symptoms include lethargy, muscle cramps, and dizziness. In severe cases, there may be a marked drop in blood pressure leading to confusion, fainting, and palpitations.

Dosage range for treating deficiency
Depends on the individual and on the nature and severity of symptoms. In extreme cases, intravenous sodium chloride may be required.

Symptoms and risks of excessive intake
Excessive sodium intake is thought to contribute to the development of high blood pressure, which may increase the risk of heart disease, stroke, and kidney damage. Other adverse effects include abnormal fluid retention, which leads to swelling of the legs and face. Large overdoses, even of table salt, may cause fits or coma and could be fatal. Table salt should never be used as an *emetic*.

THIAMINE

Other names Thiamine hydrochloride, vitamin B,

Availability
Thiamine is available without prescription in single-ingredient and a variety of multivitamin and mineral preparations. It is also available on prescription only as an injection.

Actions on the body
Thiamine plays a vital role in the activities of many *enzymes*. It is essential for the breakdown and utilization of fats, alcohol, and carbohydrates. It is important for a healthy nervous system, healthy muscles, and normal heart function.

Dietary and other natural sources
Thiamine is present in all unrefined food. Good dietary sources include wholemeal or enriched cereals and breads, brown rice, pasta, liver, kidneys, meat, fish, beans, nuts, eggs, and most vegetables. Wheat germ and bran are excellent sources.

Normal daily requirement
The recommended daily allowances (RDA) for thiamine are: 0.2mg (birth–6 months); 0.3mg (7–12 months); 0.5mg (1–3 years); 0.6mg (4–8 years); 0.9mg (9–13 years); 1.2mg (males aged over 14 years); 1mg (females aged 14–18 years); and 1.1mg (females aged over 18 years). Daily requirements rise by 0.3mg in pregnancy and when breast-feeding.

When supplements are helpful
A balanced diet generally provides adequate amounts of thiamine. However, supplements may be helpful in elderly people on poor diets or those with high energy requirements caused, for example, by overactivity of the thyroid or heavy manual work. As with other B vitamins, requirements of thiamine are increased during severe illness, surgery, serious injury, and prolonged psychological stress. Additional thiamine is usually necessary on medical advice for deficiency associated with conditions in which absorption of nutrients from the intestine is impaired, and for prolonged liver disease or severe alcoholism.

Symptoms of deficiency
Deficiency may cause fatigue, irritability, loss of appetite, and disturbed sleep, confusion, loss of memory, depression, abdominal pain, constipation, and beriberi, a disorder that affects the nerves, brain, and heart. Symptoms of beriberi include tingling or burning sensations in the legs, cramps and tenderness in the calf muscles, incoordination, palpitations, fits, and heart failure. In chronic alcoholics and in malnutrition, thiamine deficiency may lead to a characteristic deterioration of central nervous system function known as Wernicke Korsakoff's syndrome. The syndrome results in paralysis of the eye muscles, severe memory loss, and dementia, for which urgent treatment is needed.

Dosage range for treating deficiency
Depends on the nature and severity of the disorder but, in general, for mild chronic deficiency 5–30mg by mouth should be taken daily. Injections of the vitamin are sometimes given when deficiency is very severe or when symptoms have appeared suddenly.

Symptoms and risks of excessive intake
The risk of adverse effects is very low because any excess is rapidly eliminated in the urine. However, prolonged use of large doses of thiamine may deplete other B vitamins and should therefore be taken in a vitamin B complex formulation. There is a risk of allergic reactions with thiamine injections.

VITAMIN A

Other names Beta-carotene, retinol

Availability
Retinol and beta-carotene are available without prescription in various single-ingredient and multivitamin and mineral preparations. Derivatives of vitamin A (isotretinoin and tretinoin) are used in prescription-only treatments for acne and psoriasis.

Actions on the body
Vitamin A is essential for normal growth and strong bones and teeth in children. It is necessary for normal vision and healthy cell structure. It helps to keep skin healthy and protect the linings of the mouth, nose, throat, lungs, and digestive and urinary tracts against infection. Vitamin A is also necessary for fertility in both sexes. Beta-carotene is an important antioxidant (i.e., it protects the body from cell damage).

Dietary and other natural sources
Liver (the richest source), fish liver oils, eggs, dairy products, orange and yellow vegetables and fruits (carrots, tomatoes, apricots, and peaches), and leafy green vegetables are good dietary sources. Vitamin A is also added to margarine.

Normal daily requirement
The recommended daily allowances (RDA) for vitamin A are: 400mcg (birth–6 months); 500mcg (7–12 months); 300mcg (1–3 years); 400mcg (4–8 years); 600mcg (9–13 years); 900mcg (males aged 14 and over); 700mcg (females aged 14 and over); 750mcg (pregnancy); and 1250mcg (breast-feeding).

When supplements are helpful
Most diets provide adequate amounts of vitamin A. Diets very low in fat or protein can lead to deficiency. Supplements are often given to young children in developing countries. They may also be needed by people with cystic fibrosis, obstruction of the bile ducts, overactivity of the thyroid gland, and certain intestinal disorders, and by people on long-term treatment with certain lipid-lowering drugs (e.g., cholestyramine), which reduce absorption of the vitamin from the intestine. They are recommended with other vitamins for pregnant women, children under 5 years, and nursing mothers.

Symptoms of deficiency
Night blindness (difficulty in seeing in dim light) is the earliest symptom of deficiency; others include dry, rough skin, loss of appetite, and diarrhea. Resistance to infection is decreased. Eyes may become dry and inflamed. Severe deficiency may lead to corneal ulcers.

Dosage range for treating deficiency
Deficiency is treated by oral doses of up to 30,000 mcg daily in adults.

Symptoms and risks of excessive intake
Prolonged excessive intake (7.5–15mg daily) in adults can cause loss of appetite, diarrhoea, dry or itchy skin, and hair loss. Fatigue and irregular menstruation are common. Headache, weakness, and vomiting may result from increased pressure of the fluid surrounding the brain. In extreme cases, bone pain and enlargement of the liver and spleen may occur. High doses of beta-carotene may turn the skin orange but are not dangerous. Excessive intake in pregnancy may lead to birth defects (see box, below).

VITAMIN A AND PREGNANCY

Very large doses of vitamin A in the early weeks of pregnancy can, rarely, cause defects in the baby, leading to damage of the central nervous system, face, eyes, ears, or palate. Pregnant women and those considering pregnancy should keep to the prescribed dose and not take extra vitamin A or eat liver products such as pâté (one serving of liver may contain 4–12 times the dose recommended for pregnancy). No other dietary restrictions are considered necessary.

VITAMIN B12

Other names Cyanocobalamin, hydroxocobalamin

Availability
Vitamin B₁₂ is available without prescription in a wide variety of preparations. Cyanocobalamin is given only by injection under medical supervision.

Actions on the body
Vitamin B₁₂ plays a vital role in the activities of several *enzymes*. It is essential for the manufacture of the genetic material of cells and thus for growth and development. The formation of red blood cells by the bone marrow is particularly dependent on this vitamin. It is also involved in the utilization of folic acid and carbohydrates in the diet, and is necessary for maintaining a healthy nervous system.

Dietary and other natural sources
Liver is the best dietary source of vitamin B₁₂. Almost all animal products, as well as seaweed, are also rich in the vitamin, but vegetables are not.

Normal daily requirement
Only minute quantities of vitamin B₁₂ are required. Recommended daily allowances (RDA) are: 0.4mcg (birth–6 months); 0.5mcg (7–12 months); 0.9mcg (1–3 years); 1.2mcg (4–8 years); 1.8mcg (9–13 years); 2.4mcg (14 years and over); 2.8mcg (breast-feeding); and 2.6mcg (pregnancy).

When supplements are helpful
A balanced diet usually provides more than adequate amounts of this vitamin, and deficiency is generally due to impaired absorption from the intestine rather than low dietary intake. However, a strict vegetarian or vegan diet lacking in eggs or dairy products is likely to be deficient in vitamin B₁₂, and supplements are usually needed. The most common cause of deficiency is pernicious *anemia*, in which absorption of the vitamin is impaired due to inability of the stomach to secrete a special substance – known as intrinsic factor – that normally combines with the vitamin so that it can be taken up in the intestine. Supplements are also prescribed on medical advice in certain bowel disorders, such as celiac disease and various other causes of malabsorption, after surgery to the stomach or intestine, and in fish tapeworm infestation.

Symptoms of deficiency
Vitamin B₁₂ deficiency usually develops over months or years – the liver can store up to 6 years' supply. Deficiency leads to anemia. The mouth and tongue often become sore. The brain and spinal cord may also be affected, leading to numbness and tingling of the limbs, memory loss, and depression.

Dosage range for treating deficiency
Depends on the individual and on the type and severity of deficiency. Pernicious anemia (due to impaired absorption of vitamin B₁₂) is treated in adults with injections of 0.1mg–1mg (100–1,000mcg) on alternate days for 1–2 weeks, then 0.1–0.2mg per week until blood counts are normal, then 1mg every 2–3 months. Higher monthly doses of up to 1,000mcg of B₁₂, together with folic acid, may be given if the deficiency is severe. Children are treated with a total of 30–50mcg daily. Dietary deficiency is usually treated with oral supplements of 50–150mcg or more daily (35–50mcg twice daily in infants). Deficiency that results from a genetic defect preventing use of the vitamin is treated with 250mcg every three weeks throughout life.

Symptoms and risks of excessive intake
Harmful effects from high doses of vitamin B₁₂ are rare. Allergic reactions may in rare cases occur with preparations given by injection.

VITAMIN C

Other name Ascorbic acid

Availability
Vitamin C is available without prescription in a wide variety of single-ingredient and multivitamin and mineral preparations. Ascorbic acid can also be given by injection under specialized medical supervision.

Actions on the body
Vitamin C plays an essential role in the activities of several *enzymes*. It is vital for the growth and maintenance of healthy bones, teeth, gums, ligaments, and blood vessels, and is an important component of all body organs. Vitamin C is also recognized as an important antioxidant (i.e., it protects the body against cell damage and may prevent fat deposits from building up in the blood vessels) and is important for the manufacture of certain *neurotransmitters* and adrenal hormones. It is required for the utilization of folic acid and absorption of iron. This vitamin is also necessary for normal immune responses to infection and for wound healing.

Dietary and other natural sources
Vitamin C is found in most fresh fruits and vegetables. Citrus fruits, tomatoes, potatoes, and leafy green vegetables are good dietary sources. This vitamin is easily destroyed by cooking; some fresh, uncooked fruit and vegetables should be eaten daily. Adding a daily source of vitamin C, such as a glass of orange juice, is also recommended.

Normal daily requirement
The recommended daily allowances (RDA) for vitamin C are: 40mg (birth–6 months); 50mg (7–12 months); 15mg (1–3 years); 25mg (4–8 years); 45mg (9–13 years); 75mg (males aged 14–18 years); 65mg (females aged 14–18 years); 90mg (males aged over 19 years); 75mg (females aged over 19 years); 85mg (pregnancy); and 120mg (breast-feeding).

When supplements are helpful
A healthy diet generally contains sufficient quantities of vitamin C. However, it is used up more rapidly after a serious injury, major surgery, burns, and in extremes of temperature. Supplements may be necessary to prevent or treat deficiency in the elderly and chronically sick, for smokers, and in severe alcoholism. They are recommended with other vitamins for pregnant women, children under 5 years, and nursing mothers. Women taking estrogen-containing contraceptives may also require supplements. Although many people take larger doses (1g daily) for the prevention or treatment of colds, there is no convincing evidence that vitamin C in large doses prevents them, although it may reduce the severity of symptoms.

Symptoms of deficiency
Mild deficiency may cause weakness and aches and pains. Severe deficiency results in scurvy, the symptoms of which include inflamed, bleeding gums, nosebleeds, excessive bruising, and internal bleeding. In adults, teeth become loose. In children, there is abnormal bone and tooth development. Wounds fail to heal and become infected. Deficiency of vitamin C often leads to *anemia* (abnormally low levels of red blood cells), the symptoms of which are pallor, fatigue, shortness of breath, and palpitations. Untreated scurvy may cause fits, coma, and death.

Dosage range for treating deficiency
For scurvy, 100–250mg of vitamin C is given daily for several weeks.

Symptoms and risks of excessive intake
The risk of harmful effects is low, since excess vitamin C is excreted in the urine. However, doses of over 3g daily may cause diarrhea, nausea, and stomach cramps. Kidney stones may occasionally develop.

VITAMIN D

Other names Alfacalcidol, calcifediol, calciferol, calcitriol, cholecalciferol, ergocalciferol, vitamin D₂, vitamin D₃

Availability
Vitamin D and its analogs are available without prescription in a variety of multivitamin and mineral preparations. Injections are given only under medical supervision.

Actions on the body
Vitamin D (together with parathyroid hormone) helps regulate the balance of calcium and phosphate in the body. It aids in the absorption of calcium from the intestinal tract, and is essential for strong bones and teeth.

Dietary and other natural sources
Margarine (to which vitamin D is added by law), oily fish (sardines, herring, salmon, and tuna), liver, dairy products, and egg yolks are usually good sources of this vitamin. It is also formed by the action of ultraviolet rays in sunlight on chemicals naturally present in the skin. Sunlight is one main source of vitamin D for most people.

Normal daily requirement
The recommended daily allowances (RDA) for vitamin D are: 5mcg (birth–6 months); 5mcg (7 months–50 years); 10mcg (51–70 years); 15mcg (over 70 years); and 5mcg (women who are pregnant or breast-feeding). Most people do not require dietary supplements of vitamin D. 1mcg of cholecalciferol equals 40 international units (IU) of vitamin D.

When supplements are helpful
Vitamin D requirements are small and are usually adequately met by dietary sources and normal exposure to sunlight. However, a poor diet and inadequate sunlight may lead to deficiency; dark-skinned people (particularly those living in smoggy urban areas) and night-shift workers are more at risk. In areas of moderate sunshine, supplements may be given to infants. Premature infants, strict vegetarians, vegans, and the elderly may benefit from supplements of this vitamin. Supplements are usually necessary on medical advice to prevent and treat vitamin D deficiency-related bone disorders, and for conditions in which absorption from the intestine is impaired, deficiency due to liver disease, certain kidney disorders, prolonged use of certain drugs, and genetic defects. They are also used in the treatment of hypoparathyroidism. Supplements are recommended with other vitamins for pregnant women, children under 5 years, and nursing mothers, and with calcium to prevent or treat osteoporosis.

Symptoms of deficiency
Long-term deficiency leads to low blood levels of calcium and phosphate, which results in softening of the bones. In children, this causes abnormal bone development (rickets), and in adults, osteomalacia, causing backache, muscle weakness, bone pain, and fractures.

Dosage range for treating deficiency
In general, rickets caused by dietary deficiency is treated initially with 1,500–6,000 IU of vitamin D daily, depending on the age of the child, followed by a maintenance dose of 400 IU. Osteomalacia caused by deficiency of vitamin D is treated initially with 3,000–40,000 IU daily, followed by a daily maintenance dose of 400 IU. Deficiency caused by impaired intestinal absorption is treated with doses of 10,000–40,000 IU daily (adults) and 10,000–25,000 IU daily (children).

Symptoms and risks of excessive intake
Doses of over 800 IU of vitamin D daily are not beneficial in most people and may increase the risk of adverse effects. Prolonged excessive use disrupts the balance of calcium and phosphate in the body and may lead to abnormal calcium deposits in the soft tissues, blood vessel walls, and kidneys and retarded growth in children. Excess calcium may lead to symptoms such as weakness, unusual thirst, increased urination, gastrointestinal disturbances, and depression.

VITAMIN E

Other names Alpha tocopherol, alpha tocopheryl acetate, tocofersolan

Availability
Vitamin E is available without prescription in many single-ingredient and multivitamin and mineral preparations. It is also available as a component of a multivitamin injection, and is included in skin creams. Alpha tocopherol is the most powerful form of vitamin E.

Actions on the body
Vitamin E, a potent anti-oxidant, is vital for healthy cell structure, for slowing the effects of the ageing process on cells, and for maintaining the activities of certain *enzymes*. Vitamin E protects the lungs and other tissues from damage caused by pollutants, and protects red blood cells against destruction by poisons in the bloodstream. It also helps to maintain healthy red blood cells, and is involved in the production of energy in the heart and muscles. There is some evidence that vitamin E may protect against coronary heart disease and cancer, but further research is required.

Dietary and other natural sources
Some vegetable oils are good sources. Other sources rich in this vitamin include leafy green vegetables, wholemeal cereals, and wheat germ.

Normal daily requirement
Vitamin E is measured in milligrams of alpha-tocopherol equivalents (mg alpha-TE). Approximately 3–15mg daily are recommended. The recommended daily allowances (RDA) are: 4mg alpha-TE as alpha tocopherol (birth–6months); 6mg alpha-TE (7 months–3 years); 7mg alpha-TE (4–8 years); 11mg alpha-TE (9–13 years); 15mg alpha-TE (over 14 years); 15mg alpha-TE (pregnancy); and 19mg alpha-TE (breast-feeding).

When supplements are helpful
A normal diet supplies adequate amounts of vitamin E, and supplements are rarely necessary. However, people who consume large amounts of polyunsaturated fats in vegetable oils, especially if used in cooking at high temperatures, may need supplements. Supplements of vitamin E are also recommended for premature infants and people with impaired intestinal absorption, liver disease in children, or cystic fibrosis.

Symptoms of deficiency
Vitamin E deficiency leads to destruction of red blood cells (hemolysis) and eventually *anemia* (abnormally low levels of red blood cells), symptoms of which may include pallor, fatigue, shortness of breath, and palpitations. In infants, deficiency may cause irritability and fluid retention.

Dosage range for treating deficiency
Doses are generally four to five times the RDA in adults and children, for the relevant sex and age group.

Symptoms and risks of excessive intake
Harmful effects are rare, but there is a risk of diarrhoea and abdominal pain with doses of more than 1g per day. Prolonged use of over 250mg daily may lead to nausea, abdominal pain, vomiting, and diarrhea.

VITAMIN K

Other names Phtondione, vitamin K,

Availability
Vitamin K is available without prescription in several multivitamin and mineral preparations. Injectable and oral preparations of vitamin K alone are used to treat bleeding disorders, and are to be used only under close medical supervision. Oral vitamin K tablets are available through a Special Access Programme.

Actions on the body
Vitamin K is necessary for the formation in the liver of several substances that promote the formation of blood clots (blood clotting factors), including prothrombin (clotting factor II).

Dietary and other natural sources
The best dietary sources of vitamin K are leafy green vegetables and root vegetables, fruits, seeds, cow's milk, and yoghurt. Alfalfa is also an excellent source. In adults and children, the intestinal bacteria manufacture a large part of the vitamin K that is required.

Normal daily requirement
The recommended daily allowances (RDA) are: 2mcg (birth–6 months); 2.5mcg (7–12 months); 30mcg (1–3 years); 55mcg (4–8 years); 60mcg (9–13 years); 75mcg (14–18 years); 120mcg (males aged over 19 years); and 90mcg (females aged over 19 years). There are no extra requirements in pregnancy or breast-feeding.

When supplements are helpful
Vitamin K requirements are generally met adequately by dietary intake and by manufacture of the vitamin by bacteria that live in the intestine. Supplements are given routinely to newborn babies, since they lack intestinal bacteria capable of producing the vitamin and are therefore more at risk of deficiency than adults are. In adults and children, additional vitamin K is usually necessary only on medical advice for deficiency associated with prolonged use of antibiotics or sulfonamide antibacterials that destroy bacteria in the intestine, or when absorption of nutrients from the intestine is impaired. These conditions include liver disease, obstruction of the bile duct, and intestinal disorders causing chronic diarrhea. Vitamin K may also be given to reduce blood loss during labour or after surgery in people who have been taking oral anticoagulants. Vitamin K also reverses the effect of an overdose of oral anticoagulants.

Symptoms of deficiency
Vitamin K deficiency leads to low levels of prothrombin (hypoprothrombinemia) and other clotting factors, resulting in delayed blood clotting and a tendency to bleed. This may cause easy bruising, oozing from wounds, nosebleeds, and bleeding from the gums, intestine, urinary tract, and, rarely, in the brain.

Dosage range for treating deficiency
Depends on the individual and on the nature and severity of the disorder.

Symptoms and risks of excessive intake
Excess dietary intake of vitamin K has no known harmful effects. Adverse effects are extremely rare with vitamin K preparations taken by mouth.

ZINC

Other names Zinc gluconate, zinc hydroxide, zinc oxide, zinc sulfate, zinc pyrithione

Availability
Zinc supplements are available without prescription in single-ingredient and multivitamin and mineral preparations. Zinc sulfate is used in ocular solutions. Zinc is also one ingredient included in a variety of topical formulations used for the treatment of minor skin irritations, dandruff, acne, hemorrhoids, and fungal infections.

Actions on the body
Zinc plays a vital role in the activities of over 100 *enzymes*. It is essential for the manufacture of proteins and nucleic acids (the genetic material of cells), and is involved in the function of the hormone insulin in the utilization of carbohydrates. It is necessary for normal functioning of the immune system, a normal rate of growth, development of the reproductive organs, normal function of sperm, and healing of wounds and burns.

Dietary and other natural sources
Zinc is present in small amounts in a wide variety of foods. The mineral is better absorbed from animal sources than from plant sources. Protein-rich foods such as lean meat and seafood are the best sources of the mineral. Wholemeal breads and cereals, as well as dried pulses, are also good dietary sources.

Normal daily requirement
The recommended daily allowances (RDA) for zinc are: 2mg (birth–6 months); 3mg (7 months–3 years); 5mg (4–8 years); 8mg (9–13 years); 11mg (males aged over 14 years); 9mg (females 14–18 years); 8mg (females aged 19 and over); 11mg (pregnancy); and 12mg (breast-feeding).

When supplements are helpful
A balanced diet containing natural, unprocessed foods usually provides adequate amounts of zinc. Dietary deficiency is rare, and is likely only in people who are generally malnourished, such as debilitated elderly people on poor diets. Supplements are usually recommended on medical advice for those with reduced absorption of the mineral due to certain intestinal disorders, such as cystic fibrosis; for those with increased zinc requirements due to sickle cell disease or major burns; and for those with liver damage occurring, for example, as a result of excessive alcohol intake. There is evidence that zinc supplements may shorten the duration of the common cold.

Symptoms of deficiency
Deficiency may cause loss of appetite and impair the sense of taste. In children, it may also lead to poor growth and, in severe cases, to delayed sexual development and short stature. Severe, prolonged lack of zinc may result in a rare skin disorder involving hair loss, rash, inflamed areas of skin with pustules, and inflammation around the mouth, tongue, eyelids, and around the fingernails.

Dosage range for treating deficiency
Depends on the individual and on the cause and severity of the deficiency.

Symptoms and risks of excessive intake
Large overdoses of zinc salts in powder form are corrosive to tissues and may cause burns in the mouth and throat. Prolonged use of high doses may interfere with the absorption of copper, leading to deficiency, and may cause nausea, vomiting, headache, fever, malaise, and abdominal pain.

DRUGS OF ABUSE

The purpose of these pages is to clarify the medical facts concerning certain drugs (or classes of drugs) that are commonly known to be abused. Their physical and mental effects, sometimes combined with a dangerous habit-forming potential, have led to their use outside a medical context. Some of the drugs listed in this section are illegal, while others have legitimate medical uses – such as anti-anxiety and sleeping drugs – and are also discussed in other parts of the book. Alcohol, nicotine, and solvents, although not medical drugs, are all substances that have drug-like effects and high abuse potential. These substances are not illegal, but the sale of alcohol and tobacco products to young people is regulated by law, and the sale of solvents by voluntary agreement.

The individual profiles are designed to instruct and inform the reader, enabling him or her to understand how these drugs affect the body, to become more aware of the hazards of drug abuse, and to be able to recognize signs of drug abuse in other people.

Since a large proportion of drug abusers are young people, the following pages may serve as a useful source of reference for parents and teachers who are concerned that young people in their charge may be taking drugs.

The drugs of abuse profiles

The profiles are arranged in alphabetical order under their medical names, with street names, drug categories, and cross-references to other parts of the book where appropriate. Each profile contains information on that drug under standard headings. Topics covered include the various ways it is taken, its habit-forming potential, its legitimate medical uses, its legal status, its effects and risks, the signs of abuse, and interactions with other drugs.

HOW TO UNDERSTAND THE PROFILES

Each drug of abuse profile contains standard headings under which you will find information covering important aspects of the drug.

Other common names
Lists the usual, alternative, and street names of each drug.

How taken
Tells you the various forms in which each substance is taken.

Short-term effects
Explains the immediate mental and physical effects of the drug.

Signs of abuse
Describes the outward effects of taking the drug, both short- and long-term, that concerned observers may notice.

Practical points
Gives tips on how to avoid abuse of the drug and suggests ways to stop or reduce intake.

Drug category
Categorizes the drug according to its principal effects on the body, with cross-references to other parts of the book where relevant.

BENZODIAZEPINES

Other common names Tranquillizers, benzies
Drug category Central nervous system depressants (see Sleeping drugs, p.66, and Anti-anxiety drugs, p.67)

Habit-forming potential
The addictive potential of benzodiazepines is much lower than that of some other central nervous system depressants such as barbiturates. However, use of these drugs can lead to physical and psychological *dependence* on their sedative effects, especially when taken regularly long-term and in higher than normal doses.

How taken
By mouth as tablets or capsules, or by injection.

Legitimate uses
Benzodiazepines are commonly prescribed mainly for short-term treatment of anxiety and stress, as well as for relief of sleeplessness. They are also used in anesthesia, both as *premedication* and for induction of general anesthesia. Other medical uses include the management of alcohol withdrawal, control of epileptic fits, and relief of muscle spasms. Benzodiazepines are listed under the Benzodiazepines and Other Targeted Substances schedule (Controlled Drugs and Substances Act, Part IV) of the Food and Drugs Act.

Short-term effects
Benzodiazepines can reduce mental activity. In moderate doses, they may also cause unsteadiness, reduce alertness, and slow the body's reactions, thus impairing ability as well as increasing the risk of accidents. Benzodiazepines may also cause amnesia (loss of memory regarding events that occurred while the person was under the influence of the drug). Any benzodiazepine in a high-enough dose induces sleep. Very large overdoses may cause depression of the breathing mechanism and death can occur.

Long-term effects and risks
Benzodiazepines tend to lose their sedative effect with longterm use. This may lead the user to increase the dose progressively, a manifestation of tolerance and physical dependence. Older people may become apathetic or confused when taking these drugs. On stopping the drug, the chronic user may develop *withdrawal symptoms* that may include anxiety, panic attacks, palpitations, shaking, insomnia, headaches, dizziness, aches and pains, nausea, loss of appetite, and clumsiness. Symptoms can last for days or weeks. This can be minimized by stopping the drug gradually. Babies born to women who use benzodiazepines regularly may suffer withdrawal symptoms during the first week of life.

Signs of abuse
Abuse can occur by injection in young people. Another type of abuser is a middle-aged or elderly person who may have been taking these drugs by prescription for months or years. He or she is usually unaware of the problem, and may freely admit to taking "nerve" or sleeping pills in normal or large quantities. Problems usually occur if people attempt to cut down or stop taking the drugs without medical advice.

Interactions
Benzodiazepines increase the risk of sedation with any drug that has a sedative effect on the central nervous system. These include other anti-anxiety and sleeping drugs, alcohol, *opioid* analgesics, antipsychotics, tricyclic antidepressants, and antihistamines.

Practical points
Benzodiazepines should normally be used for courses of two weeks' duration or less. If these drugs have been taken for longer than two weeks, it is usually best to reduce the dose gradually to minimize the risk of withdrawal symptoms. If you have been taking benzodiazepines for many months or years, it is best to consult your physician to work out a dose reduction programme. If possible, it will help to tell your family and friends and enlist their support.

CANNABIS

Other common names Marijuana, marihuana, grass, pot, dope, reefers, weed, hash, ganja, skunk, skunkweed
Drug category Central nervous system depressant, hallucinogen, anti-emetic.
Cannabis sativa extract; brand name Sativex

Habit-forming potential
There is evidence that regular users of cannabis can become physically and psychologically *dependent* on its effects.

How taken
Usually smoked, either like tobacco or through a "bong" pipe. May be eaten, often in cakes or biscuits, or brewed like tea and drunk.
Sativex (cannabidiol) a spray formulation to be used under the tongue or inside of the cheek. Approved for neuropathic pain management in patients with multiple sclerosis (MS).

Legitimate uses
Preparations of the leaves and resin of the cannabis plant have been in use for over 2,000 years. Introduced into Western medicine in the mid-19th century, cannabis was formerly taken for many complaints, including anxiety, insomnia, rheumatic disorders, migraine, painful menstruation, strychnine poisoning, and *opioid* withdrawal. Today, cannabis derivatives – for example, nabilone – can be prescribed with certain restrictions for the relief of nausea and vomiting caused by treatment with anticancer drugs. Cannabis is listed under the Food and Drugs Act, Restricted Drugs, Part J (Controlled Drugs and Substances Act). An exception to this is under the Marihuana Medical Access Regulations, where an application can be placed to receive an authorization to possess cannabis for medical illness, such as terminal illness.

Short-term effects
In small doses, the drug promotes a feeling of relaxation and well-being, enhances auditory and visual perception, and increases talkativeness. Appetite is usually increased. However, in some individuals the drug may have little or no effect.
Under the influence of the drug, short-term memory may be impaired and driving ability and coordination are disrupted. Confusion, emotional distress, and loss of the sense of time can result. Hallucinations may occur in rare cases. The effects last for one to three hours after smoking cannabis and for up to 12 hours or longer after it is eaten, but reaction times remain slowed for 24 hours after a single use of the drug so that driving ability may remain impaired without the person being aware of it.

Long-term effects and risks
Cannabis smoking increases the risk of bronchitis and lung cancer. Regular users may become apathetic and lethargic, and neglect their work or studies and personal appearance. In susceptible people, heavy use may trigger depression or psychotic illness such as schizophrenia. Cannabis is thought by some physicians to increase the likelihood of experimentation with other drugs.
Since cannabis may increase the heart rate and lower blood pressure, people with heart disorders may be at risk from adverse effects of this drug. Regular use of cannabis may reduce fertility in both men and women and, if used during pregnancy, may contribute to premature birth.

Signs of abuse
The cannabis user may appear unusually relaxed or drunk under the influence of the drug. Appetite is increased. The user may become defensive or aggressive when challenged about use of the drug.
Cannabis smoke has a distinct herbal smell that may linger in the hair and clothes. Burns may occur on clothing as a result of pieces of lighted cannabis falling from the cigarette.

Interactions
Cannabis may increase the risk of sedation with any drugs that have a sedative effect on the central nervous system. These include anti-anxiety drugs, sleeping drugs, *general* anesthetics, opioid analgesics, antipsychotics, tricyclic antidepressants, antihistamines, and alcohol.

487

Habit-forming potential
Explains to what extent the drug is likely to produce physical or psychological *dependence.*

Legitimate uses
Describes the accepted medical uses of the substance, if any.

Long-term effects and risks
Explains the serious long-term effects on health and the risks involved with regular use of the drug.

Interactions
Describes interactions that may occur with other drugs.

ALCOHOL

Other common names Booze, drink (includes beer, wine, alcopops, hard liquor, and spirits); also known as ethyl alcohol or ethanol
Drug category Central nervous system depressant; sedative

Habit-forming potential
It is difficult to measure the habit-forming potential of alcohol because individual responses vary so widely. There is certainly a disease called alcoholism that is characterized by a person's inability to control intake. Regular drinking and heavy drinking do not cause alcoholism so much as indicate that it may be present. Alcoholism involves psychological and physical dependence, evidenced by large daily consumption, heavy weekend drinking, or periodic binges.

How taken
Orally, in the form of wines, beers and cider, and a wide range of spirits and liqueurs. Alcopops, the lemonade or fruit juice-based drinks, actually contain as much alcohol (5%) as beer or cider.

The alcohol content of drinks
Glasses vary in the amount they hold, so approximate volumes are quoted to help comparisons:

1 UNIT of alcohol =	1 glass of wine (125ml)
	½ pint of alcopops (250ml)
	½ pint of beer or cider (250ml)
	¼ pint of super strong lager (125ml)
	1 pub glass of port or sherry
	1 single shot of whisky, gin, vodka or brandy

Pub measures of sherry, port, and spirits are usually less generous than drinks at home.

Legitimate uses
The legal age to possess, consume, or purchase alcohol varies with each province, with many, such as Ontario, having the legal age for all of these three categories as 19 years. The manufacture and sale of alcoholic drinks is closely regulated by both provincial and federal laws.

Absorption of alcohol
Alcohol is rapidly absorbed from the stomach and particularly from the small intestine. Very strong drinks such as neat spirits are actually absorbed more slowly than weaker ones (as the alcohol reduces stomach movements that would push it into the intestine). Very dilute drinks are absorbed relatively slowly due to the large amount of water. In between these extremes, the stronger drinks will give higher blood levels; sherry and port are at about the "optimum" concentration. The presence of bubbles of carbon dioxide (in champagne, lemonade, and lager) may help to speed up absorption. So will mixing drinks; for example, drinking a glass of spirits as a "chaser" after drinking beer will produce a higher concentration that is absorbed more quickly.

Food in the stomach slows the rate of absorption of alcohol. Full cream milk, in which the fat is present in small droplets with a large surface area, seems particularly efficient for this purpose. Even the amount of carbohydrate in beer slows alcohol absorption a little, compared to a solution of alcohol in water at the same strength. Slowing the rate of absorption means that some of the alcohol can be broken down (metabolized, detoxified) before the rest is absorbed. Blood levels will thus not be so high, and the effects of the consumed alcohol will be less pronounced.

One unit of alcohol is the equivalent of about 15ml of pure alcohol, which is the amount that the average human adult male can break down in 1 hour. If you drink at a faster rate, your blood alcohol level will continue to rise. It will then take as many hours for your body to rid itself of all the alcohol as you have drunk units. For example, if you had five pints of beer (10 units) in a few hours, it will, on average, take around 10 hours to be removed from your blood. However, there is much variation in these figures. Women achieve higher blood levels than men after drinking the same amount (because women's bodies contain a lower percentage of water, into which the alcohol is distributed). A large-framed adult will have a lower blood level of alcohol than a smaller person after they have had the same amount to drink.

Short-term effects
Alcohol acts as a central nervous system depressant, reducing anxiety, tension, and inhibitions. In moderate quantities, it creates a feeling of relaxation and confidence, and increases sociability and talkativeness, but does not improve mental performance. Moderate amounts also dilate small blood vessels, especially in the skin, leading to flushing and a feeling of warmth. Increasing amounts progressively impair concentration and judgement and the body's reactions are increasingly slowed. Accidents, particularly driving accidents, are more likely. As blood alcohol levels rise, violent or aggressive behaviour is possible. Speech is slurred, and the person becomes unsteady, staggers, and may experience double vision and loss of balance. Nausea and vomiting are frequent; incontinence may also occur. Loss of consciousness may follow if blood alcohol levels continue to rise, and there is a risk of death occurring as a result of choking on vomit or cessation of breathing.

In addition to alcohol's effects on the central nervous system, where it depresses the higher functions such as judgement and co-ordination first, the drug has a number of other effects. The most noticeable to the drinker is its diuretic action. Beer drinkers will be particularly aware of this, but dehydration after drinking any kind of alcohol is responsible for much of the headache and other symptoms described as a "hangover" because the water removed comes from organs such as the brain. The best means of prevention is to drink less, or at least to drink a glass of water for each glass of alcohol, during the same time period.

Alcoholic drinks are not the same as "alcohol". They contain other chemical ingredients that might have side effects; for example, the juniper oil in gin is also diuretic, adding to the alcohol's action. It is thought that many of the ingredients in drinks can add to the hangover experience perhaps by delaying alcohol metabolism. Congeners – complex organic molecules such as polyphenols, higher alcohols, and histamine, which occur in varying amounts in different alcoholic drinks – may also have their own toxicity.

Long-term effects and risks
Heavy drinkers risk developing liver diseases, such as alcoholic hepatitis, liver cancer, cirrhosis, or fatty liver (excess fat deposits that may lead to cirrhosis). High blood pressure and strokes may also result from heavy drinking. Inflammation of the stomach (gastritis) and peptic ulcers are more common in alcoholics, who also have a higher than average risk of developing dementia (irreversible mental deterioration).

Long-term heavy drinking is generally associated with physical dependence. An alcoholic may appear to be sober, even after heavy drinking, because of built-up tolerance. But a reverse tolerance effect is frequently seen in alcoholics, where relatively little alcohol can rapidly produce a state of intoxication. As well as health problems, alcohol dependence is associated with a range of personal and social problems. Alcoholics may suffer from anxiety and depression, and because they often eat poorly, they are at risk of various nutritional deficiency diseases, particularly deficiency of thiamine (see p.479).

Drinking during pregnancy can cause fetal abnormalities and poor physical and mental development in infants; even taking moderate amounts of alcohol can lead to miscarriage, low birth weight, and mental retardation. As little as two units of alcohol taken by the mother may lead to behavioural and physiological effects in babies.

About 4 per cent of breast cancers in women may be related to alcohol intake. In developed countries, the risk of breast cancer rises with increased alcohol consumption.

Signs of abuse

Alcohol consumption may be getting out of control if any or all of the following signs are noted:

- changes in drinking pattern (for example, early morning drinking or a switch from beer to spirits);
- changes in drinking habits (such as drinking alone or having a drink before an appointment or interview);
- neglect of personal appearance;
- personality changes;
- poor eating habits;
- furtive behaviour;
- increasingly frequent or prolonged bouts of intoxication with memory lapses (blackouts) about events that occurred during drinking episodes.

Physical symptoms of heavy drinking may include nausea, vomiting, or shaking in the morning, abdominal pain, and cramps. The face may look red due to enlarged blood vessels. There may also be weakness in the legs and hands, general unsteadiness, poor memory, and incontinence.

Attempts to stop heavy drinking should always be made under medical supervision. The sudden stopping of heavy drinking, if not treated, can lead to delirium tremens (severe shaking, confusion, hallucinations, and occasionally fatal convulsions). These symptoms begin after one to four days of abstinence and last for up to three days. Drugs such as atenolol and benzodiazepines (for example, diazepam) given short term under medical supervision, can control these withdrawal symptoms.

Practical points

If you drink alcohol, know what your limits are. They vary from person to person, and your capacity depends a good deal on your body weight, age, experience, and mental and emotional state. However, you can use a "rule of thumb" guide to judge the body's ability to break down alcohol. Generally, the body can break down only about one unit of alcohol per hour, which means that alcoholic drinks should be spaced about one hour apart. If you drink faster than this, your blood alcohol is likely to rise above the "legal limit" for driving. But lower levels than this can affect judgement and reaction times, so the safest advice is not to drink at all if you plan to drive.

Drinking guidelines suggest that men should have no more than a total of 14 drinks a week, and women should have no more than nine each week. The weekly allowance of units should not be "saved up" in order to have a binge at the weekend. The usual recommendation is for no more than two standard drinks at each occasion. If you are a woman and are pregnant, or you are trying to conceive, the safest course of action is complete abstinence.

If you find that you are having trouble controlling your drinking, seek help and advice from your physician or from an organization, such as Alcoholics Anonymous, which is dedicated to helping people with this particular problem.

Even if you do not have a control problem with alcohol, you should still avoid drinking heavily because alcohol can have harmful effects on many parts of your body, including your liver and brain.

INTERACTIONS WITH OTHER DRUGS

Alcohol interacts with a wide variety of drugs and it is important to be aware of the interactions if you are on medication and want to have a drink. The main drug categories and their effects when taken with alcohol are shown below.

Type of drug	For example	Effects
Anti-anxiety drugs	Diazepam, lorazepam	Increased risk of sedation
Sleeping drugs	Temazepam, zopiclone	Increased risk of sedation
General anesthetics	Thiopental	Increased risk of sedation
Antipsychotics	Chlorpromazine, haloperidol	Increased risk of sedation
Tricyclic antidepressants	Amitriptyline, desipramine, trimipramine	Increased risk of sedation
Antihistamines	Chlorpheniramine, promethazine	Increased risk of sedation
Antimuscarinics	Hyoscine	Increased risk of sedation
Muscle relaxants	Baclofen, tizanidine	Increased risk of sedation
Cannabis derivatives	Nabilone	Increased risk of sedation
Opioid analgesics	Morphine, dihydrocodone, meperidine	Increased risk of sedation, fall in blood pressure, coma, death
Antidepressants, SSRIs	Citalopram, paroxetine	Possibly increased alcohol effects
Antihypertensives	Nifedipine, atenolol, losartan, captopril	Fall in blood pressure
	Clonidine,	Increased risk of sedation
Drugs of abuse	Barbiturates, heroin, solvents	Coma, death
Salicylates	ASA	Risk of stomach bleeding
Antibacterials	Metronidazole	Unpleasant reactions, including nausea, vomiting, headache, palpitations, flushing
Cytotoxics	Procarbazine	Unpleasant reactions, including nausea, vomiting, headache, palpitations, flushing
Antidiabetics	Insulin	Increased hypoglycemia
	Sulfonylureas	Possibly increased effects
	Chlorpropamide	Skin flushing, burning
MAOIs	Phenelzine, tranylcypromine	Dangerous rise in blood pressure with tyramine in red wine; fall in blood pressure with other alcoholic drinks
Anticoagulants	Warfarin	Increased risk of bleeding
Antiepileptics	Carbamazepine	CNS side effects increased
Dopamine-boosters	Bromocriptine	Reduced tolerance to drug

AMPHETAMINE

Other common names Speed, uppers, bennies, whizz, blues
(see also Ecstasy, p.488)
Drug category Central nervous system stimulant (see p.72)

Habit-forming potential
Regular use of amphetamine or methamphetamine rapidly leads
to the development of *tolerance*, so that larger and larger
doses are required to achieve the same effect. Users become
psychologically dependent on the drug's effects. Toxic effects
can occur at relatively low doses.

How taken
Usually swallowed as tablets or powder. Sometimes sniffed
or mixed with water and injected.

Legitimate uses
During the 1950s and 1960s, amphetamine was widely given
as an appetite suppressant. This use of the drug to suppress
appetite has been stopped because of the risk of *dependence*
and abuse. Amphetamine was used to maintain wakefulness by
drivers and pilots. It is still prescribed as dexamphetamine for
attention deficit disorder (hyperactivity) and narcolepsy (see
also Nervous system stimulants, p.72). Amphetamine is
classified under the Food and Drugs Act, Part 3 (controlled
Drugs and Substances Act). Possession without a prescription
is illegal.

Short-term effects
In small doses, amphetamine increases mental alertness
and physical energy. Breathing and heart rate speed up, the
pupils dilate, appetite decreases, and dryness of the mouth is
common. As these effects wear off, depression and fatigue may
follow. At high doses, amphetamine may cause tremor,
sweating, anxiety, headache, palpitations, and chest pain. Large
doses may cause delusions, confusion, hallucinations, delirium,
collapse, aggressive behaviour, convulsions, coma, and death.

Long-term effects and risks
Regular use frequently leads to muscle damage, weight loss,
and constipation. People who use amphetamine regularly may
also become emotionally unstable; psychosis may develop.
Severe depression and suicide are associated with withdrawal.
Heavy long-term use reduces resistance to infection and also
carries a risk of damage to the heart and blood vessels, leading
to strokes and heart failure.

    Use of amphetamine in early pregnancy may increase the
risk of birth defects, especially in the heart. Taken throughout
pregnancy, amphetamine leads to premature birth and low
birth weight.

Signs of abuse
The amphetamine user may appear unusually energetic,
cheerful, and excessively talkative while under the influence of
the drug. Restlessness, agitation, and a lack of interest in food
are typical symptoms; personality changes, psychotic
reactions, and paranoid delusions may also occur. Regular
users may exhibit unusual sleeping patterns, staying awake for
two or three nights at a stretch, then sleeping for up to 48 hours
afterwards. Mood swings are common.

Interactions
Amphetamine interacts with a variety of drugs. It causes an
increase in blood pressure, thus opposing the effect of
antihypertensive drug treatments. Taken with monoamine
oxidase inhibitors (MAOIs), it may lead to a dangerous rise
in blood pressure. It also increases the risk of abnormal
heart rhythms with digitalis drugs, levodopa, and certain
anesthetics that are given by inhalation. Amphetamine
counteracts the *sedative* effects of drugs that depress the
central nervous system.

BARBITURATES

Other common names Barbs, downers
Drug category Central nervous system depressant (see also
Sleeping drugs, p.66), sedative

Habit-forming potential
Long-term, regular use of barbiturates can be habit-forming.
Both physical and psychological *dependence* may occur.

How taken
By mouth in the form of capsules or tablets. Occasionally mixed
with water and injected.

Legitimate uses
In the past, barbiturates were widely prescribed as sleeping
drugs. Since the 1960s, however, they have been almost
completely replaced by benzodiazepines, which may also be
addictive but are less likely to cause death from overdose.

    The widest uses of barbiturates today are in *anesthesia*
(thiopental) and for epilepsy (phenobarbital).

    Most barbiturates are listed under Schedule G of the Food
and Drugs Act (Controlled Drugs and Substances Act, Part IV).

Short-term effects
The short-term effects are similar to those of alcohol. A low
dose produces relaxation, while larger amounts make the
user more intoxicated and drowsy. Coordination is impaired
and slurred speech, clumsiness, and confusion may occur.
Increasingly large doses may produce loss of consciousness,
coma, and death caused by depression of the person's
breathing mechanism.

Long-term effects and risks
The greatest risk of long-term barbiturate use is physical
dependence. In an addicted person, sudden withdrawal of
the drug precipitates a withdrawal syndrome that varies in
severity, depending partly on the type of barbiturate, its dose,
and the duration of use, but primarily on the availability and
administration of supportive treatment, including appropriate
medication. Symptoms may include irritability, disturbed sleep,
nightmares, nausea, vomiting, weakness, tremors, and extreme
anxiety. Abrupt withdrawal after several months of use may
cause convulsions, delirium, fever, and coma lasting for up to
one week. Long-term, heavy use of barbiturates increases the
risk of accidental overdose. The risk of chest infections is also
increased because the cough reflex is suppressed by long-
term, heavy use of these drugs.

    Use of barbiturates during pregnancy may cause fetal
abnormalities and, used regularly in the last three months,
may lead to *withdrawal symptoms* in the newborn baby.

Signs of abuse
Long-term heavy use of barbiturates may cause prolonged
bouts of intoxication with memory lapses ("blackouts"), neglect
of personal appearance and responsibilities, personality
changes, and episodes of severe depression.

Interactions
Barbiturates interact with a wide variety of drugs and increase
the risk of sedation with any drug that has a *sedative* effect on
the central nervous system. These include anti-anxiety drugs,
opioid analgesics, antipsychotics, antihistamines, and tricyclic
antidepressants. High doses taken with alcohol can lead to a
fatal coma.

    Barbiturates also increase the activity of certain enzymes
in the liver, leading to an increase in the breakdown of certain
drugs, thus reducing their effects. Tricyclic antidepressants,
phenytoin, griseofulvin, and corticosteroids are affected in this
way. However, the toxicity of an acetaminophen overdose is
likely to be greater in people taking barbiturates.

BENZODIAZEPINES

Other common names Tranquillizers, temmies
Drug category Central nervous system depressants (see Sleeping drugs, p.66, and Anti-anxiety drugs, p.67)

Habit-forming potential
The addictive potential of benzodiazepines is much lower than that of some other central nervous system depressants such as barbiturates. However, use of these drugs can lead to physical and psychological *dependence* on their *sedative* effects, especially when taken regularly long-term and in higher than normal doses.

How taken
By mouth as tablets or capsules, or by injection.

Legitimate uses
Benzodiazepines are commonly prescribed mainly for short-term treatment of anxiety and stress, as well as for relief of sleeplessness. They are also used in *anesthesia,* both as *premedication* and for induction of general anesthesia. Other medical uses include the management of alcohol withdrawal, control of epileptic fits, and relief of muscle spasms. Benzodiazepines are listed under the Benzodiazepines and Other Targeted Substances schedule (Controlled Drugs and Substances Act, Part IV) of the Food and Drugs Act.

Short-term effects
Benzodiazepines can reduce mental activity. In moderate doses, they may also cause unsteadiness, reduce alertness, and slow the body's reactions, thus impairing driving ability as well as increasing the risk of accidents. Benzodiazepines may also cause amnesia (loss of memory regarding events that occurred while the person was under the influence of the drug). Any benzodiazepine in a high-enough dose induces sleep. Very large overdoses may cause depression of the breathing mechanism and death can occur.

Long-term effects and risks
Benzodiazepines tend to lose their sedative effect with longterm use. This may lead the user to increase the dose progressively, a manifestation of tolerance and physical dependence. Older people may become apathetic or confused when taking these drugs. On stopping the drug, the chronic user may develop *withdrawal symptoms* that may include anxiety, panic attacks, palpitations, shaking, insomnia, headaches, dizziness, aches and pains, nausea, loss of appetite, and clumsiness. Symptoms can last for days or weeks. This can be minimized by stopping the drug gradually. Babies born to women who use benzodiazepines regularly may suffer withdrawal symptoms during the first week of life.

Signs of abuse
Abuse can occur by injection in young people. Another type of abuser is a middle-aged or elderly person who may have been taking these drugs by prescription for months or years. He or she is usually unaware of the problem, and may freely admit to taking "nerve" or sleeping pills in normal or large quantities. Problems usually occur only if people attempt to cut down or stop taking the drugs without medical advice.

Interactions
Benzodiazepines increase the risk of sedation with any drug that has a sedative effect on the central nervous system. These include other anti-anxiety and sleeping drugs, alcohol, *opioid* analgesics, antipsychotics, tricyclic antidepressants, and antihistamines.

Practical points
Benzodiazepines should normally be used for courses of two weeks' duration or less. If these drugs have been taken for longer than two weeks, it is usually best to reduce the dose gradually to minimize the risk of withdrawal symptoms. If you have been taking benzodiazepines for many months or years, it is best to consult your physician to work out a dose reduction programme. If possible, it will help to tell your family and friends and enlist their support.

CANNABIS

Other common names Marijuana, marihuana, grass, pot, dope, reefers, weed, hash, ganja, skunk, skunkweed
Drug category Central nervous system depressant, hallucinogen, anti-emetic.
Cannabis sativa extract; brand name Sativex

Habit-forming potential
There is evidence that regular users of cannabis can become physically and psychologically *dependent* on its effects.

How taken
Usually smoked, either like tobacco or through a "bong" pipe. May be eaten, often in cakes or biscuits, or brewed like tea and drunk.
   Sativex (cannabidiol): a spray formulation to be used under the tongue or inside of the cheek. Approved for neuropathic pain management in patients with multiple sclerosis (MS).

Legitimate uses
Preparations of the leaves and resin of the cannabis plant have been in use for over 2,000 years. Introduced into Western medicine in the mid-19th century, cannabis was formerly taken for many complaints, including anxiety, insomnia, rheumatic disorders, migraine, painful menstruation, strychnine poisoning, and *opioid* withdrawal. Today, cannabis derivatives – for example, nabilone – can be prescribed with certain restrictions for the relief of nausea and vomiting caused by treatment with anticancer drugs. Cannabis is listed under the Food and Drugs Act, Restricted Drugs, Part 4 (Controlled Drugs and Substances Act). An exception to this is under the Marihuana Medical Access Regulations, where an application can be placed to receive an authorization to possess cannabis for medical illness, such as terminal illness.

Short-term effects
In small doses, the drug promotes a feeling of relaxation and well-being, enhances auditory and visual perception, and increases talkativeness. Appetite is usually increased. However, in some individuals the drug may have little or no effect.
   Under the influence of the drug, short-term memory may be impaired and driving ability and coordination are disrupted. Confusion, emotional distress, and loss of the sense of time can result. Hallucinations may occur in rare cases. The effects last for one to three hours after smoking cannabis and for up to 12 hours or longer after it is eaten, but reaction times remain slowed for 24 hours after a single use of the drug so that driving ability may remain impaired without the person being aware of it.

Long-term effects and risks
Cannabis smoking increases the risk of bronchitis and lung cancer. Regular users may become apathetic and lethargic, and neglect their work or studies and personal appearance. In susceptible people, heavy use may trigger depression or psychotic illness such as schizophrenia. Cannabis is thought by some physicians to increase the likelihood of experimentation with other drugs.
   Since cannabis may increase the heart rate and lower blood pressure, people with heart disorders may be at risk from adverse effects of this drug. Regular use of cannabis may reduce fertility in both men and women and, if used during pregnancy, may contribute to premature birth.

Signs of abuse
The cannabis user may appear unusually talkative or drunk under the influence of the drug. Appetite is increased. The user may become defensive or aggressive when challenged about use of the drug.
   Cannabis smoke has a distinct herbal smell that may linger in the hair and clothes. Burns may occur on clothing as a result of pieces of lighted cannabis falling from the cigarette.

Interactions
Cannabis may increase the risk of sedation with any drugs that have a *sedative* effect on the central nervous system. These include anti-anxiety drugs, sleeping drugs, *general anaesthetics*, opioid analgesics, antipsychotics, tricyclic antidepressants, antihistamines, and alcohol.

COCAINE

Other common names Coke, crack, nose candy, snow
Drug category Central nervous system stimulant and local anesthetic (p.64)

Habit-forming potential
Taken regularly, cocaine is habit-forming. Users may become psychologically dependent on its physical and psychological effects, and may step up their intake to maintain or increase these effects or to prevent the feelings of severe fatigue and depression that may occur after the drug is stopped. The risk of *dependence* is especially pronounced with the form of cocaine known as "freebase" or "crack" (see below).

How taken
Smoked, sniffed through a tube ("snorted"), or injected.

Legitimate uses
Cocaine was formerly widely used as a *local anesthetic*. It is still sometimes given for *topical* anesthesia in the eye, mouth, and throat prior to minor surgery or other procedures. However, because of its *side effects* and potential for abuse, cocaine has now been replaced in most cases by safer local anesthetic drugs. Cocaine is classified under the Narcotic Control Act.

Short-term effects
Cocaine is a central nervous system stimulant. In moderate doses it overcomes fatigue and produces feelings of wellbeing. Appetite is reduced. Physical effects include an increase in heart rate and blood pressure, dilation of the pupils, tremor, and increased sweating. Large doses can lead to agitation, anxiety, paranoia, and hallucinations. Paranoia may cause violent behaviour. Very large doses may cause convulsions and death due to heart attacks or heart failure.

Long-term effects and risks
Heavy, regular use of cocaine can cause restlessness, anxiety, hyperexcitability, nausea, insomnia, and weight loss. Continued use may cause increasing paranoia and psychosis. Repeated sniffing also damages the membranes lining the nose and may eventually lead to the destruction of the septum (the structure separating the nostrils). Regular cocaine use leads to increased atheroma (fatty deposits in the arteries) and consequent risk of heart attacks.

Signs of abuse
The cocaine user may appear unusually energetic and exuberant under the influence of the drug and show little interest in food. Heavy, regular use may lead to disturbed eating and sleeping patterns. Agitation, mood swings, aggressive behaviour, and suspiciousness of other people may also be signs of a heavy user.

Interactions
Cocaine can increase blood pressure, thus opposing the effect of antihypertensive drugs. Taken with monoamine oxidase inhibitors (MAOIs), it can cause a dangerous rise in blood pressure. It also increases the risk of adverse effects on the heart when taken with certain general anesthetics.

CRACK
This potent form of cocaine is taken in the form of crystals that are smoked by vaporizing with a flame and inhaling the fumes. Highly addictive, crack appears to have more intense effects than other forms of cocaine and it is associated with an increased risk of abnormal heart rhythms, high blood pressure, heart attacks, stroke, and death. Other consequences of crack abuse include coughing of black phlegm, wheezing, irreversible lung damage, hoarseness, and parched lips, tongue, and throat from inhaling the hot fumes. Mental deterioration, personality changes, social withdrawal, paranoia or violent behaviour, and suicide attempts may occur.

ECSTASY

Other common names E, MDMA, XTC, methylenedioxymethamphetamine. Other slang names vary from place to place
Drug category Central nervous system stimulant

Habit-forming potential
As with other amphetamines, regular use leads to tolerance, so that higher doses are required to achieve the same effect. Users may become psychologically dependent on the effects of the drug and the lifestyle that surrounds its use.

How taken
By mouth in tablet or capsule form.

Legitimate uses
Although there have been claims that ecstasy may have a place in psychotherapy, it currently has no legitimate medical use. The drug is classified under the Food and Drugs Act, Restricted Drugs (Part 4).

Short-term effects
Ecstasy is most commonly used as a dance drug at "raves" or parties to increase the emotional effects of dancing to fast music and to enable users to dance for many hours. Adverse effects are more commonly due to "recreational" doses rather than to an overdose. Ecstasy stimulates the central nervous system, leading to increased wakefulness and energy and suppression of thirst, tiredness, and sleep. It can produce tight clenching of the jaw muscles (sometimes leading to involuntary tooth grinding) and stiffness in other muscles. The drug also increases the heart rate and raises the blood pressure. Various complications may occur, in particular, heatstroke due to prolonged dancing without replacing fluids lost by sweating. Heatstroke can lead to muscle breakdown, kidney failure, problems with the blood clotting mechanism, convulsions, and death. In some cases there may be low sodium levels and brain swelling due to excessive intake of fluid in the absence of sufficient exertion to sweat it off. These patients may experience vomiting, headaches, and drowsiness.
Liver damage and stroke have also occurred.

Long-term effects and risks
There is increasing evidence that ecstasy can reduce memory. In addition, some cases of psychiatric illness have been reported, such as schizophrenia and depression. Sleep disturbances and a craving for chocolate have also been reported. There may be an increased likelihood of developing depression even years after stopping the drug.

Signs of abuse
Ecstasy causes dilated pupils. Behaviour may be excitable or agitated. The ecstasy user may experience weight loss, tooth damage as a result of jaw-clenching, and anxiety.

Interactions
Ecstasy interacts with a variety of drugs. If it is taken with monoamine oxidase inhibitors (MAOIs), ecstasy may lead to a dangerous rise in blood pressure. It also increases the risk of abnormal heart rhythms with digoxin, levodopa, and certain anesthetics given by inhalation. Ecstasy tends to counteract the *sedative* effects of drugs that depress the central nervous system, and its effect on the mind is reduced by these drugs.

GHB

Other common names Liquid X, GBH, Liquid E, gamma hydroxybutyrate, sodium oxybate
Drug category Central nervous system depressant

Habit-forming potential
GHB is addictive if taken regularly in large doses.

How taken
By mouth. Often sold as a liquid in bottles, but it may be presented in a capsule or as a powder that is commonly dissolved in water to produce a clear, colourless liquid.

Legitimate uses
GHB is a naturally occurring chemical produced in the body in small amounts. Originally developed as an anesthetic, it has been used in the treatment of narcolepsy, insomnia, and alcohol and *opioid* withdrawal, but currently has no recognized medical use. Possession of GHB is illegal.

Short-term effects
GHB is a central nervous system depressant. Its effects are somewhat similar to alcohol, with talkativeness, cheerfulness, and euphoria occurring soon after taking an average dose. Most people become drowsy but recover within 4–8 hours of ingestion. Some users may experience confusion, headache, or gastrointestinal symptoms such as vomiting or stomach pain. Excessive doses may cause unconsciousness, and seizures, slowed heart rate, low blood pressure, and respiratory arrest have been reported. Recovery may take 96 hours, and hospital treatment may be necessary. Deaths have occurred after taking excessive doses of GHB.

Long-term effects and risks
Users may suffer a "hung-over" state for 2–3 days, and insomnia and dizziness may linger for up to 2 weeks. Longer-term effects of the drug have not been well studied. Stopping after prolonged use may cause a withdrawal syndrome.

Signs of abuse
As the drug is taken in liquid form it is difficult to estimate the correct dose, and the response to a low dose varies widely. Many abusers simply "guzzle" it until they reach an adequate high. This is often achieved only shortly before becoming unconscious, so sudden unconsciousness on the dance floor, for example, may be caused by GHB intoxication. Abnormally long-lasting hangovers and dizziness may be signs of abuse.

Interactions
The effects will be increased by other central nervous system depressants – for example, alcohol, benzodiazepines, and antipsychotics. GHB may also add to the effects of opioid analgesic drugs and muscle relaxants. It is sometimes mixed with amphetamines to prolong the "high" for several hours.

KETAMINE

Other common names Kit-Kat, Special K, Super K, vitamin K
Drug category General anesthetic with analgesic properties (see p.64)

Habit-forming potential
Likely to lead to psychological addiction if taken regularly.

How taken
Usually swallowed as the liquid pharmaceutical preparation or as tablets/capsules, produced mainly by heating the liquid anesthetic to evaporate the water, leaving ketamine crystals. Sometimes smoked or sniffed as a powder.

Legitimate uses
A *general anesthetic* with analgesic properties, used both in human and veterinary medicine. It is related to phencyclidine.

Short-term effects
The effects may depend on mood and environment, but have a rapid onset. Ketamine stimulates the cardiovascular system, producing a racing heart. There are a number of psychological effects that may occur, including hallucinations and a feeling of paralysis in which the user cannot move or speak but is still fully conscious and can see and hear. Actions or words may be repeated persistently, or the user may have an "out of body" experience. Users may be unconcerned whether they live or die. Due to the analgesic effects, the user is unlikely to feel pain. Severe reactions, usually due to overdose, may include convulsions, depression of the breathing mechanism, or heart failure.

Long-term effects and risks
The long-term use of ketamine may interfere with memory, learning, and attention span. Users may also experience flashbacks. Psychosis may occur.

Signs of abuse
Strange behaviour may suggest the psychological effects of ketamine. Painful injuries (such as cigarette burns) appear to go unnoticed.

Interactions
Barbiturates lengthen the duration of action that results from ketamine use, and in combination there is a risk of respiratory depression. Use of ketamine together with theophylline or aminophylline may increase the likelihood of convulsions. Alcoholics tend to be resistant to ketamine, although the psychological effects may be exaggerated during the recovery period.

KHAT

Other common names Cat, chaat, mriaa, quat
Drug category Central nervous system stimulant

Habit-forming potential
Dependence on khat is exclusively psychological.

How taken
Khat is composed of the leaves and small twigs of a plant (*Catha edulis*) that grows on high ground in many tropical countries. A large amount of the leaves or stems are chewed, and the plant material is kept in the cheek while the juice is swallowed. Occasionally it is brewed and drunk as tea.

Legitimate uses
The drug is widely used as a social stimulant in many Middle East and African countries, and is often taken at celebrations and gatherings. It has also been used as a traditional remedy to treat depression, fatigue, obesity, and gastric ulcers. However, the authorities in these countries are increasingly concerned about its adverse effects on health.

Short-term effects
Khat produces appetite suppression, dry mouth, euphoria, increased alertness, talkativeness, and hyperactivity. Gastrointestinal *side effects* are common, as well as a mild rise in the blood pressure, pulse, respiratory rate, and temperature. Insomnia, poor concentration, and malaise are also common side effects. Aggressive verbal outbursts and hallucinations may occur as a result of khat use, and psychosis has occurred. Mental depression and sedation may follow withdrawal after heavy or regular use.

Long-term effects and risks
Constipation is a very common side effect and stomach ulcers are quite common in regular users of khat. Men may experience impotence and reduced sex drive. Khat use may contribute to the risk of high blood pressure in young adults. Chronic use during pregnancy may lead to low birth weight, and the drug is excreted in breast milk.

Signs of abuse
The drug causes a brown staining of the teeth. Weight loss may occur as a result of appetite suppression.

Interactions
It may interact with amphetamine to cause mental stimulation, a fast heart rate and high blood pressure.

LSD

Other common names Lysergide, diethylamide, lysergic acid, lysergic acid diethylamide, acid, haze, microdots
Drug category Hallucinogen

Habit-forming potential
Although it is not physically addictive, LSD may cause psychological *dependence*. After several days of regular use, a person develops a tolerance to its actions. A waiting period must pass before resumption of the drug will produce the original effects.

How taken
By mouth, as tiny coloured tablets (known as "microdots"), or absorbed onto small squares of paper, gelatin sheets, or sugar cubes.

Legitimate uses
None. Early interest of the medical profession in LSD focused on its possible use in psychotherapy, but additional studies suggested that it could lead to psychosis in susceptible people. LSD is listed under the Food and Drugs Act, Restricted Drugs, Part 4 (Schedule III, Controlled Drugs and Substances Act).

Short-term effects
The effects of usual doses of LSD last for about 4–12 hours, beginning almost immediately after taking the drug. Initial effects include restlessness, dizziness, a feeling of coldness with shivering, and an uncontrollable desire to laugh. The subsequent effects include distortions in vision and, in some cases, in the perception of sound. Introspection is often increased and mystical, pseudoreligious experiences may occur. Loss of emotional control, unpleasant or terrifying hallucinations, and overwhelming feelings of anxiety, despair, or panic may occur (a "bad trip"), particularly if the user is suffering from underlying anxiety or depression. Suicide may be attempted. Driving and other hazardous tasks are extremely dangerous. Some people under the influence of this drug have fallen off high buildings, mistakenly believing they could fly.

Long-term effects and risks
The effects of long-term LSD use include an increase in the risk of mental disturbances, including severe depression. In those with existing psychological difficulties, it may lead to lasting mental problems (e.g., permanent psychosis). In addition, for months or even years after last taking the drug, some frequent users experience brief but vivid recurrences of LSD's effects ("flashbacks"), which cause anxiety and disorientation. There is no evidence of lasting physical ill-effects from LSD use.

Signs of abuse
A person under the influence of LSD may be behaving strangely but rarely shows any other outward signs of intoxication. Occasionally, a user who is drugged with LSD may seem overexcited, or appear withdrawn or confused.

Interactions
Chlorpromazine reduces the effects of LSD, so it can be used to treat a person who is acutely disturbed. Interactions with other drugs acting on the brain, such as alcohol, may increase the likelihood of unpredictable or violent behaviour. Lysergide abusers who are given SSRI antidepressants (e.g., fluoxetine, paroxetine, or sertraline) may experience onset or worsening of flashbacks.

MESCALINE

Other common names Peyote, cactus buttons, big chief
Drug category Hallucinogen

Habit-forming potential
Mescaline has a low habit-forming potential; it does not cause physical *dependence* and does not usually lead to psychological dependence. After several days of taking mescaline, the user develops a tolerance for further doses of the drug, thus discouraging regular daily use.

How taken
By mouth as capsules, or in the form of peyote cactus buttons, eaten fresh or dried, drunk as tea, or ground up and smoked with cannabis.

Legitimate uses
The peyote cactus has been used by Native Mexicans for over 2,000 years, both in religious rituals and as a herbal remedy for various ailments ranging from wounds and bronchitis to failing vision. Mescaline is listed under the Food and Drugs Act, Restricted Drugs, Part 4 (Schedule III, Controlled Drugs and Substances Act).

Short-term effects
Mescaline alters visual and auditory perception, although true hallucinations are rare. Appetite is reduced under the influence of this drug. There is also a risk of unpleasant mental effects, particularly in people who are anxious or depressed.

Peyote may have additional effects caused by several other active substances (in addition to mescaline) in the plant. Strychnine-like chemicals may cause nausea, vomiting, and, occasionally, tremors and sweating, which usually precede the perceptual effects of mescaline by up to 2 hours.

Long-term effects and risks
The long-term effects of mescaline have not been well studied. It may increase the risk of mental disturbances, particularly in people with existing psychological problems. Studies have shown that, after taking mescaline, most of the drug concentrates in the liver rather than in the brain, and it may therefore have special risks for people with impaired liver function.

Signs of abuse
Mescaline or peyote abuse may not have obvious signs. Users might sometimes appear withdrawn, disoriented, or confused.

Interactions
The combination of alcohol and peyote, although common, is recognized to be dangerous. There is a risk of temporary derangement, leading to disorientation, panic, and violent behaviour. Vomiting is likely to occur.

NICOTINE

Other common names Found in tobacco products
Drug category Central nervous system stimulant (see also p.367)

Habit-forming potential
The nicotine in tobacco is largely responsible for tobacco *addiction* in over one-third of the population who are cigarette smokers. Most are also probably psychologically *dependent* on the process of smoking. Most people who start go on to smoke regularly, and most become physically dependent on nicotine. Stopping can produce temporary *withdrawal symptoms* that include nausea, headache, diarrhea, hunger, drowsiness, fatigue, insomnia, irritability, depression, inability to concentrate, and craving for cigarettes.

How taken
Usually smoked in the form of cigarettes, cigars, and pipe tobacco. Sometimes sniffed (tobacco snuff) or chewed (chewing tobacco).

Legitimate uses
There are no legal restrictions on tobacco use. Its sale, however, is restricted to those over the age of 18. Nicotine chewing gum or slow-release patches may be prescribed on a temporary basis, along with behaviour modification therapy to help people who want to give up smoking.

Short-term effects
Nicotine stimulates the sympathetic nervous system (see p.63). In regular tobacco users, it increases concentration, relieves tension and fatigue, and counters boredom and monotony. These effects are short-lived, thus encouraging frequent use. Physical effects include narrowing of blood vessels, increase in heart rate and blood pressure, and reduction in urine output. First-time users often feel dizzy and nauseated, and may vomit.

Long-term effects and risks
Nicotine taken regularly may cause a rise in fatty acids in the bloodstream. This effect, combined with the effects of the drug on heart rhythm and blood vessel size, may increase the risk of diseases of the heart and circulation, including angina, high blood pressure, peripheral vascular disease, stroke, and coronary thrombosis. In addition, its stimulatory effects may lead to excess production of stomach acid, and thereby increase the risk of peptic ulcers.

Other well-known risks of tobacco smoking, such as chronic lung diseases, adverse effects on pregnancy, and cancers of the lung, mouth, and throat, may be due to other harmful ingredients in tobacco smoke. It is now believed that the cancer-causing chemical in tobacco smoke is benzo (a) pyrene diol epoxide (a tarry substance).

Signs of abuse
Regular smokers often have yellow, tobacco-stained fingers and teeth and bad breath. The smell of tobacco may linger on hair and clothes. A smoker's cough or shortness of breath are early signs of lung damage or heart disease.

Interactions
Cigarette smoking reduces the blood levels of a variety of drugs and reduces their effects. Such drugs include the benzodiazepines, tricyclic antidepressants, theophylline, propranolol, heparin, and caffeine. Diabetics may require larger doses of insulin. The health risks involved in taking oral contraceptives are increased by smoking.

Practical points
▼ Don't start smoking; nicotine is highly addictive.
▼ If you smoke already, give up now even if you have not yet suffered *adverse effects*. There are various strategies to help you with this.
▼ Ask your physician for advice and support.
▼ Inquire about self-help groups in your neighbourhood for people trying to give up smoking.

NITRITES

Other common names Amyl nitrite, butyl nitrite, poppers, snappers
Drug category Vasodilators (see also p.84)

Habit-forming potential
Nitrites do not seem to cause physical *dependence*; major *withdrawal symptoms* have never been reported. However, users may become psychologically dependent on the stimulant effect of these drugs.

How taken
By inhalation, usually from small bottles with screw or plug tops or from small glass ampules that are broken.

Legitimate uses
Amyl nitrite was originally introduced as a treatment for angina but has now largely been replaced by safer, longer-acting drugs. It is still available as an *antidote* for cyanide poisoning. Butyl and isobutyl nitrites are not used medically.

Short-term effects
Nitrites increase the flow of blood by relaxing blood vessel walls. They give the user a rapid "high", felt as a strong rush of energy. Less pleasant effects include an increase in heart rate, intense flushing, dizziness, fainting, pounding headache, nausea, and coughing. High doses may cause fainting, and regular use may produce a blue discoloration of the skin due to alteration of hemoglobin in the red blood cells.

Long-term effects and risks
Nitrites are very quick-acting drugs. Their effects start within 30 seconds of inhalation and last for about 5 minutes. Regular users may become *tolerant* to these drugs, thus requiring higher doses to achieve the desired effects. Lasting physical damage, including cardiac problems, can result from chronic use of these drugs, and deaths have occurred.

The risk of *toxic* effects is increased in those with low blood pressure. Nitrites may also precipitate the onset of glaucoma in susceptible people, by increasing pressure inside the eye.

Signs of abuse
Nitrites have a pungent, fruity odour. They evaporate quickly; the contents of a small bottle left uncapped in a room usually disappear within 2 hours. Unless someone is actually taking the drug or is suffering from an overdose, the only sign of abuse is a bluish skin discoloration. Overdose is usually through swallowing rather than inhaling, and can result in collapse, convulsions, and coma.

Interactions
The blood pressure-lowering effects of these drugs may be increased by alcohol, beta blockers, calcium channel blockers, and tricyclic antidepressants, thus increasing the risk of dizziness and fainting.

OPIOIDS (HEROIN)

Other common names Horse, junk, smack, scag, H, diamorphine, morphine, opium
Drug category Central nervous system depressant

Habit-forming potential
Opioid analgesics include not only those drugs derived from the opium poppy (opium and morphine) but also synthetic drugs whose medical actions are similar to those of morphine (meperidine, methadone, and dextropropoxyphene). Frequent use of these drugs leads to *tolerance*, and all have a potential for *dependence*. Among them, heroin is the most potent, widely abused, and dangerous. It is also associated with criminal behaviour.

After only a few weeks of use, *withdrawal symptoms* may occur when the drug is stopped; fear of such withdrawal effects may be a strong inducement to go on using the drug. In heavy users, the drug habit is often coupled with a lifestyle that revolves around its use.

How taken
A white or speckled brown powder, heroin is smoked, sniffed, or injected. Other opioids may be taken by mouth.

Legitimate uses
Heroin is widely used in countries such as Britain and Belgium for the treatment of acute severe pain. Although Canadian drug regulations were changed in the 1980s to allow heroin to be prescribed in hospital, it is rarely used. Heroin and morphine are powerful cough suppressants. Other opioids, such as morphine and methadone, are used as analgesics. Most opioids are listed under Schedule I of the Controlled Drugs and Substances Act of the Food and Drugs Act. Mild opioids such as codeine are also sometimes included in cough suppressant and antidiarrheal medications.

Short-term effects
Strong opioids induce a feeling of contentment and well-being. Pain is dulled and the activity of the nervous system is depressed; breathing and heart rate are slowed and the cough reflex is inhibited. First-time users often feel nauseated and vomit. With higher doses, there is increasing drowsiness, sometimes leading to coma and, in rare cases, death from respiratory arrest.

Long-term effects and risks
The long-term regular use of opioids leads to constipation, reduced sexual drive, disruption of menstrual periods, and poor eating habits. Poor nutrition and personal neglect may lead to general ill health.

Street drugs are often mixed ("cut") with other substances, such as caffeine, quinine, talcum powder, and flour, that can damage blood vessels and clog the lungs. There is also a risk of abscesses at the injection site. Dangerous infections, such as hepatitis, syphilis, and human immunodeficiency virus (HIV), may be transmitted via unclean or shared needles.

After several weeks of regular use, sudden withdrawal of opioids produces a flu-like withdrawal syndrome beginning 6–24 hours after the last dose. Symptoms may include runny nose and eyes, hot and cold sweats, sleeplessness, aches, tremor, anxiety, nausea, vomiting, diarrhea, muscle spasms, and abdominal cramps. These effects are at their worst 48–72 hours after withdrawal and fade after 7–10 days.

Signs of abuse
An opioid abuser may exhibit such signs as apathy, neglect of personal appearance and hygiene, loss of appetite and weight, loss of interest in former hobbies and social activities, personality changes, and furtive behaviour. Users resort to crime to continue financing their habit. Signs of intoxication include pinpoint pupils and a drowsy or drunken appearance.

Interactions
Opioids dangerously increase the risk of sedation with any drug that has a sedative effect on the central nervous system, including benzodiazepines and alcohol.

PHENCYCLIDINE

Other common names PCP, angel dust, crystal, ozone
Drug category General anesthetic (see p.64), hallucinogen

Habit-forming potential
There is little evidence that phencyclidine causes physical *dependence.* Some users become psychologically dependent on this drug and *tolerant* to its effects.

How taken
May be sniffed, used in smoking mixtures (in the form of angel dust), eaten (as tablets), or, in rare cases, injected.

Legitimate uses
Although it was once used as an anesthetic, it no longer has any medical use. Its only legal use now is in veterinary medicine. Phencyclidine's effects on behaviour (see below) make it one of the most dangerous of all drugs of abuse.

Short-term effects
Phencyclidine taken in small amounts generally produces a "high", but sometimes leads to anxiety or depression. Coordination of speech and movement deteriorates, and thinking and concentration are impaired. Hallucinations and violent behaviour may occur. Other possible effects include increases in blood pressure and heart rate, dilation of the pupils, dryness of the mouth, tremor, numbness, and greatly reduced sensitivity to pain, which may make it difficult to restrain a person who has become violent under the influence of the drug. Shivering, vomiting, muscle weakness, and rigidity may also occur. Higher doses lead to coma or stupor. The recovery period is often prolonged, with alternate periods of sleep and waking, usually followed by memory blackout of the whole episode.

Long-term effects and risks
Repeated phencyclidine use may lead to paranoia, auditory hallucinations, violent behaviour, anxiety, severe depression, and schizophrenia. While depressed, the user may attempt suicide by overdosing on the drug. Heavy users may also develop brain damage, which may cause memory blackouts, disorientation, visual disturbances, and speech difficulties.

Deaths due to prolonged convulsions, cardiac or respiratory arrest, and ruptured blood vessels in the brain have been reported. After high doses or prolonged coma, there is also a risk of mental derangement, which may be permanent.

Signs of abuse
The phencyclidine user may appear drunk while under the influence of the drug. Hostile or violent behaviour and mood swings with bouts of depression may be more common with heavy use.

Interactions
Using phencyclidine may inhibit the effects of *anticholinergic* drugs, as well as beta blockers and antihypertensive drugs.

SOLVENTS

Other common names Inhalants, glue
Drug category Central nervous system depressant

Habit-forming potential
There is a low risk of physical *dependence* with solvent abuse, but regular users may become psychologically dependent. Young people with family and personality problems are at particular risk of becoming habitual users of solvents.

How taken
By breathing in the fumes, usually from a plastic bag placed over the nose and/or mouth or from a cloth or handkerchief soaked in the solvent.

Legitimate uses
Solvents are used in a wide variety of industrial, domestic, and cosmetic products. They function as aerosol propellants for spray paints, hair lacquer, lighter fuel, and deodorants. They are used in adhesives, paints, paint stripper, lacquers, petrol, and cleaning fluids.

Short-term effects
The short-term effects of solvents include lightheadedness, dizziness, confusion, and progressive drowsiness; loss of coordination occurs with increasing doses. Accidents of all types are more likely. Heart rhythm might be disturbed, sometimes fatally. Large doses can lead to disorientation, hallucinations, and loss of consciousness. Nausea, vomiting, and headaches may also occur.

Long-term effects and risks
One of the greatest risks of solvent abuse is accidental death or injury while intoxicated. Some products, especially aerosol gases, butane gas, and cleaning fluids, may seriously disrupt heart rhythm or cause heart failure and sometimes death. Aerosols and butane gas can also cause suffocation by sudden cooling of the airways and these are particularly dangerous if squirted into the mouth. Butane gas has been known to ignite in the mouth. Aerosol products, such as deodorant and paint, may suffocate the user by coating the lungs. People have suffocated while sniffing solvents from plastic bags placed over their heads. There is also a risk of death from inhalation of vomit and depression of the breathing mechanism.

Long-term misuse of solvent-based cleaning fluids can cause permanent liver or kidney damage, while long-term exposure to benzene (found in plastic cements, lacquers, paint remover, petrol, and cleaning fluid) may lead to blood and liver disorders. Hexane-based adhesives may cause nerve damage leading to numbness and tremor. Repeated sniffing of leaded petrol may cause lead poisoning.

Regular daily use of solvents can lead to pallor, fatigue, and forgetfulness. Heavy use may affect the student's school performance and lead to weight loss, depression, and general deterioration of health.

Signs of abuse
Most abusers are adolescents between the ages of 10 and 17, although the average age, 14–15, for this type of drug abuse is thought to be falling.

Obvious signs of solvent abuse include a chemical smell on the breath and traces of glue or solvents on the body or clothes. Other signs include furtive behaviour, uncharacteristic moodiness, unusual soreness or redness around the mouth, nose, or eyes, and a persistent cough.

Interactions
Sniffing solvents increases the risk of sedation with any drug that has a *sedative* effect on the central nervous system. Such drugs include anti-anxiety and sleeping drugs, *opioids*, tricyclic antidepressants, antipsychotics, and alcohol.

ALTERNATIVE MEDICINE

Alternative, or complementary, medicine has become increasingly popular in recent years. A growing number of people consult alternative practitioners as well as, or instead of, their own physicians, and the use of alternative remedies has become considerably more widespread. Physicians are also more likely to refer some patients to alternative practitioners or to recommend the use of alternative treatments. However, there is little evidence of how alternative medicines work or of the safety and effectiveness of many of these remedies.

Many of these alternative medicine products will be better regulated in Canada over the next few years once the Natural Health Products Regulations are fully implemented.

Although many medicines are derived from plant matter, the use of plants and other natural substances to aid healing can be found in different cultures all around the world. Many modern alternative remedies are based on these traditional therapies. Most alternative practitioners believe that an illness is caused by an imbalance in the body, which must be restored to treat the illness. Many aim to treat the whole body rather than just certain symptoms.

Natural Health Products Regulations
Health Canada defines Natural Health Products as including vitamins, minerals, herbal remedies, and homeopathic medicines. Natural Health Products Regulations have come into effect as of January 1, 2004, with a transition period of 6 years, during which time all natural products will be required to receive a product licence so that they are legally authorized for sale in Canada by the Natural Health Products Directorate. All products will be required to display a product identification number preceded by NPN or, in the case of a homeopathic medicine, preceded by DIN-HM on their labels. Standard labelling requirements for natural products should include information on product name, quantity of product in the bottle, recommended conditions of use, and any special storage conditions. Recommended conditions of use include its recommended use or purpose, dose, dosage form, route of administration, warnings, cautions, contraindications, and possible adverse effects. Health Canada also requires that these products be monitored for adverse reactions and that these be reported to Health Canada.

Buying alternative medicines
Most alternative medicines are available over the counter from pharmacists and health shops. Only buy products from a reputable manufacturer, who will usually provide information leaflets and instructions for use. Other medicines can only be dispensed by suitably trained and registered practitioners. Some alternative practitioners are also medically trained and qualified.

Using alternative medicines
You may be able to treat yourself for minor, short-lived conditions, such as a cold, but professional advice should always be sought for more serious or persistent complaints. Always follow the instructions given when taking alternative medicines, and never exceed the recommended dose. Certain herbs and preparations contain ingredients that can be harmful if not used with care.

Some alternative medicines can interact with other drugs or affect pre-existing disorders in an adverse way. You should therefore tell your practitioner about any drugs you are taking as well as any pre-existing illnesses. You should also inform your physician or pharmacist about any alternative remedies you are taking before you start taking conventional drugs. Do not stop or reduce conventional treatment without asking your physician's advice.

HOMEOPATHY

The aim of homeopathy is to stimulate the body's powers of self-healing. Treatment is based on the concept of "like cures like" and uses the principle that the body can be stimulated to overcome illness if a patient is given extremely dilute doses of a substance that, at full strength, would produce symptoms of the illness. For example, minute doses of pollen are used to treat hayfever and allergic asthma.

Creating homeopathic remedies
There are at least 2000 homeopathic remedies. They are made from extracts of plants, animals, or minerals. These extracts are then infused in alcohol and water to make a tincture. This is then diluted repeatedly, in a process that is known as potentiation.

Homeopathic practitioners believe that the more dilute the remedy, the stronger the effect it will have. A few drops of the tincture are usually added to sugar tablets, creams, or other substances for administration.

How homeopathy works
One theory of how homeopathy works is that an electromagnetic imprint of the homeopathic substance remains after dilution, even though no molecules of the original substance are present. This imprint is believed to stimulate a response in the body. Some homeopathic practitioners believe that the imprint acts on the flow of energy in the body rather than on physical processes.

However, these findings are not reproducible and the basic principles underlying homeopathy are still generally regarded with scepticism.

Using homeopathic remedies
Homeopathic remedies are available as sugar tablets, powders, tinctures, oils, creams, and ointments. Tablets should be sucked or chewed. Tinctures are usually diluted in water and taken internally or applied externally. Ointments, oils, and creams are applied externally to the skin. Your homeopathic practitioner can provide specific recommendations on how to take the remedy; usually they are taken at least 30 minutes before or after eating or drinking.

COMMON HOMEOPATHIC REMEDIES

Coughs, colds, and 'flu
Aconite
Bryonia
Gelsemium

Hayfever
Allium
Arsen. alb.
Euphrasia
Nat. mur.

Indigestion
Acid. phos.
Bryonia
Carbo veg.
Nux vom.

Irritable bowel syndrome
Argent. nit.
Arsen. alb.
Cantharis
Nux vom.

Headaches and migraine
Aconite
Belladonna
Hypericum
Nat. mur.

Eczema and dermatitis
Graphites
Nat. mur.

Bruises, sprains, and minor injuries
Arnica
Hypericum
Ruta.grav.

Menopause
Calcarea
Graphites
Sepia
Sulfur

Insomnia and exhaustion
Arnica
Arsen. alb.
Coffea
Nux vom.

Stress
Ignatia
Nux vom.
Sepia

Depression
Lycopodium
Nat. mur.
Pulsatilla
Sulfur

Anxiety
Argent. nit.
Arsen. alb.
Gelsemium
Phos.

Many homeopathic medicines are taken every few hours at the start of treatment. The interval between successive doses is then increased as symptoms improve.

Homeopathic remedies have a good safety record and do not interact with conventional medicines. Because the remedies are highly diluted, they are very unlikely to cause side effects. However, in some cases, symptoms being treated may worsen briefly at the start of treatment before getting better.

WESTERN HERBAL MEDICINE

Western herbal medicines are extracted from the leaves, flowers, roots, seeds, berries, fruits, or bark of whole plants. They differ from modern drugs derived from herbs in that they use parts of the whole plant instead of isolating a single active ingredient. Many herbalists believe that the therapeutic effect of the whole plant is greater and safer than that of its isolated constituents. Several herbs may be combined in one remedy, and products should indicate which part of the plant has been used. The World Health Organization acknowledges that Western herbal medicine plays an important role in healthcare.

How Western herbal medicine works
The use of specific herbs is based on their recognized actions on the body. Although research into the use of herbal medicines is limited, evidence supports the claims made for the effectiveness of several herbal medicines. These include echinacea, which appears to stimulate the immune system, and St John's wort (hypericum perforatum), which seems to be effective in treating mild depression.

Using Western herbal remedies
Herbal remedies are available in a range of forms including infusions or teas, decoctions, tinctures, tablets, creams, lotions, ointments, and oils. Treatment is individually prescribed by a herbal practitioner, although you can treat yourself for simple, short-lived illnesses.

Remedies are most often taken three times a day. They should only be taken for short periods as the effects of long-term use are not known. Side effects are not common, although allergic reactions may occur. In general, herbal remedies should be avoided during pregnancy or breast-feeding, and they should not be taken by young children or by elderly people without professional advice.

Some interactions between herbal medicines and conventional drugs have been reported, with some causing serious problems; some combinations are dangerous. Their potential interactions can be predicted from the known effects of a plant. Plant remedies that could interfere with conventional drugs include liquorice,

COMMON WESTERN HERBAL REMEDIES

Minor injuries and bruises
Comfrey
Marigold
St John's wort

Coughs and colds
Echinacea
Garlic
Ginger

Nausea and vomiting
Chamomile
Fennel
Ginger
Peppermint

Headaches and migraine
Chamomile
Feverfew
Lavender

Acne
Echinacea
Dandelion root
Nettle

Premenstrual syndrome
Agnus castus
Cramp bark
Dandelion
Gamolenic acid
Marigold

Chronic fatigue
Astragalus
Echinacea
Ginseng
Goldenseal
Yellow dock root

Stress
Chamomile
Ginseng
Hops
Motherwort
Passion flower
Valerian
Vervain

blue cohosh, broom, ginger, and St John's Wort. It is important that you discuss potential interactions between herbal medicines and conventional drugs with your pharmacist or physician before use.

CHINESE HERBAL MEDICINE

Chinese herbal medicine is part of the ancient system of healing known as Traditional Chinese Medicine (TCM). Medicines are derived from hundreds of different plant species. Parts used may include the flowers, leaves, fruits, stalks, seeds, or bark. Chinese herbal medicine is different from Western medicine in that it regards symptoms as being due to disharmony in the body and tries to treat the underlying cause in order to restore balance. Western medicine tends to concentrate on specific symptoms. In China, TCM is taught at university level and practised in all hospitals.

How Chinese herbal medicine works
TCM is based around the concepts of *ying* and *yang*, two complementary but opposing forces. If these forces are disturbed, disease occurs. Different symptoms indicate excess *ying* or *yang*. Another belief is that of the five elements – fire, earth, metal, water, and wood. Each internal organ is associated with one of these elements.

Herbal remedies are used to restore balance between all these forces within the body. Herbs are classified under one of the five elements and according to their *ying* and *yang* qualities.

Although some studies have shown an improvement in symptoms following the use of Chinese herbal medicines, the concepts underlying traditional Chinese medicine cannot be explained by Western science and many Western physicians are still sceptical.

Using Chinese herbal remedies
Herbs are generally prescribed by the practitioner as a formula containing several different ingredients, usually up to 15 in combination. Each herb performs a particular function and is used for a specific purpose. The herbs are usually boiled in water to make a decoction or tea but may also be available as tablets, pills, powders, pastes, ointments, creams, and lotions. Medicine is usually taken daily at the start of treatment.

A large range of Chinese herbal medicines for minor conditions can be bought over-the-counter from health shops, pharmacists, Chinese herbalists, or Chinese medicine centres. More complex remedies and formulas are prescribed by a practitioner.

Although side effects are uncommon, some Chinese medicinal plants can have toxic effects. In particular, some remedies have been associated with liver damage. Additionally, recent analysis of a small sample of Chinese herbal cream showed that a significant proportion contained potent corticosteroids, which can be harmful if used inappropriately.

COMMON CHINESE HERBAL REMEDIES

Coughs and colds
Astragalus root
Balloon flower
Fritillary
Plantain

Eczema
Chinese gentian
Chinese wormwood
Peony root
Rehmannia

Irritable bowel syndrome
Chinese angelica
Chinese rhubarb
Dandelion
Magnolia bark
Poria

Arthritis
Aconite
Chinese angelica
Cinnamon
Ginger
Liquorice

Headaches and migraine
Cassia
Chrysanthemum

Menopause
Chinese angelica
Ginseng
Peony
Rehmannia
Thorowax root

Insomnia
Fleeceflower
Poria
Wild jujube

AIDS
Chinese bitter melon
Ginseng
Lentinan
Red sage
White peony

DRUGS IN SPORT

The use of drugs to improve athletic performance has been universally condemned by sporting authorities. Certain drugs give the athlete an unfair advantage and may also endanger health. On 1 January 2000, the whole of the International Olympic Movement adopted a common Olympic Movement Antidoping Code. Now the World Anti-Doping Agency (WADA) is responsible for the preparation and publication of the prohibited list of substances. If traces of a prohibited substance are found by means of a urine test, the athlete is banned from the competition and risks lifelong exclusion from the sport. Not only strong, prescribed medications affect athletic performance; everyday items such as cigarettes, alcohol, tea, and coffee can also have an effect. Drugs of any kind should be taken by athletes only under strict medical supervision and must be declared in writing to the relevant medical authority before the competition.

Many drugs affect the performance of athletes who are taking them. Some have been prescribed by physicians to treat specific medical conditions but are abused by athletes who want to benefit from the body-building and general performance-improving effects of these drugs. Others are everyday non-prescribed substances, such as caffeine and nicotine, which have a relatively minor effect on performance. However, even these substances can cause drug levels in the athlete's body to rise to unacceptable levels if taken in excess.

Detecting drugs
Drugs can be detected in the urine and other body fluids. Increasingly sensitive tests are constantly being devised to check for prohibited substances. These tests are performed frequently in most sports, during competitions and in training.

Prohibited substances
WADA includes several classes of drugs that are prohibited, some at all times and some during competition. These include: stimulants, narcotics (*opioids*), diuretics, anabolic agents (steroids), peptide hormones, mimetics, and analogues and all releasing factors. Hormones and related substances include erythropoietin (used to boost blood), growth hormone, and gonadotrophins. Many other drugs are banned in most sports – for example, alcohol, cannabis, *local anesthetics*, corticosteroids, and beta blockers. In addition, substances and methods that alter the validity of tests are illegal.

Legitimate medications
Certain prescribed drugs are allowed to be taken legitimately by athletes for certain medical disorders, such as asthma or epilepsy. Prescribed medicines must be declared in writing to the appropriate medical authority before any competition. Other prescribed drugs, such as antibiotics, may not make any noticeable difference to athletic performance, but the underlying disorder for which the drugs are being taken may make strenuous exercise inadvisable. The athlete should also be careful when using certain over-the-counter preparations, as many contain low doses of prohibited substances.

TYPES OF DRUGS AND PRACTICES
Antibiotics
These drugs may occasionally impair ability by causing nausea or diarrhea.

Antihistamines
Preparations containing chlorpheniramine or diphenhydramine may cause drowsiness, dizziness, or blurred vision.

Anti-inflammatory drugs
Using anti-inflammatory drugs to relieve pain in muscles, tendons, or ligaments can be dangerous; masking pain may result in aggravation of an injury.

Asthma drugs
An asthma drug should not contain isoprenaline, ephedrine, or phenylephrine, which are prohibited stimulants. However, inhalers containing salbutamol and specific required medicines may be used under the Therapeutic Use Exemption.

Blood doping
This illegal practice involves removing blood from an athlete during training and replacing it shortly before a competition. After the blood is removed, the volume and number of red blood cells in the remaining blood is naturally replenished. When stored blood is reinfused, the hemoglobin content of the blood is increased, enhancing the blood's ability to deliver oxygen to muscles. A similar effect is achieved by erythropoietin (epoietin), which stimulates extra blood production.

Caffeine
Although caffeine is listed as a prohibited stimulant, disqualification results only if large quantities (more than 12mg/litre) are detected in the urine sample.

Cocaine
This illegal and highly addictive stimulant is prohibited in sport. Dangerous side effects include heart arrhythmias, negative personality changes, and damage to the nasal lining after regular inhalation. A high dose can trigger convulsions or psychosis and may cause death.

Cough and cold remedies
Avoid preparations that contain codeine, ephedrine, pseudoephedrine, or phenylephrine for 12 hours before a competition. Drugs that can be used legally include antibiotics and antihistamines, steam inhalations, dextromethorphan, guaifenesin, and acetaminophen.

Diarrhea remedies
Any preparation containing opioids, such as morphine, must be avoided. However, diphenoxylate, loperamide, or electrolytes may be used.

Dieting drugs
Most diet drugs contain a prohibited stimulant or diuretic.

Hay fever remedies
Many remedies contain the prohibited stimulants ephedrine, pseudoephedrine, or phenylephrine. However, nasal sprays that contain steroids or xylometazoline and sodium cromoglycate eye drops can be used legally. See also Antihistamines, p.110.

Liniment
Used as a counter irritant on the pain receptors in the skin, it is important that application of liniment does not mask pain to the point where further damage to an injury may result after exertion.

Nicotine
Available from tobacco products as well as from nicotine transdermal patches, nicotine reduces the flow of blood through the muscles. Carbon monoxide from smoking decreases the available oxygen carried round the body, thereby reducing the capacity for exercise.

Painkillers
Strong painkillers such as meperidine and morphine, known as opioid analgesics, are prohibited in sport. Weaker painkillers, – for example, acetaminophen, ibuprofen, ASA, and local anesthetics in spray, ointment, or cream form – are permitted, but their use can mask pain, resulting in the aggravation of an injury.

Sleeping drugs
Many sports authorities ban sedatives, so a sleeping drug should not be taken less than 24 hours before a competition.

MEDICINES AND TRAVEL

Low cost air transport has resulted in enormous growth in international travel for both business and pleasure in recent years. This expansion has been paralleled by a more adventurous approach to leisure destinations. Few areas of the world are not on someone's itinerary and travellers are more likely than ever before to visit destinations with health hazards they have not encountered before and with poorly developed health services. Although few travellers run into serious medical problems, it is worth paying a little attention to the health aspects of travel when planning a trip. This should help to prevent problems later on and to ensure that any that do arise will not be serious. Risks can be minimized by seeking information about the country you are visiting, checking out facilities before you travel, and being prepared for both minor and major medical emergencies.

BEFORE YOU GO

If you take medicines regularly
Pack sufficient supplies to last for the entire trip. Some drugs may not be available at your destination or may require a local prescription. If any of your medicines are opioid or controlled drugs (see p.13), check with your physician or pharmacist as these may be stopped by Customs in some countries. It might be helpful for your physician to give you a letter with details of the drugs you have been prescribed to show to Customs abroad and to Canadian Customs on your return. If you are worried about taking a prescription medicine into another country, you could ask the relevant embassy whether there might be a problem.

... and even if you don't
Take a few everyday medicines with you, including:
• a motion sickness remedy
• simple painkillers
• an antidiarrheal and rehydration salts for traveller's diarrhea
• a laxative for constipation caused by changes in diet or routine
• an antiseptic cream for small injuries
• a bite/sting relief spray or cream for insect bites
• a high-protection factor (SPF 25+) sunscreen lotion
• an insect repellent

If you are going to a high risk area for malaria, start taking antimalarial drugs (p.123) a week or two before going to ensure that any intolerable side effects become apparent before departure.

If you are going outside the usual tourist routes, backpacking, or living among the local people, you might need to carry an emergency sterile syringe and needle kit. If you are intending to stay away for a long time, see your dentist for a check-up before you leave.

Vaccinations
Vaccinations are not normally necessary when travelling to Western Europe, the U.S., Australia, or New Zealand (although you should make sure that your tetanus and poliomyelitis boosters are up to date). However, consult your physician if you are visiting other destinations. If you are taking children with you, check that they have had the full set of routine childhood vaccinations as well as any vaccinations that are necessary for the areas you will be travelling in.

If you are visiting an area where there is yellow fever, an International Certificate of Vaccination will be needed. You may also need this certificate in the future. Many countries that you might want to visit require an International Certificate of Vaccination if you have already been to a country where yellow fever is present.

You are at risk of other infectious diseases in many parts of the world and appropriate vaccinations are a wise precaution. For example, there is a zone across northern India, Nepal, Bhutan, Pakistan, continuing in a wide band across Africa from the Sahara down to Kenya, that is called the "Meningitis Belt". Meningococcal vaccine A and C should be given to anyone who intends to visit this zone. Visitors who are going to Saudi Arabia at certain times of the year may also be required to have had the meningitis group A and C vaccine.

You may need extra vaccinations if you are planning to stay for a long time or backpacking. For example, hepatitis A vaccine would be sensible for anyone travelling to a developing country, but a long-stay traveller should consider having hepatitis B vaccine and BCG (tuberculosis) as well. Anyone travelling into remote areas is recommended to have rabies vaccination.

All immunization should be completed well before departure as the vaccinations do not give instant protection (BCG needs 3 months), and some need more than one dose to be effective.

Health Canada (see Further Information p.501) provides information and Travel Health Advisories to Canadians. Their Travel Medicine Program (TMP) lists travel clinics across Canada, specific diseases prevalent in parts of the world, and other relevant information.

Outbreaks of disease
Some infectious diseases are endemic (constantly or generally present). For example, dengue fever is found throughout the tropics; only the severity of the illness varies. Other diseases appear as definite outbreaks or epidemics; influenza is an example. While we are accustomed to think of influenza as a winter illness, it may occur at any time, especially in the tropics. If you or family members are likely to be at special risk and did not get the latest influenza booster, it would be worth checking whether there is an outbreak of influenza (or any other serious infectious disease) in the area you are planning to visit.

You could ask your physician or travel insurance company about the risk of disease in the country you are visiting. If you have access to the Internet, the best source of information on serious outbreaks of disease is the website of the Centers for Disease Control and Prevention (www.cdc.gov).

Insurance
Being taken ill when you are abroad can be expensive. Even if you are only travelling to the U.S., in the event of serious illness or accident you will need to show your insurance coverage in order to receive medical treatment. You should always take out travel health insurance, which can be inexpensive, before you leave. If you have a regular annual policy, check that it is kept up to date and is valid for the entire travel period and for any activities that you may be planning (such as skiing or watersports).

WHILE YOU ARE TRAVELLING

Travel sickness
If you are prone to travel sickness, take a travel sickness medicine about half an hour before you start your journey. Ask your physician or pharmacist for advice on which drug to choose. Do not drink alcohol if taking travel sickness drugs as alcohol can interact with the drugs and may make you excessively sleepy.

Dehydration and other cabin problems
The dry atmosphere inside the cabin of a passenger plane makes it very easy to become dehydrated, especially if you over-indulge in alcoholic drinks. Drink plenty of non-alcoholic fluids and limit alcoholic drinks, and you will feel fresher when you reach your destination.

Sitting still during a long-haul flight may lead to thrombosis (a blood clot) in the leg veins. A single tablet of soluble ASA taken with food before a long-haul flight may give protection. Discuss this with your physician before taking it and ensure that this is an appropriate medication for you. Once on the flight, get up and walk around the cabin now and again; also practise ankle- and knee-flexing exercises to try to help your circulation. Flight socks can help, too.

Taking medicines

International travel, in which time zones are crossed and airline meals are served at apparently random intervals, may make it difficult to decide when to take your regular medicines. Fortunately, precise timing is not critical with most medicines;

take them at the correct intervals (e.g. every 8 hours for a drug normally taken 3 times a day) regardless of the clock time, then adjust to the original schedule upon arrival at your destination.

However, the timing of some drugs is much more crucial. For example, progestin-only oral contraceptives (p.149), must be taken at intervals of almost exactly 24 hours in order to remain effective; a delay of more than 3 hours will interfere with contraceptive protection. Timing is less critical with the combined (estrogen and progestin) oral contraceptive drugs.

People with insulin-dependent diabetes also face problems when travelling as their insulin dosage regimen is governed by the clock and by the timing of their meals (p.128). Such individuals should

always consult their physician or diabetic educator before travelling long distances.

Jet lag

Rapid travel across time zones can cause physical and psychological stress. Business travellers should try to avoid major decisions on the first day after arrival, and all travellers should have a quiet adjustment period of at least a day to settle into the new day/night timing. Those on regular medication should seek advice from their physician about dosage adjustment before travelling.

Melatonin can shift the body clock when taken 15–30 minutes before bedtime in the new time zone, and repeated for the following 2–4 days. Melatonin is now available as a Natural Health Product in Canada.

TRAVEL IMMUNIZATION

The immunizations that you will need before travelling depend on the area of the world you intend to visit, although some diseases can be contracted almost anywhere. Wherever you are

planning to go, make sure that you have been immunized against tetanus and polio and have had booster doses if necessary. Advice on other necessary immunizations may change from time to

time. Before you travel, it is advisable to ask your physician, pharmacist, or travel clinic about vaccination for specific areas of the world as they should have the most up-to-date information.

Disease	Number of doses	When effective	Period of protection	Who should be immunized
Diphtheria	1 injection	Immediately	10 years	People travelling to countries where it is endemic and expatriates living in developing countries.
Hepatitis A	2 injections 6–12 months apart	2–4 weeks after 1st dose	10 years	Frequent travellers to the Mediterranean or developing countries.
Hepatitis B	3 injections, 1 month between 1st and 2nd doses, 5 months between 2nd and 3rd doses	Immediately after 2nd dose	3–5 years	People travelling to countries in which hepatitis B is prevalent; those who might need medical or dental treatment while travelling in a developing country; and people likely to have unprotected sex.
Japanese B encephalitis	2–3 injections 1–2 weeks apart	10–14 days after last dose	About 2 years	People staying for an extended period in rural areas of the Indian subcontinent, China, Southeast Asia, and the Far East.
Meningitis A and C	1 injection	After 15 days	3–5 years	People travelling to sub-Saharan Africa, Nepal, Bhutan, Pakistan, and Brazil; quadrivalent vaccine and immunization certificate needed if travelling to Saudi Arabia for the Hajj at Mecca.
Rabies	3 injections, 1 week between 1st and 2nd doses, 3 weeks between 2nd and 3rd doses	Immediately after 3rd dose	2–3 years	People travelling to areas where rabies is endemic and who are at high risk (veterinary surgeons, people working with animals, and those travelling into remote country).
Typhoid	1 injection or 3 oral doses	10 days after last dose or injection	3 years	People travelling to areas with poor sanitation.
Yellow fever	1 injection	After 10 days	10 years	People travelling to parts of South America and Africa.
Cholera	No satisfactory vaccine exists. Travellers to countries where cholera exists must pay scrupulous attention to food, water, and personal hygiene.			

ON ARRIVAL

Insect bites
Many microbial and viral diseases are spread by insect bites; taking steps to prevent these bites can help minimize risks. Ticks, sand flies, simulium flies, tsetse flies, and mosquitoes are among the insect carriers of disease. Although usually thought of as tropical problems, ticks, sand flies, and mosquitoes may spread some of the diseases mentioned here as far from the tropics as Europe, North America and the Mediterranean.

Viral diseases borne by insects include dengue fever, yellow fever, Japanese encephalitis, phlebotomus fever (sand fly fever), Colorado tick fever, and many others. Insects also transmit protozoal parasitical diseases, for example: malaria, filariasis, leishmaniasis, Lyme disease, river blindness, and trypanosomiasis (African sleeping sickness).

To reduce the chance of being bitten wear long sleeved shirts and trousers, apply insect repellent regularly, and sleep under an insecticide-impregnated mosquito bed net or in screened accommodation sprayed with an insecticide just before bedtime and protected by an insecticide vaporizer.

Malaria prevention
Travellers to malaria-affected areas should protect themselves by taking antimalarial tablets regularly (p.123) and taking steps to prevent mosquito bites (see above).

Traveller's diarrhea
This unpleasant, although usually short-lived, condition affects up to 50 per cent of all travellers to the developing world and is usually the result of different local bacteria. The condition is largely avoidable by drinking only mineral water and other bottled beverages or sterilized water and avoiding ice in drinks, uncooked and unpeeled fruit and vegetables, salads, and meat that is not freshly and thoroughly cooked. Be cautious about shellfish, even if it seems to have been cooked. Avoid buying cooked food from street vendors. When brushing teeth, rinse with bottled water, not tap water. People who are careful about water often overlook this.

If you do get traveller's diarrhea, it normally disappears quickly without medicines, and so your primary concern should be on preventing the dehydration that may accompany it, especially in young children, by using rehydration salts. Commercial packs of oral rehydration salts are available from pharmacies in Canada.

Although antidiarrheal drugs are of no value in reducing the overall duration of traveller's diarrhea, they might be useful for people who wish to reduce the frequency of bowel movements. Loperamide (p.332) and diphenoxylate are often used for this purpose. Remember that severe diarrhea can reduce both the absorption and the effectiveness of medicines that are taken by mouth. Discuss with your physician and pharmacist when it may be appropriate to take antidiarrheal drugs.

Typhoid and cholera are two serious diseases spread by contaminated food and drink that may start like traveller's diarrhea. No effective vaccine is available for cholera. If you are going to a country where typhoid is endemic, you should be vaccinated against it before you travel, but you must still observe all precautions. Do not hesitate to call local medical help if diarrhea seems to be getting worse.

Eating raw, salted, dried, or pickled fish may lead to liver fluke or tapeworm infestations, particularly in the Far East.

Sun
In North America, thousands of people develop skin cancer each year, and these numbers are increasing by 8 per cent annually. Sun-induced skin damage can be avoided by following a few simple precautions. Travellers, especially those with fair skins, should avoid exposure to the hottest sun (from 11 am to 3 pm), apply a high-protection factor (25+) sunscreen protecting against both UVA and UVB to exposed skin, and use a wide-brimmed hat and clothing for additional sun protection. There is no such thing as a healthy tan.

A traveller who is unaccustomed to hot climates may experience heat exhaustion and even sunstroke, causing weakness, dizziness, nausea, muscle cramps, and eventually unconsciousness. Rarely, severe sunstroke may be fatal. Drinking plenty of non-alcoholic fluids, limiting exposure to the sun, especially during the hottest part of the day, and avoiding physical exertion until you are acclimatized can usually prevent this developing.

Bites and stings
Seek expert advice if stung or bitten by any unfamiliar wildlife or by any mammal, and try to avoid such incidents by following local advice on where it is safe to walk or swim. Tropical and subtropical rivers and lakes may contain parasitic flukes such as bilharzia that will infest visitors who drink, bathe, or swim in them. Walking outdoors with bare feet is a bad idea in many areas; hookworms and threadworms in the soil are able to penetrate the skin and enter the body, passing through tissues, the bloodstream, and the lungs before parasitizing the intestines to suck blood. If hiking, always wear good walking shoes or boots and long trousers with the bottoms tucked into your socks. Keep to paths and avoid walking in long grass.

ON RETURN
If you have any unusual symptoms such as persistent diarrhea or unexplained fever after you have travelled, see your physician right away and inform him or her of which country or countries you have visited. If you were taking anti-malarial drugs while you were travelling, you should continue to take them for 4 weeks after your return.

INTERACTIONS OF TRAVEL DRUGS
Two or more drugs taken at the same time may interact and therefore, if you are taking regular medication, it is advisable to consider what the potential interaction might be when it is combined with some common drugs that may be taken while you are travelling. For more details on the interactions of particular drugs consult your physician or pharmacist.

Travel (motion) sickness drugs
• **Dimenhydrinate** Nitrates (taken sublingually) may have a reduced effect because of dry mouth, which is a side effect of dimenhydrinate. Alcohol and sedative drugs increase the sedative effect of dimenhydrinate.
• **Antihistamines** These drugs may negate the effect of anti-arrhythmics and increase the effect of sedatives.

Painkillers
• **Acetaminophen** The effect of anticoagulant drugs may be increased if taken with acetaminophen.
• **ASA and other NSAIDs** When taken with other NSAIDs, the effect is increased; there is an increased risk of bleeding if these drugs are taken with anticoagulants. ASA and NSAIDs increase the toxicity of methotrexate. When taken with ACE inhibitors, these drugs may reduce their antihypertensive effects. The effects of lithium may be increased when combined with ASA and other NSAIDs.

Antidiarrheal drugs
Alcohol increases the sedative effects of opioid analgesics when they are taken as antidiarrheals. Antidiarrheal drugs may increase the adverse effects of MAOIs and the overall effects of anti-epileptic drugs. There is a greater risk of toxicity when antiviral (HIV) drugs are taken with antidiarrheal drugs.

Drugs for malaria prevention
• **Chloroquine and mefloquine** The effect of amiodarone and quinidine may be decreased with chloroquine, and mefloquine may antagonize antiepileptic drugs. Chloroquine and mefloquine may increase digoxin levels and toxicity.
• **Proguanil** This may increase the effects of warfarin.

PART

5

GLOSSARY
AND INDEX

FURTHER INFORMATION
GLOSSARY
GENERAL INDEX
DRUG POISONING EMERGENCY GUIDE

FURTHER INFORMATION

It is important to have as much information as possible about any medications that you, or someone that you are caring for, are taking. All medications, whether prescribed or bought over-the-counter should come with a patient information leaflet. Always read these leaflets. If you are still in doubt about anything to do with a medication, you should ask your physician or pharmacist.

Organizations should be able to provide general information on medications. Some of these societies are listed below. Further information is usually also available from your local hospital, as well as social services and local libraries. If you have access to the Internet you will also be able to find hundreds of websites that offer information.

Although much of the available advice on medications and drugs is useful and reliable, some information may sometimes be misleading, oversimplified, or even wrong. Always be careful of following advice that does not appear to be from a qualified source, and discuss the matter with your physician or pharmacist if you are unsure.

GENERAL INFORMATION
Canadian Health Network
Online: www.canadian-health-network.ca

Canadian Medical Association
1867 Alta Vista Drive
Ottawa, ON   K1G 3Y6
Tel: (800) 457-4206
Online: www.cma.ca

Canadian Pharmacists Association
1785 Alta Vista Drive
Ottawa, ON   K1G 3Y6
Tel: (800) 917-9489
Online: www.pharmacists.ca

Food and Drug Administration (US)
5600 Fishers Lane
Rockville, MD 20857
USA
Tel: 001 888 463 6332
E-mail: webmail@oc.fda.gov
Online: www.fda.gov

HealthAnswers (US)
Online: www.healthanswers.com

Canadian Public Health Association
1565 Carling Avenue
Suite 400
Ottawa, ON   K1Z 8R1
Tel: (613) 725-3769
Online: www.cpha.ca

Kid's Health (US)
Online: www.kidshealth.org/

Canadian Red Cross
170 Metcalfe Street
Suite 300
Ottawa, ON   K2P 2P2
Tel: (613) 740-1900
Online: www.redcross.ca

College of Family Physicians of Canada
2630 Skymark Avenue
Mississauga, ON L4W 5A4
Tel: (905) 629-0900
Online: www.cfpc.ca

Health Canada
A.L. 0900C2
Ottawa, ON   K1A 0K9
Tel: (613) 957-2991
Online: www.hc-sc.gc.ca

Health Canada
Therapeutics Products Directorate
Online: http://www.hc-sc.gc.ca/hpfb-dgpsa/tpd-dpt/index_e.html

World Health Organization
Avenue Appia 20
1211 Geneva 27
Switzerland
Tel: 0041 22 791 2111
Online: www.who.int

DRUG DEPENDENCE
Alcoholics Anonymous
Online: www.alcoholics-anonymous.org

Canadian Centre for Substance Abuse
75 Albert Street
Suite 300
Ottawa, ON   K1P 5E7
Tel: (613) 235-4048
Online: www.ccsa.ca

Centre for Addiction and Mental Health
24 Hour Information Line (800) 463-6273
Online: www.camh.net

Narcotics Anonymous
Online: www.na.org

DRUG REACTIONS
Adverse Drug Reaction Reports
Health Canada
Online: www.hc-sc.gc.ca

Asthma Society of Canada
4950 Yonge Street, Suite 2306
Toronto, Ontario
M2N 6K1
1-866-787-4050
Online: www.asthma.ca

Canadian MedicAlert Foundation
National Office
2005 Sheppard Avenue East
Suite 800
Toronto, ON   M2J 5B4
Tel: (416) 696-0267
or 1-800-668-1507

Motherisk
The Hospital for Sick Children
555 University Avenue
Toronto, ON
M5G 1X8
Tel: (416) 813-6780
Online: www.motherisk.org

SPECIFIC CONDITIONS
Alzheimer Society of Canada
20 Eglinton Avenue West
Suite 1200
Toronto, ON
M4R 1K8
Tel: (416) 488-8772
Online: www.alzheimer.ca

Arthritis Society
393 University Avenue
Suite 1700
Toronto, ON
M5G 1E6
Tel: (416) 979-7228
Online: www.arthritis.ca

Canadian AIDS Society
190 O'Connor Street
Suite 800
Ottawa, ON   K2P 2R3
Tel: (613) 230-3580
Online: www.cdnaids.ca

Canadian Association of the Deaf
251 Bank Street
Suite 203
Ottawa, ON
K2P 1X3
(613) 565-2882
Online: www.cad.ca

Canadian Cancer Society
10 Alcorn Avenue
Suite 200
Toronto, ON
M4V 3B1
Tel: (416) 961-7223
Online: www.cancer.ca

The Canadian Continence Foundation
P.O. Box 417,
Peterborough, ON
K9J 6Z3
Tel: (705) 750-460
Online: www.continence-fdn.ca

Canadian Diabetes Association
1400-522 University Avenue
Toronto, ON
M5G 2R5
Tel: (800) BANTING
Online: www.diabetes.ca

Canadian Lung Association
3 Raymond Street
Suite 300
Ottawa, ON   K1R 1A3
Tel: (613) 569-6411
or 1-888-566-5864
Online: www.lung.ca

Canadian Mental Health Association
8 King Street East
Suite 810
Toronto, ON   M5C 1B5
Tel: (416) 484-7750
Online: www.cmha.ca

Canadian National Institute for the Blind
1929 Bayview Avenue
Toronto, ON
M4G 3E8
Tel: (416) 486-2500
Online: www.cnib.ca

Canadian Pain Society
268 Grosvenor Street
London, ON
N6A 4L6
Tel: (519) 646-6388
Online: www.canadianpainsociety.ca

Heart & Stroke Foundation of Canada
222 Queen Street
Suite 1402
Ottawa, ON
K1P 5V9
Tel: (613) 569-4361
Online: www.heartandstroke.ca

Menopause Canada
Online: www.menopausecanada.com

Osteoporosis Canada
1090 Don Mills Road
Toronto, ON   M3C 3R6
Tel: (800) 463-6842
www.osteoporosis.ca

ALTERNATIVE MEDICINE
Canadian Naturopathic Association
1255 Sheppard Avenue East
North York, ON
M2K 1E2
Tel: (800) 551-4381
Online: www.naturopaticassoc.ca

Chinese Medicine & Acupuncture Association of Canada
154 Wellington Street
London, ON
N6B 2K8
Tel: (519) 642-1970
www.cmaac.ca

Homeopathic Medical Council of Canada
20 Eglinton Avenue East
Suite 340
Toronto, ON
M4P 1A9
Tel: (877) 722-4622
Online: www.hmcc.ca

DRUGS IN SPORT
Canadian Olympic Committee
21 St. Clair Avenue East
Suite 900
Toronto, ON
M4T 1L9
Tel: (416) 962-0262
Online: www.olympic.ca

Sport Canada
16th Floor,
15 Eddy
Gatineau, QC
K1A 0M5
Tel: (819) 956-8003
Online: www.pch.gc.ca/sportcanada/

MEDICINES AND TRAVEL
Canadian Society for International Health
1 Nicholas Street
Suite 1105
Ottawa, ON
K1N 7B7
Tel: (613) 241-5785
Online: www.csih.org

Centers for Disease Control and Prevention (US)
1600 Clifton Road NE
Atlanta
GA 30333
USA
Tel: 404 639 3534
Online: www.cdc.gov/travel

Department of Foreign Affairs and International Trade
125 Sussex Drive
Ottawa, ON
K1A 0G2
Tel: (800) 267-8376
Online: www.dfait.gc.ca

McGill Centre For Tropical Diseases Montreal General Hospital
1650 Cedar Avenue
Room D7-153
Montreal, QC
H3G 1A4
Tel: (514) 934-8049
Online: www.medicine.mcgill.ca/tropmed/

Travel Medicine Program Health Canada
Online: www.travelhealth.gc.ca

Centre for Travel and Tropical Medicine
Travel Clinic
123 Edward Street
Toronto, ON
M5G 1E2
Pre Travel Tel: (416) 730-5700
Post Travel Tel: (416) 340-3675
Online:
www.uhn.ca/programs/clinics/travel_tropical_medicine.asp

GLOSSARY

The following pages contain definitions of drug-related terms whose technical meanings are not explained in detail elsewhere in the book, or for which an easily located precise explanation may be helpful. These are words that may not be familiar to the general reader, or that have a slightly different meaning in a medical context from that in ordinary use. Some of the terms included refer to particular drug actions or effects; others describe methods of drug administration. A few medical conditions that may occur as a result of drug use are also defined. All words printed in *italics* in the main text are included as entries in this glossary.

The glossary is arranged in alphabetical order. To avoid repetition, where relevant, entries include cross-references to further information on that topic located in other sections of the book, or to another glossary term.

A

Activator
See *Agonist*.

Addiction
Addiction or psychological dependence refers to the use of substances, including opioid medications, to alter mood. It is usually associated with compulsive use, continued use, and craving.

Adjuvant
A drug or chemical that enhances the therapeutic effect of another drug. One example of an adjuvant is aluminium, which is added to certain vaccines in order to enhance the immune response, thereby increasing the protection that is given by the vaccine.

Adrenergic
See *Sympathomimetic*.

Adverse effect
Like side effect and adverse reaction, this is a term that refers to any unwanted effects of a drug. When drugs are taken they are distributed throughout the body and their actions are unlikely to be restricted to just the intended organ or tissue. Other parts of the body contain *receptors* like those at which the drug is aimed. The drug molecule may fit other, different receptors well enough to affect them as well. Most of these unwanted effects are dose-related, increasing as the dose is increased, and are commonly referred to as "side effects". Other unwanted adverse effects appear not to be dose-related, such as an *idiosyncrasy* or an *allergic reaction*. See also Adverse effects (p.15).

Adverse reaction
See *Adverse effect*.

Agonist
A term meaning to have a stimulating effect. An agonist drug (often called an activator) is one that binds to a *receptor*, and triggers or increases a particular activity in that cell.

Allergic reaction
An allergic reaction or allergy is one that appears not on first exposure to a drug but on a subsequent occasion. Causes and symptoms are similar to a reaction caused by other allergens. See Allergy (p.109) and *Anaphylaxis*.

Amoebicide
A drug that kills amoebae (single-celled microorganisms). See also Antiprotozoal drugs (p.122).

Anemia
A condition in which the concentration of the oxygen-carrying pigment of the blood, hemoglobin, is below normal. Many different disorders may cause anemia, and it may sometimes occur as a result of drug treatment. Severe anemia may cause fatigue, pallor, and occasionally, breathing difficulty.

Anesthetic, general
A drug or drug combination given to produce unconsciousness before and during surgery or potentially painful investigative procedures. General anesthesia is usually induced initially by injection of a drug such as thiopental, and maintained by inhalation of the fumes of a volatile liquid such as halothane or a gas such as nitrous oxide mixed with oxygen. See also *Premedication*.

Anesthetic, local
A drug applied topically or injected to numb sensation in a small area. See also Local anesthetics (p.64).

Analeptic
A drug given in hospital that stimulates breathing. See also Respiratory stimulants (p.72).

Analgesia
Relief of pain, usually by drugs. See also Analgesics (p.64).

Anaphylaxis
A severe reaction to an allergen such as a bee sting or a drug (see Allergy, p.109). Symptoms may include rash, swelling, breathing difficulty, and collapse. See also Anaphylactic shock (p.528).

Antagonist
A term meaning to have an opposing effect. An antagonist drug (often called a blocker) binds to a *receptor* without stimulating cell activity and prevents any other substance from occupying that receptor.

Antibiotic
A substance that kills particular bacteria or fungi. Originally, antibiotics were produced by microorganisms such as moulds, but most are now produced synthetically. See also Antibiotics (p.114), Antifungal drugs (p.124), and Antibacterial drugs (p.117).

Antibody
A protein manufactured by lymphocytes (a type of white blood cell) to neutralize an antigen (foreign protein) in the body. The formation of antibodies against an invading microorganism is part of the body's defence against infection. *Immunization* carried out to increase the body's resistance to a specific disease involves either injection of specific antibodies or administration of a *vaccine* that stimulates antibody production. See also Vaccines and immunization (p.120).

Anticholinergic
A drug that blocks the action of acetylcholine. Acetylcholine, a neurotransmitter secreted by the endings of nerve cells, allows certain nerve impulses to be transmitted, including those that relax some involuntary muscles, tighten others, and affect the release of saliva. Anticholinergic drugs are used to treat urinary incontinence because they relax the bladder's squeezing muscles while tightening those of the sphincter. Anticholinergic drugs also relax the muscles of the intestinal wall, helping to relieve irritable bowel syndrome (p.98). See also Autonomic nervous system (p.63).

Antidote
A substance used to neutralize or counteract the effects of a poison. Very few poisons have a specific antidote.

Antineoplastic
An anticancer drug (p.140).

Antioxidant
A substance that delays deterioration due to free radicals (unstable oxygen atoms). free radicals are generated by the body's normal processes and are thought to play a role in aging and disease. Vitamins A, C, and E are antioxidants. See also Vitamins (p.135).

Antiperspirant
A substance that is applied to the skin to reduce excess sweating. Antiperspirants

reduce the activity of the sweat glands or block the ducts carrying sweat to the skin surface.

Antipyretic
A type of drug that reduces fever. The most commonly used antipyretic drugs are ASA and acetaminophen.

Antiseptic
A chemical that destroys bacteria and sometimes other microorganisms. Antiseptics may be applied to the skin or other areas to prevent infection. See also Anti-infective skin preparations (p.163).

Antispasmodic
A drug that reduces spasm (abnormally strong or inappropriate contraction) of the digestive-tract muscles. The pain caused by intestinal spasm is known as colic. These drugs may be used to relieve irritable bowel syndrome (p.98).

Antitussive
A drug that prevents or relieves a cough. See also Drugs to treat coughs (p.80).

Aperient
A mild laxative. See Laxatives (p.97).

Astringent
A substance that causes tissue to dry and shrink by reducing its ability to absorb water. Astringents are used in a number of antiperspirants and skin tonics to remove excessive moisture from the skin surface. They are also used in ear drops for inflammation of the outer ear because they promote healing of inflamed tissue.

B

Bactericidal
A term used to describe a drug that kills bacteria. See also Antibiotics (p.114) and Antibacterials (p.117).

Bacteriostatic
A term used to describe a drug that stops the growth or multiplication of bacteria. See also Antibiotics (p.114) and Antibacterials (p.117).

Balm
A soothing or healing preparation applied to the skin.

Bioavailability
The proportion of a dose of a drug that enters the bloodstream and so reaches the body tissues, usually expressed as a percentage of the dose given. Injection of a drug directly into a vein produces 100 per cent bioavailability. Drugs given by mouth generally have a lower bio-availability because some of the drug may not pass through the gut wall, and some may be broken down in the liver before reaching the rest of the body.

Blocker
See *Antagonist*.

Body mass index (BMI)
An indicator of healthy body weight. BMI is calculated by dividing a person's weight in kilograms by the square of his or her height in metres. The normal range is 20–25.

Body salts
Also known as electrolytes, these are minerals that are present in body fluids such as blood, urine, and sweat, and within cells. These salts play an important role in regulating water balance, the acidity of the blood, conduction of nerve impulses, and muscle contraction. The balance between the various body salts can be upset by such conditions as diarrhea and vomiting. The balance may also be altered by the action of drugs such as diuretics (p.85).

Bronchoconstrictor
A substance that causes the airways in the lungs to narrow. An attack of asthma may be caused by the release of bronchoconstrictor substances such as histamine or certain prostaglandins.

Bronchodilator
A drug that widens the airways. See Bronchodilators (p.76).

C

Capsule
See p.19.

Cathartic
A drug that stimulates bowel action to produce a soft or liquid bowel movement. See also Laxatives (p.97).

Chelating agent
A chemical used in the treatment of poisoning by metals such as iron, lead, arsenic, and mercury. The chelating agent combines with the metal to form a less poisonous substance and, in some cases, increases excretion of the poison in the urine. Penicillamine is a commonly used chelating agent.

Chemotherapy
The drug treatment of cancer or infections. *Cytotoxic* drugs (see also p.140) and *antibiotics* (see also p.114) are examples of drugs used in chemotherapy.

Cholinergic
A drug, also called *parasympathomimetic*, that acts by stimulating the parasympathetic nervous system. See also Autonomic nervous system (p.63).

Coma
A state of unconsciousness and unresponsiveness to external stimuli such as noise and pain. Coma results from damage to or disturbance of, part of the brain, which may occur, for example, through trauma or drug overdose.

Contraindication
A factor in a person's current condition, medical history, or genetic make-up that may increase the risks of an *adverse effect* from a drug, to the extent that the drug should not be prescribed (called an absolute contraindication), or should only be prescribed with caution (called a relative contraindication).

Counter-irritant
Another term for *rubefacient*.

Cycloplegic
The action of paralysing the ciliary muscle in the eye. This muscle alters the shape of the lens when it contracts, enabling the eye to focus on objects. A cycloplegic drug prevents this action, thereby making both examination of, and surgery on, the eye easier. See also Drugs affecting the pupil (p.158).

Cytotoxic
A drug that kills or damages cells. Drugs with this action are most commonly used to treat cancer. Although these drugs are primarily intended to affect abnormal cells, they may also kill or damage healthy ones. See also Anticancer drugs (p.140).

D

Dependence
Psychological dependence is also referred to as addiction. This is a term referring to compulsive use of a drug that can cover anything from intense, habitual cravings for caffeine (the stimulant drug in coffee, tea, and cola drinks) to physical and psychological dependence on drugs such as nicotine (in tobacco) and *opioids*. Psychological dependence involves intense mental cravings if a drug is unavailable or withdrawn. Physical dependence causes physical withdrawal symptoms (such as sweating, shaking, abdominal pain, and convulsions) if the substance is not taken. The term dependence also implies loss of control over intake. See also Drug dependence (p.23).

Depot injection
Injection into a muscle of a drug that has been specially formulated to provide for a slow, steady absorption of its active ingredients by the surrounding blood vessels. The drug may be mixed with oil or wax. Alternatively, some drugs may be injected under the skin using an applicator. This is known as an implant injection. The release period can be made to last up to several weeks. See also Methods of administration (p.17).

Designer drugs
A group of unlicensed substances whose only purpose is to duplicate the effects of certain illegal drugs of abuse or to provide even stronger ones. Designer drugs differ chemically in some minor degree from the original drug, enabling the user and supplier to evade prosecution for dealing in, or possession of, an illegal drug. They are very dangerous because their effects are unpredictable, they are often highly potent, and they may contain impurities.

Double-blind
A test used to determine the effectiveness of a new drug compared to an existing medicine or a *placebo*. Neither patients nor the physicians administering the drug know who is receiving which substance. Only after the test is completed and the patients' responses are recorded is the identity of those who received the new drug revealed. Double-blind trials are performed for almost all new drugs. See also Testing and approving new drugs (p.12).

Drip
A non-medical term for *intravenous infusion*.

E

Electrolyte
See *Body salts*.

Elixir
A clear, sweetened liquid, often containing alcohol, that forms the base for many liquid medicines such as those used to treat coughs.

Embrocation
An ointment or liniment rubbed on to the skin to relieve joint pain, muscle cramp, or muscle injury. An embrocation usually contains a *rubefacient*.

Emetic
Any substance that causes a person to vomit. An emetic may work by irritating the lining of the stomach and/or by stimulating the part of the brain that controls vomiting. Emetics such as ipecac (ipecacuanha) may be used in the treatment of drug overdose but are not generally very effective. See also Drug poisoning emergency guide (p.526).

Emollient
A substance having a soothing, softening effect when applied to the skin. An emollient also has a moisturizing effect, preventing loss of water from the skin surface by forming an oily film. See also Bases for skin preparations (p.163).

Emulsion
A combination of two liquids that do not normally mix together but, on addition of a third substance (known as an emulsifying agent), can be mixed to give a complex liquid consisting of droplets of one liquid suspended in the other. An example of an emulsion is liquid paraffin. The medicine bottle may have to be shaken well before use to ensure that the two liquids are thoroughly mixed.

Endorphins
A group of substances occurring naturally in the brain. Released in response to pain, they bind to specialized receptors and reduce the perception of pain. *Opioid* analgesics such as morphine work by mimicking the action of endorphins. See also Analgesics (p.64).

Enteric coated
Treatment of a drug to give it a coating so that, after being taken orally by the individual, it passes safely and unaltered through the stomach and is released in the intestine. This can minimize stomach upsets caused by the drugs.

Enzyme
A protein that controls the rate of one or more chemical reactions in the body. There are thousands of enzymes active in the body. Each type of cell produces a specific range of enzymes. Cells in the liver contain enzymes that stimulate the breakdown of nutrients and drugs; cells in the digestive tract release enzymes that help digest food. Some drugs work by altering the activity of enzymes – for example, certain anticancer drugs halt tumour growth by altering enzyme function in cancer cells.

Excitatory
A term meaning having a stimulating or enhancing effect. A chemical released from a nerve ending that causes muscle contraction is having an excitatory effect. See also *Inhibitory*.

Expectorant
A type of cough remedy that enhances the production of sputum (phlegm) and is used in the treatment of a productive (sputum-producing) cough. See also Drugs to treat coughs (p.80).

F

Formula, chemical
A way of expressing the constituents of a chemical in symbols and numbers. Every known chemical substance has a formula. Water has the formula H_2O, indicating that it is composed of two hydrogen atoms (H_2) and one oxygen atom (O). All drugs have much more complicated formulae than that of water.

Formulary
A list of drugs produced as a guide to prescribers and other health professionals with the aim of aiding choice. Local formularies are frequently found in hospitals and are sometimes used by groups of physicians.

G

Generic name
The official name for a substance that is therapeutically active. The term generic is distinct from a *product name*, which is a term chosen by a manufacturer for its version of a product containing a generic drug. For example: nitrazepam is a generic name; Mogadon is a brand name for a product that contains nitrazepam. See also How drugs are classified (p.13).

H

Half-life
A term used in *pharmacology* for the time taken to reduce the concentration of the drug in the blood by half. Knowledge of the half-life of a drug helps to determine frequency of dosage.

Hallucinogen
A drug that causes hallucinations (unreal perceptions of surroundings and objects). Common hallucinogens include the drugs of abuse LSD (p.490) and cannabis (p.487). Alcohol taken in large amounts may have an hallucinogenic effect; hallucinations may also occur during withdrawal from alcohol (p.484). Certain prescribed drugs may in rare cases cause hallucinations.

Hormone
A chemical released directly into the bloodstream by a gland or tissue. The body produces numerous hormones, each of which has a specific range of functions – for example, controlling the *metabolism* of cells, growth, sexual development, and the body's response to stress or illness. Hormone-producing glands make up the endocrine system; the kidneys, intestine, and brain also release hormones. See also Hormones and endocrine system (p.126).

I

Idiosyncrasy
Some *adverse effects* appear not to be dose related. Where such an effect happens on the first use of a drug and is pharmacologically unexpected, the phenomenon is called idiosyncrasy, or an idiosyncratic reaction. This happens because people are different genetically; they may lack a particular enzyme or an enzyme may be less active than usual. In normal life this may not cause any problems. Because of this difference, they may react differently to a drug.

Immunization
The process of inducing immunity (resistance to infection) as a preventive measure against

the spread of infectious diseases. See Vaccines and immunization (p.120).

Indication
The term used to describe a disorder, symptom, or condition for which a drug or treatment may be prescribed. For example, indications for the use of beta blockers include angina and high blood pressure (hypertension).

Infusion pump
A machine for administering a continuous, controlled amount of a drug or other fluid through a needle inserted into a vein or under the skin. It consists of a small battery-powered pump that controls the flow of fluid from a syringe into the needle. The pump may be strapped to the patient and pre-programmed to deliver the fluid at a constant rate. See also Methods of administration (p.17).

Inhaler
A device used for administering a drug in powder or vapour form. Inhalers are used principally in the treatment of respiratory disorders such as asthma and chronic bronchitis. The kinds of drugs that are often administered by this method include corticosteroids and bronchodilators. See also Methods of administration (p.17) and Inhalers (p.77).

Inhibitory
A term meaning to have a blocking effect on cell activity, e.g., a chemical that prevents muscle contraction has an inhibitory effect. See also *Antagonist* and *Excitatory*.

Inoculation
A method of administering biological substances, such as microorganisms, to produce immunity to disease by scratching the *vaccine* into the skin. See also Vaccines and immunization (p.120).

Interaction
See p.16.

Intramuscular injection
Injection of a drug into a muscle, usually located in the upper arm or buttock. The drug is absorbed into the bloodstream from the muscle. See also Methods of administration (p.17).

Intravenous infusion
Prolonged, slow injection of fluid (often a solution of a drug) into a vein. The fluid flows at a controlled rate from a bag or bottle through a fine tube inserted into an opening in a vein. An intravenous infusion may also be administered via an *infusion pump*.

Intravenous injection
Direct injection of a drug into a vein, putting the drug immediately into the circulation. Because it has a rapid effect, intravenous injection is useful in an emergency. See also Methods of administration (p.17).

JL

Jaundice
A condition in which the skin and whites of the eyes take on a yellow coloration. It can be caused by an accumulation in the blood of the yellow-brown bile pigment bilirubin. Jaundice is a sign of many disorders of the liver. A drug may cause jaundice as an *adverse effect* either by damaging the liver or by causing an increase in the breakdown of red blood cells in the circulation. See also Liver and kidney disease, p.22.

Liniment
A liquid medicine for application to the skin with friction, that is, to be rubbed in. See also *Embrocation*.

Lotion
A liquid preparation that may be applied to large areas of skin. See also Bases for skin preparations (p.163).

M

Medication
Any substance prescribed to treat illness. See *Medicine*.

Medicine
A medication or drug that is taken in order to maintain, improve, or restore health.

Metabolism
The term used to describe all chemical processes in the body that involve either the formation of new substances or the breakdown of substances to release energy or detoxify foreign substances. The metabolism provides the energy that is required to keep the body functioning at rest – that is, to maintain breathing, heart beat, and body temperature and to replace worn tissues. It also provides the energy needed during exertion. This energy is produced by the metabolism from the breakdown of foods.

Miotic
A drug that constricts (narrows) the pupil. *Opioid* drugs such as morphine have a miotic effect, and someone who is taking one of these drugs has very small, pinpoint pupils. The pupil is sometimes deliberately narrowed by other miotic drugs, such as pilocarpine, in the treatment of glaucoma. See also Drugs for glaucoma (p.156) and Drugs affecting the pupil (p.158).

Mucolytic
A drug that liquefies mucus secretions in the airways. See also Drugs to treat coughs (p.80).

Mydriatic
A drug that dilates (widens) the pupil. *Anticholinergic* drugs, such as atropine, have this effect and they may cause *photophobia*

as a consequence. Mydriatic drugs may occasionally provoke the onset of glaucoma. These drugs are also used to facilitate examination of the retina at the back of the eye. See also Drugs affecting the pupil (p.158).

N

Narcotic
Originating from the Greek word for numbness or stupor and once applied to drugs derived from the opium poppy, the word narcotic no longer has a precise medical meaning; some American sources use the term to mean any potent abused drug. Narcotic analgesic, a term largely replaced by *opioid* analgesic, is used to refer to opium-derived and synthetic drugs that have pain-relieving properties and other effects similar to those of morphine (see Analgesics, p.64). See also Opioids (p.492)

Nebulizer
A method of administering a drug to the airways and lungs in aerosol form through a facemask. The apparatus includes an electric or hand-operated pump that sends a stream of air or oxygen through a length of tubing into a small canister containing the drug in liquid form. This inflow of gas causes the drug to be dispersed into a fine mist, which is then carried through another tube into the facemask. Inhalation of this drug mist is much easier than inhaling from a pressurized aerosol. See also *Inhaler*.

Neuroleptic
A drug used to treat psychotic illness. See Antipsychotic drugs (p.69).

Neurotransmitter
A chemical released from a nerve ending after receiving an electrical impulse. A neurotransmitter may carry a message from the nerve to another nerve so that the electrical impulse passes on, or to a muscle to stimulate contraction, or to a gland to stimulate secretion of a particular hormone. Acetylcholine and noradrenaline are examples of neurotransmitters. Many drugs either mimic or block the action of neurotransmitters. See also Brain and nervous system (p.62).

O

Opioid
A group of drugs (also called *narcotic analgesics*) that are given to relieve pain, treat diarrhea, and suppress coughs. See Opioids (p.492).

Orphan drug
A drug that is effective for a rare medical condition, but that may not be marketed by a drug manufacturer because of the small profit potential compared with the high costs of

development and production. These drugs can usually be obtained by special request.

OTC
The abbreviation for over-the-counter. Over-the-counter drugs can be bought from a pharmacy without a prescription. See also Managing your drug treatment (p.25).

P

Parasympathomimetic
A drug that is prescribed to stimulate the parasympathetic nervous system (see Autonomic nervous system, p.63). These drugs (also called *cholinergic* drugs) are used as *miotics* and to stimulate bladder contraction in urinary retention (see Drugs used in urinary disorders, p.154).

Parkinsonism
Neurological symptoms including tremor of the hands, muscle rigidity, and slowness of movement that resemble Parkinson's disease. Parkinsonism may be caused by prolonged treatment with an antipsychotic drug. See Drugs for parkinsonism (p.71).

Patch
See *Transdermal patch*.

Pharmacist
A registered health professional (often called a "chemist") concerned with the preparation, manufacture, and dispensing of drugs. Pharmacists can advise on the correct use of drugs and can help detect potential interactions between your medications.

Pharmacodynamics
A word used to describe the effects or actions that a drug produces in the body. For example, bronchodilation and pain relief are some pharmacodynamic effects that may stem from a drug.

Pharmacokinetics
The term used to describe how the body deals with a drug, including how it is absorbed into the bloodstream, distributed to different tissues, broken down, and excreted from the body.

Pharmacologist
A scientist concerned with the study of the actions and *pharmacokinetics* of drugs. Pharmacologists form one of the groups responsible for scientific research into new drugs and new uses for existing drugs. Clinical pharmacologists are usually qualified physicians.

Pharmacology
The science of the origin, appearance, chemistry, and action of drugs.

Pharmacopoeia
A publication (in book or electronic form) that describes the drugs used in medicine. The term pharmacopoeia usually refers to an official national publication (such as the U.S. Pharmacopoeia) that sets standards and describes the methods used to identify drugs and determine their purity. These publications are used for reference by the medical profession.

Pharmacy
A term that is used to describe the science and technology involved in the study of drugs. The term is also used to refer to the place where the practise of preparing drugs, making up prescriptions, and dispensing the drugs is carried out.

Photophobia
Dislike of bright light. Certain drugs (notably *mydriatics*) and diseases may induce photophobia.

Photosensitivity
An abnormal reaction of the skin to light, often causing reddening. Photosensitivity may be caused by certain drugs.

Placebo
A "medicine", often in tablet or capsule form, that contains no medically active ingredient. Placebos are frequently used in clinical trials of new drugs (see *Double-blind*). See also Placebo response (p.15).

Poison
A substance that, in relatively small amounts, disrupts the structure and/or function of cells, causing harmful and sometimes fatal effects. Many drugs are poisonous if taken in overdose.

Premedication
The term applied to drugs given to patients between one and two hours before an operation. The premedication usually contains an *opioid* analgesic to help relieve pain and anxiety and to reduce the dose of anesthetic needed to produce unconsciousness (see also *Anesthetic, general*). In some cases, an *anticholinergic* drug is also included to reduce secretions in the airways.

Prescription
A written instruction from the physician to the pharmacist, detailing the name of the drug to be dispensed, the dosage, how often it has to be taken, and other instructions as necessary. A prescription is written and signed by a physician and carries the name and address of the patient for whom the drug is prescribed. The pharmacist keeps a record, often computerized, of all prescriptions dispensed to each patient. See also Managing your drug treatment (p.25).

Product name
The name chosen by a manufacturer for its particular version of a product containing a generic drug, e.g., Viagra is a product name for the generic drug sildenafil. See also *Generic name* and How drugs are classified (p.13).

Prophylactic
A drug, procedure, or piece of equipment used to prevent disease. The process of prevention is called prophylaxis. For example, a course of drugs given to a traveller to prevent malarial infection is known as malaria prophylaxis.

Proprietary
A term now applied to a drug that is sold over-the-counter and having its name registered to a private manufacturer, i.e., a proprietor.

Prostaglandin
A fatty (organic) acid that acts in a similar way to a hormone. Prostaglandins occur in many different tissues and have various effects. These include causing inflammation in damaged tissue, lowering blood pressure, and stimulating contractions in labour.

Purgative
A drug that helps eliminate feces from the body, to relieve constipation or to empty the bowel/intestine before surgery. See also *Cathartic* and Laxatives (p.97).

Pyrogen
A substance that causes a rise in temperature.

R

Receptor
A specific site on the surface of a cell with a characteristic chemical and physical structure. Natural body chemicals such as *neurotransmitters* bind to cell receptors to initiate a response in the cell. Many drugs also have an effect on cells by binding to a receptor in the same way. They may promote cell activity or may block it. See also *Agonist* and *Antagonist*.

Replication
The duplication of genetic material (DNA or RNA) in a cell as part of the process of cell division that enables a tissue to grow or a virus to multiply.

Rubefacient
A preparation, also known as a counter-irritant, that, when applied to an area of skin, causes it to redden by increasing blood flow in vessels in that area. A rubefacient such as methyl salicylate may be included in an *embrocation* or a *liniment*.

S

Sedative
A drug that dampens the activity of the central nervous system. Sleeping drugs (p.66) and anti-anxiety drugs (p.67) have a sedative effect, and many other drugs, including antihistamines (p.110) and antidepressants (p.68), can produce sedation as a side effect.

Side effect
See *Adverse effect*.

Sterile
A term meaning free from living micro-organisms. Drugs that are administered by certain methods, such as by injection and *bladder irrigation/instillation*, must be sterile to avoid causing infection. See also *Pyrogen*.

Subcutaneous injection
A method of giving a drug by which the drug is injected just under the skin. It is then slowly absorbed over a few hours into surrounding blood vessels. Insulin is given in this way. See also Methods of administration (p.17).

Sublingual
A term meaning under the tongue. Some drugs are administered sublingually in tablet or spray form. The drug is rapidly absorbed through the lining of the mouth. Nitrate drugs may be given this way to provide rapid relief of an angina attack. See also Methods of administration (p.17).

Suppository
A bullet-shaped pellet usually containing a drug for insertion into the rectum or vagina. See also Methods of administration (p.17).

Sympatholytic
A term that means blocking the effect of the sympathetic nervous system. Sympatholytic drugs work either by reducing the release of the stimulatory *neurotransmitter* norepinephrine (noradrenaline) from nerve endings, or by occupying the receptors to which the neurotransmitters epinephrine (adrenaline) and noradrenaline normally bind, thereby preventing their normal actions. Beta blockers are examples of sympatholytic drugs. See also Autonomic nervous system (p.63).

Sympathomimetic
Having the same effect as stimulation of the sympathetic nervous system to cause, for example, an increase in the heart rate and widening of the airways. A drug having a sympathomimetic action may work either by causing the release of the stimulatory *neurotransmitter* noradrenaline from the nerve endings or by mimicking neuro-transmitter action (see Autonomic nervous system, p.63). The sympathomimetic drugs include certain bronchodilators (p.76) and decongestants (p.79).

Syrup
A solution of sucrose (sugar) in water. Syrup is used as a basis for some liquid medicines because it acts as an *antioxidant*; bacteria, fungi, and moulds do not grow in it; and its sweetness hides the taste of some drugs. Syrups are not suitable for diabetics.

Systemic
Having a generalized effect, causing physical or chemical changes in tissues throughout the body. For a drug to have a systemic effect it must be absorbed into the bloodstream, usually via the digestive tract, by injection or by rectal suppository.

Tablet
See p.19.

Tardive dyskinesia
Abnormal, uncontrolled movements, mainly of the face, tongue, mouth, and neck, that may be caused by prolonged treatment with antipsychotic drugs. This condition is distinct from *parkinsonism,* which may also be caused by such drugs. See also Antipsychotic drugs (p.69).

Tolerance
The need to take a higher dosage of a specific drug to maintain the same physical or mental effect. Tolerance occurs during prolonged treatment with *opioid* analgesics and benzodiazepines. See also Drug dependence (p.23).

Tonics
A diverse group of remedies prescribed or bought over-the-counter for relieving vague symptoms such as malaise, lethargy, and loss of appetite, for which no obvious cause can be found. Tonics sometimes contain vitamins and minerals, but there is no scientific evidence that such ingredients have anything other than a *placebo* effect. Nevertheless, many individuals feel better after taking a tonic for a few weeks.

Topical
The term used to describe the application of a drug to the site where it is intended that it should have its effect. Disorders of the skin, eye, outer ear, nasal passages, anus, and vagina are often treated with drugs applied topically.

Toxic reaction
Unpleasant and possibly dangerous symptoms caused by a drug, the result of an overdose. See also The effects of drugs (p.15).

Toxin
A poisonous substance such as a harmful chemical released by bacteria.

Tranquillizer, major
A drug used to treat psychotic illness such as schizophrenia. See Antipsychotic drugs (p.69).

Tranquillizer, minor
This is an older term for a sedative drug used to treat anxiety and emotional tension. See Anti-anxiety drugs (p.67).

Transdermal patch
An adhesive patch that is impregnated with the drug and placed on the skin. The drug is slowly absorbed through the skin into the underlying blood vessels. Drugs administered in this way include nicotine, nitrates, travel sickness remedies, and estrogens. See also Methods of administration (p.17).

Vaccine
A substance administered to induce active immunity against a specific infectious disease (see Vaccines and immunization, p.120).

Vasoconstrictor
A drug that narrows blood vessels, often prescribed to reduce nasal congestion (see Decongestants, p.79). These drugs are also frequently given with injected local anesthetics (p.64) (see also *Anesthetic, local*). Ephedrine is a commonly prescribed vasoconstrictor.

Vasodilator
A drug that widens blood vessels. See Vasodilators (p.84).

W

Wafer
A thin wafer that is impregnated with a drug and placed on the tongue. The wafer slowly dissolves and the drug is absorbed through the lining of the mouth into the surrounding blood vessels.

Withdrawal symptom
Any symptom caused by abrupt stopping of a drug. These symptoms occur as a result of physical *dependence* on a drug. Drugs that may cause withdrawal symptoms after prolonged use include *opioids*, benzo-diazepines, and nicotine. Withdrawal symptoms vary according to each drug, but common examples include sweating, shaking, anxiety, nausea, and abdominal pain. See also Drug dependence (p.23).

THE GENERAL INDEX

This General Index contains references to the information in all sections of the book. It can be used to look up topics such as groups of drugs, individual drug names, diseases, and conditions. References for generic and brand-name drugs are also listed, with references to the listing in the Drug Finder (pp.33–59).

Entries that contain a page reference followed by the letter "g" indicate that the entry is defined in the Glossary on the page specified (pp.503–508).

A

abacavir 33
abatacept 33
abciximab 33
Abdominal infections 117
Abelcet 33
Abenol 33
Abortion 153
acarbose 33
Accolate 33
Accutane Roche 33
acebutolol 33
Acellular pertussis, vaccine 121
acetaminophen 33
acetazolamide 33
Acetazone Forte 33
Acetoxyl 33
acetylcholine 33
acetylcysteine 33
acetylsalicylic acid 33
Acid, drugs for disorders caused by antacids 94
anti-ulcer drugs 95
acitretin 33
Aclasta 33
Acne
drugs used to treat 165
herbal remedies 495
Acromegaly 131
Actifed 33
Action of drugs 14
affecting the pupil 158
analgesics 65
antacids 94
anti-angina drugs 87
anti-anxiety drugs 67
antibiotics 114
anticancer drugs 141
anticoagulant drugs 91
anticonvulsant drugs 86
antidepressant drugs 68
antidiabetic drugs (oral) 128
antidiarrheal drugs 96
anti-emetics 74
antifungal drugs 124
antihypertensive drugs 88
antiplatelet drugs 90
antipruritics 161
antipsychotic drugs 69
anti-ulcer drugs 95
antiviral drugs 119
benzodiazepines 67
bronchodilators 92

corticosteroids
on inflamed joints 104
on the skin 162
cough remedies 80
cytotoxic drugs see Anticancer drugs 141
decongestants 79
digitalis 82
diuretics 85
drugs for parkinsonism 87
drugs for thyroid disorders 130
drugs for ulcerative colitis 98
drugs affecting urination 170
drugs used for migraine 73
fertility drugs 152
glaucoma drugs 157
immunosuppressant drugs 143
laxatives 97
lipid-lowering drugs 89
monoclonal antibodies 142
muscle relaxants (centrally acting) 106
in myasthenia gravis 107
nervous system stimulants 72
non-steroidal anti-inflammatory drugs in osteoarthritis 102
sulfonamides 117
sulfonylurea drugs 128
sunscreens 169
thrombolytic drugs 91
uricosuric drugs 105
vasodilators 84
Action, sites of drug
analgesics 64
anti-arrhythmics 86
antihistamines 110
muscle relaxants 106
in rectal disorders 99
Activase 33
Activated charcoal 48
Activator see Agonist
Actonel 33
Actonel Plus 33
Actos 33
Acular 33
acyclovir 33
Adalat XL 33
adalimumab 33
adapalene 33
Adasept Skin Cleanser 33
Adderall 33
Addiction 503g
Addison's disease see
Corticosteroids 127
Tuberculosis 118
Adefovir 33

Adenocard 33
adenosine 33
Adjuvant 503g
Administration, methods of 17
Adrenal gland disorders, drugs for see Corticosteroids 127
Adrenaline see Epinephrine 272
Adrenergic see Sympathomimetic
Adriamycin PFS 33
Adrucil 33
Adsorbent agents 96
Advair 33
Adverse effect 503g
Adverse reaction see Adverse effect
Advicor 33
Advil 33
Aerius 33
Aerosol inhalers 19, 77
African sleeping sickness see Trypanosomiasis
Agonist 503g
AIDS
drugs for 144
herbal remedies 493
Airways 75
clearance of, essential first aid 527
Airomir 33
Akineton 33
Alcohol 484
interactions with other drugs 485
Alcohol abuse deterrent 24
Alcomicin 33
Aldactazide 33
Aldactone 33
alendronate 33
Alertec 33
Alesse 33
alfacalcidol 33
alfuzosin 33
alginates/alginic acid 33
Alka-Seltzer Morning Relief 33
Alkeran 33
allantoin 33
Allegra 33
Allerdryl 33
Allergic reaction 503g
severe see Anaphylaxis, dealing with response 109
rhinitis, drugs for
antihistamines 110
decongestants 79
homeopathic remedies 494
Allergies, drugs for
antihistamines 110

antipruritics 161
bronchodilators 92
decongestants 79
Allergy 109
Alloprin 33
allopurinol 33
almotriptan 33
Alomide 33
Alpha blockers 84, 88, 154
Alphagan 34
alpha tocopheryl 34
alprazolam 34
alprostadil 34
Altace 34
Altace HCT 34
alteplase 34
Alternative medicine 494
Alti-Beclomethasone 34
aluminum acetate 34
Aluminum compounds 94
aluminum hydroxide 34
Alvesco 34
amantadine 34
Amaryl 34
AmBisome 34
Amcinonide 34
Amenorrhea 131, 133
Amerge 34
amethocain 34
Ametop 34
amikacin 34
Amikin 34
amiloride 34
aminobenzoic acid 34
aminoglycosides 115, 116
and skin infections 163
aminophylline 34
aminosalicylates 98
amiodarone 34
amitriptyline 34
amlodipine 34
ammonium chloride 34
amoxicillin 34
amoxicillin/clavulinic acid 34
Amoebiasis 122
Amoebicide 503g
Amphetamine 72
as drug of abuse 486
Amphojel 34
amphotericin B 34
ampicillin 34
amprenavir 34
Anabolic steroids 132
prohibited substances in sport 496
Anafranil 34
anakinra 34

Anal disorders, drugs for 99
Analeptic 503g
Analgesia 503g
Analgesics 64
  use in labour 153
  use in sport 496
  use of when travelling 497
Anaphylaxis 503g
  dealing with 528
  See also Allergy 109
Anaprox 34
anastrozole 34
Andriol 34
Androcur 34
Androderm 34
AndroGel 34
Androgens 132
Anemia 503g
  and anabolic steroids 132
  hemolytic 450, 471, 481
  iron deficiency 473
  pernicious 138, 480
  sideroblastic 477
  and vitamin C deficiency 480
Anesthesia, general 503g
Anesthesia, local 503g see
  Local anesthetics 64
  as antipruritics 161
  use in labour 153
  use in rectal and anal
    disorders 99
  See also Epinephrine 272
Angina 87, 84
Angiotensin II blockers 84
Ansaid 34
Antacids 94
Antagonist 503g
Anthelmintic drugs 125
Anthraforte 34
anthralin 34
Anthranol 34
Anthrascalp 34
Anti-acne drugs 165
Anti-allergy drugs 111
Anti-angina drugs 87
Anti-anxiety drugs 67
Anti-arrhythmics 86
Antibacterial drugs 96, 117
Antibiotic 503g
Antibiotics 114
  actions of 114
  classes of 116
  resistance to 114
  in skin preparations 163
  use in sport 496
  uses of 115
Antibody 503g
  See also Malignant and
    immune disease 138;
  Vaccines and Immunization 120
Anticancer drugs 140
  as immunosuppressants 143
Anticholinergic 503g
  drugs used for urinary
    disorders 154
  mydriatics 158

uses of
  as bronchodilators 76, 78
  in irritable bowel syndrome 96
  for parkinsonism 71
  See also Autonomic nervous
    system 63
Anticoagulants 90, 91
  and drug interactions 16
  and Vitamin K 482
Anticonvulsant drugs 86
Antidepressant drugs 68, 68
  in urinary disorders 154
Antidiabetic drugs 128
Antidiarrheal drugs 96, 499
Anti-D immunoglobulin 50
Antidote 503g
  See also Chelating agents
Anti-emetics 74
Antifibrinolytic drugs 90, 91
Antifoaming agents 94
Antifungal drugs 124, 168
antihemophilic factor 35
Antihistamines 82, 110, 499
  and allergic rhinitis 111
  as anti-emetics 74
  as antipruritics 161, 167
  comparison of 111
  use in sport 496
Antihypertensive drugs 88
Anti-infective skin preparations
  163
Anti-inflammatory drugs,
  non-steroidal 102
  use in sport 496
Antimalarial drugs 123
  malaria prophylaxis 498, 499
Antimanic drugs 69
Antimetabolites 141, 142
Antimicrobials see Antibacterials
  117
Antineoplastic 503g
Antioxidant 503g
Antiparasitic drugs 164
Antiparkinsonism drugs 71
Antiperspirant 503g
Antiplatelet drugs 90, 91
Antiprotozoal drugs 122
Antipruritics 161
Antipsychotic drugs 69
Antipyretic 504g
Antiretroviral drugs 145
Antirheumatic drugs 103
Antiseptic 504g
  See also Anti-infective skin
    preparations 163
Antispasmodic 504g
  See also Antidiarrheal drugs 96
Antithyroid drugs 130
Antituberculous drugs 118
Antitussive 504g
Anti-ulcer drugs 95
Antiviral drugs 119
Anugesic-HC 34
Anus, disorders of 99
Anusol 34
Anuzinc HC Plus 34

Anxiety
  homeopathic remedies 494
  drugs for 67
Anxiolytics 67
Anzemet 34
Apnea 72
Apo-Acetaminophen 34
Apo-Acyclovir 34
Apo-Allopurinol 34
Apo-Alpraz 34
Apo-Alpraz TS 34
Apo-Amitriptyline 34
Apo-Amoxi 34
Apo-Amoxi-Clav 34
Apo-Atenolol 34
Apo-Azathioprine 34
Apo-Baclofen 34
Apo-Benztropine 34
Apo-Bromocriptine 34
Apo-Buspirone 34
Apo-Capto 34
Apo-Carbamazepine 34
Apo-Cefaclor 34
Apo-Cefuroxime 34
Apo-Cephalex 34
Apo-Cetirizine 34
Apo-Chlorax 34
Apo-Chlordiazepoxide 34
Apo-Chlorpromazine 34
Apo-Chlorpropamide 34
Apo-Chlorthalidone 34
Apo-Cimetidine 34
Apo-Citalopram 34
Apo-Clindamycin 34
Apo-Clomipramine 34
Apo-Clonazepam 34
Apo-Clonidine 34
Apo-Clorazepate 34
Apo-Cloxi 34
Apo-Clozapine 34
Apo-Cyclobenzaprine 34
Apo-Desipramine 34
Apo-Diazepam 34
Apo-Diclo 34
Apo-Diflunisal 35
Apo-Diltiaz 35
Apo-Dipivefrin 35
Apo-Divalproex 35
Apo-Domperidone 35
Apo-Doxazosin 35
Apo-Doxepin 35
Apo-Doxy 35
Apo-Erythro-ES 35
Apo-Erythromycin 35
Apo-Fenofibrate 35
Apo-Feno-Micro 35
Apo-Fluconazole 35
Apo-Flunisolide 35
Apo-Fluoxetine 35
Apo-Fluphenazine 35
Apo-Flurazepam 35
Apo-Flurbiprofen 35
Apo-Flutamide 35
Apo-Fluvoxamine 35
Apo-Gabapentin 35
Apo-Gain 35

Apo-Gemfibrozil 35
Apo-Glimepiride 35
Apo-Haloperidol 35
Apo-Hydroxyzine 35
Apo-Ibuprofen 35
Apo-Imipramine 35
Apo-Indapamide 35
Apo-Ipravent 35
Apo-ISDN 35
Apo-Keto 35
Apo-Ketoconazole 35
Apo-Ketotifen 35
Apo-lactulose 35
Apo-levobunolol 35
Apo-Levocarb 35
Apo-Loperamide 35
Apo-Loratadine 35
Apo-Lorazepam 35
Apo-Lovastatin 35
Apo-Loxapine 35
Apo-Metformin 35
Apo-Methyldopa 35
Apo-Metoclop 35
Apo-Metoprolol 35
Apo-Methotrimeprazine 35
Apo-Minocycline 35
Apo-Misoprostol 35
Apo-Moclobemide 35
Apo-Nabumetone 35
Apo-Naproxen SR 35
Apo-Nifed 35
Apo-Nifed PA 35
Apo-Nortriptyline 35
Apo-Orciprenaline 35
Apo-Oxazepam 35
Apo-Oxtriphylline 35
Apo-Pen VK 35
Apo-Perphenazine 35
Apo-Pioglitazone 35
Apo-Piroxicam 35
Apo-Pravastatin 35
Apo-Prazo 35
Apo-Prednisone 35
Apo-Primidone 35
Apo-Procainamide 35
Apo-Prochlorazine 35
Apo-Propafenone 35
Apo-Propranolol 35
Apo-Quinidine 35
Apo-Salvent 35
Apo-Salvent-HFA 35
Apo-Selegiline 35
Apo-Sertraline 35
Apo-Sotalol 35
Apo-Sulfatrim 36
Apo-Sulfinpyrazone 36
Apo-Sulin 36
Apo-Temazepam 36
Apo-Tenoxicam 36
Apo-Terazosin 36
Apo-Terbinafine 36
Apo-Tetra 36
Apo-Theo LA 36
Apo-Thioridazine 36
Apo-Tiaprofenic 36
Apo-Trazodone 36

Apo-Trazodone D 36
Apo-Triazo 36
Apo-Trifluoperazine 36
Apo-Trihex 36
Apo-Trimethroprim 36
Apo-Trimip 36
Apo-Zopiclone 36
Appetite suppressants see
  Nervous system stimulants
  72
apraclonidine 36
Apresoline 36
aprotinin 36
Aptivus 36
Aranesp 36
Arava 36
Arenalin 36
Aricept 36
Arimidex 36
Aristocort 36
Aristospan 36
Arixtra 36
Arrhythmias, types of 86
Arthritis
  herbal remedies 495
  rheumatoid 103
Arthrotec 36
Artificial tear preparations 158
ASA 36
Asacol 36
Asaphen 36
Asaphen EC 36
ascorbic acid 36
Aspirin 36
Aspirin Backache 36
Asthma, drugs for 77
  antihistamines 110
  bronchodilators 92
Asthma, drugs for
  corticosteroids 127
  use in sport 496
Astringent 504g
  in rectal and anal disorders 99
Atacand 36
Atarax 36
Atasol 36
Atazanavir 36
atenolol 36
Atherosclerosis 89
Athlete's foot 124
Athletic performance
  legitimate medications 496
  prohibited drugs 496
Ativan 36
atomoxetine 36
atorvastatin 36
atovaquone 36
Atripla 36
atropine 36
Atrovent 36
attapulgite 36
auranofin 36
Autoimmune disorders see
  Malignant and immune
  disease 138
Autonomic nervous system 63

Avalide 36
Avamys 36
Avandamet 36
Avandia 36
Avandaryl 36
Avapro 36
Avastin 36
Avelox 36
avobenzone 36
Avodart 36
Avonex 36
Axert 36
azatadine 36
azathioprine 36
Azilect 36
azithromycin 36
Azopt 36
AZT see Zidovudine 145, 466

B

Babies, drug treatment in 20
Baciguent 36
bacitracin 36
Back pain 102
baclofen 36
Bacteria 112, 113
Bacterial infections, drugs for
  antibacterial drugs 117
  antibiotics 114
  antituberculous drugs 118
Bactericidal 504g
Bacteriostatic 504g
Bactigras 36
Bactroban 36
Balantidiasis 122
Baldness, male pattern 168
Balm 504g
Balminil Codeine Night-Time
  and Expectorant 36
Balminil DM 36
Balminil DM-D-E 36
Baraclude 36
Barbiturates 66
  as drugs of abuse 486
Barrier creams 163
Basalgel 36
Bases for skin preparations 163
basiliximab 36
BCG vaccination 118
beclomethasone 36
Bedsores, infected 163
Bedwetting see Enuresis
Beech Nut Cough Drops
  Honey-Lemon 36
Beech Nut Cough Drops
  Menthol 36
Beech Nut Cough Drops Wild
  Cherry 36
belladonna 37
Bellergal Spacetabs 37
Benadryl 37
Benoxyl 37

benserazide 37
Bentylol 37
Benuryl 37
Benylin DM 37
Benylin DM-E Extra Strength 37
Benylin First Defence Syrup 37
Benzac AC 37
Benzac W Wash 37
Benzaclin 37
Benzalip 37
Benzalip-SR 37
Benzamycin 37
benzocaine 37
Benzodiazepines 66, 67
  as drugs of abuse 487
  as sleeping drugs 66
benzophones 37
benzoyl peroxide 37
benztropine 37
Benztropine Mesylate 37
Benztropine Omega 37
benzylpenicillin 37
Beriberi 479
Berotec 37
Beta blockers 83, 86
  as anti-anxiety drugs 67
  as antihypertensives 88
  in glaucoma 157
  prohibited substances in sport
  496
Beta-carotene 479
Betadine Topical 37
Betagan 37
betahistine 37
Betaject 37
Betaloc 37
Betaloc Durules 37
betamethasone 37
Beta receptors, types of 83
Betaseron 37
betaxolol 37
bethanechol 37
Betnesol 37
Betoptic S 37
Bevacizumab 37
bezafibrate 37
Biaxin 37
Biaxin BID 37
Biaxin XL 37
Bile salts, drugs that bind to 89
Bilharzia 125, 499
bimatoprost 37
biotin 37
Bioavailability 504g
Biquin Durules 37
bisacodyl 37
Bismutal 37
bismuth 37
Bites 499
  allergic reaction to 110
Bladder
  cancer, drugs for 140
  disorders 154
Bleeding, control of see Blood
  clotting; Labour
Blephamide 37

Blocker see Antagonist
Blood
  cancer see Leukemias
  cells 138
  circulation 81
  clotting, drugs that affect 90, 91
  doping 496
  glucose, monitoring of 129
  infections 115
  pressure, high see
    Hypertension
  transfusions, allergic reactions
    to 110
Body mass index (BMI) 504g
Body salts 504g
Boils see Infection, bacterial
Bonamine 37
Bone 101
  cancer, drugs for 140
  disorders, drugs for 108
  infections 114
  pain 102
  wasting disorders 108
Bone marrow
  blood cell production in 138
  cancer, drugs for 140
Botox 37
Botox Cosmetic 37
botulism 209
botulinum toxin 37
Bowel
  disease, inflammatory 98
  infections, drugs for
    antibiotics 114
    antifungal drugs 124
    antiprotozoal drugs 122
Brain 62
  effect of drugs that act on 22
  infections, drugs for
    antibiotics 114
    antifungal drugs 124
    antiprotozoal drugs 122
Breast cancer, drugs for 140
Breast discomfort, premenstrual
  64
Breast-feeding, during drug
  treatment 21
Breathing, drugs to improve
  bronchodilators 92
  respiratory stimulants 72
  See also Respiratory system 75
Breathlessness see
  Bronchodilators 92
bretylium 37
Bretylium Tosylate 37
Brevibloc 37
Brevicon 0.5/35 37
Bricanyl Turbuhaler 37
brimonidine 37
brinzolamide 37
bromocriptine 37
brompheniramine 37
Bronchitis, drugs for
  antibacterial drugs 117
  antibiotics 114
  bronchodilators 92

Bronchoconstrictor 504g
Bronchodilator 504g
Bronchodilators 92
Bruises, alternative medicines
   for 494, 495
buclizine 37
budesonide 37
Bulk-forming agents
   as antidiarrheal drugs 96
   as laxatives 97
bupivacaine 37
bupropion 37
Burinex 37
Burns, infected 163
Buro-Sol 37
Bursitis 104
buserelin 37
BuSpar 37
buspirone 37
butaconazole 37
Butyrophenones see Anti-
   emetics 74; Antipsychotic
   drugs 69

C

cabergoline 37
Caduet 37
Caelyx 37
Cafergot 37
Cafergot-PB 37
caffeine 37, 72
   use in sport 496
calamine 37
calcifediol 37
Calcimar 37
calcipotriol 37
calcitonin 37
calcitriol 37
Calcium 500 37
calcium 37, 136, 469
calcium acetate 37, 52
calcium carbonate 37, 469
Calcium channel blockers 87
   as anti-arrhythmics 86
   as antihypertensive drugs 88
   as vasodilators 84
calcium chloride 37, 469
Calcium citrate 469
Calcium D 500 37
Calcium fluoride 471
Calcium gluconate 38, 469
Calcium lactate 469
Calcium Oyster Shell 38
Caltine 38
camphor 38
Camptosar 38
Cancer see Malignant and
   immune disease 138
   drugs for 140
Cancidas 38

Candesartan 38
Candida infections 124
Candistatin 38
Canesten 38
cannabidiol 38
cannabis 487
Capex shampoo 38
Capoten 38
capreomycin 38
Capsule 18, 19
captopril 38
carbachol 38
carbamazepine 38
carbidopa 38
carbocysteine 38
Carbolith 38
Carbonic anhydrase inhibitors
   157
carboplatin 38
Cardiac
   compression 527
   glycosides see Digitalis drug 82
   See also Heart
Cardizem 38
Cardizem CD 38
Cardura 38
carnitine 38
cascara 38
caspofungin 38
Castor oil 38
Catapres 38
Cathartic 504g
Caverject 38
Cedocard SR 38
cefaclor 38
cefadroxil 38
cefamandole 38
cefazoline 38
cefepime 38
cefixime 38
Cefizox 38
Cefotan 38
cefotaxime 38
cefoxitin 38
cefprozil 38
ceftazidime 38
Ceftin 38
ceftriaxone 38
Cefuroxime 38
Cefzil 38
Celebrex 38
celecoxib 38
Celestone 38
Celexa 38
CellCept 38
Celontin 38
Celsentri 38
Central nervous system 78
   infections, drugs for 115
   stimulants 72
cephalexin 38
Cephalosporins see Antibiotics
   114, 115, 116
Cerebral palsy 106
Cerebyx 38
C.E.S. 38

Cesamet 38
cetirizine 38
cetrimide 38
Chagas' disease see
   Trypanosomiasis 122
Champix 38
Chelating agent 504g
Chemotherapy 504g
   anticancer drugs 140
   See also Antibiotics 114
Cheracol 38
Chest infections see Respiratory
   system infections
Chickenpox, drugs for
   antihistamines 110
   antipruritics 161
   antiviral drugs 119
Childbirth see Labour
Childhood infectious diseases
   see Antiviral drugs 119
   vaccines for 120
Children
   drug treatment in 20
   giving medicines to 27
      dos and don'ts concerning 31
Chinese herbal
      medicine 495
Chlamydial infections 117
Chloral derivatives 66
chloral hydrate 38
chlorambucil 38
chloramphenicol 38
chlordiazepoxide 38
chlorhexidine 38
Chloromycetin 38
chloroquine 38
chlorpheniramine 38
chlorpromazine 38
chlorpropamide 38
chlorthalidone 38
Chlor-Tripolon 38
Chlor-Tripolon N.D. 38
Choledyl 38
Cholera 498, 499
Cholesterol
   drugs to reduce level of 89
   stones 100
cholestyramine 38
Cholinergic 504g
Choriocarcinoma 140
Christmas disease 90
Chromium 38, 136, 470
Chromium picolinate 470
Chronic fatigue 495
Cialis 38
Cicatrin 38
Ciclesonide 38
Ciclopirox 38
Ciloxan 38
cimetidine 38
Cipralex 38
Cipro 38
Ciprodex 38
ciprofloxacin 38
Cipro HC 38
Circulation 81

Cirrhosis, liver
   and alcohol abuse 484
   use of diuretics 85
cisplatin 38
citalopram 38
Citrate 600 38
Citro-Mag 38
Claforan 38
Classification of drugs 13
clarithromycin 38
Claritin 38
Claritin Allergic Congestion
   Relief 38
Claritin Extra 38
Claritin Eye Allergy
   Relief 38
Claritin Liberator 38
Claritin Skin Itch Relief 38
Clarus 38
clavulinic acid 38
Clavulin 39
clemastine 39
clindamycin 39
Clindets 39
Clindoxyl 39
clioquinol 39
Clioquinol 39
clobazam 39
clobetasol 39
clobetasone 39
Clomid 39
clomiphene 39
clomipramine 39
clonazepam 39
Clopixol 39
Clopixol-Acuphase 39
Clopixol-Depot 39
clonidine 39
clopidogrel 39
Clotting of blood, drugs that
   affect 90
Clotrimaderm 39
clotrimazole 39
cloxacillin 39
clozapine 39
Clozaril 39
CoActifed Tablets 39
Coal tar 39, 53
Coated Aspirin 39
Cobalamin 480
Cocaine 39, 488
   use in sport 496
codeine 39
Codeine Contin 39
Codeine Phosphate 39
Co-enzyme Q_{10} 39, 470
Coenzyme R 469
CO Fluoxetine 39
Cogentin 39
Co-Glimepiride 39
Colace 39
colchicine 39
Cold cures 80
   alternative medicines 494, 495
   use in sport 496
Cold sores 119

colecalciferol 39
colestipol 39
colistin 39
Colitis, ulcerative see Ulcerative
    colitis
collodion 39
Colon, cancer of 140
Colorado tick fever 499
Coma 504g
Combigan 39
Combivent 39
Complementary medicine see
    Alternative medicine 494
Comtan 39
Concerta 39
Condyline 39
Congest 39
Congestive heart failure see
    Heart failure
Conjugated estrogens 39
Conjunctivitis, drugs for
    antibiotics 114
    antihistamines 110
Constipation see Laxatives 97
Contac Cold 12 Hour Relief
    Non Drowsy 39
Contact Head and Chest
    Congestion 39
Contraception
    comparison of reliability of
        different methods of 149
    postcoital 151
Contraceptives, oral 149
    balancing the risks and
        benefits of 150
    hormone content of 149
    and menstrual disorders
        148
    minimizing health risks while
        taking 150
    and missing a pill 151
    reliability of 149
Contraindication 504g
Co-Pioglitazone 39
Copper 39, 136, 471
Cordarone 39
Cornea, ulceration of 479
Coronary thrombosis see Heart
    attack
Cortate 39
Cortef 39
Cortenema 39
Corticosteroids 127
    use in allergies 110
    as bronchodilators 76
    in ear disorders 159
    ending treatment with 28
    locally acting 104
    topical 161, 162
    use in inflammatory bowel
        disease 98
    prohibited substances in sport
        496
corticotropin 39
Cortifoam 39
Cortimyxin ointment 39

cortisol 39
Cortisone 39
Cortisone acetate 39
Cortisporin ointment 39
Cortoderm 39
Cosopt 39
co-trimoxazole 39
Cough drugs 80
    alternative medicines 494, 495
    use in sport 496
Coumadin 39
Counter-irritant see Rubefacient
Coversyl 39
Coversyl Plus 39
Coversyl Plus LD 39
COX-2 inhibitors 102
Cozaar 39
Crack see Cocaine 488
Cramps, muscle 106
Creams 19, 161, 163
Creeping eruption 125
Creon 39
Crestor 39
Crinone 39
Crixivan 39
Crohn's disease 98
Cromolyn 39
crotamiton 39
Cryptosporidosis 122
Crystapen 39
Cubicin 39
Cuprimine 39
cyanocobalamin 39, 480
cyclizine 39
Cyclogyl 39
Cyclomen 39
cyclopentolate 39
cyclophosphamide 39
Cycloplegic 504g
cyclosporine 39
Cyklokapron 39
cyproheptadine 39
cyproterone 39
Cystic fibrosis 100
    Drugs to treat coughs 80
    sodium supplements for 478
Cystitis 154
cytarabine 40
Cytokines 141, 142
Cytomel 40
Cytotoxic 504g
    See also Anticancer drugs 140
Cytotoxic antibiotics 141, 142
Cytovene 40
Cytoxan 40

D

daclizumab 40
Dalacin C 40
dalfopristin 40
Dalmacol 40
dalteparin 40, 305

danazol 40
Dandruff, treatment for 168
Dantrium 40
dantrolene tizanidine 40
dapsone 40
Daptomycin 40
Daraprim 40
darbepoetin 40
darifenacin 40
darpoeitin see erythropoeisis
darunavir 40
Darvon-N 40
Daypro 40
DDAVP 250
ddC see Zalcitabine 145
ddI see Didanosine 145
Deca-Durabolin 40
Decongestants 77
    use in ear disorders 159
Dehydration 497
Delatestryl 40
delavirdine 40
Delestrogen 40
Demerol 40
Dementia drugs 71
Demerol 40
Denavir 40
Dengue fever 499
Denorex 40
Depakene 40
DepoCyt 40
Depo-Medrol 40
Depo-Provera 40
Depo-Testosterone 40
Depot injection 504g
    See also Methods of
        administration 17
Depression
    drugs for see Antidepressant
        drugs 68
    homeopathic remedies 494
    manic see Antipsychotics 69
Dermatitis, drugs for
    antihistamines 110
    antipruritics 161
    homeopathic remedies 494
    topical corticosteroids 162
    See also Drugs and other
        treatments for eczema 167
Dermatomyositis 200
Derma-Smooth/FS 40
Dermovate 40
desipramine 40
Desensitization 110
Designer drugs 505g
Detoxification see Treating drug
    dependence 24
desloratadine 40
desmopressin 40
desogestrel 40
desonide 40
Desoxi 40
desoximetasone 40
Desquam-X 40
Desyrel 40
Desyrel Dividose 40
Detrol 40

dexamethasone 40
dexedrine 40
dextromethorphan 40
dextrophetamine 40
Diabeta 40
Diabetes
    insipidus, drugs for 131
    mellitus, drugs used in 128
Diabetic ketoacedosis 476
Dialysis see Kidney dialysis
Diamicron 40
Diamicron MR 40
diamorphine 40
    opioids, abuse of 492
Diamox 40
Diane-35 40
Diarrhea, drugs for 96
    use in sport 496
    traveller's 499
Diastat 40
Diazemuls 40
diazepam 40
Diclectin 40
diclofenac 40
dicyclomine 40
didanosine 40
Didrocal 40
Didronel 40
diethylcarbamazine 40
diethylstilbestrol 40
Dieting drugs, use in sport 496
Differin 40
Diflucan 40
diflucortolone 40
diflunisal 40
Digestion of fats 100
Digestive system see
    Gastrointestinal tract
Digitalis 82
    as anti-arrhythmic 86
digoxin 40
Digoxin Injection C.S.D. 40
dihydroergotamine 40
Dihydroergotamine Mesylate
    Injection 40
dihydrotachysterol 40
Dilantin 40
Dilaudid 40
diloxanide 40
diltiazem 40
dimenhydrinate 40
dimercaprol 40
Dimetapp Cold Liquid 40
Dimetapp-C Syrup 40
Dimetapp Daytime Cold 40
Dimetapp Oral Infant Cold
    Drops 40
Dimetane Expectorant-DC 40
dimethyl sulfoxide 40
dinoprost 40
dinoprostone 40
Diophenyl-T 40
Diovan 40
Diovan HCT 40
Diovol 41
Diovol Plus 41

Dipentum 41
diphenhydramine 41
diphenoxylate 41
diphenylpyraline 41
Diphtheria, vaccine for 121, 498
Diprolene Glycol 41
Diprosalic 41
Diprosone 41
dipyridamole 41
disopyramide 41
dithranol 41
Ditropan 41
Ditropan XL 41
Diuretics 85, 88
  prohibited substances in sport
    496
divalproex 41
Dixarit 41
Doak Oil 41
docetaxel 41
docusate sodium 41
dolasetron 41
Dom-Indapamide 41
Dom Lindane 41
domperidone 41
donepezil 41
dopamine 41
dornase alfa 41
dorzolamide 41
Doses
  exceeding 30
  missed 28
Dostinex 41
Double blind 505g
  See also Testing and
    approving new drugs 12
Dovobet 41
Dovonex 41
doxazosin 41
doxepin 41
doxorubicin 41
doxycycline 41
doxylamine succinate 41
Doxylar 41
DPT vaccination 121
Drip 505g
Drisdol 41
Dristan Long Lasting Nasal
  Mist/Spray 41
Dristan N.D. 41
Dristan Decongestant 41
dronabinol 41
Drospirenone 41
Drug
  abuse 483
  actions see Action of drugs
  administration, methods of 17
  classification 13
  dependence 23
  dose and response 15
  effects 15
  forms 19
  interactions 16
    with alcohol 485
    with travel medication 499
  marketing 12

misuse 24
overdose 30
placebo response 15
poisoning emergency guide
  526
receptor sites 14
sources 12
testing 12
tolerance 23
withdrawal symptoms 24
See also Drugs; Drug
  treatment; Medication
Drugs
  of abuse 483
  controlled 13
  effects of on sleep
    patterns 66
  effects of overdose on body
    30
  high danger of overdose 528
  how they accumulate 30
  how they pass through the
    body 17
  incorrect use of 22
  over-the-counter 25
  prescription 26
  storing 29
  when to dispose of 29
  use in sport 496
  and travel 497
  See also Drug; Drug
    treatment; Medication
Drug treatment
  in the elderly 22
  ending 28
  exceeding the dose 30
  in infants and children 20
  in kidney and liver disease 22
  long-term 29
  managing 25
  in pregnant and breast-
    feeding women 21
  and travel 497
  See also Drug; Drugs;
    Medication
Dry eye 158
Dulcolax 41
Duovent 41
Duragesic 41
Duralith 41
Duricef 41
Dutasteride 41
Dysentery, amoebic 122
Dysmenorrhea 148
Dyspepsia see Antacids 94

E

Ear(s) 151
  disorders, drugs for 17
  drops, how to use 17
  infections of 115
  wax removal 17
Ebixa 41

econazole 41
Ecostatin 41
Ecstasy 488
Eczema, drugs and other
  treatments for 167
  alternative medicines
    494, 495
  antihistamines 110
  antipruritics 161
    topical corticosteroids 162
  infected 163
edrophonium 41
EES 41
efavirenz 41
Effexor 41
Effexor XR 41
Efudex 41
Egg cells, cancer affecting 140
Elaboration see What are
  drugs? 12
Elbow, tennis 104
Elderly, drug treatment in 22
Electrolyte see Body salts
eletriptan 41
Elixir 19, 505g
Elocom 41
Eltor 120 41
Eltroxin 41
Emend 41
EMLA Cream 41
EMLA Patch 41
Emocort 41
Emollient 505g
  creams, as antipruritics
    161, 167
Emphysema 92
Emtricitabine 41
Emtriva 41
Emulsion 19, 505g
Enablex 41
enalapril 41
Enbrel 41
Endantadine 41, 185
Endocet 41
Endocrine system 126
Endometrial cancer 140
Endometriosis 148, 248
Endorphins 505g
enfuvirtide 41
Enlon 41
enoxaparin 41, 305
Entacapone 41
entecavir 41
Enteric coated 505g
Enteritis, regional 98
Entocort 41
Entrophen 41
Enuresis 154
Enzyme 505g
  pancreatic 100
ephedrine 41
Ephedrine Sulfate 41
Epidural anesthesia 153
Epilepsy 86
epinephrine 41
EpiPen 41

epirubicin 41
Epival 41
Epival ER 41
epoetin see erythropoietin
epoprostenol 41
Eprex 42
Ergamisol 42
ergocalciferol 42
Ergodryl 42
ergometrine 42
ergonovine 42
Ergonovine maleate 42
ergotamine 42
ertapenem 42
Erybid 42
Eryc 42
Erythro Base 42
erythromycin 42
erythropoietin 42
Escitalopram 42
esmolol 42
Estalis 42
Estalis-Sequi 42
Estar 42
Estrace 42
Estracomb 42
Estraderm 42
estradiol 42
Estring 42
estrone estropipate 42
etanercept 42
ethambutol 42
ethinyl estradiol 42
Ethopropazine 42
ethosuximide 42
Ethynodrol diacetate 42
Etibi 42
etidronate 42
etodolac 42
etomidate 42
Etonogestrel 42
etoposide 42
eucalyptus 42
Euflex 42
Euglucon 42
Eumovate 42
Eurax 42
Evista 42
Evra 42
Excitatory 78, 505g
Exdol-8 42
Exdol-15 42
Exdol-30 42
Exelon 42
Exhaustion, homeopathic
  remedies for 494
Exophthalmos 130
Expectorant 505g
  See also Drugs to treat
    coughs 80
Eye(s) 155
  disorders
    see Drugs for glaucoma 156;
    Drugs affecting the pupil 158
  drops 19
    applying in glaucoma 157

infections, drugs for
    antibiotics 115
    antiviral drugs 119
    inflammation 155
    See also Infection
Ezetimibe 42
Ezetrol 42

F

5-ASA 42
famciclovir 42
famotidine 42
Famvir 42
Farmer's lung 109
Fat levels in blood 89
Fat-soluble vitamins 137
Fats, digestion of 100
felodipine 42
Female reproductive system 147
Female urinary system 147
Female sex hormones 133
Femara 42
FemHRT 42
fenofibrate 42
fenoprofen 42
fenoterol 42
fentanyl 42
Ferrlecit 42
ferrous fumarate 42
ferrous gluconate 42
ferrous sulfate 42
Fertility drugs see Drugs for
    infertility 152
Fever see Antipyretic 504g
fexofenadine 42
Fibrates 89
Fibrillation 86
Fibrocystic disease, of
    breasts 248
Fibrinolytics see
    Thrombolytics 91
Filariasis 113, 125, 499
filgrastim 42
finasteride 42
Fiorinal-C 42
First aid, essential 527
Fits see Seizures
Flagyl 42
Flagystatin 42
flavoxate 42
flecainide 42
Flexeril 42
Flolan 42
Flomax 42
Flonase 42
Florazole ER 42
Florinef 42
Flovent Diskus 42
Flovent HFA 42
Fluanxol 42
Fluanxol Depot 42
fluconazole 42
flucytosine 42

fludrocortisone 42
Fluid retention see Diuretics 85
Flukes 113, 125
flumazenil 42
flumethasone 42
flunarizine 42
flunisolide 42
fluocinolone 42
fluocinonide 42
Fluoderm 42
fluoride 42
fluorometholone 42
Fluorosis 471
fluorouracil 42
Fluotic 42
fluoxetine 42
flupentixol 42
fluphenazine 42
Fluphenazine Omega 42
flurazepam 42
flurbiprofen 42
flutamide 42
fluticasone 43
fluvastatin 43
fluvoxamine 43
folates 472
folic acid 43, 135, 136, 472
folinic acid 43
Follicle-stimulating hormone 152
follitropin alpha 43
follitropin beta 43
Fondaparinux 43
Food allergy see Antihistamines
    110
    See also Nutrition 134
Foradil 43
formoterol 43
Formula, chemical 505g
Formulary 505g
Fortaz 43
Forteo 43
Fortovase 43
Fosamax 43
Fosamprenavir 43
Fosavance 43
fosfomycin tromethamine 43
fosinopril 43
Fosphenytoin 43
Fragmin 43
framycetin 43
Fraxiparine 43
Frisium 43
Froben SR 43
Frozen shoulder 104
FSH (follicle-stimulating
    hormone) 43
Fucidin 43
Fucidin H 43
Fucithalmic 43
Fulvicin U/F 43
Fungal infections 124
Fungizone Intravenous 43
furosamide 293
fusidic acid 43
Fuzeon 43

G

GABA 67
gabapentin 43
Galactorrhea 131
galantamine 43
Gallstones, drug treatment for
    100
Gamma-aminobutyric acid
    (GABA) 67
gamma benzene hexachloride 43
ganciclovir 43
ganirelix 43
Garamycin 43
Gardasil 43
Gastrointestinal tract 92
    infections 114, 115
    movement of food through 93
Gasulsol 43
gatifloxacin 43
Gaviscon Heartburn Relief
    Formula 43
Gelusil 43
gemfibrozil 43
Gen-Acyclovir 43
Gen-Alprazolam 43
Gen-Amantadine 43
Gen-Amoxicillin 43
Gen-Atenolol 43
Gen-Azathioprine 43
Gen-Baclofen 43
Gen-Buspirone 43
Gen-Carbamazepine 43
Gen-Cimetidine 43
Gen-Clindamycin 43
Gen-Clobetasol 43
Gen-Clomipramine 43
Gen-Clonazepam 43
Gen-Cyclobenzaprine 43
Gen-Cyproterone 43
Gen-Diltiazem 43
Gen-Doxazosin 43
Generic name 505g
    classification of drugs13
    prescribing 26
Genetic engineering see What
    are drugs? 12
Gen-Fenofibrate Micro 43
Gen-Fluoxetine 43
Gen-Gemfibrozil 43
Gen-Gliclazide 43
Gen-Indapamide 43
Gen-Ipratropium 43
Genital tract infections, drugs for
    antibacterial drugs 117
    antibiotics 115
    antiprotozoal drugs 122
    antiviral drugs 119
Gen-Lovastatin 43
Gen-Medroxy 43
Gen-metformin 43
Gen-Metoprolol 43
Gen-Minocycline 43
Gen-Mirtazepine 43
Gen-Nabumetone 43

Gen-Nortriptyline 43
Gen-Oxybutynin 43
Gen-Pioglitazone 43
Gen-Piroxicam 43
Gen-Salbutamol 43
Gen-Selegiline 43
Gen-Sertraline 43
Gen-Sotalol 43
gentamicin 43
Gen-Temazepam 43
Gen-Terbinafine 43
Gentlax 43
Gentlax.S 44
Gen-Trazodone 44
Gen-Triazolam 44
Gen-Valproic 44
Gen-Verapamil 44
Gen-Zopiclone 44
German measles, vaccine for 121
Germ cell tumours 140
Germicides see Antiseptics 163
Giardiasis 122
Gigantism, pituitary 131
Glaucoma 156
    use of diuretics 85
    action of drugs for 157
    applying eye drops in 157
    what happens in 156
Gleevec 44
gliclazide 44
glimepiride 44
Glomerulonephritis 127
glucagon 44
Glucobay 44
GlucoNorm 44
Glucophage 44
Glucosamine 44
Glucose
    blood levels of in diabetes 128
    monitoring 129
glyburide 44
Glycosides, cardiac see Digitalis
    drug 82
Goitre 130, 473
Gold 60
Gold-based drugs 103
Golden Eye 60
gold sodium thiomalate 44
gonadorelin 44
Gonadotropin, human
    chorionic 44
Gonal-F 44
Goodpasture's syndrome 143
goserelin 44
Gout 105
Gouty arthritis 105
gramicidin 44
granisetron 44
Graves' disease see
    Hyperthyroidism
Gravol Preparations 44
griseofulvin 44
Growth factor inhibitors 141, 142
Growth hormone 44
    disorders, drugs for 131
guaifenesin 44

Gynazole-I 44
Gynecomastia 248

H

H1 blockers 110
H1 receptors 110
H2 blockers 95
H2 receptors 95
5HT1 agonists 73
Hair follicles, blocked 165
Hair loss, treatment for 168
halcinonide 44
Halcion 44
Half-life 505g
Hallucinogen 505g
halobetasol 44
Halog 44
haloperidol 44
Haloperidol LA 44
Haloperidol-LA Omega 44
halothane 44
Hansen's disease, drugs for 117
Hashimoto's disease 138
    See also Drugs for thyroid
        disorders 130
Hay fever, drugs for
    alternative medicines 494, 495
    Antihistamines 110
    Decongestants 79
Headaches, drugs for
    alternative medicines 494, 495
    non-opioid analgesics 64
    See also Migraine
Head and neck cancer 140
Head lice 164
Heart and circulation 81
Heart attack, drugs for
    beta blockers 83
    thrombolytics 91
Heart beat disorders, drugs for
    see Anti-arrhythmics 86
Heart block, drugs for see Types
    of arrhythmia 86
Heartburn see Dyspepsia
Heart disorders, drugs for
    anti-angina drugs 87
    anti-arrhythmics 86
    antihypertensive drugs 88
    beta blockers 83
    digitalis drug 82
    diuretics 85
    drugs that affect blood clotting
        90
    lipid-lowering drugs 89
    vasodilators 84
Heart failure, drugs for
    digitalis drug 82
    diuretics 85
    vasodilators 84
Heart infections 115
Helicobacter pylori 95
Hemochromatosis 473
Hemolytic anemia 477, 481

Hemophilia 90
Hemophilus influenzae
    meningitis, drugs for 116
    vaccinations for 121
Hemorrhoids 99
Hemostatic drugs see Drugs
    used to promote blood
    clotting 90, 91
Hepalean 44
Hepalean-Lok 44
heparin 44
Heparin Leo 44
Hepatitis
    and alcohol abuse 484
    vaccine for 121, 498
Hepsera 44
Heptovir 44
Herbalism see What are drugs?
    12, Alternative medicines 495
herceptin 44
Heroin 44
    withrawal 24
Herpes infections 119
Herplex-D 44
hexachlorophene 44
Histamine and histamine
    receptors 109
Histamine blockers 95
Histanil 44
Hives (urticaria) 161
HIV, drugs for 144
Hivid 44
Hodgkin's disease 156
homatropine 44
Homeopathy 494
Hookworm 125
Hormone 505g
    anticancer treatment 141, 142
    effects of replacement therapy
        in the menopause 133
    in diabetes 128
    in pituitary disorders 131
    replacement therapy
        in adrenal gland disorders 127
        in menopause see Female
            sex hormones 133
    in thyroid disorders 130
Hormones 143
    kidney 146
    pituitary 131
    sex
        female 133
        male 132
    thyroid 130
Hot flushes see Menopause 133
HRT see Menopause 133
Hp-PAC 44
Humalog 44
Humatrope 44
Humira 44
Humulin 44
Humulin N 44
hyaluronidase 44
Hycodan 44
Hycomine 44
Hycomine-S 44

Hycort 44
Hydatid disease 125
Hyderm 44
hydralazine 44
hydrochlorothiazide 44
hydrocodone 44
hydrocortisone 44
Hydromorph Contin 44
hydromorphone 44
Hydromorphone HP 44
Hydromorphone HP Forte 44
hydroxocobalamin 44
hydroxychloroquine 44
hydroxyzine 44
Hygroton 44
Hyperglycemia 128
Hyperlipidemia 89, 475
Hypermagnesemia 474
Hyperphosphatemia 200
Hypertension 88
Hyperthyroidism 146
    and beta blockers 83
Hyperuricemia 198
    See also Drugs for gout 105
Hypnotics 66
Hypoglycemia 128
Hypokalemia 85
Hypoparathyroidism 481
Hypoprothrombinemia 482
Hypothyroidism 130, 473
Hypurin 44
Hytrin 44

I

ibuprofen 44
ibutulide 44
ichthammol 44
Idiosyncrasy 505g
idoxuridine 44
imatinib 44
Imdur 44
imipenem-cilastin 44
imipramine 44
Imitrex 44
Immune
    deficiency, drugs for 144
    disease 138
    globulins 120
    responses 139
    system, drugs that suppress
        143
Immunization 505g
    See also Vaccines and
        immunization 120; Medicines
        and travel 497
Immunoglobulins 61
Immunosuppressant drugs 143
    as antirheumatic drugs 103
    in inflammatory bowel disease
        98
Imodium 44
Imovane 44
Impetigo 163

Implants 18
Impotence 152, 429
Imuran 44
Incontinence 170
indapamide 44
Inderal-LA 44
Indication 506g
Indigestion, drugs for
    antacids 94
    homeopathic remedies 494
indinavir 44
Indocid P.D.A. 44
indomethacin 44
Induction of labour 153
Infants, drug treatment in 20
Infection 112
    bacterial, drugs for
        antibacterial drugs 117
        antibiotics 114
    fungal 124
    immunization for 120
    protozoal 122
    transmitting 113
    tuberculous 118
    viral 119
    See also Childhood
        infectious diseases; specific
        areas of body
Infertility, drugs for 152
Infestations 112, 499
    drugs for 125
Inflammation, drugs for
    analgesics 64
    corticosteroid drugs 127
    locally acting 104
    non-steroidal anti-
        inflammatory drugs 102
Inflammatory bowel disease,
    drugs for 98
infliximab 44
Influenza
    antiviral drugs 119
    homeopathic remedies 494
    vaccine for 120
Infusion
    intravenous 506g
    pump 506g
Inhalation 18
Inhaler 19, 506g
    how to use 78
    types of 77
    See also Bronchodilators 92;
        Methods of administration 18
Inhibitory 78, 506g
Injection
    administration of 18
    depot 504g
    intramuscular 506g
    intravenous 506g
    of joints, common sites 104
    solutions 19
    subcutaneous 508g
Injection sites
    insulin 129
    locally acting corticosteroids 104
Innohep 44

Inoculation 506g
inosiplex 45
Insecticides 164
Insect bites 499
Insomnia
    alternative medicine 494,
        495
    sleeping drugs 66
insulin 45
    administration of 128
    sites of injection 129
    and travel 498
insulin aspart 45
insulin detemir 45
insulin glargine 45
insulin NPH 45
insulin ultralente 45
Insurance, travel 497
Intal 45
Interactions 16
Interferon 45
    See also Malignant and
        immune disease 139
Interferon alfa-2b 45
Interferon beta-1a 45
Interferon beta-1b 45
Intestinal disorders see
    Gastrointestinal tract 92
Intestine, cross section of
    92
Intramuscular injection 506g
Intrinsic factor 480
Intron-A 45
Invirase 45
iodine 45
iopidine 45
ipecac 45
ipratropium bromide 45
irbesartan 45
irinotecan 45
Iris, inflamed see Uveitis
Iron 45
Iron deficiency anemia 473
Irritable bowel syndrome
    alternative medicines 494,
        495
    drugs for 96
Isentress 45
isoflurane 45
isoniazid 45
isoproterenol 45
Isoproterenol Hydrochloride
    45
Isoptin 45
Isopto Atropine 45
Isopto Carbachol 45
Isopto Carpine 45
Isopto Homatropine 45
isosorbide dinitrate 45
isosorbide mononitrate 45
Isotamine 45
isotretinoin 45
Itching 161
    in rectal and anal disorders
        99
itraconazole 45

J

Januvia 45
Japanese B encephalitis 498,
    499
Jaundice 506g
Jet lag 498
Jock itch 124
Joints 101
    infected 114, 115
    inflamed, see
        antirheumatic drugs 103
    locally acting corticosteroids
        104
    non-steroidal anti-
        inflammatory drugs 102

K

Kadian 45
Kaletra 45
Kaolin 45
Kaopectate 45
Kefzol 45
Kenalog 45
Keppra 45
Keratolytic drugs see Drugs
    used to treat acne 165
ketamine 45
Ketek 45
ketoconazole 45
Ketoderm 45
ketoprofen 45
ketorolac 45
ketotifen 45
Kidney
    corticosteroids 127
    disease, prescribing drug
        treatment in 22
    dialysis, drugs to prevent
        formation of blood clots
        during 91
    diuretics, action on 85
    hormone 143
    infections, drugs for
        antibiotics 114
        antifungal drugs 124
    stones 105
    See also Nephrotic syndrome
Kineret 45
K-Lyte 45
Koffex DM 45
Kwellada-P 45
Kytril 45

L

Labour
    drugs used in 147, 153
Lactation, suppressing 131
lactic acid 45

lactulose 45
Lamictal 45
Lamisil 45
lamivudine 45
lamotrigine 45
Lanoxin 45
lansoprazole 45
Lariam 45
Lasix 45
latanoprost 45
Laxatives 97, 99
Leflunomide 45
Leishmaniasis 122, 499
Leprosy see Hansen's disease
Lescol 45
letrozole 45
Leukemias 140
Leukeran 45
Leukotriene antagonists 78,
    110
Leutinizing hormone 152
Levaquin 45
Levetiracetam 45
Levitra 45
levobunolol 45
levocabastine 45
levodopa 45
levodopa/benserazide 45
levodopa/carbidopa 45
levofloxacin 45
levonorgestrel 45
levothyroxine 45
Levsin 45
Libido, reduced 132
Librax 45
Lice infestation 113, 164
Lidemol 45
Lidex 45
lidocaine 45
Lidocaine Parenteral 45
Lidodan Endotracheal 45
Lin-Buspirone 45
lindane 45
linezolid 45
Liniment 496, 506g
Lipidil EZ 45
Lipidil-Micro 45
Lipidil Supra 45
Lipid-lowering drugs 89
Lipitor 45
Lioresal 45
liothyronine 45
Liquid medication 19
Liquid paraffin 45
lisinopril 45
Lithane 45
lithium 46
Liver
    disease, drug treatment in 22
    drugs acting on 89
    infections, protozoal 122
Livostin 46
LMWH 46
Locacorten Vioform 46
Local anesthetics see
    Anesthesia, local

Locally acting corticosteroids
    104
Iodoxamide 46
Loestrin 46
Lomine 46
Lomotil 46
Loniten 46
Loop diuretics 85
loperamide 46
Lopid 46
lopinavir/ritonavir 46
Lopresor 46
loratadine 46
lorazepam 46
losartan 46
Losec 46
Lotion 19, 506g
    See also Bases for skin
        preparations 163
Lotriderm 46
Lovastatin 46
Lovenox 46
Lovenox HP 46
Low molecular weight heparin
    46
Loxapac 46
loxapine 46
Lozide 46
Lugol's solution 46
Lumigan 46
Lung
    cancers 140
    infection
        bacterial 114
        fungal 124
        protozoal 124
Lupus erythematosus see
    Systemic lupus erythematosus
Lutein 46
Luteinizing hormone (LH) 63
Lutropulse 46
Luvox 46
Lyderm 46
Lyme disease 499
Lymphatic cancers 140
Lymph nodes, cancer of 140
Lymphomas 140
Lyrica 46
Lysergic acid see LSD 490

M

Maalox 46
Maalox Antacid with Anti-Gas
    46
Maalox Antacid with Anti-Gas
    Extra Strength 46
Maalox Quick Dissolve 46
Maalox TC 46
Macrolides 115, 116
magnesium 46
magnesium carbonate 46
magnesium citrate 46

magnesium hydroxide 46
magnesium oxide 46
magnesium sulfate 46
magnesium trisilicate 46
Major tranquillizer see
  Tranquillizer, major 508g
Malabsorption 134
Malaria 499
  drugs for 123
  prevention 499
Malarone 46
Male infertility 152
Male pattern baldness, hair
  regrowth 168
Male reproductive system 146
Male sex hormones 132
Malignant disease 138
  See also Cancer
Manerix 46
Manic depression
  drugs for 69
mannitol 46
MAOIs see Antidepressant
  drugs 68
maprotiline 46
Maraviroc 46
Marcaine 46
Marijuana see Cannabis 487
Marinol 46
Marvelon 46
Maxidex 46
Maxitrol 46
Maxalt 46
Maxalt RPD 46
mebendazole 46
Measles, vaccine for 121
meclizine 46
Medication 506g
  dos and don'ts concerning 31
  ending treatment 28
  exceeding the dose 30
  giving to children 27
  how to take 27
  missed doses 28
  remembering your 28
  and sport 496
  and travel 497
  when to take 27
  See also Drug
Medicine 506g
  and travel 497
  See also Medication
Medrol 46
medroxyprogesterone 46
mefloquine 46
Mefoxin 46
Megace 46
Megace OS 46
megestrol 46
meloxicam 46
melphalan 46
memantine 46
menadiol 46
Ménière's disease 74, 85, 205,
  258
Meningitis see Antibiotics 116

"Belt" 497
  cryptococcal 124
  meningococcal 121
  tuberculous 118
  vaccine for 498
Menke's syndrome 471
Menopause
  alternative medicines 494, 495
  hormone replacement therapy
    133
Menorrhagia 148, 248
menotropins 46
menthol 46
Menstrual
  cycle 147
  disorders, drugs for 148
menthyl anthranilate 46
mepacrine 46
meperidine 46
mepivacaine 46
Mepron 46
mercaptopurine 46
Meridia 46
meropenem 46
Mersyndol with Codeine 46
mesalamine/5-ASA 46
Mesasal 46
M-Eslon 46
Mestinon 46
Mestinon-SR 46
Metabolism 506g
  disorders of see Nutrition 134
Metadol 46
Metamucil 46
metformin 46
methadone 46
Methazolamide 46
methenamine 46
methimazole 46
methocarbamol 46
methotrexate 46
methotrimeprazine 46
Methoxacet-C 46
Methoxisal 47
methoxsalen 47
Methsuximide 47
methylcellulose 47
methyldopa 47
methylphenidate 47
methylprednisolone 47
methyl salicylate 47
methysergide 47
metoclopramide 47
Metoclopramide Omega 47
metolazone 47
metoprolol 47
Metreton 47
MetroCream 47
MetroGel 47
metronidazole 47
Mevacor 47
mexiletine 47
mexoryl SX 47
Miacalcin NS 47
micafungin 47
Micardis 47

Micatin 47
miconazole 47
Micozole 47
Micronor 47
Midamor 47
Midol Regular 47
Migraine
  alternative medicines 494, 495
  drugs used for 73
Migranal 47
Milk production, suppressing 131
Minerals 137
  main food sources of 136
mineral oil 47
Minestrin 47
Minims Atropine 47
Minims Cyclopentolate 47
Minims Phenylephrine 47
Minims Tetracaine 47
Minims Tropicamide 47
Minipress 47
Minitram 47
Minocin 47
minocycline 47
Minor injuries, alternative
  medicines 494, 495
Minor tranquillizers see
  Tranquillizers, minor 508g
Min-Ovral 47
minoxidil 47
Mintezol 47
Miostat 47
Miotic 506g
  See also Drugs affecting the
    pupil 158; use in glaucoma
    157
Mirapex 47
Mirena 47
mirtazapine 47
misoprostol 47
Misuse of drugs 24
Mixture 19
Mobicox 47
moclobemide 47
modafinil 47
Modecate 47
Modified-release preparations 18
Mogadon 47
molybdenum 47
mometasone 47
Monistat 47
Monoamine oxidase inhibitors
  (MAOIs) 68
  and drug interactions 16, 486
Monoclonal antibodies 141,
  142, 143
montelukast 47
Monurol 47
morphine 47
  abuse of see Opioids 492
  use in labour 153
Morphine Sulfate 47
M.O.S. 47
Motion sickness see Travel
  sickness
Motrin 47

Mouth
  infection
    bacterial 115
    fungal (thrush) 124
  -to-mouth resuscitation 527
moxifloxacin 47
MS Contin 47
MSD Enteric Coated ASA 47
MS-IR 47
Mucaine 47
Mucolytic 506g
  See also Drugs to treat
    coughs 80
Multiple sclerosis 106
Mumps 119
  vaccine for 121
mupirocin 47
Muscle 101
  injury, drugs for
    analgesics 64
    locally acting corticosteroids
      104
  in myasthenia gravis 107
  relaxants 106
  spasm 106
  strength, drugs to improve see
    Anabolic steroids 132
  uterine 153
MUSE 47
Myasthenia gravis 107, 200
Mycamine 47
Mycobutin 47
mycophenolate mofetil 47
Mycostatin 47
Mydfrin 47
Mydriacil 47
Mydriatic 506g
  See also Drugs affecting the
    pupil 158
Mylanta Double Strength Plain
  47
Mylanta Extra Strength 47
Myocet 47
Myochrysine 47
Myotonachol 47
Mysoline 47
Myxedema see
  Hypothyroidism

N

nabilone 47
nabumetone 47
nadolol 47
nadroparin 47
nafarelin 47
Nails, fungal infections
  of 124
nalbuphine 47
Nalcrom 47
Nalfon 47
naloxone 47
naltrexone 47

nandrolone 47
Naprosyn 47
naproxen 47
naratriptan 47
Narcan 47
Narcolepsy see Nervous system
    stimulants 72
Nardil 48
Nasacort AQ 48
Nasal drops/spray 19
Nasal passages 79
Nasonex 48
nateglinide 48
Nausea
    anti-emetics 74
    herbal remedies 495
Navane 48
Nebcin 48
nedocromil 48
nelfinavir 48
Neo-Laryngobis 48
Neo-Medrol Acne Lotion 48
neomycin 48
Neoral 48
neostigmine 48
NeoStrata Canada Blemish
    Spot Gel 48
Neo-Synephrine Parenteral 48
Nephrotic syndrome see
    Diuretics 85
Nerisalik 48
Nerisone 48
Nerve signals, how they are
    transmitted 78
Nervous system 78
    infections 115
    stimulants 72
Neulasta 48
Neuleptil 48
Neupogen 48
Neuroleptic 506g
    See also Antipsychotic drugs
    69
Neurological disorders see
    Muscle relaxants 106
Neurontin 48
Neurotransmitter 78, 63, 506g
nevirapine 48
niacin 48
niacinamide 48
Nicoderm 48
Nicorette 48
nicotinamide 48
nicotine 48
    as a drug of abuse 491
    use in sport 496
nicotinic acid 48
nicotinyl alcohol tartrate 48
Nicotrol 48
NidaGel 48
Nidazol 48
nifedipine 48
Night blindness 479
Nit infestation 164
Nitrates see Vasodilators 84
    See also Anti-angina drugs 87

nitrazepam 48
Nitrazodon 48
Nitro-Dur 48
nitrofurantoin 48
nitroglycerin 48
Nitrol 48
Nitrolingual Pumpspray 48
Nitrostat 48
nitrous oxide 48
Nits 164
Nix 48
nizatidine 48
Nizoral 48
Non-opioid analgesics 64, 65
    cough suppressants 80
Non-nucleoside transcriptase
    inhibitors 144, 145
Non-steroidal anti-inflammatory
    drugs (NSAIDs) 64, 65, 102,
    499
    use in sport 496
    and digestive tract irritation 64
nonacog alfa 48
nonoxynol '9' 48
noradrenaline 48
Norelgestromin 48
norepinephrine 48
norethindrone 48
Norflex 48
norfloxacin 48
Norgesic Forte 48
norgestimate 48
norgestrel 48
Noritate 48
Normo Gastryl 48
Norpramin 48
nortriptyline 48
Norvasc 48
Nose
    blocked 79
        nasal drops/spray 19
        infections of 115
Novahistex DH 48
Novahistine DH 48
Novamoxin 48
Novasen 48
Novo-Alprazol 48
Novo-Amiodarone 48
Novo-Atenol 48
Novo-Azathioprine 48
Novo-Buspirone 48
Novo-Carbamaz 48
Novo-Cefaclor 48
Novo-Chloroquine 48
Novo-Chlorpromazine 48
Novo-Cholamine 48
Novo-Clindamycin 48
Novo-Clobetasol 48
Novo-Clobazam 48
Novo-Clonazepam 48
Novo-Clonidine 48
Novo-Clopamine 48
Novo-Clopate 48
Novo-Cloxin 48
Novo-Cycloprine 48
Novo-Cyproterine 48

Novo-Desipramine 48
Novo-Difenac 48
Novo-Diflunisal 48
Novo-Diltiazem 48
Novo-Divalproex 49
Novo-Domperidone 49
Novo-Doxazosin 49
Novo-Doxepin 49
Novo-Doxylin 49
Novo-Fluoxetine 49
Novo-Flutamide 49
Novo-Fluprofen 49
Novo-Fluvoxamine 49
Novo-Gabapentin 49
Novo-Gemfibrozil 49
Novo-Gesic C8 49
Novo-Gesic C-15 49
Novo-Gliclazide 49
Novo-Hydroxyzin 49
Novo-Ipramide 49
Novo-Ketoconazole 49
Novo-Ketotifen 49
Novo-Levodicarbidopa 49
Novo-Levobunolol 49
Novo-Lexin 49
Novolin ge NPH 49
Novo-Loperamide 49
Novo-Lorazem 49
Novo-Maprotiline 49
Novo-Medrone 49
Novo-Metformin 49
Novo-Methacin 49
Novo-Metoprol 49
Novo-Mexiletine 49
Novo-Minocycline 49
Novo-Misoprostol 49
Novo-Moclobemide 49
Novo-Naprox 49
Novo-Nifedin 49
Novo-Nortriptyline 49
Novo-Oxybutynin 49
Novo-Pen-VK 49
Novo-Peridol LA 49
Novo-Pirocam 49
Novo-Prazin 49
Novo-Profen 49
Novo-Purol 181
Novo Rapid 49
Novo-Salmol 49
Novo-Selegiline 49
Novo-Sertraline 49
Novo-Sotalol 49
Novo-Spiroton 49
Novo-Spirozine 49
Novo-Sundac 49
Novo-Temazepam 49
Novo-Terazosin 49
Novo-Terbinafine 49
Novo-Tetra 49
Novo-Theophyl SR 49
Novo-Tiaprofenic 49
Novo-Trazodone 49
Novo-Trimel 49
Novo-Tripramine 49
Novo-Valproic 49
Novo-Veramil 49

Novo-Zopiclone 49
Nozinan 49
NSAIDs see Non-steroidal anti-
    inflammatory drugs
Nu-Acyclovir 49
Nu-Alpraz 49
Nu-Amoxi 49
Nu-Ampi 49
Nu-Atenol 49
Nu-Baclo 49
Nubain 49
Nu-Buspirone 49
Nu-Cefaclor 49
Nu-Cephalex 49
Nucleoside analogues 144, 145
Nucleoside reverse
    transcriptase inhibitors 144
Nucleotide analgogues 144, 145
Nu-Clonazepam 49
Nu-Clonidine 50
Nu-Cloxi 50
Nu-Cotrimox 50
Nu-Cyclobenzaprine 50
Nu-Desipramine 50
Nu-Diclo 50
Nu-Diflunisal 50
Nu-Diltiaz 50
Nu-Divalproex 50
Nu-Doxycycline 50
Nu-Fenofibrate 50
Nu-Fluoxetine 50
Nu-Flurbiprofen 50
Nu-Fluvoxamine 50
Nu-Gemfibrozil 50
Nu-Ibuprofen 50
Nu-Indo 50
Nu-Ipratropium 50
Nu-Ketoprofen 50
Nu-Levocarb 50
Nu-Loraz 50
Nu-Loxapine 50
Nu-Megestrol 50
Nu-Metoclopramide 50
Nu-Metop 50
Nu-Moclobemide 50
Nu-Naprox 50
Nu-Nifed 50
Nu-Nifedipine-PA 50
Nu-Nortriptyline 50
Nu-Oxybutyn 50
Nu-Pen-VK 50
Nu-Pirox 50
Nu-Pravastatin 50
Nu-Prazo 50
Nu-Prochlor 50
Nu-Propranolol 50
Nu-Salbutamol 50
Nu-Selegiline 50
Nu-Sotalol 50
Nu-Sulfinpyrazone 50
Nu-Sulindac 50
Nu-Temazepam 50
Nu-Terazosin 50
Nu-Tetra 50
Nu-Tiaprofenic 50
Nu-Trazodone 50

Nu-Trazodone-D 50
Nutrients see Nutrition 134
Nu-Trimipramine 50
Nutropin 50
Nu-Valproic 50
Nu-Verap 50
Nu-Zopiclone 50
Nyaderm 50
nystatin 50
Nytol 50

O

Obesity see Nutrition 134
  See also Appetite
    suppressants
octocrylene 50
octoxynol 50
octreotide 50
Ocufen 50
Oesclim 50
ofloxacin 50
Ogen 50
Ointments 19, 163
olanzapine 50
olopatadine 50
olsalazine 50
omalizumab 50
omega-3 fatty acids 50
omeprazole 50
ondansetron 50
Opiates see Opioids
Opioid 506g
  abuse of 492
  as analgesics 64, 65
  as antidiarrheals 96
  as cough suppressants 80
  and drug interactions 16
  use in labour 153
  prohibited substances in sport
    496
opium 50
Opticrom 50
Optimine 50
Optimyxin ointment 50
Oracort 50
Oral antidiabetic drugs 128
Oral contraceptives see
  Contraceptives, oral
Oral medication 17, 27
Oral rehydration 499
Orap 50
orciprenaline 50
Orencia 50
Orgalutran 50
Organ transplants,
  immunosuppresant drugs to
    prevent rejection 143
orlistat 50
Orphan drug 506g
orphenadrine 50
Ortho 0.5/35 50
Ortho 7/7/7 50
Ortho-Cept 50

Ortho-Novum 51
Os-Cal 51
Oseltamavir 51
Osmotic diuretics 85
Osmotic laxatives 97
Osteoarthritis, drugs for
  locally acting corticosteroids
    104
  non-steroidal anti-
    inflammatory drugs 102
Osteomalacia 108
Osteoporosis 108, 133, 195,
  469
Ostoforte 51
OTC (Over-the-counter drugs)
  507g
Otitis externa 159
Otitis media 159
Otrivin 51
Ovaries 147
  cancer of 140
  failure of 133
  underdeveloped 133
    See also Ovulation
Overdose 30
  emergency guide 526
Over-the-counter drugs see
  OTC 507g
  buying and using 25
Ovol 51
Ovulation, stimulating see Drugs
  for infertility 152
oxaprozin 51
oxazepam 51, 380
oxcarbazepine 51, 70
Oxeze Turbuhaler 51
Oxipar Lotion 51
oxprenolol 51
Oxsoralen 51
Oxsoralen-Ultra 51
oxtriphylline 51
oxybenzone 51
oxybuprocaine 51
oxybutynin 51
oxycodone 51
OxyContin 51
Oxyderm 51
Oxygen 153
Oxy.IR 51
oxymetazoline 51
oxymorphone 51
oxytocin 51
Oxytrol 51
Ozonol 51

P

paclitaxel 51
padimate-O 51
Paget's disease 279
Painkillers see Analgesics
Pain, relief of see Analgesics
palivizumab 51
pamidronate 51
pancrealipase 51

Pancreas 126
  agents used in disorders of 100
  cancer of 140
Pancrease 51
Pancreatic
  cancer 140
  enzymes 100
pancreatin 51
Pancreatitis, chronic 100
panthenol 51
PANTO IV 51
Pantoloc 51
pantoprazole 51, 382
pantothenic acid 51
papaverine 51
paraldehyde 51
Paraplatin-AQ 51
Parasites 164
Parasympathomimetic 507g
  See also Autonomic nervous
    system 63
Parasympathomimetic drugs,
  used for urinary disorders 154
Parkinsonism 507g
  due to antipsychotic drugs 69
  drugs for 71
Parkinson's disease 71
Parlodel 51
Parnate 51
paroxetine 51
Parsitan 51
Parvolex 51
Pastes 163
Patanol 51
Patch see Transdermal patch
Patch testing 167
Paxil 51
Pecliapred 51
Pediapred 51
Pediatrix 51
Pediazole 51
Pegetron 51
peginterferon alfa-2a 51
peginterferon alfa-2b 51
Peg-Intron 51
Pellagra 475
Pelvic infections, drugs for
  antibacterial drugs 117
Penbritin 51
penciclovir 51
penicillamine 51
penicillin 51
penicillin G 51
penicillin V 51
Penlac 51
Pentacarinat 51
pentamidine 51
Pentamycetin 51
Pentasa 51
pentazocine 51
pentoxifylline 51
Pepcid 51
Pepcid Complete 51
Peppermint 495
Peptic ulcers 111
Peptide hormones, prohibited

  use in sport 496
Pepto-Bismol 51
Percocet 51
Percodan 51
pergolide 51
Pergonal 51
pericyazine 51
Peridex 51
perindopril 51
Periods, menstrual see
  Menstrual cycle; Menstrual
    disorders
Peripheral nervous system 62
Peripheral vascular disease 84
permethrin 51
Pernicious anemia 138, 480
perphenazine 51
Persantine 51
Pertussis, vaccine for 121
Peru balsam 51
Pessaries see vaginal
  suppositories 19
Pharmacist 507g
Pharmacodynamics 507g
Pharmacokinetics 507g
Pharmacologist 507g
Pharmacology 507g
Pharmacopeia 507g
Pharmacy 507g
Pharmorubicin PFS 52
Phazyme 51
phenelzine 51
phenobarbital 51
phenol 51
Phenothiazines
  as anti-emetics 74
  as antipsychotics 69
phentolamine 51
phenylephrine 51
phenytoin 51
Phillips Preparations 51
pHisoHex 51
PHL-Cholestyramine Light 51
PHL-Procyclidine 51
Phlebotomus fever 499
Phobias, drugs for see
  Monoamine oxidase
    inhibitors 68
  See also Anti-anxiety drugs 67
phosphorus 51
Photophobia 507g
Photosensitivity 507g
Phyllocontin 51
phytomenadione 51
Piles see hemorrhoids 115
Pill see Contraceptives, oral
pilocarpine 51
Pilopine HS 51
pimozide 51
pioglitazone 51
piperacillin 51
piperazine 51
piperonyl butoxide 51
Piportil L4 51
pipotiazine 51
Pipracil 51

piroxicam 51
Pituitary disorders, drugs for 131
Pituitary hormones 131
pizotifen 52
Placebo 507g
  response 15
Placenta
  How drugs cross 21
Plan B 52
Plaquenil 52
Plavix 52
Plendil 52
PMS-Atenolol 52
PMS-Baclofen 52
PMS-Bezafibrate 52
PMS-Bromocriptine 52
PMS-Buspirone 52
PMS-Cefaclor 52
PMS-Chloral Hydrate 52
PMS-Clonazepam 52
PMS-Desipramine 52
PMS-Dexamethasone 52
PMS-Diclofenac 52
PMS-Dipivefrin 52
PMS-Dopazide 52
PMS-Fluoxetine 52
PMS-Fluphenazine 52
PMS-Flutamide 52
PMS-Fluvoxamine 52
PMS-Gabapentin 52
PMS-Gemfibrozil 52
PMS Hydroxyzine 52
PMS-Indapamide 52
PMS-Isoniazid 52
PMS-lactulose 52
PMS-Levobunolol 52
PMS Lindane Lotion 52
PMS-Loperamide 52
PMS-Loxapine 52
PMS-Mefenamic Acid 52
PMS-Methylphenidate 52
PMS-Metoprolol-B 52
PMS-Moclobemide 52
PMS-Nortriptyline 52
PMS-Nystatin 52
PMS-Oxybutynin 52
PMS-Sodium Cromoglycate 52
PMS-Sotalol 52
PMS-Temazepam 52
PMS-Terazosin 52
PMS-Terbinafine 52
PMS-Tiaprofenic 52
PMS-Trazodone 52
PMS-Valproic Acid 52
Pneumocystis pneumonia 122
  See also Drugs for AIDS and immune deficiency 144
Pneumonia, drugs for see Respiratory tract infection 115
  pneumocystis 122, 144
  vaccine for 119
podophyllin 52
Poison 507g
Poisoning, drug 526

Polio, vaccine for 121
Polycitra-K 52
Polymyositis 200
polymyxin B 52
Polysporin ear drops 52
Polysporin ointment 52
polyvinyl alcohol 52
Pontocaine 52
posaconazole 52
Postcoital contraception 151
potassium 52
potassium bicarbonate 52
potassium citrate 52
potassium iodide 52
potassium permanganate 52
povidone-iodine 52
pralidoxime mesylate 52
pramipexole 52
Pramox HC 52
Pramoxine 52
Pravachol 52
Pravasa 52
pravastatin 52
praziquantel 52
prazosin 52
Pred Forte 52
Pred Mild 52
Prednicarbate 52
prednisone 52
prednisolone 52
pregabalin 52
Pregnancy
  drug treatment in 21
  hormone levels during 133
  nausea and vomiting in see Anti-emetics 74
  termination of 153
  and Vitamin A 479
Pregnyl 52
Premarin 52
Premature labour, delaying 153
Premedication 507g
Premenstrual syndrome 148
  use of diuretics in 85
  herbal remedies 494
Premplus 52
Prescription 507g
  See also Managing your drug treatment 26
Prevacid 52
Prevex HC 52
Prezista 52
prilocaine 52
primaquine 52
Primaquine sulfate 52
Primaxim 53
primidone 53
Prinivil 53
probenecid 53
Probeta 53
procainamide 53
Procan-SR 53
prochlorperazine 53
Proctodan HC 53
Proctofoam HC 53

procyclidine 53
Procytox 53
Prodium Plain 53
Prodium Plus 53
Product name 507g
Profasi HP 53
Progesterones 133
Progestins 133
  See also Oral contraceptives 149, 151
Prograf 53
proguanil 53
Prolactin levels, drugs to reduce 131
Prolopa 53
Proloprim 53
promethazine 53
Prometrium 53
Pronestyl-SR 53
propafenone 53
Prophylactic 507g
Propecia 53
Propine 53
propoxyphene 53
propranolol 53
propylthiouracil 53
Propyl-Thyracil 53
Proscar 53
Prostaglandin 507g
Prostaglandins see Drugs used in labour 153; Drugs for glaucoma 157
Prostin VR 53
Protease inhibitors 144, 145
Prothrombin 482
protirelin 53
Proton pump inhibitors 95
Protopic 53
Protozoa 112, 122
Protozoal diseases, summary of 122
Provera 53
Proviodine 53
Prozac 53
Pruritus 161
Pruritus ani 99
pseudoephedrine 53
Pseudofrin 53
Psoriasis, drugs for 166
  See also Antipruritics 161
Psychotic disorders see Antipsychotic drugs 69
Psyllium 53
Puberty, delayed
  female see Female sex hormones 133
  male see Male sex hormones 132
Puffers see Inhalers
Pulmicort 53
Pulmozyme 53
Pulse, checking 526
Pump, infusion 506g
Pupil, drugs affecting 158
Puregon 53
Purgative 507g

Purinethol 53
Pyelonephritis see Kidney infections
pyrantel 53
pyrazinamide 53
pyridostigmine 53
pyridoxine 53
pyrimethamine 53
pyrvinium pamoate 53

Q

quetiapine 53
quinapril 53
quinidine 53
quinidine sulfate 53
quinine 53
Quinine-Odan 53
Qvar 53

R

Rabies, vaccine for 498
Radiation therapy, nausea and vomiting caused by 74
Radiocative iodine 53, 473
Ralivia 53
raloxifene 53
raltegravir 53
ramipril 53
R and C II Shampoo/Conditioner 53
R and C II Spray 53
ranitidine 53
rasagiline 53
Rash, allergic see Antihistamines 110
  and itching see Antipruritics 161
ratio-Aclavulanate 53
ratio-Amiodarone 53
ratio-Atenolol 53
ratio-Baclofen 53
ratio-Brimonidine 53
ratio-Buspirone 53
ratio-Calmydone 53
ratio-Clindamycin 53
ratio-Clobazam 53
ratio-Clobetasol 53
ratio-Clonazepam 53
ratio-Codeine 53
ratio-Colchicine 53
ratio-Coristex-DH 53
ratio-Cyclobenzapine 53
ratio-Desipramine 53
ratio-Dexamethasone 53
ratio-Doxazosin 53
ratio-Flunisolide 53
ratio-Fluoxetine 53
ratio-Fluvoxamine 53
ratio-Gentamicin 53

ratio-Indomethacin 53
ratio-Ipratropium UDV 53
ratio-Lovastatin 54
ratio-Methotrexate 54
ratio-methylphenidate 54
ratio-Morphine 54
ratio-MPA 54
ratio-Nortriptyline 54
ratio-Nystatin 54
ratio-Oxycodone 54
ratio-Prednisolone 54
ratio-Salbutamol HFA 54
ratio-Sertraline 54
ratio-Terazosin 54
ratio-Theo-Brone 54
ratio-Topilene 54
ratio-Trazodone 54
ratio-Triacomb 54
ratio-Valproic 54
ratio-Zopiclone 54
Reactine 54
Rebif 54
Rebound congestion 77
Receptor 507g
    sites 14
Recovery position 527
Rectal administration of drugs
    18
Rectal disorders, drugs for 99
Rectogel HC 54
Reflux, acid 94
Rejuva-A 54
Relenza 54
Relpax 54
Remeron 54
Remicade 54
Reminyl 54
Renedil 54
Renova 54
repaglinide 54
Replication 507g
Reproductive tract 146
ReQuip 54
Rescriptor 54
Resistance, antibiotic 114
Respiratory stimulants 72
Respiratory system 75
    infection, drugs for
        antibacterial drugs 117
        antibiotics 115
resorcinol 54
Restoril 54
Resuscitation, mouth-to-mouth
    527
Retention, urinary 154
Reticular activating system 67, 72
Retin-A 54
Retin-A Micro 54
retinoic acid 54
Retinoids 479
    See also Drugs to treat acne
        165
retinol 54
Retrovir 54
Revatio 54
Reyataz 54

Reye's syndrome 65, 195
Rheumatoid arthritis 103
Rhinocort Aqua 54
Rhodacine 54
Rho-Nitro Pumpspray 54
Rhovane 54
Rhoxal-loperamide 54
Rhoxal-Sotalol 54
Rhythmol 54
ribavirin 54
riboflavin 54
Rickets 108, 469, 481
Ridaura 54
rifabutin 54
rifampin 54
Rifater 54
Rimso-50 54
Ringworm infections 124
risedronate 54
Risperdal 54
risperidone 54
Ritalin 54
Ritalin SR 54
ritodrine 54
Rituxan 54
rituximab 54
Riva-Loperamide 54
Rivanase AQ 54
rivastigmine 54
River blindness 499
Rivotril 54
rizatriptan 54
Robaxacet-8 54
Robaxin 54
Robaxisal 54
Robaxisal Extra Strength 54
Robitussin DM 54
Robitussin Honey Cough
    DM 54
Rocaltrol 54
Rocky Mountain spotted fever
    447
Rofact 54
Rogaine 54
Ropinirole 54
rosiglitazone 54
rosuvastatin 54
Roundworm infestation 113, 125
Royvac 54
Rubefacient 507g
Rubella, vaccine for 121
Rythmodan 54
Rythmodan-LA 54

S

642 Tablets 54
Sabril 54
Saizen 54
Salagen 55
Salazopyrin 55
Salazopyrin En-Tabs 55
salbutamol 55

salicylic acid 55
salmeterol 55
Salofalk 55
Salts, body 504g
Sand fly fever 499
Sandimmune IV 55
Sandomigran 55
Sandomigran DS 55
Sandostatin 55
Sandostatin LAR 55
Sandoz Glimepiride 55
Sandoz Pioglitazone 55
Sansert 55
Saquinavir 55
Sarna HC 55
Sativex 55
Scabene Aerosol 55
Scabies infestation 113, 164
Scalp, fungal infections of 124
Scheduled drugs 13
Schistosomiasis see Bilharzia
Schizophrenia 69
scopolamine 55
Scurvy 480
Sebcur 55
Sebivo 55
Sedative 507g
Seizures
    dealing with 528
    drugs for see Anticonvulsant
        drugs 86
Select 1/35 55
Selective serotonin re-uptake
    inhibitors (SSRIs) 68
selegiline 55
selenium 55
selenium sulfide 55
Self-treatment see Over-the-
    counter drugs
Selsun 55
senna 55
Sensorcaine 55
Sensorcaine with Epinephrine
    55
Septra 55
Serc 55
Serevent 55
Serophene 55
Seroquel 55
Serostim 55
sertraline 55
Sex
    drive, reduced 132
    hormones
        female 133
        male 132
Sexual development, delayed
    see Puberty, delayed
Sexually transmitted diseases
    see Genital tract infections
Shingles (herpes) 119
Short stature 131
Shoulder, frozen 104
Sibelium 55
sibutramine 55
Side effect see Adverse effect

sildenafil 55
silver sulfiadiazine 55
simethicone 55
Simply Sleep 55
simvastatin 55
Simulect 55
Sinemet 55
Singulair 55
Sinomet CR 55
Sinutab with Codeine 55
Sinutab Sinus and Allergy 55
Sitagliptin 55
Sjögren's syndrome 158
Skin 160
    action of corticosteroids on
        162
    allergic reactions involving
        110
    cancer, drugs for 140
    infections 115, 122, 163
    inflammation 162
    itchy 161
    parasites 164
    preparations 19, 161
Sleeping drugs 66
    use in sport 496
Sleeping sickness see
    Trypanosomiasis 122
Slow-Fe 55
Slow-Fe Folic 55
Slow-K 55
Slow-release preparations 18
sodium 55
sodium cellulose phosphate 55
sodium chloride 55
sodium cromoglycate 55
sodium ferric gluconate 55
sodium fluoride 55
Sofracort 55
Soframycin 55
sofra-Tulle 55
Soft tissue
    cancer 140
    infection 115
    injuries, drugs for 102
Softening agents 97
solifenacin 55
Solugel 55
Solu-Medrol 55
Soluver 55
Solvents, abuse of 493
Somatostatin 55
somatropin 55
Soriatane 55
sotalol 55
Spacer, how to use 78
Spasm, muscle 106
Spasticity 106
Sperm
    abnormal 152
    cancer affecting 140
    production 146
Spinal cord injury 106
Spiriva 55
spironolactone 55, 433
Sporanox 55

Sport, drugs used in 496
  legitimate medications 496
  prohibited substances 496
Sprains, drugs for 102
Spriafil 55
SSRIs 68
Staphylococcal infections 114
Starlix 55
Statins 89
stavudine 55
Steam inhalations 80
Sterile 508g
Steroid flare 104
Steroids see Corticosteroids 127
Stieva-A 55
Stilamine 55
stilboestrol 55
Stimulant laxatives 97
Stimulants
  nervous system 72
  prohibited substances in
    sport 496
  respiratory 72
  uterine 153
Stings 499
St John's Wort 71
Stones
  gallbladder 100
  kidney 105
Strains, drugs for 102
Strattera 55
Streptase 55
Streptococcal infections 114
streptokinase 55
streptomycin 55
Stress
  alternative medicines 494,
  495
  See also Anxiety
Stress incontinence 154
Strokes
  preventing 90
  relieving spasticity in 106
Subcutaneous injection 508g
Sublingual 508g
  tablets 17
sucralfate 55
Sudafed Decongestant
  12 Hour 55
Sulcrate 55
sulfacetamide 56
sulfadiazine 56
Sulfa drugs see Antibacterial
  drugs 117
sulfamethoxazole 56
sulfasalazine 56
sulfinpyrazone 56
Sulfonamides see Antibacterial
  drugs 115, 117
Sulfonylurea (oral antidiabetic)
  drugs 128, 129
sulindac 56
sumatriptan 56
Sunburn
  avoiding 499
  drugs for 161

sun protection factors 169
  sunscreens 169
Sun protection factors 169
Sunscreens 169
  and travel 499
Supeudol 56
Suppository 19, 508g
Suprax 56
Suprefact 56
Suprefact Depo 56
Surgam 56
Surgam SR 56
Surgery
  pain relief following 64
  prevention of blood clots
    following 90
Surmontil 56
Sustiva 56
Swelling see Inflammation
Symbicort Turbuhaler 56
Symmetrel 56
Sympathetic nervous system 63
Sympatholytic 508g
  See also Autonomic nervous
    system 63
Sympatholytic drugs
  use in hypertension 88
  vasodilators 84, 154
Sympathomimetic 508g
  See also Autonomic nervous
    system 63
Sympathomimetic drugs
  as bronchodilators 76, 78
  as decongestants 79
  as mydriatics 157, 158
  in urinary disorders 154
Synagis 56
Synalar 56
Synarel 56
Synphasic 56
Synthroid 56
Syrup 508g
Systemic 508g
Systemic lupus erythematosus
  127, 138, 143, 200

T

222 Tablets 56
282/292 Tablets 56
282 MEP C8 56
Tablets 19
tacrolimus 56
Tachycardia 86
tadalafil 56
Talwin 56
Tambocor 56
Tamiflu 56
Tamofen 56
tamoxifen 56
tamsulosin 56
Tapazole 56
Tapeworm infestations 113, 125

Tardan 56
Tardive dyskinesia 508g
Tarka 56
Taro-Sone 56
Taxol 56
Taxotere 56
Tazidime 56
tazarotene 56
tazobactam 56
Tazocin 56
Tazorac 56
Tears Naturale 56
Tear preparations, artificial 158
Tebrazid 56
Tegretol 56
telbivudine 56
telithromycin 56
telmisartan 56
Telzir 56
temazepam 56
Tempra 56
Tendinitis 104
Tendons, strained 104
tenecteplase 56
Tennis elbow 104
tenofovir 56, 72
Tenoretic 56
Tenormin 56
tenoxicam 56
Tequin 56
Terazol 56
terazosin 56
terbinafine 56
terbutaline 56
terconazole 56
teriparatide 56
Tersaseptic 56
Testis, cancer 140
Testosterone 56, 132
Tetanus, vaccine for 121
tetracaine 56
Tetracycline 56
  See also Uses of antibiotics
    115; Classes of antibiotics
    116
Thalidomide 72
Theolair 56
theophylline 56
Therapeutic range 15
thiamine 135, 136, 479
Thiazides 85
thiopental 56
thiothixene 56
Threadworm infestation 125
Throat, bacterial infections of 115
Thrombolytics 91
Thrombosis 91
  and travel 498
Thrush 124
Thyroid disorders 130
Thyroid hormones 130
Tiamol 56
tiaprofenic acid 56
Tiazac 56
ticarcillin 56
tigecycline 56

Tilade 56
timolol 56
Timoptic 56
Timoptic-XE 56
Tinea infections 124
tinidazole 56
tinzaparin 56, 305
tiotropium 56
tipranavir 56
Tissue, disorders of soft see
  Soft tissue
Tissue plasminogen
  activator 73
Tissue transplants 143
titanium dioxide 56
tizanidine 56, 451
TNKase 56
TOBI 56
Tobradex 56
tobramycin 56
tocopherol 56
tocopheryl acetate 56
Tofranil 56
Tolerance 508g
  See also Drug dependence 23
tolnaftate 56
tolterodine 56
Tonics 508g
Toothache 64
Tooth decay 471, 478
Topamax 56
Topical 508g
  application of drugs 18
    corticosteroids 99, 162
    skin preparations 19, 161, 165
Topicort 57
topiramate 57
Topsyn 57
Toxic reaction 508g
Toxin 508g
Toxocariasis 125
Toxoplasmosis 122
Traditional Chinese Medicine
  (TCM) 495
Tramacet 57
tramadol 57, 454
tranexamic acid 57
Tranquillizer
  major 508g
  minor 508g
Tranquillizers, abuse of see
  Benzodiazepines 487
Transdermal patch 18, 47,
  508g
Transderm-Nitro 57
Transfusions, allergic reactions
  to 110
Trans-Plantar 57
Transplants, drugs to prevent
  rejection 143
Trans Ver Sal 57
tranylcypromine 57
trastuzumab 57
Travatan 57
Travel, drugs used in 497
Traveller's diarrhea 499

Travel immunization 498
Travel insurance 498
Travel sickness 497, 499
  drugs for 74
travoprost 57
trazodone 57
Trelstar 57
Trental 57
tretinoin 57
triamcinolone 57
Triaderm 57
Triaminic Pediatric Oral Cold
  Drops 57
triamterene 57
Triatec-8 57
Triatec-30 57
Triavil 57
Trichinosis 125
Trichomoniasis 122
triclosan 57
Tricyclic antidepressants 68
  in urinary disorders 154
Tridural 57
trifluoperazine 57
trifluridine 57
Trilafon 57
Trileptal 57
trimeprazine 57
trimethoprim 57
trimipramine 57
Trinalin 57
Triphasil 57
triptorelin 57
tropicamide 57
Trosec 57
trospium 57
Trusopt 57
Trypanosomiasis 122, 499
tryptophan 57
T-Stat 57
Tuberculosis 118
  vaccination for 121
Tumours see Cancer
Tussionex 57
Tygacil 57
Tylenol 57
Tylenol Allergy Sinus 57
Tylenol Cold Suspension
  Children's 57
Tylenol Elixir with Codeine 57
Tylenol No. 1 57
Tylenol No. 1 Forte 57
Tylenol No. 2 with Codeine 57
Tylenol No. 4 with Codeine 57
Typhoid 499
  vaccine 121, 498

U

Ulcerative colitis 98
Ulcers
  peptic 95
  skin, infected 163
Ultradol 57
Ultramop capsules 57
Ultramop lotion 57
Ultraviolet light treatment
  (PUVA) 166
Uniphyl 57
Unisom 57
Unisom-2 57
Urea 74
Urethritis 154
Urispas 57
Urgency see Drugs for urinary
  incontinence 154
Uric acid levels, high 105
Uricosuric drugs 105
Urinary system 146
Urinary tract 146
  disorders, drugs for 154
  infections 115
Urticaria 161
urofollitropin 57
Uromax 57
Urso 57
ursodeoxycholic acid 57
Ursodiol 57
Uterine
  muscle relaxants 153
  stimulants 153
Uterus, cancer of 140

V

Vaccinations
  common 121
  and travel 497, 498
Vaccine 508g
  See also Vaccines and
    immunizations 120
Vagifem 57
Vagina
  dryness of 133
  infections of 124
Vaginal suppositories 19
valacyclovir 57
Valcyte 57
valganciclovir 57
Valisone 57
Valium Roche Oral 57
valproic acid 57
valsartan 57
Valtrex 57
Vancocin 57
vancomycin 57
vardenafil 57
varenicline 57
Vaseline Petroleum Jelly 74
Vasoconstrictor 508g
Vasoconstrictor drugs 99
Vasodilator 508g
Vasodilator drugs 84, 88
Vasopressin 74
Vasotec 57
venlafaxine 57
Ventodisks 57
Ventolin 57
Vepesid 57
Veramil 57
verapamil 57
Vermox 57
Vertigo 74
Vesanoid 58
Vesicare 58
Vfend 58
Viaderm-K.C. 58
Viagra 58
Vibramycin 58
Vibramycin-D 58
Vibra-Tabs 58
Videx 58
vigabatrin 58
Vigamox 58
vinblastine 58
vincristine 58
Vioform Hydrocortisone
  58
Viral infections 119
  immunization against
  120
Virazole 58
Viread 58
Viroptic 58
Viruses 112
  See also Viral infections
Visine Workplace Eye
  Drops 58
Vitamin A 135, 136, 479
Vitamin A Acid 58
Vitamin B1 479
Vitamin B2 477
Vitamin B3 475
Vitamin B5 476
Vitamin B6 477
Vitamin B9 472
Vitamin B12 135, 136, 480
Vitamin C 135, 136, 480
Vitamin D 108, 135, 136, 481
Vitamin D2 481
Vitamin D3 481
Vitamin E 135, 136, 481
Vitamin G 456
Vitamin H 449
Vitamin K 90, 91, 135, 136,
  482
Vitamin K1 482
Vitamin K2 482
Vitamin K3 482
Vitamins
  calculating daily requirements
    of 137
  fat-soluble and water-soluble
    137
  main food sources of 136
  primary functions of 135
  supplements 134
Voltaren 58
Voltaren Ophtha 58
Vomiting
  dealing with 528
  drugs for 74
  herbal remedies 495
voriconazole 58

W

Wafers 19, 508g
warfarin 58
Water retention 85
Water-soluble vitamins 137
Weight
  gain see Anabolic steroids 132
  loss see Nervous system
    stimulants 72
  See also Obesity
Wellbutrin SR 58
Westcort 58
Western herbal medicine 495
Whipworm infestation 125
Whooping cough see Pertussis
Wilm's tumour 140
Wilson's disease 471
Withdrawal symptom 508g
  See also Drug dependence 23
Worm infestations 125
  life cycle of 113
Wounds, infected 163

X

Xalatan 58
Xanax 58
Xanax TS 58
Xanthines 76, 78
Xatral 58
Xenical 58
Xolair 58
Xylocaine 58
Xylocaine Jelly 2% 58
Xylocaine Parenteral with
  Epinephrine 58
Xylocard 58
xylometazoline 58

Y

Yasmin 58
Yeast infections 124
Yellow fever, vaccine for 498,
  499

Z

Zaditen 58
zafirlukast 58
Zanaflex 58
zanamivir 58
Zantac 58
Zarontin 58
ZeaSorb AF 58
Zenapax 58
Zestoretic 58
Zestril 58
zidovudine (AZT) 58

Zinc 58, 136
Zincofax 58
zinc oxide 58
zinc pyrithione 58
zinc sulfate 58
Zithromax 58
Zocor 58
Zofran 58
Zofran ODT 58
Zoladex 58
Zoladex LA 58
zoledronic acid 58

Zollinger-Ellison syndrome
  324
zolmitriptan 58
Zoloft 58
Zomig 58
Zomig Rapimelt 58
zopiclone 58
Zovirax 58
Z-Pak 58
Zuclopenthixol 58
Zyban 58
Zyloprim 58

Zyprexa 58
Zyprexa Zydis 58
Zytram 58
Zyvoxam 58

DRUG POISONING EMERGENCY GUIDE

The information on the following pages is intended to give practical advice for dealing with a known or suspected drug poisoning emergency. Although many of the first-aid techniques described can be used in a number of different types of emergency, these instructions apply specifically to drug overdose or poisoning.

Emergency action is necessary in any of the following circumstances:
- If a person has taken an overdose of any of the high-danger drugs listed in the box on p.528.
- If a person has taken an overdose of a less dangerous drug, but has one or more of the danger symptoms listed (right).
- If a person has taken, or is suspected of having taken, an overdose of an unknown drug.
- If an infant or child has swallowed, or is suspected of having swallowed any medications or any drug of abuse.

What to do

If you are faced with a drug poisoning emergency, it is important to carry out first aid and arrange immediate medical help in the correct order. The Priority Action Decision Chart (below left) will help you to assess the situation and to determine your priorities. The following information should help you to remain calm in an emergency if you ever need to deal with a case of drug poisoning.

DANGER SYMPTOMS

Take emergency action if the person has one or more of the following symptoms:
- Drowsiness or unconsciousness
- Shallow, irregular, or stopped breathing
- Vomiting
- Seizures

PRIORITY ACTION DECISION CHART

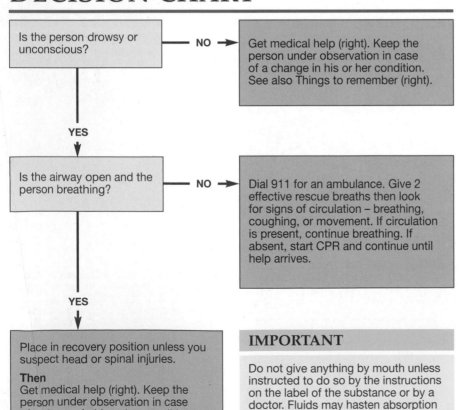

Is the person drowsy or unconscious? — **NO** → Get medical help (right). Keep the person under observation in case of a change in his or her condition. See also Things to remember (right).

YES

Is the airway open and the person breathing? — **NO** → Dial 911 for an ambulance. Give 2 effective rescue breaths then look for signs of circulation – breathing, coughing, or movement. If circulation is present, continue breathing. If absent, start CPR and continue until help arrives.

YES

Place in recovery position unless you suspect head or spinal injuries.
Then
Get medical help (right). Keep the person under observation in case of a change in his or her condition.

IMPORTANT

Do not give anything by mouth unless instructed to do so by the instructions on the label of the substance or by a doctor. Fluids may hasten absorption of the drug, increasing the danger.

GETTING MEDICAL HELP

In an emergency, a calm person who is competent in first aid should stay with the victim, while others summon help. However, if you have to deal with a drug poisoning emergency on your own, use first aid (see the Priority Action Decision Chart, left) before getting help.

Calling an ambulance may be the quickest method of transport to hospital. Then call your physician or a hospital emergency department for advice. If possible, tell them what drug has been taken and how much, and the age of the victim. Follow the physician's or hospital's instructions precisely.

THINGS TO REMEMBER

Effective treatment of drug poisoning depends on the physician making a rapid assessment of the type and amount of drug taken. Collecting evidence that will assist the diagnosis will help. After you have carried out first aid, look for empty or opened medicine (or other) containers. Keep any of the drug that is left, together with its container (or syringe), and give these to the nurse or physician. Save any vomit for analysis by the hospital.

ESSENTIAL FIRST AID

AIRWAY CLEARANCE AND MOUTH-TO-MOUTH RESUSCITATION

When there is no rise and fall of the chest and you can feel no movement of exhaled air, open the airway and immediately start mouth-to-mouth resuscitation.

1 Lay the victim on his or her back on a firm surface. Place one hand on the victim's forehead and gently tilt the head back. Wipe any vomit from around the mouth and clear the mouth of any obvious obstruction that might block the airway.

2 Then place two fingers under the point of the victim's chin and lift his or her jaw.

3 Pinch the victim's nostrils closed with the hand that is placed on the forehead. Take a deep breath, seal your mouth over that of the victim, and give a breath twice in succession. Look for signs of circulation (below). If signs are present, continue by giving one breath every 5 seconds.

4 After each breath, turn to watch the chest falling while you listen for the sound of air leaving the victim's mouth. Continue until the victim starts to breathe regularly on his or her own, or until medical help arrives. Check for signs of circulation after every 10 breaths.

CARDIAC COMPRESSION

This technique is used in conjunction with mouth-to-mouth resuscitation to continue output of blood from a stopped heart. It does not usually restart a heart that has stopped.

Cardiac compression involves putting repeated pressure on the centre of the chest with the heels of both hands, at a rate of 100 compressions per minute for adult victims (right). After each set of 30 compressions, two breaths should be given using mouth-to-mouth resuscitation (above). Continue this sequence until breathing restarts.

CHECKING CIRCULATION

After you have given two breaths of mouth-to-mouth resuscitation, check for signs of circulation such as breathing, coughing, or movement for no more than 10 seconds. If not present, start cardiac compression.

THE RECOVERY POSITION

The recovery position is the safest for an unconscious or drowsy person as long as you do not suspect head or spinal injuries. It allows the person to breathe easily and helps to prevent choking if vomiting occurs. A drug poisoning victim should be placed in the recovery position if more urgent first aid, such as mouth-to-mouth resuscitation, is not needed. Place the victim on his or her side with one leg bent. Tilt the head back to keep the airway open, and support it in this position by placing the victim's hand under the cheek. Cover him or her with a blanket.

DEALING WITH A SEIZURE

Certain types of drug poisoning may provoke seizures. These may occur whether the person is conscious or not. The victim usually falls to the ground twitching or making uncontrolled movements of the limbs and body. If you witness a seizure, remember the following points:

● Do not try to hold the person down.

● Loosen clothing around neck if possible.

● Do not attempt to put anything into the person's mouth.

● Try to ensure that the person does not suffer injury by keeping him or her away from dangerous objects or furniture.

● Once the seizure is over, place the person in the recovery position (p.527).

HIGH-DANGER DRUGS

The following is a list of drugs given a high overdose rating in the drug profiles or included in the drugs of abuse. If you suspect that someone has taken an overdose of any of these drugs, seek immediate medical attention.

Acetaminophen	Pseudoephedrine
Amitriptyline	Pyridostigmine
ASA	
Atropine	Quinidine
	Quinine
Betahistine	
Bupropion	Rosiglitazone
Chloroquine	Selegiline
Clomipramine	Theophylline/
Codeine	aminophylline
Colchicine	Timolol
Digoxin	Venlafaxine
Epinephrine	Warfarin
(adrenaline)	
	Drugs of abuse
Fentanyl	Alcohol
Gliclazide	Amphetamines
Glyburide	Barbiturates
	Benzodiazepines
Heparin	Cannabis
Hydrocodone	(marijuana)
Hydromorphone	Cocaine
	(including crack)
Imipramine	Ecstasy
Insulin	GHB
Isoniazid	Ketamine
	Khat
Lithium	LSD
	Mescaline
Mefloquine	Nicotine
Metformin	Nitrites
Methadone	Opioids
Methylphenidate	(including heroin)
Metoprolol	Phencyclidine
Morphine	Solvents
Orphenadrine	
Phenobarbital	
Procyclidine	
Propranolol	

DEALING WITH ANAPHYLACTIC SHOCK

Anaphylactic shock can occur as the result of a severe allergic reaction to a drug (such as penicillin). Blood pressure drops dramatically and the airways may become narrowed. The reaction usually occurs within minutes of taking the drug. The main symptoms are:

● Breathing difficulty

● Pallor

● Blotchy red rash

● Anxiety

● Swelling of tongue or throat

1 If the person is consious but having breathing difficulties, he or she is usually more comfortable sitting up. If the breathing is normal, lay him or her down, face up, with legs raised above the level of the heart to ensure adequate circulation of the blood.

2 If the person becomes unconsious, ensure that he or she is breathing. If breathing has stopped, immediate mouth-to-mouth resuscitation should be carried out as described on p.527.

3 Phone for medical help. While waiting, cover the person with a blanket or other article of clothing. If you have to leave the person, place him or her in the recovery position. Do not attempt to administer anything by mouth.

DEALING WITH VOMITING

Vomiting is the body's response to many things, including contaminated food, viral infections, and severe pain. It also occurs as an adverse effect of some drugs and as a result of drug overdose.

Do not attempt to provoke vomiting by pushing fingers down the victim's throat. When vomiting does occur, remember the following:

● Vomiting can be a sign of poisoning.

● Vomiting due to drugs is usually a result of an overdose rather than a side effect. Check in the relevant drug profile whether vomiting is a possible adverse effect of the suspected drug. If vomiting appears to be due to an overdose, get medical help urgently.

● Even if vomiting has stopped, keep the person under observation in case he or she loses consciousness or has a seizure.

● If the person is drowsy and is vomiting, place him or her in the recovery position (p.527).

1 Ensure that the victim leans well forward to avoid either choking or inhaling vomit. If the victim appears to be choking, encourage coughing.

2 Keep the vomit for later analysis (see Things to remember, p.526).

3 Give water to rinse the mouth. This water should be spat out; it should not be swallowed.